Rossi's Principles of Transfusion Medicine

Rossi's Principles of Transfusion Medicine

Fifth Edition

Edited by

Toby L. Simon, MD
Senior Medical Director, Plasma Product Development and CSL Plasma, CSL Behring, King of Prussia, Pennsylvania; and
Clinical Professor of Pathology, University of New Mexico School of Medicine, Albuquerque, New Mexico, USA

Jeffrey McCullough, MD
Professor, Department of Laboratory Medicine and Pathology, University of Minnesota Medical School, Minneapolis, Minnesota, USA

Edward L. Snyder, MD, FACP
Professor, Department of Laboratory Medicine, Yale University School of Medicine; and
Director, Blood Bank/Apheresis Service, Yale-New Haven Hospital, New Haven, Connecticut, USA

Bjarte G. Solheim, MD, PhD, MHA
Professor Emeritus, Institute of Immunology, Oslo University Hospital–Rikshospitalet, and University of Oslo, Oslo, Norway

Ronald G. Strauss, MD
Professor Emeritus, Departments of Pathology and Pediatrics, University of Iowa College of Medicine, Iowa City, Iowa, USA;
Associate Medical Director, LifeSource/Institute for Transfusion Medicine, Chicago, Illinois, USA

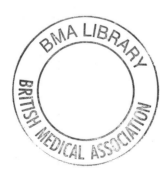

WILEY Blackwell

This edition first published 2016 © 2016 by John Wiley & Sons, Ltd.
Previous edition © 2009 by AABB, published by Blackwell Publishing Ltd.

Registered office: John Wiley & Sons, Ltd, The Atrium, Southern Gate, Chichester, West Sussex, PO19 8SQ, UK

Editorial offices: 9600 Garsington Road, Oxford, OX4 2DQ, UK

    The Atrium, Southern Gate, Chichester, West Sussex, PO19 8SQ, UK

    111 River Street, Hoboken, NJ 07030-5774, USA

For details of our global editorial offices, for customer services and for information about how to apply for permission to reuse the copyright material in this book please see our website at www.wiley.com/wiley-blackwell

Library of Congress Cataloging-in-Publication Data

Rossi's principles of transfusion medicine / edited by Toby L. Simon, Jeffrey McCullough, Edward L. Snyder, Bjarte G. Solheim, Ronald G. Strauss. – Fifth edition.

    p. ; cm.

  Principles of transfusion medicine

  Includes bibliographical references and index.

  ISBN 978-1-119-01299-3 (cloth)

  I. Simon, Toby L., editor. II. McCullough, Jeffrey, 1938- , editor. III. Snyder, Edward L. (Edward Leonard), 1946- , editor. IV. Solheim, Bjarte G., editor. V. Strauss, Ronald G., editor. VI. Title: Principles of transfusion medicine.

  [DNLM: 1. Blood Transfusion. 2. Blood Banks–organization & administration. 3. Blood Grouping and Crossmatching. WB 356]

  RM171

  615.3'9–dc23

                              2015031868

A catalogue record for this book is available from the British Library.

Wiley also publishes its books in a variety of electronic formats. Some content that appears in print may not be available in electronic books.

Set in 9/11pt, MinionPro-Regular by Thomson Digital, Noida, India
Printed and bound in Malaysia by Vivar Printing Sdn Bhd

1 2016

Contents

Contributors

Amin Alousi, MD
Associate Professor of Medicine
Department of Stem Cell Transplantation
and Cellular Therapy
The University of Texas
MD Anderson Cancer Center
Houston, TX, USA

Arna Andrews, PhD
Director, Cell Line Development, CSL Behring
Broadmeadows, VIC, Australia

Donald M. Arnold, MD, MSc, FRCPC
Associate Professor, Division of Hematology and
Thromboembolism, Department of Medicine, Michael
G. DeGroote School of Medicine, McMaster
University, Hamilton, ON, Canada

Jeffrey A. Bailey, MD, PhD
Assistant Professor, Departments of Medicine
and Pathology, Division of Transfusion Medicine;
Program in Bioinformatics and Integrative Biology
University of Massachusetts Medical School; and UMass
Memorial Medical Center, Worcester, MA, USA

Jenna Balestrini, PhD
Postdoctoral Fellow in Anesthesiology
Department of Biomedical Engineering, Department of
Anesthesiology, Yale University School of Medicine
New Haven, CT, USA

**Richard J. Benjamin, MD, PhD,
FRCPath**
Chief Medical Officer, Cerus Corp, Concord CA, USA

Melvin Berger, MD, PhD
Senior Director, Medical Research Strategy
CSL Behring, King of Prussia, PA, USA

Alexey Bersenev, MD, PhD
Associate Research Scientist, Department of Laboratory
Medicine, Yale University School of Medicine, and
Blood Bank, Yale-New Haven Hospital, New Haven
CT, USA

Joseph Bertolini, PhD
R&D Director, CSL Behring
Broadmeadows, VIC, Australia

Morris A. Blajchman, MD, FRCP(C)
Professor Emeritus, Departments of Pathology and
Medicine, McMaster University, Hamilton
ON, Canada

Martin H. Bluth, MD, PhD
Professor, Department of Pathology
Wayne State University School of Medicine
Detroit, MI, USA

Kevin Boehm, MD
Student, Department of Biomedical Engineering
Department of Anesthesiology, Yale University School
of Medicine, New Haven, CT, USA

José O. Bordin, MD
Associate Professor, Department of Hematology and
Transfusion Medicine, Universidade Federal de São
Paulo, São Paulo, Brazil

Anneke Brand, MD, PhD
Professor of Transfusion Medicine, Sanquin Blood Bank
and Department of ImmunoHematology and Blood
Transfusion, Leiden University Medical Center, Leiden
The Netherlands

Emanuela Bruscia, PhD
Assistant Professor of Pediatrics, Yale University School
of Medicine and Blood Bank, Yale-New Haven Hospital
New Haven, CT, USA

Edwin A. Burgstaler, MT, HP(ASCP)
Development Technologist, Therapeutic Apheresis
Treatment Unit, Mayo Clinic, Rochester
MN, USA

Jeffrey L. Carson, MD
Richard C. Reynolds Professor of Medicine
Chief, Division of General Internal Medicine; and
Provost— New Brunswick, Rutgers Robert Wood
Johnson Medical School, Rutgers Biomedical Health
Sciences, Rutgers University, New Brunswick, NJ, USA

Richard Champlin, MD
Professor and Chairman, Department of Stem Cell
Transplantation and Cellular Therapy, University of
Texas-MD Anderson Cancer Center, Houston, TX, USA

Jocelyn Chandler, MD
Chief Resident, Department of Pathology
Yale University School of Medicine; and Blood Bank
Yale-New Haven Hospital, New Haven, CT, USA

Robert D. Christensen, MD
Presidential Professor and Chief, Division of
Neonatology, University of Utah School of Medicine
Salt Lake City, UT, USA

Leanne Clifford, BM, MSc
Resident, Department of Anesthesiology, Mayo Clinic
Rochester, MN, USA

Laura Cooling, MD
Associate Professor
Department of Pathology
University of Michigan
Ann Arbor, MI, USA

Michael W. Cripps, MD
Assistant Professor of Surgery, Department of Surgery
Division of Burn/Trauma/Critical Care, University of
Texas Southwestern Medical Center, Dallas, TX, USA

Kendall P. Crookston, MD, PhD
Professor, Departments of Pathology and Medicine
University of New Mexico School of Medicine; Regional
Medical Director, United Blood Services of
New Mexico; and Associate Medical Director, TriCore
Reference Laboratories, Albuquerque, NM, USA

Robertson D. Davenport, MD
Associate Professor, Department of Pathology
The University of Michigan Medical School
Ann Arbor, MI, USA

Sarah M. Drawz, MD
Fellow, Department of Laboratory Medicine and
Pathology, University of Minnesota
Minneapolis, MN, USA

Amy L. Dunn, MD
Associate Professor, Department of Pediatrics
The Ohio State University; and Director, Hemophilia
and Bleeding Disorder Program, Hemophilia Treatment
Center, Division of Hematology/Oncology/BMT
Columbus, OH, USA

Anne F. Eder, MD, PhD
Vice President, National Medical Affairs; Biomedical
Services, American Red Cross, Adjunct Associate
Professor, Georgetown University Medical Center
Washington DC, USA

**Lise Estcourt, MA(MEL), MSc, DPhil,
MRCP, FRCPath**
Consultant Hematologist, NHS Blood and Transplant
and The National Institute for Health Research (NIHR)
Oxford Biomedical Research Centre, Oxford University
Hospitals, NHS Foundation Trust and the University of
Oxford, Oxford, UK

Emmanuel A. Fadeyi, MD
Associate Professor, Department of Pathology
Wake Forest University School of Medicine
Winston-Salem, NC, USA

Øystein Flesland, MD, PhD
Head of Section, Patient Reporting and Learning Systems Unit, Norwegian Knowledge Centre for the Health Services, Oslo, Norway

Sameh Gaballa, MD
Assistant Professor of Medical Oncology
Division of Hematological Malignancies and Bone Marrow Transplantation
Thomas Jefferson University
Philadelphia, PA, USA

Susan A. Galel, MD
Senior Director of Scientific Affairs, Blood Screening Roche Molecular Systems, Pleasanton, CA; and Associate Professor Emeritus, Department of Pathology Stanford University School of Medicine, Palo Alto CA, USA

Ashley Gard, PhD cand.
Department of Biomedical Engineering, Department of Anesthesiology, Yale University School of Medicine New Haven, CT, USA

Eric A. Gehrie, MD
Instructor, Department of Laboratory Medicine Yale University School of Medicine
and Blood Bank, Yale-New Haven Hospital
New Haven, CT, USA

Sergio Giralt, MD
Professor of Medicine, Weill Cornell Medical College Chief, Adult BMT Service, Memorial Sloan Kettering Cancer Center, New York, NY, USA

Lawrence Tim Goodnough, MD
Professor of Pathology and Medicine, Co-Director Transfusion Medicine Program, Director, Transfusion Medicine Fellowship Program, Associate Medical Director, Stanford Blood Center
Stanford University Medical Center
Stanford, CA, USA

Morten Grönn, MD
Consultant Neonatologist, Department of Child and Adolescent Medicine, Akershus University Hospital Nordbyhagen, Norway

Thor Willy Ruud Hansen, MD, PhD
Professor of Pediatrics, Consultant Neonatologist Neonatal Intensive Care, Women and Children's Division, Oslo University Hospital; and Institute for Clinical Medicine, Faculty of Medicine, University of Oslo, Oslo, Norway

Paul Hébert, MD
Professor of Medicine, University of Montreal; and Physician-in-Chief, Centre Hospitalier de L'Université de Montréal (CHUM), Montreal, Canada

Peter Hellstern, MD
Director and Professor, Institute of Hemostaseology and Transfusion Medicine, Academic City Hospital Ludwigshafen, Germany

Jeanne E. Hendrickson, MD
Associate Professor, Departments of Laboratory Medicine and of Pediatrics, Yale University School of Medicine, and Associate Director, Transfusion Medicine Service, Yale-New Haven Hospital, New Haven CT, USA

Tor Hervig, MD, PhD
Professor, Department of Clinical Science
Department of Immunology and Transfusion Medicine Haukeland University Hospital, Bergen, Norway

John R. Hess, MD, MPH
Professor, Department of Laboratory Medicine and Hematology, University of Washington
School of Medicine; and Medical Director, Transfusion Service, Harborview Medical Center
Seattle, WA, USA

John B. Holcomb, MD
Professor of Surgery; Chief, Division of Acute Care Surgery; and Director, Center for Translational Injury Research, University of Texas Health Science Center Houston, TX, USA

Iris Jacobs, MD
Global Clinical Program Director, CSL Behring
King of Prussia, PA USA

Cassandra D. Josephson, MD
Professor, Pathology and Pediatrics, Emory University School of Medicine, Medical Director, Children's Healthcare of Atlanta, Blood Tissue & Apheresis Services, Atlanta, GA, USA

Karen E. King, MD
Associate Professor, Department of Pathology and Oncology, Director, Hemapheresis and Transfusion Support, Associate Director, Transfusion Medicine, The Johns Hopkins University School of Medicine Baltimore, MD, USA

Joseph E. Kiss, MD
Medical Director, Hemapheresis and Blood Services The Institute for Transfusion Medicine; and Associate Professor of Medicine, Division of Hematology-Oncology, Department of Medicine, The University of Pittsburgh, Pittsburgh, PA, USA

Daryl J. Kor, MD, MSc
Associate Professor, Department of Anesthesiology Mayo Clinic, Rochester, MN, USA

Mark J. Koury, MD
Professor of Medicine, Division of Hematology/ Oncology, Vanderbilt University, Nashville, TN, USA

Diane Krause, MD, PhD
Professor, Laboratory Medicine, Pathology and Cell Biology, Yale University School of Medicine and Blood Bank, Yale-New Haven Hospital, New Haven, CT, USA

David J. Kuter, MD, DPhil
Chief of Hematology, Massachusetts General Hospital Professor of Medicine, Harvard Medical School, Boston MA, USA

Jeanne V. Linden, MD, MPH
Director, Blood and Tissue Resources, Wadsworth Center, New York State Department of Health Albany, NY, USA

Jeffrey McCullough, MD
Professor, Department of Laboratory Medicine and Pathology, University of Minnesota Medical School Minneapolis, MN, USA

Janice G. McFarland, MD
Medical Director, Platelet and Neutrophil Immunology Laboratory, Blood Center of Wisconsin; and Professor Department of Medicine, Medical College of Wisconsin Milwaukee, WI, USA

Andrea M. McGonigle, MD
Assistant Professor, Department of Pathology and Laboratory Medicine, Associate Medical Director Transfusion Medicine, David Geffen School of Medicine at UCLA, Los Angeles, CA USA

David H. McKenna, MD
Associate Professor of Laboratory Medicine and Pathology, Director, Division of Transfusion Medicine University of Minnesota Medical School
Minneapolis, MN, USA

Jeffrey S. Miller, MD
Department of Medicine
Division of Hematology, Oncology and Transplantation Blood and Marrow Transplantation Program
University of Minnesota, Minneapolis, MN, USA

Paul D. Mintz, MD
Director, Division of Hematology Clinical Review Office of Blood Research and Review, Center for Biologics Evaluation & Research, US Food and Drug Administration, Silver Spring, MD, USA

Shanna Morgan, MD
Medical Director,
American Red Cross-North Central Region
Adjunct Assistant Professor
Laboratory Medicine and Pathology
Division of Transfusion Medicine
University of Minnesota
Assistant Medical Director Blood Bank
Veterans Affairs Hospital, Minneapolis, MN, USA

Michael F. Murphy, MD, FRCP, FRCPath
Professor of Transfusion Medicine and Consultant Haematologist, NHS Blood & Transplant, National Institute of Health Research (NIHR)
Oxford Biomedical Research Centre
Oxford University Hospitals and the
University of Oxford, UK

Christian Naper, MD, PhD, MHA
Senior Consultant, Institute of Immunology
Oslo University Hospital–Rikshospitalet and
University of Oslo, Oslo, Norway

Andrew Nash, PhD
Senior Vice President, Research, CSL Behring
Broadmeadows, VIC, Australia

Ishac Nazi, PhD
Assistant Professor, Department of Medicine, Michael G. DeGroote School of Medicine, McMaster University Hamilton, ON, Canada

Paul M. Ness, MD
Professor, Pathology, Medicine and Oncology, Director Transfusion Medicine Division, The Johns Hopkin University School of Medicine Baltimore, MD, USA

Laura Niklason, PhD, MD
Professor of Anesthesiology and Biomedical Engineering, Department of Anesthesiology, Yale University School of Medicine, New Haven, CT, USA

Tho D. Pham, MD
Assistant Medical Director of Clinical Services, Stanford Blood Center; and Clinical Instructor, Department of Pathology, Stanford University School of Medicine, Palo Alto, CA, USA

Gregory J. Pomper, MD
Associate Professor, Department of Pathology Wake Forest School of Medicine, Winston-Salem NC, USA

Ralph M. Powers, DDS
Senior Manager, Scientific Affairs, Institute of Regenerative Medicine, LifeNet Health Virginia Beach, VA, USA

Aaron E. Pritchard, MD
Assistant Professor of Pathology, University of New Mexico School of Medicine, Albuquerque, NM, USA

Keith Quirolo, MD
Formerly Department of Hematology/Oncology, UCSF Benioff Children's Hospital, Oakland, Oakland, CA USA

Lawrence Rice, MD
Chief, Division of Hematology, Houston Methodist Hospital; Professor of Medicine, Weill Cornell Medical College; and Adjunct Professor of Medicine, Baylor College of Medicine, Houston, TX, USA

Henry M. Rinder, MD
Professor of Laboratory Medicine and Internal Medicine (Hematology), Yale University School of Medicine and Director, Hematology Laboratories, Yale-New Haven Hospital, New Haven, CT, USA

Ennio C. Rossi, MD
Professor Emeritus of Medicine, Northwestern University School of Medicine, Chicago, IL, USA

Nathan J. Roth, PhD
Director, Global Pathogen Safety, CSL Behring King of Prussia, PA, USA

Alex B. Ryder, MD
Assistant Professor, Departments of Pediatrics and Pathology, University of Tennessee Health Science Center, Le Bonheur Children's Hospital Memphis, TN, USA

Ulrich J. Sachs, MD, PhD
Head and Professor, The Platelet and Granulocyte Laboratory, Institute for Clinical Immunology and Transfusion Medicine, Justus Liebig University Giessen, Germany

Michael Schmidt, MD
Professor, Institute of Transfusion Medicine and Immunohematology, German Red Cross, Frankfurt/M Germany

Wade L. Schulz, MD, PhD
Resident, Department of Laboratory Medicine Yale University School of Medicine and Blood Bank Yale-New Haven Hospital, New Haven, CT, USA

Jerard Seghatchian, MD
Senior Consultant, International Consultancy in Blood Components Quality/Safety Improvement, Audit/Inspection and DDR Strategies, London, UK

Erhard Seifried, MD, PhD
Director and Professor
Institute of Transfusion Medicine and Immunohematology, German Red Cross, Frankfurt/M Germany

Neil Shah, MD
Clinical Assistant Professor of Pathology and Transfusion Medicine, Medical Director of Referral Testing, Departments of Pathology and Medicine Stanford School of Medicine Stanford, CA, USA

Sujit Sheth, MD
Professor of Clinical Pediatrics, Department of Pediatrics, Weill Cornell Medical College New York, NY, USA

Don L. Siegel, PhD, MD
Professor, Pathology and Laboratory Medicine; and Director, Division of Transfusion Medicine and Therapeutic Pathology, Department of Pathology and Laboratory Medicine, Perelman School of Medicine at the University of Pennsylvania, Philadelphia, PA, USA

Joshua Siewert, MSc
School of Management, Department of Biomedical Engineering, Yale University; Department of Anesthesiology, Yale University School of Medicine New Haven, CT, USA

Toby L. Simon, MD
Senior Medical Director, Plasma Product Development and CSL Plasma, CSL Behring, King of Prussia PA; Clinical Professor of Pathology, University of New Mexico School of Medicine,Albuquerque, NM, USA

James W. Smith, MT, BSc
Technical Director, Platelet Immunology Laboratory Michael G. DeGroote School of Medicine McMaster University, Hamilton, ON, Canada

Edward L. Snyder, MD
Professor, Department of Laboratory Medicine Yale University School of Medicine, Director Blood Bank/Apheresis Service, Yale-New Haven Hospital, New Haven, CT, USA

Martha C. Sola-Visner, MD
Associate Professor of Pediatrics, Harvard Medical School, Harvard University; and Attending Neonatologist, Division of Newborn Medicine, Boston Children's Hospital, Boston, MA, USA

Bjarte G. Solheim, MD, PhD, MHA
Professor Emeritus, Institute of Immunology Oslo University Hospital–Rikshospitalet and University of Oslo, Oslo, Norway

Bryan R. Spencer, MPH
Research Scientist, American Red Cross Dedham, MA, USA

Simon J. Stanworth, MA, FRCP, DPhil, FRCPath
Consultant Haematologist, NHS Blood and Transplant and The National Institute for Health Research (NIHR) Oxford Biomedical Research Centre, Oxford University Hospitals, NHS Foundation Trust and the University of Oxford, Oxford, UK

Jill R. Storry, PhD
Blood Group Immunology, Clinical Immunology and Transfusion Medicine, University and Regional Laboratories Region Skåne, Lund University Hospital; and Associate Professor, Division of Hematology and Transfusion Medicine, Department of Laboratory Medicine, Lund University Lund, Sweden

Ronald G. Strauss, MD
Professor Emeritus, Departments of Pathology and Pediatrics, University of Iowa College of Medicine, Iowa City, IA, USA, Associate Medical Director, Life Source/Institute for Transfusion Medicine, Chicago, IL, USA

James R. Stubbs, MD
Chairman, Division of Transfusion Medicine, Department of Laboratory Medicine and Pathology Mayo Clinic, Rochester, MN, USA

Sumati Sundaram, PhD
Post Doctorate Associate in Cell Biology, Department of Biomedical Engineering, Yale University; Department of Anesthesiology, Yale University School of Medicine New Haven, CT, USA

Miho Teruya, MD, MPH
Postdoctoral Fellow, Department of Hematology/Oncology, Baylor College of Medicine, Houston, TX USA

Alan T. Tinmouth, MD, MSc (Clin Epi), FRCPC
Assistant Professor, Departments of Medicine, and Laboratory Medicine & Pathology, University of Ottawa; Head, General Hematology and Transfusion Medicine, Division of Hematology, The Ottawa Hospital; and University of Ottawa Centre for Transfusion Research Ottawa Hospital Research Institute Ottawa, ON, Canada

Christopher A. Tormey, MD
Associate Professor, Department of Laboratory Medicine, Yale University School of Medicine, New Haven, CT; and Director of Transfusion Medicine Veterans Affairs Medical Center West Haven, CT, USA

Darrell J. Triuzi, MD
Professor of Pathology
Director, Division of Transfusion Medicine
University of Pittsburgh Medical Center
Medical Director
Institute for Transfusion Medicine
Pittsburgh, PA, USA

Marc L. Turner, PhD
Professor, Department of Cellular Therapy, University
of Edinburgh; and Medical Director, Scottish National
Blood Transfusion Service, Edinburgh, Scotland, UK

Eleftherios C. Vamvakas, MD, PhD
Formerly, Rita and Taft Schreiber Chair in Transfusion
Medicine; Professor of Pathology and Director of
Clinical Pathology, Department of Pathology
Cedars-Sinai Medical Center Los Angeles, CA, USA

Jos J.M. van Roosmalen, MD, PhD
Professor of International Safe Motherhood and Health
Systems, Department of Obstetrics, Leiden University
Medical Center, Leiden; and Section of Health Care and
Culture, Athena Institute, VU University, Amsterdam
The Netherlands

Ralph R. Vassallo, Jr., MD
EVP/Chief Medical and Scientific Officer
Blood Systems, Inc., Scottsdale AZ, USA and
Adjunct Associate Professor of Medicine, University of
Pennsylvania School of Medicine, Philadelphia, PA
USA

Marieke B. Veenhof, MD
Senior Resident, Obstetrics and Gynaecology
Department of Obstetrics, Leiden University Medical
Center, Leiden, The Netherlands

Elliott Vichinsky, MD
Medical Director, Hematology/Oncology, UCSF Benioff
Children's Hospital Oakland, Oakland, CA; and
Professor of Pediatrics, University of California San
Francisco, San Francisco, CA, USA

**Jonathan P. Wallis, BA oxon, MB.
BS. lond., FRCP(UK), FRCPath**
Consultant Haematologist, Department of
Haematology, Freeman Hospital, Newcastle upon
Tyne, UK

**Theodore E. Warkentin, MD, BSc
(Med), FRCPC, FACP, FRCP(Edin)**
Professor, Departments of Pathology, Medicine and
Molecular Medicine, Michael G. DeGroote School of
Medicine, McMaster University, Hamilton, ON, Canada

Jonathan H. Waters, MD
Chief, Department of Anesthesiology
Magee-Womens Hospital of UPMC, Professor of
Anesthesiology and Bioengineering, University of
Pittsburgh, Medical Director, Patient Blood
Management Program of UPMC
Pittsburgh, PA, USA

Mark J. Weinstein, PhD
Associate Deputy Director for Science, Office of Blood
Research and Review, Center for Biologics Evaluation &
Research, US Food and Drug Administration, Silver
Spring, MD, USA

Robert Weinstein, MD
Professor, Departments of Medicine and Pathology, and
Chief, Division of Transfusion Medicine, University of
Massachusetts Medical School; and UMass Memorial
Medical Center, Worcester, MA, USA

Connie M. Westhoff, SBB, PhD
Director, Laboratory of Immunohematology and
Genomics, New York Blood Center, New York
NY, USA

**Johanna C. Wiersum-Osselton,
PhD**
TRIP National Hemovigilance and Biovigilance Office
Leiden, The Netherlands

Elise Wilcox
Student, Department of Biomedical Engineering
Yale University; Department of Anesthesiology
Yale University School of Medicine, New Haven, CT
USA

Michael Wilson, PhD
Senior Director, Molecular Biology, CSL Behring
Broadmeadows, VIC, Australia

Jeffrey L. Winters, MD
Medical Director, Therapeutic Apheresis Treatment
Unit, Mayo Clinic, Rochester, MN, USA

Steven E. Wolf, MD
Professor of Surgery and Chairman for Research
Department of Surgery, Division of Burn/Trauma/
Critical Care, University of Texas Southwestern Medical
Center, Dallas, TX, USA

Gary M. Woods, MD
Assistant Professor, Department of Pediatrics
Eastern Virginia Medical School, Division of Pediatric
Hematology/Oncology, Children's Hospital of the
King's Daughters, Norfolk VA, USA

Mark H. Yazer, MD
Professor of Pathology, University of Pittsburgh
Associate Medical Director, Centralized Transfusion
Service, Institute for Transfusion Medicine
Pittsburgh, PA, USA

Preface

After an interval of six years, we have again focused on the task of updating *Rossi's Principles of Transfusion Medicine* in order to support the continually evolving disciplines of transfusion medicine, blood banking, and cellular therapies. Many of the trends we identified and covered in the last edition have continued to evolve. More extensive use of molecular techniques, increased focus on hemovigilance and donor vigilance, continued maturation of pathogen inactivation technologies, and advances in cellular therapy are but some examples. Many controversies remain, such as the impact of red cell storage on patient well-being and the best approach to follow for the treatment of severe bleeding, particularly in the acute trauma setting.

As before, we welcome back authors from the prior editions as well as introduce new authors to strategically deal with changes in the field, including as a new editor Dr. Jeffrey McCullough. Keeping abreast of changing technology in publishing, we have provided a web connection for all purchasers of the book—both the print and electronic editions. To keep the size of the book manageable, the full list of numbered references is available on the web. Additionally, after each chapter, authors have provided a short list of major reviews or key articles.

We have made one significant organizational change. We removed the section at the end that was called "Delivery of Transfusion and Transplantation Services." Instead, the first section of the book is titled "Contemporary issues in donation and transfusion." After the historical perspective, a new chapter on patient blood management explores in greater detail than before what has been arguably the most transformative movement in the field since the last edition. Teaching the responsible and cautious use of blood components has long been a major part of the role of the transfusion medicine expert. But, somehow in the last five years, the message has resonated as never before and the resulting decline in blood utilization has revolutionized the business model of community and national blood programs as well as reduced dramatically the frequency of blood shortages in the developed world. Recruitment techniques have been refined so that the right number of donors for the right component with the right blood type at the right time has become more important than total numbers. Of course, we do need to remember that the situation in countries with underdeveloped economies is much different. There, the lack of adequate quantities of safe blood components and transfusion services for lifesaving needs is still all too common.

In this same section, there is a new chapter on the technical aspects of transfusion as well as an updated chapter on collection of blood. In consideration of the increased attention focused on both preventing the acute problem of loss of consciousness after donation and the chronic problem of iron depletion in red cell donors, a new separate chapter on adverse effects of donation has been added. Chapters on hemovigilance and donor vigilance and regulatory oversight complete the section. The latter chapter combines material from several chapters in the prior edition covering quality and regulation from both the manufacturing and hospital perspectives on a global basis.

In the second section on transfusion medicine practice, new data on blood components are added and the restrictive use of red cells is further documented. In addition, the chapters on plasma are expanded given the growth in use of plasma derivatives—a trend opposite to the declining use of most cellular components. The third section on apheresis, transplantation, and new therapies has been expanded to keep up with increased activity, particularly in cell and gene therapy. Section IV is devoted to specialized clinical practice, with coverage of the new approaches to treatment of trauma and massive bleeding. The last section covers the hazards of transfusion. As the "big three" viruses (hepatitis B and C and HIV) have come under better control, that material has been placed in one chapter. A new chapter on testing for pathogens complements an expanded chapter on pathogen reduction to highlight approaches to containing infectious threats. The book concludes with chapters on non-infectious hazards of transfusion.

Our publisher, Wiley-Blackwell, was able to provide full support for the coordination and production of this edition. We appreciate all of their efforts, which they have provided efficiently and with high quality.

As we publish the fifth edition, we simultaneously celebrate both the continuity in the field and the new developments and once again emphasize the teamwork of the transfusion medicine professionals at all levels, including medical specialists in all fields who utilize transfusion medicine, technologists, administrators, nurses, and donors. We hope that a new upcoming generation of transfusion medicine specialists will carry on its proud traditions and bring about exciting innovation.

Most importantly, it is our ability to provide help to the patient—who, as the recipient of transfusion medicine products and services, is better able to extend his or her life, improve the quality of that life, or both—that constantly motivates us to move the field forward throughout the world.

We, as an editorial group, recognize the contribution of our invaluable authors and thank our families, colleagues, employers, teachers, and students for their understanding and support during the intense period of time needed for preparation and execution of this, the fifth edition of *Rossi's Principles of Transfusion Medicine*.

List of abbreviations

2-ME	2-mercaptoethanol	aPCC	activated prothrombin complex concentrate
2RBC	double red cell collection	APS	antiphospholipid antibody syndrome
AA	aplastic anemia	aPTT	activated partial thromboplastin time
AABB	(Not spelled out; originally founded as the American Association of Blood Banks)	ARDS	acute respiratory distress syndrome
		ARITI	Age of Red Blood Cell in Premature Infants
AAP	American Academy of Pediatrics	ASP	antibody specificity prediction
aAPC	artificial antigen presenting cell	ASRI	American Society for Reproductive
AAV	adeno-associated virus		Immunology
Ab	antibody	Atf4	activating transcription factor-4
ABC	America's Blood Centers	ATG	antithymocyte globulin
ABLE	Age of Blood Evaluation (trial)	ATP	adenosine triphosphate
ABT	allogeneic blood transfusion	AUC	area under the ROC curve
ACCP	American College of Chest Physicians	AvWS	acquired von Willebrand syndrome
ACD	acid–citrate–dextrose	BAGP	bicarbonate, adenine, glucose, and phosphate
ACE	angiotensin-converting enzyme	B-ALL	B-cell acute lymphoblastic leukemia
ACEI	angiotensin-converting enzyme inhibitor	BART	Blood Conservation Using Antifibrinolytics
ACh	acetylcholine		in a Randomized Trial
AChR	acetylcholine receptor molecule	BasoEB	basophilic erythroblast
ACI	anemia of chronic inflammation	B-CAM	basal cell adhesion molecule
ACOG	American College of Obstetricians and Gynecologists	BDD	B-domain-deleted
		BECS	blood establishment computer software
ADCC	antibody-dependent cellular cytotoxicity	BFU-E(s)	burst-forming unit(s)-erythroid
ADF	actin depolymerizing factor	BFU-MK	MK burst-forming unit
ADP	adenosine diphosphate	BiKE	bispecific killer engager
ADSC	adipose-derived stem cell	BMD	Becker muscular dystrophy
AFSA	American Society for Apheresis	BMP	bone morphogenetic protein
AGM	aortogonadomesonephros	BMSC	bone marrow stem cell
AHF	antihemophilic factor	BNP	B-type natriuretic peptide
AHG	antihuman globulin	BOS	bronchiolitis obliterans syndrome
AHRQ	Agency for Healthcare Research and Quality	BRN	Blood Regulators Network
AHSP	alpha-hemoglobin stabilizing protein	BSA	body surface area
aHUS	atypical hemolytic uremic syndrome	BSS	Bernard Soulier syndrome
AIDS	acquired immune deficiency syndrome	BTHC	butyryl-tri-hexyl citrate
AIHA	autoimmune hemolytic anemia	BVDV	bovine viral diarrhea virus
AIS	absent iron stores	CABG	coronary artery bypass graft
ALAS2	5-aminolevulinic acid synthase	CAD	cold agglutinin disease
ALCL	anaplastic large-cell lymphoma	CAEV	arthritis-encephalitis virus of goats
ALK	anterior lamellar keratoplasty	CAFC	cobblestone area-forming cell
ALL	acute lymphoblastic leukemia	CAP	College of American Pathologists
ALT	alanine aminotransferase	CAR	CXCL12 abundant reticular (cell)
AMKL	acute megakaryoblastic leukemia	CARS	compensatory anti-inflammatory response syndrome
AML	acute myelogenous leukemia		
AMP	adenosine monophosphate	CAR-T cell	T cell expressing a chimeric antigen receptor
AMR	Ashwell–Morell receptor	CBC	complete blood count
ANC	absolute neutrophil count	CBER	Center for Biologics Evaluation and Research
ANCA	anti-neutrophil cytoplasmic antibody		
ANH	acute normovolemic hemodilution	CCAD	Central Cardiac Audit Database
APC	antigen-presenting cell	CCI	corrected count increment
API	alpha$_1$-proteinase inhibitor	CCPD	complement control protein domain

CDA	congenital dyserythropoietic anemia	DBA	Diamond–Blackfan anemia
CDC	Centers for Disease Control and Prevention	DC	dendritic cell
CDER	Center for Drug Evaluation and Research	DCASGPR	dendritic cell asialoglycoprotein receptor
CDR	complementarity-determining region	DDAVP	desmopressin acetate
CDRH	Center for Devices and Radiologic Health	DEA	diethyleneamine
CD–P–TS	European Committee on Blood Transfusion	DEAE	dietlylaminoethyl
CDSS	clinical decision support software	DEHP	diethylhexyl phthalate
cffDNA	cell-free fetal DNA	DFPP	double-membrane filtration plasmapheresis
CFR	US Code of Federal Regulations	DFSD	dry fibrin sealant dressing
CFU-GM	progenitor cells with the capacity to generate neutrophils in vitro	DHF	dihydrofolate
		DHFR	dihydrofolate reductase
CGD	chronic granulomatous disease	DHSt	dehydrated stomatocytosis
cGMP	current good manufacturing practice	DIC	disseminated intravascular coagulation
CH2-THF	methylenetetrahydrofolate	DITP	drug-induced immune thrombocytopenia
CH3-THF	methyltetrahydrofolate	DMD	Duchenne muscular dystrophy
CHCM	cell hemoglobin concentration mean	DMS	demarcation membrane system
ChLIA	chemiluminescent immunoassay	dsDNA	double-stranded DNA
CHMP	Committee for Medicinal Products for Human Use	dsRNA	double-stranded RNA
		DTT	dithiothreitol
CHO-THF	formyltetrahydrofolate	DVT	deep vein thrombosis
CHr	cellular hemoglobin in reticulocytes	EACA	ε-aminocaproic acid
CI	confidence interval	EBA	European Blood Alliance
CIBMTR	Center for International Blood and Marrow Transplant Research	EBI	erythroblastic island
		ECBS	Expert Committee on Biological Standardization
CIDP	chronic inflammatory demyelinating polyneuropathy	ECM	extracellular matrix
CJD	Creutzfeldt–Jakob disease	ECP	extracorporeal photopheresis
CLET	cultured limbal epithelial transplantation	EDQM	European Directorate for the Quality of Medicines
CLIA	Clinical Laboratory Improvement Amendments	EDTA	ethylenediaminetetraacetic acid
CM	carboxymethyl	EFIC	exception from informed consent
CML	chronic myelogenous leukemia	EIA	enzyme immunoassay
CMP	common myeloid precursor	ELISA	enzyme-linked immunosorbent assay
CMS	Centers for Medicare and Medicaid Services	EMP	erythroblast–macrophage protein
CMV	cytomegalovirus	EPO	erythropoietin
CNS	central nervous system	EPO-α	erythropoietin alpha
COBLT	Cord Blood Transplant (study)	EPO-R	erythropoietin receptor
COM	All Common Checklist	EEA	European Economic Area
CPB	cardiopulmonary bypass	EIA	enzyme immunoassay
CPD	citrate–phosphate–dextrose	EIAV	infectious anemia virus of horses
CPDA	citrate–phosphate–dextrose–adenine	ELISA	enzyme-linked immunosorbent assay
CPOE	computerized physician order entry	EMA	European Medicines Agency
CPSI	Canadian Patient Safety Institute	ERMAP	erythrocyte membrane-associated protein
CRASH-2	Clinical Randomization of an Antifibrinolytic in Significant Hemorrhage trial	ESC	embryonic stem cell
		ET	essential thrombocythemia
CREG	cross-reactive group	EU	European Union
CRM	cross-reactive material	EUHASS	European Hemophilia Safety Surveillance
CRISPR	clustered regularly interspaced short palindromic repeat	EVA	ethylene vinyl acetate
		EXM	electronic crossmatch
CRPS II	chronic regional pain syndrome type 2	FACT	Foundation for the Accreditation of Cellular Therapy
CSA	cyclosporine	
CSF	circulating steel factor	FADH	reduced flavin adenine dinucleotide
CTA	cancer-testis antigen	FAST	focused ultrasonographic survey for trauma
CTL	cytotoxic T-cell	FBS	fetal blood sampling
CVAD	central venous access device	FCR	fraction of cells remaining
CXCL12	stromal-cell derived factor 1	FcRn	neonatal Fc receptor
DAF	decay accelerating factor	FDA	US Food and Drug Administration
DARC	Duffy antigen receptor for chemokines	FDAAAA	Food and Drug Administration Amendments Act
DART	Danish Registration of Transfusion Accidents	
		FDAMA	Food and Drug Administration Modernization Act
DAT	direct antiglobulin test	

FDA cGMP	US Food and Drug Administration current good manufacturing practice	HE	hereditary elliptocytosis
FDASIA	Food and Drug Administration Safety and Innovation Act	HELLP	syndrome of hemolysis, elevated liver enzymes, and low platelet count
FDC	follicular dendritic cell	HES	hydroxyethyl starch
FDP	fibrin degradation product	hESC	human embryonic stem cell
FEIBA	factor VIII inhibitory bypass activity	HEV	hepatitis E virus
FEP	free erythrocyte protoporphyrin	HFMEA	Healthcare Failure Mode and Effect Analysis
FFP	fresh frozen plasma	HH	hereditary hemochromatosis
FGS	focal glomerulosclerosis	HHV	human herpesvirus
FH	familial hypercholesterolemia	HIF	hypoxia-inducible transcription factor
FLAER	fluorescent aerolysin	HIPA	heparin-induced platelet activation assay
FNAIT	fetal/neonatal alloimmune thrombocytopenia	HIT	heparin-induced thrombocytopenia
		HIV	human immunodeficiency virus
FNHTR	febrile nonhemolytic transfusion reaction	HIV-1	human immunodeficiency virus type 1
FT/RA	first-time and reactivated (donors)	HIV-2	human immunodeficiency virus type 2
G6PD	glucose-6-phosphate dehydrogenase	HLA	human leukocyte antigen
GABA	γ-amino butyric acid	HMW	high molecular weight
GAD-65	65-kD isoform of glutamic acid decarboxylase	HO1	heme oxygenase-1
		HPC	hematopoietic progenitor cell
GAG	glycoslyaminoglycan	HRI	heme-regulated inhibitor
GBM	glomerular basement membrane	HSC	hematopoietic stem cell
G-CSF	granulocyte colony-stimulating factor	HSCT	hematopoietic stem cell transfusion
GDP	guanosine diphosphate	HSV	herpes simplex virus
GEN	Laboratory General Checklist	HTA	health technology assessment
GI	gastrointestinal	HTLV-I	human T-cell lymphotropic virus, type I
GLUT1	glucose transporter 1	HTLV-II	human T-cell lymphotropic virus, type II
GM-CSF	granulocyte macrophage colony-stimulating factor	HTR	hemolytic transfusion reaction
		HUS	hemolytic uremic syndrome
GMP	good manufacturing practice	%HYPOm	percentage of hypochromic mature red blood cells
GP	glycoprotein		
GPA	glycophorin A	%HYPOr	percentage of hypochromic red blood cells
GPB	glycophorin B	IAT	indirect antiglobulin testing
GPI	glycosylphosphatidylinositol	IBCT	incorrect blood component transfused
GPS	Goodpasture syndrome	IBR	intraoperative blood recovery
GRADE	Grading of Recommendations Assessment, Development and Evaluation	ICAM4	interstitial cell adhesion molecule-4
		ICH	International Conference on Harmonization (of Technical Requirements)
GSH	glutathione		
GSL	glycospingolipid	ICH	intracranial hemorrhage
GSS	Gerstmann–Sträusler–Scheinker (disease)	ICU	intensive care unit
GTP	guanosine triphosphate	IDA	iron-deficiency anemia
GTX	granulocyte transfusion	IDE	iron-deficient erythropoiesis
GVHD	graft-versus-host disease	IDSA	Infectious Disease Society of America
GVL	graft-versus-leukemia	IDT	individual testing
GWA	genome-wide association	IFAT	immunofluorescent antibody test
HA	hydroxyapatite	IFN	interferon
HAM (test)	(Not an abbreviation; named after its creator, Thomas Ham)	IGF1	insulin-like growth factor-1
		IgG	immunoglobulin G
HBc	hepatitis B core (antigen)	IgSF	immunoglobulin superfamily
HBcAg	hepatitis B core antigen	IHN	International Hemovigilance Network
HBeAg	hepatitis B e antigen	IL	interleukin
HBSAg	hepatitis B virus surface antigen	IND	investigational new drug
HBV	hepatitis B virus	iNKT	invariant natural killer T cell
HCEC	human corneal endothelial cell	IPD	individual-patient data
HCT	hematopoietic cell transplant	INR	international normalized ratio
HCT/P	human cells, tissues, and cellular and tissue-based product	IPFA	International Plasma Fractionation Association
		iPSC	induced pluripotent stem cell
HCV	hepatitis C virus	IPSS	International Prognostic Scoring System
HDL	high-density lipoprotein	IQPP	International Quality Plasma Program
HDFN	hemolytic disease of the fetus and newborn	IRE	iron-responsive element
HDV	hepatitis D virus	IRP	iron regulatory protein

ISBT	International Society of Blood Transfusion	NAAT	nucleic acid amplification testing
ISTARE	International Surveillance Database for Transfusion Adverse Reactions and Events	NAD	nicotinamide adenine dinucleotide
		NADH	reduced nicotinamide adenine dinucleotide
ISTH	International Society on Thrombosis and Hemostasis	NADP	nicotinamide adenine dinucleotide phosphate
IT	information technology	NAIT	neonatal alloimmune thrombocytopenia
ITI	immune tolerance induction	NAPTT	non-activated partial thromboplastin time
ITP	immune thrombocytopenic purpura	NAT	nucleic acid testing
IV	intravenous	NATA	Network for Advancement of Transfusion Alternatives
IVD	in vitro diagnostic		
IVIG	intravenous immunoglobulin	NBCUS	(AABB) National Blood Collection and Utilization Survey
JAK2	Janus tyrosine kinase-2		
KIR	killer immunoglobulin-like receptor	NCA	national competent authority
KLF1	Krüppel-like factor-1	NCI	National Cancer Institute
LAK	lymphokine-activated killer	NET	neutrophil extracellular trap
LCL	lymphoblastoid line	NHLBI	National Heart, Lung, and Blood Institute
LCR	locus control region	NIBSC	National Institute of Biological Standards and Control
LCT	lymphocytotoxicity		
LDL	low-density lipoprotein	NICU	neonatal intensive care unit
LEMS	Lambert–Eaton myasthenic syndrome	NIH	National Institutes of Health
LESC	limbal epithelial stem cell	NOD	non-obese diabetic
LGL	large granular lymphocyte	NPO	*nil per os*
LHR	long homologous repeat	NSAID	nonsteroidal anti-inflammatory drug
LIC	liver iron concentration	NTBI	non-transferrin-bound iron
LISS	low-ionic-strength saline	NYHA	New York Heart Association
LMAN	lectin mannose binding	OBI	occult hepatitis B infection
LMW	low molecular weight	OBRR	Office of Blood Research and Review
LR	leukocyte-reduced *or* leukoreduction	OCS	open canalicular system
LSC	limbal stem cell	OHI	occult hepatitis infection
MAG	myelin-associated glycoprotein	OHSt	overhydrated stomatocytosis
MAHA	microangiopathic hemolytic anemia	OMCL	Official Medicines Control Laboratory
MAIPA	monoclonal antibody-specific immobilization of platelet antigens	OR	odds ratio
		OrthoEB	orthochromatic erythroblast
MAP	mean arterial pressure	PAI-1	plasminogen activator inhibitor type 1
MAPK	mitogen-activated protein kinase	PAIgG	platelet-associated IgG
MART	melanoma antigen recognized by T cells	PANDAS	pediatric autoimmune neuropsychiatric disorders associated with streptococcal infections
MBP	myelin basic protein		
MCFD	multiple coagulation factor deficiency gene		
MCH	mean cell hemoglobin	PAS	platelet additive solution
MCHC	mean corpuscular hemoglobin concentration	PASSPORT	Post Approval Surveillance Study of Platelet Outcomes, Release Tested (protocol)
MCP	macrophage chemoattractant protein	PBM	patient blood management
MCV	mean corpuscular volume	PBMC	peripheral blood mononuclear cell
MDS	myelodysplastic syndrome	PBPC	peripheral blood progenitor cell
MEP	megakaryocytic-erythroid progenitor	PBR	postoperative blood recovery
MGSA	melanocyte growth-stimulating activity	PBSC	peripheral blood stem cell
MGUS	monoclonal gammopathy of undetermined significance	PC	platelet concentrate
		PCAM	platelet-endothelial cell adhesion molecule-1
MHC	major histocompatibility complex		
MIRL	membrane inhibitor of reactive lysis	PCC	prothrombin complex concentrate
MK	megakaryocyte	PCH	paroxysmal cold hemoglobinuria
MMP	matrix metalloproteinase	PCL	polycaprolactone
MODS	multiple-organ dysfunction syndrome	PCP	*Pneumocystis carinii*
MOF	multiple-organ failure	PCR	polymerase chain reaction
MOG	myelin oligodendrocyte glycoprotein	PDMP	plasma-derived medicinal product
MPP	multipotent progenitor	PEG	polyethylene glycol
MPV	mean platelet volume	PEG-rHuMGDF	pegylated recombinant human mega karyocyte growth and development factor
MRI	magnetic resonance imaging		
MSC	mesenchymal stem (or stromal) cell	PEI	Paul Ehrlich Institute
MTP	massive transfusion protocol	PF	platelet factor
MTX	methotrexate	PF24	24-hour frozen plasma

PFA-100	platelet function analyzer 100	RBM15	RNA binding motif protein 15
PfEMP	*Plasmodium falciparum* erythrocyte membrane protein	RCAS1	receptor-binding cancer antigen expressed on SiSo cells
PGA	polyglycolic acid	RECESS	Red Cell Duration Study
PhEur	European Pharmacopeia	REF	febrile nonhemolytic transfusion reaction
PHSA	Public Health Service Act	RFLP	restriction fragment length polymorphism
PICC	peripherally inserted central catheter	RhAG	Rh-associated glycoprotein
PIC/S	Pharmaceutical Inspection Co-operation Scheme and Pharmaceutical Inspection Convention	RhIG	Rh immune globulin
		RING	Safety and Effectiveness of Granulocyte Transfusion in Resolving Infection in People with Neutropenia (study)
PIG-A	phosphatidylinosital glycan class A		
PIVKA	proteins induced in vitamin K absence or antagonism	RIPA	radioimmunoprecipitation assay
		RIR	replication-incompetent retrovirus
PK	penetrating keratoplasty	RISE	REDS-II Donor Iron Status Evaluation
PKD	pyruvate kinase deficiency	RLS	reporting and learning systems
PLA	polylactic acid	ROC	receiver operating characteristic
PLADO	Optimal Platelet Dose Strategy to Prevent Bleeding in Thrombocytopenia Patients	ROS	reactive oxygen species
		RP	reticulated platelet
PLGA	polylactic-co-glycolic acid	RSV	respiratory syncytial virus
PMMA	polymethylmethacrylate	SAA	severe aplastic anemia
PMN	neutrophil	SABM	Society for the Advancement of Blood Management
PNH	paroxysmal nocturnal hemoglobinuria		
PNM	polymorphonuclear	SAG	saline, adenine, and glucose
POEMS	polyneuropathy, organomegaly, endocrinopathy, monoclonal protein, and skin changes (syndrome)	SAG-M	saline, adenine, glucose, and mannitol
		SCD	sickle cell disease
		SCF	stem cell factor
POISE	Perioperative Ischemic Evaluation (trial)	scFv	single-chain variable fragment
PolyEB	polychromatophilic erythroblast	SCL	stem cell leukemia
PPH	postpartum hemorrhage	SCN	severe congenital neutropenia
PPi	pyrophosphate	sc-TPA	single-chain tissue plasminogen activator
PPTA	Plasma Protein Therapeutics Association	sc-UPA	single-chain urokinase plasminogen activator
PRA	panel-reactive antibody		
PRAC	Pharmacovigilance Risk Assessment Committee	S/D	solvent and detergent (*or* solvent–detergent)
		SDS-PAGE	sodium dodecyl sulfate–polyacrylamide gel electrophoresis
ProEB	pro-erythroblast		
PRP	platelet-rich plasma	serpin	serine protease inhibitor
PRPP	phosphoribosyl pyrophosphate	SIRS	systemic inflammatory response syndrome
PRV	pseudorabies virus	SLE	systemic lupus erythematosus
PS	phosphatidylserine	SMC	smooth muscle cell
PSA	prostate-specific antigen	SNP	single nucleotide polymorphism
PSGL1	platelet sialoglycoprotein ligand-1	SoGAT	International Working Group on the Standardization of Genomic Amplification Techniques for the Virological Safety Testing of Blood and Blood Products
PSO	patient safety organization		
PT	prothrombin time		
PTFE	polytetrafluoroethylene		
PTLD	posttransplant lymphoproliferative disease	SOP	standard operating procedure
PTP	posttransfusion purpura	SP	sulfopropyl
PTR	platelet transfusion refractoriness	SPRCA	solid-phase red cell adherence
PT/PTT	prothrombin time and partial thromboplastin time	SPS	stiff-person syndrome
		SQUID	superconducting quantum interference device
PUP	previously untreated patient		
PVC	polyvinyl chloride	SRA	serotonin release assay
pVHL	von Hippel–Lindau protein	SRF	serum response factor
QA	quality assurance	ssDNA	single-stranded DNA
QAE	quaternary amino ethyl	SSOPH	sequence-specific oligonucleotide probe hybridization
QALY	quality-adjusted life year		
QC	quality control	ssRNA	single-stranded RNA
RA	rheumatoid arthritis	STAT5	signal transduction and activator of transcription-5
RANTES	regulated on activation, normal T-cell expressed and secreted		
		sTfR	soluble transferrin receptor
RBC	red blood cell	TACO	transfusion-associated circulatory overload
RBC(s), LR	red blood cell(s), leukocytes reduced	TAD	transfusion-associated dyspnea

TAFI	thrombin-activatable fibrinolysis inhibitor	TRICC	Transfusion Requirements in Critical Care
TA-GVHD	transfusion-associated graft-versus-host disease	TRICK	transfusion-related inhibition of cytokines
TALENS	transcription activator–like effector nucleases	TRIM	transfusion-related immunomodulation
		TRS	(WHO) Technical Report Series
TA-MC	transfusion-associated microchimerism	TSO	Transfusion Safety Office
TAMMv	timed average mean maximum velocity	TT	thrombin time
TAPS	twin anemia–polycythemia sequence	TTI	transfusion-transmissible infection
TCD	transcranial Doppler	TTP	thrombotic thrombocytopenic purpura
TCP	tricalcium phosphate	TTTS	twin-to-twin transfusion syndrome
tc-TPA	two-chain tissue plasminogen activator	TWEAK	TNF-like weak inducer of apoptosis
tc-UPA	two-chain urokinase plasminogen activator	TXA	tranexamic acid
TEE	thromboembolic event	UDHQ	Uniform Donor History Questionnaire
TEG	thromboelastography	ULR	universal leukocyte reduction
TEVG	tissue-engineered vascular graft	UTR	untranslated region
TFPI	tissue factor pathway inhibitor	VATS	Viral Activation by Transfusion Study
TGA	thrombin generation assay	VCAM1	vascular cell adhesion molecule 1
Th	T helper (cell)	vCJD	variant Creutzfeldt–Jakob disease
THA	total hip arthroplasty	VEGF	vascular endothelial growth factor
THF	tetrahydrofolate	VEGFR	vascular endothelial growth factor receptor
TI	tincture of iodine	VGKC	voltage-gated potassium channel
TIL	tumor-infiltrating lymphocyte	VKA	vitamin K antagonist
TLR	toll-like receptor	VLBW	very-low-birthweight
TM	thalassemia major	VLDL	very-low-density lipoprotein
TMA	thrombotic microangiopathy	VMV	visna-maedi virus of sheep
TMAA	thrombotic micro-angiopathic anemia	VWD	von Willebrand disease
TNC	total nucleated cell count	WAIHA	warm-type autoimmune hemolytic anemia
TNF	tumor necrosis factor	WAS	Wiskott–Aldrich syndrome
TNF-α	tumor necrosis factor alpha	WBC	white blood cell
TOP	Transfusion of Prematures	WBD	whole blood derived
TOTM	triethyl hexyl trimellitate	WBIT	wrong blood in tube
tPA	tissue plasminogen activator	WCC	WHO Collaborating Center
TPMT	thiopurine methyltransferase	WFH	World Federation of Hemophilia
TPO	thrombopoietin	WHIM (syndrome)	warts, hypogammaglobulinemia, infections, and myelokathexis
TRAIL	TNF-related apoptosis-inducing ligand	WHO	World Health Organization
TRALI	transfusion-related acute lung injury	ZFN	zinc finger nuclease
TRAP	Trial to Reduce Alloimmunization to Platelets	ZnPP	zinc protoporphyrin

About the companion website

This book has a companion website:

> **www.wiley.com/go/simon/transfusion**

The website features the figures from the book, the full text of the book, and all references.

The password for the website is the first word of Chapter 2. Please use all lowercase.

CHAPTER 1

Transfusion in the new millennium

Ennio C. Rossi[1] & Toby L. Simon[2]

[1]Northwestern University School of Medicine, Chicago, IL, USA
[2]Plasma Product Development and CSL Plasma, CSL Behring, King of Prussia, PA; and Department of Pathology, University of New Mexico School of Medicine, Albuquerque, NM, USA

Prehistoric man left drawings of himself pierced by arrows.[1] This means he was as aware of blood as he was of his own limbs. The flint implements he used as tools and weapons distinguished him from other creatures and contributed to the violence of his era. As he hunted food and fought enemies, he observed bleeding and the properties of blood. A cut, received or inflicted, yielded a vivid red color. If the cut was shallow, there was little blood. But if the cut was deep, a red torrent flowing from the stricken victim quickly led to death, with shed blood congealed and darkening in the sun. Fatal hemorrhage was commonplace. Nonetheless, the sight must have been fearful and possibly existential as life flowed red out of the body of an enemy or a wounded animal.[2] It is no wonder, then, that at the dawn of recorded history, blood was already celebrated in religious rites and rituals as a life-giving force.

The cultural expressions of primitive and ancient societies, although separated by time or space, can be strikingly similar. Whether these expressions emerged independently or were diffused about the world by unknown voyagers will probably always remain clouded in mystery.[2] Nonetheless, there is a common thread in the ancient rituals that celebrate blood as a mystical vital principle. In Leviticus 17:11, "the life of the flesh is in the blood," and the Chinese Neiching (ca. 1000 BC) claims the blood contains the soul.[2] Pre-Columbian North American Indians bled their bodies "of its greatest power" as self-punishment,[3] Egyptians took blood baths as a recuperative measure, and Romans drank the blood of fallen gladiators in an effort to cure epilepsy.[4] The Romans also practiced a ceremony called taurobolium—a blood bath for spiritual restoration. A citizen seeking spiritual rebirth descended into a pit, or *fossa sanguinis*. Above him on a platform, a priest sacrificed a bull, and the animal's blood cascaded down in a shower upon the beneficiary. Then, in a powerful visual image, the subject emerged up from the other end of the pit, covered with blood and reborn.[1]

The legend of Medea and Aeson taken from Ovid's *Metamorphoses* and quoted in Bulfinch's *Mythology*[5] also ascribed rejuvenating powers to blood. Jason asked Medea to "take some years off his life and add them to those of his father Aeson." Medea, however, pursued an alternative course. She prepared a cauldron with the blood of a sacrificed black sheep. To this, she added magic herbs, hoarfrost gathered by moonlight, the entrails of a wolf, and many other things "without a name." The boiling cauldron was stirred with a withered olive branch, which became green and full of leaves and young olives when it was withdrawn. Seeing that all was ready,

Medea cut the throat of the old man and let out all his blood, and poured into his mouth and into his wound the juices of her cauldron. As soon as he had imbibed them, his hair and beard laid by their whiteness and assumed the blackness of youth; his paleness and emaciation were gone; his veins were full of blood, his limbs of vigour and robustness. Aeson is amazed at himself and remembers that such as he now is, he was in his youthful days, 40 years before.

This legend seems to echo the apocryphal story of Pope Innocent VIII, who is said to have received the blood of three young boys in 1492 while on his deathbed. As the story goes, a physician attempted to save the pope's life by using blood drawn from three boys 10 years of age, all of whom died soon thereafter. Some 19th-century versions of this tale suggest the blood was transfused. However, earlier renditions more plausibly suggest that the blood was intended for a potion to be taken by mouth. In any event, there is no evidence the pope actually received any blood in any form.[6,7]

The folklore that flowed with blood was not accompanied by a great deal of accurate information. The ancient Greeks believed that blood formed in the heart and passed through the veins to the rest of the body, where it was consumed. Arteries were part of an independent system transporting air from the lungs. Although Erasistratos (circa 270 BC) had imagined the heart as a pump, his idea was ahead of its time. As long as veins and arteries were dead-end channels transporting blood and air, there was little need for a pump in the system. Although Galen (131–201 AD) finally proved that arteries contain blood, communication with the venous system was not suspected. Blood, formed in the liver, merely passed through the blood vessels and heart on its way to the periphery.[1] These teachings remained in place for 1400 years until they were swept away in 1628 by Harvey's discovery of the circulation.

The realization that blood moved in a circulating stream opened the way to experiments on vascular infusion. In 1642, George von Wahrendorff injected wine[8]—and, in 1656, Christopher Wren and Robert Boyle injected opium and other drugs[9]— intravenously into dogs. The latter studies, performed at Oxford, were the inspiration for Richard Lower's experiments in animal transfusion.

The first animal transfusion

Richard Lower (1631–1691) was a student at Oxford when Christopher Wren and Robert Boyle began their experiments on infusion. In due course, Lower joined their scientific group and studied the

Rossi's Principles of Transfusion Medicine, Fifth Edition. Edited by Toby L. Simon, Jeffrey McCullough, Edward L. Snyder, Bjarte G. Solheim, and Ronald G. Strauss.
© 2016 John Wiley & Sons, Ltd. Published 2016 by John Wiley & Sons, Ltd.

intravenous injection of opiates, emetics, and other substances into living animals.[10] In time, the transfusion of blood itself became the objective. The announcement of the first successful transfusion, performed by Richard Lower at Oxford in February 1665, was published on November 19, 1666, in the *Philosophical Transactions of the Royal Society* in a short notation titled, "The Success of the Experiment of Transfusing the Blood of One Animal into Another."[11] The entire notation is as follows:[11]

> This experiment, hitherto look'd upon to be of an almost insurmountable difficulty, hath been of late very successfully perform'd not only at Oxford, by the directions of that expert anatomist Dr. Lower, but also in London, by order of the R. Society, at their publick meeting in Gresham Colledge: the Description of the particulars whereof, and the Method of Operation is referred to the next opportunity.

The December 17, 1666, issue of the *Transactions* contained the full description as promised.[12] It was taken from a letter[13] written by Lower to Robert Boyle on July 6, 1666, in which Lower described direct transfusion from the carotid artery of one dog to the jugular vein of another. After describing the insertion of quills into the blood vessels of the donor and recipient dogs, Lower wrote:[13]

> When you have done this you may lay the dogs on their side and fasten them densely together as best you may to insure the connection of the two quills. Quickly tighten the noose around the neck of the receiving animal as in venasection, or at all events compress the vein on the opposite side of the neck with your finger, then take out the stopper and open the upper jugular quill so that while the foreign blood is flowing into the lower quill, the animal's own blood flows out from the upper into suitable receptacles—until at last the second animal, amid howls, faintings, and spasms, finally loses its life together with its vital fluid.
>
> When the tragedy is over, take both quills out of the jugular vein of the surviving animal, tie tightly with the former slipknots, and divide the vein. After the vessel has been divided, sew up the skin, slacken the cords binding the dog, and let it jump down from the table. It shakes itself a little, as though aroused from sleep, and runs away lively and strong, more active and vigorous perhaps, with the blood of its fellow than its own.

These studies inevitably led to the transfusion of animal blood to humans. In England, this occurred on November 23, 1667, when Lower and Edmund King transfused sheep blood into a man named Arthur Coga.[14] Described by Samuel Pepys as "a little frantic," Coga was paid 20 shillings to accept this transfusion, with the expectation that it might have a beneficial "cooling" effect. One week later, Coga appeared before the Society and claimed to be a new man, although Pepys concluded he was "cracked a little in the head."[13] However, this was not the first transfusion performed in a human. The credit for that accomplishment belongs to Jean-Baptiste Denis (1635–1704), who had performed the first human transfusion several months earlier in Paris.

The first animal-to-human transfusion

The founding of the Royal Society in London in 1662 was followed in 1666 by the establishment of the Academie des Sciences in Paris under the patronage of King Louis XIV. The new Academie reviewed the English reports on transfusion with great interest. Denis probably read of Lower's experiments in the *Journal des Savants* on January 31, 1667, and he began his own studies approximately one month later.[15,16] The first human transfusion was then performed on June 15, 1667, when Denis administered the blood of a lamb to a 15-year-old boy (Figure 1.1).

(489) Numb. 27.

A LETTER

Concerning a new way of curing sundry diseases by Transfusion of Blood, Written to Monfieur de MONTMOR, Counsellor to the French King, and Master of Requests.

By J: DENIS Professor of Philosophy, and the Mathematicks.

Munday July 22. 1667.

SIR,

HE project of causing the Blood of a healthy animal to passe into the veins of one diseased, having been conceived about ten years agoe, in the illustrious Society of *Virtuosi* which assembles at your house; and your goodness having received M. *Emmeriz*, & my self, very favorably at such times as we have presum'd to entertain you either with discourse concerning it, or the sight of some not inconsiderable effects of it : You will not think it strange that I now take the liberty of troubling you with this Letter, and design to inform you fully of what pursuances and successes we have made in this Operation; wherein you are justly intitled to a greater share than any other, considering that it was first spoken of in your *Academy*, & that the Publick is beholding to you for this as well as for many other discoveries, for the benefits & advantages it shall reap from the same. But that I may give you the reasons of our procedure & convince

Ccc   vince

Figure 1.1 The first human transfusion. Source: Denis (1967).[17]

Although discovery of the circulation had suggested the idea of transfusion, indications for the procedure remained uninformed. Transfusion was still thought to alter behavior and possibly achieve rejuvenation. The blood of young dogs made old dogs seem frisky; the blood of lions was proposed as a cure for cowardice; and, five months later, Arthur Coga would receive a transfusion of sheep blood because of its presumed "cooling" effect. Denis used animal blood for transfusion because he thought it was "less full of impurities":[17]

> Sadness, Envy, Anger, Melancholy, Disquiet and generally all the Passions, are as so many causes which trouble the life of man, and corrupt the whole substance of the blood: Whereas the life of Brutes is much more regular, and less subject to all these miseries.

It is thus ironic that the symptoms of the first transfusion recipient may have been explained in part by profound anemia; the single transfusion of lamb blood may have produced temporary amelioration owing to increased oxygen transport. Denis described the case as follows:[17]

> On the 15 of this Moneth, we hapned upon a Youth aged between 15 and 16 years, who had for above two moneths bin tormented with a contumacious and violent fever, which obliged his Physitians to bleed him 20 times, in order to asswage the excessive heat.

Before this disease, he was not observed to be of a lumpish dull spirit, his memory was happy enough, and he seem'd chearful and nimble enough in body; but since the violence of this fever, his wit seem'd wholly sunk, his memory perfectly lost, and his body so heavy and drowsie that he was not fit for anything. I beheld him fall asleep as he sate at dinner, as he was eating his Breakfast, and in all occurrences where men seem most unlikely to sleep. If he went to bed at nine of the clock in the Evening, he needed to be wakened several times before he could be got to rise by nine the next morning, and he pass'd the rest of the day in an incredible stupidity.

I attributed all these changes to the great evacuations of blood, the Physitians had been oblig'd to make for saving his life.

Three ounces of the boy's blood were exchanged for 9 ounces of lamb arterial blood. Several hours later the boy arose, and "for the rest of the day, he spent it with much more liveliness than ordinary." Thus the first human transfusion, which was heterologous, was accomplished without any evident unfavorable effect.

This report stimulated a firestorm of controversy over priority of discovery.[18,19] The letter by Denis was published in the *Transactions* on July 22, 1667, while the editor, Henry Oldenburg, was imprisoned in the Tower of London. Oldenburg, following some critical comments concerning the Anglo-Dutch War then in progress (1665–1667), had been arrested under a warrant issued June 20, 1667. After his release 2 months later, Oldenburg returned to his editorial post and found the letter published in his absence. He took offense at Denis's opening statement, which claimed that the French had conceived of transfusion "about ten years agoe, in the illustrious Society of Virtuosi" (Figure 1.1). This seemed to deny the English contributions to the field. Oldenburg cited these omissions in an issue of the *Transactions* published September 23, 1667, "for the Months of July, August, and September." By numbering this issue 27 and beginning pagination with 489, Oldenburg attempted to suppress the letter by Denis.[18] However, as is evident, this did not ultimately succeed. Nonetheless, subsequent events created even greater difficulties for Denis.

Although the first two subjects who underwent transfusion by Denis were not adversely affected, the third and fourth recipients died. The death of the third subject was easily attributable to other causes. However, the fourth case initiated a sequence of events that put an end to transfusion for 150 years.

Anthony du Mauroy was a 34-year-old man who suffered from intermittent bouts of maniacal behavior. On December 19, 1667, Denis and his assistant Paul Emmerez removed 10 ounces of the man's blood and replaced it with 5 or 6 ounces of blood from the femoral artery of a calf. Failing to note any apparent improvement, they repeated the transfusion 2 days later. After the second transfusion, du Mauroy experienced a classic transfusion reaction:[20]

His pulse rose presently, and soon after we observ'd a plentiful sweat over all his face. His pulse varied extremely at this instant, and he complain'd of great pains in his kidneys and that he was not well in his stomach.

Du Mauroy fell asleep at about 10 o'clock in the evening. He awoke the following morning and "made a great glass full of urine, of a colour as black, as if it had been mixed with the soot of chimneys."[20] Two months later, the patient again became maniacal, and his wife again sought transfusion therapy. Denis was reluctant but finally gave in to her urgings. However, the transfusion could not be accomplished, and du Mauroy died the next evening.

The physicians of Paris strongly disapproved of the experiments in transfusion. Three of them approached du Mauroy's widow and encouraged her to lodge a malpractice complaint against Denis. She instead went to Denis and attempted to extort money from him in return for her silence. Denis refused and filed a complaint before the Lieutenant in Criminal Causes. During the subsequent hearing, evidence was introduced to indicate that Madame du Mauroy had poisoned her husband with arsenic. In a judgment handed down at the Chatelet in Paris on April 17, 1668, Denis was exonerated, and the woman was held for trial. The court also stipulated "that for the future no Transfusion should be made upon any Human Body but by the approbation of the Physicians of the Parisian Faculty."[21] At this point, transfusion research went into decline, and within 10 years it was prohibited in both France and England.

The beginnings of modern transfusion

After the edict that ended transfusion in the 17th century, the technique lay dormant for 150 years. Stimulated by earlier experiments by Leacock, transfusion was "resuscitated" and placed on a rational basis by James Blundell (1790–1877), a London obstetrician who had received his medical degree from the University of Edinburgh.[22] Soon after graduation, Blundell accepted a post in physiology and midwifery at Guy's Hospital. It was there that he began the experiments on transfusion that led to its rebirth. The frequency of postpartum hemorrhage and death troubled Blundell. In 1818, he wrote:[23]

A few months ago I was requested to visit a woman who was sinking under uterine hemorrhage. . . . Her fate was decided, and notwithstanding every exertion of the medical attendants, she died in the course of two hours.

Reflecting afterwards on this melancholy scene . . . I could not forbear considering, that the patient might very probably have been saved by transfusion; and that . . . the vessels might have been replenished by means of the syringe with facility and promptitude.

This opening statement introduced Blundell's epoch-making study titled "Experiments on the Transfusion of Blood by the Syringe"[23] (see Figure 1.2). Blundell described in detail a series of animal

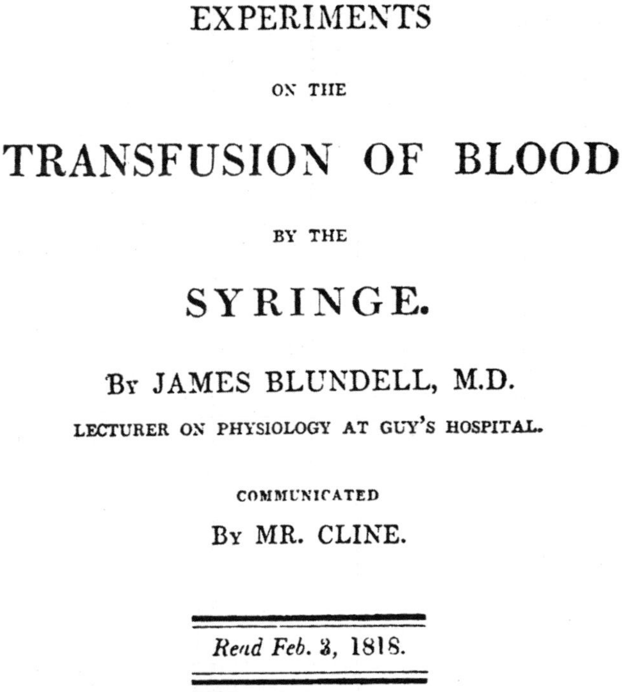

EXPERIMENTS

ON THE

TRANSFUSION OF BLOOD

BY THE

SYRINGE.

By JAMES BLUNDELL, M.D.

LECTURER ON PHYSIOLOGY AT GUY'S HOSPITAL.

COMMUNICATED

By MR. CLINE.

Read Feb. 3, 1818.

Figure 1.2 The beginnings of modern transfusion. Source: Blundell (1818).[23]

experiments. He demonstrated that a syringe could be used effectively to perform transfusion, that the lethal effects of arterial exsanguination could be reversed by the transfusion of either venous or arterial blood, and that the injection of 5 drams (20 cc) of air into the veins of a small dog was not fatal but transfusion across species ultimately was lethal to the recipient.[23] Thus, Blundell was the first to state clearly that only human blood should be used for human transfusion. The latter conclusion was confirmed in France by Dumas and Prevost, who demonstrated that the infusion of heterologous blood into an exsanguinated animal produced only temporary improvement and was followed by death within 6 days.[24] These scientific studies provided the basis for Blundell's subsequent efforts in clinical transfusion.

The first well-documented transfusion with human blood took place on September 26, 1818.[25] The patient was an extremely emaciated man in his mid-thirties who had pyloric obstruction caused by carcinoma. He received 12 to 14 ounces of blood in the course of 30 or 40 minutes. Despite initial apparent improvement, the patient died two days later. Transfusion in the treatment of women with postpartum hemorrhage was more successful. In all, Blundell performed 10 transfusions, of which five were successful. Three of the unsuccessful transfusions were performed on moribund patients, the fourth was performed on a patient with puerperal sepsis, and the fifth was performed on the aforementioned patient with terminal carcinoma. Four of the successful transfusions were given for postpartum hemorrhage, and the fifth was administered to a boy who bled after amputation.[22] Blundell also devised various instruments for the performance of transfusion. They included an "impellor," which collected blood in a warmed cup and "impelled" the blood into the recipient via an attached syringe, and a "gravitator"[26] (Figure 1.3), which received blood and delivered it by gravity through a long vertical cannula.

The writings of Blundell provided evidence against the use of animal blood in humans and established rational indications for transfusion. However, the gravitator (Figure 1.3) graphically demonstrated the technical problems that remained to be solved. Blood from the donor, typically the patient's husband, flowed into a funnel-like device and down a flexible cannula into the patient's vein "with as little exposure as possible to air, cold and inanimate surface."[25] The amount of blood transfused was estimated from the amount spilled into the apparatus by the donor. In this clinical atmosphere, charged with apprehension and anxiety, the amount of blood issuing from a donor easily could be overstated. Clotting within the apparatus then ensured that only a portion of that blood actually reached the patient. Thus, the amount of blood actually transfused may have been seriously overestimated. This may explain the apparent absence of transfusion reactions. Alternatively, reactions may have been unrecognized. Patients who underwent transfusion frequently were agonal. As Blundell stated, "It seems right, as the operation now stands, to confine transfusion to the first class of cases only, namely, those in which there seems to be no hope for the patient, unless blood can be thrown into the veins."[26] Under these circumstances, "symptoms" associated with an "unsuccessful" transfusion might be ascribed to the agonal state rather than the transfusion itself. For a time, the problem of coagulation during transfusion was circumvented by the use of defibrinated blood. This undoubtedly increased the amount of blood actually transfused. However, there were numerous deaths. Interestingly, these deaths were attributed to intravascular coagulation when in actuality they were probably fatal hemolytic reactions caused by the infusion of incompatible blood.[27]

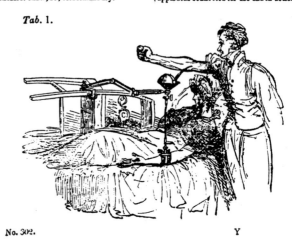

VOL. II.]   LONDON, SATURDAY, JUNE 13.   [1828-9.

OBSERVATIONS
ON
TRANSFUSION OF BLOOD.
BY DR. BLUNDELL.

With a Description of his Gravitator.*

STATES of the body really requiring the infusion of blood into the veins are probably rare; yet we sometimes meet with cases in which the patient must die unless such operation can be performed; and still more frequently with cases which seem to require a supply of blood, in order to prevent the ill health which usually arises from large losses of the vital fluid, even when they do not prove fatal.

* The instrument is manufactured by Messrs. Maw, 55, Aldermanbury.

In the present state of our knowledge respecting the operation, although it has not been clearly shown to have proved fatal in any one instance, yet not to mention possible, though unknown risks, inflammation of the arm has certainly been produced by it on one or two occasions; and therefore it seems right, as the operation now stands, to confine transfusion to the first class of cases only, namely, those in which there seems to be no hope for the patient, unless blood can be thrown into the veins.

The object of the Gravitator is, to give help in this last extremity, by transmitting the blood in a regulated stream from one individual to another, with as little exposure as may be to air, cold, and inanimate surface; ordinary venesection being the only operation performed on the person who emits the blood; and the insertion of a small tube into the vein usually laid open in bleeding, being all the operation which it is necessary to execute on the person who receives it.

The following plate represents the whole apparatus connected for use and in action :—

Tab. 1.

No. 302.   Y

Figure 1.3 Blundell's gravitator. Source: Blundell (1828).[26]

Transfusion at the end of the 19th century, therefore, was neither safe nor efficient. The following description, written in 1884, illustrates this point:[28]

> Students, with smiling faces, are rapidly leaving the theatre of one of our metropolitan hospitals. The most brilliant operator of the day has just performed immediate transfusion with the greatest success. By means of a very beautiful instrument, the most complex and ingenious that modern science has yet produced, a skilful surgeon has transfused half a pint, or perhaps a pint, of blood from a healthy individual to a fellow creature profoundly collapsed from the effects of severe hemorrhage. Some little difficulty was experienced prior to the operation, as one of the many stop-cocks of the transfusion apparatus was found to work stiffly; but this error was quickly rectified by a mechanic in attendance. Towards the close of the operation the blood-donor, a powerful and heavy young man, swooned. Two porters carried him on a stretcher into an adjoining room.

In the latter half of the 19th century, there were many attempts to render transfusion a more predictable and less arduous procedure. In 1869, Braxton-Hicks,[29] using blood anticoagulated with phosphate solutions, performed a number of transfusions on women with obstetric bleeding. Many of the patients were in extremis, and ultimately all died. Unfortunately, a detailed description of terminal symptoms was not provided.[29] Some investigators attempted to rejuvenate animal-to-human transfusion, and Oscar Hasse persisted in this approach despite disastrous results. Studies by Emil

Ponfick and by Leonard Landois finally put an end to this practice. Ponfick, in carefully controlled studies, confirmed the lethality of heterologous transfusion and identified the resulting hemoglobinuria along with its donor erythrocyte source. Landois documented the poor results of animal-to-human transfusion and demonstrated the lysis of sheep erythrocytes by human serum in vitro.[8]

Frustration with blood as a transfusion product led to even more bizarre innovations. From 1873 to 1880, cow, goat, and even human milk was transfused as a blood substitute.[30] The rationale derived from an earlier suggestion that the fat particles of milk could be converted into blood cells. Milk transfusion was particularly popular in the United States,[30] where the practice of animal-to-human transfusion was recorded as late as 1890.[31] Fortunately, these astonishing practices were discontinued when saline solutions were introduced as "a life-saving measure" and "a substitute for the transfusion of blood."[32] A passage from an article written by Bull in 1884[32] is particularly instructive:

> The danger from loss of blood, even to two-thirds of its whole volume, lies in the disturbed relationship between the calibre of the vessels and the quantity of the blood contained therein, and not in the diminished number of red blood-corpuscles; and. . . . This danger concerns the volume of the injected fluids also, it being a matter of indifference whether they be albuminous or containing blood corpuscles or not.

Mercifully, volume replacement with saline solutions deflected attention from the unpredictable and still dangerous practice of blood transfusion. Accordingly, transfusions were abandoned until interest was rekindled by the scientific and technical advances of the early 20th century.

The 20th century

The 20th century was ushered in by a truly monumental discovery. In 1900, Karl Landsteiner (1868–1943) observed that the sera of some persons agglutinated the red blood cells of others. This study, published in 1901 in the *Wiener Klinische Wochenschrift* [33] (Figure 1.4), showed for the first time the cellular differences in individuals from the same species. In his article, Landsteiner wrote:[34]

> In a number of cases (Group A) the serum reacts on the corpuscles of another group (B), but not, however, on those of group A, while, again, the corpuscles of A will be influenced likewise by serum B. The serum of the third group (C) agglutinates the corpuscles of A and B, while the corpuscles of C will not be influenced by the sera of A and B. The corpuscles are naturally apparently insensitive to the agglutinins which exist in the same serum.

With the identification of blood groups A, B, and C (subsequently renamed group O) by Landsteiner and of group AB by Decastello and Sturli,[35] the stage was set for the performance of safe transfusion. For this work, Landsteiner somewhat belatedly received the Nobel Prize in 1930. But even that high recognition does not adequately express the true magnitude of Landsteiner's discovery. His work was like a burst of light in a darkened room. He gave us our first glimpse of immunohematology and transplantation biology and provided the tools for important discoveries in genetics, anthropology, and forensic medicine. Viewed from this perspective, the identification of human blood groups is one of only a few scientific discoveries of the 20th century that changed all of our lives.[34] Yet the translation of Landsteiner's discovery into transfusion practice took many years.

At the turn of the 20th century, the effective transfer of blood from one person to another remained a formidable task. Clotting, still uncontrolled, quickly occluded transfusion devices and frustrated most efforts. In 1901, the methods used in transfusion were too primitive to demonstrate the importance of Landsteiner's discovery. Indeed, the study of in vitro red cell agglutination may have seemed rather remote from the technical problems that demanded attention. An intermediate step was needed before the importance of Landsteiner's breakthrough could be perceived and the appropriate changes could be incorporated into practice. This process was initiated by Alexis Carrel (1873–1944), another Nobel laureate, who developed a surgical procedure that allowed direct transfusion through an arteriovenous anastomosis.

Carrel[36] introduced the technique of end-to-end vascular anastomosis with triple-threaded suture material. This procedure brought the ends of vessels in close apposition and preserved luminal continuity, thus avoiding leakage or thrombosis. This technique paved the way for successful organ transplantation and brought Carrel the Nobel Prize in 1912. It was also adapted by Carrel[37] and others[38,39] to the performance of transfusion. Crile[38] introduced the use of a metal tube to facilitate placement of sutures, and Bernheim[39] used a two-piece cannula to unite the artery to the vein (Figure 1.5). Because all of these procedures usually culminated in the sacrifice of the two vessels, they were not performed frequently. Direct transfusion was also fraught with danger. In a passage written two decades later, the procedure was recalled in the following manner:[40]

> The direct artery to vein anastomosis was the best method available but was often very difficult or even unsuccessful. And, what was almost as bad, one never knew how much blood one had transfused at any moment or when to stop (unless the donor collapsed). (I remember one such collapse in which the donor almost died—and the surgeon needed to be revived.)

Aus dem pathologisch-anatomischen Institute in Wien.

Ueber Agglutinationserscheinungen normalen menschlichen Blutes.

Von Dr. **Karl Landsteiner,** Assistenten am pathologisch-anatomischen Institute.

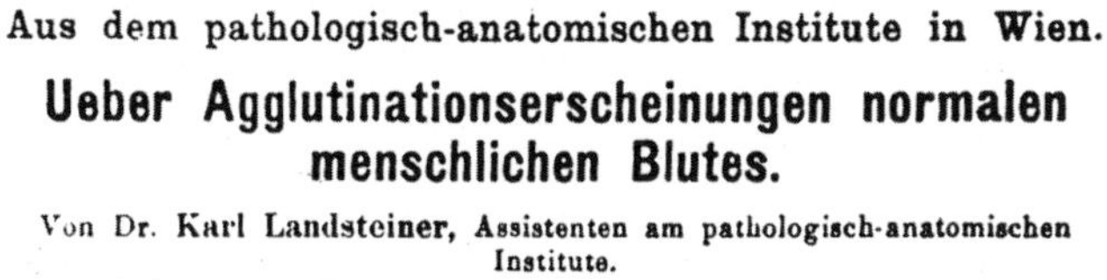

Figure 1.4 Landsteiner's description of blood groups. Source: Landsteiner (1901). [33]

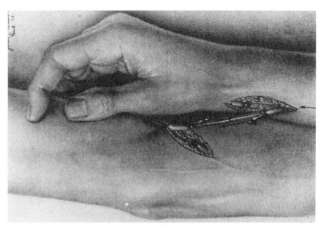

Figure 1.5 Direct transfusion by means of arteriovenous anastomosis through the two-pieced cannula of Bernheim. Source: Bernheim (1917). [39]

A CASE OF FATAL HEMOLYSIS FOLLOWING DIRECT TRANSFUSION OF BLOOD BY ARTERIOVENOUS ANASTOMOSIS.*

WILLIAM PEPPER, M.D.
Instructor in Medicine, University of Pennsylvania.
AND
VERNER NISBET, M.D.
Assistant Instructor in Medicine, University of Pennsylvania; Assistant Director of the William Pepper Laboratory of Clinical Medicine.
PHILADELPHIA.

Figure 1.6 Report of a fatal transfusion reaction. Source: Pepper and Nisbet (1907). [41]

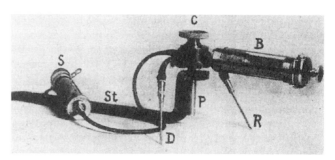

Figure 1.8 Apparatus for Unger's two-syringe, four-way stopcock method of indirect transfusion. Source: Unger (1915). [49]

Despite these many difficulties, direct transfusion through an arteriovenous anastomosis for the first time efficiently transferred blood from one person to another. The process also disclosed fatal hemolytic reactions that were undeniably caused by transfusion[41] (Figure 1.6). However, the relation of these fatal reactions to Landsteiner's discovery was not recognized until Reuben Ottenberg (1882–1959) demonstrated the importance of compatibility testing.

Ottenberg's interest in transfusion began in 1906 while he was an intern at German (now Lenox Hill) Hospital in New York. There, Ottenberg learned of Landsteiner's discovery and in 1907 began pretransfusion compatibility testing.[42] Ottenberg accepted an appointment at Mount Sinai Hospital the next year and continued his studies on transfusion. In 1913, Ottenberg published the report that conclusively demonstrated the importance of preliminary blood testing for the prevention of transfusion "accidents"[43] (Figure 1.7). This was not Ottenberg's only contribution. He observed the Mendelian inheritance of blood groups,[44] and he was the first to recognize the relative unimportance of donor antibodies and consequently the "universal" utility of type O blood donors.[45]

Further advances in immunohematology were to occur in succeeding decades. The M, N, and P systems were described in the period between 1927 and 1947.[46] The Rh system was discovered in connection with an unusual transfusion reaction. In 1939, Levine and Stetson[47] described an immediate reaction in a group O woman who had received her husband's group O blood soon after delivery of a stillborn fetus with erythroblastosis. This

ACCIDENTS IN TRANSFUSION

THEIR PREVENTION BY PRELIMINARY BLOOD EXAMINATION: BASED ON AN EXPERIENCE OF ONE HUNDRED TWENTY-EIGHT TRANSFUSIONS *

REUBEN OTTENBERG, M.D.
AND
DAVID J. KALISKI, M.D.
NEW YORK

Accidents following transfusion have been sufficiently frequent to make many medical men hesitate to advise transfusion, except in desperate cases. It has been our opinion since we began making observations on this question in 1908 that such accidents could be prevented by careful preliminary tests, leading to the exclusion of agglutinative or hemolytic donors. Our observations on over 125 cases have confirmed this view and we believe that untoward symptoms can be prevented with absolute certainty.

Figure 1.7 Report of the importance of testing before transfusion. Source: Ottenberg and Kaliski (1913). [43]

sequence of events suggested that the infant had inherited a red cell agglutinogen from the father that was foreign to the mother. At about the same time, Landsteiner and Wiener[48] harvested a rhesus monkey red cell antibody from immunized guinea pigs and rabbits. This antibody agglutinated 85% of human red cell samples (Rh-positive) and left 15% (Rh-negative) unaffected. When the experimentally induced antibody was tested in parallel with the serum from Levine's patient, a similar positive and negative distribution was observed, and the Rh system had been discovered. Other red cell antigen systems were subsequently described, but when Rh immunoglobulin was introduced as a preventive measure for hemolytic disease of the newborn, it became one of the major public health advances of the century.

Despite the introduction of compatibility testing by Ottenberg, transfusion could not be performed frequently as long as arteriovenous anastomosis remained the procedure of choice. Using this method, Ottenberg needed five years (Figure 1.7) to accumulate the 128 transfusions he reported in his study on pretransfusion testing.[43] New techniques, such as Unger's two-syringe method introduced in 1915[49] (Figure 1.8), eventually put an end to transfusion by means of arteriovenous anastomosis. However, transfusions did not become commonplace until anticoagulants were developed and direct methods of transfusion were rendered obsolete.

Anticoagulants, the blood bank, and component therapy

The anticoagulant action of sodium citrate completely transformed the practice of transfusion. Early reports from Belgium[50] and Argentina[51] were followed by the work of Lewisohn[52] that established the optimal citrate concentration for anticoagulation. The work of Weil[53] then demonstrated the feasibility of refrigerated storage. Subsequently, Rous and Turner[54] developed the anticoagulant solution that was used during World War I.[55] Despite its very large volume, this solution remained the anticoagulant of choice until World War II, when Loutit and Mollison[56] developed an acid–citrate–dextrose (ACD) solution. Used in a ratio of 70 mL ACD to 450 mL blood, ACD provided 3 to 4 weeks of preservation of a more concentrated red cell infusion. Thus, the two world wars were the stimuli for the development of citrate anticoagulants and the introduction of indirect transfusion.[46] For the first time, the donation process could be separated, in time and place, from the actual transfusion. Blood drawn and set aside now awaited the emergence of systems of storage and distribution. Again, it was the provision of medical support during armed conflict that stimulated these developments.

A blood transfusion service, organized by the Republican Army during the Spanish Civil War (1936–1939), collected 9000 L of blood in citrate–dextrose anticoagulant for the treatment of battle casualties.[57] At about that same time, Fantus[58] began operation of the first hospital blood bank at Cook County Hospital in Chicago. His interest had been stimulated by Yudin's report[59] on the use of cadaveric blood in Russia. Apart from certain scruples attached to the use of cadaveric blood, Fantus reasoned that a transfusion service based on such a limited source of supply would be impractical. Accordingly, he established the principle of a "blood bank" from which blood could be withdrawn, provided it had previously been deposited. As Fantus[58] himself stated, "[J]ust as one cannot draw money from a bank unless one has deposited some, so the blood preservation department cannot supply blood unless as much comes in as goes out. The term 'blood bank' is not a mere metaphor." The development of anticoagulants and the concept of blood banks provided an infrastructure upon which a more elaborate blood services organization could be built. World War II was the catalyst for these further developments.

At the beginning of World War II, blood procurement programs were greatly expanded.[46] In Great Britain, an efficient system had been developed through the organization of regional centers. When the war started, these centers, already in place, were able to increase their level of operation. In the United States, the use of plasma in the management of shock had led to the development of plasma collection facilities.[60] The efficient long-term storage of plasma had been further facilitated by the process of lyophilization developed by Flosdorf and Mudd and the introduction of ABO-independent "universal" plasma produced by pooling several thousand units of plasma.[61] In 1940, the United States organized a program for the collection of blood and the shipment of plasma to Europe. The American Red Cross, through its local chapters, participated in the project, which collected 13 million units by the end of the war.[46]

The national program of the American Red Cross ceased at the end of the war. However, many of the local chapters continued to help recruit donors for local blood banks, and in 1948, the first regional Red Cross blood center was begun in Rochester, New York. By 1949–1950 in the United States, the blood procurement system included 1500 hospital blood banks, 1100 of which performed all blood bank functions. There were 46 nonhospital blood banks and 31 Red Cross regional blood centers. By 1962, these numbers had grown to 4400 hospital blood banks, 123 nonhospital blood banks, and 55 American Red Cross regional blood centers, and the number of units collected had grown to between 5 and 6 million per year.[62]

During this time, blood was collected through steel needles and rubber tubing into rubber-stoppered bottles. After washing and resterilization, the materials were reused. On occasion, "vacuum bottles" were used to speed up the collection. However, the high incidence of pyrogenic reactions soon led to the development of disposable plastic blood collection equipment.

In a classic article written in 1952, Walter and Murphy[63] described a closed, gravity technique for whole blood preservation. They used a laminar flow phlebotomy needle, an interval donor tube, and a collapsible bag of polyvinyl resin designed so that the unit could be assembled and ready for use after sterilization with steam. The polyvinyl resin was chemically inert to biologic fluids and nonirritating to tissue. Soon thereafter, Gibson et al.[64] demonstrated that plastic systems were more flexible and allowed removal of plasma after sedimentation or centrifugation. In time, glass was replaced with plastic, and component therapy began to emerge. This development was enhanced by the US military's need to reduce the weight and breakage of blood bottles during shipment in the Korean War.

Component and derivative therapy began during World War II, when Edwin J. Cohn and his collaborators developed the cold ethanol method of plasma fractionation.[65] As a result of their work, albumin, globulin, and fibrinogen became available for clinical use. As plastic equipment replaced glass, component separation became a more widespread practice, and the introduction of automated cell separators provided even greater capabilities in this area.

Clotting factor concentrates for the treatment of patients with hemophilia and other hemorrhagic disorders also were developed during the postwar era. Although antihemophilic globulin had been described in 1937,[66] unconcentrated plasma was the only therapeutic material until Pool discovered that Factor VIII could be harvested in the cryoprecipitable fraction of blood.[67] This resulted in the development of cryoprecipitate, which was introduced in 1965 for the management of hemophilia. Pool showed that cryoprecipitate could be made in a closed-bag system and urged its harvest from as many donations as possible. The development of cryoprecipitate and other concentrates was the dawn of a golden age in the care of patients with hemophilia. Self-infusion programs, made possible by technologic advances in plasma fractionation, allowed early therapy and greatly reduced disability and unemployment. This golden age came abruptly to an end with the appearance of the AIDS virus.

Transfusion in the age of technology

In contrast to the long ledger of lives lost in previous centuries because of the lack of blood, transfusion in the 20th century saved countless lives. In 1937, during those early halcyon days of transfusion, Ottenberg wrote:[40]

> Today transfusion has become so safe and so easy to do that it is seldom omitted in any case in which it may be of benefit. Indeed the chief problem it presents is the finding of the large sums of money needed for the professional donors who now provide most of the blood.

It is ironic that Ottenberg's statement should refer to paid donors and foreshadow difficulties yet to come. However, experience to that point had not revealed the problem of viral disease transmission. More transfusions would have to be administered before that problem would be perceived.

After the introduction of anticoagulants, blood transfusions were given in progressively increasing numbers. At Mount Sinai Hospital in New York, the number of blood transfusions administered between 1923 and 1953 increased 20-fold[68,69] (Table 1.1). This increase was particularly notable after the establishment of blood banks. It was during this period that Beeson wrote his classic description of transfusion-transmitted hepatitis.[70] He had been alerted to the problem by the outbreaks of jaundice that followed inoculation programs with human serum during World War II. Thus blood transfusion entered a new era. Blood components not only saved lives but also transmitted disease. The discovery of the Australian antigen[71] and the subsequent definition of hepatitis A virus and B virus (HBV) still left residual non-A and non-B disease,[72] a gap that has been largely filled by the discovery of the hepatitis C virus (HCV).[73] However, it was the outbreak of AIDS that galvanized public attention to blood transfusion.

The AIDS epidemic was first recognized in the United States, and the first case of AIDS associated with transfusion was observed in a 20-month-old infant.[74] Subsequently, the suspicion that AIDS could be transmitted by means of transfusion was confirmed.[75]

Table 1.1 Increase in the Number of Blood Transfusions at Mount Sinai Hospital, New York, 1923–1953

Year	Number of Transfusions
1923	143
1932	477
1935	794
1938	(Blood bank started)
1941	2097
1952	2874
1953	3179

Source: Lewisohn (1955).[68] Adapted with permission of Elsevier.

The human immunodeficiency virus (HIV) was identified,[76] and an effective test to detect the HIV antibody was developed.[76]

Concern for blood safety

Since 1943, transfusion therapy has been shadowed by the specter of disease transmission. In that year, Beeson described posttransfusion hepatitis and unveiled a problem that has grown with time. As transfusion increased, so did disease transmission. In 1962, the connection between paid donations and posttransfusion hepatitis was made.[77] A decade later, the National Blood Policy mandated a voluntary donation system in the United States. And yet, blood usage continued to increase.

Concern about posttransfusion hepatitis was not sufficient to decrease the number of transfusions. Although the use of whole blood declined as blood components became more popular, total blood use in the United States doubled between 1971 and 1980 (Table 1.2).[78–85] This pattern changed as the emergence of AIDS exposed all segments of society to a revealing light.

AIDS probably arose in Africa in the 1960s and spread quietly for years before it was detected. By 1980, an estimated 100,000 persons were infected, and by 1981, when the first cases were reported, a worldwide pandemic lay just beneath the surface. The initial response of the public and officials seemed trifling and insufficient as the outbreak grew to proportions few had foreseen. Criticism was levied against the news media for initially ignoring the story, the government for delay in acknowledging the problem, gay civil rights

groups for resistance to epidemiologic measures, research scientists for unseemly competition, blood services for delayed response in a time of crisis, and the US Food and Drug Administration (FDA) for inadequate regulatory activity. Historians with the perspective of time will determine whether there really were more villains than the virus itself.[86]

The realization that transfusion can transmit an almost invariably fatal disease had a chilling effect on the public. Two major changes in blood services have occurred in the aftermath of the AIDS epidemic. The FDA, using pharmaceutical manufacturing criteria not "tailored to . . . blood banks," became more aggressive in regulatory actions against blood collection establishments.[87] And, finally, blood use moderated for approximately 10 years. Through the 1980s and early 1990s, red cell and plasma transfusion peaked and began to stabilize (Table 1.2). Only platelet use and human progenitor cell transplantation, driven by the demands of cancer chemotherapy, continued to increase.[78–85] Educational programs to encourage judicious use of blood have been initiated, and they have been favorably received by practicing physicians. Use of red cells and plasma fell from 2008 to 2011. This was a combined impact of the great recession reducing healthcare utilization and the widespread use of patient blood management programs intended to reduce blood transfusion. This represents the first time since the end of the Second World War that the growth in transfusion of blood products in the United States and other developed countries stopped and was reversed for a sustained period.

Relentless public pressure for a "zero-risk" blood supply resulted in dividends through continued scientific and technologic improvements. Enhanced sensitivity and better use of serologic testing, along with improved scrutiny of donors, resulted in major reductions in risk of transmitted disease by the mid-1990s.[88] Discovery that pools of units subjected to nucleic acid testing almost closed the window for HIV and HCV virus resulted in application of this testing for both whole blood and plasma donations beginning between 1998 and 2000.[88,89] This, combined with virus reduction and inactivation of the final product, resulted in plasma derivatives that have not transmitted AIDS or hepatitis since 1994.[90] For whole blood and platelet components, risks have become low. A solvent/detergent-treated fresh frozen plasma component has been used in Europe and recently became available in the United States.

With the reduction in the risk of viral transmission, the focus in the developed world has shifted to transfusion-related acute lung injury (TRALI)—possibly from recipient-directed leukocyte antibodies and lipid mediators in transfused plasma—and bacterial infection primarily occurring in room-temperature stored platelets. So that incremental gains can be made against these risks, the use of male plasma only and the culture of platelets before they are released have been implemented. The 2011 blood utilization survey indicated a 28.8% reduction in TRALI, suggesting a significant breakthrough with regard to this risk.[85] Geographic exclusions have been aimed at reducing the potential for variant Creutzfeldt–Jakob disease (vCJD) transmission by transfusion, although in the United States such occurrence seems highly unlikely. In many countries, universal leukocyte reduction has been a response to the vCJD risk. Ironically, universal application of leukocyte reduction is probably ineffective for vCJD but has stimulated controversy over its use for preventing other problems.[91]

Finally, focus on the understanding, management, and prevention of medical errors in general might lead to progress against remaining nemesis hemolytic transfusion reactions caused by

Table 1.2 Transfusions in the United States (in Millions of Units)[78–85]

Year	Whole Blood and Red Blood Cells	Platelets	Plasma	Total**
1971	6.32	0.41	0.18	6.91
1979	9.47	2.22	1.29	12.98
1980	9.99	3.19	1.54	14.72
1982	11.47	4.18	1.95	17.60
1984	11.98	5.53	2.26	19.77
1986	12.16	6.30	2.18	20.64
1987	11.61	6.38	2.06	20.05
1989	12.06	7.26	2.16	21.48
1992	11.31	8.33	2.26	21.90
1994	11.11	7.87	2.62	21.60
1997	11.52	9.04	3.32	23.88
1999	12.39	9.05	3.32	24.76
2001	13.90	10.20	3.93	28.03
2004	14.18	9.88	4.09	28.15
2006	14.65	10.39	4.01	29.05
2008	15.02	2.28*	4.48	23.24
2011	13.79	3.16*	3.88	20.93

* Platelets reported in apheresis units.

** Includes other components.

mistransfusion. Bar code technology at the bedside, commonly applied to prevent errors in medication administration, has shown efficacy in reducing transfusion errors.[92] Radiofrequency identification shows further promise in error-prone situations such as operating rooms.[93] Transfusion safety officers and hemovigilance systems are other initiatives that have been instituted.

"Zero risk" has still not been achieved. Emerging global infections such as West Nile virus, Chagas disease, and Chikungunya virus remain future potential threats and have encouraged further test development and implementation of strategies for pathogen reduction (see Chapter 56).

Current megatrends

In the developed world, no cost has usually been spared in meeting public demands for blood safety. Service fees charged to hospitals by independent blood centers in the United States (Figure 1.9) illustrate the effect each new safety development has had on the cost of red blood cells (RBCs) (see also Table 1.3). As the new millennium began, the mean payment for RBC units was $100, and a leukocyte-reduced unit was $126. By 2005, those had risen to $157 and $188, respectively, with significant annual increases.[95]

One group of researchers (committed to programs to reduce blood use) has published data suggesting that the societal cost of a unit of RBCs is $1400 per unit, taking into account not only the blood center fee but also hospital-related costs, costs of treating adverse reactions, litigation, lost productivity of donors, and hemovigilance.[96] Although the figure might be inflated, such work does highlight the ever increasing cost of this form of therapy to the patient and society.

In the underdeveloped world, the picture is quite different. The greatest blood need is for women hemorrhaging during childbirth, infants and children with anemia caused by malaria, and victims of trauma. In 80 of 172 countries responding to a World Health Organization (WHO) survey, less than 1% of the population donate blood. In sub-Saharan Africa, fewer than 3 million units of blood are collected annually for a population of more than 700 million. Of the 148 countries reporting data to WHO, 41 are unable to screen for minimum safety (HIV, HBV, HVC, and syphilis). WHO estimates that unsafe blood in these countries results in 16 million new infections with HBV, 5 million with HCV, and 160,000 with HIV each year (accounting for 5–10% of the world's HIV infections). Fortunately, there is progress in some nations in achieving an all-volunteer supply and minimum screening. Thus, there are two drastically different pictures of blood safety and availability worldwide.[97,98]

Even in the developed world, availability has been a challenge in the past.[98] A clear need is for more group O red cells; populations of non-European ethnicity generally have an increased proportion of group O.[99]

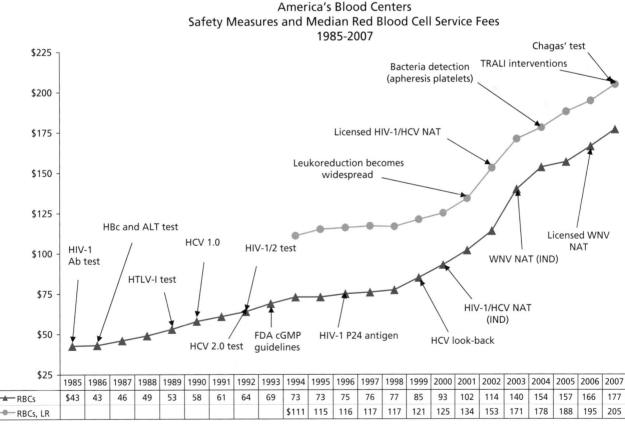

America's Blood Centers
Safety Measures and Median Red Blood Cell Service Fees
1985-2007

	1985	1986	1987	1988	1989	1990	1991	1992	1993	1994	1995	1996	1997	1998	1999	2000	2001	2002	2003	2004	2005	2006	2007
RBCs	$43	43	46	49	53	58	61	64	69	73	73	75	76	77	85	93	102	114	140	154	157	166	177
RBCs, LR										$111	115	116	117	117	121	125	134	153	171	178	188	195	205

Figure 1.9 Red blood cell service fees charged by community blood centers from 1985 to 2007, correlated with safety measures. Courtesy of America's Blood Centers (modified). RBCs, red blood cells; RBCs, LR, RBCs, leukocytes reduced; HIV, human immunodeficiency virus (−1/2 = types 1 and 2); Ab, antibody; HBc, hepatitis B core (antigen); ALT, alanine aminotransferase; HTLV-I, human T-cell lymphotropic virus, type I; HCV, hepatitis C virus; FDA cGMP, US Food and Drug Administration current good manufacturing practice; NAT, nucleic acid testing; IND, investigational new drug; WNV, West Nile virus.

Table 1.3 Risk Estimates per Unit of Red Blood Cells Transfused in the United States, Ranked by Frequency as of 2007

Type of Risk	Estimated Occurrence
Urticaria	1 in 50–100
Red cell allommunization	1 in 100
Febrile reaction	1 in 300
TRALI	1 in 5000
Hemolytic reaction	1 in 6000
Transfusion to the wrong recipient	1 in 14,000–19,000
Anaphylaxis	1 in 20,000–50,000
Hepatitis B virus	1 in 100,000–200,000
HTLV-I/II	1 in 641,000
Hepatitis C virus	1 in 1–2 million
HIV	1 in 2–3 million
Malaria	1 in 4 million
Bacterial contamination	1 in 5 million
GVHD	Very rare, no estimates

TRALI, transfusion-related acute lung injury; HTLV-I/II, human T-cell lymphotropic virus, types I and II; HIV, human immunodeficiency virus; GVHD, graft-versus-host disease.

Source: Klein *et al.* (2007).[94] Adapted with permission of Elsevier.

Another approach to maintain adequate availability is to control usage by ensuring that blood is used appropriately. Some US blood centers have been successful in bringing their transfusion medicine expertise into the patient care setting by providing transfusion services to hospitals. The model in Seattle, Washington, has operated for decades.[100,101] In the United Kingdom, liaison systems for blood centers to hospitals employing web-based technology for supply chain management have been introduced.[102,103] In Denmark, success has been reported using the Thromboelastograph (Haemoscope, Niles, IL) hemostatic system to manage coagulopathy in conjunction with treating physicians—something also done in many US hospitals.[104] Other point-of-care tests to assess the state of the coagulation system and tissue oxygenation could also result in more accurately targeted component transfusion. Transfusion medicine specialists in hospitals—whether from pathology groups, blood center staff, or other areas such as anesthesiology or hematology—are critical to the successful use of blood transfusion in patient care. Today, patient blood management has become a new standard for assuring transfusion is indicated based on best evidence. This has significantly reduced blood utilization in developed countries and has been supported by indications that restrictive blood transfusion strategy does not impair outcomes in most cases, although certain subsets of patients such as cancer patients might require a higher hemoglobin threshold.[105,106] At the same time, the treatment of trauma is returning to what is in effect whole blood for massive bleeding by administering plasma and platelets in proportion to red cells early in the care of victims.[107]

Although some advances in transfusion medicine at the end of the last millennium have been difficult to implement, such as the use of hemoglobin solutions, the field has continued to advance into new areas of stem cell biology, regenerative medicine, and cord blood banking. In addition, transfusion medicine specialists increasingly function in collaboration with surgeons, oncologists, and hematologists in treating the acutely ill patient with complex medical problems. With all the added sophistication, the optimal hemoglobin and platelet triggers and endpoints for transfusion remain unsettled. Clinicians are less likely to use oxygenation transport endpoints to determine the need for red cell transfusion but are beginning to look for other means to assess tissue oxygenation. If a patient's hemoglobin is too high (even when below normal), complications such as thromboembolism can result. Too low an endpoint exposes some patients to the risk of tissue hypoxia. The clearest trend has been away from autologous transfusion, although some medical centers seek bloodless medicine and surgery combining pharmacotherapy (mainly erythropoietin and iron), blood recovery and reinfusion, and conservative triggers and endpoints.[94] More conservative triggers and endpoints for platelet transfusion are becoming accepted, but approaches to alloimmunized patients and bacterial contamination are still in question.[108] Also debatable is whether transfusion, through some poorly quantifiable mechanism such as immunomodulation, confers a poorer prognosis on acutely ill patients.[105]

From ancient times into the new millennium, blood has been a substance that fascinates mankind. Despite unresolved controversies, blood transfusion remains of critical importance in the care of sick patients throughout the world.

Disclaimer

The authors have disclosed no conflicts of interest.

Key references

A full reference list for this chapter is available at: http://www.wiley.com/go/simon/transfusion

4 Zimmerman LM, Howell KM. History of blood transfusion. Ann Med Hist 1932; **4**: 415–33.

8 Maluf NSR. History of blood transfusion. J Hist Med 1954; **9**: 59–107.

31 Schmidt PJ. Transfusion in America in the eighteenth and nineteenth centuries. N Engl J Med 1968;**279**:1319–20.

46 Diamond LK. The story of our blood groups. In: Wintrobe MM, ed. Blood, pure and eloquent. New York: McGraw-Hill, 1980. 658–717.

62 Diamond LK. History of blood banking in the United States. JAMA 1965;**193**:40–5.

85 The 2011 National Blood Collection and Utilization Survey report. Bethesda, MD: AABB, 2012.

86 Starr D. Blood: an epic history of medicine and commerce. New York: Alfred A Knopf, 1998;147–357.

Contemporary issues in donation and transfusion

CHAPTER 2

Patient blood management

Darrell J. Triulzi,[1] Mark H. Yazer,[1] & Jonathan H. Waters[2]

[1]Department of Pathology, University of Pittsburgh Medical Center, Pittsburgh, PA, USA
[2]Departments of Anesthesiology and Bioengineering, University of Pittsburgh, Pittsburgh, PA, USA

Introduction

Patient blood management (PBM) is a multidisciplinary approach to improve patient outcomes using evidence-based strategies in patients who may need transfusion. The goal is not only to improve outcomes by transfusing blood appropriately, but also to introduce strategies to prevent patients from needing a transfusion in the first place. Avoiding and/or minimizing transfusion certainly leads to fewer transfusion reactions, fewer donor exposures, and in some cases lower cost. It has been stated that transfusions are also associated with worse patient outcomes, including bacterial infections, increased length of stay, prolonged ventilation, and mortality.[1] Such statements are based primarily on observational data or meta-analyses[2] and are controversial because of potential confounding and/or methodologic issues.[3] Even in the absence of serious morbid events causally related to transfusion, if a transfusion does not confer a benefit, it should be avoided. In a 2011 survey of 1342 US hospitals, 30% of respondents stated they offered some components of a PBM program.[4] Undoubtedly, that proportion has risen since then. Several professional organizations have focused on PBM; AABB, the Society for the Advancement of Blood Management (SABM), and, in Europe, the Network for Advancement of Transfusion Alternatives (NATA). Each of these organizations has annual meetings with PBM content and abundant written resources, including published PBM program standards.[5,6] An effective PBM program combines multiple approaches that span patient care from prehospitalization to intrahospitalization and even after discharge. Furthermore, the techniques of PBM are not limited to surgical patients. The features of a comprehensive PBM program are listed in Table 2.1 and will be discussed in this chapter.

Table 2.1 Features of a patient blood management program

1. Evidence-based guidelines for transfusion indications and dose
2. Physician education and monitoring
3. Preoperative anemia evaluation and management
4. Intraoperative and postoperative autologous salvage
5. Intraoperative normovolemic hemodilution
6. Point-of-care hemostasis testing
7. Use of hemostatic agents
8. Limiting phlebotomy blood loss for laboratory testing

Implementing a PBM program

There is not a single approach to implementing a PBM program that is appropriate for all hospitals. The approach will vary depending on the size of the hospital, patient populations, and hospital resources. Strategies common to a successful program have been described.[7-9] By its nature, a PBM program is multidisciplinary, and thus a program should start by identifying and recruiting the relevant physician, nursing, and administration "champions" from a variety of specialties. Once identified, these champions can form the basis for a PBM oversight committee with representatives from transfusion medicine, surgery, anesthesia, critical care medicine, hematology-oncology, nursing, and information technology (IT). Some PBM committees also include representatives from perfusion, pharmacy, laboratory medicine, internal medicine, risk management, or hospital administration. Many institutions have created a coordinator position called a Transfusion Safety Office (TSO) or PBM coordinator. This position is analogous to an Infection Control Officer but focuses on transfusion and PBM. The TSO is typically a nurse but could be a person with a laboratory or a quality systems background. Such individuals act as a liaison between the PBM committee and clinical services focusing on education, auditing, monitoring, data collection, and reporting. The PBM committee should have a medical director or co-directors responsible for direction, organization, and oversight of committee activities and representing the committee within the hospital. Ideally, the chair should be a clinician with credibility among the physicians who order blood. A transfusion medicine physician may also serve well in this role. The most important point is that it is a physician who is committed and passionate about creating a successful PBM program.

Essential to the success of the PBM committee is visible and vocal support of the hospital leadership. This includes the hospital CEO and senior management as well as the departmental chairs of the key clinical services who utilize blood. Effective leadership drives physicians and staff to participate in PBM initiatives. Some PBM initiatives may require financial investment, such as hiring a TSO or making IT enhancements. Such vital investment will require institutional leaders to "buy in" to the notion of investing now in order to improve patient care and ultimately reduce future costs. A lack of hospital leadership support is the most common reason why PBM programs fail to achieve their goals.

Many hospitals have an existing transfusion committee or similarly tasked committee that reports to the hospital medical executive

Rossi's Principles of Transfusion Medicine, Fifth Edition. Edited by Toby L. Simon, Jeffrey McCullough, Edward L. Snyder, Bjarte G. Solheim, and Ronald G. Strauss.
© 2016 John Wiley & Sons, Ltd. Published 2016 by John Wiley & Sons, Ltd.

committee or in some cases through the hospital quality assurance structure. Traditional transfusion committee activities will include some, but not all, PBM activities. For example, transfusion committees typically monitor blood usage and adverse event reports, but not the management of preoperative anemia or the use of point-of-care testing. It is prudent for the PBM committee to work closely with the transfusion committee to complement but not replicate their activities. When the transfusion committee is a standing committee, it can be a useful conduit for the approval of PBM policy proposals and education, and an additional source of resources for PBM activities. It is also feasible to roll the oversight of PBM activities into the responsibilities of the existing transfusion committee.

Once the PBM committee has been constituted, it should define the scope of activities it will address. Table 2.1 presents a comprehensive list of PBM activities, but rarely can all be addressed and almost certainly not simultaneously. The goal is to achieve measurable and visible success. Thus, initially it would be wise to address those aspects that are the most feasible and will have the greatest impact on patient care. In this way, the program can attract positive attention to itself, and perhaps flush out additional PBM champions, and continued administration support. Later, as the program matures and circumstances change, other aspects of the program can be addressed. Monitoring, measurement, and metrics are vital components of a PBM program.[10] The metrics should be meaningful, quantitative, and feasible to measure. This is where IT support and having a TSO/PBM coordinator to collect the data are so important. As part of defining its scope of activities, the PBM committee should define the metrics for each activity, definition of success (goals), and the IT resources (e.g., for reports) or staff needed for chart review.

Transfusion guidelines

There is no doubt that evidence-based transfusion guidelines derived from review of the current literature are a key component of a PBM program. They do not, however, solely constitute a PBM program. If the transfusion committee does not already have such guidelines in place, the PBM committee should develop a set of transfusion guidelines for the hospital. A number of organizations have conducted careful literature reviews based on Grading of Recommendations Assessment, Development and Evaluation (GRADE) methodology and published suggested guidelines.[5,11–13] The multidisciplinary membership of the committee lends itself to the adoption of the guidelines across the clinical services. The guidelines should address the indications for each blood component *and* the recommended dosing. Transfusing one unit of red cells at a time for an appropriate indication and reevaluating a stable patient are mainstays of optimal red cell transfusion practice.[9] Other chapters in this textbook will provide transfusion guidelines and dosage recommendations for each component and a detailed review of the evidence for these guidelines. Once guidelines have been established, physician education, implementation, and auditing of transfusion practice are the next steps. These steps, particularly implementation and auditing, are far more difficult than developing the guidelines.

Physician education and monitoring

To implement the various aspects of PBM, detailed information on baseline practices is required.[8,14] Although some of this information might be obtainable through a manual review of patient charts, large-scale data mining is really only possible by implementing electronic monitoring programs. These programs not only can serve to harvest data to elucidate the state of practice, but also can be used to advise clinicians about potentially unnecessary transfusions before the order to transfuse is placed. Broadly known as clinical decision support software (CDSS), these automated programs can be designed to accomplish several tasks that would otherwise be impossible to achieve using a manual system once they are integrated into the computerized physician order entry (CPOE) system. Once installed, the CDSS can operate continuously, and dispassionately provide suggestions every time that it detects a blood product order on a patient whose laboratory values do not indicate that a transfusion is necessary—a task that, although potentially successful,[15] would otherwise require a significant time commitment from the blood bank staff. Several large meta-analyses have shown practice improvements following the implementation of CDSS in various clinical areas.[16,17]

As it pertains to transfusion, a CDSS can be very basic or highly complex. A basic system would, for example, consider only one parameter (e.g., a hemoglobin or platelet value) in its analysis of whether a transfusion order was in accord with the institutional guidelines. Several studies have reported on using a single pretransfusion hemoglobin value to evaluate the suitability of the impending transfusion order.[18–20] However, this "one-size-fits-all" or static approach to laboratory-based transfusion threshold values is not amenable to the needs of physicians who are caring for patients with specialized disorders or for patients in specific clinical situations. Different patients can benefit from transfusion at different hemoglobin concentrations.[21–23] Thus, the evolution of the CDSS can be toward an "adaptive alert" system. This type of CDSS often requires the prescriber to first select an indication for the transfusion; associated with each indication is an evidence-based threshold for the product (Table 2.2). If the patient's most

Table 2.2 List of transfusion indications in the computerized physician order entry screen at the authors' Institutions

---

RBC (Hb values in g/dl)
Acute bleeding with blood pressure instability*
HB ≤7.0 in stable ICU patient
Hb ≤8.0 non-ICU patient with signs and symptoms of anemia
Hb ≤10.0 with acute cardiac ischemia
Hb ≤8.5 in an outpatient setting
Surgical blood loss anticipated*
Other (alert generated if Hb ≥8)

Plasma
INR ≥1.6 with bleeding
INR ≥1.6 and the patient is about to undergo an invasive procedure
Therapeutic exchange*
Massive bleeding*
Other (alert generated if INR <1.6)

Cryoprecipitate (fibrinogen level in mg/dl)
Fibrinogen ≤100 and the patient is bleeding or about to undergo an invasive procedure
Massive bleeding*
Other

PLT (Platelet count in ×10^6)
PLT ≤10 k stable patient
PLT ≤20 k with PLT consumption
PLT ≤50 k and the patient is bleeding or about to undergo an invasive procedure
Bleeding on anti-PLT medications*
Massive bleeding*
Other

---

* Indicates that an antecedent laboratory value is not required to order the product, and an alert will not be triggered if a blood product is ordered using this indication.

recent laboratory values are higher than the recommended guideline values (or lower, in the case of plasma transfusion and an INR threshold), a warning will appear on screen to inform the prescriber that, based on their patient's laboratory values, the transfusion does not appear to be indicated. The prescriber can again override the warning and proceed to order the product or can cancel the transfusion altogether. Baer *et al.*[24] reported on the implementation of a CDSS that displayed their neonatal intensive care units' (ICU) transfusion thresholds when the prescriber was ordering a blood product in the CPOE.

Compared to a period before the implementation of a CDSS, most studies have demonstrated a statistically significant improvement in institutional transfusion threshold compliance after one was implemented.[25-34] Although the exact reason for the improved compliance is unclear, it is reasonable to assume that being repeatedly presented with the institution's transfusion guidelines at the time of blood product ordering is sufficient to change some practices. Having adaptive alerts also helps to improve compliance by facilitating a patient-specific approach to transfusion decision making. At the authors' institutions, there were statistically significant decreases in the number of RBC orders that were placed and the number of orders that generated an alert after the "static" alert was changed to an adaptive alert. There was a trend toward a reduction in the median number of RBCs ordered per month after the adaptive alerts were implemented compared to the four months preceding the implementation of the adaptive alerts ($p = 0.089$).[35] Similarly, several other studies have reported a trend toward reduced RBC transfusions after a CDSS was implemented,[18,20,25,26,28,31] whereas others showed a statistically significant reduction in usage.[24,29,30,33,34,36]

There are fewer studies that have analyzed the effect of a CDSS on plasma or platelet orders. This might well relate to the paucity of randomized controlled trials (RCTs) on transfusion thresholds for these products, which makes establishing evidence-based thresholds difficult. At the authors' institutions, when the static alert for plasma transfusion (i.e., an alert was generated for any plasma order on a patient whose most recent international normalized ratio [INR] value was <1.6) was replaced with an adaptive alert (Table 2.2), there was a 15% decrease in the number of orders that generated an alert ($p < 0.0001$ compared to the period when a static alert was in place), and the percentage of alerts that were heeded increased significantly.[37] The implementation of the adaptive alerts for plasma in a neonatal ICU led to a significant reduction in the number of patients that received a plasma transfusion.[24] Similarly, when the CPOE displayed one institution's plasma transfusion guidelines, there was a decrease in the total number of plasma orders, inappropriate plasma orders, and plasma units transfused,[38] although the CDSS was not as successful in reducing "invalid" plasma orders at a different hospital.[39] As mentioned above, a CDSS that made recommendations for the number of plasma units to be transfused based on the recipient's demographics and the intended goal of the transfusion led to the transfusion of 68 additional plasma units.[25] Two studies demonstrated that there were non–statistically significant reductions in the number of patients who received platelet transfusion after a CDSS was implemented,[24,40] whereas there was a trend toward fewer platelet units transfused after the CDSS was implemented in one study.[40] To date, only two studies have analyzed the effect of a CDSS on cryoprecipitate orders.[24,41] A CDSS resulted in 49% of cryoprecipitate orders generating an alert, of which 14.9% were cancelled.[41]

In addition to potentially realizing cost savings by transfusing fewer blood products and having patients experience fewer transfusion reactions, the CDSS can also inform the selection of charts for the audits that are performed by transfusion committees. It is important to note that laboratory values alone are sometimes insufficient to indicate why a patient might require a blood product. Thus, permitting the physician to add a free-text explanation to an order that might not appear warranted based on laboratory parameters is a useful feature in a CPOE system. Explanatory comments can also suggest other legitimate blood product order indications for the CDSS. Thus, although high-quality evidence should form the basis when establishing transfusion thresholds, the input of the blood product users should also be sought in order to achieve consensus threshold values for the alerts.

In the absence of a CDSS, other metrics can be followed to ensure compliance with institutional guidelines. Once a restrictive RBC transfusion threshold is in place, evaluating the number of single-unit RBCs transfusions and the recipients' mean pretransfusion hemoglobin values over time by service or by individual provider can identify non-evidence-based practices and focus interventional efforts to achieve higher compliance rates. Benchmarking between providers of similar procedures or between hospitals or national databases can also be employed to identify non-evidence-based practices.[42-46] All of these methods require significant support from the institution's IT department.

Targeted prescriber education can occur after the decision to transfuse a patient has been made, and the use of the electronic medical record can facilitate this sort of audit. Benchmarking of blood use between surgeons who perform the same procedures can be a useful way of establishing the current state of practice and permit the identification of any practitioners whose transfusion habits appear to be aberrant. For example, the RBC transfusion practice among orthopedic surgeons performing total hip arthroplasties (THAs) can be highly variable. This variability can range between a few surgeons who rarely transfuse their patients with RBCs (and, when they do, it is typically a small quantity) to others who routinely transfuse most of their patients with large quantities of RBCs.[47] The publication of the FOCUS study served as the benchmark against which these surgeons' transfusion practice could be evaluated.[23] To this end, a "bubble graph" can be generated (Figure 2.1). This graph plots all surgeons who perform THA surgeries by the frequency with which they transfuse RBCs to their patients and the mean number of RBCs that are transfused per patient. The size of the bubble reflects the number of cases. By identifying those who repeatedly transfuse greater than average quantities of RBCs, the transfusion committee or hospital transfusion service can provide focused feedback and education where and when it is required.

It is clear that automated prescriber education alone is insufficient to eliminate non-evidence-based transfusions. Surely, the best way to reduce aberrant transfusion practice is though a multimodal approach involving automated alerts, presentations at grand rounds, and informal discussions with the house staff and faculty when apparently non-evidence-based transfusion practices are detected, and by providing easy access to the most up-to-date and well-executed research studies. By providing a consistent message about transfusion thresholds, waste reduction strategies, and techniques to avoid transfusion, the most optimum effects of PBM can be realized.

Preoperative anemia management

The World Health Organization (WHO) defines anemia as a hemoglobin <13 g/dl in men and <12 g/dl in women.[48]

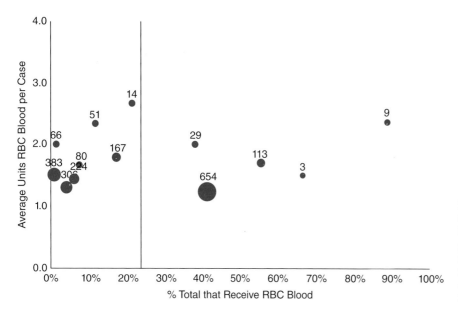

Figure 2.1 An example of a *bubble plot*. Each bubble represents a surgeon who performs total hip arthroplasties, and the size of the bubble represents the relative number of cases performed over a set time period. The *x*-axis represents the percentage of patients who received at least one RBC unit during the case, and on the *y*-axis the average number of RBCs transfused is plotted.

Preoperative anemia is common in surgical patients with an incidence ranging from 5 to 76% depending on the type of surgery, comorbidities, patient age, and gender.[49] A systematic review of patients undergoing hip and knee surgery reported a range of 24–44%,[50] which is very similar to the 28–36% observed in patients undergoing coronary artery bypass grafting.[51] Multiple studies have shown that preoperative anemia in the orthopedic patient population is associated with a 5–12-fold higher risk of transfusion, prolonged length of stay, and higher readmission rates.[50,52,53] Preoperative anemia has also been associated with increased morbidity and mortality in surgical patients.[50,54,55] Carson *et al.*[54] reported a retrospective study of 1958 patients who refused blood transfusion and underwent noncardiac surgery, and found that perioperative mortality was significantly increased when the preoperative hemoglobin was ≤10 g/dl. Wu *et al.*[55] reported a retrospective study of over 310,000 men >65 years old who underwent noncardiac surgery in the American Veterans' Affairs system showing that postoperative mortality and cardiac events progressively increased as the preoperative hematocrit fell below 39%. In a systematic review of the literature, Spahn *et al.*[50] found that preoperative anemia in orthopedic surgery patients was associated with more infections and higher mortality. A recent study in orthopedic surgery patients, however, calls into question whether anemia is causally related to these outcomes.[56] It is clear, however, that anemia does increase the risk of transfusion. That reason alone would justify implementing measures to manage preoperative anemia.

Patient blood management programs have been developed to manage preoperative anemia primarily in orthopedic surgery patients,[52,57,58] although these programs have also been applied to other patients who are undergoing elective surgery that is expected to feature significant blood loss. These programs consist of identifying patients undergoing elective procedures ideally 4 weeks, but not less than 2 weeks, prior to surgery and performing a screening hemoglobin. This practice was suggested by the Joint Commission as a performance measurement initiative.[59] Using the WHO definition of anemia, patients would be referred to a hematologist, preoperative clinic, or other physician for evaluation and management of the anemia. Several algorithms for the evaluation

and management of preoperative anemia have been published, including one by the NATA group using GRADE methodology (Figure 2.2).[58] This algorithm uses serum ferritin and transferrin saturation to triage patients to appropriate management strategies that may include oral iron, intravenous (IV) iron, folic acid, vitamin B_{12}, and/or erythropoietin (EPO). Other algorithms use the red cell mean corpuscular volume (MCV)[57] or ferritin alone[52] as screening tests. There are no studies demonstrating that one particular strategy is superior to another.

The pharmacologic therapies for the management of preoperative anemia have been recently reviewed.[58] Oral iron may be sufficient to correct the anemia in patients who have iron-restricted erythropoiesis due to absolute iron deficiency. Oral preparations include ferrous gluconate, ferrous fumarate, ferrous sulfate, and iron polysaccharide. The advantage to oral iron replacement is that it is inexpensive and easy to administer. There are several limitations, however, including gastrointestinal side effects and compliance issues. It also takes 2–4 weeks to increase hemoglobin levels. Oral iron is not very effective in patients with anemia of inflammation (chronic disease).

IV iron therapy is becoming a more common strategy for management of preoperative anemia as safer preparations are now available in the United States. IV iron bypasses absorption, tolerance, and compliance issues. It is also effective in patients with anemia of chronic disease in whom inflammation and subsequent elevated hepcidin levels prevent iron mobilization.[58] The total dose is typically 1 g, independent of the patient's weight. The number of doses required to deliver 1 g and achieve a therapeutic effect depends on the preparation used. An increase in hemoglobin is apparent at one week after starting IV iron therapy, and reaches its apogee after two weeks.[57] Serious acute adverse events (i.e., anaphylaxis) have been associated with high-molecular-weight (HMW) dextran IV iron preparations but appear to be lower with low-molecular-weight (LMW) dextran preparations. These iron dextran preparations have a US Food and Drug Administration (FDA) "black box" warning and require a test dose before infusion. LMW dextran preparations can be given as a single 1 g infusion and are less costly than other preparations. Other IV iron preparations that are approved in the United States include iron gluconate, iron

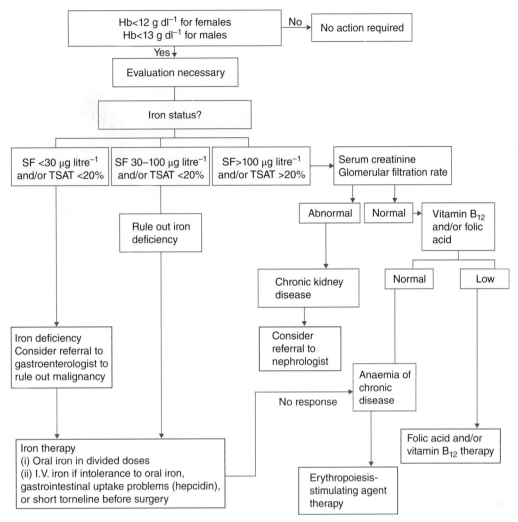

Figure 2.2 Proposed algorithm for the detection, evaluation, and management of preoperative anemia. SF, serum ferritin; TSAT, transferrin saturation. Source: Goodnough *et al.*, 2011 [58]. Reproduced with permission of Oxford University Press.

sucrose, iron isomaltose, iron carboxymaltose, and iron carboxymethyl dextran. None of these preparations have a "black box" warning, and they do not require a test dose as they do not contain HMW dextrans. The iron gluconate and sucrose preparations are not approved for an infusion dose of more than 500 mg and thus would require the patient to return for one or more infusions. The other preparations can be given as a single total dose infusion.

Erythropoietic stimulating agents are FDA approved for use in patients with anemia due to chronic kidney disease, in oncology patients with chemotherapy-induced anemia, for HIV-therapy-related anemia, and in patients with anemia undergoing elective surgery.[58] There are two approved preparations: epoietin alfa and, more recently, darbepoietin alfa. Only the former is approved for use in elective surgery, and it is intended for patients with a preoperative hemoglobin >10 to ≤13 g/dL who are at high risk for perioperative blood loss from elective, noncardiac, nonvascular surgery.[60,61] In this setting, EPO has been shown to be effective in reducing the need for transfusion.[62] Subsequent RCTs in patients undergoing hip or knee arthroplasty reported similar results[63,64] and did not find a difference in the rates of deep venous thrombosis between the EPO-α and control groups. The preoperative dosing schedule for EPO-α is typically 600 U/kg weekly for 3 weeks and a fourth dose on the day of surgery. A daily regimen is also available but requires dosing for 10 consecutive days before surgery, on the day of surgery, and for four days after surgery. It is mainly of use in patients who have <2 weeks before scheduled surgery. The onset of action of EPO, indicated by a rise in hemoglobin, is 4–6 days. Concomitant iron therapy is necessary during EPO-α therapy due to increased demand for iron as it is incorporated into hemoglobin. EPO should not be used in patients with a hemoglobin >13 g/dl. Safety concerns about EPO in elective surgery patients have recently been raised. In 2007, the results of an RCT of EPO versus no EPO in 681 adult patients who underwent spine surgery without prophylactic anticoagulation was reported to the FDA.[60] Patients in the EPO arm received 4 weekly EPO doses of 600 U/kg Epoetin alfa (21, 14, and 7 days before surgery, and the day of surgery). An increased incidence of deep vein thrombosis (DVT) in patients receiving EPO was observed (4.7%) compared to the control group (7 patients [2.1%]). Based on this study and a higher incidence of DVT in other patient populations treated with EPO, the FDA recommended that prophylactic anticoagulation be "strongly considered" when EPO-α is used in surgical patients. EPO is not approved for use in patients undergoing cardiac or vascular surgery due to FDA concerns about increased mortality.[60,61]

Cell salvage

The process of collecting shed autologous blood, its processing, and it re-administration has been termed *cell salvage, autotransfusion, intraoperative blood recovery*, as well as *cell saving*. For the purpose of this chapter, the term *cell salvage* will be used. Cell salvage can take place either in the intraoperative period or in the postoperative period. Salvage can also involve washing of the collected blood, or it can be simply re-administered with microaggregate filtration.

Unwashed cell salvage

To this day, both washed and unwashed salvage devices are used. Postoperative unwashed blood salvage has been utilized in a wide variety of surgical procedures,[65] but it is predominantly used after cardiac[66] and orthopedic procedures (Figure 2.3).[67] Estimates of postoperative blood loss after cardiac surgery range from 371 mL to 553 mL,[68–70] whereas volumes following total joint replacement range from 166 mL to 750 mL.[71–73] The average hemoglobin of this shed blood is reported to range from 20 to 30%.[74,75] At best, the volume returned to a patient would equal the red cell mass present in one unit of allogeneic red cells so the efficacy of this unwashed product in avoiding allogeneic transfusion is limited. Controversy arises as to whether the risks of retransfusion of this blood warrant the minimal amount of blood that is returned to the patient.

When one considers that this salvaged blood is laden with various inflammatory mediators,[76,77] fibrin split products,[78–80] complement fractions,[81–83] interleukins,[84–86] tumor necrosis factor α (TNF-α),[87] and fat particles,[88] which are multiple degrees higher than circulating levels, it is easy to believe that there is risk from re-administration of this shed, unwashed blood. This being said, the reported risks appear to be minimal. The most frequently reported complication following unwashed postoperative shed blood reinfusion relates to febrile reactions, which is a complication frequently seen following allogeneic transfusion. Dependent upon the study, the rates of febrile reactions after postoperative salvage re-administration vary from 4 to 12%.[89–92] This complication is generally the

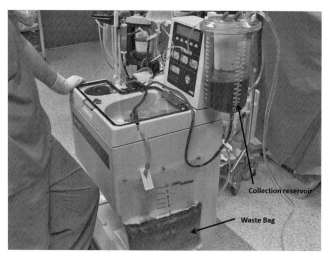

Figure 2.4 A device for salvaging and washing blood is shown.

only reported complication following re-administration of unwashed, shed blood; however, all of these reports are small case series.

In a Cochrane systematic review, Carless *et al.* reviewed complications of all available studies on perioperative salvage.[93] They evaluated total complications, wound infections, and thromboembolic events that included nonfatal myocardial infarction. They found no difference in any of these events, but they mixed washed with unwashed salvage and the vast preponderance of studies was from cardiac surgery. A simple solution to the perceived hazards of the contaminants of unwashed, postoperative cell salvage would be to wash the blood (Figure 2.4).

Washed cell salvage

In a washed salvaged product, the blood is collected via suction into a reservoir where it is stored until processing. When adequate amounts of blood are collected, the blood is pumped into a centrifuge bowl where it is concentrated. During the concentration of the erythrocytes, plasma and anticoagulant are spilled into a waste bag. Following the concentration of the erythrocytes, normal saline or Ringers' Lactate solution is percolated through the red cell pack with the goal to wash out tissue factor and the inflammatory mediators mentioned previously. Following washing, the blood is leukoreduced by filtration and re-administered to the patient. Washing comes with its own set of problems, which include air embolism[94] and washing with non-isotonic solutions.[95] When the processing is completed, the blood is pumped into a reinfusion bag, and preceding the blood is a column of air. When multiple units of blood are processed, the air can accumulate in the reinfusion bag, which then presents a hazard to the patient if the patient's intravenous line is connected directly to this bag. In order to prevent this problem, the reinfusion bag should never be directly connected to the patient. Washing can also be problematic if an isotonic wash solution is not chosen. For instance, if blood is washed with sterile water, the cells will all be lysed. If the free hemoglobin is administered to the patient, it could potentially result in renal failure or be fatal.

Maximizing washed salvage efficiency

Washed cell salvage can provide multiple units of autologous erythrocytes for a bleeding patient.[96] Small changes in the collection

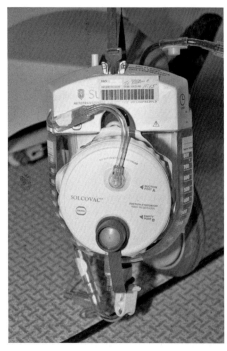

Figure 2.3 An unwashed salvage device in use for a knee replacement.

and processing of shed red cells can make large differences in the volume of blood returned to the surgical patient. Mathematical modeling illustrates this point.[97] Assuming a 70-kg patient with a 5-L blood volume and preoperative hemoglobin of 15 gm/dL, and using a transfusion trigger of 7 gm/dL, a theoretical patient can avoid transfusion of allogeneic blood up to a blood loss of 9600 mL if salvages return 60% of lost red cells. However, the tolerable blood loss rises to 13,750 mL if 70% of the red cells are captured and returned. The most important factors in increasing efficiency of these systems are regulating the suction imposed on the red cells and washing bloody surgical sponges.

Suction

For blood recovery systems to work, it is necessary to deliver shed blood to a collection reservoir where the blood awaits processing. Collection is done through suction from the site of surgery or a salvage system can be connected to a surgical drain. The way this suction pressure is applied affects the shear forces applied to the red cells. In general, turbulence and high negative pressure destroy red cells. Shear force occurs anytime a fluid moves in contact with a solid surface.[98] High suction pressure leads to increased mechanical force, hemolysis, and subsequently fewer salvageable erythrocytes. As such, the lowest tolerable suction pressure should be applied when removing blood from the surgical field.

Suction pressure should be regulated to −80 to −120 mmHg, which is generally adequate to clear blood from the surgical field.[99,100] If massive blood loss occurs, it is important to increase the suction pressure so that the surgeon can clearly see the surgical field. Following control of the blood loss, the suction pressure can be lowered.

Sponge rinsing

Fully soaked surgical sponges may contain up to 100 mL of blood.[101] Of this blood, approximately 95% of these erythrocytes can be captured by rinsing the sponge in a basin of normal saline or Ringer's Lactate solution. The bloody rinse solution is then intermittently sucked into the salvage collection reservoir at a point when the rinse solution appears to be grossly bloody. This practice has been reported to increase erythrocyte retrieval rates by 28%.[102]

Indications

Determining when to salvage erythrocytes depends upon anticipated blood loss. Prediction of anticipated blood loss is difficult. With this lack of predictability, a cell salvage program should be assessed in composite rather than for a single case. Some cases might generate 20 units of blood, whereas other cases will not generate any. If the sum of salvaged units achieves one allogeneic red cell unit equivalent on average, then the program is generally considered successful, although financial success may dependent upon whether the service is provided in-house or whether an external perfusion service is hired.[103] Major vascular, cardiac, and transplantation surgery tend to be procedures that generate a large amount of blood loss.[104] Blood loss can also be surgeon dependent. Surgeons will have widely varying blood loss performing the same procedure. So, the type of procedure and who is performing it are primary criteria for determining need.

Given the lack of predictability of blood loss, an important feature of washed salvage is recognizing that the cost of the disposables can be staged through the use of a "standby" system. A standby system involves simply collection of shed blood. The standby system utilizes a collection reservoir, a suction line, and anticoagulant.

This represents approximately half of the cost of the disposables of a salvage system. If processing is indicated, then a processing bowl and tubing system are utilized that double the cost. In this way, half of the cost is not expended if inadequate blood is captured.

Contraindications

Absolute contraindications to cell salvage involve contamination of the blood with anything that will lyse the erythrocyte. This would include hypotonic solutions like sterile water, hydrogen peroxide, and alcohol. Topical collagen hemostatic agents when incorporated into a salvaged blood product can also be hazardous if the topical agent is infused. Heavy metals (chromium and cobalt) can be found in blood salvaged from metal on metal hip prostheses.[105] Accumulation of metal debris in the surrounding joint tissue can be suctioned into blood during replacement. Neuropathy and cardiomyopathy can result from high heavy metal blood levels.

Traditionally, cell salvage has been avoided in obstetrics where the blood might be contaminated with amniotic fluid, malignant surgery where cancer cells might be entrained into the blood, and "dirty" surgery where blood might be contaminated with bacteria. All of these areas are recommended to be contraindicated by the machine manufacturers; however, a striking lack of evidence is available to support these contraindicated areas. Theoretical concerns regarding risk of amniotic fluid embolism when using salvaged blood in obstetrical hemorrhage have not been substantiated. Due to the lack of evidence to support an obstetric contraindication, national and international bodies including the American College of Obstetricians and Gynecologists (ACOG)[106–108] have promoted the use of cell salvage in obstetrics.

Similarly, a fear of generating a diffuse metastasis when salvaging blood around a tumor site has not been borne out. In 2008, the British National Institute of Clinical Excellence[109] approved use of salvage during urological malignancies. Systematic reviews have also been performed evaluating salvage use during malignant surgery[110] as well as surgery involving tumors of the spine.[111] In neither of these reviews was there support for avoiding the salvage in these surgeries for malignancy. Lastly, blood that might be contaminated with bacteria has been a further contraindication. Surprisingly, bacterial contamination of recovered blood appears to be common. Bland et al.[112] reported that bacterial contamination of recovered blood in cardiac surgery approaches 30% of the units processed. Kang et al.[113] reported that 9% of the blood returned to liver transplant patients contained bacterial contaminants, usually of skin origin. In these circumstances of bacterial contamination, no clinical effects were seen. Although it would be prudent to avoid use of blood that has been grossly contaminated with stool, blood salvage during support of abdominal trauma would appear to be safe. In these contraindicated circumstances, the use of leukocyte depletion filters has been advocated.[114] Leukocyte depletion filters have been demonstrated to remove many contaminants, including cancer cells, cellular contaminants associated with amniotic fluid, and bacteria. Although these filters have not been demonstrated to produce better outcomes, theoretically additional safety may be provided by their use.

Acute normovolemic hemodilution (ANH)

Acute normovolemic hemodilution (ANH) is a technique intended to minimize or decrease the need for allogeneic transfusion. With ANH, blood is phlebotomized from a surgical patient at the start of surgery, generally shortly after the induction of anesthesia. The blood that is taken off is replaced with a colloid or crystalloid volume expander in order to maintain isovolemia. At the end of surgery, the phlebotomized blood is given back to the patient. The central tenet of ANH is that the patient will bleed blood that is less concentrated in terms of its erythrocytes. Although this theoretical savings sounds substantial, the savings appear to be small clinically.[115]

Given that the phlebotimized blood is whole blood, the effectiveness in transfusion avoidance applies to both erythrocytes and coagulation products. The real value of ANH is in the preservation of platelets and plasma. If sufficient whole blood is collected prior to surgery, a dilutional coagulopathy can be reversed.[116,117] Pairing of ANH and cell salvage provides a comprehensive hematologic approach to avoiding allogeneic transfusion. Cell salvage provides erythrocytes for treating anemia, whereas the ANH provides the coagulation product avoidance. In addition, the anemia created by hemodilution exposes fewer red cells to the mechanical trauma of salvage, thus providing a higher rate of erythrocyte return.[118]

A number of mechanisms allow the patient to tolerate aggressive phlebotomy. Increased cardiac output resulting from increases in heart rate and cardiac contractility, and a reduction in whole blood viscosity, lead to maintenance of oxygen delivery.[119,120] In addition, tissue oxygen needs are reduced during hemodilution from anesthesia and mechanical ventilation.

The practice of ANH is relatively limited due to a lack of understanding in how it is performed. In general, multiple units of blood are withdrawn into a standard donor bag containing 63 mL of citrate anticoagulant. The goal is to remove 450 mL of whole blood into each donor bag. The 63 mL of citrate is adequate to anticoagulate this volume of blood. Typically, the blood is removed through an arterial or venous catheter. Optimally, the shortest catheter should be used in order to minimize resistance to flow and to minimize activation of platelets. Double- or triple-lumen catheters with their long catheter lengths are likely to fail because flow rates are slow. As a result of the slow flow rate, blood clotting may result. Blood flow should be greater than 30 mL/min in order to prevent clotting in the collection bag. Periodic agitation of the collected blood should take place in order to optimally mix the citrate anticoagulant with the blood.[121] Once the blood is collected, it should be maintained in the operating room close to the patient, and it should be maintained at room temperature. Once the blood has been mixed with the anticoagulant, there is no need to continuously agitate it.[122] Units should be reinfused in the reverse order of collection.

Point-of-care testing

Point-of-care or near-care laboratory testing involves the placement of laboratory equipment near or at the patient bedside. A number of point-of-care devices are available with available laboratory information, including hemoglobin concentration, PT/PTT (prothrombin time and partial thromboplastin time), glucose, blood gas and electrolyte concentrations, and whole blood clotting function.

The advantage to using point-of-care devices instead of centralized laboratory testing relates to the speed of getting data for management decisions. In the acute care setting, such as the operating room or the intensive care unit where critically ill, dynamically changing patients are being cared for, the tendency is to make empiric care decisions based on guesses regarding the patient condition. When laboratory information is obtained at the patient bedside, more informed patient care decisions are made.

Another advantage to point-of-care testing involves the use of microsampling. Generally, these devices require blood samples in the microliter size, whereas traditional laboratory based testing requires milliliter-sized samples. It is well recognized that repeated, large-volume samples can quickly result in an iatrogenic anemia, most prominently in the critical care setting.[123] It has been estimated that the average ICU patient will have a fall in hemoglobin concentration of 0.5 gm/dL/day with 80% of the fall related to blood draws.[124]

One of the drawbacks to point-of-care testing is that the methodology for measurement is frequently different than that of laboratory-based testing, which will sometimes give values that are viewed as not being accurate. In many of these circumstances, there is no gold standard by which to say one methodology is better than another. As such, it is important to understand the biases of each device and react accordingly.

For PBM programs, whole blood clotting assays using thromboelastography such as TEG (Haemonetics, Braintree, MA, USA) or ROTEM (TEM Systems Inc., Durham, NC, USA) have become increasingly popular in managing perioperative coagulopathic bleeding and blood product therapy. In addition to the advantage of rapid results and point-of-care availability, these assays have the theoretical advantage of providing assessment of the interactions between the various components of hemostasis. Traditional laboratory measures of hemostasis such as aPTT (activated partial thromboplastin time), PTT, fibrinogen, and platelet count provide a limited assessment of only that aspect of hemostasis and not their interaction. The use of TEG- and ROTEM-based algorithms for assessing hemostasis and managing blood component therapy has been shown to reduce transfusions and bleeding in the settings of massive trauma, liver transplantation, and cardiac surgery,[125–131] and it is discussed extensively in this volume.

Use of hemostatic agents

The hemostatic management of patients has been advanced through better understanding of the mechanism of coagulaopathy, availability of point-of-care testing, and a growing array of hemostatic agents. The clinical use and description of these agents have been reviewed[132,133] and will be described here.

Solvent/detergent plasma

Physicians are familiar with using plasma from a single donation of whole blood or apheresis collection to treat a coagulopathy. A pooled solvent detergent (S/D)-treated plasma called Octaplas (Octapharma AG, Vienna Austria) is now approved in the United States.[134] This product is manufactured from plasma pools of 630–1520 donors, which are ultrafiltered (1 micron pore size) and then subject to solvent (1% Tri(n-butyl)phosphate [TNBP]) and detergent (1% Octoxynol-9) treatment for 1–1.5 hours.[134] This processing inactivates lipid membrane-bound viruses. The product is further processed through an affinity column to remove prions. Protein-coated non-enveloped viruses such as HAV or parvovirus B19 are resistant to S/D treatment. Transmission is prevented by screening for low virus loads in the starting plasma units, dilution through pooling, and the presence of neutralization antibodies introduced by pooling. The risk of transfusion-related lung injury appears to be dramatically reduced, if not eliminated, which is likely due to pooling and screening for HLA antibodies.[135] Octaplas LG is provided as a standard 200 ml bag of type-specific S/D plasma. It is maintained frozen at −18 °C and thawed when requested. Once thawed,

Octaplas LG is stored up to 12 hours at 2–4 °C.[134] The content of Octaplas LG is similar to that of plasma with the exception of lower levels of protein S (0.61; normal range, 0.56–1.68) and α2-antiplasmin (0.48; normal range, 0.72–1.32).[136] Prior S/D plasma formulations approved in the United States had lower levels of protein S and α2-antiplasmin, and were associated with reports of enhanced fibrinolysis and thrombosis during liver transplant.[137] It does not appear to be the case with current Octaplas LG formulations.[135] Octaplas LG can be used clinically interchangeably with plasma,[135] including for thrombotic thrombocytopenic purpura as ADAMTS-13 levels are adequate.[138]

Prothrombin complex concentrates (PCC)

Three-factor nonactivated PCC containing lyophilized factor II, IX, and X but low levels of factor VII (Profilnine–Grifols, Bebulin VH-Baxter) and an activated PCC, FEIBA (factor VIII inhibitory bypass activity; Baxter), have been available in the United States for years. These have been used primarily for the treatment of hemophilia. Their use for warfarin reversal is controversial.[139] In April 2013, the FDA approved the first four-factor nonactivated PCC, K-Centra (CSL Behring GmbH, Marburg,Germany).[140] K-Centra contains hemostatic levels of factors II, VII, IX, and X. It is indicated for the urgent reversal of acquired coagulation factor deficiency induced by vitamin K antagonist (VKA; e.g., warfarin) therapy in adult patients with acute major bleeding. Dosing is based on weight and baseline INR values. The dose calculation uses the factor IX content, which is approximately 500 IU/vial. For INR 2–4, use 25 IU/kg not to exceed 2500 IU; for INR 4–6, use 35 IU/kg not to exceed 3500 IU; and, for INR>6, use 50 IU/kg not to exceed 5000 IU. Patient should receive vitamin K concomitantly with K-Centra. Repeated dosing is not recommended. The primary US study upon which the US Food and Drug Administration (FDA) approval was based was an open-label RCT comparing K-Centra to plasma for urgent VKA reversal in 202 patients with major bleeding.[141] The study demonstrated that K-Centra was equivalent to plasma in achieving the hemostatic endpoint and did so more rapidly (17 minutes vs 148 minutes). There was no difference in thromboembolic rates (7.8% PCC vs 6.4% FFP) or serious adverse events, although the mortality rate at 45 days was 9.7% in the PCC group versus 4.6% in the FFP group. There are limited studies of the use of four-factor PCC for treatment of coagulopathy in other settings. It has been suggested as a treatment for reversal of anti-Xa inhibitors and direct thrombin inhibitors but with limited supportive evidence.[142,143] K-Centra contains trace amounts of heparin and thus should not be used in patients with heparin-induced thrombocytopenia. Clinical trials of four-factor PCCs with regard to their efficacy, safety (thrombotic risk), and cost-effectiveness in patients not on VKAs are needed.

Antifibrinolytics

The fibrinolytic system contributes to the balance between bleeding and thrombosis by controlling clot formation and extension, and dissolving unnecessary clots. In patients with excessive bleeding, inhibiting fibrinolysis can improve hemostasis by delaying clot dissolution. The two most commonly used agents, epsilon aminocaproic acid (EACA) and tranexamic acid (TXA), are lysine analogs that inhibit the conversion of plasminogen to its active form, plasmin.[133] With the removal of aprotinin from the US market in 2007, these agents have been shown to be efficacious in reducing bleeding in cardiac surgery.[144] TXA interest was greatly promoted by the trauma study, Clinical Randomization of an Antifibrinolytic in Significant Hemorrhage (CRASH-2).[145] This was an RCT involving 20,211 adult trauma patients assigned to receive TXA versus placebo within 8 hours of injury. The primary endpoint, all-cause mortality, was reduced in the TXA arm (14.5% vs 16.0%), as was death due to bleeding (4.9% vs 5.7%). A follow-up analysis showed that the benefit was strongest when TXA was given within one hour of injury; it was still apparent at 1–3 hours after injury, but TXA actually increased mortality if given 3–8 hours after injury.[146] There was no difference in bleeding or transfusions. A recent review and meta-analysis of RCTs of TXA versus no TXA found 129 trials involving more than 10,000 patients who underwent cardiac, orthopedic, hepatic, urologic, gynecologic, cranial, or vascular surgery published between 1972 and 2011 and showed that transfusion risk is consistently reduced by one-third.[147] The effects of TXA on thromboembolic events and mortality were, however, unclear. The results of a large international RCT of TXA in 15,000 women with postpartum hemorrhage (the WOMAN Trial) are expected in 2015.[148]

Desmopressin

Desmopressin (DDAVP) is a synthetic analog of vasopressin that is primarily used for the treatment of patients with von Willebrand disease (VWD), hemophilia A, some platelet disorders, and uremic bleeding. DDAVP is known to increase the plasma levels of von Willebrand factor, factor VIII, and tissue plasminogen activator. The hemostatic effect of DDAVP is well understood.[149] DDAVP has been used to enhance hemostasis in patient undergoing surgery with expected high blood loss. A meta-analysis of 38 trials involving 2488 patients undergoing mostly cardiac surgery but also orthopedic, vascular, and plastic surgery found a statistically reduction in bleeding (80 ml) and transfusion (0.3 units), but the clinical relevance of these finding is questionable.[150] Due to its limited efficacy, DDAVP is not routinely used in surgical patients.

Fibrinogen concentrates

A heat-treated virally inactivated fibrinogen concentrate derived from pooled human plasma is available in the United States (RiaSTAPP, CSL Behring GmbH, Marburg, Germany).[151] The labeled indication is to replace fibrinogen in bleeding patients with congenital afibrinogenemia or hypofibrinogenemia. Vials contain 900–1300 mg of fibrinogen, equivalent to 4–5 units of cryoprecipitate. Fibrinogen concentrates have been used widely in Europe for patients with perioperative bleeding and acquired hypofibrinogenemia.[152] The fibrinogen level at which replacement is recommended in the perioperative setting has evolved from 100 mg/dl[153] to more recently 150–200 mg/dl in the European trauma guidelines.[130] In the perioperative setting, the recommended dose is 2–4 g (25–50 mg/kg) of fibrinogen concentrate with an expect increment of 25–28 mg/dl per gram of fibrinogen concentrate.[132] The reported side effects include allergic reactions chills, fever, nausea, vomiting, and thrombosis. There is a paucity of published RCT data in the United States. A non-US industry-sponsored multicenter RCT of fibrinogen concentrate in 152 patients with complex cardiac surgery was recently completed.[154] The efficacy and safety of these products in the perioperative setting await these results and those of ongoing trials.

Recombinant activated factor VII

Recombinant activated factor VII (rfVIIa, NovoSeven, Novo Nordisc A/S, Bagsvaerd, Denmark) is structurally similar to plasma-derived factor VIIa and is intended to promote hemostasis through the activation of the extrinsic pathway of the coagulation cascade.[155]

rfVIIa binds to tissue factor, which then converts factor X to factor Xa, as well as coagulation factor IX to factor IXa. The factor VII gene was cloned and expressed in Chinese hamster kidney cells where the expressed protein is auto-activated during chromatographic purification.[156] The labeled indication for rVIIa is to treat or prevent bleeding in hemophilia A or B patients with inhibitors or patients with congenital factor VII deficiency.[155] Dosing in hemophilia patients with bleeding is 90 μg/kg every 2 hours until hemostasis is achieved (t ½ is 2.3 hours). It is available as a lyophilized powder requiring reconstitution in 1 mg, 2 mg, or 5 mg vials.

There has been extensive interest in using rVIIa off label to promote hemostasis in trauma, surgery, intracranial bleeding, and other patient populations.[157] Early enthusiasm based on largely observational data or small RCTs[158,159] was not confirmed by RCTs in penetrating trauma,[158] pediatric cardiac surgery,[160] intracranial bleeding,[161] liver resection,[162] or variceal bleeding.[163] rfVIIa has also been suggested as a potential therapy for reversal of new anticoagulants, warfarin, Xa inhibitors, and direct thrombin inhibitors. With the availability of four-factor PCC, rfVIIa should not be used for warfarin reversal. Data on its use to reverse dabigitran or rivaroxaban are mixed.[164–167] Given the uncertainty regarding clinical effectiveness in off-label settings, safety issues must be carefully considered. A systematic review of 35 clinical trials involving 4468 patients who received rfVIIa for an off-label indication reported significantly higher risk of arterial (but not venous) thromboembolic events (CI 1.68 [1.20–2.36]).[168] A recent meta-analysis of six clinical trials involving 470 cardiac surgery patients reported a higher risk of stroke (OR 3.69 [1.1–12.38], $p = 0.03$) in those treated with rfVIIa.[169] Taken together the literature suggests that use of rfVIIa in an off-label setting has unproven efficacy, should be entertained with caution, and, if used, should be limited to patients with life-threatening bleeding.

Limiting phlebotomy blood loss for laboratory testing

Although it might seem like a trivial amount of blood loss, repetitive phlebotomy for laboratory testing can result in a significant decrease in the patient's hemoglobin concentration and can result in anemia. A computerized model of blood loss predicted that it would take a healthy adult of average weight and blood volume about 40–70 days of 53 ml daily blood draws to reach a hemoglobin concentration of 7 g/dl, whereas a sick patient in the ICU would require only 9–14 days to reach the same level.[170] The volume of phlebotomy has been correlated with the decrease in the recipient's hemoglobin or RBC transfusion requirements,[171–174] and one Canadian study found that for every 100 ml of blood lost by phlebotomy, the recipient's hematocrit decreased by nearly 2%.[171] Several studies have demonstrated that the amount of blood that is collected for diagnostic purposes is far in excess of that which is actually necessary to complete the testing,[174,175] suggesting that measures to reduce the volume of blood collected for laboratory testing should be implemented. To this end, the AABB has suggested several steps that can be implemented.[7] Some of these suggestions involve educating the providers about the potential problems caused by reduced hemoglobin and anemia that can arise from excessive phlebotomies, and changing their practices when ordering laboratory testing; limiting the number of phlebotomies to the absolute minimum number required for patient care should reduce the amount of blood lost to testing, as will eliminating standing orders for certain laboratory tests, that is, laboratory tests should only be ordered when there is a change in the patient's condition or when a diagnostic or therapeutic intervention based on their results is being considered. Other recommendations involve making changes in the way that laboratory tests are ordered, such as by electronically limiting the number of times that a test can be ordered during a defined time period,[176] and redesigning the electronic or paper forms on which laboratory tests are ordered to discourage ordering unnecessary testing. If a laboratory test is indeed required, then the smallest volume possible should be phlebotomized. This means that special small-volume tubes must be easily accessible on the ward and that the laboratory's diagnostic equipment must be able to process these kinds of tubes, which might have different dimensions than standard tubes. Furthermore, point-of-care testing should be performed when available (and when validated) as the volume of blood required to perform the testing is usually much smaller than that required by the machinery in the main laboratory.

Summary

PBM has become a major clinical and research focus for not only the field of transfusion medicine but also any discipline in which patients are transfused. It is designed to be patient care focused and requires a multidisciplinary approach. A PBM program requires resources, effort, and institutional support but can be implemented gradually by initially capitalizing on the obvious opportunities. IT has provided unprecedented opportunity to systematically influence ordering and monitoring of physician practices. A PBM program is one of the most powerful ways to optimize patient care in a cost-effective manner.

Acknowledgments

Parts of the section on physician education and monitoring were adapted, with the kind permission of Elsevier, from SP Hibbs, ND Nielsen, S Brunskill, C Doreed, **MH Yazer**, RM Kaufman, MF Murphy. The impact of electronic decision support on transfusion practice: a systematic review. Transfusion Medicine Reviews 2015; 29:14-23.

Key references

A full reference list for this chapter is available at:
http://www.wiley.com/go/simon/transfusion

3 Yazer MH, Triulzi DJ. Things aren't always as they seem: what randomized trials of red blood cell transfusion tell us about adverse outcomes. *Transfusion* 2014; **54**: 3243–6.

5 Society for the Advancement of Blood (SABM). *The administrative and clinical standards for patient blood management programs.* 2nd ed. Englewood, NJ: SABM, 2013.

6 AABB. *AABB standards for a patient blood management program.* Bethesda, MD: AABB, 2014.

8 Yazer MH, Waters JH. How do I implement a hospital-based blood management program? *Transfusion* 2012; **52**: 1640–5.

13 Kaufman RM, Djulbegovic B, Gernsheimer T, *et al.* Platelet transfusion: a clinical practice guideline from the AABB. *Ann Intern Med* 2015; **162** (3): 205–13.

CHAPTER 3

Clinical and technical aspects of blood administration

Eric A. Gehrie, Jocelyn Chandler, & Edward L. Snyder

Department of Laboratory Medicine, Yale School of Medicine; and Blood Bank, Yale-New Haven Hospital, New Haven, CT, USA

Introduction

Errors in pretransfusion specimen collection, omission of appropriate transfusion filters, or co-administration of incompatible fluids with blood products could transform blood transfusion from a lifesaving measure into a life threatening event. In this chapter, we will summarize key aspects of blood component administration, with an emphasis on processes and technologic advances that promise to improve the quality of patient care and patient safety. The paragraphs below are only general guidance based on current guidelines and regulations. In addition to this information, the reader is directed the latest version of the AABB Standards, local standards of practice, and institutional requirements.

Pretransfusion considerations

Prior to transfusion, there are several steps that should be taken to ensure that patient safety is protected. First, unless the request for blood is emergent, it is essential to obtain informed consent for blood transfusion. Per the *AABB Standard* (5.26.1.1), at minimum, informed consent requires the inclusion of the following: (1) a description of the risks, benefits, and alternatives (including non-treatment); (2) the opportunity to ask questions; and (3) the right to accept or refuse transfusion.[1] In some parts of the United States, there is also a legal requirement (e.g., the Paul Gann Blood Safety Act in California) to discuss alternatives to transfusion. Furthermore, it is recommended that this discussion between healthcare provider and patient be properly documented.[2,3]

Second, unless the indication for transfusion is emergent, pretransfusion compatibility testing should be performed prior to component issue. Determining a transfusion recipient's blood type and identifying whether any unexpected antibodies are present in the recipient's plasma can prevent hemolytic transfusion reactions and conserve limited resources (e.g., group O RBCs and group AB plasma).[4] To begin the pretransfusion compatibility testing process, the clinical staff must obtain a blood sample from a correctly identified patient. The specimen should be labeled with a minimum of two patient identifiers (e.g., name and date of birth), the date of the blood draw, and the identification of the person who drew the blood (e.g., phlebotomist initials). Samples can be rejected by the blood bank if they are improperly labeled, if the requisition form is missing key identifying information, or if the sample was drawn in the incorrect tube.[1,5] Studies have consistently shown that human errors throughout the pretransfusion process occur at substantial rates and can lead to fatal incompatible transfusions.[5–7]

Venipuncture for intravenous (IV) access

Blood components are most often transfused intravenously through peripheral veins, but central venous access can also be used in critically ill patients.[8] A previously established IV line can be used for blood transfusion. However, prior to use, the line should always be examined for patency and signs of infection. Ideally, the line should be flushed with normal saline to ensure that any incompatible fluid is removed prior to blood component infusion. The line should also be of sufficient bore to prevent hemolysis.

Component issue, release, storage, and transport

Component issue and release

Before a component is issued from the blood bank, safeguards should be established to ensure that the correct component is released to the intended patient. The verification process between the blood bank laboratory technologist and the transportation courier includes checks of donor and recipient identifying information as well as ABO group and Rh type, expiration date of the unit, crossmatch results, satisfaction of any special transfusion requirements (e.g., irradiated or washed), and a check for any visual abnormalities of the unit.[1] Once this checklist is complete, the date and time of issue should be noted, and the component can then be taken to the patient's bedside.

Component storage

Blood bank storage devices include freezers, refrigerators, and platelet incubators. Maintaining proper component storage and equipment monitoring systems is critical to protect the quality of blood products. All storage devices must also be equipped with an emergency power supply and a continuous alarm monitoring system. In the absence of such a system, the temperature must be monitored and documented every four hours. Alarms should continue to function even in the event of a power failure. Scheduled alarm checks should occur at least quarterly.[9]

Red blood cells (RBCs)

RBCs must be stored within refrigerators in the blood bank and continuously maintained at 1–6 °C to limit their metabolic activity while ensuring cell viability.[10] During the transport process, warming of blood a few degrees (up to 10 °C) is acceptable. Historically, studies have demonstrated that RBC units change temperature quickly when

Rossi's Principles of Transfusion Medicine, Fifth Edition. Edited by Toby L. Simon, Jeffrey McCullough, Edward L. Snyder, Bjarte G. Solheim, and Ronald G. Strauss.

removed from refrigeration and that this temperature increase can affect the cellular viability of the component.[11] These findings led to the so-called 30-minute rule, whereby blood stored outside of the recommended storage temperatures for greater than 30 minutes could not be placed back into the blood bank inventory. However, current studies have questioned the validity of this rule.[12,13] According to the 2014 CAP (the College of American Pathologists) checklist (TRM.42470), blood components can be reintroduced into the inventory if the unit has not exceeded 10 °C and if steps have been taken to "verify the integrity and appearance of the container."[9]

Platelets

Current *AABB Standards* recommend platelet storage at room temperature (20–24 °C) with continuous gentle agitation.[1,14] Room temperature storage is favored because platelets stored at 20–24 °C have good posttransfusion in vivo recovery, and exposure to cold results in platelet inactivation.[15] Although room temperature storage puts platelets at increased risk of bacterial contamination, changes in regulations seen in the *AABB Standards* in 2004 introduced a requirement to limit and detect bacterially contaminated platelet components in an effort to mitigate this potential hazard.[16]

Platelets are sensitive to pH changes and must be adequately agitated.[17] Importantly, platelet agitation promotes gas exchange through the plastic storage container, helping to effectively maintain pH.[18] Platelet agitation devices have been extensively studied.[15,19,20] Results of these studies show that horizontal agitation (circular or flatbed agitators moving side to side) maintain platelet functionality better than do more vigorous, vertical (end over end) methods of agitation.[21] Studies have also demonstrated that deleterious effects on platelet components can begin to take place after one day or longer of interrupted agitation.[21,22] Accordingly, *AABB Standards* permit a maximum 24-hour period during product transport when platelets do not need to be agitated.[1]

Plasma

There are several different preparations of plasma that are differentiated based on the manner and timing of the plasma separation and freezing processes. The most familiar product for many blood centers is fresh frozen plasma (FFP), which is separated from whole blood and placed in a freezer within eight hours of collection. Generally, if plasma is frozen within 24 hours of collection, it can be labeled either as plasma frozen within 24 hours (PF24) or plasma frozen within 24 hours after phlebotomy held at room temperature up to 24 hours after phlebotomy (PF24RT24), although specific manufacturing requirements must be met in order to qualify for these labels. FFP, PF24 and PF24RT24 can generally be maintained in a freezer at ≤−18 °C for 12 months after collection. Plasma that is separated from whole blood and is never frozen can be labeled as *liquid plasma*, which expires five days after the whole blood from which it was derived. These variations in labeling are due to concern that plasma that is not separated and frozen within eight hours could have diminished levels of coagulation factors.[23]

After thawing, FFP should subsequently be stored at 1–6 °C. Temperatures up to 10 °C are acceptable during transport. If the component is not transfused within 24 hours, it can be relabeled as thawed plasma and stored in a refrigerator for an additional four days. Trauma centers, which treat patients emergently requiring plasma transfusion, may use some thawed plasma units in order to avoid wasting FFP that has already been thawed, as well as to avoid delays in the provision of plasma due to the time required for thawing. Outside of the United States, there is limited availability of freeze-dried plasma, which has a 15–24-month shelf life and can be reconstituted in 5–10 minutes.[24]

Cryoprecipitate

Cryoprecipitate is derived from FFP thawed slowly in an ice bath or in a refrigerator at 1–6 °C. At this low temperature, insoluble cryoprecipitable proteins can be collected by centrifugation, and all but 10–15 mL of the thawed plasma is removed and relabeled as cryoprecipitate-reduced plasma. The remaining 10–15 mL of plasma and insoluble precipitate is labeled *cryoprecipitate*. According to current AABB Standards, cryoprecipitate must contain at least 150 mg of fibrinogen and a factor VIII activity level of 80 IU. This component also contains other plasma proteins, including fibronectin, factor XIII, and von Willebrand factor. Cryoprecipitate, once collected from thawed FFP, must be frozen within one hour and can be maintained at ≤−18 °C for up to 12 months. When the product is requested for clinical use, it should be thawed at 30–37 °C, and then stored and transported at room temperature to prevent re-precipitation of the component. A pooled component expires within four hours unless the pooling occurred with the use of a sterile connection device. In this case, and in the case of single pools, the product shelf life is extended to six hours.[1,25,26]

Granulocytes

Although controversial, septic patients with severe neutropenia may require transfusion with granulocytes. From a blood component administration perspective, granulocytes must be irradiated and infused within 24 hours of collection. Because the RBC content of a granulocyte collection usually exceeds 2% (typically approximately 6%), granulocyte products must also be ABO and crossmatch-compatible with the recipient. Granulocytes should be maintained at room temperature without agitation and must never be leukoreduced.[25,26]

Hematopoietic progenitor cells

Once infused, hematopoietic progenitor cells are intended to engraft in the recipient's bone marrow. For this reason, infused hematopoietic progenitor cells must never be irradiated. In an effort to minimize prevent hematopoietic progenitor cell loss, many transplant centers infuse hematopoietic stem cells into the recipient without the use of a standard infusion set, a microaggregate filter, or a leukoreduction filter. After infusion, sterile saline may be injected into the empty stem cell container to rinse the bag in an effort to maximize stem cell recovery. Specific standards for cellular therapy products are established and maintained by the US Food and Drug Administration (FDA; www.fda.gov), AABB (www.aabb.org), CAP (www.cap.org), and the Foundation for the Accreditation of Cellular Therapy (FACT; www.factwebsite.org).

Prothrombin complex concentrates and recombinant clotting factors

Some transfusion services are responsible for dispensing prothrombin complex concentrates (PCCs) and recombinant clotting factors, which are increasingly utilized in patients with uncontrolled bleeding.[27] These products are often lyophilized and must be reconstituted with sterile water or another diluent prior to infusion. Administration of these drugs should always be in compliance with the package insert. In general, recombinant factors can be administered by a slow intravenous push, whereas multifactor pooled plasma products (e.g., factor VIII inhibitor bypassing agent [FEIBA] and the four-factor PCC) must be administered much more slowly. For hospitals that regularly infuse FEIBA or four-factor PCC, use of a syringe pump or infusion pump can help to ensure that the product is administered safely and at the recommended rate.

Storage equipment

Automated equipment for blood component storage includes refrigerators, freezers, cell washers, platelet agitators, and plasma thawing devices. One example of new equipment for blood storage is the Hemosafe refrigeration system (Haemonetics Corp, Braintree, MA). The Hemosafe device maintains a temperature of 4 °C and acts as a "vending machine" for RBC units, allowing them to be stored and dispensed remotely. Hemosafe's computer system interfaces with that of the hospital's blood bank and relies on an electronic crossmatch to issue compatible blood to patients. If a particular patient cannot receive an electronically crossmatched unit, the system also allows for the emergency release of uncrossmatched blood. A similar system, the HemoNine (Haemonetics Corp, Braintree, MA), contains nine locking drawers, one for each blood type–Rh type combination, plus one additional drawer for crossmatched RBC units. The utility of these systems in hospitals of varying sizes is still undergoing evaluation.

Component transport

Considerations for component transportation are critical to maintaining the integrity of the component to be transfused. Many medical centers rely on validated portable containers or coolers to transport blood products in order to maintain RBC and plasma temperatures below 10 °C. These coolers should have the capability of being temperature monitored at least every four hours with the expectation that the transfusion should occur quickly and before substantial temperature shifts have taken place.[1] Temperature-sensitive adhesive labels that attach directly to the component or the containers can also be used to monitor transport temperatures. These labels have indicators that change color when the temperature limit is exceeded.[28] Therefore, when a blood component is not transfused, either the label can be checked for a color change or the temperature of the unit can be taken to determine whether it can be safely returned to the blood bank inventory.[9]

Novel transport and storage devices

Portable refrigerator technology has improved with some portable refrigerators being capable of maintaining a refrigerated temperature for up to 24 hours after leaving the blood bank. Some models incorporate tracking devices, so that the location of the cooler can be tracked by the blood bank at all times. In addition, some coolers maintain a temperature log during use. These types of technologies have the potential to increase cost savings and limit product waste, but they require a substantial capital investment. However, more studies are needed to evaluate these devices and their utility before widespread implementation is likely.

Component modification and preparation

When ordering blood components, physicians should also stipulate any specific product modification requirements. Leukoreduction, washing, irradiation, and volume reduction are common component manipulations that take place in the blood bank to enhance safety for special populations. As these component modifications often influence the expiration date of the component, the time of outdate must be noted as well.

Leukoreduction

Prestorage leukoreduction, the process of removing leukocytes from whole blood prior to storage, is utilized to prevent the transfusion-mediated transmission of cytomegalovirus (CMV),[29] human leukocyte antigen (HLA) alloimmunization,[30] platelet refractoriness,[31] and febrile nonhemolytic transfusion reactions.[32] Importantly, certain blood components, such as granulocytes and hematopoietic progenitor cells, must never be processed through a leukoreduction filter (Table 3.1).[26] Leukoreduction filters, which work by interception and adhesion of white blood cells to filter fiber media, should not be confused with the 170–260 micron screen filters incorporated into standard blood administration tubing sets. These screen filters work by clot or debris interception and are used for all blood component infusions (see Table 3.1). The 40 micron microaggregate filters, which also work by interception, are used in cell salvage devices.

In the United States, leukoreduction of units of RBCs requires removal of leukocytes to less than 5.0×10^6 leukocytes/unit. Notably, this requirement is less stringent than current European requirements, which stipulate that less than 1×10^6 leukocytes should remain.[14,33] There is a clear move toward universal leukoreduction in the United States, and the FDA advisory committee specifically recommended leukoreduction in 2001. According to 2011 estimates, only 70.5% of whole blood–derived RBCs and 80.1% of apheresis platelets transfused in the United States were leukoreduced.[34] The American Red Cross, which supplies ~50% of the US blood needs, does report universal leukoreduction of blood components manufactured in their facilities.[33] However, because leukoreduction policies differ by blood bank and blood supplier, it is

Table 3.1 Considerations in the preparation and administration of various blood components

Component	Transfuse through Standard Transfusion Set and filter?	Need for Leukoreduction?	Need for Irradiation?
Red blood cells	Always	Desirable—to reduce risk of CMV transmission, febrile nonhemolytic transfusion reactions, platelet refractoriness, and HLA alloimmunization	Yes, to prevent TA-GVHD in vulnerable populations
Platelets	Always	Desirable—to reduce risk of CMV transmission, febrile nonhemolytic transfusion reactions, platelet refractoriness, and HLA alloimmunization	Yes, to prevent TA-GVHD in vulnerable populations
Plasma	Always	Not applicable	No
Cryoprecipitate	Always	Not applicable	No
Granulocytes	Always	Never	Always, to prevent TA-GVHD
Hematopoietic precursor cells	No	Never	Never

important for healthcare providers to be aware of their hospital-based practices.

Irradiation

Irradiation of cellular blood components (i.e., granulocytes, platelets, and RBCs) is necessary when transfusing patients determined to be at high risk for transfusion-associated graft-versus-host disease (TA-GVHD). Irradiation of donor units is also performed when the blood donor is known to be a blood relative or an HLA match with the recipient.[1,25] Ensuring proper irradiation is especially critical because there is no known effective treatment of TA-GVHD, which is generally fatal.[35] To prevent TA-GVHD, a radiation dose of 25 Gy (2500 cGy/rads) directed at the central portion of the blood canister, with no less than 15 Gy to any part of the canister is required in the US. This dose of irradiation damages the DNA of T cells contained within the cellular blood component, thereby preventing T-cell engraftment and TA-GVHD. The irradiation of noncellular blood components, such as plasma and cryoprecipitate, is not required.

The source of radiation used by blood banks is typically ^{137}Cs, ^{60}Co, an X-ray generator, or a linear accelerator. Irradiators that utilize ^{137}Cs or ^{60}Co contain the isotope within chambers made of lead to prevent escape of γ rays from the irradiator device. Typically, ^{137}Cs irradiators contain 1–4 pencil-shaped rods of cesium and a rotating platform or cylinder.[36] During irradiation of blood products, the blood component is placed on the rotating platform to ensure an even dose of radiation to the unit. In contrast, ^{60}Co irradiators usually contain rods of cobalt arranged in a circular configuration, and do not generally utilize a rotating platform.[36] Linear accelerator irradiators generate a beam of X-rays, allowing blood components being irradiated to lay flat during the irradiation procedure.[36] An X-ray tube generating device can also be used. All of these types of irradiators require periodic maintenance and quality assurance programs, and irradiators using ^{137}Cs or ^{60}Co must periodically be recalibrated to account for the gradual radioactive decay of the radioactive isotopes.[36] The US government is reviewing the possibility of eliminating hospital or blood center irradiators that use ^{137}Cs or ^{60}Co and replacing them with X-ray tube devices that pose less of a target for bioterrorism.

Regardless of the source, irradiation reduces the expiration date of RBCs to 28 days from the date of irradiation or the original expiration date, whichever is sooner.[14,37] Irradiation, however, does not alter the expiration date or the function of platelets, and as a result, some hospitals with large oncology wards irradiate all platelets at the time that they are placed in hospital inventory. Special radiographic indicator labels are recommended in order to confirm that an irradiated blood component has received an appropriate dose of radiation.

Washing

The washing process for RBCs or platelets is usually performed with isotonic saline in an automated, centrifuge-based machine housed in the blood bank or blood center. Once the RBCs or platelets are centrifuged into a "packed" state, isotonic saline flows through the packed, cellular mass, washing out the plasma and preservative solution, and replacing it with isotonic saline. There should be a clear clinical indication for cell washing, as the automated washing process can result in loss of as much as 20% of the RBCs or platelets being washed. Furthermore, cells are generally washed in an open

system, and as a result, RBCs expire 24 hours after washing and platelets expire four hours after washing, regardless of the original product expiration dates.[14] Some washing devices may induce more RBC destruction during the washing process than others, resulting in higher supernatant potassium levels.[38] For these reasons, washing RBCs and platelets immediately prior to use is preferred.

Volume reduction via aliquoting

In an effort to prevent transfusion-associated circulatory overload (TACO) in at-risk patients, RBC, platelet, and plasma units can be split into smaller aliquots using transfer bags and a sterile connecting device. Sterile connecting devices work by connecting sterile tubing segments with copper wafers heated to more than 500 °F, melting the plastic tubing and juxtaposing the severed ends together. The heating process prevents bacterial contamination. As long as the system remains closed throughout the process, the shelf life of the transfer bag will remain the same as the shelf life of the primary unit. Similar technology is employed by heat sealers, which melt plastic tubing and generate a seal that can be detached without opening the blood component.

For neonates requiring very small transfusion volumes (sometimes as little as 10–30 mL), aliquoting of cellular components into a syringe with a connecting device can help to maintain an aseptic environment, and can preserve the remainder of the blood component, which can be stored properly in the blood bank, for future transfusions.[39] Because transferring to a syringe is not generally performed within a closed system, blood components transferred to syringes must also be transfused to the recipient within four hours or be discarded.[14]

Thawing plasma

Compared to warming procedures for other blood components, plasma thawing is relatively complex. FFP and PF24 are stored at −18 °C or below, and can take 20–30 minutes to thaw in a 37 °C water bath. Microwave ovens are more expensive than water baths, but may be more suitable for urgent plasma requests. Indeed, specially designed microwave ovens have been shown to thaw components more quickly, in approximately 5–10 minutes, without affecting the function of the coagulation proteins in the plasma.[40] Unlike microwave ovens, 37 °C water baths have the potential to introduce bacterial contamination into the component if the component is not properly sealed and protected in a waterproof bag.[41] Water-based warmers, which circulate warm water through a plastic attachment inserted next to the plasma bag rather than requiring the plasma bag to be submerged in the water bath, may also protect against this risk.

Although both water baths and microwave ovens must be properly maintained, microwave ovens have the added risk of damaging the component plasma proteins in the event of malfunction or the development of "hot spots."[25] Indeed, some experiments with early microwave ovens identified areas of overheating within the plasma bag, such as at the junction where the tubing segment connects to the bag.[41] More recent experiments with specially designed microwave blood warmers have not identified overheating during normal function.[42] Nonetheless, it appears that the state of the art may be moving away from microwave technology and toward radiofrequency-based thawing, which uses longer wavelengths to achieve a more uniform distribution of energy, thus minimizing temperature gradients within the plasma during rapid warming.[43]

At the bedside: transfusion administration

Pretransfusion

Once a blood product that has been modified as necessary is issued by the blood bank and reaches the patient's bedside, the next step is to ensure that the transfusion recipient is properly identified. The transfusionist as well as a second person must verify pertinent information before the transfusion is initiated. Required elements of the process include identification of the patient by two unique identifiers as well as confirmation of the patient's blood group and Rh type. Similarly, the donor unit should be crosschecked for ABO group and Rh type. The results of the crossmatch, any special component modifications, and the expiration date of the component must also be reviewed.[1] Before the transfusion begins, there should be a documented set of pretransfusion vital signs e.g., (temperature, pulse, blood pressure, and oxygen saturation). If the patient experiences any clinical changes during the transfusion, these initial vital signs will serve as baseline values.

Blood administration sets and filters

Once blood components leave the blood bank, transfusion should be initiated as quickly as possible to avoid the risk of bacterial overgrowth.[44] All blood component transfusions must be completed within four hours. Institution specific criteria should be followed, but Standard blood administration infusion sets are required for infusion of all blood products (except hematopoietic precursor cells). These sets consist of three main parts: inline filters, drip chambers, and tubing that can be attached directly to a previously established IV line. The inline filters of the administration sets have a 170–260 micron pore size and are responsible for removing large fibrin clots and cellular debris from all blood components immediately before they enter the patient.[8,45] The filters should be used and replace according to manufacturers recommendations.

Historically, it was found that smaller aggregates of cellular debris and fibrin strands could also develop within stored blood. It was thought that these microaggregates played a role in the development of acute respiratory distress syndrome (ARDS), but a causal link was never established.[46] Currently, microaggregate filters of 20–40 μm sizes are primarily used to transfuse autologous blood that has been salvaged from cardiac surgery procedures. Previously, leukoreduction filters were also available for bedside use, but with the trend toward universal prestorage leukoreduction, these filters are less frequently used at the bedside.[8,34] The drip chamber is a standard component of the infusion set that allows the transfusionist to control the rate of infusion and serves to avoid infusion of air. Prior to use, the infusion set and tubing can be rinsed or primed with either 0.9% sodium chloride or the component to be transfused.[14]

When the aliquoting technique is employed for small-volume infusions in neonates, as previously discussed in this chapter, a special syringe administration set is used. Typically, during the aliquoting procedure in the blood bank, the blood component is passed through a filter.[14]

Co-administration of fluids and blood components

Considerations as to whether other IV solutions can be administered in parallel with a blood component through the same IV line are often raised. According to the *AABB Standards*, the only compatible fluid is 0.9% normal saline. However, allowances are made for FDA-approved drugs or solutions that have been shown to be isotonic and that do not contain enough calcium to neutralize the citrate anticoagulant in the blood component.[1] Lactated Ringer's solution and other solutions that contain high calcium concentrations should be avoided as they can cause clotting of the blood component if they overwhelm the ability of the citrate to effectively anticoagulate the product.[14] Hypotonic or hypertonic solutions should be avoided because of the risk of osmotic hemolysis.

Co-administration of medications

Although this practice has not been extensively studied, in general, medications should not be administered simultaneously through the same IV line as the blood component.[14] This is for several reasons, including the fact that, in the event of simultaneous administration of a blood component and a medication, it would be difficult to differentiate a reaction to the medication from a reaction to the blood component. In addition, if a transfusion needed to be stopped, then the patient may not receive the intended dose of the co-administered medication. Furthermore, some medications may not be compatible with the blood components and may cause hemolysis or clotting. For these reasons, it is best to use a second IV line for medication administration. In the event that additional IV access has not been established, then the IV line used for the blood component should be clamped and flushed with 0.9% saline before infusing any medications.[8] When blood components must be administered concomitantly, as in the setting of trauma or surgery, this can be accomplished with the use of separate IV lines. In emergent cases, multiple blood components (e.g., RBCs and plasma) can be transfused through the same tubing and IV line.[14]

Patient monitoring

After the transfusion has begun, the patient's vital signs should be evaluated and documented 15 minutes after the start of the transfusion. If the patient has any suspected adverse reactions, then the transfusion should be stopped until the patient can be clinically evaluated. Depending on the scenario, the transfusion may need to be discontinued altogether. If a patient has a mild allergic reaction (hives) without signs of vasomotor instability, laryngeal edema, or tongue or lip swelling, it is permissible to restart the transfusion if the symptoms resolve with antihistamine therapy. However, a transfusion should not be restarted if the recipient has a drop in blood pressure, fever, chills, an anaphylactoid reaction as just described, or an increase in temperature (even if there was a preexisting fever). Symptoms of this type should trigger a transfusion reaction workup by the physician responsible for the transfusion, the blood bank and the blood bank consulting physician.

Infusion flow rates

Optimal infusion rates vary with the component being transfused and the patient's ability to tolerate increased intravascular volume. Components should generally be infused slowly at first, and then the rate can be increased as tolerated by the patient. Patients at risk for volume overload, such as those with poor cardiac status, should receive a slow infusion rate with close monitoring, if feasible. In general, RBCs and plasma have volumes ranging from 200 to 400 mL and are typically infused over 1–2 hours. Platelets range in volume from 200 to 300 mL and are also generally infused over 1–2 hours.[14,26] Cryoprecipitate can be given as rapidly as tolerated and should be infused as soon after the thawing procedure as is clinically acceptable.[14]

There is a paucity of evidence to make specific recommendations regarding blood component flow rates in neonatal and pediatric patients. Although concern exists that increased rates can cause intraventricular hemorrhage or electrolyte imbalances in neonates, there is limited high quality evidence to support this theory. Therefore, in this patient population, for routine blood component administration, transfusions are usually administered over 2–4 hours.[14] Recommended infusion rates range from 5 ml/kg/h (RBCs) to 10–20 ml/kg/h (platelets) and 15 ml/kg/h (plasma).[47]

In certain clinical scenarios, there is a need to transfuse a unit of RBCs, plasma, or platelets at a slower rate than would allow for completion of a transfusion in a four-hour period. As mentioned in the "Volume Reduction via Aliquoting" section, one strategy to accomplish this relies on the blood bank's ability to split units using a sterile tubing welder, so that half units can be issued to the patient, with the remaining sterile half unit properly stored in the blood bank. The transfusionist can administer the split unit over a four-hour period, and then contact the blood bank to request the other half of the unit. This practice allows for a unit of RBCs, plasma, or platelets to be divided and effectively infused over eight hours, or more.

RBC salvage devices

RBC salvage refers to the concept of reclaiming and processing blood lost in the surgical field for the purpose of autologous transfusion. There are two types of devices. One type of device works by combining blood salvaged from the surgical field with an anticoagulant solution. The blood–anticoagulant mixture is then fed into a storage chamber before being centrifuged, washed, and infused back into the patient through a microaggregate filter. These salvage devices, which incorporate a washing step, are usually confined to the operating room. Other salvage devices without a washing feature are intended for patients undergoing orthopedic surgery, and they also act as a surgical drain. These devices remain connected to the patient even after leaving the operating room. Salvage devices have been shown by some studies to reduce allogeneic RBC transfusions for both adult and pediatric patients undergoing cardiac surgery.[48,49] Due to the minimum amount of blood loss needed for any of the RBC salvage devices to function effectively and due to their extracorporeal volume, these devices are not useful in children under six months of age.[50]

Rapid infusion practices

Blood products are occasionally requested on an urgent basis when a patient is deemed to have a life-threatening condition that does not allow for sufficient time for a full crossmatch prior to blood component issue. Conspicuously labeled un-crossmatched units can be stored in blood bank–monitored refrigerators in critical areas throughout the hospital such as the emergency department, operating rooms, labor and delivery suites, and intensive care units. Most hospitals reserve Rh-negative units for women of childbearing age and infants, because of the limited supply. When Rh-negative trauma patients (male or female) receive Rh-positive blood components, they are at risk of alloimmunization to the D antigen.[51] However, if the patient's ABO and Rh type is known with certainty, but there is no time for crossmatch compatibility testing, then the patient should reasonably receive type-specific products, rather than defaulting to universally compatible products (O-negative RBCs and AB plasma). Most importantly, any un-crossmatched unit that is issued should be clearly labeled as such.[1] In urgent circumstances, blood components often need to be transfused as quickly as possible, and large-bore intravenous catheters can be used for this purpose.

In addition, when blood losses are substantial, blood infusers can be utilized to rapidly infuse blood components. Rapid infusers can deliver warmed blood components at infusion rates exceeding 500 mL per minute through a pump, which is far faster than the rate that a standard infusion can be programmed to deliver.[52] Given this rapid rate of infusion, it is essential that blood components are warmed in order to prevent hypothermia-induced coagulopathy.[53] Rapid infusers are frequently credited with providing lifesaving delivery of blood, although care should be taken to avoid air emboli.[54] Newer models of infusion pumps are reported to have improved safety features to prevent infusion of air emboli, which can cause a fatal tricuspid valve occlusion.[55]

Blood warming and bedside blood pumps

Stand-alone blood warmers may be utilized when large volumes of blood components are transfused (without a rapid infuser) or when patients have cold agglutinins detected during compatibility testing. Only validated, approved blood warmers should be used for this process in order to ensure patient safety. Such approved blood warmers often consist of tubing coiled around a central heating core that is temperature monitored. Blood must never be warmed by holding the unit in a hot water stream under a faucet or by heating it in a standard microwave oven. Hemolysis is a real danger with either of these methods. Monitored blood warmers are frequently used during lengthy apheresis procedures to promote patient comfort. Importantly, nonwarmed blood has been shown to lower the core temperature of transfusion recipients, possibly contributing to cardiac arrest.[56] Interestingly, it has been reported that repeated plasma exchanges using a blood warmer may actually result in clinically significant blood loss.[57] Blood warmers must be maintained regularly to prevent malfunction and possible hemolysis. Blood can also be administered through medication infusion pumps if they have been shown to not cause shear stress–induced hemolysis. These devices are often used for neonatal or pediatric transfusions when precise infusion volumes are needed. Not all pumps are compatible with red cell infusions, so each device needs to be evaluated to ensure red cell compatibility.

Post transfusion

At the completion of the transfusion, the patient should be checked again for any signs of an adverse reaction to the blood component, and a final set of vital signs should be taken. Because transfusion reactions can occur several hours after the completion of the transfusion, inpatients should be monitored for at least 4–6 hours after a transfusion is completed. If a patient will be discharged from an ambulatory care setting after receiving a transfusion, then written documentation of signs and symptoms of transfusion reactions and a telephone number of a responsible practitioner should be provided to the patient prior to leaving the clinic.[14]

Key references

A full reference list for this chapter is available at: http://www.wiley.com/go/simon/transfusion

5 Maskens C, Downie H, Wendt A, *et al.* Hospital-based transfusion error tracking from 2005 to 2010: identifying the key errors threatening patient transfusion safety. *Transfusion.* 2014 Jan; **54**(1): 66–73. PubMed PMID: 23672511.

6 Karim F, Moiz B, Shamsuddin N, Naz S, Khurshid M. Root cause analysis of non-infectious transfusion complications and the lessons learnt. *Transfusion Apheresis Sci* 2014 Feb; **50**(1): 111–7. PubMed PMID: 24239270.

36 Moroff G, Luban NL. The irradiation of blood and blood components to prevent graft-versus-host disease: Technical issues and guidelines. *Transfusion Med Rev* 1997 Jan; **11**(1): 15–26. PubMed PMID: 9031487.

38 O'Leary MF, Szklarski P, Klein TM, Young P.P. Hemolysis of red blood cells after cell washing with different automated technologies: clinical implications in a neonatal cardiac surgery population. *Transfusion* 2011 May; **51**(5): 955–60. PubMed PMID: 21091957.

48 Wang G, Bainbridge D, Martin J, Cheng D. The efficacy of an intraoperative cell saver during cardiac surgery: A meta-analysis of randomized trials. *Anesth Analg* 2009 Aug; **109**(2): 320–30. PubMed PMID: 19608798.

CHAPTER 4

Recruitment and screening of donors and the collection, processing, and testing of blood

Kendall P. Crookston,[1,2] Aaron E. Pritchard,[1] & Toby L. Simon[1,3]

[1]Department of Pathology, University of New Mexico School of Medicine, Albuquerque, NM, USA
[2]United Blood Services of New Mexico, Albuquerque, NM, USA
[3]Plasma Product Development and CSL Plasma, CSL Behring, King of Prussia, PA, USA

The blood donation and transfusion chain

Although much effort has been expended to find suitable replacements for blood components, the best source continues to be blood collected from healthy, human donors. The process of supplying sufficient blood components and derivatives for patient needs is complex and highly regulated. At the same time, it must be dynamic in adapting to the local and regional needs for providing blood products that may have a short shelf life. Other chapters have detailed descriptions of how to prepare and preserve red blood cells (RBCs; Chapter 9), platelets (Chapter 19), granulocytes (Chapter 23), and plasma and plasma derivatives (Chapter 27). This chapter focuses on the donation and collection process, from recruitment of donors to the receipt of products in the hospital inventory. Physician involvement is essential to this process.[1]

An overview of the entire blood donation and transfusion chain is seen in Figure 4.1.[2]

The role of hemovigilance as the last step of the chain has become increasingly emphasized over the past decade (see Chapter 6). Hemovigilance is "a set of surveillance procedures covering the whole transfusion chain from the collection of blood and its components to the follow-up of its recipients, intended to collect and assess information on unexpected or undesirable effects resulting from the therapeutic use of labile blood products, and to prevent their occurrence and recurrence."[3] The entire process is typically under intense regulatory scrutiny from governmental agencies and industry groups such as AABB (formerly known as the American Association of Blood Banks, see www.aabb.org) and the Plasma Protein Therapeutics Association (www.pptaglobal.org). Details on the regulatory aspects are addressed in Chapter 7. In many countries, there are dual systems for supplying blood for patient transfusion in the hospital, and for collecting *source plasma* for derivatives. This is due to parallel development of these systems during the latter half of the 20th century. This is reflected in the arrangement of this chapter, with separate sections for collection of transfusable products and source plasma.

In this chapter, an introduction to the organization of blood services responsible for managing this complex process will be covered first. Recruitment of blood donors will then be described, followed by a detailed analysis of the donation process from the perspective of the donor and also of the component prepared. Finally, source plasma donation will be addressed. Donor adverse events are considered in Chapter 5.

Organization of blood services to meet global needs

In 2012, 108 million units of blood were collected worldwide.[4] The use of blood is very heterogeneous among countries. For instance, in low-income countries, two-thirds of transfusions are given to children under 5 years of age; whereas in high-income countries, three-fourths of all transfusions are given to patients over 65.[4] In high-income countries, blood is most commonly used for supportive care in cardiovascular surgery, transplant surgery, massive trauma, and cancer therapy. In other countries, it is used more often to manage complications of pregnancy and severe anemia in children.[4]

Various successful models have been developed to deliver blood products. The worldwide spectrum of blood service organization is diverse, and it varies based on local health initiatives, government intervention, historical development, and available resources. In this section, a brief history of blood collection services will be addressed first, followed by a discussion about the organization of blood services in the United States and then an introduction to blood services outside of the United States. A more extensive history of transfusion medicine is detailed in Chapter 1.

The British Red Cross is credited with establishing the first organized blood donor service in 1921, identifying a panel of potential donors who would provide fresh blood at the time it was needed.[5] In 1935, the International Society of Blood Transfusion (ISBT) was established as a scientific and educational society to bring together professionals involved in blood transfusion and transfusion medicine worldwide (www.isbt-web.org). By 1935, a number of blood centers had been established in Russia, at least two of which were providing blood for patient care.[6] Cook County Hospital in Chicago became the first blood bank in the Western world to store blood for future use in 1937.[5] The first community blood center was established in 1941 in San Francisco, California. Significant advances in transfusion medicine occurred over the next decade, when the National Blood Service was established in the United Kingdom (1946) and the American Red

Rossi's Principles of Transfusion Medicine, Fifth Edition. Edited by Toby L. Simon, Jeffrey McCullough, Edward L. Snyder, Bjarte G. Solheim, and Ronald G. Strauss.

BLOOD DONOR RECRUITMENT (goal is to collect the right kind of blood at right time, to anticipate needs and avoid shortages and wastage)
- voluntary versus paid donors
- physician referral required for autologous or directed donation

PRE-DONATION INFORMATION (screening is intended to protect both the recipient and the donor)
- donor interview (health history, medication use, lifestyle risk factors, travel history. TRALI risk assessment)
- directed physical examination, hemoglobin screening

COMPONENT COLLECTION (procedure selection depends on local needs and maximizing the components the donor is eligible to donate)
- whole blood (maximum volume ~500 mL)
- apheresis collection (maximum units collected from a single donor for RBC = 2, platelets = 3, plasma = 4, combinations possible)
- additional blood specimens collected for donor testing

PREPARATION AND TESTING (testing of donor and appropriate preparation of the blood component to ensure a safe and effective product)

COMPONENT PREPARATION AND TESTING
- component separation (i.e. packed RBC, whole blood-derived platelets, plasma, cryoprecipitate)
- component modification (e.g. pre-storage leukocyte reduction to reduce febrile reactions, HLA sensitization and CMV transmission)
- quality assurance testing
- bacterial testing (platelets)
- plasma fractionation and pathogen inactivation (to produce intravenous immune globulin, coagulation factor concentrates, etc.)

BLOOD DONORTESTING
- ABO/RhD typing
- screening for donor RBC antibodies (to prevent hemolytic reactions in recipient)
- infectious disease testing
    - → serologic (HBV, HCV, HIV, syphilis, Chagas, etc.)   → nucleic acid (HCV, HIV, West Nile Virus, etc.)
- other testing (such as screening for HLA antibodies to minimizeTRALI)

POST-DONATION INFORMATION (incorporates any new information to ensure safety of product)
- donor illness notification or self-deferral via confidential unit exclusion
- review and follow-up of any donor reaction
- positive infectious disease testing on subsequent donations may prompt notification of prior recipients ("look back")

LABELLING OF PRODUCTS FOR DISTRIBUTION (all legal and industry standards are met and testing is satisfactory)
- inventory management to ensure sufficient stock when and where needed and to minimize blood product expiration

BLOOD PRODUCTS IN HOSPITAL INVENTORY (the hospital can further modify the product and must ensure compatibility with patient)
- antibody screening of blood recipients
- selection of suitable product for appropriate indication (based on crossmatch, clinical status of patient, etc.)
- local component modification before transfusion
    - → gamma irradiation (to prevent graft-vs-host disease)   → plasma reduction/washing (to reduce allergens and antibodies)
    - → pooling (whole blood-derived platelets, cryoprecipitate)   → preparation for special procedures (baby aliquots, neonate exchange, etc.)
- documentation of recipient's clinical information (antibodies present, component modifications required, etc.)

BLOOD TRANSFUSED INTO PATIENT BY CLINICAL STAFF (indication depends on patient oxygenation/coagulation needs for given situation)
- positive identification of patient and blood product
- monitoring for reactions and treatment of transfusion complications

HEMOVIGILANCE SURVEILLANCE / CLINICAL QUALITY IMPROVEMENT (outcomes and benchmarking data collected to improve practice)

Figure 4.1 The blood donation and transfusion chain: from donor arm to patient vein. The bold arrows outline nine important stages in the system that assures safe and effective patient blood transfusions. Graphic design by Kimberly E. Crookston. Source: Crookston *et al.* (2015).[2] Reproduced with permission of Lippincott, Williams & Wilkins.

Cross began its National Blood Program for civilians (1948). World War II provided a great stimulus for the development of blood donor services. The extraordinary efforts of a number of individuals in different countries to provide this lifesaving resource have been documented elsewhere.[7]

Organization of blood services in the United States

Blood collection for transfusion in the United States is accomplished by an eclectic system that has evolved since World War II. Close to half of the blood for transfusion in the United States has historically been collected by the American Red Cross (www.redcross.org). Community blood centers were established nationwide in areas where the Red Cross did not operate. Most of these nonprofit collection agencies are now loosely affiliated with a trade organization known as America's Blood Centers. Members range from very large blood programs such as Blood Systems (founded in 1943—see www.unitedbloodservices.org), New York Blood Center, and OneBlood (Florida based), to very small one-county programs. In addition to community blood centers, a number of hospitals also started collecting blood for their own use.

The concept of regionalization of blood services emerged from the assumption that a blood center should serve the surrounding areas that referred patients to major city medical centers. This allows the entire geographic area to support the needs of its patients, whether they are cared for in the community or a referral center. By managing the blood within a region in a systematic way, waste can be reduced through the use of technological innovations and careful inventory management. There are resource-sharing arrangements that allow organizations to move blood around to different centers that are in need of blood.

In response to the transfusion-transmitted acquired immune deficiency syndrome (AIDS) epidemic of the 1980s, the US Food and Drug Administration (FDA) increased blood industry accountability to levels similar to that of pharmaceutical regulation (see Chapter 7). Blood centers found themselves implementing quality assurance programs with dedicated personnel to assure compliance within the new regulatory framework. The voluntary AABB accreditation program likewise moved from an inspection and accreditation focus to one on quality systems. As organizations struggled to conform to this new paradigm, a number of blood centers were placed under judicial consent decree for failing to meet regulations—including three of the largest collection organizations in the United States. A significant portion of the blood used in the United States today is provided by organizations that still remain under court supervision due to judicial consent decree.[8]

Competition for market share was not well received by many of the nonprofit monopolies that felt blood was more of a gift than a commodity.[9] These centers viewed their mission primarily as community service, linking donors with recipients.[10] This view of blood as a commodity did not diminish as mergers, acquisitions, and consolidations affected blood collection agencies in parallel with the changing healthcare industry. By the end of the 20th century, competition had lessened and the relationship of blood centers with hospitals began shifting from a commodity-based relationship to one valuing service, medical expertise, and patient outcomes. However, it was soon realized that healthcare expenses were rising more quickly than other parts of the economy, particularly in the United States. Through aggressive reorganization and cost control strategies, the price of blood has decreased. This has been accompanied by a decrease in demand for RBCs (see Figure 4.2):[11] 13.8 million units were transfused in the United States in 2011, which was 8.2% fewer than in 2008.[11] The annual blood *transfusion rate* in the United States (RBCs/whole blood) decreased from 54 allogeneic units per 1000 people in 2004, to 49 in 2008, and to 44 in 2011.[11,12] The *donation rate* per unit population of 76.2 was the lowest reported since 1997.[11] Although these trends correlate with the global financial crisis of 2008 and the growth of patient blood management programs, the specific cause of the decline is not fully understood.[8] *Patient blood management* is discussed in Chapter 2. In brief, it is a multidisciplinary approach to improve patient outcomes using evidence-based strategies in patients who may need transfusion. The goal is to improve outcomes, not only by transfusing blood appropriately but also by introducing strategies to prevent patients from needing a transfusion in the first place.

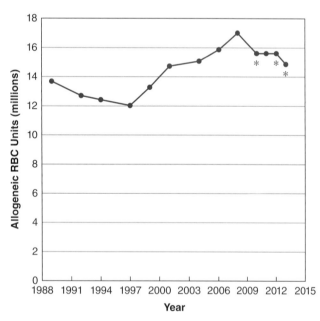

Figure 4.2 Allogeneic red blood cell (RBC) units drawn in the United States by year. Note the steady increase over the decade leading to the maximum draw in 2008 and then the sharp decline. The data are taken from the 2011 National Blood Collection and Utilization Survey.[11] The points indicated by asterisks (∗) have been extrapolated from cumulative member data supplied by Blood Centers of America (courtesy of Bill Block). Graphic design by Joshua E. Crookston.

Many blood centers are affiliated with national blood banking organizations, including AABB (founded in 1947—see www.aabb.org). The "voluntary" standards set by the AABB are so well regarded that these often become the standard of care in North America and in other areas of the world, even without government regulatory intervention.

Many hospitals have found it impractical to maintain hospital-based collections. Although hospital-based collection still exists in the United States, the increasing cost, external regulation, shortage of medical technologists, and variable supply and demand have progressively shifted collection activities to blood centers. However, the proportion of blood collected by hospitals in 2011 remained relatively constant when compared to 2004 (6.6 vs 6.4%, respectively)[11,12] Even hospitals that collect their own blood usually do not perform donor testing, and out of necessity they maintain a supplemental blood contract with the local blood supplier. The US Department of Defense continues to operate an independent blood services organization for its hospitals as well as its military mission.

Blood components collected for transfusion in the United States are from volunteer donors; in contrast, most plasma for fractionation is collected from paid donors, as discussed later in this chapter.[4]

Organization of blood services outside the United States

Most high-income countries have adequate blood services, maintaining a full range of donor screening and quality assurance procedures, while producing most of the components needed in the region. However, there exists a wide variety of dissimilar organizational structures that are successful in meeting the transfusion needs of areas served. These models can be centralized or decentralized, governmental, military, private, hospital based, or mixed. For the most part, the local transfusion system reflects the administrative system of each country. For instance, in countries that have strong governmental control, there is often a centralized transfusion system operated by government-run institutions. The World Health Organization (WHO) encourages strong governmental leadership in establishing national transfusion networks.[13] Many countries outside the United States have instituted national blood programs. Overall, the provision of blood services worldwide is heterogeneous and varies with historical development, the socioeconomic development of the region, and the influence of national scientific and political factors.[13]

Donor recruitment is sometimes performed externally to the blood collection agencies. Recruitment is sometimes carried out by independent organizations that have a special relationship with the procurement agency, such as a country's national Red Cross. The International Federation of Blood Donor Organizations was established in 1955 as a support network for donor recruitment (www.fiods-ifbdo.org). Seventy-two nations participate, although there is a notable absence of many English-speaking countries. The goal of the organization is member state self-sufficiency in blood from voluntary, unpaid blood donors, while also improving safety and, in turn, confidence in the national blood supplies by developing minimum standards for donations, inspection, and quality assurance.

In 1975, the 28th World Health Assembly passed a resolution recognizing the value of voluntary blood donation and called on member states to promote national blood transfusion services based on voluntary unpaid donations.[13] Voluntary donation has been a goal for some time, as it is perceived as a safer alternative. In 2002, the European Union approved legislation that established comprehensive standards for blood products that included a requirement for voluntary donation.[13] The WHO Global Database on Blood Safety 2011 report presents data from 164 countries representing 92% of the global population.[14] It shows that half of the global blood collection occurs in high-income countries, home to only 15% of the world population. Global blood donations from voluntary unpaid donors increased from 2004 to 2012. Seventy-three countries collect over 90% of their blood supply from voluntary unpaid blood donors. However, 72 countries collect more than 50% of their blood supply from family/replacement or paid donors. Around 1.5 million donations intended for transfusion were collected from paid donors.[4] Nevertheless, countries are increasingly moving toward voluntary blood donation.

WHO recommends that, at minimum, all blood for transfusion should be screened for HIV, hepatitis B, hepatitis C, and syphilis. Twenty-five countries are not able to screen all donated blood for one or more of these infections. Irregular supply of test kits is one of the most commonly reported barriers to screening.[4] Yet, even in countries that are able to screen all of their blood, the risk of transfusion-transmitted infections (TTIs) varies. The prevalence of TTIs in blood donations in high-income countries is considerably lower than in low- and middle-income countries.[4] External quality control assessment is often lacking: whereas 97% of blood-screening laboratories in high-income countries are monitored, only 33% of middle-income and 16% of low-income countries have external quality assessment.[4]

There is still heterogeneity in the practices that are taken for granted as mandatory in North America, even among the most effective blood services. For instance, in Norway, nucleic acid testing for HIV is not performed on repeat blood donors due to the low incidence in the recruited donor population and the effectiveness of the serological screening.

Low- and middle-income countries often struggle to provide the same level of safety as high-income countries with established blood procurement systems. The costs of procurement and testing of the blood are often prohibitive. For instance, in sub-Saharan Africa, although blood transfusion has a long history,[15] collection services are fragmented. Blood is sometimes in short supply, and safety seldom can be guaranteed.[4]

Some high-income countries such as the United States have implemented a "precautionary principle" that has meant extreme costs for marginal added safety when measured by standards such as quality-adjusted life-years.[16] Many countries simply do not have resources to implement this strategy, even if it were medically justified. In stark contrast to the precautionary principle, blood in some parts of the world is still transfused without testing. In addition, when testing can be done, there may not be resources to notify and counsel donors about positive test results, such as HIV. This provides an opportunity for the world community to make a great impact on global health through collaboration and collegiality. In response, WHO established the Global Collaboration for Blood Safety in 1994, a voluntary partnership of organizations, institutions, associations, agencies, and experts that are concerned with the safety and availability of blood. Many of these functions are now carried out by the WHO Global Blood Safety Network and the WHO Global Forum for Blood Safety (http://www.who.int/bloodsafety/collaboration/en/).

Recruitment of blood donors

The first task of a regional blood center is to recruit adequate numbers of donors to provide for patient needs. Traditionally, this requires a strong association between the blood center and the population in an area, as well as the cultivation of an altruistic spirit and a sense of social responsibility within the community.[17,18] As described by Titmuss, the act of giving blood clearly demonstrates the integration of individuals into society.[19] However, there exists a fragile balance between blood supply and blood demand in the United States. Previous calculations estimated this number at 177 million eligible blood donors.[20] These findings come at the same time that the baby boomers, a mainstay of the donor base, approach those years when exclusionary factors increase and only a small fraction of eligible donors donate the "gift of life." The recruitment of blood donors is now the most challenging task at the blood center. Blood donation is one of few "gifts" that involves physical insult to the body, conceivably offering a higher level of service than giving of one's time or money. The gift of blood is most often given to an unknown individual with no direct thanks or appreciation or knowledge of the transfusion outcome. The thanks and appreciation must come from the blood center, the steward of the community's blood supply. Data from the following discussion of donor recruitment have been derived mainly from the volunteer donor populations in the United States and Canada. The blood donation rate in high-income countries such as these is 36.8 donations per 1000 population. The rates in middle- and low-income countries are 11.7 and 3.9 donations, respectively.[4]

Many studies have attempted to explain why people do, or do not, become blood donors.

Other studies have sought to determine the motivation to repeat the donation process. These studies have evaluated demographic and sociological/psychological characteristics as well as donor motivation for giving or not giving blood. The challenge is to use these findings and apply them to the everyday recruitment of blood donors.

Donor demographics

The demographics of current blood donors provide the blood center with insights into where and to whom they might focus marketing and recruiting efforts. As expected, individuals who are integrated into American society at upper socioeconomic ranges are more likely to volunteer in community efforts, give money to charitable causes, and donate blood than individuals in marginalized populations who are struggling at lower socioeconomic levels.[21-25] Donors who are older (>50 years) and who have more education (college graduates) are more likely to return as repeat donors than those who are younger and who have not gone to college.[26-30] Other studies have observed differences in donation rates among minority groups that exist apart from socioecomomic status. Thus, as the population at large continues to become more diverse, blood donor organizations are ever more challenged to recruit a more widely representative group of donors who are not reflected in the traditional donor pool.

Current donors in the United States included a significantly higher proportion of females aged 45 or older, white, college graduates, repeat donors, persons married or living as married, and born in the United States. When comparing the demographics of a group of donors who had donated five gallons or more with a group of randomly selected donors, the five-gallon-or-more donors tended to be white, male, college graduates, and regular voters with an average age of 52.[26] First-time donor demographics at five US blood centers between 1991 and 1996 noted a continuing high proportion of first-time donors younger than 35 years of age who were white non-Hispanic and US-born with a college degree or higher. There was, however, a significant increase in the proportion of non-US-born first-time donors at each blood center over the six-year period with a concurrent decrease in the proportion of white donors.[27]

Return behaviors of blood donors in comparison to donor demographics have also been evaluated. In general, younger donors were the least likely to return. With increases in age, return rates increased to over 40% for those aged 50 and older. Multiple-return rates were highest among college graduates and lowest among donors with no more than a high school education.[28] In evaluating older volunteer blood donors with a mean age of 68 years, the majority was married, well educated, and somewhat affluent.[29] Additionally, when returning first-time donors were compared with nonreturning donors, returning donors were more likely US born, white, better educated, and older.[30]

Donor motivation

Studies continue to show that the concept of altruism has been associated most often as the reason for giving blood.[31–33] In volunteer blood programs across the globe, the unselfish act of giving blood for the welfare of others remains the centerpiece of blood donor recruitment initiatives. But other motivators include the concepts of community need, and social pressure to conform to expectations or desires of an individual or group. People may donate because someone asked them to, they have heard about an emergent need for blood, or others are doing it. Convenience to donate has also been identified as an important factor, and blood centers understand the value of strategically located fixed donation sites and the need for mobile operations.[34]

More recent studies have examined the role that incentives have on donor motivation. Blood credits (e.g., credit toward blood units required by members of a family or community group) were most attractive to donors as incentives, as well as cholesterol screening and a prostate-specific antigen (PSA) screen in men. In general, small incentives or tokens of appreciation were more likely to appeal to younger donors than older donors.[35] In a follow-up study, first-time donors were positively influenced with incentives, but this finding was also related to the younger age of these donors.[36] In another study, first-time donors were more likely than repeat donors to be encouraged to donate and less likely to be discouraged if offered cash, event or lottery tickets, or merchandise. Donors attracted by cash were more likely to have a risk for TTIs. Medical testing and blood credits were attractive to both first-time and repeat donors.[37]

Nonetheless, blood shortages have continued to raise the question of compensation for donation. The concept of targeted and selective nonmonetary incentives for certain populations, such as lapsed donors during times of shortages, continues to be raised.

Younger and first-time donors also decided to donate because of a family member, friend, or coworker. Younger and first-time donors were also motivated to donate because of testing for infections. When compared to donors with a high school education or less, donors with a college or higher degree were more likely to donate because it was *the right thing to do*, and less likely to donate to improve their health (e.g., by receiving a PSA or cholesterol screening) or because of family or peer influence. Men tended to donate more often than women because it is good for their health, they wanted to be tested, or they wished to receive an item or gift. Women tended to donate because it was *the right thing to do* or because they had heard about a need for more blood.[32]

More than 90% of respondents to a questionnaire administered to Asian, black, Hispanic, and white donors cited a desire, responsibility, or perceived duty to help others as an important or very important motivator to donation. Being asked to participate in a work-related blood drive was also an important motivator, and not being asked was a deterrent. Getting the results of a health screen appealed to many and was most important to black and Hispanic donors. More than 50% of respondents did not find any of the incentives (gifts, tickets, time off work, or reward) important at all in their decision to donate.[38]

In a 2005 Canadian study, the importance of altruism as a motivator to donation was noted along with family and social influences.[39] Blood centers need to identify potential donors who are more likely to be motivated by the message to "make it available for themselves if required" versus a message to "make it available for someone close to you."[40] In another randomized controlled trial, donors received information about the indication for transfusion of their blood and the recipient's status. Donors were enthusiastic about receiving this information. However, as the study was performed in a highly committed blood type O-negative donor population, no significant increase in donation frequency could be demonstrated.[41]

Deterrents to donation

There are many deterrents to blood donation. Some deterrents, such as inconvenience, perceived incompetence of personnel performing blood collection activities, and the lack of cleanliness of a given facility or operation, are clearly within the control of the blood center. But some deterrents, including the perception that blood donation is not important, the belief that one can contract a disease by donating, and the desire to remain ignorant of any positive results from infectious disease testing on the donation, are more difficult to overcome.

The most frequently mentioned negative motivator to donation is fear,[39,42,43] including fear of needles, seeing blood, weakness, dizziness, and discomfort. In some individuals, these types of fears may never be overcome. Education programs tailored to overcome fear and heighten the awareness of need may be helpful.

Medical disqualification is also a frequently given reason for nondonation. However, several studies have shown that many perceived reasons for nondonation have been invalid or imagined.[31,42] At least for some individuals, invoking a medical disqualification is more appealing than admitting to some type of "fear" relative to blood donation.

Treatment by blood center staff and the donor's perception of staff competence, coupled with donor sense of well-being during and after donation, influence the likelihood of donor return, although highly committed donors are generally not deterred by the occasional bad experience during donation.[23,26,34,44] Blood donation–related symptoms including dizziness, nausea, and fainting are a significant reason for donor nonreturn.[45] Several strategies have been proposed to mitigate symptoms and increase donor returns.[46,47]

Temporary deferral has a significant impact; deferred donors return less frequently than nondeferred donors and are more likely to lapse from donation.[48–50] In a further study, repeat donors who reported a previous temporary deferral were more likely to lapse, but the association disappeared when other factors such as accessibility, satisfaction with last donation, and perceived need for blood were adjusted.[44] Of interest, several lapsed donors incorrectly viewed themselves as permanently deferred for temporary conditions such as low hemoglobin or hematocrit.[43]

Sociological and psychological theories of blood donation

Many theories exist about donor motivation, and several excellent reviews are available with more detail on this complex aspect of blood donor recruitment.[48,51–53] Opponent-process theory has been used to explain why some individuals repeat the process of donation and become committed, habitual blood donors. Donors experience a "warm glow" after donation, which may represent an opponent process in response to negative feelings experienced before and during initial donations.

Attribution theory suggests that people who have taken an action (e.g., donating blood) without external coercion or large reward are likely to attribute to themselves a predisposition toward that action. Once they have attributed such a tendency to themselves, or once they decide that they are "the kind of people who do such things," they are more likely to act in ways consistent with that attribution in the future.

In the model of commitment, four processes are proposed: coping with and neutralizing the negative aspects of donation; developing internalized motives for donation and integrating them into one's self-concept; developing a behavioral intention to continue giving blood; and, finally, developing a self-sustaining habit of donation.

The theory of reasoned action states that all behavior is preceded by a behavioral intention that can be measured by seeking an estimate of the probability of acting on that specific behavior. Intention is a function of two additional factors: the individual's attitude toward performing the act, and the perceived expectations of others for what one should do in a particular situation. This theory has been, in general, effective in explaining donor action related to blood donation. For example, donors who verbally expressed their intention to donate when recruited were more likely to attend the drive than those who were merely reminded that a drive was occurring. Likewise, when donors are informed of a bloodmobile and also sent a checklist of dates to which they could commit (forming an intention), they were more likely to give blood when compared to donors who were merely informed of the drive through the media.

The attitudes of donors and nondonors in three areas including affect, cognition, and behavior have been reported.[54] In terms of affect, donors were more likely to indicate that blood donation made them feel generous, assured, relaxed, and useful. Nondonors were more likely to indicate that donation made them feel uncomfortable and ill. On cognition scores, more nondonors believed that blood donation was dangerous and appeared to know little about the process. Donors were more likely to cite that blood donation is worth any inconvenience and is an important civic duty. For behaviors, donors ranked more favorably those behaviors that reflected the donation process. The authors concluded that blood donor behaviors may be more strongly determined by affective and emotional processes rather than by carefully reasoned decisions.[54]

It appears from the literature that the model most likely to predict future blood donation behavior is the theory of planned behavior.[55,56] This model postulates that behavior can be determined by intentionality, which in turn is affected by attitude (positive or negative evaluation of the behavior), subjective norm (perception of social pressure), and perceived behavioral control (perceived ease or difficulty in performing the behavior). Several studies involving nondonors concluded that this model predicted 31–72% of the variance in intention to future blood donation. In a study based on the theory of planned behavior and experienced donors, 65% of the variance in donation intention and 50% of the variance in attitude were accounted for.[56] Self-efficacy showed the strongest positive relationship to donation intention, followed by attitude, subjective norm, satisfaction, and personal moral norm. Prior vasovagal reactions related negatively to intention to donation.[57]

Once a recruited donor presents to donate at a blood or plasma center, a highly regulated process ensues. This process will first be outlined for volunteer donors, followed by a separate section for plasma donors

The collection process for blood components for transfusion: screening, phlebotomy, choice of product, collection, testing, and distribution of blood and apheresis components

Donor evaluation

The twofold purpose of blood donor screening is to minimize the risks to both the blood recipient and the donor (see Figure 4.1 and Chapter 5). Donors should be informed as early as possible about all aspects of the donation procedure and about the importance of critical self-evaluation and self-exclusion for those who do not qualify. Pre-recruitment information about donor qualifications and pre-donation information about risk factors for transmitting infections through transfusion should lead to self-deferral by some donors. When the donor presents for donation, written educational material is given, including a list of deferral medications.

Answers to donor history questions in a confidential setting provide another opportunity to obtain information about potential risk. Only three years after the founding of AABB, a list of 21 diseases and conditions were introduced on the "donor record card" that was intended to be used nationwide for screening criteria.[58] This was based more on the medical judgment of the day than on clear-cut data or evidence. Many of the current medical deferrals are still based less on data and more on a combination of opinion, tradition, and "conventional wisdom."[58] With the advent of HIV, a second phase in the development of the questionnaire was based on epidemiologic evidence and included direct questions about sexual risks. The FDA stressed a face-to-face interview, rather than filling out a questionnaire, in hopes of ensuring complete honesty in answering the questions. Such data as history of hepatitis and possible exposure to HIV are used to deter donations from persons with potentially infectious exposures. This is done in order to reduce the pretest probability of finding true-positive results during laboratory testing. In other words, the precollection donor-screening process reduces the amount of blood collected that can transmit infectious diseases. Although laboratory testing is very sophisticated, it can never completely eliminate the risk of an infected unit. Reducing the number of infectious units that make it to the testing laboratory will reduce the number of infectious units that make it through the testing process undetected (i.e., false-negative test results).

The donor questionnaire is a dynamic document that is updated as new risks become apparent.[58,59] The interview process will be ineffective if it becomes too onerous or lengthy. If there are too many questions, important issues about high-risk behavior might be obscured, and the ultimate purpose of the interview process would be defeated. In the United States, an effort has gone toward creating a Uniform Donor History Questionnaire (UDHQ) to standardize criteria used for all tissue and blood donations and reduce the complexity, burden, and possible confusion. Donors are queried using broad-based capture questions to make screening more efficient. Certain questions are designed to eliminate the need for further exploration of the subject if the answer is no. The questions are asked reverse chronologically. Questions start with the day of presentation, proceeding backward, and query about donor health status, travel, medications, and other items associated with increased risk to either donor or recipient (e.g., "In the past 48 hours . . . ," "In the past 6 weeks . . . ," "In the past 12 months . . . ," or "Have you *ever* . . ."). Some medications are deferring because the indication for use increases the donor's risk in donating (e.g., antiseizure medications), and others are deferring in order to protect blood recipients (e.g., the use of potentially teratogenic medications such as isotretinoin). Still other medications might suggest a condition where the donor may not be able to give informed consent (e.g., Alzheimer's disease).

A comprehensive treatment of the screening process has been published.[59] Questions deal with items such as the following:

- Current state of health;
- Medication use (including aspirin);
- Pregnancy;
- Recent blood donations or immunizations;
- Receipt of a transfusion, transplant, or graft;
- Sexual practices that may increase the risk of HIV;
- Body piercing or tattoos;
- Incarceration;
- Exposure to hepatitis;
- Travel to areas where certain diseases are endemic (e.g., malaria, variant Creutzfeldt–Jacob disease, and Chagas disease);
- Use of clotting factor concentrates;
- Injection of any drugs not prescribed by a physician; and
- History of diseases such as malaria, Chagas disease, babesiosis, cancer, cardiovascular disease, a bleeding condition, or a family history of Creutzfeldt–Jakob disease.

The most recent questionnaire and accompanying educational materials may be found online by following this path on the AABB website: http://www.aabb.org > Give Blood > Donor History Questionnaires > Blood Donor History Questionnaire. An abbreviated questionnaire has been developed for recent repeat donors that eliminates nonrepeatable events from the questionnaire.[59] Most US blood centers have adopted the UDHQ.

During the interview, prospective donors might become aware of disqualifying factors in the health histories but feel too embarrassed or coerced to admit to disqualifications. Provisions must be made at all collection sites for persons to exit at any time without examination, and the opportunity must be provided for the donor to easily indicate that collected blood not be used for transfusion. Mechanisms have been established for confidential unit exclusion that provide for this, either at the donation site using a confidential form or barcode, or by anonymous telephone call after donation.

Donors also receive an abbreviated physical examination, including monitoring for symptoms of current disease processes, body temperature, heart rate and rhythm, and the ability to comprehend the screening questions and give informed consent. Informed consent for donation should also include the possibility that the donor will be listed in a deferral registry if the history or testing precludes donation. In some areas, laws may require that public health authorities be notified when donors test positive for certain diseases.

A blood sample is tested before donation to make sure the hemoglobin is at least 12.5 g/dL using an instrument, or a spun hematocrit $\geq$38%, to screen for anemia (recently increased to 13.0 g and 39% for male donors). This is the minimum requirement for allogeneic whole blood donation in the United States and many countries. Other automated procedures such as red cell, platelet, and plasma collection by apheresis technology may require more rigorous hemoglobin cutoffs and have minimum height and weight guidelines. Blood centers in the past most often measured red cell mass using copper sulfate, but recently more objective measurement methods that measure hemoglobin or hematocrit have been employed. In the copper sulfate method, a drop of capillary blood from a fingerstick sample is dropped into a copper sulfate solution with a specific gravity of 1.053. Sinking of the drop indicates a hemoglobin of 12.5 g or above. The copper sulfate method, although well accepted for decades, suffers from problems with both specificity and sensitivity. Because of the former, donors who fail are often retested with a spun hematocrit. This test can also err in accepting individuals who are proven anemic by a venous sample taken at the same time.[60,61]

A prospective donor with a diagnosis of chronic, degenerative, or infectious disease should be deferred from blood donation. Donors whose histories carry significant risk and those who have tested positive for infectious diseases are placed on deferral registries. For some deferrals, "reentry" pathways back into the donor pool have been made available when the risk is no longer present. On occasion, donors attempt to donate in spite of permanent deferral. Reasons include a desire to obtain results of infectious disease testing, to receive credit for community service, a misunderstanding about the reason for deferral, and erroneous recruitment by the blood center staff.[62]

The effectiveness of the donor interview in deferring individuals who have risk factors that could impact the safety of the product has been a subject of investigation. The Retrovirus Epidemiology Donor Study has shown areas where improvement is needed. Younger donors (less than 25 years of age) have a higher behavioral risk factor than older donors. Educational reinforcement is needed for this group.[63] Most donors skim the educational material and fail to assimilate the information. Thus, more effective materials are needed. However, some high-risk donors seem resistant to any attempt at education, and test-seeking behavior is a particular problem.[64–66] Computer-assisted self-interviewing (typically using a touch screen) has become an increasingly popular vehicle for donor screening. Data from this group suggest that it is probably able to reduce the number of high-risk donors by increasing self-deferral.[67]

Acceptable donor age is 17 and above in most centers, but there is considerable variation in practice. Recent efforts have convinced some governments to allow 16 year olds to donate. Experience with healthy donors over the age of 65 has generally been favorable; thus, the need for an upper age limit is questionable.[29]

In 2011, 18.0 million individuals presented to donate in the United States, 93.5% of whom were at blood centers; 31% were first-time donors, and 2.46 million of these donors were deferred (13.7%, an increase from 12.6% in 2008). Of these, 48.8% were deferred for low hemoglobin and 1.4% for high-risk behaviors; 1.1% of successful donors had the units destroyed due to abnormal disease markers.[11] Once the donor has been appropriately evaluated to insure that the risk to the donor and to the recipient is acceptable, then blood collection may occur.

Blood collection

This section will first address the traditional collection of whole blood and its separation into components, followed by discussion of newer automated apheresis technology.

Whole blood collection

Despite the many technologies for automated collection, some blood centers—indeed, entire countries—are able to produce the bulk of needed inventory from whole blood collections. A typical whole blood collection takes 45–60 minutes, including the interview, physical exam screening, aseptic scrub, antecubital vein venipuncture, and monitoring for postdonation reactions in a canteen area where refreshments are offered. The blood draw itself should be accomplished in approximately 10 minutes, with periodic agitation to mix the fresh blood with the anticoagulant in the draw bag to reduce clotting. The tubing is clamped before the needle is removed so that air is not drawn into the blood bag. Blood samples are taken into pilot tubes for testing. This is normally done from the blood tubing at the conclusion of the donation or from a diversion pouch filled from the first blood collected, a process that captures contaminating skin organisms. The tubing is sealed, and the needle is discarded without recapping. The donor holds firm pressure over the venipuncture site, and then a pressure bandage is applied. The donor is instructed to keep the pressure bandage on and avoid strenuous activity for a prescribed amount of time, to increase fluid intake for the next day or two, and to spend at least 15 minutes in the canteen area. Reactions usually occur at the end of donation in the donor chair or in the area where refreshments are served. If the donor leaves immediately against advice, risk of injury might be increased. Staff monitoring the postdonation canteen area must be vigilant in assessing for signs of reactions and proactive in preventing fall injuries.

Whole blood collection has the longest cumulative experience and requires fewer resources than automated collection. For countries in the process of developing simple, reliable collection networks, whole blood is the logical first step, with or without component separation.

Component separation

Whole blood may generally be stored for up to 21 days. Whole blood may be separated by centrifugation into RBC, platelet, and plasma components according to density. This allows longer shelf life, better inventory management, and more choices and resources for patient care. The capacity to provide patients with the different blood components they require is still limited in low-income countries: 45% of the blood collected in low-income countries is separated into components, 80% in middle-income countries, and 95% in high-income countries.[4]

Using a "closed" separation system that is not ever open to outside air is important to prevent contamination with microorganisms during collection and component separation. Centrifuge-separated components are transferred from the original whole blood draw container to satellite bags through integrally connected plastic tubing. Adding nutrients and saline to the RBCs permits storage at 1–6 °C for up to 42 days (see Chapter 9). The preservative solution may be held sterilely in one of the integral transfer bags until the plasma is separated off into a third bag after centrifugation. Then the solution may be added back to the packed RBCs in the original bag.

Platelets may be separated from the whole blood or allowed to degenerate without being separated. In Europe and many areas of the world outside the United States, "buffy-coat" platelets are produced by using a "hard" spin initially to separate all cellular elements from the plasma. Then the buffy coat containing the platelets, white blood cells, and a significant contaminant of RBC is further processed to isolate the platelets. In the United States, an initial "soft" spin separates platelet-rich plasma from the RBCs, and then a "hard" spin separates the platelets from the plasma. Additional information about platelet preparation and storage may be found in Chapter 19. Platelets are typically stored for 5 days at controlled room temperature before expiration. In 2011, 3.9 million platelet apheresis/pools were transfused in the United States—a decrease of 13.4% from 2008.[11] The ratio of doses of apheresis platelets to whole blood–derived platelets rose from 7:1 to 10:1 during the same period. About 12.8% of platelets produced in 2011 expired, due to the short half-life and logistical challenges.[11]

Plasma separated and frozen within 8 hours is called *fresh frozen plasma* (FFP), whereas that frozen up to 24 hours is known as FP24. Each contains coagulation factors in quantities adequate for most patient indications. FP24 represented only 15% of the 4.1 million units of plasma transfused in the United States in 2004[12] but 47% of the 5.9 million units of plasma produced in 2011.[11] This increase may be in part due to the concern about transfusion-related acute lung injury (TRALI) and the exclusion of women who have been pregnant from plasma donation. Blood centers are attempting to make plasma from all eligible donors of the needed types, even though the plasma logistically cannot always be frozen within eight hours. More volunteer plasma is typically drawn than needed for transfusion. Plasma stored for as long as 72 hours before freezing may be sold for fractionation (discussed further in this chapter).

After separation from the RBCs, plasma may be pooled and treated with solvent and detergent (S/D) to decrease the risk of transfusion-transmitted disease. In addition, the pooling enables quality control of coagulation factors per lot, and the dilution dramatically decreases the risk of TRALI.[68,69] Other pathogen reduction techniques may be applied (see Chapter 56). Only a small amount of S/D-treated plasma is used in the United States due to political and economic factors, and possible safety concerns regarding pooled products.[69] However, some countries in Europe rely on this process for the majority of plasma transfused.[68]

Preparation of cryoprecipitate involves thawing frozen plasma at 4 °C in a circulating water bath, followed by centrifugation so that the supernatant plasma can be drained into an integrally attached storage bag (see Chapter 26). The remaining cold-precipitated material is then refrozen at ≤ -18 °C and stored for up to 1 year. Approximately 1.7 million units of cryoprecipitate were prepared in the United States in 2011, an increase of 16% since 2008.[11] In some regions in Europe, cryoprecipitate is not produced, as the use of factor concentrates for inherited bleeding disorders and plasma or fibrinogen concentrate for hypofibrinogenemia has proven satisfactory.

Leukocyte reduction is accomplished by passing whole blood or RBCs through filters that reduce the number of white blood cells (WBCs) (see Chapter 24). Ideally, this should be done as soon after collection as possible, but no longer than 72 hours. Leukoreduction has been shown to be more effective when done before storage because some of the adverse effects of transfusion are caused by factors produced or released by leukocytes during storage. Although leukocyte reduction can reduce untoward events, significant amounts of WBCs still remain in leukoreduced products (up to 5×10^{-6} WBCs/unit in the United States and 1×10^{-6} in Europe). Automated apheresis collections often have technology that produces leukocyte-reduced products during the collection process.

Automated collection

Over the first decade of the 21st century, advances in technology combined with a desire to optimize donations have led to a dramatic increase in automated collection of blood components. The collection of single-donor platelets using apheresis has increased coincident with the greater availability of automation and implementation of bacterial testing of platelet products. In 2011, 91.1% of platelets produced in the United States were from automated collection, up from 83.7% in 2008 and 67.7% in 2001.[11] Eight of 30 European countries reporting for the same year collected >50% of their platelets by apheresis (the United Kingdom was the highest at 83%).[70]

Choice of which automated product(s) to collect depends on a number of factors, including blood type, height, weight, sex, risk of having antibodies that could cause TRALI, platelet count, hematocrit, the available collection technology, distance from manufacturing laboratories, and the time the donor has available to donate. Minimum donor qualification requirements for the various automated collection methods have developed historically—often independently. Therefore, some procedures have minimum requirements and length of deferrals that may differ from those of other procedures. A *double RBC* product is produced by an apheresis procedure where two units of RBC are collected at the same time, while returning donor plasma and often additional saline solution. In the United States, there is a 112-day deferral for donation of a double RBC product that also precludes platelet and plasma donation on some instrumentation. At the same time, a donor of a combined automated platelet, plasma, and RBC is deferred only 56 days for RBCs, but may often continue donating platelets and plasma again during the RBC deferral.

Product selection

Selection of which product(s) to draw from a given donor may be complex in a center with many choices. Obviously, the first concern is which product is most needed for patient care at that time. In addition, an underlying theme in blood banking is to maximize collection of universal donor AB plasma and universal donor group O RBCs. Many centers avoid collection of RBC units from group AB donors because many of these RBC units are wasted, since only AB recipients may use this blood. Recently, risk of antibodies that may cause TRALI has also disqualified donors from plasma and platelet donation who are at risk of having these antibodies. Finally, there may also be minimum height, weight, and hematocrit requirements that vary by technology and by sex. Therefore, a large male with a high platelet count might donate three units of platelets by apheresis, whereas a small woman who has TRALI risk might only donate an RBC unit.

With proper attention to donor interviewing and care of the donor, the blood donation process can be a pleasant and safe experience for the donor, while providing a safe and efficacious product to the recipient—the goal of the entire blood donation and transfusion chain.

Testing

Blood specimens drawn from the donor at the time of collection are sent for blood typing and infectious disease testing. Many hospitals that still collect their own blood find it more economical to send out the testing and receive the results electronically. Bacterial testing of platelet units is sometimes also done centrally.

ABO and RhD testing

Donor centers routinely test blood from each donation for ABO and RhD type (and K in some countries). "Forward" typing occurs by addition of antibody directed toward the A, B, and D antigens on donor red cells to obtain the blood type. "Reverse" grouping is performed by adding donor plasma to reagent red cells bearing A or B antigens to detect naturally occurring donor antibody to A and B. Algorithms ensure concordance of forward and reverse typing.

RhD is a special case (see Chapter 14). "Rh-negative" donors lacking RhD antigen undergo an additional step in the blood-screening process to determine if their cells possess the weak-D antigen. As a rule, when in doubt, blood centers err on the side of calling a donor RhD-positive, to avoid the chance of giving RhD-positive blood to an RhD-negative patient. At the transfusion service (recipient) level, the patient is typed, and, if in doubt, the transfusion service errs on the side of calling recipients RhD-negative, so they will not inadvertently be stimulated to make an alloantibody to D. The processes are optimized for these two divergent purposes. This is the reason that discrepancies may sometimes be discovered when blood donors become patients and their D typing may appear to change from positive in the blood donor setting to negative in the blood recipient setting.

Antibody screening

Donor plasma is also added to reagent red cells bearing an array of clinically significant RBC antigens. This is to screen for unexpected alloantibodies to epitopes in the Rh, Kell, Kidd, Duffy, and other antigen systems. Plasma from donors bearing alloantibodies is not used for transfusion; however, since RBCs contain so little plasma, these may be made available from donors with alloantibodies with the appropriate labeling. The screening of the donor for alloantibodies eliminates the need for the transfusion service to screen for donor antibodies to red cells and eliminates the need to perform a "minor" crossmatch (donor plasma mixed with patient red cells).

Infectious disease testing

Serological and nucleic acid testing for infectious disease is carried out in most high-income countries. The exact tests performed in a center depend on the incidence of the diseases in the population and also on availability of resources for testing (see Chapter 55). Testing requirements have changed frequently in recent years. Currently, infectious agents for which serologic screening is performed in the United States include human immunodeficiency virus-1 and -2 (HIV 1/2), hepatitis C virus (HCV), hepatitis B virus (HBV; HBV surface antigen [HBS-Ag] and HBV core [HBc]), human T-cell lymphotropic virus-1 and -2 (HTLV-I/II), Chagas disease, and syphilis. Nucleic acid amplification testing (NAAT) is performed for HIV 1/2, HCV, HBV, and West Nile virus. Supplemental or confirmatory testing is often done when licensed tests are available. This is useful for donor counseling and to potentially allow the donor to be eligible for a "reentry" protocol (which in the United States must conform to FDA guidance). In the United States, a donor is generally deferred even if the screening test is known to give a false-positive result. This is because the test has become uninformative for that donor (i.e., it cannot discriminate whether the donor has the disease). This often happens when blood-testing laboratories change from one testing platform to another (e.g., switching to a different instrument or reagent manufacturer). It is not unusual to have a higher number of deferrals concurrent with the implementation of the new technology due to the false-positive tests. Some countries—such as England—may be more donor centered in their testing algorithms. For instance, if a donor is known to be false positive on a certain screening platform, subsequent specimens may be routed to an alternate platform, rather than deferring the donor. If a donor is known to have visited a malaria-endemic area, the donor might become eligible to donate after a short deferral period if a supplemental malaria test is performed, rather than be deferred as long as US donors. In 2011 in the United States, 1.1% of blood donors had abnormal disease marker results, resulting in a destruction of 102,000 units of blood.[11]

In addition to serological and nucleic acid testing of blood, bacterial culture is becoming widely used to test platelet products (see Chapter 53). Because platelets are stored at room temperature, rather than refrigerated or frozen, there is a greater chance that bacteria in the product might grow. These organisms may come from normal skin flora that contaminate the bag during phlebotomy, or they may be transiently circulating in the donor's blood during collection.

Component modification and distribution

When a blood component has successfully completed processing, testing, and record review, then it is "labeled," meaning that it has met all standards and is ready for infusion. Many countries have adopted ISBT 128, an identification system developed by the International Society of Blood Transfusion, that incorporates comprehensive barcode labels intended to set a global safety standard for the identification, labeling, and information processing of human blood, tissue, and organ products across international borders and disparate healthcare systems.[71]

The majority of a typical area's blood supply is stored in hospitals for use when it is needed, rather than at the blood center. Availability and turnaround time are key components for determining allocations to each hospital; these depend on usage patterns and transportation distance from the blood center, and often the temperament of the clinical staff. Even a very small hospital that is a great distance from its blood supplier might have 10 or 20 units of RBCs on its shelves in preparation for the acute motor vehicle trauma that might occur every year or two. Unfortunately, this means that the vast majority of products shipped to this location will never be used. This leads to increased "outdating" of the products, and a disproportionally large effort to track the rotating inventory. Many blood centers monitor inventories in the hospitals. The center can then rotate out blood that may be expiring soon from the hospitals that use less blood to large hospitals and trauma centers that will be able to use the blood before expiration. In the United States in 2011, only 2.1% of allogeneic RBC donations outdated.[11] The mean age of RBC units was 17.9 days at the time of transfusion.[11] The low outdate rate suggests that blood centers have become more efficient at delivering the appropriate product when needed. However, when the expiration rate drops too low, then the safety margin of having enough blood at any particular time is reduced. The same year, 3.3% of US hospitals reported at least one day of cancelled elective surgeries due to blood inventory shortages, the lowest percentage reported since 1997.[11]

In the United States in 2011, 12% percent of transfused RBC units were modified by irradiation, an increase from 10% in 2008. Irradiation of platelets was higher: 46% of apheresis and 34% of whole blood–derived platelets were irradiated. At the same time, 53% of all transfused components were leukocyte reduced: 71% of RBC/whole blood, 80% of apheresis platelets, and 37% of whole blood–derived platelets.[11] Leukoreduction in Europe remains variable. In 2011, 17 of 31 European countries responding to a survey used >95% leukoreduced blood.[70]

Plasma that is separated during component preparation and not needed for patient use becomes "recovered" plasma, and it is often used to supplement the supply of source plasma, as discussed in the "The Collection Process for Source Plasma" section.

Autologous and directed donation

The volunteer donor collection process also facilitates the collection of nonvolunteer blood donations. Many of the processes are similar. Autologous blood donation is the donation of one or more units of blood to oneself, usually in the preoperative setting. This practice rose in the 1980s and 1990s chiefly in response to concern over the risk of transfusion-transmitted viral infections. Since that time, preoperative autologous blood donation has been in decline while viral marker testing has improved significantly.[72] Many other factors have converged to contribute to this downward trend in autologous blood donation, including recognition of the high cost, increased waste, and risk when compared to allogeneic blood donation, as well as the widespread adoption of patient blood management. Figure 4.3 illustrates the decreasing collection of autologous blood over the past decade in the United States.

A study published in the *New England Journal of Medicine* reported that the additional cost of autologous blood ranged from $68 to $4783 per unit of blood and resulted in "little expected health benefit" based on quality-adjusted years of life saved,[73] which may reach tens of millions of dollars.[74] The increased cost of autologous blood donation is not only related to the increased labor involved in collecting and storing the units, because a significant percentage of autologous donation units that are donated are ultimately discarded. A randomized study of preoperative autologous donation prior to hip surgery found that

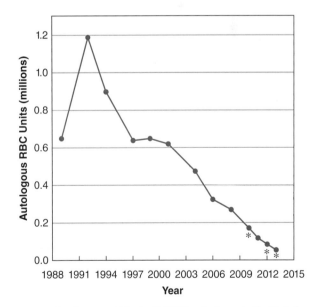

Figure 4.3 Autologous red blood cell (RBC) units drawn in the United States by year. Note the dramatic decline after the maximum reached in 1992 (greater than a 21-fold decrease). The data are taken from the 2011 National Blood Collection and Utilization Survey.[11] The points indicated by asterisks (∗) have been extrapolated from cumulative member data supplied by Blood Centers of America (courtesy of Bill Block). Graphic design by Joshua E. Crookston.

41% of the autologous units donated were not transfused.[75] The choice of autologous blood donation has in the past been guided by the perceived increased risk associated with allogenic blood transfusion. However, the risk of transfusion-transmitted viral infection in the modern era of viral testing is lower than the risk associated with administrative error.[76] Autologous blood donations have also been shown to be associated with an increased risk of developing adverse reactions when compared with the risks associated with donations from healthy volunteers.[77] Finally, the concept of patient blood management has increasingly taken hold. This practice includes interventions that decrease the likelihood of transfusion, such as addressing anemia in the preoperative setting, intraoperative blood recovery, and restrictive use of transfusion overall.

Only 58% of the 113,000 autologous units collected in the United States in 2011 were transfused.[11] This was a 59% decrease from 2008. The high outdate rate illustrates the high cost and inefficiency of autologous blood collection. These only accounted for <0.5% of all units transfused. Certain patients with rare blood types and alloantibodies that are difficult to match may benefit from autologous blood donation; however, it is not indicated for most transfusions. Some jurisdictions, such as the State of California, may require that a physician discuss the option of autologous blood donation when consenting patients for blood transfusion. However, clinicians may also point out that following a conservative transfusion practice and using allogeneic blood only when needed remains the best choice for the majority of patients.

The collection process for source plasma: screening, phlebotomy, choice of product, collection, and testing of source plasma donors

The handling of source plasma donors differs in several respects from the handling of whole blood and apheresis donors providing blood products for hospital transfusion. Source plasma is collected by apheresis specifically for further manufacture into biological derivatives, in contrast to "recovered plasma," which is the plasma remaining after RBC production from whole blood donation. About half of the recovered plasma collected for fractionation comes from Europe. Many European countries have maintained national programs that fractionate plasma from recovered plasma from volunteer donors. However, the demand for biological therapies worldwide requires the additional supply from remunerated or compensated (paid) donors. Source plasma is collected (in order of amount per population) in the United States, Austria, the Czech Republic, and Germany from compensated donors. Smaller programs are found for collections from noncompensated donors (in order of number per population) in Australia, the Netherlands, Denmark, France, Sweden, and Belgium and more recently Hungary. In 2010, source plasma accounted for approximately 75% of plasma for further manufacturing worldwide, with recovered plasma accounting for the remainder. In 2012, approximately 28 million L of source plasma was fractionated along with approximately 9 million L of recovered plasma. The number of collection centers in 2014 by Plasma Protein Therapeutics Association (PPTA) members was 467 and constantly increasing. US source plasma collections have been steadily increasing from more than 23.5 million L in 2011 to 26 million L in 2012 to 29 million L in 2013. The requirement for immune globulins have largely driven this increase (data from www.pptaglobal.org). The United States

provides a large proportion of the world's source plasma requirements for two reasons: First, under FDA regulations, source plasma donors can donate more plasma, more frequently, than is the case in most countries. Second, the United States has a well-developed source plasma industry that has invested in a network of centers that compensate donors for their time and inconvenience.

In both the United States and the European countries, source plasma is collected in fixed sites without mobile collections. Either the Autopheresis-C (Fresenius) or the PCS-2 (Haemonetics) is used for most collections. Recruitment is typically by word of mouth, newspapers, radio, and posters. The donor groups are heterogeneous. Sites near campuses that can attract student donors are common. Medium-sized cities and towns are favored over larger metropolitan areas. Payment varies between $25 and $50 for normal source plasma. More money is paid for donations from immunized donors for hyperimmune plasma (rabies immune plasma, tetanus immune plasma, hepatitis B immune plasma, anti-D plasma, etc.) and by those from donors with disease-state antibodies needed for diagnostic manufacture.

In addition to specific national regulations and guidance, in the United States and Europe an International Quality Plasma Program (IQPP) of the PPTA is also followed. The program has been judged successful because the major manufacturers in Europe and the United States will only use plasma from these programs. This self-regulation includes the following:

- *Community-based donors:* Donors must have a permanent address in the vicinity of the center.
- *Qualified donor standard:* Each donor's plasma is used only after two medical screenings and required viral testings are successful and less than six months has elapsed between the two donations.
- *National Donor Deferral Registry (NDDR):* All donors deferred for viral marker testing are entered into an NDDR that must be checked before each *applicant* (i.e., not qualified) donor is accepted.
- *Viral marker standard:* This requires centers to keep their viral marker rates below established levels.
- *60-day inventory hold:* This is so that units from a donor with a subsequent positive test or disqualifying information can be removed before being pooled (part of the Q-SEAL Standards for fractionators).

The community-based donor standard discourages transient individuals from donating, as this population has been associated with an increased incidence of infectious disease markers. Under-the-nail photosensitive nail coloring is applied to ensure the donor only donates at one program at a time. A minimum weight of 50 kg (110 lbs.) must be met. At each donation, the hematocrit and total protein are determined from a fingerstick blood sample. The hematocrit must be 38% or greater (recently increased by FDA to 39% for males), and protein 6.0 g/dL or greater. The protein is measured using a refractometer (the only device currently available to meet the FDA requirement).

Initially, the donor is subjected to an extensive interview similar to that used for blood donors, followed by physical examination by a physician. In the United States, a physician substitute may be used, such as a nurse, paramedic, or other health professional trained to do the physical exam and operating under the guidance of the center medical director. The physical examination consists of an external eye, ear, and nose exam, with an examination of the throat with a tongue blade and light. Lymph nodes in the neck area are palpated. Auscultation of the back and front of the chest for lung abnormalities is followed by auscultation of the heart. The abdomen is examined for liver and spleen enlargement. A short neurological and extremity review completes the examination. In some centers, a urine dipstick for protein and glucose is also performed. After passing these initial tests, the donor can donate as an *applicant* donor. Collected units are held until the donor has two successful donations without any positive infectious disease markers. If the donor does not return for the second donation, the plasma is considered an "orphan" unit and cannot be used for injectable product. The donor must pass initially, and every four months, tests that include serum protein electrophoresis, total protein, and syphilis. The physical examination with full interview is repeated annually or if the donor has not presented in the past six months. An informed consent must be executed on the first donation and again whenever the consent is changed.

The donor donates according to a nomogram: body weights of 50–67.5, 68–79, and greater than 79 kg can donate 625, 750, and 800 ml plasma, respectively, not counting anticoagulant. Some centers infuse saline at the end of the donation. After a brief rest in the donation chair, the donor is allowed to collect the compensation (usually electronically added to a debit card) and leave. Refreshment and recovery areas are not common in plasma donor centers. In the United States, donors are allowed to donate no more than twice in seven days, with at least two days between donations. A donor could theoretically donate 104 times per year (65–83 L, depending on donor weight). The Council of Europe recommendations limit the amount of plasma collected per session to 600 mL, not counting anticoagulant.[78,79] There is a also a 15 L annual limit. German national guidelines set in 1999 allowed donations of up to 650 ml plasma twice weekly with an annual limit of 25 L. Donors must weigh a minimum of 50 kg and have a hemoglobin level of 12.5 g/dL in females and 13.5 g/dL in males. Immunoglobulin G (IgG) is measured at every 15th donation and must be at least 115 g/L.

To determine if less restrictive donation standards (closer to those in the United States) were safe, 21 German plasma donor centers participated in a study known as SIPLA. They found that donors weighing greater than 70 kg could donate 850 mL each session up to 60 times per year with appropriate monitoring (up to 51 L total per year). Currently, there is an effort to change European requirements to be consistent with these findings.[80,81]

Each donation by a source plasma donor is tested serologically for HIV antibody, HBS-Ag, and hepatitis C antibody. Nucleic acid testing is done on each donation for HBV, HCV, and HIV. A positive test results in deferral. This is usually regardless of results of confirmatory tests that are performed for donor counseling. In addition, tests for hepatitis A and parvovirus are also performed. If positive, the units are discarded, but donor status is not affected and there is no counseling.

Due to the investment in the applicant's first donation, donor centers cultivate long-term donors who donate often. Some very dedicated donors are given vaccines to provide rabies immune plasma, tetanus immune plasma, hepatitis B, or other immune plasma in order to make specialty immunoglobulins. Rh-negative donors who are not of childbearing potential can become donors of Rh-immune plasma for manufacture into Rh immune globulin. This is done by immunization with carefully "qualified" D-positive red cells. Long-term consistent donation is particularly important for these specialty donors.

There are additional requirements for donors receiving red cell immunizations, including physician performance of the initial physical examination and a separate informed consent, physician presence when immunizations are given, and a specific physician approval of the red cells to be injected. Meticulous preparation of the red cells for immunization occurs. Red cells from whole blood donors are frozen and collected over a year. Only when a year's viral marker testing remains negative can the cells be deglycerolized and used to immunize a donor. When the red cells from a specific whole blood donor are first used, they are given to 1–3 recipients for a year. When viral marker testing is negative throughout the year for those recipients as well as the donor, the cells are then "qualified." Plasma from these donors is used to manufacture Rh immune globulin, and the pool must contain a sufficient concentration (titer) of antibody to allow acceptable product to be made.

Rates of viral marker test positivity in donors are monitored, and plasma centers are expected to take steps to reduce levels when they rise above predetermined alert levels. Source plasma donors tend to be more likely male, younger, and larger in size than volunteer donors, probably reflecting the more demanding donation program frequency. In addition, they are more ethnically diverse. Some of these factors act to increase prevalence and incidence of viral diseases. Socioeconomic status and compensation programs might play a role as well. With the push toward voluntary donations worldwide, the payment of plasma donors has been criticized. Nevertheless, monetary compensation of source plasma donors has had an enviable safety record for the last 15 years since many of the additional controls have been put in place. The viral reduction and inactivation treatment of the final product provides additional safety. Thus, the layers of protection operate differently in source plasma programs than in the volunteer programs, but are still highly effective in preventing infectious units from entering plasma pools and in assuring safety of the final product.[82–84]

The blood collection and transfusion chain is heterogeneous

In summary, the recruitment and screening of donors and the collection, processing, and testing of blood have developed dramatically over the past half-century. The blood donation and transfusion chain describes a highly regulated and technology-rich field. Much of the global blood supply is collected by procurement agencies that may differ greatly in structure and organization. Systems that are very different may still be successful in collecting and delivering a beneficial, life-saving product to patients when they need it. At the same time, the disparity between resources used in high-income countries and low-income countries for procurement of safe blood is perhaps greater than in any other area of healthcare.[16]

Key References

A full reference list for this chapter is available at:
http://www.wiley.com/go/simon/transfusion

2 Crookston KP, Koenig SC, Reyes MD. Transfusion reaction identification and management at the bedside. *J Infusion Nurs* 2015; **38** (2): 104–13.

4 World Health Organization (WHO). *Blood safety and availability factsheet*. Geneva: WHO, 2014.

7 Starr DP. *Blood: an epic history of medicine and commerce*. New York: Alfred A. Knopf, 1998.

8 Wald ML. Blood industry shrinks as transfusions decline. New York Times, August 22, 2014. http://www.nytimes.com/2014/08/23/business/blood-industry-hurt-by-surplus.html?_r=0.

10 Crookston KP. The pledge of the community blood center. *Transfusion* 2010; **50**: 2768.

11 Whitaker B, Hinkins S. *2011 National Blood Collection and Utilization Survey.* Rockville, MD: States Department of Health and Human Services, 2011.

14 World Health Organization (WHO). *Global Database on Blood Safety summary report 2011.* Geneva: WHO, 2011.

19 Titmuss RM. *The gift relationship: from human blood to social policy.* New York: Pantheon, 1971.

59 Eder A, Bianco C, AABB. *Screening blood donors: science, reason, and the donor history questionnaire.* Bethesda, MD: AABB Press, 2007.

70 van Hoeven L, Janssen MP, Rautmann G. The collection, testing and use of blood and blood components in Europe: 2011 report. Strasbourg: European Directorate for the Quality of Medicines and HealthCare, 2011.

72 Brecher ME, Goodnough LT. The rise and fall of preoperative autologous blood donation. *Transfusion* 2001; **41**: 1459–62.

76 Goodnough LT. Autologous blood donation. *Anesthesiol Clin North America* 2005; **23**: 263–70.

79 European Committee on Blood Transfusion. *Guide to the preparation, use and quality assurance of blood components.* 17th ed. Strasbourg, France: European Directorate for the Quality of Medicines and HealthCare, 2013.

83 Klamroth R, Groner A, Simon TL. Pathogen inactivation and removal methods for plasma-derived clotting factor concentrates. *Transfusion* 2014; **54**: 1406–17.

CHAPTER 5

Adverse reactions and iron deficiency after blood donation

Anne F. Eder[1] & Joseph E. Kiss[2]

[1] National Medical Affairs; Biomedical Services, National Headquarters, American Red Cross and Adjunct Associate Professor, Georgetown University Medical Center, Washington, DC, USA

[2] Hemapheresis and Blood Services, The Institute for Transfusion Medicine; and Associate Professor of Medicine, Division of Hematology-Oncology, Department of Medicine, The University of Pittsburgh, Pittsburgh, PA, USA

A safe and adequate blood supply depends on healthy, altruistic volunteers who are willing to donate blood without expecting personal gain despite the potential risk of discomfort or adverse reaction. Blood donation has an impressive safety record, and most donors have a good experience or only mild symptoms after donation. But with over 9 million blood donations each year in the United States,[1] even a low rate of reactions may negatively affect the health and well-being of many people and influence their willingness to donate again. Adverse reactions can occur immediately or soon after a blood collection procedure or become apparent only after multiple, regular blood donations over an extended period of time. Immediate or acute reactions after blood donation typically are minor symptoms such as dizziness and fainting or phlebotomy-related bruises, but also the less common and more serious injuries; long-term or chronic complications include iron depletion and its sequelae. Blood collection agencies must inform prospective donors about the possible risks at each encounter and monitor adverse reactions during and after the collection procedure as part of ongoing continuous improvement efforts to reduce donation-related complications. Although blood centers cannot completely eliminate all risks associated with blood donation, the systematic analysis of adverse reactions has led to changes in collection procedures and policies that have significantly improved safety for the most susceptible groups of blood donors.

Adverse reactions after blood donation

Most acute reactions (>90%) that occur immediately or within a few hours after donating blood are mild or minor symptoms such as dizziness, lightheadedness, or phlebotomy-related bruises and hematomas that resolve promptly but are still unpleasant for the donor. More serious complications are uncommon, but typically result from a loss of consciousness, from injuries after blood donation, or from a needle-related nerve injury.[2] Young donors are much more likely to experience immediate adverse reactions after blood donation than older donors, with loss of consciousness affecting about 4 in 1000 donations and injury resulting in 0.6 in 1000 donations among donors age 16 to 17 years.[3] Not surprisingly, blood donors who have an adverse reaction are less likely to return to donate blood again than those who have an uneventful

donation.[4–6] Even minor reactions and transient symptoms discourage return donation by 36%, with more severe reactions further decreasing the likelihood by 66%.[4] The potential loss in annual donations resulting from donor attrition after adverse reactions has been estimated as 1.6% per year.[5] Donor retention has far-reaching implications for the blood supply, for not only availability but also safety because repeat donors account for about 70% of the US blood supply and are less likely than first-time donors to have positive infectious disease markers, such as hepatitis and HIV.

Many studies of reactions after allogeneic blood donation published since the 1940s have reported various incidence rates and associated risk factors.[7] The observed reaction rates in different blood centers span a wide range (<1% to >20%). Many factors contribute to this variability, including different reaction definitions, subjective assessments of reaction severity, disparate donor demographics, and various methods of data collection and analysis. Reactions may be captured at the site by collection staff or identified only after the donor calls the center back to report a reaction. Higher reaction rates are generally observed when donors complete surveys asking them about mild subjective symptoms or are directly interviewed days to weeks after a donation.[8,9] Many studies of donor reactions are limited by methodological problems, including retrospective design, poorly controlled comparisons, or the use of univariate methods to detect associations of various factors with donor reactions. Consequently, any conclusions about the possible association of donation-related reactions with various risk factors should be evaluated in conjunction with an assessment of the study design and analytical methods.

In recent years, blood centers have focused on the practical application of donor hemovigilance, which is an effort to monitor, track, and trend reactions after blood donation, in order to design and implement preventive measures. An example of such a program in the American Red Cross is shown in Table 5.1, which captures reactions managed by collection staff at the blood drives and calls back to the blood center about delayed reactions after whole blood and automated (apheresis) blood donation. AABB has also launched a voluntary national program for donor hemovigilance in the United States, which encourages centers to use common reaction definitions and may facilitate analysis of complicated data

Rossi's Principles of Transfusion Medicine, Fifth Edition. Edited by Toby L. Simon, Jeffrey McCullough, Edward L. Snyder, Bjarte G. Solheim, and Ronald G. Strauss.
© 2016 John Wiley & Sons, Ltd. Published 2016 by John Wiley & Sons, Ltd.

Table 5.1 Adverse reactions after allogeneic whole blood and apheresis donations in the American Red Cross, 2006–2007

Reaction Category and Description		Whole Blood Donations (12.0 Million)				Automated Procedures (1.42 Million)			
		All Reactions		Outside Medical Care		All Reactions		Outside Medical Care	
		n	Rate	n	Rate	n	Rate	n	Rate
Systemic (syncopal)	Presyncope (prefaint)	324,129	269	69	0.06	14,919	104	4	0.03
	LOC (<1 min)	11,081	9.20	107	0.09	521	3.65	4	0.03
	Major (includes callbacks)								
	LOC (≥1 min)	2050	1.70	251	0.21	206	1.44	14	0.10
	Prolonged recovery	4228	3.51	829	0.69	424	2.97	48	0.34
	LOC with Injury	2181	1.81	680	0.57	98	0.69	18	0.13
Phlebotomy	Small hematoma	125,082	104	87	0.07	49,304	345	13	0.09
	Major (includes callbacks)								
	Large Hematoma	4932	4.09	556	0.46	2850	19.9	103	0.72
	Suspected nerve injury	3858	3.20	513	0.43	572	4.00	47	0.33
	Suspected arterial puncture	1644	1.37	112	0.09	82	0.57	1	0.01
Citrate reactions	Citrate (minor symptoms)	—	—	—	—	16,556	116	3	0.02
	Citrate (major, includes callbacks)	—	—	—	—	406	2.84	21	0.15
Allergic reactions	Local (minor) allergic reactions	123	0.10	19	0.02	49	0.34	8	0.06
	Systemic (major) allergic reactions (includes callbacks)	17	0.01	11	0.01	42	0.29	8	0.06
	TOTAL	479,325	398	3234	2.69	86,029	602	292	2.04

Rate per 10,000 donations. LOC, loss of consciousness; small hematoma, 2 × 2 in. or less; large hematoma, more than 2 × 2 in. Prolonged recovery (>30 minutes) after presyncope
Automated collections include plateletpheresis, plateletpheresis with concurrent plasma or other co-component, 2-unit red cell collections, and plasmapheresis procedures
Minor reactions (e.g., presyncope, small hematoma) are documented at the collection site; Major reactions are documented at the collection site or reported after donation, require follow-up with the donor, and receive a follow-up call, and are reviewed by a blood center physician.

sets. Although the absolute incidence of donor complications varies dramatically among centers for all the reasons mentioned previously, the practical value of hemovigilance activities lies not in the casual comparison or "benchmarking" of reported rates across blood centers, but in the careful analysis of rates within a blood system as part of continuous process improvement efforts to monitor and ultimately reduce the risk of reactions over time.

Acute reactions after blood donation: immediate symptoms and delayed complications

Most systemic reactions (95%) to blood donation are acute symptoms such as pallor, lightheadedness, dizziness, diaphoresis, and nausea, occurring in about 2–15% of whole blood donations.[2] The term *vasovagal* is often used to describe these reactions, to refer to physiologic changes that may be associated with syncope (i.e., increased vagal tone and bradycardia). The more general term *presyncope* captures the spectrum of reactions that result from various mechanisms involving not only peripheral baroreceptor activity, but also susceptibility to acute blood loss and orthostatic changes, as well as anxiety and psychological stress. Ultimately, syncope results from an insufficient supply of oxygen to the brain and a transient loss of consciousness. About one in every 20 presyncopal reactions (Table 5.1) progresses to loss of consciousness immediately or soon after the blood donation, and may be associated with seizure-like movements or loss of bowel and bladder function.

Presyncopal symptoms typically have rapid onset and short duration, and they resolve spontaneously. Although most of these reactions are self-limiting and transient, they are still distressing for many donors and some require prolonged recovery periods of more than 30 minutes.[2] Syncope-related falls may be associated with serious injuries. Most (90%) fainting events occur with the

phlebotomy or soon afterward at the blood drive, but delayed hypotensive reactions after the donor left the collection site comprised about 10% of the episodes in one series.[10,11] Young donors (16 to 17 years old) accounted for almost half of all injuries at collection sites among whole blood donors, and some of the injuries (e.g., concussions, lacerations, and dental injuries) required urgent medical care.[3]

Risk factors associated with reactions after blood donation

Many studies have evaluated donor characteristics and other variables that influence the risk of immediate and delayed reactions after allogeneic blood donation, and the strength of the conclusions depends on the study design and statistical analysis to control for confounding variables. An overview of risk factors and the strength of the available evidence that supports a possible association with syncopal reactions after allogeneic blood donation is summarized in Table 5.2.[7] The strongest, independent risk factors for both immediate and delayed reactions consistently identified in several well-controlled studies of whole blood donation are young age (<23 years old), first-time donation status, total blood volume (<3.5 L) and estimated blood loss (>15%), and, in most studies, female sex.[12–14] Young age had the strongest association with complications even after controlling for first-time donation status in one study that showed 16 and 17 year olds were threefold more likely to experience an adverse reaction than older donors.[3] Although regulations in some countries restrict the upper age limit of blood donation, many studies have confirmed the lower observed rates of reactions among elderly donors compared to younger donors.[15,16] A multivariate analysis predicted that young donors (<23 years) with low blood volume contributed about 3% of all donations but disproportionately accounted for about 10% to 15% of presyncopal reactions and syncope-related complications after whole blood

Table 5.2 Variables associated with syncopal reactions after blood donation

Independent variables strongly associated with increased risk (strong evidence based on multivariate analysis in multiple studies):
- First-time vs. repeat donation status
- Young (<23 years) vs. older age
- Low body weight/total blood volume (<3.5 L) with standard WB donation (~525 mL)
- Female vs. male sex
- Caucasian vs. African ethnicity

Variables associated with increased risk (weak or no association in some studies, inconsistent or low-quality evidence, and poorly controlled or univariate analysis)
- Admitted anxiety
- Collection volume
- Greater than 4 hours since last meal
- Temperature/season
- Wait time
- Duration of phlebotomy
- History of fainting not related to blood donation
- Mobile blood drive
- History of prior reactions after blood donation

Variables not associated with reactions (strong evidence, multivariate analysis)
- Predonation blood pressure

Table 5.3 Strategies to reduce reactions among young blood donors

Predonation education
Drive setup and environment
Staff supervision and phlebotomist skills
Selection criteria (e.g., estimated blood volume) for whole blood donors
Automated red cell collection
Interventions
- Water ingestion before donation and within 10–20 min of phlebotomy
- Distraction during phlebotomy
- Muscle tension during phlebotomy
Postreaction instructions to donors and parents

donation.[14] Many other variables related to the donor, environment, or staff have been reported to have weaker associations with immediate adverse reactions after blood donation, although the supporting data are generally weak and often not consistent among studies.[7] Finally, autologous blood donors might have significant medical conditions that potentially increases their risk for postdonation reactions compared to healthy, allogeneic blood donors.[17]

Most publications report on immediate donation-related reactions or reactions that occur soon after the blood donation, and less information is available on possible chronic complications. But in a recent study, allogeneic blood donation did not have a long-term effect on the risk of cardiac ischemia.[18] Germain *et al.* compared a group of 50,889 eligible blood donors who made 0.36 donations/year to 12,357 donors disqualified for false-positive infectious disease markers as a control group of healthy donors during a 17-year study in Canada.[18] There was no statistical difference in the incidence of hospitalizations or deaths attributable to coronary heart disease in the group of donors who remained eligible (3.60/1000 person-years) compared to the control group of disqualified donors (3.52/1000 person-years; rate ratio 1.02; 95% confidence interval, 0.92–1.13).

Preventing syncopal reactions at blood drives

Focusing on the factors that most strongly predict immediate and delayed reactions, blood centers have recently applied strategies to improve safety for the youngest and most susceptible group of blood donors. In 2008, an AABB Task Force recommended that blood centers adopt one or more of the measures in Table 5.3 to reduce reactions among young donors, and develop monitoring programs to continually assess donation safety.[19] Operational tactics to improve donation safety aim to recruit donors less likely to have reactions, to modify the drive environment, or to use automated (apheresis) procedures instead of whole blood collection. Physiologic strategies may reduce an individual blood donor's risk of a reaction, such as having the donor drink water shortly before the phlebotomy or perform applied muscle tension maneuvers.[20]

Psychological aspects of the donation experience may be addressed by gauging donors' fear and anxiety, providing donors with information about coping strategies before blood donation, or distracting their attention during the phlebotomy. Each measure is supported to varying degrees by controlled trials or by observational data and predictive models.

In 2009, the American Red Cross and Blood Systems Inc. independently made operational changes in their standard practice in an effort to reduce syncopal reactions among young whole blood donors.[21,22] Both centers introduced precautionary measures, which included new donor selection criteria that required individuals to have an estimated blood volume greater than 3.5 L to prevent loss of more than 15% of their total blood volume with a standard whole blood donation. The AABB Standards define the minimum donor weight (50 kg or 110 lbs.) and maximum collection volume (10.5 mL/kg) in order to limit acute blood loss. These measures protect most but not all donors, especially young female donors who have an estimated blood volume less than 3.5 L based on the Nadler equation that takes into account sex, height, and weight. These young, female donors with low blood volume disproportionately account for the presyncopal reactions and syncope-related complications. The programs at both American Red Cross and BSI also addressed donor education, drive environment and supervision, predonation water, and muscle tension during collection.

In the American Red Cross, full implementation of the new donor selection criteria and other preventive measures resulted in a 33%, 25%, and 18% reduction in reactions among 16-, 17- and 18-year-old donors, respectively, compared to the baseline rates before the operational changes.[21] The benefit was most pronounced for the youngest, most susceptible donors. When the data were stratified for first-time donation status and sex, 16-year-old girls had the same relative risk of presyncopal reactions as their 19-year-old counterparts (Figure 5.1). Moreover, a significant 14% decrease in syncope was observed among 16-year-old donors with the new selection criteria. The rate of injuries at the collections sites was low in each year, but no consistent changes were observed over time for any age group. The most encouraging result, however, has been the sustained reduction in the overall reaction rates among 16–18-year-old donors observed over the subsequent two years, despite the dynamic nature of operations on high school drives, and the increased recruitment of young donors each year (Figure 5.1).[21]

Similarly, Tomasulo and colleagues at Blood Systems reported that using the new selection criteria to ensure an estimated blood volume of at least 3.5 L for 17- to 22-year-olds and other

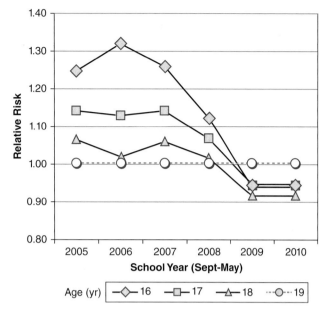

Figure 5.1 Relative risk of reactions among female, novice (first-time) whole blood donors by age (16 to 19 years), comprising different age groups (16 to 18 years compared to 19 years; relative risk = 1.0). Before implementing the safety measures (2005–2007), the overall rate of reactions was highest among 16-year-olds compared to their older peers. The new selection criteria for estimated blood volume became effective in the 2009 school year, and eliminated the excess risk for the young donors compared to 19-year-olds. The benefit has been sustained over 2 years.

interventions decreased the aggregate reaction rates in male and female donors by 24%.[22] In addition, the measures were associated with a 25% decrease in delayed reactions occurring more than four minutes after the phlebotomy was completed, and a 38% decrease in off-site reactions among female donors. Falls were infrequent in all donor groups, occurring at a rate of 1.4 per 1000 donations before the interventions. Multivariate analysis clearly showed that the interventions decreased the occurrence of reactions in susceptible groups, but the known risk factors (young age, first-time donation status) were still associated with relatively higher reaction rates than the comparison groups.[22]

These data from the American Red Cross and Blood Systems independently support the benefit of the selection criteria for estimated blood volume to mitigate reactions among young donors, largely to the extent predicted by statistical models.[21,22] In both reports, the aggregate effect of the selection criteria for estimated blood volume reduced reactions by at least 20% in susceptible groups. As expected, the measures did not eliminate the risk of reactions after whole blood donation. Both blood centers noted that the inconsistent or incomplete implementation of the provision of water and use of applied muscle tension likely limited the effectiveness of these interventions. Both studies also documented a low rate of falls or injuries at the collection sites in all donor groups, which did not change after introducing the operational changes. These studies were large enough to detect a 20% reduction in these uncommon events but may have missed a smaller difference. Alternate approaches to predict and prevent presyncopal reactions that show promise in small trials evaluate collecting smaller volumes (350 mL rather than 450 mL) from young (16- to 18-year-old) first-time donors, screening to identify and educate fearful donors, and predonation measurements of hemodynamic responses to

standing before and after water ingestion.[23–26] Unfortunately, no single preventive measure has been shown to have a significant effect on the rare but potentially serious injuries resulting from syncope after whole blood donation. Future operational efforts and research studies should evaluate other possible evidence-based approaches to reduce the risk of syncope after whole blood donation.

Phlebotomy-related complications

Whole blood and apheresis collections utilize large-bore (16-gauge needles) for phlebotomy, which achieve rapid blood flow and minimize clotting and hemolysis but also introduce a risk of injury.[27] General guidelines for phlebotomy emphasize the importance of staff training, technique, and experience, as well as knowledge of the anatomy of the antecubital area and careful selection of the vein.[28] The median cubital vein, in the center of the antecubital space near the elbow crease, is often prominent and well-anchored lying between muscles, making it a good first choice for phlebotomy. The basilic vein, located on the medial aspect (i.e., closest to the body) of the forearm, runs close to the brachial artery and nerve and is less likely to be visible or palpable, which increases the risk of nerve injury or arterial puncture. Although these generalizations are useful guides, the anatomic relationships are more complex and variable than depicted in textbooks.[29] Cutaneous nerve branches are closely associated with veins and anatomic variation is common, making it impossible to avoid them completely during phlebotomy. Needle adjustment after insertion should be limited to no more than one forward-to-backward maneuver, with careful attention to the donor's comfort level. The phlebotomy should be discontinued if the donor cannot tolerate the venipuncture, and the needle should be removed if it is readily apparent that the venipuncture was not successful. Despite adherence to these general guidelines and good technique, phlebotomy as with any invasive procedure carries with it inherent risk that cannot be completely eliminated.

Adverse reactions such as sore arms, hematomas, or bruises are relatively common but usually self-limiting; rarely, more severe nerve injuries or chronic complications occur after phlebotomy. Hematomas are raised areas of localized swelling, and bruises (contusions) are flat areas of discoloration. Both result from local injury and blood leaking from the punctured blood vessel that accumulates in the subcutaneous tissue and spreads along fascial planes. As the swelling subsides, the extravasated blood is broken down and reabsorbed, and the area can change in shape, size, and discoloration over a spectrum of blue, black, purple, yellow, and green before resolving completely within a few weeks.

Hematomas or bruises may be noted by the staff at the collection site, but more often develop after the donor leaves the drive, complicating about 1% of whole blood and 3.5% of apheresis donations (Table 5.1). When donors were questioned about bruises or other symptoms several weeks after a donation, additional information was elicited about minor complications and the rate of bruises reached 8% to 22%.[8,9] Although this suggests that some minor reactions are not routinely captured, the available blood center data still serve as a relevant gauge of the more severe or concerning reactions, and identify hematomas that cause such discomfort, pain, or distress that about 1 in 10,000 whole blood and apheresis blood donors seek outside medical care (Table 5.1).

Hematomas may be alarming to donors, especially if they extend along the arm or progress through the various stages of discoloration, but typically resolve completely within a few weeks. Treatment of the area with ice immediately and intermittently for

24 hours after the phlebotomy, followed by warm compresses or soaks, may provide symptomatic relief and promote healing. Over-the-counter medications such as acetaminophen may also be taken as directed for pain. In very rare cases, the phlebotomy site may show signs of infection or septic phlebitis (e.g., redness, swelling, or "red streaks" extending up the arm), which may be treated with antibiotics or resolve on its own. In case reports, superficial venous thrombosis in the upper extremity has occurred after blood donation, although a causal relationship with the donation may not be clearly established.

Arterial puncture is suspected in about 1.4 in 10,000 whole blood donations (Table 5.1). Signs of an arterial puncture are rapid filling of the collection bag, often within 3 minutes; bright red blood; and pulsatile flow. All of these signs might not be present, making some arterial sticks difficult to distinguish from venous draws. Possible arterial punctures are more often reported in young, male donors, but can occur in other donors because of anatomical variation in the location of the artery in the forearm. Whenever a possible arterial puncture is suspected, staff should discontinue the collection, remove the needle, and apply direct pressure to the site for 10 minutes or more, until bleeding has stopped. Donors typically recover without rebleeding or further consequences, but about 7% of donors with a suspected arterial puncture sought additional medical care, likely related to the resultant hematoma or bruise. In extremely rare cases, an arterial puncture has resulted in complications that required surgical intervention, such as pseudoaneurysm (three published reports), arteriovenous fistula (four published reports), or compartment syndrome (two published reports), after whole blood donation.[27]

Phlebotomy-related nerve injury

Phlebotomy-related nerve injuries are uncommon and typically resolve without sequelae within weeks, but in rare cases have long-term debilitating consequences. Most patients experience characteristic symptoms when the needle is advanced in the arm suggestive of direct nerve trauma, often described as sharp, shooting pain or tingling that radiates to the hands or fingers. Donors may also report immediate numbness or tingling that persists after removing the needle or intense pain with burning, lancinating, or electrical sensations. The relationship of hematoma formation to the development of nerve damage and symptoms is unclear, and most hematomas do not cause symptoms suggestive of nerve irritation. However, hematomas may aggravate nerve dysfunction and pain possibly by impinging on damaged nerves or traumatized areas.[29,30]

Based on hemovigilance data from the American Red Cross, suspected nerve injuries occurred in about 3 in 10,000 whole blood donors; of those, 13% sought additional medical care after the event (Table 5.1). Almost all (>90%) donors who report symptoms of nerve injuries will recover completely within three months.[30] Some donors may report mild residual numbness that persists over an extended duration. Permanent nerve injury after phlebotomy is an extremely uncommon but potentially debilitating outcome, and reliable estimates on its incidence are not available because it is so infrequently encountered among blood donors. Given the close association of nerves with veins and the unavoidable possibility of direct injury to nerves with phlebotomy, factors other than direct nerve contact by the needle appear to be necessary for the chronic pain syndrome to occur. Chronic regional pain syndrome type 2 (CRPS II, previously called causalgia or reflex sympathetic dystrophy) describes neuropathic pain after confirmed nerve injuries. CRPS symptoms vary in severity and duration, but most cases are mild and individuals recover gradually with time. In more severe cases, individuals may have long-term disability. Treatment options for CRPS neuropathic pain include rehabilitation and occupational therapy, psychotherapy to treat associated depression and psychological symptoms, medications, sympathetic nerve block, and surgical sympathectomy. No drugs have yet been approved by the US Food and Drug Administration (FDA) to treat CRPS, but several different classes of drugs such as nonsteroidal anti-inflammatory drugs, corticosteroids, opioids, and botulinum toxin injections have been used to effectively treat some patients, especially early in the course of disease.

Reactions after automated collection of blood components

Advances in apheresis (automated) technology now allow simultaneous collection of multiple standard blood components during a single procedure, yielding various combinations of plasma and blood components such as two units of red blood cells (double red cell collection [2RBC]) or two or three units of platelets (double or triple plateletpheresis), often with a concurrent unit of plasma from one donation. Blood centers have increasingly relied on apheresis donors to optimize the collection process, and increase operational efficiency and cost-effectiveness. Continuing on an upward trend in recent years, apheresis platelets accounted for over 90% of the platelet units produced in the United States in 2011.[1] Triple plateletpheresis contributes substantially to that increase, accounting for about 15% of the apheresis platelet units distributed by the American Red Cross. Similarly, 2RBC collections continue to increase each year, now accounting for 12.6% of the total US supply of red cell units in 2011.[1]

As with whole blood donation, automated (apheresis) procedures are generally well tolerated, but some donors will experience phlebotomy-related or syncopal complications (Table 5.1). In addition, apheresis complications may result specifically from the device or anticoagulant (e.g., citrate reactions), preparatory regimens (e.g., G-CSF and/or corticosteroids for neutrophil collection), or frequency of procedures. The available data from several different blood centers, however, suggest that automated collections have a favorable safety profile compared to whole blood donation.[31,32] Hematomas are the most frequent complication and are more commonly reported after apheresis than WB donation because automated collections often use both arms for venous access (Table 5.1). The overall rate of minor complications at the collection site is higher for automated procedures than WB collections, reflecting primarily minor citrate reactions and small hematomas. Automated collection procedures had lower rates of presyncope and syncope than whole blood donation, which likely reflects donor demographics, more stringent selection criteria, and the use of saline replacement with automated procedures.

Medically serious complications are less likely after apheresis than WB collection, with observed rates of major complications at the collection site of 7.4, 5.2, and 3.3 per 10,000 donations for WB, plateletpheresis, and automated red cell procedures, respectively.[2] Similar rates of reactions requiring additional medical care occurred after WB donation (3.2 per 10,000) compared to automated procedures (2.9 per 10,000).[2] Hospitalization after donation was reported for 46 whole blood donors (1 in 130,749 donations) and eight apheresis donors (1 in 84,722 donations); a causal relationship between the donation and the hospitalization was not established in all cases.

As observed for whole blood donation, multivariate analysis reveals that young age, first-time donation status, female gender, and low weight are independently associated with the risk of reactions after automated red cell collection and plateletpheresis. Yuan *et al.* reported moderate to severe adverse events in 47 per 10,000 plateletpheresis or automated red cell collections over a 2-year period in a hospital-based donor center, and found that small, female donors with lower predonation hematocrit were at higher risk of moderate to severe vasovagal-type reactions than other donors, especially when RBCs were collected.[33] Reactions had a similar dampening effect on return donation by first-time apheresis donors comparable to that observed for whole blood donors. Among experienced donors, however, reactions had less of an effect on retention and decreased the rate of return by about 28% for whole blood donors but only about 4% for 2RBC donors.[6]

Citrate reactions and other immediate complications during apheresis procedures

Citrate is used as an anticoagulant during apheresis procedures because it effectively chelates divalent cations such as calcium to transiently and immediately inhibit the coagulation cascade. Citrate causes minimal side effects in donor plasmapheresis because the citrate is mostly in the retained plasma. Plateletpheresis, large-volume leukapheresis, and hematopoietic progenitor cell collection are more likely to expose the donor to the effects of citrate toxicity. Greater exposure to citrate during triple plateletpheresis was associated with an increase in mild citrate reactions compared to double plateletpheresis, but did not substantially affect donor safety or product quality in one study.[34] Symptoms are usually transient and rapidly reversible because of citrate metabolism occurs within minutes in the liver, kidneys, and muscles. In addition, release of parathyroid hormone mobilizes calcium from body stores and increases its absorption from the kidney to restore calcium hemostasis. Despite these compensatory mechanisms, citrate infusion can acutely decrease the concentration of ionized calcium to cause symptoms such as perioral tingling and paresthesias, chills, nausea, twitching, and tremors during the apheresis procedure. If severe, citrate toxicity can progress to carpopedal spasm, seizures, tetany, and cardiac arrhythmia.

Prompt attention to mild symptoms usually requires only pausing the procedure, slowing the re-infusion rate, or decreasing the amount of citrate infused by increasing the whole blood-to-citrate ratio and allowing for dilution and clearance of citrate. In addition, donors may be given oral calcium in the form of calcium-containing antacids (e.g., Tums), or the procedure may be stopped if symptoms persist or worsen. Intravenous calcium is rarely if ever needed to reverse the citrate effect during donor apheresis procedures and should not be used in routine practice. Donors who have had severe or unusual citrate reactions during automated procedures should be evaluated for possible underlying factors or medications such as loop diuretics that could predispose to these adverse events. The propensity for citrate reactions depends not only on donor characteristics, but also on device-related factors, such as the citrate infusion rate or extracorporeal volume of the device.

Oral calcium supplementation during automated collection procedures may reduce the severity of parasthesias and improve ionized and total calcium levels.[35] However, multivariate analysis revealed that oral administration of calcium was not associated with a reduction in overall symptom development and did not prevent the occurrence of more severe symptoms during donor apheresis procedures.[35] The possible significance of long-term metabolic effects of repeated citrate exposure on bone mobilization and calcium metabolism are not well characterized and remain an area of study.

Equipment and disposables used in apheresis collections may cause unusual reactions in rare cases, such as allergic reactions among repeat donors linked to plateletpheresis collection sets sterilized with ethylene oxide.[31,32] Preventive measures include avoiding use of certain disposables if sensitization is suspected, or minimizing exposure to ethylene oxide by repeatedly priming the disposable collection set or using kits closest to their expiration dates. Air embolism is a very rare complication of apheresis procedures because the instruments have sensors to detect air within the extravascular circuit that stop the procedure. But symptoms of air embolism are still possible if more than 3–8 mL/kg of air enters the donor's venous system through either a leak in the access, instrument failure, or operator's error. These symptoms of air embolism include dyspnea, tachypnea, cyanosis, tachycardia, and hypotension as air enters the right ventricle and pulmonary artery with obstruction of the right ventricular output and pulmonary artery vasoconstriction. If collection staff expect air embolism, they should stop the procedure and place the donor in the Trendelenberg position (i.e., lay the donor on their back and raise their feet higher than their head) on their left side. If the air does not dissipate or symptoms worsen, surgical intervention to aspirate the air through a pulmonary artery catheter may be necessary.

Procedure-related complications related to donation frequency or multiple component collection

The high volume and efficiency of apheresis collection procedures, as well as the frequency and allowable interval for repeat donations, pose potential acute and long-term risks to donors, such as cellular depletion, iron depletion, and serum protein loss. The current regulations that govern donor selection define precautions for adequate pre- and postprocedure cell counts and serum protein values before donation, as well as limits on the donation interval and frequency for apheresis procedures.

After plateletpheresis, a donor's platelet count may decrease by 20–30% but quickly returns to baseline within about four days.[31] Current FDA-approved apheresis devices have different methods to ensure that the donor's platelet count remains above a predefined set value at the completion of the procedure, typically 100 platelet/μL, which have been validated in practice by blood centers. An intensive schedule of serial plateletpheresis procedures (e.g., 5–15 procedures within 10–30 days) was associated with only transient decreases in platelet counts, which in some cases rebounded to above baseline values about a week after the final procedure. The transient platelet count decrease and recovery after serial collection procedures are generally larger and last longer for female donors than male donors, but changes are transient and recovery occurred promptly after donation.

Recently, evidence of progressive decreases in platelet counts after years of donation in some individuals raised concerns about possible long-term effects of frequent apheresis platelet donation.[36–38] Lazarus *et al.* retrospectively examined platelet counts from 939 individuals who had 11,464 plateletpheresis donations over four years, and described sustained decreases in platelet counts in some donors that correlated with donation frequency. However, these observations were not observed by other large blood centers. A retrospective review of plateletpheresis records at a regional blood center revealed no clinically important decrease in platelet counts among individuals donating multiple platelet components up to 24 times per year, regardless of interdonation interval.[38] These observations were confirmed by several other facilities, and the available data do not demonstrate clinically important changes in platelet or lymphocyte counts in frequent plateletpheresis donors. Plateletpheresis procedures collect negligible red cells in the component, but frequent plateletpheresis donors lose as much as 80–100 mL of whole blood with each donation as a result of samples taken for infectious disease testing and residual red cell loss in the collection sets. Chronic, small-volume red cell losses sufficient to cause iron depletion have been described in case reports of frequent plateletpheresis donors.

Several studies have examined the long-term effects of intensive plasmapheresis regimens on donor serum protein, albumin, and immunoglobulin levels. Serial plasmapheresis donors can give 625–800 mL of plasma twice weekly in the United States, provided they meet all selection criteria. Serum protein, albumin, and IgG concentration are statistically lower in frequent plasmapheresis donors compared to nondonors, but their levels do not correlate with the intensity of donation and remain stable over time in most donors.[39,40] Moreover, plasmapheresis donors who gave up to 45 L of plasma per year did not develop impaired humoral and cellular immunity, maintained adequate iron stores, and did not show signs of increased cardiovascular risk by biochemical measures.[39] Only 4–16% of regular donors discontinued plasma donation when IgG, total serum protein, or hemoglobin fell below acceptable values; most donors stopped for socioeconomic or medical reasons unrelated to plasma donation.[40] Taken together, these studies support the safety of long-term intensive donor plasmapheresis under the current regulations, and provide some reassurance about the reasons that donors discontinue participation in the programs. Finally, none of the 12 deaths following source plasma donation that were reported to the FDA in 2005–2006 were determined to have a causal relationship with the plasmapheresis procedure.[41]

Special considerations: granulocyte collection

Granulocyte collection (leukapheresis) poses unique risks for donor complications.[1] To collect sufficient numbers of granulocytes for an adequate therapeutic dose, healthy donors are given corticosteroids (e.g., dexamethasone) and/or granulocyte colony-stimulating factor (G-CSF) prior to the leukapheresis procedure. G-CSF may cause short-term side effects such as bone pain, myalgia, and headache in granulocyte donors. The rare complication of splenic rupture seen with hematopoietic progenitor cell collection has not been reported in G-CSF-stimulated granulocyte donors, likely because of the lower dose and shorter course of treatment. To date, the available data support the use of G-CSF stimulation in volunteer donors and have not detected long-term cardiac, inflammatory, or malignant consequences among granulocyte donors who received G-CSF on three or more occasions.[42]

The risk of subcapsular cataracts in granulocyte donors who received corticosteroids has been evaluated in two controlled studies. Differences between the treatment and the control (unstimulated) groups were not significant, but the tendency for bilateral occurrence of cataracts was observed exclusively among glucocorticoid-stimulated granulocyte donors. The relatively small size of both studies suggests that ongoing surveillance is prudent to better define the prevalence of posterior subcapsular cataracts in this donor population.[43,44]

Iron deficiency after blood donation

The impact of blood donation on depleting donor iron stores has been recognized for well over 30 years.[45,46] With each whole blood collection of 500 ml, an average of 200–250 mg of iron from

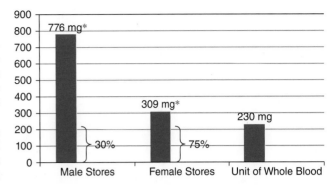

Figure 5.2 Iron stores versus iron removed from donation. Source: Cook *et al.* (2003).[53] Reproduced with permission of the American Society of Hematology.

RBC hemoglobin is removed. This amount represents about 25% of the average iron stores in men but almost 75% of the iron stores in women (Figure 5.2). The acute iron loss is replenished by gastrointestinal (GI) absorption of dietary iron, which occurs gradually over many months. However, individuals may donate blood as frequently as every 56 days (in North America), an insufficient time for a donor to replace the iron that is lost. The cumulative effects of repetitive blood donation at shorter intervals than iron can be replenished eventually results in a deficit in body iron that is dependent primarily on donation intensity and gender, as well as other factors to be discussed in this chapter. In addition, the consequences of iron depletion in terms of donor well-being and potential strategies to manage donor iron loss, including extending the minimum required donation interval, decreasing donation frequency, testing of iron status, and iron supplementation, will be considered.

Brief review of iron physiology

Iron is an essential element involved in several key physiologic processes. In association with heme, it facilitates the reversible binding of oxygen by red blood cells and the binding of oxygen to muscle myoglobin and mitochondrial cytochromes. Nonheme iron is involved in the actions of a number of cellular enzymes. Dietary iron is absorbed by enterocytes in the duodenum and proximal jejunum. Absorption is tightly regulated because iron in excessive amounts is toxic to cells (e.g., by generation of ferric peroxides and free radicals) and there is no defined mechanism of excretion. Iron from animal sources (heme iron) is more bioavailable (~35% absorbed) than nonheme iron (vegetable sources: ~10% absorbed).[47] Men normally absorb ~1 mg/day, equaling basal losses from the GI tract and skin. Iron absorption in premenopausal women is ~0.5 mg/day greater, because of additional losses from menstruation. Absorption capacity increases in proportion to the level of iron deficiency (Figure 5.3), reaching a maximum that averages 4–5 mg/day in frequent donors,[48,70] and is enhanced with supplemental iron.[49]

Hepcidin has been recognized as the master regulator of iron homeostasis. This 25-amino-acid peptide hormone produced in the liver controls iron absorption and release of iron from storage sites through inhibition of the transmembrane iron receptor, ferroportin.[50,51] In iron deficiency, hepcidin decreases, permitting ferroportin to shuttle iron into enterocytes from the intestinal lumen and out of hepatic and other storage sites, to be transported by transferrin for cellular uptake via transferrin receptors located on early erythroid and, to a lesser extent, other nucleated cells. Iron not

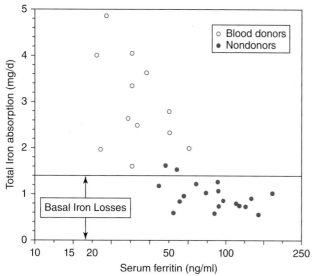

Figure 5.3 Iron absorption in blood donors. Modified from Hallberg *et al.* (1997).[47] Reproduced with permission of American Society for Nutrition.

Table 5.4 Assessment of Iron Status in Blood Donors

- Ferritin
- Soluble transferrin receptor (sTfR)
- Soluble transferrin receptor/ferritin ratio
- Zinc (Free Erythrocyte) Protoporphyrin (ZPP)
- Red blood cell parameters (HYPOm, CHr)

HYPOm % hypochromic mature RBC; CHr, hemoglobin content of reticulocytes.

directly utilized in physiologic pathways is stored in tissues as ferritin; small amounts present in blood are in equilibrium with tissue ferritin, which is considered a reliable indicator of available storage iron, especially in healthy blood donors, who have low rates of inflammatory conditions that can result in elevated ferritin values irrespective of iron status.[52] The total body iron content in men averages approximately 50 mg/kg (~4000 mg), whereas women have 35 mg/kg (~2500 mg). The majority of the total (70–80%) exists in red blood cells bound to hemoglobin. Approximately 10% of body iron is engaged in other cellular physiologic functions, such as enzymes and cytochromes, or bound to transferrin. Only 10–20% of the total is present in the form of tissue iron stores that are available for erythropoiesis and metabolic use. Cook *et al.* estimated tissue iron stores of 776 ± 313 mg in men and 309 ± 346 mg in women.[53] The loss of approximately 230 mg iron with each whole blood donation along with the limited stores and capacity for absorption lead to a high incidence of iron deficiency in frequent donors, especially women.

Measurement of iron status

The only point-of-care screening test currently used to qualify a blood donor is the capillary (fingerstick) hemoglobin $\geq$12.5 g/dL in both women and men in the United States and Canada. Some countries have adopted a higher standard in men (e.g., 13.0 or 13.5 gm/dl) that reflects the higher range of normal for hemoglobin.[54] The minimum hemoglobin threshold is intended to prevent collection of blood from donors with anemia (this is approximate, because according to WHO the lower range of normal hemoglobin in women is 12.0, and the lower range for men is 13.0 gm/dl), but does not prevent collection of blood from donors who are iron deficient. Various laboratory tests have been used to assess the iron status of blood donors and are listed in Table 5.4.

Serum (or plasma) ferritin

Ferritin, a protein that stores excess iron and releases it in a controlled way, reflects the level of tissue iron stores and can be assayed in either serum or plasma. Using EDTA

(ethylenediaminetetraacetic acid) plasma, ferritin concentration is ~5% lower than serum.[55] Blood levels are believed to result from passive equilibration from cell or tissue sites. Each ng/ml of ferritin in blood equals 8–10 mg of iron in the storage compartment.[56,57] Normal population values differ by gender and age, with adult males age 20–60 years reaching a plateau between 134 and 150 ng/ml, and females 20–59 years between 32 and 53 ng/ml.[58] Ferritin increases in women after menopause, so that after age 60 the average is 86 ng/ml. The "classic" cutoff value, 12 ng/ml, has been utilized as a specific but insensitive indicator of absent iron stores in the clinical setting[59] and in blood donors.[60] One study found that this cutoff failed to identify iron depletion in over one-third of cases in blood donors.[61] Two clinical studies based largely on bone marrow staining for iron have found 15 ng/ml to more accurately reflect iron deficiency anemia.[62,63] Studies based on increased levels of soluble transferrin receptor (sTfR), a truncated form of the transferrin receptor that is released into blood when early erythroid cells become deprived of iron, suggest a ferritin concentration of 22–40 ng/ml is more sensitive as an indication of iron-deficient erythropoiesis.[64,65]

The classic description by Finch correlated a drop in ferritin levels with blood donation activity, showing that a ferritin level of less than 12 ng/mL increased with the number of donations in the previous year.[45] Simon *et al.*, in an observational study of blood donors, showed that the frequency of iron depletion as measured by serum ferritin $\leq$12 ng/ml was zero in male first-time donors but 12% in female first-time donors, reflecting the impact of menstrual blood loss.[46] The frequency in men increased to 2% and in women increased to 20% with three blood donations in one year. A direct effect of donation intensity on iron stores has been shown in multiple studies, which indicate a stronger effect of donation frequency (i.e., donations/year) rather than lifetime donations (Figure 5.4).[66,67]

Soluble transferrin receptor

The highest density of transferrin receptors exists on the surface of erythroid cells. A reduction in iron availability leads to increased TfR synthesis and shedding of soluble transferrin receptors (hence sTfR) into the blood. Levels greater than the normal reference range (95% CI) suggest tissue iron deficiency in the absence of conditions that are also known to increase sTfR levels, including accelerated erythropoietic proliferative activity (e.g., hemolytic anemia and thalassemia), race (~9% higher in black subjects), and altitude (also ~9% higher).[56] Because of the lack of a reference standard for transferrin, the results vary according to the assay used. However, research studies indicate sTfR levels reflect the functional iron compartment and correlate with depleted iron stores in bone marrow preparations[59] and the response to oral iron therapy in otherwise healthy females with anemia.[68]

As iron depletion progresses to the stage of tissue iron deficiency, sTfR continues to increase as ferritin levels reach the lower limit of

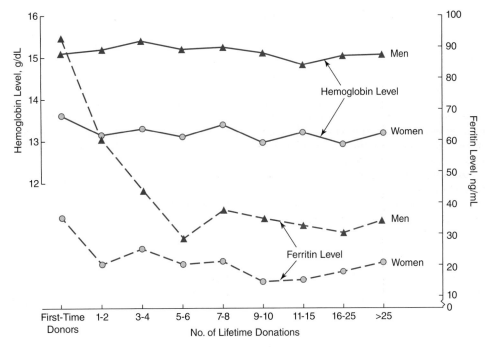

Figure 5.4 Changes in hemoglobin and ferritin with successive blood donations.[46]

detection. sTfR values (representing functional iron deficiency) have been combined with ferritin measurements (representing storage iron levels) into a ratio, log sTfR/ferritin.[61,69,71] A sTfR/ log ferritin "index" has also been utilized to distinguish iron-deficient erythropoiesis from storage iron depletion.[59,68] However, an advantage to using the log sTfR/ferritin construct was demonstrated by Skikne and Cook,[53,64] who were able to assess iron stores quantitatively by performing careful measurements of iron loss in serial phlebotomy subjects bled until they became iron depleted, as expressed by the formula:

$$\text{Body iron(mg/kg)} = -[\log(\text{sTfR}/\text{Ferritin}) - 2.8229]/0.1207$$

This methodology allows an estimation of tissue iron stores, which can be uniquely expressed as the iron surplus in stores (positive values) or the iron deficit (negative values) in tissues, and also permits an estimation of iron absorption in blood donors in longitudinal studies.[49,70]

In the REDS-II Donor Iron Status Evaluation (RISE) study (described in the "Other Measures" section), sTfR did not correlate with iron-deficient erythropoiesis (IDE) as well as plasma ferritin, R^2 0.54 versus R^2 −0.96.[69] A log sTfR/ferritin value of 2.07 (97.5% of the upper limit of the reference range) equated to a ferritin level of 26.7 µg/L by multivariate regression, suggesting this ferritin level reflected iron-deficient erythropoiesis in healthy blood donors. At this threshold, ferritin had 95.1% sensitivity and 89.6% specificity in identifying IDE, and sTfR added little additional diagnostic information.

Other measures

A limitation with ferritin testing in blood donors is that results may not be available for several days. A point-of-care test using capillary (fingerstick) samples is being evaluated to assess blood donor iron status. Zinc protoporphyrin (ZnPP), also called free erythrocyte protoporphyrin (FEP), can be measured in capillary samples using a portable hematofluorometer. During the last step of porphyrin ring

synthesis, zinc is chelated by protoporphyrin IX if iron is limited, resulting in increased levels of erythrocyte ZnPP–mole Heme (ferrous protoporphyrin).[72] Lead intoxication and thalassemia, conditions that have a low prevalence in blood donors, also result in elevated values.[73] A study of over 5000 accepted blood donors found that 6.9% of male donors and 9.8% of female donors had subclinical iron deficiency as defined by ZnPP levels of ≥100 mmol/ molheme.[74] Some studies show early detection of iron deficiency and correlation with hemoglobin deferral in blood donors. One trial showed that a positive predictive value of ZnPP in predicting deferral of the donor after one or two donations was 75%, and a serum ferritin concentration ≤12 µg/L of only 26%.[75] Another trial reported that elevated ZnPP levels (using venous, not capillary, blood) aided in the prediction of subsequent hemoglobin deferral when added to other variables, including previous hemoglobin value, age, gender, time since previous visit, and total number of blood donations over two years.[74] However, an attempt to validate this model in another donor population using different hemoglobin eligibility criteria was unsuccessful.[76]

Changes in conventional red blood cell morphologic parameters, including mean corpuscular volume (MCV), mean cell hemoglobin (MCH), and mean corpuscular hemoglobin concentration (MCHC), occur late in the development of iron depletion and are insensitive, resulting in low correlation with reduced iron levels (R^2 minus 0.08–0.17).[78] RBC parameters including MCHC (<330 g/l; $R^2 = 0.12$) and MCV (<80 fl; $R^2 = 0.00$) were inferior to hemoglobin ($R^2 = 0.63$) in predicting subsequent hemoglobin deferral in another study.[79]

Although not a point-of-care test, measurement of RBC indices by laser light scatter using specialized hematology analyzers (ADVIA 120, Siemens Healthcare Diagnostics, Deerfield, IL, USA; and Sysmex XE-5000, Kobe, Japan), with "same-day" results available within hours, has also been evaluated in blood donors.[77,80] Selected RBC subpopulations have been found to be more sensitive indicators of functional iron deficiency than biochemical iron tests in renal failure patients who are treated with erythroid stimulating agents, in pregnancy, and in pediatric patients with iron deficiency.[80,81–83] In young women with iron deficiency anemia, the percentage of hypochromic mature red blood cells (%HYPOm) was found to correlate with sTfR (area under the receiver operating characteristic [ROC] curve, or AUC, of −0.98) and returned to normal after oral iron therapy.[81] CHr (cellular hemoglobin content in reticulocytes) measures incorporation of iron into developing reticulocytes that can be detected within their three-day lifespan.[84] %HYPOm is a time-averaged indicator of iron that is incorporated within the three-month lifespan of mature RBCs. These parameters are analogous to monitoring glucose levels and HbA1c levels in diabetics, respectively. Using the ADVIA 120 analyzer, one study in blood donors found adequate sensitivity of CHr at 32 pg cutoff and HYPOm at 0.3% cutoff individually (57.5% for both measures) and combined (69%) in donors with iron-deficient erythropoiesis, along with excellent specificity (~90%).[61] A smaller study found 81% sensitivity and 89% specificity for a HYPOm equivalent parameter, RBC-Y, and lower sensitivity (69%) versus 93% specificity for CHr at 28 pg level.[71] Each study used the log [sTfR/ferritin] ratio as the "gold standard" to identify iron deficiency. Despite logistical issues, the investigators felt that RBC indices were superior to hemoglobin in the assessment of iron status blood donors.

In the multicenter RISE study, plasma ferritin and sTfR were evaluated in relation to RBC indices, including CHr and the % HYPOm red cells, to characterize absent iron stores (AIS) and IDE in blood donors.[69] The RBC index that performed the best overall was %HYPOm. At a %HYPOm cutoff value of 0.55%, sensitivity/specificity was 85%/57% for AIS and 72%/68% for IDE. CHr had lower diagnostic usefulness than HYPOm or other indices. The RBC assays were better (greater AUC) at identifying more severe iron depletion (i.e., ferritin < 12 ng/ml). In a single-center study in blood donors, CHr using a cutoff value of 28 pg was reported to have excellent specificity for AIS (defined by sTfR/log ferritin >97.5th percentile, or 1.5); however, CHr was not sensitive for detecting "latent" iron-depleted donors.[85] An important limitation in using RBC indices is the manufacturer recommendation for testing within six hours of draw because cell swelling may affect the accuracy of the parameters, including HYPOm, hypochromic red blood cells (HYPOr), cell hemoglobin concentration mean (CHCM), and MCV but not CHr.[69,77]

The RISE study and the other studies summarized above found that RBC indices had only a modest value in assessing the iron status of blood donors. Ferritin provided the most useful laboratory information overall. In the two largest studies, a plasma ferritin value of 26.7 μg/L[69] in one and a serum value of 22 ng/ml[61] in the other provided the optimum discrimination between iron-depleted and iron-replete blood donors, regardless of gender.

Given the central role it plays in regulating iron homeostasis, serum hepcidin levels have also been evaluated in selected populations of blood donors. In non-anemic premenopausal women donors, hepcidin was found to correlate closely with ferritin levels (coefficient 0.66, $p < 0.001$).[86] As a diagnostic test for iron deficiency (defined as ferritin <15 ng/ml), hepcidin compared similarly to other biomarkers such as sTfR, and had an AUC^{ROC} of 0.87 (95% CI 0.82, 0.92). The reference range in non-iron-depleted women was 8.2–199.7 ng/ml. Using ROC analysis, a hepcidin level of 8 ng/ml had a sensitivity of 41.5% and high specificity of 97.6%; at a cut point of 18 ng/ml, sensitivity increased to 79.2% while maintaining specificity of 85.6%. In a longitudinal follow-up study, low baseline hemoglobin (AUC^{ROC} 0.88), ferritin (AUC^{ROC} 0.86), and hepcidin

(AUC^{ROC} 0.81) values were predictive of future low hemoglobin deferrals.[86] Hepcidin and ferritin levels were also reported to be highly correlated in a study of first-time female donors and frequent male donors (Spearman r^2 0.74), and the predicted hemoglobin decline between donations varied according to hepcidin and ferritin. Hemoglobin was found to be 0.51 g/dL lower for subjects with low (≤45.7 ng/mL) or decreasing hepcidin and low ferritin (≤26 ng/mL), and hemoglobin was stable in donors with high (>45.7 ng/mL) or increasing hepcidin and low ferritin (≤26 ng/mL) levels ($p < 0.001$).[87] Based on these findings, hepcidin may provide a useful diagnostic tool in addition to ferritin to assess blood donor iron status.

Prevalence and risk factors for iron deficiency in blood donors

Iron depletion begins with the gradual loss of storage iron, a relatively small compartment as indicated above. Once stores are exhausted, a phase of IDE ensues, which then progresses to iron-deficiency anemia (IDA).[68] Iron deficiency is prevalent in the US population as a whole, especially among premenopausal women, in whom survey data reveal ferritin values <15 ng/ml in 14% of women aged 12–49.[58] In first-time blood donors, iron deficiency (defined as ferritin ≤12 ng/ml) is rare in men (under 1%) and reported in 6.6–12% overall.[46,66] Nearly 70% of the 9 million blood donors who donate annually in the United States are repeat donors, who are especially subject to iron depletion.[1] The prevalence of iron deficiency (using ferritin ≤12 ng/ml) reported in repeat donors ranges from 6 to 16% in men and from 28 to 63% in women.[60,66] Overall, using the most sensitive laboratory measures, iron depletion (defined as iron levels associated with impaired erythropoiesis; see below) is estimated to affect as much as 25–35% of the entire donor population.[88,89] Even individuals who exclusively donate by plateletpheresis may develop low iron because of the increased frequency allowed and fixed red blood cell losses occurring with each procedure (50–80 ml in samples and tubing).[90]

Low hemoglobin, a late consequence of iron deficiency, is the most common reason for donor deferral, with nearly 7% of presenting donors not allowed to donate because they cannot meet the minimum capillary hemoglobin standard of 12.5 gm/dl.[1] Hemoglobin deferral disproportionately affects women, with 17.7% of presenting women and 1.6% of men deferred.[91] Using the WHO defined thresholds of 13 gm/dl in men and 12 gm/dl in women, by definition, all men who are deferred are anemic, as are those women with hemoglobin values below 12 mg/dl. Prevalence estimates of iron depletion are high in hemoglobin-deferred donors. In one study, 53% of women and 61% of the men had iron measurements below lower gender-based limits.[92] The prevalence of iron depletion in controls (nondeferred donors) was also quite high in the study, reflecting the poor correlation of hemoglobin with iron status. Consistent with these findings, an Australian study of premenopausal women found mean ferritin to be lower in hemoglobin-deferred donors, 8.4 ng/ml, versus 27 ng/ml in women who were not deferred ($p < 0.0001$).[93]

Several large observational studies have evaluated risk factors for iron depletion in blood donors. The RISE study[66,89] enrolled and tracked individuals who had not previously donated or not within the prior two years (first-time and reactivated donors, FT/RA), and another cohort consisting of frequent repeat donors (females with >2 donations or males with >3 donations in prior year) longitudinally over a 15–24-month period. At enrollment, female donors of reproductive age were 3–7 times more likely to have AIS, or plasma ferritin ≤12 ng/ml, than menopausal women or male donors. The prevalence of AIS was 0% in FT/RA male donors and 6.6% in FT/RA female donors; IDE was found in 2.5% males and 24% females. In the frequent donors, AIS was found in 16% males and 28% females; iron-deficient erythropoiesis (IDE) was found in 49% of male donors and 67% female donors. In statistical models controlling for demographic, behavioral, and other factors, donation intensity stood out as the most important predictor by far, with those donating 10 or more times over the prior two years 19 times more likely to have AIS than first-time donors and 50 times more likely to have IDE, an intermediate degree of iron depletion. The importance of donation frequency as a contributor to iron depletion in blood donors was highlighted at follow-up nearly two years later, when the prevalence of AIS in the FT/RA donor cohort had tripled in women (from 6.6 to 20%) and rose from 0 to 8% in men; higher increases were noted for IDE.[89] At the end of the study, the overall prevalence of AIS and IDE remained the same within frequent repeat donor cohorts. Donation intensity and female sex were found to be the strongest independent predictors of AIS and/or IDE. Age, weight, smoking, HFE genotype, menstrual, and pregnancy status were less strongly associated. Waiting longer intervals between donations (up to 14 weeks) was associated with lower risk for AIS compared to donations made at shorter intervals, as was taking self-directed iron supplements alone or in a multivitamin combination (reported in 39%). Diet had little or no impact.

A Danish study of nearly 15,000 blood donors also found high rates of iron depletion (ferritin < 15 ng/ml) in individuals donating three times per year for several years: 9% of men, 39% of premenopausal women, and 22% of postmenopausal women.[94] Iron deficiency was strongly associated with sex, menopausal status, blood donation frequency, and the time since the previous donation. The risk of iron depletion was only weakly associated with body weight, intensity of menstruation, and dietary and supplemental iron intake.

Genetic assessment of iron status in blood donors

A novel area of research that may help guide blood donor management in the future involves identifying common molecular polymorphisms that impact iron homeostasis.[52] In hereditary hemochromatosis (HH), defects in several iron pathway mediators or hepcidin leads to excessive accumulation of iron in the body. The FDA has approved a variance allowing blood centers to collect blood from individuals with HH for allogeneic transfusion, if certain requirements are met.[95] In addition, a transferrin polymorphism (G277S mutation) has been described that predisposes individuals to the development of iron deficiency.[96] Despite these considerations, no appreciable effect has been observed involving the transferrin G277S or heterozygous HFE mutations and iron status in blood donors.[97] A variant polymorphism of hypoxia-inducible factor-1α (HIF1α) has been reported to allow more donations without being deferred for low hemoglobin in male donors.[98] Novel polymorphisms involving TMPRSS6 are also being investigated.[99]

Adverse effects of iron depletion

It is well established that iron deficiency anemia results in fatigue and diminished exercise and work capacity. However, there is now increasing evidence that iron deficiency may have adverse effects even without anemia, related to the role of iron in metabolic pathways in the central nervous system and muscle tissue. Fatigue,[100] decreased exercise capacity,[101] pica,[102] restless legs syndrome (RLS),[103] and decreased cognitive performance[104,105] have been reported in association with non-anemic iron deficiency. A survey following blood donation found that fatigue was the third most common adverse event, resulting in a 20% reduction in donor return rates at one year.[106] Women who are fatigued but non-anemic have benefited from iron therapy.[100,107] In one study, premenopausal women with ferritin levels less than 50 ng/ml were randomized to receive intravenous iron or placebo.[100] Fatigue scores were significantly improved after therapy in the subgroup of women with ferritin under 15 ng/ml. In a study of oral iron therapy (80 mg/day elemental iron, ferrous sulfate), non-anemic women with unexplained fatigue in a general practice were found to have reduced fatigue scores after one month of treatment, but only in those with a baseline ferritin level <50 ng/ml.[107]

Fatigue has not been extensively studied in blood donors; however, in a study of 154 non-anemic female blood donors given 80 mg elemental iron versus placebo, fatigue scores were no different in the iron and no-iron groups when measured one month after blood donation and treatment.[108] However, it should be noted that this study was designed to evaluate the acute effect of low ferritin after blood donation. Pre-donation ferritin levels were 36.3 and 34.1 ng/ml in the iron and placebo groups, respectively (i.e., not in the iron-deficient range). Thus, the study did not evaluate the chronic effects of low iron and fatigue in blood donors.

Pica is an eating disorder characterized by the compulsive ingestion of nonfood substances—mostly ice (pagophagia), but including other substances such as chalk, clay, or uncooked starch—that also has been strongly associated with iron deficiency.[109] In the RISE study, pica symptoms were found in 6% of donors when surveyed at end of study, and in a multivariate analysis was eight times more common in women who had ferritin ≤12 ng/ml than in iron-replete women.[103] At the NIH, pica was found in 11% of iron-depleted or -deficient donors (ferritin < 20 ng/ml in women and <30 ng/ml in men) compared to 4% of iron-replete donors (p < 0.0001). Pica symptoms resolved generally within two weeks of starting oral iron therapy.[102] Pica symptoms predominated in female donors in these studies.

RLS is a neuromuscular movement disorder in which patients complain of crawling, aching, or burning sensations in their legs, associated with a compelling urge to move their extremities to relieve the discomfort. Because the symptoms may appear or intensify at rest, the movement disorder may result in sleep disturbances. RLS has been associated with both iron deficiency anemia and non-anemic iron deficiency, which suggests a role for iron in dopaminergic pathways and metabolism.[110] A study in Sweden found the prevalence to be 15% in male donors and 25% in female donors, significantly higher than the prevalence of 6% in men and 11% in women reported in the general population.[111] Using questionnaire data, the RISE study found probable RLS in 9% of donors and possible RLS in 20%; however, there was no correlation with low ferritin levels.[103] At the National Institutes of Health (NIH), restless legs syndrome was reported in 16% of iron depleted or deficient donors and 11% of iron-replete donors (p = 0.012). Clinical improvement took longer than in donors with pica, requiring at least 4 to 6 weeks of therapy.[102]

Evidence of neurocognitive impairment resulting from iron deficiency and reversal with iron treatment suggests an important role of iron in central nervous system function.[104,112] In addition, long-term studies of teenaged subjects have shown that iron depletion during adolescence is associated with micro- and macro-neuroanatomical changes measured by high-resolution magnetic resonance imaging (MRI) scanning in early adulthood,[113] reinforcing concern about possible effects of iron deficiency on fetal neurological development in female blood donors who become pregnant. Iron supplementation has also been shown to improve maximal and submaximal exercise performance in premenopausal women.[114] Taken together, these studies suggest that iron depletion may have deleterious consequences in blood donors and that measures to monitor and prevent iron depletion are warranted.

Iron present in excessive amounts in the body may be toxic due to the formation of iron-induced free radicals and lipid peroxidation.[115] Some studies of adults have reported that high iron stores are associated with increased risk for coronary heart disease,[116] implying that low iron levels may be salutary and that blood donation may be beneficial. However, this notion has not been substantiated in large population-based ferritin studies or epidemiological studies of blood donors.[117,118] The age-adjusted relative risk (RR) of myocardial infarction for men in the highest category of blood donations (>30 lifetime; mean ferritin from subset of subjects, 64 ng/ml) compared with never donors (mean ferritin, 187 ng/ml) was 1.2 (95% CI, 0.8 to 1.8), and this risk was not significantly changed after adjustment for coronary risk factors or subgroup analyses limited to men with hypercholesterolemia or those who never used antioxidant supplements or aspirin.[118] In a trial of serial phlebotomy to lower ferritin levels in men with peripheral arterial disease, there was no effect on all-cause mortality (HR, 0.85; 95% CI, 0.67–1.08) or the incidence of myocardial infarction and stroke (HR, 0.88; 95% CI, 0.72–1.07).[119] A comprehensive review of epidemiologic and intervention studies concluded that existing evidence does not indicate a link between ferritin and cardiovascular disease risk.[120]

Mitigation of iron deficiency

Increased interdonation interval

Observational studies suggest that prolonging the interdonation interval reduces the risk of iron depletion in blood donors. The RISE study found that interdonation intervals of less than 14 weeks were associated with increased risk of low hemoglobin deferral (OR ~ 2–2.5) and iron deficiency (OR ~ 3–4.4 for ferritin <12 µg/L), and concluded that lengthening the minimum interval would reduce the risk of iron depletion.[89] However, because 39% of donors in RISE acknowledged taking some form of iron supplements, iron ingestion (and not simply waiting longer between donations) may also have played a role in shortening the period of iron recovery. A Norwegian study in non-iron-supplemented donors followed for 1 year also described decreased ferritin levels in both sexes and decreased hemoglobin levels in females, suggesting in their model that increased donation intervals (from a three-month minimum) may protect against iron deficiency.[121] However, studies also show that prolonging the minimum donation interval (changing from 8 weeks to 12 or 16 weeks) might reduce the blood supply (especially for critically needed O-negative blood type) in the United States by as much as 5–7%.[122]

Although intended to protect blood donors from iron deficiency and anemia, there is wide variation in international standards that regulate the allowable frequency of blood donation involving red blood cells.[54] Previous studies that led to the establishment of an eight-week interdonation interval were based on research using small numbers of young, iron-replete subjects,[123] or on limited data on regular blood donors before the availability of reliable iron measurements.[124] A more contemporary study using a quantitative carboxyhemoglobin technique found that hemoglobin from 550 ml donated blood was replenished in 36 +/− 11 days after donation, but it also lacked generalizability because it was restricted to iron-replete young men.[125] Recovery of hemoglobin and iron after donating a unit of whole blood with and without iron supplementation was tested directly in the Hemoglobin and Iron Recovery Study (HEIRS) protocol.[126] The investigators enrolled over 200 blood donors (men and women, 18 to 79 years old) who had not donated for at least four months, measured their iron (ferritin) levels, and divided them into two groups: a low-ferritin group (iron-depleted, plasma ferritin ≤26 ng/ml) and higher ferritin group (non-iron-depleted, plasma ferritin >26 ng/ml). They randomized half of each group to take low-dose iron tablets, 37.5 mg daily, for 24 weeks, and monitored hemoglobin and ferritin levels at regular intervals to see how fast they recovered. Hemoglobin and ferritin recovery were delayed in both untreated ferritin groups (Figures 5.5 and 5.6): the low-ferritin group required a mean of 158 days and the higher ferritin group required a mean of 78 days to recover 80% of the hemoglobin they lost at the time of donation. Without iron, two-thirds of the donors did not recover the iron they lost by 24 weeks. Thus, although extension of the minimum interval would by definition allow for more complete recovery between donations, an increase in the interdonation interval to as long as 24 weeks would still not provide adequate time for hemoglobin and iron recovery in many donors.

Ferritin testing

Studies examining the impact of providing ferritin results to blood donors are limited. Investigators in Switzerland conducted a large single-center longitudinal study to evaluate routine ferritin testing in blood donor management.[127] Serum ferritin was assessed at each blood donation in over 160,000 donations (approximately 24,000 donors) from 1996 to 2009 starting in 2004. Ferritin below 10 ng/ml was the threshold considered to be iron depleted, leading to medical counseling by a blood bank physician to assess other potential medical reasons for low iron or to be referred to their physician, and to considering measures to improve iron status such as reducing donation frequency and/or taking supplemental iron. Comparing groups before and after institution of screening ferritin in donors revealed (1) increased hemoglobin levels, 0.26 g/dl in women and 0.19 g/dl in men; (2) reduced prevalence of anemia: using WHO criteria, hemoglobin <12 g/dl (women) or 13 g/dl (men), from 3.6% to 2.2% in women, and from 0.7% to 0.5% in men; and (3) using reduced hemoglobin deferrals (using hemoglobin <12.3 g/dl in women, and <13.3 g/dl in men), deferral rate went from 2.8% to 1.9% in women. The donor return rate declined as well, from 72–75% before to 60–64% after institution of ferritin screening. This study shows that ferritin monitoring can reduce anemia and hemoglobin deferral in blood donors; however, some donors stop donating when informed of their ferritin results. Of some interest, the investigators have discontinued routine ferritin screening, deciding on a more targeted strategy incorporating annual ferritin testing.[128]

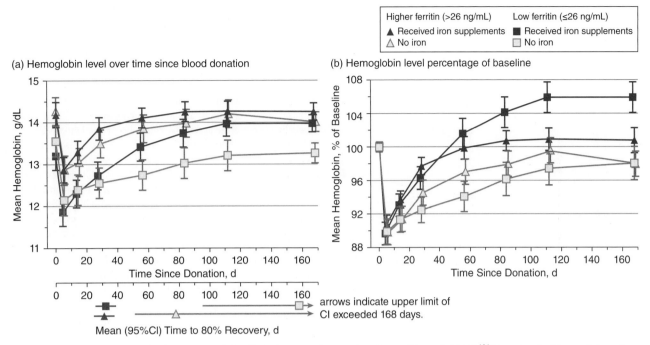

Figure 5.5 Hgb recovery after a blood donation and the effect of iron supplementation. Source: Kiss *et al.* (2015).[126] Reproduced with permission of American Medical Association.

In a multivariable analysis, the Danish Blood Donor Study Group found the strongest predictors of low hemoglobin concentration and risk of declining hemoglobin (at least 0.5 gm/dl) were low ferritin (<15 ng/mL) and current use of iron supplementation (an unexpected association with *lower* hemoglobin was considered to be because of routine iron prescription in the event of low hemoglobin deferral).[129] As the strongest predictor of hemoglobin level, "regular" ferritin measurement was felt to be the most informative tool for blood donor management; however, additional studies are needed to evaluate how often ferritin testing should be performed and what treatment should be offered. A pivotal study, Strategies to Reduce Iron Deficiency (STRIDE), is designed to determine the effectiveness of donor education (two arms: "Thank you" or ferritin result) and oral iron supplementation (three arms: placebo, 19 mg, or 38 mg iron tablets) for mitigating iron deficiency in frequent blood donors.[130] In the preliminary results, withdrawals within two months of enrollment occurred more frequently among donors receiving tablets than those receiving letters, with iron status outcomes pending publication of final results.

Iron supplementation

A number of trials have shown that iron deficiency can be prevented and/or ameliorated by providing iron supplements to blood donors.[131–135] Many studies have targeted premenopausal women because of the disproportionate prevalence of iron deficiency in this donor population. A study performed in Australia reported that, for female donors aged 18–45 who had mean baseline ferritin values ~31 ng/ml and who took 45 mg elemental carbonyl iron daily for eight weeks, ferritin levels at week 12 were significantly higher in donors receiving carbonyl iron (17.0 ± 10.9 ng/mL) compared with those receiving placebo (10.6 ± 8.4 ng/mL; $p < 0.001$), and the proportion of iron-deficient donors (ferritin ≤15 ng/ml) was significantly lower in the carbonyl iron group (51.9%) compared to the

placebo (80.5%; $p < 0.001$).[133] Excluding darker stool color, 31.2% of the carbonyl iron group reported at least one GI side effect, compared with 25.5% of the placebo group. 85% of the participants responded that they would be willing to take iron supplementation in the future. An additional study of iron replacement in female blood donors <50 years old with iron deficiency without anemia showed that four weeks of oral ferrous sulfate, 80 mg of elemental iron/day, resulted in a significantly lower prevalence of a ferritin <12 ng/mL compared to donors given placebo.[134] A study in very frequent blood donors of both sexes (men up to six times and women up to four times per year) who were randomized to 40 mg, 20 mg, or placebo ferrous gluconate found that the ferritin levels remained low but were maintained in donors who received 20 mg daily but declined in the placebo controls.[135] Positive iron balance (increased ferritin) was observed only in donors taking 40 mg daily. In the HEIRS trial, compared to donors who did not take iron, donors taking iron supplements had a significantly shorter time to hemoglobin recovery in *both* the low-ferritin (mean 32 days vs. 158 days) and higher ferritin groups (31 days vs. 78 days).[126] The accelerated hemoglobin recovery from iron supplements was seen in donors with ferritin values up to 50 ng/ml, or higher than expected based on pre-donation ferritin. This is because of the iron deficit induced by blood donation, essentially lowering ferritin in some donors to iron-deficient levels post donation (ferritin <26 ng/ml; Figure 5.6), thus delaying their erythropoietic recovery. Above a ferritin of 50 ng/mL, donors no longer recovered hemoglobin any faster on iron supplements. With iron tablets, iron stores recovered in about 11 weeks, slightly longer than the current eight-week waiting period for donors to be eligible to donate again. Without iron, two-thirds of the donors did not recover the iron they lost by the end of the study in 24 weeks.

A meta-analysis of iron supplementation has reported results of 30 randomized controlled trials involving 4704 blood donors to

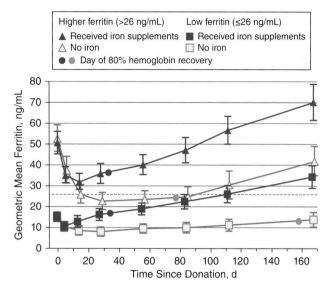

Figure 5.6 Ferritin recovery after blood donation. Source: Kiss *et al.* (2015).[126] Reproduced with permission of American Medical Association.

reduce low hemoglobin deferral, anemia, and iron deficiency.[136] The systematic review concluded there was moderate-quality evidence of "considerably lower" rates of deferral (RR, 0.34; 95% CI, 0.21, 0.55; $n = 1194$, $p < 0.0001$) and improved hemoglobin levels (mean increase, 0.24 gm/dl; 95% CI, 0.01, 0.47; $n = 847$, $p = 0.04$) and iron stores (mean ferritin increase, 14.0 ng/ml; 95% CI, 8.9, 19.0; $n = 640$, $p < 0.00001$) in supplemented donors at the first donation, which persisted at subsequent donations. Adverse effects (constipation, diarrhea, nausea, vomiting, and taste disturbance) were also higher (RR, 1.60; 95% CI, 1.23, 2.07; $n = 1748$, $p = 0.0005$), which prompted the authors to caution about potential limitations in widespread supplementation programs. However, the dosage, frequency (up to tid), and duration of therapy (up to one year) in some studies were high, and this may have increased the incidence of adverse events. The investigators concluded that targeted use of supplements (in those at highest risk) should be considered, with tailored donation schedules and dietary advice in others. The compelling reduction in hemoglobin deferral rate by approximately two-thirds should translate into improved donor retention and decreased donor recruitment resource expenditures at blood centers.

Studies targeting hemoglobin-deferred donors have also been reported. At the NIH, approximately 1200 blood donors deferred for a low hemoglobin and 400 nondeferred donors were evaluated for iron depletion (defined as a ferritin level of 9–19 mg/L in women and 18–29 mg/L in men) and deficiency (as defined by serum ferritin levels below the institutional reference range of 9 ng/ml in women and 18 ng/ml in men).[92] Iron depletion or deficiency was found in 53% of females and 61% of males who were deferred versus 39% of female and 39% of male nondeferred donors. Individuals who were iron deficient or deferred received 60 tablets of 325 mg oral ferrous sulfate (65 mg elemental iron) and instructed to take one daily (and again at subsequent donations). Iron-related laboratory measurements improved in all donors despite continued blood donations. An operationalized approach to implementing an iron replacement program to mitigate iron deficiency in deferred female donors has also been described.[137]

Although more blood centers have begun to advise frequent donors to take supplements to replace iron lost with the donation,

iron supplementation may not be more widely recommended for several reasons. First, it may be that side effects (or simply taking a pill regularly) have a limiting effect on a donor's willingness to ingest oral iron. Conventional doses as used in clinical iron deficiency anemia have been poorly tolerated with up to 80% GI side effects and frequent donor dropout.[138] Several studies have suggested that a 2000 mg elemental iron total dose for short-term replacement after blood donation is effective[139–142] and that a 40 mg daily dose given as ferrous iron salt over an eight-week period can achieve this therapeutic outcome.[106] Doses of 18–45 mg elemental iron daily (regardless of congener, e.g., sulfate, gluconate, and carbonyl) are generally tolerated with occasional GI symptoms such as nausea, bloating, cramps, and constipation, and with advance notice about having darker stools.[126,133,135] In the NIH study, initial use of 65 mg elemental iron as ferrous sulfate resulted in unacceptable side effects in 21% of donors, with successful resolution in some individuals after switching to 38 mg elemental iron tablets (ferrous gluconate).[92] Concern by blood center personnel also remains in regard to recommending or providing iron to individuals with undiagnosed hemochromatosis and potentially masking anemia due to occult blood loss from the GI tract, possibly delaying the discovery of a GI illness.[143] Steps to address these important issues, especially donors with a family history of iron overload, a personal or family history of colon polyps or cancer, and severe anemia or failure to improve hemoglobin after taking oral iron, should be considered as part of donor education and informed consent.

In summary, iron deficiency is widespread in blood donors, and certain groups of donors are particularly likely to become iron depleted, including premenopausal women (with ongoing menstrual blood losses), and "frequent" blood donors including women who donate two or more times a year, and men who donate three or more times a year. Although questions remain regarding how best to manage this problem, solutions are beginning to emerge. It is evident that simply waiting longer between donations (i.e., increase the interdonation interval) is not particularly effective, because the amount of iron removed in the 10 minutes or so it takes to donate a unit of blood requires over 24 weeks to replace on a "standard" diet (i.e., without added iron in the form of supplements). The cumulative effect of repeat blood donations without adequate iron replacement results in iron deficiency in many donors and anemia in some. On the other hand, low-dose iron supplements (18–45 mg elemental iron, available over the counter) accelerate hemoglobin and iron recovery, reduce hemoglobin deferrals, and appear to be tolerated fairly well by most blood donors. Ferritin screening has also been shown to improve hemoglobin levels and iron status; however, iron supplementation has also been recommended in conjunction with this approach and is likely to account for the salutary benefits reported in these studies.

Conclusion

Whole blood donation and apheresis procedures to collect blood components have an impressive safety record, and most volunteer blood donors have uneventful donations and feel good about donating blood to help others. Still, blood donation is a procedure associated with risk of minor discomfort and pain, iron depletion, and, in rare cases, serious injury. Recent operational trials and research programs identify possible ways to reduce the risk of complications and iron depletion after blood donation. Ongoing efforts and continued vigilance are necessary to further improve safety for volunteer blood donors.

Key references

A full reference list for this chapter is available at: http://www.wiley.com/go/simon/transfusion

3 Eder AF, Hillyer CD, Dy BA, *et al.* Adverse reactions to allogeneic whole blood donation by 16- and 17-year-olds. *JAMA* 2008;**299**(19): 2279–86.

7 Skeate RC, Wahi MM, Casanova RJ, Burch JW, Janas JS, Troughton MC. Syncope and vasovagal reactions: Risk factors, recognition and treatment. In: *Blood donor health and safety;* Eder AF, Goldman M, Eds. Bethesda, MD: AABB Press, 2009; 39–70.

21 Eder AF, Dy BA, Kennedy JM, *et al.* Improved safety for young whole blood donors with new selection criteria for total estimated blood volume. *Transfusion* 2011;**51;** 1522–31.

27 Newman B. Arm complications after manual whole blood donation. In: Eder A, Goldman M eds. *Blood donor health and safety.* Bethesda, MD: AABB Press, 2009.

32 Winters JL. Complications of donor apheresis. *J Clin Apher* 2006;**21:** 132–41.

66 Cable RG, Glynn SA, Kiss JE, *et al.* Iron deficiency in blood donors: analysis of enrollment data from the REDS-II Donor Iron Status Evaluation (RISE) study. *Transfusion* 2011;**51**(3): 511–22.

89 Cable RG, Glynn SA, Kiss JE, *et al.* Iron deficiency in blood donors: the REDS-II Donor Iron Status Evaluation (RISE) study. *Transfusion* 2012 Apr; **52**(4): 702–11.

92 Bryant BJ, Yau YY, Arceo SM, *et al.* Iron replacement therapy in the routine management of blood donors. *Transfusion* 2012;**52**: 1566–75.

126 Kiss JE, Brambilla D, Glynn SA, *et al.* Oral iron supplementation after blood donation: a randomized clinical trial. *Jama* 2015;**313**(6):575–83 doi: 10.1001/jama.2015.119 [published Online First: Epub Date].

136 Smith GA, Fisher SA, Doree C, Di Angelantonio E, Roberts DJ. Oral or parenteral iron supplementation to reduce deferral, iron deficiency and/or anaemia in blood donors. *Cochrane Database Syst Rev* 2014 Jul 3; 7: CD009532. doi: 10.1002/14651858.CD009532.pub2

CHAPTER 6

Donor vigilance and hemovigilance

Øystein Flesland[1] & Johanna C. Wiersum-Osselton[2]

[1]Patient Reporting and Learning Systems Unit, Norwegian Knowledge Centre for the Health Services, Oslo, Norway
[2]TRIP National Hemovigilance and Biovigilance Office, Leiden, The Netherlands

Introduction

Reporting and learning systems in general

The ability to learn from adverse events and near misses is a cornerstone for improving safety in different high-risk areas such as the aviation and oil industries. Commercial passenger aviation has become extremely safe partly due to extensive use of reporting and learning systems (RLS).[1]

A system for reporting adverse events and learning from these events is a general requirement in all quality work today, and a written procedure (standard operating procedure [SOP]) for reporting deviations is one of six required SOPs in ISO 9001 standards.

In healthcare, it has been more difficult to prove that RLS have improved safety.[2] A World Health Organization (WHO) guideline on adverse event reporting and learning systems[3] emphasized that the effectiveness of an adverse event reporting system is measured not only by accurate collection and analysis of data, but also by its use for making recommendations that improve patient safety. The guideline outlined the following core concepts:

- The fundamental role of patient safety reporting systems is to enhance patient safety by learning from failures of the healthcare system.
- Reporting must be safe. Individuals who report incidents must not be punished or suffer other ill effects from reporting.
- Reporting is of value only if it leads to a constructive response. At a minimum, this entails feedback of findings from data analysis. Ideally, it also includes recommendations for changes in healthcare procedures and systems.
- Meaningful analysis, learning, and dissemination of lessons learned require expertise and other human and financial resources. The agency that receives reports must be capable of disseminating information, making recommendations for changes, and informing the development of solutions.

When Canada prepared for a reporting and learning system in Canadian healthcare, the Canadian Patient Safety Institute (CPSI) performed a review of RLS to better understand such systems.[4] The review found that for RLS to be successful, healthcare workers need incentives to use the systems and these incentives must be stronger than the disadvantages. The systems should be voluntary and confidential. They should be transparent, but at the same time protect the reporter. The users should be invited to take part in the development and maintenance of the system. The system should prove to be able to prevent, detect, and reduce the effect of adverse events due to bad planning, bad practice, or other unfavorable circumstances.

In well-functioning RLS, one commonly found that:

- Adverse events and near misses were analyzed by an independent organization with enough competence;
- Feedback to the reporter was given in a timely manner;
- Suggestions on how to improve the system were given;
- The healthcare system is open for suggestions for system improvement; and
- The system is nonpunitive.

Reporting and learning systems in blood transfusion

The term *hemovigilance* has become widely used over the past decade to describe the systematic surveillance of adverse transfusion reactions and events, encompassing the whole transfusion chain and aimed at improving the safety of the transfusion process, from donor to recipient, or "vein to vein."[5,6] The term was coined in France in the early 1990s, has been developed and adopted internationally, and is now an integral part of transfusion practice. Today it is unthinkable not to have a system for reporting deviations in transfusion medicine and to use such reports in the ongoing quality improvement work. The hemovigilance system should be an integral part of the risk management or clinical governance framework of the institution.

The concepts mentioned above for RLS are directly relevant to hemovigilance systems and are applicable both at the hospital level and nationally. The scope of the system must be clear to reporters. The system should be robust, easily understood, and user friendly. Collection of complete data on adverse reactions and events requires local awareness and vigilance. There must be a "reporting and learning culture" within which events are viewed as learning opportunities. Such a culture takes time to develop, and it should be developed within a framework of professional competence and accountability.

At the regional or national level, the hemovigilance scheme must be seen as impartial, independent, supportive, and professionally credible. Data should be validated, analyzed, and reported within a predictable time frame, and published in a format that can be used to support education and training. Active involvement and "ownership" by professional bodies will help to ensure that recommendations are incorporated into clinical practice.

Rossi's Principles of Transfusion Medicine, Fifth Edition. Edited by Toby L. Simon, Jeffrey McCullough, Edward L. Snyder, Bjarte G. Solheim, and Ronald G. Strauss.
© 2016 John Wiley & Sons, Ltd. Published 2016 by John Wiley & Sons, Ltd.

History and development

Pharmacovigilance was the first surveillance system in the arena of health care, covering medicinal products of all kinds. Hemovigilance, as a separate surveillance system, was implemented in France in 1994, as required by the updated French regulation on blood in a response to a "blood scandal."[7,8] *Hemovigilance* has been defined as "a set of surveillance procedures covering the whole transfusion chain from the collection of blood and its components to the follow-up of its recipients, intended to collect and assess information on unexpected or undesirable effects resulting from the therapeutic use of labile blood products, and to prevent their occurrence and recurrence."[9]

In the United Kingdom, anticipation of forthcoming European legislation, together with concerns regarding transfusion safety, led to the establishment of the SHOT (Serious Hazards of Transfusion) scheme in 1996. Hemovigilance systems at the regional or national level were seen in numerous countries both within Europe and elsewhere by the end of the 1990s (Table 6.1) and have continued to develop thereafter. According to data reported to WHO, in 2008 a national hemovigilance system existed in 57 of 164 countries that supplied data, and 24 were preparing a system.[10] As might be expected, the percentage is highest in developed countries: a national hemovigilance system had been implemented in 13% of low-income countries, 30% of middle-income countries, and 78% of high-income countries providing data. At the other end of the spectrum, the same survey showed that in 39 countries donated blood is not routinely tested for transfusion-transmissible infections.

The initiative to start hemovigilance as well as the governance of systems varies considerably. Several well-known systems were initiated by professional societies and were subsequently modified to meet new legislative requirements (see under the "Legal Framework" section). Thus, in Norway, a voluntary, anonymous reporting system for complications related to blood donation or blood transfusion was started in 2004 by the Norwegian Society for Immunology and Transfusion Medicine. It received reports on mild, moderate, and severe complications. From 2007, when the EU directive was implemented in Norwegian law, this system has continued, but it has to report serious transfusion reactions, serious donor reactions and serious near misses to the Directorate of Health together with an evaluation of the steps taken by the reporting hospital to prevent recurrence. Although the voluntary system receives hundreds of reports yearly, only approximately 10 reports are serious enough to be sent on to the Directorate of Health.

Within hemovigilance systems, the importance of national definitions has been recognized, but inevitably there was a lack of commonality of definitions, terminology, structure, and scope of reporting. In the course of development, variable strategies were followed to address organizational difficulties, need for funding, mandates, training, and so on.

The development of hemovigilance systems was primarily driven by a desire for early detection of harm to patients and for transparency about safety of the blood components. The Danish system was early to emphasize the importance of reporting donor adverse reactions.

Descriptions of several more national hemovigilance systems can be found on the International Haemovigilance Network (IHN) website (www.ihn-org.com).[11]

Hemovigilance working methods
Investigations and assessment

As part of clinical care, transfusion adverse reactions should be investigated to establish the diagnosis and guide future treatment of the patient. Where there may be implications for other components (e.g., from the same donor), the producer must be informed. Reporting to the hemovigilance system should be accompanied by sufficient information to allow the assessors to verify the type of reported reaction. Commonly also, reports are rated for severity as well as for "imputability," the likelihood with which a reaction can be attributed to the transfused component.

For donor complications, such as a hematoma or a vasovagal reaction, this is usually no problem. For transfusion reactions, it may be obvious as in a hemolytic transfusion reaction due to the transfusion of incorrect blood. It may, however, be difficult when a severely ill patient on antibiotics and fluid treatment experiences fever, a rash, or fluid overload. Similarly, if a blood donor suffers a cerebrovascular accident less than 24 hours after an uncomplicated blood donation, the possibility of a causal relation is difficult to prove or to exclude.

Root cause analysis

As discussed in the introduction, the objective of reporting to a centralized system is to derive recommendations for the

Table 6.1 Examples of Hemovigilance Systems

Country	Date of Initiation, Scope of Reporting (Voluntary at Inception Unless Otherwise Mentioned)	Governance
Japan	1993: Transfusion-associated adverse reactions and infectious diseases	Japanese Red Cross Society
France	1994: Mandatory system created by national legislation; all severity levels	Inspectorate for Healthcare Products (currently: Agence Nationale de Sécurité du Médicament et des Produits de Santé)
United Kingdom	1996: Serious Hazards of Transfusion (SHOT); serious reports	Professional societies
Denmark	1999: Danish Registration of Transfusion Accidents (DART): modeled on SHOT	Society for Clinical Immunology. Early emphasis on donor adverse reactions (Danish Donor Society)
South Africa	2000: All severity levels; donor reactions included from 2010	South African National Blood Service
Netherlands	2002: Transfusion and transplantation reactions in patients (TRIP): "all"	Professional societies
Norway	2004: TROLL. Reports on transfusion reactions and complications of blood donation from 2004. Reports on other adverse events from 2007.	From 2004 to 2007: The Norwegian Society for Immunology and Transfusion Medicine (Professional Society). From 2007: The Norwegian Directorate of Health is responsible for hemovigilance, but the system is operated by the Norwegian Knowledge Centre for the Health Services.
New Zealand	2005: All severity levels	New Zealand Blood Service
United States	2006: National Healthcare Safety Network, Biovigilance reporting system. Gradual increase of participation; incorporated donor vigilance from inception	US Biovigilance Network (public–private collaboration between the US Department of Health and Human Services, including the Centers for Disease Control and Prevention, and organizations involved in blood collection, transfusion, tissue and organ transplantation, and cellular therapies)

improvement of practice and prevention of future errors and incidents. Underlying a mistake at the moment of transfusion may be several latent causes, such as lack of training, badly designed IT processes, or understaffing. Facilities should assess such causes and supply sufficient information to the hemovigilance system to allow analysis of recurrent problems and weak "links" in the transfusion chain.[12,13] A number of methods for analyzing and classifying contributing causes have been developed;[12] a practical toolkit based on techniques recommended by the (former) UK National Patient Safety Agency is available on the SHOT website (www.shotuk.org).[14]

Risk assessment

An in-depth root cause analysis takes considerable time and effort,[13,15] so this is usually performed for selected reports of errors or incidents in the transfusion chain. When an event has occurred, assessment of the potential for harm (even if the worst did not happen) and the likelihood of recurrence can be combined to support prioritization of a particular problem for detailed analysis and preventive measures. A risk matrix based on this principle has been developed, following similar examples that are in use in aviation and high-risk industries, for use in the vigilance of tissues and cells.[16] In hemovigilance, such a tool has not been widely implemented.

A prospective risk assessment of the transfusion chain can indicate possible improvement measures, even if no error has been reported (yet). For instance, analysis of the process of blood transfusion in pediatric emergency using the Healthcare Failure Mode and Effect Analysis (HFMEA) indicated that training and audit could be the main tools for improvement.[17,18] Another method for prospective analysis is the Bowtie method developed by the UK Civil Aviation Authority.[19,20]

Hemovigilance report

In order for learning and improvement to take place, the collected information must be made available to the professionals of the transfusion chain. Recommendations for improvement can be made, and ideally these will be incorporated in practice through changes in blood donor care, the production of blood components, recommended practices laid down in transfusion guidelines, or other mechanisms. Through the ongoing reporting, the effects of measures can be evaluated and trends can be tracked. Where possible and relevant, peer-reviewed publication should also be pursued to strengthen rigor and ensure international accessibility of the results for incorporation in meta-analyses.

Rapid alerts

Rapid spread of information about new risks is difficult to manage but potentially very useful. Examples can be problems with disposables or reagents that are discovered in one blood bank and where it may take some time before it is detected in other blood banks. Before an alert is circulated, the finding must be verified; the manufacturer must be informed, and relevant advice or actions in response to the notification included in the alert.

Things to consider when establishing a hemovigilance system

In practice, a reporting and learning system like a hemovigilance system may be organized in several ways. It may be local, regional, or national. It may be voluntary or compulsory. It may be sanction-free or have the possibility of sanctions. It may be anonymous. It may report only serious complications or include mild or moderate complications. It may include near misses. It may be passive or active (see the "Passive or Active Systems" subsection). It is important to identify the goals of the system before deciding how it should be organized. The available resources should be taken into account.

National, regional, or local systems

Transfusion reactions vary in frequency. Because some are rare, such as transfusion-associated acute lung injury (TRALI), graft-versus-host disease (GvHD), and posttransfusion purpura (PTP), a national system is most often required to get big enough numbers to monitor the incidence and to measure improvements after action has been taken to reduce the incidence further. Other transfusion reactions like FNHTR and mild allergic reactions can be monitored on a regional or local level.

Voluntary or compulsory systems

The Canadian Patient Safety Institute (CPSI) found that voluntary systems were best, and some established hemovigilance systems, like SHOT and the Danish Registration of Transfusion Accidents (DART), are voluntary. When establishing a system on a voluntary basis, some enthusiasts will start using the system and the less enthusiastic will follow. Voluntary systems are often started by the professions or by scientific bodies, and participants may therefore feel more ownership and, hence, more willingness to participate. Compulsory systems are more often initiated by governments and supported by laws or directives.

Anonymous, confidential, and nonpunitive systems

Both WHO and CPSI recommend nonpunitive systems. Many adverse events and near misses involves human error to some extent.[21] To encourage reporting and maximize learning from such cases, the hemovigilance system should be nonpunitive. This should not mean that if you make a mistake and then report it in an RLS, you are guaranteed not to suffer any sanctions. The adverse event or near miss will most probably also be detected in other ways, by other staff or by the patient, and complaints from patients and the like will have to be acted on. Staff are always accountable for their actions, and professional competence is of the highest importance, but competence should be assessed in other ways than by reports in an RLS.

Anonymous reporting may be a way to ensure potential reporters that the reporting is nonpunitive. At the local level anonymous reporting is often an illusion, and at the regional or national level it may be irrelevant, but anonymous reporting sends a signal that the person involved is not important. We know that people make mistakes, and it is the system in which they work that is our focus for improvement.[21]

Confidentiality is always important. When reports are used for learning purposes, it is important that details that could be used to identify people or places are removed or changed.

What should be reported?

Legislation often only requires reporting of serious adverse events. In theory, one may have several less serious adverse events, or near misses, before one serious adverse event, and it is better to analyze these and ideally prevent the more serious event. The number of reports the hemovigilance system will receive will, however, increase dramatically if all adverse events and near misses are reported. The resources available must therefore be taken into consideration. In an ideal system, all adverse reactions and adverse events will be reported, including near misses. The number of reports increases as the benefits of reporting are seen, whereas the number of serious adverse reactions decreases due to quality improvement because of learning from the reports.

In pharmacovigilance, the focus is on reporting only new or very serious complications, and in reporting systems for cells and tissues the focus is on product-related problems. Hemovigilance usually has a wider scope and in this respect may be more similar to a quality registry than a traditional RLS.

Background data

For understanding and analysis of the hemovigilance data from a country or region, it is useful or necessary to have some background data, such as the age group and sex of a patient, and whether universal leukodepletion of blood components is in place. Background data should be limited to parameters that can be analyzed across organizations, regions, or countries because all registration takes time and effort. A frequent problem is that the numerator (e.g., the number of reactions in a particular category) is known, but the denominator (the total number of patients or donors in that group) is not. An example may be that vasovagal reactions are reported more frequently in young women, but if we do not know what proportion of donors are young females, this information has limited value.

Typical background data that are registered for reporting donor complications are the donors' age and sex, the donation type (whole blood or apheresis), the date and time of donation, and if it was a first-time donation or not. Typical background data for transfusion reactions are patient age and sex, the indication for transfusion, department and/or ward, time from transfusion to reaction, and so on.

In certain cases, more background information may be useful, such as a female donor's parity in cases of TRALI and the patient's coronary status when transfusion-associated cardiac overload (TACO) or transfusion-associated dyspnea (TAD) is suspected. Usually, it is better to collect such data only when relevant. A rule of thumb may be "Record what you need to know, not what is nice to know."

Passive or active systems

A passive system is a system where only the adverse events or near misses are reported to the system. In an active system, the fact that a transfusion (or blood donation) was uncomplicated is also reported. On a local level, active systems are preferable because underreporting is less likely. On a regional or national level, passive systems are sufficient. Active systems may also have drawbacks as the findings depend on when the active reporting takes place. If it takes place shortly after the transfusion, the reactions that come later may not be reported. This may include reactions occuring hours, days, or even weeks later. An example is delayed hemolytic transfusion reactions, which typically are detected some 10 days after the transfusion. Conversely, if active reporting takes place a long time after transfusion, the immediate but mild reactions that occurred may be forgotten. In donors, adverse reactions that occur while the blood donor still is present in the blood bank are fairly easy to capture, whereas some serious complications, like faints that occur after leaving the blood bank, may not be reported till the time of the next donation, if ever.

Contact persons

At the hospital level, there is a need for a point of contact for clinical staff to report reactions and adverse events. This may be a transfusion practitioner or safety officer, hematologist, transfusion medicine specialist, the blood transfusion laboratory, or a hospital blood bank manager. A national system will also benefit from having a designated contact person in the blood establishment(s) (a blood establishment, blood service, or blood operator is the organization responsible for collecting, processing, and testing blood and can be located in a hospital or outside the hospital). Depending on the situation in a country, these may be the same person. Responsibilities vary but may include teaching, assisting in investigation of adverse reactions and adverse events, and sending reports to the regional or national hemovigilance system.

Cooperation with other reporting and learning systems, quality registers, and indicators

When running a hemovigilance system, it is useful to be aware of other sources of information on transfusion safety. Reporting and learning systems in general use in health care may have relevant information. An example from Norway is that the hemovigilance system rarely receives reports of blood transfusion laboratories (hospital blood banks) issuing blood too late, whereas the general RLS has several reports from clinicians about this. Other useful information can be found by looking at patient safety indicators. Frequent ordering of blood during surgery, instead of before surgery, may be an indicator of poor ordering routines. This will probably not be picked up in a hemovigilance system, but is useful information in quality improvement work. Large administrative databases and electronic health records are often the source for quality indicators and can also be used to study transfusion reactions.[22]

Cooperation with reporting and learning systems for cells and tissues and for organ transplantation may be useful as many problems are similar. Systems for vigilance relating to devices may have relevant information, and there is a need to ensure communication between these two areas.

Plasma derivatives

Plasma derivatives are covered by pharmacovigilance. Both blood banks and pharmacies may issue these products, and in some cases it may be useful to include these products in the hemovigilance system. An example is solvent detergent plasma that is blood group specific and may have similar complications to blood components; in many countries, it has been decided that it should be issued by the blood bank. If plasma derivatives are included in the hemovigilance system, an agreement between the different parties is strongly recommended.

Approvals and registrations

In some countries, approval for data registration is required, under data protection legislation, by ethical committees and the like. There may be specific requirements for electronic reporting. Different types of data may have different requirements just as different countries may have different requirements. Relevant laws and regulations should be identified before establishing a hemovigilance system.

New or not previously recognized side effects of blood donation or transfusion

Sometimes, donors or patients report complications that are not one of the known complications. This may be difficult to handle, and often the conclusion will be that it was not related to the donation or the transfusion. It may, however, be useful to collect the data because it can lead to the detection of complications that we hitherto were not aware of.

Other considerations

Patient blood management is an important topic. Monitoring over- and undertransfusion may be considered a relevant domain of hemovigilance. It is important to decide if this falls within the scope of your system.

Similarly, it is necessary to consider if complications caused by blood from cell savers, re-infusion drains, and so on should be reported in the hemovigilance system.

International reporting and collaboration

The system should be able to report its results internationally to further analysis and learning on an international level. Currently, the EU, WHO, the Council of Europe, and the IHN (see the "International Hemovigilance Network" subsection) collect data yearly.

Variation in organization, working methods, and definitions is a problem when comparing data from different countries. A number of international organizations are relevant in this respect and play a role in promoting international collaboration and harmonization of hemovigilance activity.

International Hemovigilance Network (www.ihn-org.com)

Founded in 1998 (at first under the name of European Hemovigilance Network) as a nonprofit foundation, the objectives of the IHN are to promote and engage in:

- the exchange of information that is of importance among the members of the network;
- a swiftly functioning alarm system or warning system among members of the network;
- joint activities among the members of the network; and
- educational activities relating to hemovigilance.

The members of the network are the national or, in some cases where there is no national system, regional hemovigilance systems. From 2004, the IHN has worked on development of definitions for transfusion reactions as well as for complications of blood donation. As of 2015, the network has over 30 member systems.

The IHN hosts a database for the capture of aggregate data on transfusion adverse reactions, errors, and failures as well as donor adverse reactions: the International Surveillance Database for Transfusion Adverse Reactions and Events (ISTARE).[23] Despite the limitations of comparisons owing to variations in definitions and working methods, the database allows national systems to anonymously compare their data to those of other member organizations.[11]

International Society for Blood Transfusion (ISBT; www.isbtweb.org)

This international voluntary society has individual professionals as its members. Its first objective is to promote and to maintain a high level of ethical, medical, and scientific practice in blood transfusion medicine, science, and related therapies throughout the world. The hemovigilance working party, in which over 50 members participate, formally collaborates with the IHN in the process of developing tools and definitions (publicly available on the website under Working Parties → Hemovigilance → Definitions).

The present state of the IHN–ISBT hemovigilance definitions is as follows:

- *Non-infectious transfusion reactions*: First published in 2011.
- *Complications of blood donation*: At the end of 2014, revised definitions for the surveillance of complications of blood donation were published, for the first time also in collaboration with the biovigilance working group of the AABB (formerly: American Association of Blood Banks). Further organizations have formally endorsed these definitions. This represents an important step forward in international hemovigilance collaboration.
- *Infectious transfusion complications*: Definitions and criteria for transfusion-transmitted infectious diseases are challenging to standardize—factors include the differences between the diseases and their epidemiology as well as different standards and methods of testing between countries. Work is being pursued by the ISBT transfusion-transmitted infectious diseases (TTID) working party in collaboration with the hemovigilance working party. To date, no international definitions have been adopted by the IHN or ISBT.
- *Errors, failures, and incidents*: A number of types of sentinel event have been defined by the ISBT and IHN. Nevertheless, the very term *adverse event* is used differently in different organizations, and notably the EU legislation defines *serious adverse event* differently from international pharmacovigilance legislation.[24]
- *Severity and imputability of transfusion reactions*: Incorporated in the list of noninfectious transfusion reactions.
- *Imputability of adverse reactions*: Incorporated in the list of noninfectious transfusion reactions

World Health Organization

WHO, which is in formal relations with ISBT on the subject of safe blood transfusion, has a department of blood safety that recently published an Aide-Memoire on implementing hemovigilance; a longer guidance document is in preparation. A strength of WHO is its direct links with governments and ministries of health. This can provide a strong impetus to initiate activities to implement hemovigilance and improve the safety of blood transfusion.

Within WHO, the cluster on patient safety has produced a taxonomy of terminology. At present, there are some discrepancies with other definitions (including the term *adverse event*).[24] Collaboration of clusters at WHO level could potentially contribute to reconciling the terminology.

Council of Europe

The Council of Europe has 47 member states, of which 27 are also members of the European Union. It produces a guide with recommended standards for the preparation, testing, and transfusion of blood components.[25] In this guide, both principles and standards for hemovigilance are described.

Legal framework

European hemovigilance and the EU Blood Directives

The key role of hemovigilance in blood transfusion safety is reflected in the EU Blood Directive 2002/98/EC.[26]

This Directive of the European Parliament and of the Council sets standards of quality and safety for the collection, testing, processing, storage, and distribution of human blood and blood components. An entire section is dedicated to hemovigilance, and it encompasses traceability and notification of serious adverse events and reactions. The technical details are further laid down in the so-called daughter directives:

- 2004/33/EC (Directive on donations, donors, and blood components);
- 2005/61/EC (Directive on traceability and notification—hemovigilance); and
- 2005/62/EC (Directive on a quality management system).

According to the Directives on blood, *hemovigilance* is defined as "a set of organized surveillance procedures relating to serious adverse or unexpected events or reactions in donors or recipients, and the epidemiologic follow-up of donors." It is stated that

> it is important to introduce a set of organized surveillance procedures to collect and evaluate information on the adverse or unexpected events or reactions resulting from the collection of blood or blood components in order to prevent similar or equivalent events or reactions from occurring thereby improving the security of transfusion by adequate measures. To this end a common system of notification of serious adverse events and reactions . . . should be established in member states.

See Table 6.2 for definitions for serious adverse reactions and events.

The focus of these directives is ensuring a high standard of quality and safety of human blood and of blood components for the protection of human health. They lay down standards in the context of blood matters, including hemovigilance. It is important to understand that the European Treaty (the Treaty of Amsterdam, establishing the European Community) sets limits in Article 152 that restrict the scope of European legislation to the products: the

Directives on blood apply to collection and testing of human blood and blood components, whatever their intended purpose, and their processing, storage, and distribution when intended for transfusion. The principle of subsidiarity allows other issues to be determined by individual EU member states, which may adopt regulations in addition to the provisions in the Blood Directives.

The current European legislation can therefore cover only the producers (the blood establishments) and to some extent the hospital blood banks (blood transfusion laboratories). However, the Directives do not apply to clinical activities, which are the exclusive responsibility of the individual member states. This obviously creates a complex situation in Europe with regard to hemovigilance systems. From the outset, it had been recognized that hemovigilance (including rapid alert) should encompass the whole blood chain from donor to recipient and vice versa, including both production and clinical use. The SHOT reports had shown that harm to patients, although sometimes caused by an unsafe (chiefly, infected) blood component, is more often a consequence of physiological reactions or of errors— for instance, in the 2000–2001 annual report, 71.8% of submitted reports were of incorrect blood component transfused (IBCT) and 1% were of transfusion-transmitted infections.

When the mandatory submission of annual hemovigilance reports to the European Commission commenced (2007 data), the nonbinding guidance for member states allowed for the reporting of all types of serious adverse reactions and did not restrict it to cases where the blood component was unsafe.

Because the EU directive includes minimum requirements for reporting to the health authorities, all countries in the European Union have set up hemovigilance systems. These may be comprehensive, well-staffed, and well-funded, like in France, or just the bare minimum to fulfill the requirements of the directives. In some countries, voluntary hemovigilance systems had already been

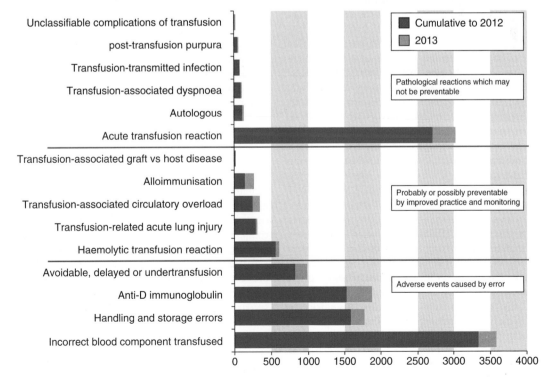

Figure 6.1 Summary of main findings and cumulative results from Annual SHOT report 2013. Source: SHOT, The 2013 annual SHOT report, 2014.[66] Reproduced with permission of SHOT.

Table 6.3 Data to Be Retained for 30 Years in EU Member States (2005/61/EU)[27]

By Blood Establishments	By Transfusing Facilities
Blood establishment identification	Blood component supplier identification
Blood donor identification	Issued blood component identification
Blood unit identification	Transfused recipient identification
Individual blood component identification	For blood units not transfused, confirmation of subsequent disposition
Date of collection (year/month/day)	Date of transfusion or disposition (year/month/day)
Facilities to which blood units or blood components are distributed, or subsequent disposition	Lot number of the component, if relevant

Source: Commission Directive 2005/61/EC,[27] http://eur-lex.europa.eu. Reproduced with permission of European Union, 1998–2015.

introduced when the EU directive came into force, and some countries therefore have two parallel systems: one voluntary, often anonymous and comprehensive run by the transfusion medicine community, and one small official system ensuring that the directive requirements are fulfilled.

Traceability

In the event of a transfusion reaction, in many cases it is necessary to trace back to the donor and investigate (e.g., does the donor have HLA antibodies?) Conversely, if a donor is found to have seroconverted, the recipients of earlier donations (tested with negative results for blood-transmissible diseases) need to be traced and tested for possible infection, if this could be clinically relevant. Traceability from donor to patient and back, the storing of data necessary to link a particular donor and donation to a particular recipient, is a prerequisite for these hemovigilance activities and is laid down in the EU directive (Table 6.3).

Although only basic data need to be retained for the 30 years specified for EU member states, it remains challenging in the face of hospital or blood establishment progression of IT technology. Of note in the legislative framework, the recommendation is that confirmation of the transfusion or of final disposal of a blood component should be obtained and recorded. In many hospitals, this is achieved using a paper form that is returned to the blood transfusion laboratory. Ideally, the confirmation of transfusion should be added to the component issue information in the laboratory computer system, enabling it to be stored electronically with the other traceability data. In the future, as electronic bedside checks of patient and unit identity become more commonplace, return of the transfusion data to the computer system can remove the need for returning paper forms. However, implementation of such technology is expensive as well as challenging, so adoption is progressing slowly.

Postdonation information (PDI)

The quality system of a blood establishment requires that if it later becomes known that the donor could have had an infection at the time of donation, the blood establishment should have a procedure for contacting the hospital to which the components manufactured from that donation were distributed. This might, for instance, be an illness with fever within 24 hours of donation, or if a blood test performed several weeks after the donation because of symptoms reveals a diagnosis of hepatitis B. Postdonation information in other cases refers to cases where the screening failed to elicit a cause for deferral and this is found out, perhaps at the donor's next attendance. If the component is still in date, it should

be retrieved. If it has already been transfused, a risk-based decision should be taken about whether it is necessary to counsel and/or test the recipient.[28]

Donor hemovigilance

Systematic surveillance of the first part of the transfusion chain—the collection of blood from the donor—is an essential element of hemovigilance, and it aims to secure and improve the safety of both the donor and the recipient. Blood establishments (including organizations that collect plasma for the production of plasma-derived medicines, often referred to as *source plasma*) should register adverse events in whole blood and component donors, actions taken as a result, and the outcomes. These events may be adverse reactions or complications resulting from donation, or adverse events—errors, incidents, and failures—related to the selection and management of donors, which may directly harm the donor or influence the quality of the product, thereby potentially harming the recipient.

Collection of blood from donors for the provision of components for clinical use is most frequently performed in the form of whole blood donation. Automated collection using apheresis technology is also used for the collection of plasma, platelets and red blood cells, depending on local or national factors and policies. The less common donations of granulocytes, as well as of lymphocytes or peripheral blood stem cells, are also collected by apheresis; space does not permit detailed discussion of vigilance relating to these procedures.

Provision of information about the risks of donation based on evidence from surveillance, together with good clinical management of any complications, indicates a high professional standard of the blood collection facility and its care of the well-being of the donors. This, in turn, will improve donor confidence and satisfaction, making it more likely that the donor will return, thus benefiting the national supply of blood.[29]

Although awareness of the complications of blood donation is probably as old as blood banking,[30,31] in the last 10–20 years this has strengthened. A joint working group from the ISBT and IHN (then, the EHN) was established in 2005, and this led to the first proposed classification with a set of definitions of complications related to blood donation[32] to form the basis for surveillance and international comparisons. A revision was concluded in 2014.[33] It is hoped that the use of this classification will enable comparisons and collaborative work to add to the available evidence to support improvements in donor care and selection.

Complications related to blood donation

Data on the occurrence of these complications were not at first included in the hemovigilance systems, but they have been reported by blood establishments. Large studies have been published by single blood centers in the United States and other countries;[34–39] comprehensive national data have now also been published (for Denmark,[40] France, New Zealand, and other countries), and data collected by the IHN with the use of the 2008 definitions have been presented at several meetings (Table 6.4).

The rate of reported donor complications varies according to the severity and range of reactions included. Preliminary data registered according to the ISBT classification suggest that the overall rate of complications in collection center practice is in the order of approximately 1 per 100 donations. The observed rate is known to be highly dependent on the method of ascertaining the reaction: A study where donors were contacted by telephone following their donation[36] elicited an overall rate of 36%.

Table 6.4 Occurrence of Complications Related to Blood Donation (Examples)

Study	Donations (Whole Blood Donations Unless Otherwise Specified; Comments)	Donor Complications (Reported Cases per 100,000 Donations)			
		Vasovagal Reaction	Hematoma	Nerve Injury or Irritation	Total
Newman[38]	1000 (interview 3 weeks after donation)	6400	1700	900	9000
Newman[38]	1000 (information obtained at donation)	2100	324	16	2440
Sorensen[40]	2,575,246 (national register of *serious* complications)	7	1	11	19
Sorensen[40]	41,274 (county register all complications)	478	274	70	822
Ounnoughene[41]	2.6 million (national data, France 2011)	107	8	1.4	116.4[a]
Eder (2008)[42]	6,014,472 whole blood donations	2721	750	7	3478
New Zealand annual hemovigilance report 2013[43]	160,211, all blood collection (national data 2013)	1340	860	70	2270
IHN (ISTARE database)[44]	18.8 million whole blood and apheresis donations (17 countries; 2012 data[b])	487	104	25[c]	616

[a] Rates derived from figures in the publication.
[b] 2012 denominator supplied by ISTARE working group, chair C. Politis.
[c] Cases of "painful arm," as defined in 2008 ISBT/IHN definitions.

Rates of reported complications are affected by differences in donor demographics—for instance, rates are higher in donors making their first donation. Studies of the occurrence of complications of blood donation have examined risk factors for their occurrence.[45–47] Such factors need to be taken into account when analyzing the effects of differences or changes in procedures. The revised ISBT–IHN definitions are accompanied by a list of recommended parameters that should be recorded if possible.

The most common complications of donation are vasovagal reactions (approximately two-thirds), whereas the needle-related complications, hematomas and injuries of tissues including nerve injury or irritation, account for most of the remainder. In centers where apheresis is performed, additional types of reactions and complications are relevant—the most frequent are the consequences of infusion of citrate-containing anticoagulant solution when the donor's blood constituents are reinfused following separation of the components that are being collected.

Vasovagal reactions

Vasovagal reaction is the most common donor complication (488 per 100,000 donations in the Danish study). The predominant symptoms are general discomfort, weakness, anxiety, dizziness, nausea, sweating, vomiting, pallor, and hyperventilation, associated with hypotension and bradycardia. The two last symptoms are essential for the diagnosis. Most vasovagal reactions are mild and transient, but some donors may lose consciousness (fainting or vasovagal syncope). In the more severe cases, this may be associated with convulsions and incontinence or may result in an accident if the donor falls. It is important to reassure the donor that these reactions do not indicate a predisposition to true epilepsy.

Vasovagal reactions are generated by the autonomic nervous system stimulated by psychologic factors and by the volume of blood removed relative to the donor's total blood volume. An increasing number of studies have shown that young age, female sex, lower blood volume (estimated from weight and height), and first-donation status are significant risk factors.[48] Based on these risk factors, a number of preventive measures have been evaluated (Table 6.5); some studies reported reductions of up to 20–25%.

Some vasovagal reactions (~10%)[40,56] occur after the donor has left the donation area; these are so-called delayed reactions. These reactions are potentially dangerous, as the donor may be at risk of a serious accident. Female sex and a low estimated blood volume are risk factors for delayed vasovagal reactions.[56]

Table 6.5 Measures to Prevent Vasovagal Reactions

Intervention	Study	Result and Remarks
Water drink shortly before donation	Newman (2007)[49] (4312 high school students <19 years of age)	21% reduction of vasovagal reactions
Applied muscle tension (AMT): The technique involves tensing the muscles in the legs and buttocks, which then raises the blood pressure.	Ditto (2003)[50] (RCT; total: 606) France (2010)[51] (intervention + full data: 342) Ditto (2013)[52] (total: 404)	Reduced presyncopal reactions in women (questionnaire studies) Possible improvement of return in male donors who adhered to instructions
Social support	Hanson (2009)[53] (n = 65 completed study)	Reduced presyncopal reactions (ascertained by questionnaire) and improved intent to donate again in inexperienced donors
Donor information addressing common donor concerns and giving tips for coping strategies	France (2010)[51] (345 undergraduate donors assigned to intervention or control brochures; 67.5% had 1–4 previous donations)	Improvements in donation attitude, confidence, and intention; more likely to volunteer to give blood
Deferral of young donors with estimated blood volume <3.5 L	Eder (2011)[54] approximately 675,000 donations <21 years annually (143,948 in 16-year-olds in 2009)	VVR rate in 16-year-olds under modified selection criteria: 10.5% vs. 7.3%; odds ratio [OR], 0.67; 95% confidence interval [CI], 0.65–0.69
Combined intervention of water drink, deferral of donors with estimated blood volume <3.5 L and encouragement to use AMT	Tomasulo (2011)[55] before-and-after study, total 213,031 donations by donors <23 years of age.	Overall reduction 24%; reduction of delayed reactions

In order to lower the risk of delayed reactions and of serious outcomes of these, it is essential to ensure that the donor feels completely well before leaving the donation area. Many facilities permanently defer donors following a severe delayed vasovagal reaction. Donors with hazardous occupations where they or others could be put at risk (e.g., pilots) should not return to work within 24 hours of donation.

Hematomas and other venepuncture-related or local complications

Hematoma is the second most common complication related to blood donation (275 per 100,000 donations).[40] The symptoms are bruising, swelling, and pain at the venepuncture site.

A hematoma may occur if the needle punctures small vessels, or if blood leaks from the vein during or after venepuncture. Blood in the soft tissues behind the biceps tendon will initially spread behind the tendon and may not produce any visible swelling or pain. As the hematoma increases in size, it tracks along the blood vessels, nerves, and tendons to the forearm, and may cause paresthesia in the fingers because of compression or irritation of the median nerve.

Accidental puncture of a large artery in the antecubital fossa carries a high risk of a hematoma and of delayed bleeding, and can lead to other rare but very serious complications such as compartment syndrome of the forearm. Donor care staff should be trained to recognize and correctly manage arterial puncture, so as to avoid the potentially very serious sequelae.

Injury to the median nerve in the antecubital fossa accounts for only a small percentage of all immediate adverse reactions, but relatively often gives rise to serious long-term complications.[40] In approximately one-third of these cases, the median nerve is directly damaged by the venepuncture needle.[40] The donor may experience immediate severe shooting pain, radiating down the forearm, sometimes associated with paresthesia in the median nerve distribution of the hand. Indirect nerve injury may be caused by pressure from an increasing hematoma, with symptoms of pain and paresthesia developing later.

Anatomical studies have shown marked individual variation in the arrangement of nerves and blood vessels in the antecubital fossa, and injuries may occur despite good venepuncture technique.[57] It is essential, however, that phlebotomists are familiar with normal anatomy of the region and are trained in correct techniques of needle insertion, together with prompt recognition and correct management of complications. To reduce the risk of direct nerve injury, the needle should be inserted only once and if the first attempt is unsuccessful, no further attempts should be made.

Hematoma should be managed by stopping the donation immediately if the donor complains of symptoms, applying pressure to the venepuncture site, and recommending that the donor rest the arm and avoid manual work with the donation arm for 24 hours. The donor should return to the blood center or seek medical treatment if there is persistent bleeding from the venepuncture site or if the swelling increases.

Complications associated with apheresis (automated) procedures

The return of donor blood, to which citrate solution has been added, causes a temporary reduction in ionized calcium in the circulation. In mild cases, this may give a tingling sensation in the mouth or extremities, a feeling of vibrations, or a metallic taste; usually, the symptoms resolve on reduction of the speed of return. Sometimes, a drink of milk or oral calcium supplement is administered.

Intravenous calcium solutions are not usually necessary for the common types of collection, but are commonly administered in longer procedures (e.g., peripheral blood stem cells). In more serious citrate reactions, if untreated, symptoms may progress to carpopedal spasms, generalized muscle contractions (tetany), or cardiac arrhythmias, including cardiac arrest. Following a small number of reports of a mixup of saline and citrate bags that led to rapid infusion of citrate solution, blood operators are working together with manufacturers of disposables to modify the connectors, which in future could (once regulatory processes have been concluded) prevent this occurrence.

Long-term effects of regular whole blood donation and apheresis

A medium-term effect is fatigue in the days following a blood donation. Reported by 7.8% of donors in Newman's interview study, it is, however, nonspecific and causality is difficult to assess. Fatigue is not currently included in the international classification system for complications of blood donation.

There has been patchy progress in monitoring and responding to longer term effects of regular whole blood donation. Most attention has been given to the iron depletion that is found in the majority of regular whole blood donors and can lead to iron-deficient erythropoiesis (with a hemoglobin level that is still normal) or to frank iron-deficiency anemia. Policies with regard to pre-donation screening of donors' hemoglobin level differ between countries and blood establishments, as well as the response if iron deficiency is suspected.[58] Some blood establishments conduct further investigations (e.g., performing a ferritin determination).[59] In other settings, such donors are directly referred to their doctor for assessment and treatment. Some blood establishments supply oral iron supplements or advise potentially iron-deficient donors—even if not anemic—to see their family doctors to discuss the possibility of iron supplementation.[60] In other countries, it is felt to be unacceptable to prescribe medication in order to obtain repeated donations—rather, the response is based on deferrals and sometimes preemptive adjustment of the interval between invitations for donation.[61]

Frequent plasmapheresis

How innocuous is frequent plasma donation? In Europe, the maximum volume of plasma collected is limited to 15 L in a year, but donors in the United States (who are often paid or compensated) are less well protected. A study in 2010 found that concentrations of total protein, albumin, immunoglobulin G (IgG), and IgM were significantly lower in plasma pools from high-frequency donors (C1-inhibitor, pre-albumin, and C-reactive protein contents were higher). It is possible that the use of citrate-containing anticoagulant solution, which leads to calcium loss, might increase the likelihood of osteoporosis. A preliminary study using Dexa scans in Dutch donors gave reassuring results.[62]

Use of growth factors, and monitoring safety of stem cell or granulocyte donors

Where donors are treated with growth factors such as granulocyte colony-stimulating factor, active follow-up is recommended for a year or longer for the ascertainment and care of conditions that could have an association with the growth factors or procedure.[63]

Blood recipient hemovigilance

The different transfusion reactions are described in detail in other chapters in this book.

The definitions used by IHN[64] and ISBT-WP[65] can be found on their websites.

Serious adverse events

The EU directives require that serious adverse events be reported, but the legal scope is formally limited to adverse events at the blood establishment or in the blood transfusion laboratory. However, different hemovigilance systems have different scopes. Adverse events can have their origin at any stage of the transfusion chain. SHOT, the ISBT and IHN, and other hemovigilance systems have raised awareness of the risks of IBCT (i.e., all episodes where a patient was transfused with a blood component that did not meet the appropriate requirements or that was intended for another patient, including when the component was ABO compatible and/or if only a small quantity of blood was transfused and/or there was no adverse event). Some systems also capture and report on all episodes where a blood component that did not meet the appropriate requirements was wrongfully released from quarantine or issued, even if it was not transfused.

What have we learned from hemovigilance systems?

We now have a better understanding of the adverse reactions that occur in both blood donors and recipients of blood transfusion. The data from hemovigilance systems generally come from a broader base than data from scientific studies. This is valuable in several ways. It gives us a much better basis for informing donors and patients about risks. It has shown that it is generally safe to donate blood, but that significant donor complications do occur, maybe as often as one per 100 donations. Hemovigilance data also give information about the frequency and seriousness of recipient complications. This is important for directing further research to the most important areas. TRALI is such an example of a transfusion reaction that was seen in hemovigilance data to be more important than previously thought. Research directed to this problem led to effective preventive measures. Similarly, some other rare complications like GvHD and PTP seem to be quite rare. Hemovigilance data can say something about the main causes for the transfusion-related harm, and most significantly there are data showing that errors in pre-administration transfusion checks are the main cause of acute hemolytic transfusion reactions due to ABO incompatibility.[66] This has led to preventive measures being identified such as computer-assisted pretransfusion bedside checking.

Hemovigilance has raised hopes that benchmarking should be possible. The European Union has already collected hemovigilance data from the member countries for several years. We have learned that benchmarking transfusion services in different countries is difficult, if not impossible. There are multiple reasons for this. The general healthcare systems in different countries vary. How the transfusion service is organized also varies, and so do the hemovigilance systems. The work done by IHN and ISBT on common definitions shows promising results in that agreement on definitions is possible, even if it takes time. Now the question is: What do we want to benchmark? When that question has been answered, the hemovigilance systems can start collecting the required data, including background data necessary to give the answers.

It is also doubtful whether hemovigilance data (e.g., the rate of reported transfusion reactions or IBCT) can be used for benchmarking hospitals or local transfusion services, because the complication rates are too low. Exceptions may be transfusion services in large countries, like the example from France mentioned in the next paragraph.

Hemovigilance data have made it possible to compare transfusion reactions to different products. The effect of introducing male-only plasma to reduce the incidence of TRALI is one such example.[42,67] The effect on transfusion reactions by switching from fresh frozen plasma (FFP) to solvent-and-detergent (S/D)-treated pooled plasma in Finland is another example.[68] In a recent health technology assessment (HTA) in Norway, comparing SD-plasma, single-donor pathogen-reduced plasma, quarantine FFP, and FFP, data from different hemovigilance systems proved to be valuable.[69] In this HTA, the data from large countries that have different plasma products in use and a comprehensive hemovigilance system like France's proved to be particularly useful in a field dominated by scientific studies too small to detect differences in infrequent complications.

Donor

Donor hemovigilance data showing the incidence of complications, together with the work[70,71] showing that donors that experience complications tend not to donate again, have led to more focus on avoiding complications. Several preventive measures have been presented, such as giving donors water or isotonic drinks, with or without salty snacks, prior to donation; teaching donors to use muscle tension; and teaching the staff about social distraction to avoid vasovagal complications.

Work has started on incorporating estimation of blood volume as an acceptance criterion for blood donors. Tables for blood volume based on donor height and weight are now incorporated in the Council of Europe guide to preparation, use, and quality of blood components.[25] One aim is to protect the donor; another is to be able to collect more from some donors.

Despite being an important complication related to whole blood donation, iron deficiency and iron deficiency anemia are frequently not reported in hemovigilance systems. There is a need for research and consensus development on the best way to capture information on this, so that this may provide background data and inform the discussion on measuring iron stores and on whether blood donors should be given iron supplementation routinely.

Recipient

Volume overload due to transfusion was not always regarded as a transfusion reaction, but since some hemovigilance systems started reporting this, it has received more attention. When the patients receive other IV fluids at the same time as blood, the volume overload was often ascribed to the other fluids, but the volume of blood components transfused should also be considered (Chapter 59).

In some cases, volume overload can result from unnecessary exposure to blood components. Both over- and undertransfusion are registered in some hemovigilance systems. These adverse events can result from (1) incorrect decision making; (2) prescribing errors, such as volume miscalculation; or (3) transfusion based on a spurious hemoglobin result from a sample diluted by intravenous infusion, from the wrong patient, or from a laboratory result that is incorrect or wrongly documented. These are relevant for a hemovigilance system, because the causes should be highlighted and preventive measures identified.

Reports to SHOT, when interpreted in the context of epidemiologic data, suggest that out of core hours, when staffing level are lover, transfusion carries an increased risk[72] compared to those administered during the day and that transfusion to pediatric patients is more likely to result in an adverse outcome than adult transfusion.[73]

Overall, however, hemovigilance systems have demonstrated that blood transfusion is safe. An example from SHOT proves this while it still points at areas for further improvement. Over a 10-year period, during which time 30 million blood components were issued from UK blood services, SHOT received 3770 reports, of which 2717 (72%) were of IBCT. Ninety-five percent of these patients survived with no serious effects, but 24 deaths were attributed wholly or in part to avoidable transfusion errors, and 100 patients suffered major morbidity.[74]

Discussion

At the regional or national level, the hemovigilance system must be seen as impartial, independent, supportive, and professionally credible. Effective hemovigilance requires not only accurate and complete collection of data, but also interpretation within a predictable timeframe of the data in the context of what is known of transfusion epidemiology and practice, and use of the data to improve patient safety, both locally and nationally. The data and the analysis should be published in a format that can be used to support education and training. Reporting in itself is not a means of reducing errors or complications. Learning from the system may lead to improved safety awareness and better adherence to protocols. For maximal nationwide improvement, recommendations need to be incorporated in national guidelines or legislation, depending on the situation. Active involvement and "ownership" by professional bodies will help to ensure that recommendations are incorporated into clinical practice.

Strengths of hemovigilance

We now have transparency that was not available 20 years ago. Awareness of error-prone areas can lead to improved working procedures. Hemovigilance results combined with published research are leading to real improvements in transfusion safety. Both SHOT and the French hemovigilance systems have reported a lower rate of ABO-incompatible red blood cell transfusions in recent years.

A national hemovigilance system can give useful information on local, regional, national, and international levels. The data can be used in local improvement work as well as in making national and international guidelines and regulations.

Limitations

Hemovigilance systems do not register harm to patients because of failure to provide blood. This may be due to failure by the clinician to order blood, failure to transfuse the issued blood, or lack of available products in the transfusion service. The latter can be due to a general shortage of blood or more specific problems like lack of red cells with certain phenotypes or lack of HLA-compatible platelets.

The current systems are poorly suited to capture of complications due to repeated donations.

A hemovigilance system will be better at detecting immediate complications than complications occurring sometime after donation or transfusion. Delayed donor complications may be discovered if returning donors are asked about any complications after the previous donation, and donors should be reminded to inform the blood bank if they have complications after leaving the donation room. Delayed hemolytic transfusion reactions, typically occurring 10 days after transfusion, are probably underreported and probably often undiagnosed.

Passive reporting system can lead to underreporting, especially if you do not have a blame-free culture.

For good analysis, it is necessary to have denominator data. This can be data on units transfused, the underlying condition of the patients, patients not transfused, and so on. Highly automated transfusion services are usually at an advantage here, as are hospitals with comprehensive administrative computer systems.

Further perspectives

An important aspect of quality work is to reduce variation.[75] At present, differences in system and in practice mean we are not properly able to investigate differences in reported incidences between countries. One must also expect that the safety culture and the reporting culture may vary a lot between countries. An example is the OECD's attempt to include wrong blood transfused as a patient safety indicator. A never event such as this was thought to have the potential of a useful safety indicator. In practice, however, it had to be abandoned because the reporting countries showed too much variation for the rates to be credible.

For a system to work, one should not register more data than will be used for analysis. International agreement on a minimum set of data to include in hemovigilance systems would be useful. This could be the next step when agreement on definitions is reached.

Conclusion

Hemovigilance systems show that both blood donation and blood transfusion are safe. The data collected has been used to improve safety further by pointing research and improvement work in the right direction. Knowing the incidence and seriousness of complications is very valuable in this respect. Giving correct information on risks to donors and patients is necessary for donors and patients to trust the transfusion service. In the future international agreement on definitions and on recommended background data to collect may make benchmarking possible.

Key references

A full reference list for this chapter is available at: http://www.wiley.com/go/simon/transfusion

24 Wiersum-Osselton JC, Wood E, Bolton-Maggs PHB, Schipperus MR. Definitions in haemovigilance: guiding principles and current state of development of international reference definitions. *ISBT Science Series* 2014;**9**: 91–7.

40 Sorensen BS, Johnsen SP, Jorgensen J. Complications related to blood donation: a population-based study. *Vox Sang* 2008;**94**: 132–7.

51 France CR, Ditto B, Wissel ME, *et al.* Predonation hydration and applied muscle tension combine to reduce presyncopal reactions to blood donation. *Transfusion* 2010;**50**: 1257–64.

54 Eder AF, Dy BA, Kennedy JM, *et al.* Improved safety for young whole blood donors with new selection criteria for total estimated blood volume. *Transfusion* 2011;**51**: 1522–31.

55 Tomasulo P, Kamel H, Bravo M, James RC, Custer B. Interventions to reduce the vasovagal reaction rate in young whole blood donors. *Transfusion* 2011;**51**: 1511–21.

56 Kamel H, Tomasulo P, Bravo M, *et al.* Delayed adverse reactions to blood donation. *Transfusion* 2010;**50**: 556–65.

66 Bolton-Maggs PHB (Ed), Poles D, Watt A, Thomas D, on behalf of the *Serious Hazards of Transfusion (SHOT) Steering Group. The 2013 annual SHOT report.* Manchester, UK: SHOT, 2014.

67 Wiersum-Osselton JC, Middelburg RA, Beckers EA, *et al.* Male-only fresh-frozen plasma for transfusion-related acute lung injury prevention: before-and-after comparative cohort study. *Transfusion* 2011;**51**: 1278–83.

CHAPTER 7

Global perspective on ensuring blood and blood product safety and availability

Paul D. Mintz & Mark J. Weinstein

US Food and Drug Administration, Silver Spring, MD, USA

Blood products are considered an essential part of medical therapy worldwide. National systems are seen in much of the developed world (e.g., Europe, Canada, Australia, and New Zealand), with the United States as an exception. (In Canada, there is one national system and a second one for the province of Quebec.) Less developed countries often have hospital-based systems (in some cases with a small national system, as in Mexico). Many are run by the International Red Cross and are government subsidized.

In the United States, a majority of the blood is collected and distributed by community blood centers that generally are part of a trade organization called America's Blood Centers (ABC). Consolidation among the members has been a recent development. The American Red Cross, which is separate from ABC, collects and distributes about 40% of the blood. The AABB (formerly the American Association of Blood Banks) is a professional society of individuals in the field, community blood centers, and hospital transfusion services. It publishes *AABB Technical Manual and Standards for Blood Bank and Transfusion Services* (as well as several publications containing standards for various specialized services) that both serve as voluntary guides to procedures and quality requirements and tend to establish a standard of care. A small percentage of blood is collected and processed by hospital-based blood banks. Testing has been centralized in large laboratories run by the American Red Cross and independent blood centers (e.g., Creative Testing Solutions and Qualtex). Blood centers have also become more active in recent years in offering transfusion services to hospitals.

Plasma collection and manufacturing organizations belong to a trade association known as the PPTA (Plasma Protein Therapeutics Association, or PPTA Source for collections), which is global and standard setting for plasma collection and fractionation. There is also an international blood transfusion society, the International Society of Blood Transfusion. In addition, the World Health Organization (WHO) has an ongoing interest in blood availability and safety worldwide. Many of these activities are overseen by national regulatory bodies that differ between the United States,

Europe, and the rest of the world but embrace similar principles related to the efficacy and safety of blood products.

US perspective on ensuring blood and blood product safety and availability

History of safety and efficacy requirements for drugs and biologics in the United States

Regulatory approval of drugs and biologics in the United States is subject to federal law. Safety and efficacy requirements related to drug and biologics approval have evolved through the 20th and 21st centuries.[1–3] In 1906, President Theodore Roosevelt included a recommendation for food and drug legislation in his annual message to Congress, which resulted in passage of the Pure Food and Drug Act (Public Law 59-384; 34 Stat. 768). The intent of the law was to prevent the manufacture, sale, and transportation of misbranded and adulterated foods and drugs. The passage of subsequent public health laws often followed several therapeutic tragedies. In 1937, the S.E. Massengill Co. introduced sulfanilamide dissolved in diethylene glycol. No drug safety testing was required by law at the time. The drug was promoted to treat streptococcal infections and caused deaths of more than 100 people in 15 states.[1,2] This and similar incidents led to the enactment of the 1938 Food, Drug, and Cosmetic Act (FDCA) (Public Law 75-717; 52 Stat. 1040).[1,2,4]

The law, which became effective in June 1939, differed substantially from the 1906 Act that it replaced. It extended coverage to include cosmetics and therapeutic devices. It required the predistribution clearance of new drugs for safety and provided authority to establish tolerances for potentially poisonous substances in foods and drugs. It added the sanctions of injunction and emergency permit control to the seizure and prosecution authority in the previous act. As the main purpose of the law was to prohibit the movement of mislabeled and adulterated food, drugs, devices, and cosmetics in interstate commerce, it authorized inspections of factories, warehouses, establishments, and vehicles used in manufacturing, processing, packing, storing, and transporting these products. The act also established a requirement that a new drug could not be introduced into interstate commerce unless an application was made. The application needed to include a full report of investigations to show whether or not the drug was safe for use; an

This book chapter reflects the views of the authors and should not be construed to represent FDA's views or policies.

Rossi's Principles of Transfusion Medicine, Fifth Edition. Edited by Toby L. Simon, Jeffrey McCullough, Edward L. Snyder, Bjarte G. Solheim, and Ronald G. Strauss.
© 2016 John Wiley & Sons, Ltd. Published 2016 by John Wiley & Sons, Ltd.

explanation of the drug's composition; a description of the methods, facilities, and controls used in manufacturing, processing, and packing; as well as samples of the drug and label. Grounds for application rejection included inadequacy of tests, failure of test results and other information to help determine the product safety, as well as inadequacy of facilities, methods, and controls used in manufacturing, processing, and packing for preserving the product's identity, strength, purity, and quality.

In the 1940s, the FDCA was amended with requirements of batch certification for certain drugs (e.g., penicillin; Public Law 79-139; 59 Stat. 463) to verify product identity, quality, purity, and strength, and thus try to ensure their safety and presumed effectiveness.[3] Thalidomide caused another public health disaster in the late 1950s and early 1960s.[1,2] Introduced in late 1957 to treat insomnia, colds, coughs, and headaches, the drug was found to relieve symptoms of so-called *morning sickness*, and was prescribed for this indication as well. At the time, drugs were not tested for their effects on the fetus. As a result, thousands of children, born in 46 countries, suffered congenital deformities. Although some pregnant women in the United States used this medication as it was distributed to physicians during the clinical testing program, the United States experienced fewer cases of birth defects, as the FDA refused to approve thalidomide. The enactment of the 1962 Amendments to the 1938 FDCA (Public Law 87-781, 76 Stat. 780; commonly known as the Kefauver–Harris Amendments) came as a response to the thalidomide disaster.[1,2] This law made regulatory approval a mandatory prerequisite for product marketing, strengthened safety regulations, and added the requirement for applicants to provide evidence of product effectiveness through adequate and well-controlled studies, including clinical investigations. Additionally, the Drug Amendments of 1962 stated that drug advertising should contain a label with the prominently printed established product name, formula with ingredient quantification, as well as information related to side effects, contraindications, and effectiveness.

Biologics-related requirements also developed gradually and roughly in parallel with drug legislation.[1–3] In 1901, 13 children in St. Louis, Missouri, and nine in Camden, New Jersey, died of tetanus after receiving contaminated diphtheria antitoxin and smallpox vaccine, respectively. In 1902, Congress passed the Biologics Control Act (Public Law 57-244; 32 Stat. 728), also known as the Virus-Toxin Law.[1,2] The law authorized the promulgation of licensing regulations for establishments involved in production of toxins, antitoxins, viruses, sera, and similar products. The act also authorized inspections at manufacturing facilities. Companies needed to be licensed for the manufacture and sale of the products. Inspectors were required to study product purity and potency. In 1934, new regulations, published under the title "Regulations for the Sale of Viruses, Serums, Toxins and Analogous Products in the District of Columbia and in Interstate Traffic," explicitly indicated that licenses for new products would not be granted without acceptable evidence of therapeutic or prophylactic efficiency.[3] In 1944, the Public Health Service Act (PHSA) was enacted (Public Law 78-410; 58 Stat. 682).[5] Section 351 of this law incorporated, with few changes, the Biologics Control Act. The document stated that licenses would be issued only upon a showing that the establishment and the products for which a license was being sought met the standards intended to ensure the continued safety, purity, and potency of the products.

> The term "biological product" means a virus, therapeutic serum, toxin, antitoxin, vaccine, blood, blood component or derivative, allergenic product, protein (except any chemically synthesized polypeptide), or analogous product, or arsphenamine or derivative of arsphenamine (or any other trivalent organic arsenic compound), applicable to the prevention, treatment, or cure of a disease or condition of human beings. (PHSA Sec. 351(i))

As noted, regulatory approval of drugs and biologics in the United States is subject to federal law. Drugs are approved under Section 505 of the Food, Drug, and Cosmetic Act (21 U.S.C. 355), as amended.[4] An order to approve an application is issued if none of the following applies: The investigations are found to be inadequate; the results either do not prove product safety or prove its unsafety; the data submitted as part of the application and other available information do not provide sufficient evidence of product safety and effectiveness; the methods, facilities, and controls used in manufacturing, processing, and packing are found to be inadequate to preserve the product's identity, strength, purity, and quality; and the application lacks the required patent information. Although biologics are also considered to be drugs, because most of them meet the definition of the term *drug* in FDCA Section 201(g)(1) (21 U.S. C. 321), they are usually licensed under authority of Section 351 of the PHSA (42 U.S.C. 262), as amended.[5] Under Section 351, which has been in effect since 1944, biologics license applications are approved following the applicants' consent to the inspection of the facilities and on the basis of a demonstration that the products are safe, pure, and potent, and the facilities in which the biologics are manufactured pass an on-site inspection.

The FDCA of 1938 has been amended dozens of times. Major amendments include the FDA Modernization Act (FDAMA) of 1997,[6] the Food and Drug Administration Amendments Act (FDAAA) of 2007,[7] and the Food and Drug Administration Safety and Innovation Act (FDASIA) of 2012.[8]

FDA regulation of blood collection establishments
Overview

Blood and blood components are used in the treatment of disease. Therefore, blood and blood components meet the definition of a drug in Section 201(g) of the FDCA; and blood products, including source plasma, must meet all statutory requirements of the FDCA. FDCA sections applicable to blood include Sections 201, Definitions; 301, Prohibited Acts; 501, Adulteration; 502, Misbranding; 510, Registration; and 704, Factory Inspection (see Ref.[26]).

The fundamental principles of the regulation of blood collection establishments are to ensure the safety, effectiveness, and availability of blood and blood products; protect the health of the donors and recipients; and ensure that the blood collected is safe for transfusion or further manufacture (see Ref.[26]). One of the means for assuring this is through the requirements for current good manufacturing practices (cGMPs). Applicable cGMP regulations are found in the US Code of Federal Regulations (CFR) within Title 21 Part 210, Manufacturing, Processing, Packing, or Holding of Drugs; Title 21 Part 211, Finished Pharmaceuticals; and 21 CFR 606s, Blood and Blood Components. Table 7.1 lists the subparts of 21 CFR Part 211 (cGMPs for finished pharmaceuticals),[9] and Table 7.2 lists the applicable sections for blood and blood products in 21 CFR Parts 600–640.

The PHSA requires licensure for biological products in interstate commerce. In this regard, each package of a biological product is plainly marked; the biological product is required to be safe, pure, potent, and effective; the facility where the product is manufactured meets standards; and the applicant consents to inspection. Licensure

Table 7.1 21 CFR Part 211 cGMP for finished pharmaceuticals[28]

- Subpart A: General Provisions
- Subpart B: Organization and Personnel
- Subpart C: Buildings and Facilities
- Subpart D: Equipment
- Subpart E: Control of Components and Drug Product Containers and Closures
- Subpart F: Production and Process Controls
- Subpart G: Packaging and Labeling Control
- Subpart H: Holding and Distribution
- Subpart I: Laboratory Controls
- Subpart J: Records and Reports
- Subpart K: Returned & Salvaged Drug Products

Table 7.2 21 CFR Parts 600–640: Applicable sections for blood and blood products[28]

- 600: Biological products: general
- 601: Licensing
- 606: Current good manufacturing practice for blood and blood components
- 607: Establishment registration and product listing for manufacturers of human blood and blood products
- 610: General biological products standards
- 630: General requirements for blood, blood components, and blood derivatives
- 640: Additional standards for human blood and blood products

signifies FDA approval of product(s) and facility. It is intended to ensure the safety, effectiveness, and availability of blood and blood products, thereby allowing shipment of product(s) in interstate commerce. It also protects the health of the donor and recipients.

In applying the requirements of cGMP to a firm, the distinction between licensure and registration is more technical than real. Licensure is required to ship products in interstate commerce or internationally. Registration is required for all blood and tissue establishments, including those located in hospitals, that manufacture (collect, store, process, or distribute) blood components for transfusion or further manufacture. Registration requirements for manufacturers of human blood and blood products are outlined in 21 CFR Part 607; license requirements are in 21 CFR Part 601. Tissue for transplantation requirements are found in 21 CFR Part 1270. Elements of cGMP are listed in Table 7.3. The division into elements is arbitrary but is based on an analysis of commonality of the requirements of Title 21 as they apply to all aspects of blood center and hospital blood bank operations. Thus, it is irrelevant whether they are applied to blood collection or to infectious disease testing; each element is applicable for each discrete blood center operation. Because blood and plasma centers are required to follow

Table 7.3 Elements of current good manufacturing practice

- Standard operating procedures
- Recordkeeping
- Personnel management
- Calibration
- Validation
- Labeling
- Error management
- Quality control and auditing
- Facilities and equipment
- Process and production change control

their own standard operating procedures (SOPs), each SOP creates unique regulatory requirements for that center. From a regulatory standpoint, this concept is significant in that compliance standards and regulatory requirements are created by individual center SOPs. cGMP describes both the production methods used by blood centers to manufacture components and the manufacturing process controls in place. Each provision of a center's SOPs must reflect the manufacturers' instructions for licensed or approved systems used in the center.

Meticulous records of compliance with cGMP elements are required to assure both executive management and the FDA that a blood establishment's manufacturing process is under control. *Control*, in this context, can be defined as compliance in every respect with the entire establishment's manufacturing SOPs and FDA requirements. It is worth emphasizing that if a firm's SOPs are more stringent than FDA requirements, it is not acceptable to deviate from the SOP, even if the FDA requirement is met, unless appropriate change control and reporting to FDA are carried out before the deviation. During inspections of blood centers, whether by the private sector or regulatory bodies such as the FDA, the overriding investigational concern is whether an establishment has this control. Records should be designed to document control of manufacturing systems.

Management of SOPs lies at the heart of quality manufacturing and cGMP compliance. Although not required by the CFR, it is generally held that the Quality Assurance (QA) unit should organizationally be distinct from manufacturing to ensure its independence, and this de facto requirement appears in FDA guidances.[10,11] In many blood centers, the director of the QA unit reports to the chief executive officer. All matters that relate to quality should funnel to a single person or group with broad knowledge of the entire blood center operation and access to the information necessary to assess the impact of proposed changes. These principles emphasize the importance with which the FDA views both the quality unit and SOPs. However, case law holds that upper management cannot avoid adverse consequences of noncompliance with regulatory requirements because a lower ranking employee is designated the authorized official.[12] QA units can be deployed to enhance the quality of blood center operations in a variety of ways. They can assume responsibility for personnel training, especially in cGMP; maintain calibration and validation records; design validation protocols; and identify trends through statistical analysis. A well-directed QA unit can be of enormous value to both the authorized officials and the staff of the facilities in which it is established. However, QA unit staff are not the ideal staff to write SOPs, because they need to be the final approval authority, and their objectivity cannot be ensured when reviewing their own work.

Although internal audits are also not specifically required by regulations, procedures to detect problems are required and internal audits are an important means of ensuring that processes remain in control. Internal audits are considered confidential by the FDA and are not available to FDA investigators unless fraud is suspected or there appears to be an imminent threat to public health. The reason for this policy is to encourage audits that are complete and detailed with no information withheld. The FDA also respects supplier audits as confidential internal audit information. However, it is critical that the center have readily available SOPs for audits, schedules demonstrating that all elements of operations are reviewed regularly (at least annually), processes for ensuring and documenting corrective and preventive action and follow-up, and formal closure notices to complete the records. It is also essential that any deviations discovered in the course of audits be properly documented in records that are available to FDA investigators. The QA system must be assessed for effectiveness by management at regular intervals. Rigorous application of cGMP principles to the production processes of blood and blood components has greatly reduced, but not completely eliminated, risks associated with the transfusion of blood components. Fortunately, the availability of industrial models broadly applicable to blood centers has facilitated cGMP implementation.

Table 7.4 lists selected QA unit responsibilities.

Inspections

Facility inspectors are instructed that the facility must have knowledgeable staff, appropriate equipment, and adequate procedures to ensure that donors are screened and units are collected, stored, and shipped in accordance with FDA regulations. The establishment's procedures must address donor screening; blood collection; unit identification; operation of all screening and collection equipment; handling of donor reactions; management of postdonation information reports; storage of product and supplies; quality control of reagents, supplies, and equipment; transport of collected units; and documentation and follow-up of any unexpected incidents. Inspections should include observations of the actual screening process and an examination of the physical layout of the facility to insure that there is limited public access to biohazardous areas, proper disposal of biohazardous materials, accessible restrooms and handwashing equipment, and clean and organized storage areas. Supplies should be examined to make certain they are used within their expiration date.

As noted, biological products are regulated under the authority of Section 351 of the PHSA and under the FDCA as drugs or devices, with the exception of certain human cells, tissues, and cellular and tissue-based products (HCT/Ps) that are regulated solely under Section 361 of the PHSA (see 21 CFR 1271.10). Blood and blood products for transfusion are prescription drugs under the FDCA.

Reporting of product deviations [21 CFR Part 211, 21 CFR 606.160(b)(7)(iii), 21 CFR 606.171, and 21 CFR 606.100(c)]

Apart from the requirement to report and investigate adverse reactions, as stipulated in 21 CFR 606.170, an organized error management process is not specifically required by the provisions of Title 21, although 21 CFR 606.171(c) mandates the reporting within 45 days of all biologic product deviations on released products. Table 7.5 provides a summary of the reporting criteria and examples of reportable and nonreportable events. Traditionally, 21 CFR 600.14 has always been interpreted to require licensed facilities to report promptly any error that may affect the safety, purity, or potency of the product, and it was understood that a system was needed for capturing these events consistently. The FDA has recognized the importance of this cGMP element in regulations finalized in 2000 (21 CFR 606.171). The rules are more broadly applicable to blood establishments than any preceding policies, although they are narrowly directed.[13,14]

The investigation and follow-up of deviations are critical to the successful improvement of blood center quality. Appropriate management of errors and deviations (accidents) forms the centerpiece of continuous improvement. Each blood center deviation should be treated as an opportunity to be used to improve center processes. All facilities must develop SOPs for reporting, managing, and correcting errors and deviations. These SOPs should form the centerpiece

---

Table 7.4 Quality unit responsibilities

Attributes of the Required Quality Unit
- Responsibilities are described in writing.
- Is independent of production.
- Is involved in all quality-related matters.
- Reviews and approves all quality-related issues.
- Has adequate analytic control facilities at its disposal.

Quality Unit Responsibilities Should Include, but Not Be Limited to, the Following
- Approve specifications.
- Approve test procedures, including process controls.
- Approve validation plans, protocols, or equipment.
- Review changes in product, process, or equipment, and determine if revalidation is required.
- Approve specification changes, sampling plans, and test procedures.
- Approve sampling procedures.
- Approve reference standards.
- Conduct analytic investigations and evaluate results.
- Approve testing materials.
- Provide analytical reports.
- Approve or reject intermediates and active pharmaceutical ingredients manufactured, processed, packed, or held under contract by another establishment.
- Gather data to support retest dates (stability testing).
- Evaluate and approve contractors.
- Review batch records.
- Review complaints.
- Dispose of materials not meeting specifications.
- Dispose of materials returned to the establishment.
- Perform internal and external audits.
- Perform periodic assessments of procedures, policies, and responsibilities within the establishment's manufacturing and control operations.

Table 7.5 Reportable biologic product deviations

- An event occurs that may affect product purity, safety, or potency.
- Postdonation information is received that potentially affects safety.
- Compatibility sample was collected from the wrong patient.
- Collection or processing materials did not meet specifications.
- FDA requirements were not met on donor deferral and screening.
- Current or subsequent viral marker test was positive.
- Donor screening (history, arm inspection, etc.) was not recorded.
- Both confidential unit exclusion stickers were not applied to unit.
- Donor deferral lists were incorrectly checked.
- Bag used for collection was outdated.
- Donor sample of unit was clotted or hemolyzed.
- Standard operating procedures for collections were inadequate or not followed.
- Collection time was not documented or extended.
- Time frame for collection or processing was incorrect.
- Use of special procedures was inappropriate.
- Testing was not performed in accordance with instructions.
- Unsuitable samples were used for testing.
- Mislabeling of ABO and the like occurred.
- Storage or shipping temperatures were incorrect.
- Unsuitable units were not quarantined.
- Special orders were not filled (e.g., cytomegalovirus-negative).

Examples of Nonreportable Biologic Product Deviations
- Transfusion errors occurred outside the blood facility.
- An error was corrected before distribution, and safety was not affected.
- Lookback, retrieval, or notification procedures were not followed.
- Donor protective measures were not met (age, colds, flu, etc).
- Previous donation records were not checked.
- Labeling errors occurred that did not affect safety (short expiration, etc).
- Shipping paperwork contained errors.
- Units were returned because of temperature deviations.

of both blood center staff training and continuous improvement. Error management efforts and results should be documented in the records of the quality unit. Monitoring corrective action outcomes to ensure effectiveness is an essential part of the system for addressing corrections.

Although error management systems are not defined in Title 21, some attributes of good systems have emerged both in blood centers and in industrial manufacturing establishments. They include:

1 Employees at all levels in the organization are encouraged to report errors. Punitive policies discourage reporting, and hence opportunities for systems improvements may be lost.

2 Employees involved in the process in which an error was made should be involved with the investigation and resolution of the error and process change. It is essential that the investigation be sufficient to determine the underlying root cause for the error rather than identifying mere "symptoms" of the root cause. The FDA also requires that staff be educated concerning the effect their errors have or potentially have on product quality; that is, it is required that they understand how their responsibilities have an effect on ensuring that only safe products are released.

3 Confirmation of the effectiveness of the corrective action is vital to ensure that the improved process continues to yield the expected results. Postchange monitoring is essential, and long-term evaluation should be performed at appropriate intervals (e.g., 3–6 months after a process improvement is completed).

CBER conducts a wide range of compliance and surveillance activities during the "life cycle" of biological products. These include:

- Conducting prelicense and preapproval inspections as well as postlicensure and postapproval inspections of manufacturing facilities and products under clinical study.
- Monitoring the safety, purity, and potency of biological products through review of:
  ○ Biological product deviation reports and HCT/P deviation reports;
  ○ Investigations into transfusion- and donation-related fatalities and other adverse events; and
  ○ Product recalls.
- Monitoring reports of biological product shortages.
- Initiating regulatory action to address noncompliance with FDA laws and regulations.
- Monitoring of research conducted on biological products and assessing the protection of the rights, safety, and welfare of human research subjects and the quality and integrity of research data.
- Monitoring import and export activities.
- Reviewing product advertising and promotional labeling.

Device regulatory controls

All classes of medical devices are subject to what are known as *general controls*. General controls are the basic provisions of the May 28, 1976, Medical Device Amendments to the FDCA. They provide the FDA with the means of regulating devices to ensure their safety and effectiveness. General controls in the FDCA apply to all medical devices. They include provisions that relate to adulteration; misbranding; device registration and listing; premarket notification; banned devices, including repair, replacement, or refund; records and reports; restricted devices; and good manufacturing practices.

Class I devices are subject to general controls and are typically exempt from submission of a premarket 510(k) notification. They are viewed as posing the lowest risk to the patient and/or user.

Class II devices are subject to what are known as *special controls* in addition to the general controls provision of the FDCA. Special controls may include compliance with a recognized standard, warning statements in the instructions for use, specific performance requirements, and/or other controls necessary to ensure a reasonable assurance of safety and effectiveness. Class II devices typically require FDA clearance of a premarket 510(k) notification to permit the device to be marketed and sold in the United States.

Class III devices are viewed as presenting a higher level of risk. They may be first-of-a-kind devices for which general and special controls are not adequate to ensure safety and effectiveness. Class III devices require FDA approval in the form of a premarket approval application prior to marketing, as well as compliance with device general controls.

The 510(k) premarket notification is a submission made to the FDA to demonstrate that the device to be marketed is at least as safe and effective as (i.e., is substantially equivalent to) a legally marketed Class I or II device of that same generic type. When determined to be substantially equivalent, the subject device may be legally marketed and sold in the United States.

The legally marketed device to which substantial equivalence is determined is known as the *predicate device*. A predicate device can be a preamendments device (legally marketed prior to the May 28, 1976, Medical Device Amendments to the FDCA) or a postamendments device that is, or was, legally marketed in the United States following the device amendments. A claim of substantial equivalence does not mean the new device must be identical to the predicate device. Substantial equivalence is based on a comparative assessment with respect to intended use, design, energy used or delivered, materials, performance, safety, effectiveness, labeling, biocompatibility, standards, and other applicable characteristics that would demonstrate the device is as safe and effective as the predicate device.

Blood establishment computer software

On December 3, 2014, the Blood Products Advisory Committee was seated as a device classification panel. In open session, the panel discussed the appropriate device classification of blood establishment computer software (BECS) and accessories to BECS. BECS is currently subject to the 510(k) premarket notification provisions of the FDCA. FDCA Section 513 established the risk-based device classification system for medical devices. BECS and BECS accessories have not been classified under this statutory provision. Currently, these devices are regulated as unclassified devices, subject to 510(k) premarket notification requirements. At this Blood Products Advisory Committee meeting, the committee also voted to recommend that BECS be designated as Class II devices.

Since the device amendments of May 28, 1976, BECS and BECS accessories have been found substantially equivalent to a device that was legally marketed prior to May 28, 1976 (i.e., a preamendments device). The preamendments devices include Advanced Medical Systems, a computer-based Blood Bank Management System used to perform compatibility testing, and the American National Red Cross (ANRC) computer-based Donor Deferral Register, which is used to determine temporary or permanent disqualification of donors.

Medical device data systems, regulated under Section 880.6310, are Class I medical devices exempt from 510(k) premarket notification, and were not included for consideration under the BECS and BECS accessories classification.

FDA Structure: Office of Blood Research and Review (OBRR)

FDA regulatory review of devices, drugs, and biologics is conducted by the Center for Drug Evaluation and Research (CDER), the Center for Devices and Radiologic Health (CDRH), and the Center for Biologics Evaluation and Research (CBER). All submissions and applications (including combination products) are assigned to one center for review. The OBRR within CBER is typically assigned biologics review (other than vaccines and cell, tissue, and gene therapies). Within OBRR, four divisions manage the review process: the Division of Hematology Clinical Review (e.g., clinical biologics and certain recombinant and transgenic analogs), the Division of Hematology Research and Review (e.g., chemistry, manufacturing, and controls), the Division of Emerging and Transfusion Transmitted Diseases (e.g., donor infectious disease testing), and the Division of Blood Components and Devices (e.g., licensing of blood establishments, immunohematology devices, and donor qualification). Policy (e.g., guidances) is developed by all four divisions along with the OBRR leadership. Numerous guidance documents (some previously titled as *guidelines* but now referred to as *guidance*) have been issued by OBRR and may be found at: http://www.fda.gov/BiologicsBloodVaccines/GuidanceComplianceRegulatoryInformation/Guidances/Blood/default.htm

Guidances represent the FDA's current thinking on a topic. They do not bind the FDA or manufacturers to any course of action. Alternative approaches are acceptable, if they satisfy the requirements of the applicable statutes and regulations.

Regulation and accreditation of hospital transfusion services
Overview

The Clinical Laboratory Improvement Act and Amendments (CLIA) stipulate requirements for the qualifications of staff who perform or supervise the testing conducted within a transfusion service. AABB standards[15] and FDA cGMP regulations also require that the transfusion service have a process for personnel training and competency evaluation.

Written SOPs are required by the FDA in 21 CFR 606.100. A system must be in place to ensure process control for the validation of processes and procedures, introduction and change of processes and procedures, proficiency testing, quality control, and the use of materials and other aspects of performance of procedures. A defined system of documentation and record retention is required by 21 CFR 606.140 and 21 CFR 606.160 and also by AABB standards.

AABB standards state that the blood bank or transfusion service shall have a medical director who is a licensed physician and qualified by education, training, and/or experience. The medical director shall have responsibility and authority for all medical and technical policies, processes, and procedures—including those that pertain to laboratory personnel and test performance—and for the consultative and support services that relate to the care and safety of donors and/or transfusion recipients. The medical director may delegate these responsibilities to another qualified physician; however, the medical director shall retain ultimate responsibility for the medical director duties. However, the standards do not require that overall executive management to be under the control of the medical director.[15] The Joint Commission also does not require that the overall direction of the laboratory be performed by a physician but does state that "a pathologist or physician qualified in immunohematology, hemotherapy, and blood banking directs blood transfusion services" (HR 1.15).[16] This often excludes the medical director from authority in personnel (other than policies

and procedures), purchasing, budgeting, and other administrative matters. The regulation states that the laboratory director must be a doctor of medicine or doctor of osteopathy licensed in the state where the laboratory is located (42 CFR 493.1443).[17]

The FDA, AABB, and the College of American Pathologists (CAP) all have requirements regarding the evaluation and reporting of adverse effects of blood transfusion. The FDA requires that records be maintained of any reports of adverse reactions to blood transfusion and that a thorough investigation of each reported reaction be conducted. All transfusion services must report deaths confirmed as being caused by a transfusion. The applicable regulation (21 CFR 606.170(b)) reads,

> When a complication of blood collection or transfusion is confirmed to be fatal, the Director, Office of Compliance and Biologics Quality, CBER, must be notified by telephone, facsimile, express mail, or electronically transmitted mail as soon as possible. A written report of the investigation must be submitted to the Director, Office of Compliance and Biologics Quality, CBER, by mail, facsimile, or electronically transmitted mail (for mailing addresses, see 600.2 of this chapter), within 7 days after the fatality by the collecting facility in the event of a donor reaction, or by the facility that performed the compatibility tests in the event of a transfusion reaction. (http://www.fda.gov/BiologicsBloodVaccines/GuidanceComplianceRegulatoryInformation/Guidances/Blood/ucm074947.htm)

The AABB requires that a transfusion service have a process for the detection, reporting, and evaluation of suspected complications of transfusion and that all suspected transfusion complications are evaluated and reviewed by the medical director.[15] The CAP requires that all transfusion reactions or incidents be reported immediately to the laboratory (TRM.41750), that documented procedures exist for actions to be taken in the event of a transfusion reaction (TRM.41700),[18] and that the results of the investigation be recorded in the patient's chart (TRM.42050).[18]

Further aspects of FDA regulations and accreditation requirements of AABB, the Joint Commission, CAP, and other accrediting organizations are described in the "FDA Regulation of Hospital Transfusion Services" section.

FDA regulation of hospital transfusion services

Total quality systems have been required for blood banks and transfusion services since 1975 when the FDA incorporated cGMP into the Code of Federal Regulations. Although the regulations were aimed primarily at blood centers, many of the provisions apply to transfusion services as well. In 1995, the Center for Biologics Evaluation and Research produced a Guidance to assist establishments in developing quality programs in accord with applicable regulations.[10]

In laboratories where clinical samples are tested, Clinical Laboratory Improvement Amendments (CLIA) requirements for quality control (QC), listed at 42 CFR Part 493, must also be followed. All personnel shall be trained in its application. The quality system shall be under the supervision of a designated person who reports to executive management. For reagents for which there are no QC requirements in Title 21, the QC testing described in the manufacturer's package insert must be followed. It is mandated that "each laboratory establish and follow written policies and procedures for a comprehensive quality assurance program. . . . The laboratory's quality assurance program must evaluate the effectiveness of its policies and procedures; identify and correct problems. . . . All quality assurance activities must be documented."[17]

For any hospital QA program to work successfully, physicians must give priority to the process, and hospital administration must make the necessary resources available to ensure its development, implementation, refinement, and continuation.

The FDA requires that errors or accidents affecting the safety, quality, integrity, purity, or potency of a blood product be reported, and this requirement extends to both licensed blood establishments and transfusion services (21 CFR 606.171).[19] However, this statutory authority extends only to the blood product itself, and does not permit FDA oversight of the actual transfusion episode. Although FDA MedWatch provides a voluntary venue for reporting adverse events, most hospitals do not voluntarily report errors to MedWatch (http://www.fda.gov/Safety/MedWatch/default.htm). Therefore, the FDA's purview extends only as far as the laboratory door, and there is no requirement to report a patient misidentification error unless it results in a death. (A transfusion-related death, however, must be reported to CBER within 24 hours.) To give an example of this regulatory lacuna, the following example suffices: Failure to irradiate a unit of RBCs that was so ordered results in an FDA reportable error. Transfusion of the same unit to the wrong patient does not result in a reportable error unless the patient dies. When a death occurs that may be related to a blood transfusion, 21 CFR 606.170 applies as described above.

The FDA considers establishments that perform certain activities that it defines as manufacturing steps to be hospital blood banks, which are required to register annually using Form FDA 2830. A hospital blood bank is an entity that routinely collects or processes whole blood or blood components. These components may be collected by means of apheresis or prepared from whole blood. Processing includes freezing, deglycerolizing, washing, irradiating, rejuvenating, or removing leukocytes from components. However, the collection and processing of blood and blood components in an emergency situation, therapeutic collection of blood or plasma, preparation of recovered plasma for further manufacture, or preparation of red blood cells for transfusion do not require registration [21 CFR 607.65(f)].[19]

Because blood and blood components are drugs under the Federal FDCA, the FDA cGMP regulations (21 CFR Parts 210 and 211) apply to the manufacture of these products.[20] In addition, cGMP regulations for blood and blood components exist in 21 CFR Part 606.[19] All of these regulations apply to FDA-defined hospital blood banks. FDA registration allows the agency to plan and perform routine cGMP inspections.

Although the FDA does not routinely inspect hospital transfusion services, these services also engage in manufacturing in the view of the FDA, because compatibility testing, blood storage, labeling, and recordkeeping are considered steps in the manufacturing process. Thus, transfusion services are also subject to cGMP regulations. Inspection of hospital transfusion services is overseen by the Centers for Medicare and Medicaid Services (CMS) through a 1980 memorandum of understanding with the FDA that addresses inspection of these establishments. In an effort to reduce duplication of inspections, it was agreed that inspection of hospital transfusion services that are approved for Medicare reimbursement and that engage in compatibility testing but that neither routinely collect nor process blood components would be subject to inspection by the CMS. This agreement pertains to responsibility for inspection only. No statutory authority transferred between the agencies. As part of the agreement, the CMS adopted FDA regulations in 21 CFR Part 606 titled "Current Good Manufacturing Practice for Blood and Blood Components" and 21 CFR Part 640 titled "Additional Standards for Human Blood and Blood Products."[19] These are the FDA requirements that have been incorporated into the CLIA regulations. Observations made by the CMS may be communicated to the FDA, which has the authority to directly inspect a hospital transfusion service.

All transfusion services, registered or unregistered and regardless of FDA nomenclature, must also comply with the regulations in 42 CFR Part 493 in accord with CLIA 1988.[17] For the purposes of CLIA certification, CMS retains responsibility for inspection of all transfusion services.

Many transfusion services may not be surveyed directly by the CMS. Some are in an exempt state or have been accredited by an organization that has been granted deemed status (discussed in the subsections below on AABB, the Joint Commission, and CAP).

FDA and transfusion service error reporting

Both registered and unregistered blood establishments, including transfusion services, must report errors and accidents in manufacturing to the FDA. *Manufacture* means "the collection, preparation, processing or compatibility testing by chemical, physical, biological, or other procedures of any blood product" and includes "manipulation, sampling, testing, or control procedures applied to the final product or to any part of the process. The term includes packaging, labeling, repackaging or otherwise changing the container, wrapper, or labeling of any blood product package in furtherance of the distribution of the blood product from the original place of manufacture to the person who makes final delivery or sale to the ultimate consumer" [21 CFR 607.3(d)]. Errors and accidents (termed *biologic product deviations*) and unexpected events in manufacturing that can affect the safety, purity, and potency of a product are deemed reportable (21 CFR 606.171 and 21 CFR 600.14).[19] Form FDA 3486 is used for reporting these deviations. The requirement to report applies only to manufacturing errors and not to transfusion errors occurring in clinical areas outside of the transfusion service. Table 7.5 provides a summary of the reporting criteria and examples of reportable and nonreportable events.

Deviations must be reported only if the product was *distributed*. This is defined as having left the control of the establishment. If the product was not distributed, the incident still must be recorded in internal records [21 CFR 606.160(b)(7)(iii)].[19] If the product was distributed, a report must be submitted to CBER within 45 calendar days from the date information is acquired that reasonably suggests a reportable event occurred. The incident must also be recorded [21 CFR 606.160(b)(7)(iii) and 21 CFR 211.198] and investigated [21 CFR 606.100(c) and 21 CFR 211.192].[19, 20] The FDA has stated that the purpose of this reporting system is to provide early warning of faulty processes as an indicator for potentially immediate problems that may be related to recalls and as surveillance for improving training and establishing guidance.

The deviation or unexpected event must occur in the facility or another facility under contract with the controlling facility. If a facility under contract to the hospital blood bank or transfusion service is responsible for a deviation, the hospital blood bank or transfusion service is responsible for reporting the problem if the product is distributed. The contract facility must perform an investigation but is not required to report. For example, if a test laboratory under contract to a hospital blood bank fails to provide viral marker testing and the unit is subsequently distributed, the blood bank must report this. If a transfusion service discovers that a unit is mislabeled with an extended outdate, the transfusion service must notify the blood center responsible for reporting to the FDA. The transfusion service would report this incident only if it further distributed the unit without correcting the label.

Deviations and unexpected events occurring within the facility or a facility under contract must be reported if they may affect the safety, purity, or potency of either licensed or unlicensed products that have been distributed. However, as noted, an error occurring after a product has left the facility need not be reported. Examples of events that would not require a report include a unit not being held at the appropriate temperature before transfusion after release from the blood bank, transfusion of a unit to the wrong patient, or failure by hospital staff to use a filter issued by the transfusion service. Reportable, unexpected events may occur even if all established procedures are followed within the transfusion service itself. An example of this would be a patient sample used for compatibility testing that was collected from the wrong patient.

The failure to report an event to the FDA within 45 days is not a reportable deviation, although a failure to report could be cited by an inspector as violative of an establishment's procedure.

A recordkeeping deviation, such as failure to include the signature of the person preparing the unit in component preparation, would not be reportable, because it would not affect the safety, purity, or potency of the product. A unit labeled with a shortened expiration date would also not be reportable, nor would a unit drawn too soon after the last donation. In addition, it would not be a reportable event if an allogeneic unit were issued when autologous blood was available. However, a unit labeled with an extended expiration date would be a reportable deviation. In summary, a deviation or unexpected event is reportable if all of the following criteria are met:

- It was associated with manufacturing.
- It occurred in the facility or at a contract facility.
- It may have affected the safety, purity, or potency of the product.
- The facility had control over the product.
- The product was distributed.

Table 7.6 presents a synopsis of the final rule on the reporting of biological product deviations.

FDA and defective product reporting

If the transfusion service determines that the transfused blood or blood component was at fault in causing the adverse event, a summary of the transfusion services' investigation and conclusions must be sent to the manufacturer or blood collection establishment, who must then maintain such copies [21 CFR 606.170(a)].

AABB

The AABB assessment incorporates evaluation of the quality system at an institution and of each operational system.[15] The quality

---

system assessment is based on the same criteria for every facility. The operational systems, however, are identified by the activities performed within an individual facility. This voluntary assessment is conducted every two years. AABB Standards for Blood Banks and Transfusion Services apply equally to member blood centers and transfusion services.[15] AABB policy includes the provision that although some requirements are based on the FDA's regulations, a committee with international expertise can review requests for variance from facilities outside the United States that involve a departure from US regulations.

In addition to standards and accreditation programs for blood banks and transfusion services, AABB has standards and accreditation programs for Cellular Therapy Services; Immunohematology Reference Laboratories; Molecular Testing for Red Cell, Platelet, and Neutrophil Antigens; Relationship Testing Laboratories; Perioperative Autologous Blood Collection and Administration; and a Patient Blood Management Program.

As noted above, AABB standards state that the blood bank or transfusion service shall have a medical director who is a licensed physician and qualified by education, training, and/or experience.[15]

In May 2014, AABB was granted deemed status for CLIA to meet CMS requirements. This status means that the CMS has determined that the AABB accreditation process provides assurance that facilities meet or exceed conditions required by federal law and regulations. A laboratory accredited by the AABB that designated AABB as its CLIA provider does not need to be inspected routinely by the CMS. However, these facilities are subject to validation surveys and surveys performed in response to complaints to the CMS or state agencies on behalf of the CMS. This deemed status applies to the following AABB Standards: Blood Banks and Transfusion Services; Cellular Therapy Services; Immunohematology Reference Laboratories; and Molecular Testing for Red Cell, Platelet, and Neutrophil Antigens.

The AABB works with CAP to coordinate the AABB assessment and CAP inspection at the same time if the institution falls under both AABB and CAP, but the activities are still separate and each organization makes their own determination of accreditation. AABB does not work with the Joint Commission in the area of accreditation. Many hospital transfusion services, especially if they are in smaller hospitals, are not members of AABB, but nearly all fall under the Joint Commission.

The Joint Commission

Since 1961, review of blood use has been an element of the accreditation process of the Joint Commission.[21] By 1970, the Joint Commission required review not only of blood utilization but also of transfusion reactions. The 1986 Standards were more comprehensive, mandating review of transfusion policies and procedures, ordering practices, and adequacy of the transfusion service generally. The standards also required evaluation of all transfusions.[22] After repeated blood utilization reviews consistently documented appropriate blood use, sampling became acceptable. Although only a minority of hospitals complied with this requirement for 100% evaluation, this standard was nevertheless the driving force behind blood utilization review in the United States.

Since 1991, the Joint Commission has made a series of modifications to this standard, and 100% review is no longer required. The actual number of transfusions to be reviewed is not mandated, although recommendations are provided. Additionally, as part of an effort to reduce medical errors, the Joint Commission has developed National Patient Safety Goals; the number one goal is to "improve

---

Table 7.6 Synopsis of final rule on reporting biological product deviations[29]

- The rule applies to all establishments: donor centers, blood banks, transfusion services.
- Reporting time is not to exceed 45 days.
- Report by mail: Director, Office of Compliance and Biologics Quality, Food and Drug Administration, 10993 New Hampshire Avenue, Silver Spring, MD 20993; or electronically via CBER's website: www.fda.gov/cber/biodev/biodev.htm.
- If the answers to the questions below are affirmative, the event is reportable:
  Was the event associated with manufacturing?
  Did the deviation affect safety, purity, or potency?
  Did it occur in a licensee's or a contract facility?
  Did the facility have control over the product when the deviation occurred?
  Was the product distributed?

the accuracy of patient identification." Although this safety goal was implemented because of the recognition that patient misidentification affects all aspects of medical care, its relevance to transfusion therapy was clearly recognized by the Joint Commission. One of the implementation expectations for the goal clearly states that "Two patient identifiers are used when administering medications or blood products" and "when collecting blood samples . . . for clinical testing." There are also explicit statements that specimens collected from a patient must be labeled at the bedside and that the patient's location may not be used as an identifier. The patient safety goal is reiterated in the body of the standards themselves.

The Joint Commission views transfusion services from a dual perspective. Standards are devoted both to the entire process of blood transfusion from blood ordering through infusion and to the laboratory procedures and practices. Two accreditation manuals have standards regarding blood transfusion. The *Comprehensive Accreditation Manual for Hospitals* [23] provides specific standards for hospitals that transfuse and monitor blood components. The *Comprehensive Accreditation Manual for Pathology and Clinical Laboratory Services* [24] contains technical standards that are patterned after the CLIA 1988 requirements and AABB standards. This dual approach provides the Joint Commission with the opportunity to assess the entire spectrum of clinical and laboratory blood transfusion practices. The Joint Commission Laboratory Accreditation Program has deemed status for CLIA to meet CMS requirements.

Standards related to blood transfusion are included in the *Comprehensive Accreditation Manual for Hospitals* in those sections addressing the medical staff, provision of care, treatment and services, management of information, improvement of organization performance, environment of care, and sentinel event review.[23] Among the salient standards, MS 3.10 states that the medical staff must have "a leadership role in hospital performance improvement activities to improve quality of care." One of the specific elements of performance for MS 3.10 requires that the medical staff be "actively involved in measurement, assessment and improvement in the use of blood and blood components." A similar provision, PI 1.10 in the section on performance improvement, states that the hospital must "collect data to monitor its performance," and this requirement includes collecting data on blood and blood product use. PI 2.20 requires that "undesirable patterns and trends in performance are analyzed," including all confirmed transfusion reactions. In addition, hemolytic transfusion reactions involving the administration of blood having major blood group incompatibilities are identified as reviewable sentinel events subject to specific review by the Joint Commission.

The *Comprehensive Manual for Laboratory and Point of Care Testing* [16] contains more specific provisions governing transfusion services. HR 1.15 requires that the director of the blood bank must be a physician, either a pathologist or other physician qualified in immunohematology and hemotherapy. Sections QC 5.10 through QC 5.260 provide guidance on what the Joint Commission regards as critical elements comprising an acceptable transfusion service. Section QC 5.10 requires that the transfusion service have written policies and procedures that "are acceptable in format, content, review process and availability." These policies and procedures must be consistent with AABB standards, and must be reviewed annually. There must also be policies and procedures governing transfusion reactions and adverse events. Every adverse event must be evaluated by the medical director and documented in the patient's medical record.

Accreditation by the Joint Commission is voluntary.

College of American Pathologists

CAP has an established accreditation program for transfusion services.[18,25,26] This program examines pre-analytical, analytical, and postanalytical aspects of quality management in the laboratory. These include the performance and monitoring of general quality control, test methodologies and specifications, reagents, controls and media, equipment, specimen handling, test reporting and internal performance assessment, and external proficiency testing. In addition, personnel requirements, safety, document management, and other administrative practices are included in the inspection process. The CAP laboratory accreditation program expects a participant laboratory to demonstrate that it is in compliance with the CAP standards for laboratory accreditation. These standards relate to requirements for laboratory direction, physical facilities and safety, quality control and performance improvement, and inspection. Assessment of whether a laboratory meets the standards is accomplished through a series of checklists. Any applicable question that cannot be answered "yes" is considered a deficiency and must be corrected within 30 days with the submission of supporting documentation for accreditation to be achieved. The inspector does not grant or deny accreditation, but makes a recommendation. The accreditation decision is made by the CAP Accreditation Committee. In addition to the on-site inspection program, the CAP laboratory accreditation program monitors the proficiency testing performance of its participant laboratories. The CAP has deemed status with the Joint Commission and for CLIA to meet CMS requirements. As requested, CAP assesses hospital blood banks and transfusion services as well as blood collection establishments every two years.

Inspection of transfusion services is not limited to the contents of the Transfusion Medicine Checklist, but includes the All Common Checklist (COM) and all applicable portions of the Laboratory General Checklist (GEN). All sections of the laboratory must be familiar with and in compliance with the requirements of the COM and GEN Checklists. The Transfusion Medicine checklist contains the following: "Note: Many of the requirements in this Checklist reflect United States regulatory requirements, particularly those of the US Food and Drug Administration (FDA). These requirements may not be applicable in other countries for purposes of CAP accreditation."[18]

Transfusion Medicine Committee

A clinical staff committee concerned exclusively with practices and policies related to transfusion and the transfusion service is not mandated by federal regulation, the Joint Commission, or other accreditation entities. However, it has become routine to have such a committee in most hospitals because a standing transfusion committee is an efficient way of meeting QA and peer review requirements.[27] In fact, one of this committee's principal activities in many institutions has been the utilization review of transfusion: both overtransfusion and undertransfusion. Assessment of transfusion practices has the potential to enhance the knowledge and judgment of healthcare professionals; provide significant information about patient care; reduce the risk of litigation; decrease costs; ensure compliance with regulatory and accreditation requirements; conserve the blood supply; provide an opportunity to demonstrate quality and value to the public; and help create, sustain, and document excellence in patient care. Many committees have also been engaged in developing informed consent practices for transfusion as well as policies related to "lookback" to find patients who may have previously been infected by a blood transfusion at the committee's institution.

This committee typically reports to the healthcare evaluation office or committee, or directly to the medical policy committee of the institution.

Conclusion: US structure and regulations

FDA and the voluntary accrediting agencies seek to advance and protect public health. Federal regulations that carry the force of law, federal guidances that contain nonbinding recommendations, and voluntary accreditation standards issued by the organizations addressed in this chapter are the instruments used to achieve these goals. Blood donor qualification and the collection of blood and blood components as well as their processing, storage, transport, and subsequent manufacturing at hospital transfusion services are FDA-regulated activities to which certain biologic and drug laws apply.

Although blood components typically represent only approximately 1% of a large hospital's budget and less in smaller hospitals, transfusion is at once a life-saving and potentially life-threatening procedure. The regulations, guidances, and standards are crafted so that compliance by the affected institutions is feasible while providing the greatest protection possible to blood donors and patients.

International perspective on ensuring blood and blood product safety and availability

From a global perspective, WHO, the European Union (EU), the Council of Europe (CoE), and the FDA are the most prominent organizations that develop guidance documents, regulations, directives, and standards, used nationally or internationally to ensure the quality, safety, efficacy, and availability of blood and blood products. Although these organizations do not co-develop their regulations, they do collaborate on common initiatives, comment on each other's public documents, and exchange ideas, all of which promotes a general convergence of their regulatory and advisory activities. The information and standards that these organizations provide are employed by many developed and developing countries to establish their own national blood programs. International trade associations, patient and professional organizations, and professional societies also contribute to global blood and blood product safety. In this section, we describe the programs and the organizational structures related to blood products of WHO, the EU, the CoE, and the FDA; and cite other major international organizations that advance global blood and blood product safety and availability.

WHO programs for blood and blood component transfusion safety

WHO is the authority within the UN system that is responsible for the coordination of health policy. It has a mandate for "providing leadership on global health matters, shaping the health research agenda, setting norms and standards, articulating evidence-based policy options, providing technical support to countries and monitoring and assessing health trends."[30]WHO is in the forefront of providing guidance for safe blood collection and transfusion. "The objective of the WHO program on Blood Transfusion Safety is to ensure provision of universal access to safe, quality and efficacious blood and blood products for transfusion, their safe and appropriate use, and also ensuring blood donor and patient safety."[31]

WHO has a 50-year history of involvement in improving blood safety and availability. In 1975, a World Health Assembly resolution urged member states to promote the development of national blood transfusion services based on voluntary non-remunerated blood donations and to take other actions to promote and protect the health of blood donors and recipients of blood and blood products. These objectives are further elaborated in WHO's strategic directions for 2008–2015[32] to: build a conducive political, social, and economic environment for the effective integration of sustainable national blood programs in health systems; respond to country needs to enhance national blood programs and improve clinical transfusion practice; build effective collaboration and partnerships for coordinated action; and strengthen systems for assessing, surveillance, vigilance, alerting, monitoring, and evaluating.

WHO has developed an extensive program to promote access to safe blood transfusion products, particularly to address the needs of less developed and transitional countries. This includes giving advice on improving blood systems by establishing a national blood system recognized through a national blood policy. Functions of the national blood system should include "policy formulation and standard setting, strategic and operational planning, provision of sufficient resources and national coordination and management to ensure an adequate supply of blood and blood products and safe clinical transfusion."[33]

WHO recommends the implementation of a quality system that "provides a framework within which activities are established, performed in a quality-focused way and continuously monitored to improve outcomes."[34] The risk associated with blood transfusion can be significantly reduced through the introduction of quality systems, external quality assessment, and education and training for staff.

Other programs supported by WHO include voluntary blood donation, donation testing, blood processing, proper clinical use of blood transfusion products, and hemovigilance.[35]

Implementation of WHO programs for access to safe blood transfusion

WHO has established a number of collaborations and partnerships to share knowledge, coordinate technical support to increase blood donations, support blood system strengthening, and promote universal access to blood transfusion. One means that WHO uses to coordinate activities related to blood is through the work of WHO Collaborating Centers (WCCs) on Blood Transfusion Safety and Blood Products, whose members currently (2014) include Iran, Thailand, the United Kingdom, China, Slovenia, Brazil, Tunisia, and Germany.[36]

Another WHO partnership is through the WHO Global Safety Network comprised of members of the WHO Expert Advisory Panel on Blood Transfusion Medicine, the WCCs on Blood Transfusion, nongovernmental officials in official relations, key developmental and implementing partners for blood safety, WHO regional focal points for blood safety, and WHO Blood Transfusion Safety staff. This group shares information from the WCCs and develops mechanisms of working together to enhance WHO strategies and objectives in the area of blood transfusion safety.

In 1998, WHO established a Global Data Base on Blood Safety to address global concerns about the availability, safety, and accessibility of blood for transfusion. The database reports the number of blood transfusions and donations in countries throughout the world, and provides information that can be used to assess where deficiencies lay and identify where progress is being made. A fact sheet[37] from 2014 provides examples of the information contained in this database:

- Of the 108 million blood donations collected globally, approximately half of these are collected in high-income countries, home to 18% of the world's population. This shows an increase of almost 25% from 80 million donations collected in 2004.
- In low-income countries, up to 65% of blood transfusions are given to children under five years of age; whereas in high-income countries, the most frequently transfused patient group is over 65 years of age, accounting for up to 76% of all transfusions.
- Blood donation rate per 1000 population in high-income countries is 36.8 donations; it is 11.7 donations in middle-income countries, and 3.9 donations in low-income countries.
- An increase of 8.6 million blood donations from voluntary unpaid donors has been reported from 2004 to 2012. In total, 73 countries collect over 90% of their blood supply from voluntary unpaid blood donors; however, 72 countries collect more than 50% of their blood supply from family/replacement or paid donors.

Only 43 of 156 reporting countries produce plasma-derived medicinal products (PDMPs) through the fractionation of plasma collected in the country, whereas the majority of the other 113 countries import PDMPs from abroad.

WHO QA and safety programs for blood products and related biologicals

In addition to programs focused on ensuring safe blood components for transfusion, WHO has an interest in providing technical guidance and QA tools to regulatory authorities, national control laboratories, and manufacturers to support implementation of quality and safety systems for the production and control of blood products and related in vitro diagnostic devices worldwide.[38] Input for the development of these tools is provided by technical experts from academia, industry, national regulatory authorities, professional societies, and WHO's Collaborating Centers for Biological Standards and Standardization (i.e., the National Institute of Biological Standards and Control [NIBSC], United Kingdom; the Paul Ehrlich Institute [PEI], Germany; and the Center for Biologics Evaluation and Research [CBER], Food and Drug Administration [FDA], United States).

As an example of these resources, WHO has issued a document entitled *Assessment Criteria for National Blood Regulatory Systems*[39] to assist "capacity building of national regulatory authorities for the regulation of blood and blood products. The document is intended to help Member States identify gaps and priorities when developing capacity building programs, and to support the introduction of regulation of blood products." This document outlines "elements and functions which may support the creation of an appropriate blood regulatory system where none exists so far, and which may also be used as a tool to assess strengths and gaps of established systems." It "identifies the essential elements and core regulatory functions that should be present in an effective national regulatory authority to assure the quality, safety and efficacy of blood and blood products, as well as associated substances and medical devices including in vitro diagnostics."

In addition to this document, WHO has produced a series of technical reports that give guidance on topics such as GMPs for blood establishments; recommendations for the production, control, and regulation of human plasma for fractionation; and guidelines on viral inactivation and removal procedures intended to assure the viral safety of human blood plasma products.

Major WHO advisory groups relevant to blood product safety, quality, and standardization

The Expert Committee on Biological Standardization (ECBS) and the WHO Blood Regulators Network (BRN) are two advisory groups associated with WHO whose work directly promotes blood product safety and quality.

ECBS was established in 1947 to provide detailed recommendations and guidelines for the manufacturing, licensing, and control of blood products and related in vitro diagnostic tests, biotechnology products, and vaccines along with the establishment of WHO Biological Reference Materials. The ECBS meets annually and reports directly to the Executive Board, the executive arm of the World Health Assembly.

Members of the ECBS are scientists from National Regulatory Agencies, academia, research institutes, and public health bodies. The decisions and recommendation of the committee are based entirely on scientific principles and considerations of public health.

Written guidelines and recommendations submitted to the ECBS are drafted through a consultative process during which WHO brings together experts from around the world on a given topic.

> Written guidelines and recommendations describe procedures for the manufacture and quality control testing of biological medicinal products to ensure safe and effective products. Guidelines provide more general information on a range of topics of interest to National Regulatory Authorities (NRAs) and manufacturers, whereas recommendations establish the technical specifications for manufacturing and quality control of specific products. By adopting these guidance documents in their pharmacopoeias or equivalent legislation, national governments ensure that the products produced and used in their country conform to current international standards. Regulatory guidance documents also advise NRAs and manufacturers on the control of biological products, with the aim of establishing a harmonized regulatory framework for products moving in international markets.[40]

In addition to guidelines and recommendations, WHO has played a key role for over 50 years in establishing the WHO Biological Reference Materials necessary to standardize biological materials. Reference materials are required to standardize potency, purity, and identity measurements for complex biological materials. "The WHO Biological Reference Materials provide a global standard against which experimental values can be compared and expressed, thereby allowing direct comparisons between products and measurements across different methodologies and assays in use around the world."[41] Reference materials are established through scientific studies involving participation of a large number of laboratories worldwide.

The proceedings of the meetings of the ECBS are published in the WHO Technical Report Series (TRS). They provide "information on the establishment, discontinuation and replacement of the WHO Biological Reference Materials as well as on the adoption of Guidelines and Recommendations. The TRS are available electronically as well as publications, and relevant topics can be searched either by the TRS number or by topic."[40]

The WHO BRN is a group whose work helps to ensure blood product safety in a timely manner. BRN was established in 2006 and is composed of leading international regulatory authorities that have responsibility for the regulation of blood, blood products, and related in vitro diagnostic (IVD) devices.

Members of the BRN exchange information and opinion on blood-related issues. The BRN focuses on scientific assessment of current and emerging threats to the safety and availability of blood

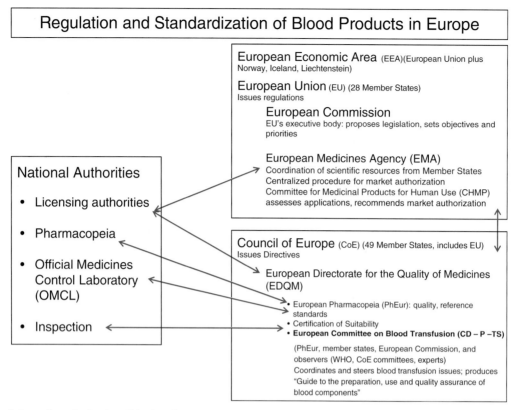

Figure 7.1 Regulation and standardization of blood products in Europe.

and blood products, assesses the impact of new blood-related technologies, and also explores opportunities for regulatory cooperation and collaboration, where possible.

> Member organizations have legal standing and well-established, demonstrated institutional capacity to regulate blood and blood products, and the necessary expertise to address emerging global public health challenges. The WHO acts as Secretariat to the BRN and coordinates network activities under the conditions of the Terms of Reference.
>
> BRN recommendations and considerations are communicated to the ECBS, through WHO. Documents published by the BRN contain the collective views of members and do not necessarily represent the decisions or the stated policy of WHO or of the participating regulatory authorities.[42]

Examples of the work of BRN are the publications *Position Paper on Collection and Use of Convalescent Plasma or Serum as an Element in Filovirus Outbreak Response* and *Potential for Use of Convalescent Plasma in Management of Ebola*. These documents were published in August and September 2014, respectively, and demonstrate BRN's ability to respond quickly to emerging threats to the blood supply.

Regulation of and guidance on blood products in Europe

The regulation of blood components for transfusion, and blood plasma derivatives and analogous recombinant analogs, in Europe is complex because of historical considerations and the balance that is needed between the role of a centralized authority and the involvement of the many independent member states that have their own medicines regulatory authorities. The functionality of

the system depends on the exchange of information among the member states and their acceptance of common standards and practices. The standards, guidance documents, and authorized medicines produced within the European framework stretch beyond its borders and have been adopted in many other parts of the world.

Organizations involved in European regulatory processes include the following (see Figure 7.1).

The European Union and associated organizations

European Union: The European Union was founded in 1948 to promote stability and economic cooperation among member states. It consists of 28 member states and "operates through a system of supranational independent institutions and intergovernmental negotiated decisions by EU Member States. The European Union has developed a single market through a standardized system of laws and the same rules and harmonized procedures apply to all the 28 Member States regarding the authorization of medicines and the supervision of the safety of medicines."[43]

European Commission: This executive arm of the European Union proposes legislation, sets objectives and priorities, and grants centralized marketing authorization.

European Economic Area (EEA): This includes the European Union plus Norway, Iceland, and Liechtenstein [44]

European Medicines Agency (EMA): The agency within the European Union responsible for the scientific evaluation of applications for marketing authorizations for human and veterinary medicines in the centralized procedure. Its main responsibility is the "protection and promotion of public and animal health, through the evaluation and supervision of medicines for human and veterinary use."[45]

Committee for Medicinal Products for Human Use (CHMP): The committee at the EMA that is responsible for preparing opinions on questions concerning medicines for human use. The members and alternates of the CHMP are nominated by EU member states in consultation with the Agency's Management Board. They are chosen on the strength of their qualifications and expertise with regard to the evaluation of medicines.[46]

Council of Europe and associated organizations

CoE: Founded in 1949, the CoE, with 49 member states, is the largest regional intergovernmental organization set up with the aim to defend human rights, parliamentary democracy, and the rule of law and acting as a political anchor and human rights watchdog for Europe at large.[47] Although the CoE is totally independent from the European Union, all 28 members of the European Union are members of the CoE, and the two organizations collaborate in certain domains.

European Directorate for the Quality of Medicines (EDQM): The EDQM is a Directorate of the CoE. Its mission is to establish and provide official standards that apply to the manufacture and quality control of medicines to member states of the CoE.

European Pharmacopeia (PhEur): Within the EDQM, the PhEur sets common standards for all the national pharmacopoeias of the member states. It is in charge of the standardization of analytical methods used for the control of substances used in medicines for human and/or veterinary use.[18] The Expert Group 6B is the entity within the PhEur that is involved with standards for blood products. Importantly, the European Pharmacopeia standards are legally binding in member states.

Official Medicines Control Laboratory (OMCL): OMCLs support regulatory authorities in controlling the quality of medicinal products for human and veterinary use available on the market. Within Europe, OMCLs are nominated by the national authority responsible for the quality control of medicines in their country. OMCLs test products in the EEA, where appropriate, and are independent of manufacturers.[48]

European Committee on Blood Transfusion (CD-P-TS): Coordinates and steers blood transfusion issues, and produces a publication entitled *Guide to the Preparation, Use and Quality Assurance of Blood Components.* Its members include PhEur, member states, the European Commission, and observers (WHO and CoE committees).

Authorization in Europe of plasma derivative and analogous recombinant products

The regulation and authorization of manufactured blood products in Europe involve an interplay among the EMA, national competent authorities (NCAs), CHMP working parties, and the EDQM that includes the PhEur and OMCLs. There are three pathways for authorizing medicines in Europe. In the "centralized" procedure, pharmaceutical companies submit a single marketing-authorization application to the EMA. For blood products, the EMA's CHMP carries out a scientific assessment of the application and gives a recommendation on whether or not to grant a marketing authorization. Once granted by the European Commission, the centralized

marketing authorization is valid in all EU member states. Most innovative medicines go through this procedure.[43]

Most medicines are not authorized through the centralized procedure. Instead, they are authorized by NCAs in member states. When a company wants to authorize a medicine in several member states, it can use one of the following procedures:

- The *decentralized procedure,* through which companies can apply for the simultaneous authorization of a medicine in more than one EU member state if it has not yet been authorized in any EU country and it does not fall within the mandatory scope of the centralized procedure; or
- The *mutual-recognition procedure,* through which companies that have a medicine authorized in one EU member state can apply for this authorization to be recognized in other EU countries.

This process allows member states to rely on each other's scientific assessments. Rules and requirements applicable to pharmaceuticals in the European Union are the same, irrespective of the authorization route for a medicine.[43]

Clinical trials

The authorization and oversight of a clinical trial is the responsibility of the Member State where the trial is taking place. Each trial must be approved by the Member State where the protocol was submitted. The European Clinical Trials Database (EudraCT) tracks which clinical trials have been authorized in the European Union. It is used by NCAs and clinical trial sponsors to enter protocol- and results-related information on clinical trials. A subset of this information is publicly available in the EU clinical trials register.[45]

Safety monitoring of medicines in Europe

EudraVigilance is an EU web-based information system within the EMA that collects, manages, and analyzes reports of suspected side effects of medicines. Information is obtained from EEA members, and these data are continuously monitored in order to identify any new safety information.

The EMA has a committee dedicated to the safety of medicines for human use—the Pharmacovigilance Risk Assessment Committee (PRAC). If there is a safety issue with a medicine that is authorized in more than one member state, patients and healthcare professionals in all member states are given the same guidance by the committee, and the same regulatory action is taken across the European Union.

The PRAC has a broad remit covering all aspects of pharmacovigilance. In addition to its role in risk assessment, the committee provides advice and recommendations to the European medicines regulatory network on risk management planning and postmarketing benefit–risk assessment for medicines.[45]

International cooperation

The EMA and the European Commission work with member states and other organizations around the world to foster international cooperation and timely exchange of information on regulatory and scientific matters. One such interaction related to blood products is the so-called Blood Cluster meeting with the FDA and Health Canada where pharmacovigilance information and other blood product–related matters are exchanged on a regular basis.

EMA works with WHO on issues such as medicines intended for markets outside of the European Union, and the quality of medicines. EMA also cooperates with the International Conference on

Harmonization of Technical Requirements (ICH) on matters related to harmonizing requirements to assure the safety, quality and efficacy of drugs.

Activities to promote blood component safety in Europe

The CoE has been actively contributing since the 1950s to the implementation of standards for blood transfusion. In 2007, the secretariat responsible for blood transfusion activities was transferred to the EDQM. Within the EDQM, the European Committee on Blood Transfusion (CD-P-TS) is in charge of steering and coordinating the actions of the CoE in this area. The membership of CD-P-TS includes the CoE member states, and parties to the Convention on the Elaboration of a European Pharmacopoeia. The European Commission, WHO, and other CoE Committees (European Public Health and Bioethics Committees) are special observers to the CD-P-TS.[49]

Activities of the CD-P-TS include, among others, addressing issues about quality and safety standards for blood transfusion, including collection, storage, distribution, and use of blood components; improving blood transfusion services; promoting the principle of voluntary non-remunerated donations; and establishing good practices in transfusion medicine and monitoring their use in Europe. These objectives are attained by setting standards and preparing guidance on professional practices (e.g., *Guide to the Preparation, Use and Quality Assurance of Blood Components*); organizing and evaluating surveys on blood components; and using resolutions to promote continuous improvement of an ethical, organizational, and regulatory approach to blood transfusion.[49]

Other major international organizations involved in the regulation or standardization of blood, blood products, and their biotechnology analogs

International Conference on Harmonization: Regulatory authorities and pharmaceutical industry experts from Europe, Japan, and the United States discuss scientific and technical aspects of product registration. The work of this organization is especially relevant to biotechnology products. Although ICH does not include the blood industry, ICH activities address blood secondarily by use of the Common Technical Document. A significant output of ICH has been guidance on informed consent for and ethical conduct of clinical trials.[50]

Pharmaceutical Inspection Co-operation Scheme and Pharmaceutical Inspection Convention (PIC/S): A collective of pharmaceutical inspectorates involved in information exchanges, training, and guideline development related to good manufacturing, device, clinical, and laboratory practices.[51]

International Working Group on the Standardization of Genomic Amplification Techniques for the Virological Safety Testing of Blood and Blood Products (SoGAT): A WHO technical discussion group that works on issues of international standardization and quality of genomic amplification techniques for the testing of products.[52]

National Institute of Biological Standards and Control (NIBSC): They prepare reference materials, for WHO among others, and organize international collaborative studies on reference preparations.[53]

Paul Ehrlich Institute (PEI): German regulatory authority that has a major influence on the development of blood products in Europe and is a WCC.[54]

Trade, professional societies, and patient-sponsored international forums

International Society on Thrombosis and Hemostasis (ISTH), Scientific and Standardization Subcommittee (SSC): This society works on the understanding, prevention, diagnosis, and treatment of thrombotic and bleeding disorders. ISTH focuses on issues about blood coagulation, hemorrhagic disorders, platelet function and regulation; the mechanisms of thrombosis, fibrinolysis and thrombolysis; and problems of thromboembolic disorders. SSC-ISTH also helps to evaluate candidate reference standards for consideration by ECBS.[55]

America's Blood Centers/European Blood Alliance (ABC/EBA): Works to harmonize requirements and decision-making processes to promote safe and high-quality blood products in North America and Europe.[56]

World Federation of Hemophilia (WFH): Works on issues involving hemophilia and other bleeding disorders, including supply, affordability, safety, and regulatory harmonization.[57]

European Hemophilia Safety Surveillance (EUHASS): This is a pharmacovigilance program to monitor the safety of treatments for people with inherited bleeding disorders in Europe.[58]

Plasma Protein Therapeutics Association (PPTA): This is the international trade association and standards-setting organization for the world's major producers of plasma-derived and recombinant analog therapies, collectively referred to as *plasma protein therapies*.[59]

International Plasma Fractionation Association (IPFA): This is an international association for nonprofit organizations involved in the manufacture of blood products made from blood collected from non-remunerated donors.[60]

International Society of Blood Transfusion (ISBT): The ISBT promotes research, new developments, and changing concepts in blood transfusion medicine.[61]

FDA role in the global regulation of blood and blood products

The activities of the FDA have a large impact on the global regulation of blood and blood products. FDA's international standing is bolstered by the substantial medical and scientific resources that it devotes to ensuring the safety, efficacy, and availability of blood and blood products. Within the FDA, the Office of Blood Research and Review (OBRR), in CBER, has the responsibility of regulating blood and blood components; plasma derivatives and analogous products; blood donor screening tests; retroviral diagnostic tests; and other medical devices, including software used to test, collect, process, or store donated blood.

FDA is strongly supportive of harmonization efforts that will maximize national and global health. A convergence of thinking on regulatory and guidance issues is important for trade as well, because many of the companies involved in blood product manufacture are international in scope; the US market for these products is extensive; and a large amount of plasma, intermediates, and manufactured products are distributed abroad.

FDA influences global regulatory and guidance norms for blood and blood product safety, through its interactions with all of the organizations cited in this chapter. For example, FDA representatives are members of the WHO's ECBS and the BRN, have Observer status with EDQM's Expert Group 6B, and routinely communicate with the EMA and Health Canada through Blood Cluster meetings. In addition to interacting with organizations that are composed of multiple international partners, FDA has bilateral memoranda of understanding and confidentiality arrangements with a number of individual countries. All of these relationships facilitate cooperative activities and the sharing of information, which support the common goal of enhancing the global safety and availability of blood and blood products.

Key references

A full reference list for this chapter is available at: http://www.wiley.com/go/simon/transfusion

4 Food, Drug, and Cosmetic Act of 1938. 21 U.S.C. Sect. 355 (2010). http://www.gpo.gov/fdsys/pkg/USCODE-2010-title21/pdf/USCODE-2010-title21-chap9-subchapV-partA-sec355.pdf

5 Public Health Service Act of 1944. 42 U.S.C. Sect. 262 (1999). http://www.fda.gov/RegulatoryInformation/Legislation/ucm149278.htm

28 Kochman SA. Overview of the regulation of blood and cGMPs. www.fda.gov/downloads/biologicsbloodvaccines/newsevents/workshopsmeetingsconferences/ucm189689.ppt

30 World Health Organization (WHO). About WHO. http://www.who.int/about/en/

32 World Health Organization (WHO). WHO Global Strategic Plan, 2008–2015: Universal access to safe blood transfusion scaling up the implementation of the WHO strategy for blood safety and availability for improving patient health and saving lives. http://www.who.int/bloodsafety/publications/UniversalAccesstoSafeBT.pdf.

37 World Health Organization (WHO). WHO blood safety and availability. Fact sheet No. 279, updated June 2014. http://www.who.int/mediacentre/factsheets/fs279/en/

43 European Medicines Agency. [Description]. http://www.ema.europa.eu/ema/index.jsp?curl=pages/about_us/general/general_content_000235.jsp&mid=

48 EDQM. OMCLs. http://www.edqm.eu/en/General-european-OMCL-network-46.html

SECTION II

Blood components and derivatives

CHAPTER 8

Red blood cell production and kinetics

Mark J. Koury

Division of Hematology/Oncology, Vanderbilt University, Nashville, TN, USA

Introduction

The main function of erythrocytes is to transport oxygen from the lungs to the other tissues of the body. Oxygen delivery is finely controlled by the number of erythrocytes circulating in the blood, which is a function of the rate of senescent erythrocyte removal and the rate of new erythrocyte (reticulocyte) entry. Circulating erythrocytes are maintained in an extremely narrow range because the normal bone marrow produces almost exactly the same number of new erythrocytes each day as is lost through senescence. This daily turnover of approximately 1% of circulating erythrocytes represents approximately 200–250 billion erythrocytes in a healthy adult. When increased numbers of erythrocytes are lost, such as with bleeding or hemolysis, the production of new erythrocytes increases rapidly, replacing the lost erythrocytes and maintaining the steady-state number of erythrocytes. The rapid expansion of erythrocyte production in response to bleeding or hemolysis is so well regulated that rebound polycythemia does not occur. This exquisitely controlled production of erythrocytes is mediated through a negative feedback mechanism that involves renal oxygen supply and utilization, the hormone erythropoietin (EPO) that is produced in the kidneys, and the erythroid progenitor cells in the bone marrow that depend upon EPO to survive. Normal red blood cell production also depends upon adequate supplies of specific nutrients, among which iron, folate, and vitamin B_{12} are the most important. Disorders of the hematopoietic system or other diseases such as those associated with chronic inflammation inhibit the erythropoietic process.

Erythropoiesis

Erythropoiesis: a component of hematopoiesis

Erythropoiesis, the process of erythrocyte production, is part of the larger process by which a pluripotent hematopoietic stem cell (HSC) proliferates and differentiates into all of the cell types of the blood and immune systems, including platelets, granulocytes, monocytes and macrophages, T lymphocytes and B lymphocytes, as well as erythrocytes. Thus, normally regulated hematopoiesis is required for effective hemostasis, inflammation, immune responses, and tissue oxygenation. Current concepts of hematopoiesis are derived mainly from studies of mice and humans. These studies

have included direct morphologic and immunologic analyses of cells in hematopoietic tissues, in vitro culture of hematopoietic cells, transplantation studies with hematopoietic cells, and genetic studies of mice with natural mutations, transgene expressions, or targeted gene knockouts.

Labeled endothelial cells in the ventral part of the aorta in developing mice have been shown to transform into HSCs[1] by a mechanism that does not require mitosis.[2] Among the various functions of blood cells, tissue oxygenation by the erythrocytes is the first one required during embryonic development and the most tightly regulated in postnatal life. Erythropoiesis has two sequential but overlapping phases during development. In the first or primitive phase, erythrocytes are produced in "blood islands" of the yolk sac during weeks 3–6 of human gestation, with primitive erythrocytes comprising the large majority of circulating erythrocytes at eight weeks but declining to undetectable levels by 12 weeks of gestation.[3] In the subsequent definitive erythropoiesis phase, erythrocytes are produced mainly in the human fetal liver from six to 22 weeks of gestation, and mostly in the bone marrow at later times.[3] Definitive erythroid cells arise from HSCs that are first detected in the aortogonadomesonephros (AGM) region of the mesoderm,[4] circulate and seed the fetal liver, and then migrate from the fetal liver to the developing bone, where they initiate marrow hematopoiesis.[5–7] The hemoglobin of the primitive erythrocytes contains embryonic ε- and ζ-globins, whereas the hemoglobin of the definitive erythrocytes contains adult α-globin and either fetal γ-globin from midgestation through the first few postnatal months and mainly adult β-globin after the first few postnatal months.[8]

Stages of erythropoiesis

Erythroid progenitor cells arise from HSCs that commit to differentiation and are termed *multipotent progenitors* (MPPs). MPPs proliferate and undergo a series of decisions based on specific transcription factor activities that determine their progeny's fate in terms of blood cell lineage (see Figure 8.1). The myeloid transcription factors PU.1 and GATA1 direct differentiation toward the nonlymphoid lineages, and, if the activity of the GATA1 transcription factor is increased, differentiation toward the bipotent megakaryocytic-erythroid progenitor (MEP) is promoted.[9,10] MEP fate, in turn, is determined by the activities of two other competing

A. Stage of Erythroid Differentiation

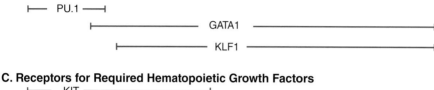

HSC → MPP → MEP → BFU-E → CFU-E → Pro EB → Baso EB → Poly EB → Ortho EB → RET → RBC

B. Transcription Factors for Erythroid Differentiation

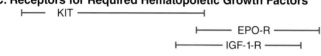

TAL1

LMO2

PU.1

GATA1

KLF1

C. Receptors for Required Hematopoietic Growth Factors

KIT

EPO-R

IGF-1-R

D. Proteins Related to Erythrocyte Structure and Function

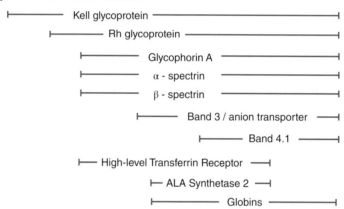

Kell glycoprotein

Rh glycoprotein

Glycophorin A

α - spectrin

β - spectrin

Band 3 / anion transporter

Band 4.1

High-level Transferrin Receptor

ALA Synthetase 2

Globins

Figure 8.1 Cellular events in erythroid differentiation. (A) The relative sizes and the known or presumed morphologic appearances of erythroid cells at various stages of differentiation: pluripotent hematopoietic stem cells (HSCs); burst-forming units–erythroid (BFU-Es); colony-forming units–erythroid (CFU-Es); proerythroblasts (ProEBs); basophilic erythroblasts (BasoEBs); polychromatophilic erythroblasts (PolyEBs); orthochromatic erythroblasts (OrthoEBs); reticulocytes (RETs); erythrocytes (red blood cells, or RBCs). (B) Erythroid transcription factors: basic helix–loop–helix factor (TAL1); Lim-domain partner of TAL1 (LMO2); factor that binds the purine-rich GAGGAA sequence (PU.1); zinc finger factor that binds GATA-containing sequences (GATA1); erythroid Krüppel-like factor (KLF1). (C) Receptors for hematopoietic growth factors: stem cell factor receptor (KIT); erythropoietin receptor (EPO-R); insulin-like growth factor-1 receptor (IGF-1-R). (D) Proteins related to erythrocyte structure and function. Periods of expression for erythroid-specific forms of proteins are shown. Transferrin receptors are present in all stages, but the period of high-level expression that characterizes hemoglobin-producing erythroblast is shown. Band 4.1 expression is for the spliced form found in circulating erythrocytes. For each transcription factor, growth factor receptor, and erythrocyte-related protein, the degree of expression can vary greatly during the period shown.

transcription factors: erythroid Krüppel-like factor-1 (KLF1), which promotes erythroid differentiation, and FLI1, which promotes megakaryocytic differentiation.[9,11]

In Figure 8.1, the hematopoietic stages committed solely to erythroid differentiation begin with the burst-forming units-erythroid (BFU-Es),[12] which produce large colonies or multiple colonies of human erythroblasts after 2–3 weeks in tissue culture. BFU-Es can circulate in the blood, but after they differentiate in marrow to the next defined stage, the colony-forming units-erythroid (CFU-Es),[12] they associate with a macrophage, forming an erythroblastic island (EBI), the basic unit of terminal mammalian erythropoiesis.[13] Coordinated KLF1 activity in both the central macrophage and the erythroid cells[14,15] of an EBI directs the development of 30 or more adherent erythroblasts at various stages of differentiation from

CFU-Es through enucleating orthochromatic erythroblasts. CFU-Es were originally defined by in vitro colony-forming activity and erythroblasts by their morphological appearances in Giemsa-stained films of aspirated marrows, but human CFU-Es and their erythroblast progeny, the pro-erythroblasts (ProEBs), basophilic erythroblasts (BasoEBs), polychromatophilic erythroblasts (Poly-EBs), and orthochromatic erythroblasts (OrthoEBs), can be identified and isolated by flow cytometry patterns of surface expressions of glycophorin A, anion transporter (Band 3), and α4 integrin.[16]

OrthoEBs enucleate forming reticulocytes, very irregularly shaped cells containing hemoglobin and residual organelles (the "reticulum") that allow them to be distinguished from the mature erythrocytes. The extruded nucleus with its thin shell of hemoglobin-containing cytoplasm, termed a *pyrenocyte*, is rapidly phagocytosed by the central macrophage, which degrades the nucleus and hemoglobin and recycles the nucleosides and iron.[17] The final stage of differentiation, the erythrocyte, is achieved after the reticulocytes have entered the circulation, lost their residual internal organelles via autophagy, and remodeled their irregular shapes by exocytosis of microvesicles to form uniform biconcave disks.[18] Reticulocyte maturation to an erythrocyte occurs within 1–2 days after entering the circulation, but mature erythrocytes continue to shed microvesicles until they are removed 110–120 days later as senescent cells.[19]

Intracellular requirements for normal erythroid differentiation

A series of intracellular and extracellular events are needed for successful completion of the erythroid differentiation scheme as shown in Figure 8.1. The intracellular events include the expression of (1) hematopoietic and erythroid-specific transcription factors; (2) specific microRNAs and long, noncoding RNAs involved in the differentiation process; (3) proteins involved in the proliferation and differentiation of the erythroid cells; and (4) proteins such as hemoglobin, intrinsic membrane, and membrane skeleton proteins that comprise the mature erythrocyte.

GATA1, KLF1, and the transcription factors complex of TAL1/SCL, LMO2, and LDB1 are essential for erythropoiesis from the pre-EPO dependent stages through late erythroblast stages.[11,20,21] In addition to regulating expression of erythroid-specific genes such as those encoding the EPO receptor, globins, and glycophorins, these transcription factors also regulate long, noncoding RNAs that can influence other erythroid gene expressions in the later stages of differentiation, such as the gene encoding Band 3.[22] The expression of transcription factors and other crucial erythroid proteins, in turn, are partially controlled by specific microRNAs, which regulate mRNA stability and translation at all stages of erythroid differentiation.[21,23] In fact, posttranscriptional regulation of protein synthesis by microRNAs allows control of the reticulocyte maturation process that occurs days after the erythroid cell has lost its nucleus.[24]

During the terminal stages of erythropoiesis in the EBI, the erythroblasts undergo progressive decreases in size, nuclear condensation, and subsequent enucleation. Decreased cell size between the ProEB and OrthoEB stages is achieved by a shortened duration of the G1 phase of the cell cycle, resulting in less protein accumulation between cytokineses.[25,26] These terminal erythroblast divisions are regulated by cyclin D3, a G1-phase cyclin,[27] and direct contact with the central macrophage shortens the G1 phase of the erythroblasts.[28] During these more rapid cell divisions, the heterochromatin/euchromatin ratio increases with a progressive condensation and reduction in nuclear size[29] that are associated with histone deacetylation[30] and DNA demethylation.[31] In the formation of the reticulocyte and pyrenocyte, the condensed erythroblast nucleus is extruded by an active process similar to cytokinesis that requires filamentous actin[32] and nonmuscle myosin IIB.[33] KLF1 regulates the phagocytosis of the pyrenocyte and subsequent degradation of its DNA and hemoglobin.[14,17]

Hemoglobin, the predominant protein of erythrocytes, is synthesized in a highly regulated process that begins in the BasoEBs and continues through the reticulocyte stage. Extremely large quantities of heme are produced without intracellular accumulations of iron or protoporphyrin. Similarly, heme is incorporated into globin chains without accumulating intracellular excesses of globin chains or heme, and 2 α-hemoglobin and 2 β-hemoglobin chains are assembled into hemoglobin A tetramers without accumulating unpaired hemoglobin chains.[34] Multiple layers of regulation that are specific to erythroid cells control hemoglobin synthesis, including (1) heme regulation of iron acquisition from endocytosed transferrin receptors;[35] (2) iron regulation of heme synthesis through a 5′ iron-responsive element (IRE) in erythroid-specific 5-aminolevulinic acid synthase (ALAS2, the first step of heme synthesis) mRNA that controls translation;[35] (3) heme regulation of erythroblast protein synthesis through inactivation of heme-regulated eIF2α kinase (heme-regulated inhibitor [HRI]), which phosphorylates the translation initiation factor eIF2α, thereby making it unable to initiate mRNA translation;[36] and (4) alpha-hemoglobin stabilizing protein (AHSP) regulation of free α-globin chain content by coordination of heme insertion, appropriate folding, and assembly of α-globin chains into hemoglobin.[37] Heme also de-represses β-globin transcription by binding and enhancing the degradation of BACH1, a transcription repressor at the locus control region (LCR). With the loss of BACH1, the NF-E2–Mafk transcription factor complex binds and activates β-globin transcription,[38,39] which combined with GATA1 and KLF1 activities leads to coordinated α-globin and β-globin transcriptions.[40]

In the terminal stages of erythroid differentiation, the plasma membrane and associated membrane skeleton undergo large changes in their composition. From the CFU-E through reticulocyte stages, several patterns of intrinsic membrane protein expression are found: (1) from a baseline of little or no expression, large increases occur in proteins that are major components of erythrocyte membranes, such as glycophorin A, glucose transporter 1 (GLUT1), and Band 3; (2) more gradual increases from low baseline levels occur in glycophorin C, and RhAG, RhD, and Lutheran antigens; (3) from a stable baseline, late declines of moderate degree occur in Kell antigen and transferrin receptor 1 (CD71); and (4) prominent declines occur in adhesion proteins such as CD36 and CD44, and integrin components α4, α5, and β1.[16] Most of the membrane skeletal proteins, including α- and β-spectrins, ankyrin, adducin, Band 4.1, Band 4.9, and tropomodulin, increase, whereas actin declines slowly during terminal erythroid differentiation.[16] This pattern of accumulation of membrane skeletal proteins during terminal erythropoiesis is related to the accumulation pattern of Band 3, to which the membrane skeleton is bound,[41] and mRNA splicing of the skeletal proteins, such as Band 4.1.[42] In addition to regulating cellular structure, alternative splicing of transcripts plays a role in the regulating cell cycle and chromatin function during terminal erythropoiesis.[43]

Extracellular requirements for erythroid differentiation

The extracellular requirements for erythroid differentiation include (1) stromal cell and matrix support within the marrow, (2) adequate supplies of required hematopoietic growth factors, and (3) sufficient supplies of nutrients required for progenitor cell proliferation and differentiation. HSCs and BFU-Es can circulate in the blood, but to complete differentiation they must adhere to and be retained in specific areas in marrow termed *niches*. HSCs home to and are retained in the marrow by cytokines and chemokines that are produced by mesenchymal stem cells, with the most prominent marrow cytokine being secreted and membrane-bound KIT ligand (SCF), which binds its receptor, KIT, on HSCs, and the most prevalent marrow chemokine being stromal-cell derived factor 1 (CXCL12), which binds its receptor, CXCR4, on HSCs.[44] In the marrow, HSCs differentiate through the MPP and MEP stages to reach the BFU-E stage. The marrow matrix protein laminin binds the p67 non-integrin receptor on circulating BFU-Es, thereby promoting their retention and proliferation in the marrow.[45] When BFU-Es differentiate to CFU-Es, they associate with stromal macrophages forming the EBIs. At least five interacting surface membrane protein pairs mediate macrophage–erythroid interactions in EBIs:[13] (1) macrophage vascular cell adhesion molecule 1 (VCAM1) binds erythroblast α4β1 integrin, (2) macrophage α_V integrin binds erythroblast interstitial cell adhesion molecule-4 (ICAM4/LW), (3) erythroblast–macrophage protein (EMP) on both macrophages and erythroblasts binds itself on the other cell type, (4) macrophage CD169–Siglec1 binds erythroblast sialated glycoproteins, and (5) macrophage hemoglobin–haptoglobin receptor (CD163) binds an unknown erythroblast ligand.

In Figure 8.1, receptors for the hematopoietic growth factors necessary for normal erythropoiesis are shown for the period when they are required. The principal growth factor regulating erythropoiesis is EPO, which is discussed in detail in the "Erythropoietin" section. Prior to EPO dependence, specific growth factors maintain progenitor cell survival and proliferation, with the most prominent being SCF and insulin-like growth factor-1 (IGF1) supplied by the marrow environment.[46] CFU-Es and ProEBs lose SCF and IGF-1 responsiveness, respectively, while they are dependent on EPO for survival. However, during periods of hypoxic stress, CFU-Es and ProEBs can expand their numbers greatly without any further differentiation. The two main mediators of this expansion are (1) glucocorticoids,[47,48] which are produced in the adrenals and appear to induce a protein in erythroid progenitors that binds the mRNAs that direct terminal erythroid differentiation;[49] and (2) bone morphogenetic protein 4 (BMP4),[50] a member of the transforming growth factor-β family of cytokines that can be produced by the central macrophage of the erythroblastic islands.[51]

Included among the vitamins and minerals that cause anemia during deficiency states are copper; cobalt; vitamins A, C, and E; pyridoxine; riboflavin; and nicotinic acid.[52] However, the most common nutritional deficiencies that cause anemia are those of folate, vitamin B$_{12}$, and iron. The roles of these last three nutrients in erythropoiesis are described in the "Nutritional Requirements" section.

Erythropoietin

Regulation of EPO production by tissue hypoxia

EPO, a glycosylated protein hormone, is a major component of the oxygenation–EPO negative feedback mechanism shown in Figure 8.2. The major determinant of oxygen delivery from the lungs to the peripheral tissues is the number of circulating erythrocytes. With anemia, when erythrocyte numbers are decreased, oxygen delivery decreases and the peripheral tissues become hypoxic. All tissues experience hypoxia during anemia, but those that respond with EPO production are the kidneys and, to a much lesser extent, the liver.[53] The kidney cells that produce EPO are a subset of interstitial fibroblasts located adjacent to proximal tubules, with EPO-producing cells in small foci of the inner cortex in slight anemia, larger areas within the inner half of the cortex in moderate anemia, and distributed throughout the cortex in severe anemia.[54,55] These progressive increases in the areas of EPO production in the kidney correspond to increasing areas of cortical hypoxia, which are a function of oxygen supply from the blood and local oxygen tissue utilization, which is determined mainly by the metabolic demands of the tubular epithelium. Rapid increases in EPO production after blood loss or hemolysis are not due to increased production by each

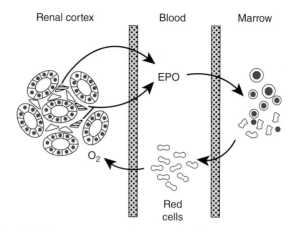

Figure 8.2 The oxygenation–erythropoietin (EPO) negative feedback mechanism. The number of circulating erythrocytes (Red Cells) determines the amount of oxygen (O$_2$) delivered from the lungs to other tissues. In the renal cortex, a specific subset of interstitial cells (hatched) produce EPO when they perceive hypoxia. The EPO is immediately secreted into the blood and acts in the bone marrow to prevent the programmed death (apoptosis) of erythroid progenitor cells. Those erythroid progenitors that survive the EPO-dependent period of differentiation mature into reticulocytes (irregularly shaped anucleate cells in marrow and blood) and subsequently into erythrocytes. Increased numbers of erythrocytes resulting from increased plasma EPO levels deliver more oxygen to the kidneys and thereby lower the amount of EPO produced as renal hypoxia is relieved.

EPO-producing cell but rather to recruitment to active EPO production of increased numbers of cells with the potential to produce EPO.[54] The number of cells actively producing EPO, and the resultant plasma EPO levels, increase exponentially with a linear decrease in hematocrit,[54,55] as was originally reported for plasma EPO levels in most clinical anemias, except for those involving patients with renal disease or malignancies.[56]

Hypoxia sensing by EPO-producing cells involves hypoxia-inducible transcription factors (HIFs), a multicomponent complex that binds hypoxia-inducible transcription enhancer elements of various genes, including *EPO*, *VEGF*, and genes encoding several glycolytic enzymes.[57,58] Under normoxic conditions, the steady-state HIF-α component of the complex does not accumulate intracellularly because it is rapidly degraded by the ubiquitin–proteasome pathway (Figure 8.3).[59] However, when a cell with EPO-producing capacity experiences hypoxia, the degradation of HIF-α ceases and intracellular levels promptly increase. Polyubiquitination of HIF-α depends upon the von Hippel–Lindau protein (pVHL) interacting with those HIF-α molecules that have hydroxylation of two specific proline residues (Figure 8.3).[60–62] These prolyl hydroxylations are directly linked to the oxygenation because they are catalyzed by a hydroxylase with nonheme iron at its active site, which uses molecular oxygen as a substrate. The transcription complex containing HIF-2α regulates renal *EPO* transcription through an enhancer that is located 6–14 kbp upstream of the *EPO* coding region.[58] Once hypoxia reaches the threshold that triggers *EPO* transcription, the resultant EPO messenger RNA is translated into the EPO glycoprotein, which is immediately secreted.[54] When an individual cell is triggered to produce EPO, it does so in an all-or-none manner.[54,63] Thus, EPO concentrations in the blood increase sharply within two hours after loss of blood, hemolysis, or a sudden decrease in atmospheric oxygen.

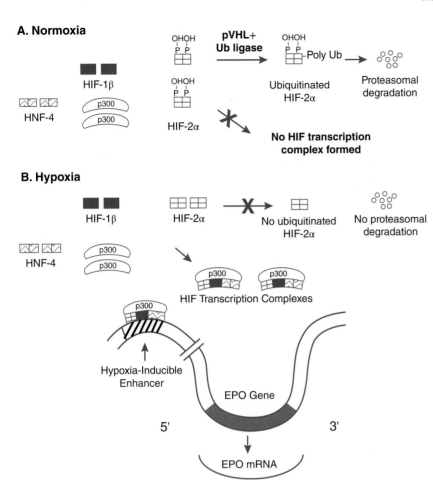

A. Normoxia

B. Hypoxia

Figure 8.3 Induction of erythropoietin (EPO) gene transcription by hypoxia in renal cortical fibroblasts. (A) In cells capable of producing EPO, two components of hypoxia-inducible factor (HIF2α and HIF1β) are constitutively produced under normoxic conditions. However, the molecular oxygen present in the EPO-producing cells under normoxic conditions is used in hydroxylation of two prolines in HIF2α. The prolyl hydroxylations (P-OH) lead to recognition by von Hippel–Lindau protein (pVHL), which targets HIF2α for polyubiquitination (Poly Ub) by ubiquitin ligase. The polyubiqitinated HIF2α is rapidly degraded by proteasomes. (B) When renal EPO-producing cells are hypoxic, HIF2α is not hydroxylated and accumulates because it is not degraded by the ubiquitin-proteasomal pathway. HIF2α forms heterodimers with HIF1β, which associates with two other components of the HIF transcription complex, hepatocyte nuclear factor-4 (HNF4) and p300. The HIF transcription complex binds to a hypoxia-inducible enhancer located 6–14 kilobase pairs upstream of the EPO coding sequences, and thereby increases EPO transcription and accumulation of EPO messenger RNAs. EPO mRNA is promptly translated and secreted into the blood such that increases in circulating EPO can be detected within two hours of experiencing hypoxia.

Effects of erythropoietin on erythroid progenitor cells

In the marrow, EPO binds to transmembrane glycoprotein erythropoietin receptors (EPO-Rs), which are first displayed on the surface of erythroid progenitor cells before the CFU-E stage and persist until the late basophilic erythroblast stage (Figure 8.1).[63] The binding of EPO to EPO-Rs leads to three major events: (1) homodimerization and conformational alterations of EPO-Rs, (2) initiation of intracellular signaling by the EPO-Rs, and (3) endocytosis of the EPO–EPO-R complexes, which are subsequently degraded.[64,65] Dimerization and structural changes of EPO-Rs after EPO binding induce both signaling and endocytosis. The endocytosis and intracellular degradation of the EPO–EPO-R complexes appear to be the normal mechanism for clearance of EPO from the blood.[66] EPO-Rs have no intrinsic enzyme activity, but they interact with several signal transduction pathways through Janus tyrosine kinase-2 (JAK2). JAK2 is physically associated with the cytoplasmic portion of EPO-Rs, chaperones EPO-Rs to the surface of the erythroid cell, and is activated by the conformational changes in the EPO-Rs produced by the binding of EPO.[67,68] Activated JAK2 phosphorylates itself and EPO-Rs as well as initiates signal transduction pathways that include signal transduction and activator of transcription-5 (STAT5), RAS–RAF–MAP kinase, and phosphoinositol-3 kinase/AKT kinase (protein kinase B).[69]

Although the mechanisms linking EPO-R signaling to the biological effects of EPO have not been determined, EPO prevents the apoptotic death of erythroid progenitor cells in CFU-E through early BasoEB stages.[70–73] During EPO dependence, individual erythroid cells at the same stage of differentiation can display wide variation in their degree of dependence on EPO for survival.[74] Such variable susceptibility to apoptosis among EPO-dependent progenitors appears to be due to expression levels of FAS, a membrane protein of the tumor necrosis factor (TNF) family, which triggers apoptosis when it binds FAS ligand.[75] EPO, in turn, acts to decrease FAS expression in erythroid progenitors. FAS-ligand, which binds and activates FAS, is produced mainly by mature erythroblasts in humans.[76] Thus, within the EBI, a negative feedback loop from the terminally differentiating erythroblasts can modulate the rate of CFU-E–ProEB apoptosis and indirectly control rates of erythrocyte production.[75] By a separate mechanism, EPO signaling also appears to protect late-stage erythroblasts from apoptosis, including in the post-EPO-dependent period, by inducing large amounts of the anti-apoptotic protein BCL-X$_{L}$.[77,78]

Erythrocyte production kinetics based on EPO levels

A model that incorporates varying plasma EPO levels and heterogeneity in EPO dependence among the EPO-dependent progenitors has been proposed to explain various physiologic and pathologic rates of erythrocyte production.[79] In an expanded version of this model, erythroid progenitors enter the EPO-dependent period of differentiation, left of the dotted line in Figure 8.4, extending from the CFU-E through the early BasoEB stage and encompassing three

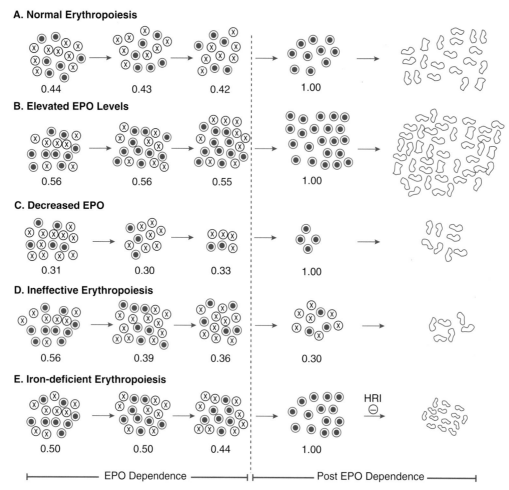

A. Normal Erythropoiesis

0.44   0.43   0.42   1.00

B. Elevated EPO Levels

0.56   0.56   0.55   1.00

C. Decreased EPO

0.31   0.30   0.33   1.00

D. Ineffective Erythropoiesis

0.56   0.39   0.36   0.30

E. Iron-deficient Erythropoiesis

HRI ⊖

0.50   0.50   0.44   1.00

├────── EPO Dependence ──────┤├────── Post EPO Dependence ──────┤

Figure 8.4 Model of erythropoiesis based on suppression of apoptosis by EPO and heterogeneity in EPO dependence among erythroid cells. From CFU-E through early basophilic erythroblast stages, erythroid progenitor/precursor cells depend on EPO for survival. The EPO-dependent period is left of the dotted line and encompasses three generations and two cell divisions. Each division is represented by an arrow. In the post-EPO-dependent period, to the right of the dotted line, two cell divisions occur. Surviving cells in each generation are shown as *circles* containing *large black dots* representing intact nuclei. Cells succumbing to apoptosis are shown as *circles* containing *Xs*. The proportion of the total cells that survive is shown below each generation. The number of surviving cells in a generation results in twice that number of total cells in the subsequent generation. The final populations of cells shown on the right represent the anucleate, irregular reticulocytes. (A) Normal erythropoiesis with average survival rates of 43% in the EPO-dependent generations. Normal erythropoiesis produces 200–250 billion reticulocytes daily, with a minority of all potential erythroid cells surviving the EPO-dependent period. (B) Elevated EPO levels as found after acute blood loss or hemolysis increase average survival rates to 56% in the EPO-dependent generation. Daily reticulocyte production shown here is increased to more than twice the normal rate. (C) Decreased EPO levels as found in renal failure decrease average survival rates to 32% in the EPO-dependent generation. Daily reticulocyte production is less than one-half of normal. (D) Ineffective erythropoiesis increases rates of apoptosis due to a pathologic process such as folate or vitamin B_{12} deficiency. High EPO levels in response to decreased erythrocyte production expand surviving cells in the early EPO-dependent generations, but the increased rates of apoptosis in the late EPO-dependent and post-EPO-dependent stages decrease daily reticulocyte production to less than one-third of normal. (E) Iron-deficient erythropoiesis with only moderately elevated EPO levels for the degree of anemia results in slightly increased average survival rates of 48% during the EPO-dependent period, but in the post-EPO-dependent period, when hemoglobin is synthesized, heme-regulated inhibitor (HRI) prevents apoptosis by inhibiting protein synthesis. The inhibited protein synthesis decreases reticulocyte numbers to about two-thirds of normal and reduces reticulocyte size and hemoglobin content.

generations of cells. The proportion of total cells that survive in a generation is shown under the population. The surviving cells are represented by circles, each of which contains a large black dot representing an intact nucleus. The cells lost to apoptosis are shown by circles containing an *X*. The number of surviving cells in a generation results in twice that number for the total cells in the subsequent generation. Most cells reaching the CFU-E stage need more EPO than the low levels found in normal plasma to sustain them and their progeny through the EPO-dependent period of

differentiation. As a result, the approximately 200–250 billion erythrocytes produced daily by a normal, healthy adult are the descendants of a minority of all the potential erythroid progenitor cells that could be generated during the EPO-dependent period (Figure 8.4A). When blood loss, hemolysis, or decreased atmospheric oxygen is encountered, plasma EPO increases, allowing the survival of many EPO-dependent progenitors that would die by apoptosis under normal conditions (Figure 8.4B). This enhanced survival increases reticulocyte production within a few days after encountering blood loss or decreased atmospheric oxygen. The increased reticulocytosis leads to increasing erythrocyte numbers until oxygen delivery recovers to normal, accompanied by declining plasma EPO levels until normal levels are achieved. In pathologic states of chronically decreased oxygen delivery, such as lung disease or cardiac diseases with right-to-left shunts, the persistently increased EPO levels (and increased glucocorticoids and BMP4) allow greater-than-normal survival of EPO-dependent cells such that the total number of erythrocytes is maintained in the polycythemic range. Likewise, the acquired somatic mutation of JAK2 (V617F) that is associated with hyperactivity of the EPO-R signaling most commonly results in polycythemia vera.[80]

When plasma EPO levels fall below normal, many erythroid progenitor cells that would survive the EPO-dependent period of differentiation under normal conditions die by apoptosis resulting in anemia from decreased reticulocyte production (Figure 8.4C). Renal disease is the major cause of decreased EPO, and, in mouse models of renal disease, EPO-producing renal cortical fibroblasts are transformed into proliferating myofibroblasts that do not produce EPO by the inflammatory cytokine, TNFα, signaling through NFκB.[81] Other clinical diseases noted to have decreased EPO levels are inflammatory disorders[82] and malignancies,[83] which are associated with increased inflammatory cytokines including TNFα, indicating that decreases in plasma EPO contribute to the anemia of chronic inflammation.

Nutritional requirements for erythropoiesis

Although erythropoiesis is finely regulated by the oxygenation–EPO feedback mechanism shown in Figure 8.2, the erythropoietic process is frequently limited by an insufficient supply of folate, vitamin B_{12}, or iron. Folate and vitamin B_{12} (cobalamin) are required for synthesis of DNA, and the daily production of very large numbers of erythrocytes results in a large DNA synthesis requirement. Although iron also is needed by all proliferating cell populations, the erythroblasts need much more iron than any other cell type because they produce hemoglobin. Through the hypoxia feedback mechanism, these nutrition-related anemias are associated with increased EPO levels,[56] but the increase in EPO is limited in iron deficiency, as described in the " Iron Deficiency and Development of Microcytic Anemia" section, and increased EPO can only partially compensate for the decreased erythropoiesis caused by a specific nutrient deficiency. Administration of the deficient nutrient, however, results in resolution of anemia in each of the deficiency states.

Deficiencies of folate or cobalamin, and development of macrocytic anemia

After reduction to tetrahydrofolate (THF), folate functions as a carrier of one-carbon molecules and becomes a cofactor in the synthesis of three deoxyribonucleosides (dGTP, dATP, and TTP) that are required for DNA synthesis.[84] In two separate reactions, formyltetrahydrofolate (CHO-THF) provides two of the carbons in the synthesis of the purine precursor of adenosyl and guanosyl deoxyribonucleosides; in both of these reactions, 10-CHO-THF is converted to THF. In a third reaction, methylenetetrahydrofolate (CH2-THF) provides a methylene group and reducing equivalents in the methylation of deoxyuridylate to form thymidylate; in the process, CH2-THF is converted to dihydrofolate (DHF). To regenerate THF, the active one-carbon acceptor–donor form, DHF must be reduced by dihydrofolate reductase (DHFR).

Thus, drugs that inhibit DHFR such as methotrexate or trimethoprim–sulfamethoxazole cause a deficiency of THF, the functional form of folate. Cobalamin is a cofactor in the conversion of methyltetrahydrofolate (CH3-THF) to THF. CH3-THF, the most prevalent form of folate in plasma, is imported into cells and retained there by addition of polyglutamates. Cobalamin deficiency results in the trapping of folate in the CH3-THF form, from which it cannot be converted to THF and subsequently to the CHO-THF and CH2-THF forms required for deoxyribonucleoside synthesis.[85,86] Furthermore, CH3-THF is the poorest THF form for polyglutamation, resulting in generalized loss of intracellular folate.[84]

Folate deficiency, cobalamin deficiency, or drugs that inhibit DHFR will decrease intracellular levels of folate coenzymes needed for de novo synthesis of all the deoxynucleosides used in DNA synthesis, except for deoxycytidine. An inadequate supply of deoxynucleosides causes accumulation of erythroid progenitors in the S phase of the cell cycle, which is rapidly followed by the induction of apoptosis.[87] Erythroid cells at the end of the EPO-dependent stage and the beginning of the period of hemoglobin synthesis appear to be most susceptible to this apoptosis. EPO-induced expansion of the EPO-dependent population at the CFU-E and proerythroblast stages leads to the presence of even greater numbers of these progenitor cells that subsequently undergo apoptosis just as they are beginning to produce hemoglobin.[88] The resultant clinical disease is megaloblastic anemia, which is characterized by ineffective erythropoiesis and macrocytic erythrocytes (Figure 8.4D). In ineffective erythropoiesis, progenitor cells in the EPO-dependent period expand due to increased EPO levels. The number of reticulocytes formed, however, is less than normal because of the increased rates of pathologic apoptosis in the EPO-dependent and post-EPO-dependent periods of differentiation.

Although the degree of ineffective erythropoiesis is prominent in megaloblastic anemia, the same process of inhibited DNA synthesis but with less apparent apoptosis is common in many macrocytic anemias. Cell size reductions during normal terminal erythroid differentiation result from shortening of the G1 phase of cell cycle while the lengths of S and G2/M phases remain unaffected.[25] Terminally differentiating erythroblasts with delayed or prolonged cell cycle durations produce larger-than-normal erythrocytes, because they accumulate larger amounts of protein during the protracted periods between cell divisions.[34] With folic acid fortification of grain products, which began in the United States in 1998, folate deficiency anemia due to dietary intake has been essentially eliminated.[89] However, cobalamin deficiency and drugs that interfere with folate metabolism such as methotrexate, trimethoprim–sulfamethoxazole, and anticonvulsants remain clinically relevant causes of macrocytic anemias.[90] Drugs that directly inhibit DNA synthesis such as antivirals (azidothymidine or zidovudine), immunosuppressives (azathioprine), and ribonucleotide reductase inhibitors (hydroxyurea) are major causes of macrocytic anemia.[90] In addition, several inherited and acquired marrow failure syndromes that cause macrocytic anemia have either directly or indirectly inhibited DNA synthesis and increased apoptotic loss of erythroid progenitors.[34] Those with direct DNA synthesis inhibition include Fanconi anemia, in which increased DNA crosslinking requires more DNA repair before cell division is completed,[91] and dyskeratosis congenital anemia, in which chromosomal telomeres cannot be maintained.[92] In addition to direct DNA damage, the induction of p53 in these erythroblasts contributes to both delayed cell cycle and apoptosis.[93] Other marrow failure diseases have indirect inhibition of DNA synthesis, such as Diamond–Blackfan anemia[94,95] and 5q-myelodysplastic syndrome anemia,[96] in which impaired ribosomal biogenesis and/or function leads to secondary inhibition of DNA synthesis and accompanying apoptosis by p53 induction.[95]

Iron deficiency and development of microcytic anemia

In addition to its function in hemoglobin, iron has essential roles in heme as part of myoglobin, mitochondrial cytochromes, and peroxidases. Among many nonheme enzymes, iron is required by three erythropoietic processes described in other sections of this chapter: aconitase in glucose metabolism, prolyl hydroxylation in HIFα stability, and ribonucleotide reductase in deoxynucleoside synthesis. Two-thirds of the body's iron is in the hemoglobin of circulating erythrocytes, and iron deficiency most commonly arises from blood loss. Two milliliters of blood contain about 1 mg of iron, which is approximately the amount absorbed daily by the duodenum, balancing the 1 mg normally lost through the gastrointestinal tract and skin. Erythroid progenitor cells are the greatest consumers of iron in the body, using about 25 mg daily under normal conditions, with the large majority of iron that is supplied to erythroid cells being recycled from macrophages that phagocytose senescent erythrocytes and degrade their hemoglobin. When erythropoietic demands are increased after bleeding or hemolysis, duodenal iron absorption is increased by erythroferrone, a hormone produced by erythroblasts that decreases hepatic production of hepcidin.[97] Hepcidin, a 25-amino-acid hormone produced in the liver, is induced by increased plasma iron and by cytokines produced in inflammation.[98] Hepcidin binds and downregulates surface expression of ferroportin, the cellular iron exporter of iron for all cells, including duodenal enterocytes, which are responsible for iron absorption.[99] The increased absorption mediated by erythroferrone is limited such that chronic blood loss of as little as 5 mL per day may cause iron deficiency.[100]

Specific regulators iron and heme metabolism protect cells from the toxic effects of iron while assuring that crucial cellular processes that rely on iron are sustained in non-erythroid cells during iron deficiency. Therefore, as iron deficiency develops, erythropoietic utilization of iron becomes restricted and anemia develops. In iron-deficient cells, iron regulatory proteins (IRP1 and IRP2) bind to iron responsive elements (IREs) in 5′- and 3′-untranslated regions (UTRs) of mRNAs controlling expression of proteins involved in cellular iron import, export, and storage.[101,102] Under iron-replete conditions, IRP1 functions as the enzyme aconitase with an iron–sulfur cluster in its active site; under iron-deficient conditions, IRP1 lacks the iron–sulfur cluster and binds IREs. IRP2 is rapidly degraded under iron-replete conditions but is stable and binds IREs during iron deficiency. IRP binding of IREs in the 5′-UTR of mRNAs inhibits their translation, decreasing their expression. Two important examples are mRNAs for ferroportin and ferritin, the intracellular storage protein, both of which decrease during iron deficiency, allowing maintenance of normal intracellular iron levels. IRP binding of IREs in the 3′-UTR of mRNAs stabilizes them and enhances their translation. An example is transferrin receptor mRNAs, where IRP binding increases transferrin receptor expression, thereby increasing cellular iron importation.

Although translation of ferroportin mRNA is controlled by the 5′-IRE in most cells, alternative splicing in duodenal enterocytes and erythroid precursor cells produces ferroportin mRNAs without 5′-IREs.[103,104] Thus, during iron deficiency, ferroportin expression is sustained in these two cell types, allowing uncompromised iron exportation into the plasma from duodenum and diminished accumulation within erythroid precursors before they begin hemoglobin synthesis.[105] During iron deficiency, IRPs increase binding to 5′-IREs of two key mRNAs involved in erythropoiesis. IRP1 binds a 5′-IRE in HIF2α mRNAs, leading to decreased translation of HIF2α messages in the renal cortical fibroblasts that are capable of producing EPO.[106–108] The decreased intracellular HIF2α protein results in less EPO production despite the hypoxia of the renal cortex from the decreased numbers of circulating erythrocytes. As a result, renal EPO production is relatively diminished in the anemia of iron deficiency when compared to other anemias of similar severity. The decreased EPO levels in iron deficiency, relative to anemia from blood loss or hemolysis, leads to relatively increased apoptosis of erythroid cells in the EPO-dependent stages that immediately precede the stages that synthesize hemoglobin (compare Figures 8.4B and 8.4E).

In the later hemoglobin-producing stages of iron-deficient erythropoiesis, IRP1 binds a 5′-IRE in mRNAs encoding ALAS2, which is the rate-controlling enzyme in porphyrin synthesis.[35] The resultant decreases in ALAS2 lead to less accumulations of protoporphyrin and heme in the erythroblasts. The decreased heme in erythroblasts increases HRI activity, which inhibits protein synthesis in general and globin syntheses in particular.[36] The combined effects of relatively decreased EPO and HRI-mediated restriction of protein synthesis in iron deficiency result in a slower rate of completion of the terminal stages of erythroblasts, with decrease rates of red blood cell production with hypochromic, microcytic anemia as shown in Figure 8.4E.

In addition to iron deficiency anemia, HRI plays a role in other microcytic anemias in which heme production is limited. Inherited disorders of ALAS2 cause sideroblastic anemia as iron accumulates in mitochondria when porphyrin synthesis does not provide sufficient protoporphyrin IX for heme formation. Likewise, mutations in ferrochelatase, the last enzyme in heme synthesis that catalyzes iron incorporation into protoporphyrin, cause decreases in intracellular heme. Mice deficient in HRI that become iron-deficient or have impaired porphyrin synthesis die from anemia when excess globin chains that cannot form hemoglobin without heme precipitate, denature, and cause oxidative damage resulting in apoptosis of erythroblasts.[109,110] Thus, HRI rescues iron-deficient erythroblasts from the thalassemia-like phenotype of oxidative damage from excess globin chains by restricting globin chain synthesis when heme synthesis is insufficient.

Thalassemia and the development of ineffective erythropoiesis and microcytosis

Thalassemia is the other major type of microcytic anemia, and, when thalassemia is severe, it is treated with chronic red cell transfusions. Thalassemias are caused by mutations or genetic deletions that decrease the synthesis of either α- or β-globin with intracellular accumulations of the excess unpaired α- and β-globin chains.[111] Compared to the excess β-globin chains in α-thalassemia, which form tetramers of hemoglobin H, the excess α-globin chains in β-thalassemia are relatively insoluble. Excess free α-globin chains in β-thalassemia are partially decreased by accumulation of γ-globin chains producing fetal hemoglobin, binding to AHSP, ubiquitination–proteasomal degradation, and autophagy of aggregated α-globins.[112] If unpaired globin chains are not removed by these intracellular adaptations, they can precipitate and denature, leading to the formation of methemoglobin and hemichromes that bind, oxidize, and disrupt the function of erythroid membrane and membrane skeletal proteins.[113] When the cytoplasmic domain of Band 3 is affected by this oxidative damage, it leads to aggregation, deposition of anti-Band 3 IgG, complement fixation, and phosphatidylserine externalization that in turn targets the cells for erythrophagocytosis.[114,115] The decreased solubility of unpaired free α-globins in β-thalassemias results in ineffective erythropoiesis due to intramedullary apoptosis of erythroblasts, whereas α-thalassemias have relatively less erythroblast apoptosis but more erythrocyte hemolysis.[116] Apoptosis in the β-thalassemias affects the late stages of erythroblast differentiation, and, because the mitigation of the EPO response due to IRP activity in iron deficiency does not occur in thalassemia, erythroid progenitors and early-stage erythroblasts expand in response to increased EPO. These early-stage erythroid populations expand extensively, with the degree of expansion directly related to the rate of apoptosis in the late-stage erythroblast populations.[117] The large expansion of erythroblast populations in the more severe cases of β-thalassemia appears to be the source of erythroferrone, which increases iron absorption and results in iron overload that complicates and limits transfusion therapy in these patients.[97]

Depending upon the severity of thalassemia, the oxidative stress due to denatured globin chains, heme, and nonheme iron can overwhelm the erythroblast's normal antioxidant enzymes such as superoxide dismutase, catalase, and glutathione peroxidase, and toxic oxygen species scavengers such as reduced glutathione and peroxiredoxin.[118] In these oxidation-stressed thalassemic erythroblasts, HRI has also been found to have an antioxidant effect that is distinct from its generalized suppression of protein synthesis. HRI increases the translation of activating transcription factor-4 (Atf4), which induces expression of antioxidant genes, including heme oxygenase-1 (HO1), the first step in degradation of heme.[119] In mice, HRI deficiency converts the moderate anemia of β-thalassemia intermedia into an embryonic lethal anemia with extensive accumulations of precipitated and denatured α-globin chains.[110] The antioxidant activity of HRI is accompanied by the general restriction of protein synthesis so that the phenotype in thalassemias is a microcytic, hypochromic anemia.[110]

Anemia of chronic inflammation

Diseases that can secondarily decrease erythropoiesis include those that directly displace the EBIs in the bone marrow, such as metastatic neoplasms, lymphoid neoplasms, and myelofibrosis.[120] However, the most common cause of secondary inhibition of erythropoiesis is anemia of chronic inflammation (ACI), which occurs in patients with chronic infections, neoplasms, and inflammatory diseases. ACI has multiple components in common with the various mechanisms shown in Figure 8.4. These components include direct and indirect inhibitory effects of specific inflammatory cytokines on erythropoietic cells and their hematopoietic progenitors. Inflammatory cytokines with recognized inhibitory mechanisms include interleukin-1 (IL1), IL6, TNFα, and interferon-γ (IFN-γ).[121] Direct inhibition of cell survival and growth by IFN-γ involves the induction of PU.1 in MEPs that suppresses erythroid differentiation and promotes megakaryocytic differentiation. In the subsequent stages of EPO dependence, IFN-γ enhances the expression of members of the apoptosis-inducing TNF receptor family, including receptors for TNFα, FAS, TNF-related apoptosis-inducing ligand (TRAIL), TNF-like weak inducer of apoptosis (TWEAK), and receptor-binding cancer antigen expressed on SiSo cells (RCAS1).[122–124] The EPO-dependent stages are also affected indirectly by decreased EPO production that is induced by TNFα. Although the concentrations of TNFα to which the EPO-producing fibroblasts in the renal cortices are exposed are lower than when the inflammation is within the renal tissue, plasma EPO levels are lower in ACI than in other anemic states without inflammation.[82,83]

The later stages of erythropoiesis when hemoglobin is produced have relatively restricted iron supplies due to IL6 and members of the bone morphogenetic protein (BMP) family that induce transcription of hepcidin in the liver.[98] Experimental models show that hepcidin induction can be mediated by IL6 signaling through the JAK2–STAT3 pathway,[125–127] or by bacterial endotoxin signaling through the BMP–Smad1/5/8 signaling pathway.[128] Hepcidin downregulates ferroportin on all cells, but its effects on three specific types of cells are most important for the inhibition of erythropoiesis in ACI. In macrophages, the decreased activity of ferroportin greatly diminishes the recycling of iron recovered from phagocytosed senescent erythrocytes. However, this sequestration of iron in macrophages is mitigated in ACI because the ferroportin-mediated loss of iron from erythroid progenitor and precursor stages prior to hemoglobin production that characterizes iron deficiency[105] does not occur in ACI due to elevated hepcidin downregulating erythroid cell ferroportin expression.[99] In severe cases of ACI, the downregulation of ferroportin on duodenal enterocytes restricts iron absorption, and eventually iron deficiency can develop. When iron deficiency complicates ACI, HRI activity causes the usually normocytic anemia to become microcytic.

Summary and outlook

Erythropoiesis is a component of the larger process of hematopoiesis, in which a pluripotent HSC gives rise through proliferation and differentiation to all the mature cells of the blood and the immune system. Within the erythroid differentiation process, the rate of erythrocyte production is regulated largely by EPO, which is produced in the renal cortex in response to the tissue hypoxia that results from decreased oxygen delivery in anemic states. The oxygen–EPO feedback mechanism results in finely controlled rates of erythrocyte production that never overshoot and result in polycythemia. This feedback mechanism, however, responds promptly to physiologic changes such as blood loss, hemolysis, or changes in atmospheric oxygen. Use of recombinant EPO is routine for patients with the anemia of renal disease. Limited responses to EPO in patients with anemias due to malignancy or myelodysplasia, combined with an increased potential for thrombotic and cardiovascular complications of EPO therapy in general, have resulted in more restricted use of recombinant EPO or its modified forms in clinical practice. In those countries that have fortified grain products, folate deficiency anemia has been largely eliminated. Although iron fortification of food has reduced the incidence of deficiency, iron deficiency remains a significant clinical problem. The identifications of hepcidin and erythroferrone and possible development of agonist or antagonist medications based on these two hormones have the potential to improve disorders related to assimilation of oral iron or macrophage recycling of iron from senescent or damaged erythrocytes.

Key references

A full reference list for this chapter is available at:
http://www.wiley.com/go/simon/transfusion

12 Gregory CJ, Eaves AC. Human marrow cells capable of erythropoietic differentiation in vitro: definition of three erythroid colony responses. *Blood* 1977; **49**: 855–64.

54 Koury ST, Koury MJ, Bondurant MC, Caro J, Graber SE. Quantitation of erythropoietin-producing cells in kidneys of mice by in situ hybridization: correlation with hematocrit, renal erythropoietin mRNA, and serum erythropoietin concentration. *Blood* 1989; **74**: 645–51.

56 Erslev AJ. Erythropoietin. *N Engl J Med* 1991; **324**: 1339–44.

60 Jaakkola P, Mole DR, Tian YM, *et al.* Targeting of HIF-alpha to the Von Hippel-Lindau ubiquitylation complex by O2-regulated prolyl hydroxylation. *Science* 2001; **292**: 468–72.

61 Ivan M, Kondo K, Yang H, *et al.* HIFalpha targeted for VHL-mediated destruction by proline hydroxylation: implications for O2 sensing. *Science* 2001; **292**: 464–8.

71 Koury MJ, Bondurant MC. Erythropoietin retards DNA breakdown and prevents programmed death in erythroid progenitor cells. *Science* 1990; **248**: 378–81.

72 Muta K, Krantz SB. Apoptosis of human erythroid colony-forming cells is decreased by stem cell factor and insulin-like growth factor I as well as erythropoietin. *J Cell Physiol* 1993; **156**: 264–71.

97 Kautz L, Jung G, Valore EV, Rivella S, Nemeth E, Ganz T. Identification of erythroferrone as an erythroid regulator of iron metabolism. *Nat Genet* 2014; **46**: 678–84.

99 Nemeth E, Tuttle MS, Powelson J, *et al.* Hepcidin regulates cellular iron efflux by binding to ferroportin and inducing its internalization. *Science* 2004; **306**: 2090–3.

109 Han AP, Yu C, Lu L, *et al.* Heme-regulated Eif2alpha kinase (HRI) is required for translational regulation and survival of erythroid precursors in iron deficiency. *EMBO J* 2001; **20**: 6909–18.

CHAPTER 9

Red blood cell metabolism, preservation, and oxygen delivery

John R. Hess[1] & Bjarte G. Solheim[2]

[1]Department of Laboratory Medicine and Hematology, University of Washington School of Medicine; and Transfusion Service, Harborview Medical Center, Seattle, WA, USA

[2]Institute of Immunology, Oslo University Hospital–Rikshospitalet, University of Oslo, Oslo, Norway

A human red cell, mature and released from the bone marrow, lacks a nucleus and mitochondria. It has a life span of 120 days, after which it is removed from the circulation in the natural course of aging.[1] It picks up oxygen in a third of a second transit of the alveolar capillary and delivers oxygen through capillaries with a smaller diameter than its own. It can neither use oxygen for the extraction of energy, nor synthesize proteins or polynucleotides. Its primary functions, transporting oxygen from the lungs to the tissues and carbon dioxide back to the lungs, do not require the expenditure of energy. However, maintaining hemoglobin in an optimal state for delivering oxygen and keeping normal cell flexibility and morphology do require active metabolism and are prerequisites for function and successful transfusion.

During standard storage at 4 °C, significant and in part reversible changes in red cell morphology and metabolism occur, called *storage lesions*. One striking example is the red cell shape change (Figure 9.1), which can be reversed to a large extent by metabolic rejuvenation of the stored cells.[2] In order to understand and improve storage, it is essential to understand basic principles of red cell metabolism.

Understanding of red cell metabolism has increased with the application of "-omic" technologies. Proteomics has identified 2200 separate proteins in the red cell that are the products of 5% of all human genes.[3] This number includes 340 proteins specifically associated with the red cell membrane. Structural proteins, membrane receptors, metabolic enzymes, heat shock proteins, chaperonins, and others have been catalogued and sorted into pathways and functional groups, and they provide the most complete overview of the molecule-by-molecule functioning of a human cell type. Metabolomics can measure simultaneously the concentrations of several hundred small molecules and follow their activities in isotopic pulse-chase experiments.[4] Lipidomics can enumerate the many forms of lipids present and their degree of oxidation.[5] Transcriptomics reveals the presence of 400 different small RNA molecules serving a variety of roles.[6] Analysis to date confirms the view that red cells are complex, metabolically active cells using glucose to make adenosine 5′-triphosphate (ATP) and reducing equivalents to ensure flexibility and oxygen delivery. The red cell may be 98% hemoglobin by weight, but it is much more than "a hapless sac of hemoglobin."[7]

Integration of biochemical metabolism and biophysical discoveries in the last two decades by several research groups shows that many molecular interactions may be missed when the red cell is considered by itself without taking into account the physiologic vascular milieu in which it performs its main biological function.[8,9] Thus, interaction of hemoglobin and the band 3 protein is influenced by conformational changes that accompany ligand binding to hemoglobin, which modulates the function of band 3, the glycolytic pathway, and the structural architecture of the red cell membrane–cytoskeletal system (Figure 9.2). During storage, concentrations of red cell ATP, DPG (also known as 2,3-bisphosphoglycerate, or BPG), and glutathione decline, leading to cell wall dysfunction and damage. Dysfunction can manifest as stiffer red cells, and damage as membrane loss. Both of these effects can in turn affect the vascular flow of transfused cells. On the arterial side, stiffer cells have trouble absorbing the energy of pulsatile flow and are projected more frequently into the normally cell-free layer of plasma at the vascular surface, where they absorb endothelium-derived nitric oxide and lead to vasoconstriction.[10] In capillaries, the close contact between hemoglobin and band 3 and carbonic anhydrase in the cell membrane promotes the production of bicarbonate with release of protons, which, via the Bohr effect (see Chapter 10), releases oxygen from hemoglobin where it is needed in the tissues.[8] On the venous side, damaged membranes can lead to procoagulant and proinflammatory events.[11] In this chapter, red cell metabolism will be discussed, taking into account intermolecular interactions of importance for the primary function of hemoglobin, which is oxygen and carbon dioxide transport, and followed by a review of the development of red cell storage systems.

Metabolism

Metabolism of glucose
Main glycolytic pathway (Embden–Meyerhof pathway)
Under physiologic circumstances, the energy that the red cell requires is derived through the breakdown of glucose to lactate or pyruvate. The sequence of reactions is generally known as *glycolysis* or the *Embden–Meyerhof pathway*.[12] This pathway is phylogenetically very old, and the sequence of reactions is the same in bacteria,

Rossi's Principles of Transfusion Medicine, Fifth Edition. Edited by Toby L. Simon, Jeffrey McCullough, Edward L. Snyder, Bjarte G. Solheim, and Ronald G. Strauss.
© 2016 John Wiley & Sons, Ltd. Published 2016 by John Wiley & Sons, Ltd.

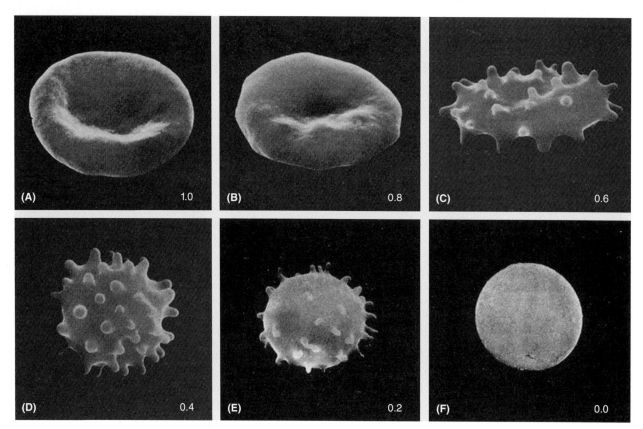

Figure 9.1 Scanning electron micrographs showing representative red blood cells in various stages of shape change typical of prolonged storage. The cells progress from discocytes (A), through several stages of echinocytes (B–D), to spheroechinocytes (E) and finally to spherocytes (F). Scores, based on the visual appearance of those shown in the lower right of the individual images, can be assigned to several hundred individual stored cells and averaged to produce a morphology score for the unit. Such scores decrease in a linear manner during storage but can be substantially reversed by rejuvenation.

yeast, and vertebrates. Except for the exaggerated production of DPG in the red cell, the pathway is the same in all tissues.

The reactions of the glycolytic pathway are shown in Figure 9.3. In this sequence of reactions, the six-carbon sugar glucose is phosphorylated, isomerized to fructose phosphate, phosphorylated again, and cleaved into three-carbon phospho-sugars. The three-carbon sugars are again phosphorylated. Finally, these

carbohydrate-bound high-energy phosphates that have been gained are transferred to adenosine diphosphate (ADP), producing the high-energy compound, ATP. The ATP synthesized is used by ATPases for the pumping of ions against concentration gradients, for the phosphorylation of membrane proteins and lipids, and, very importantly, for the phosphorylation of glucose to make more ATP in the glycolytic pathway.[13]

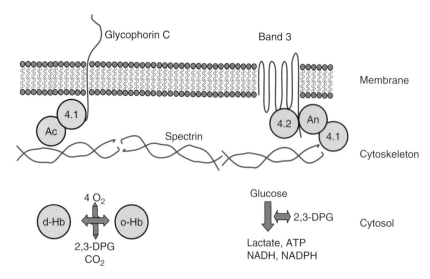

Figure 9.2 Schemata of red cell components. In the past, it was believed that oxygen transport by hemoglobin and metabolism were cytosolic functions, and that the membrane and cytoskeleton merely enclosed them. We now recognize that the attachments of the membrane to the cytoskeleton from band 3, through ankyrin (An) and proteins 4.2 and 4.1 to spectrin, and from Glycophorin C through protein 4.1 and actin (Ac) to spectrin, are destabilized by 2,3-diphosphoglycerate (2,3-DPG). 2,3-DPG released from deoxy-hemoglobin (d-Hb) binds to band 3 and partially detaches the membrane from the cytoskeleton, allowing lateral movement of membrane structures. This could have implications for red cell flexibility when slipping into peripheral capillaries. O-Hb, oxy-hemoglobin.

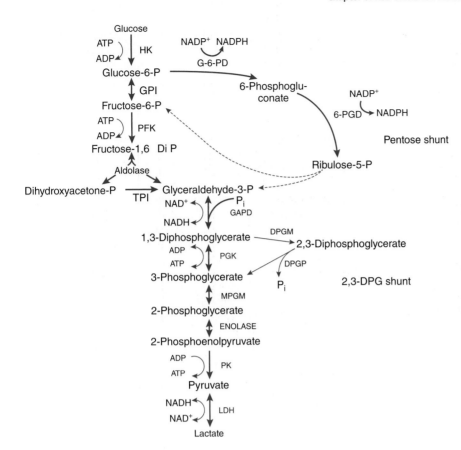

Figure 9.3 The glycolytic pathway with the pentose and 2,3-DPG shunts of red cell metabolism. *ATP*, adenosine triphosphate; *ADP*, adenosine diphosphate; *HK*, hexokinase; *NADP⁺*, nicotinamide adenine dinucleotide phosphate, oxidized form; *NADPH*, nicotinamide adenine dinucleotide phosphate, reduced form; *6-PGD*, 6-phosphogluconate dehydrogenase; *P*, phosphate; *G-6-PD*, glucose-6-phosphate dehydrogenase; *PFK*, phosphofructokinase; *TPI*, triosephosphate isomerase; *NAD⁺*, nicotinamide adenine dinucleotide, oxidized form; *NADH*, nicotinamide adenine dinucleotide, reduced form; *GAPD*, glyceraldehyde-3-phosphate dehydrogenase; *PGK*, phosphoglycerate kinase; *DPGM*, diphosphoglycerate mutase. *DPGP*, diphosphoglycerate phosphatase; *MPGM*, monophosphoglycerate mutase; *PK*, pyruvate kinase; *LDH*, lactate dehydrogenase.

The 2,3-DPG shunt (Rapoport–Luebering shunt)

Production of 2,3-DPG is the function of a shunt that branches from the main glycolytic pathway after the formation of 1,3-diphosphoglycerate (1,3-DPG) and returns to it with the formation of 3-phosphoglycerate (3-PGA) (Figure 9.3). The pathway consists of the formation of 2,3-DPG from 1,3-DPG, followed by the dephosphorylation of 2,3-DPG to 3-PGA (Figure 9.4). Both reactions are catalyzed by the same enzyme and are balanced at physiologic pH.[14] At higher pH, the enzyme acts only as a mutase moving phosphate in 1,3-DPG from position 1 to position 2 in the molecule; at low pH, it acts only as a phosphatase, transforming 2,3-DPG to 3-PG. As the 2,3-DPG shunt bypasses one of the two ATP-making steps in glycolysis, 2,3-DPG is made at the expense of ATP. In storage systems, a high pH can shut down ATP production, whereas a lower than physiologic pH leads to a burst of ATP production driven by the breakdown of 2,3-DPG.

The production of large quantities of 2,3-DPG is a unique feature of glycolysis in the red cell. Red cells contain approximately equimolar amounts of hemoglobin and 2,3-DPG. Binding of 2,3-DPG to the β subunits of deoxyhemoglobin serves to stabilize the T (tense, low oxygen affinity) state of hemoglobin and thus shifts the oxygen equilibrium curve to the right (favoring dissociation of oxygen). In the R (relaxed, high oxygen affinity) state, approximately 80% of 2,3-DPG is "free," whereas in the T state over 80% of 2,3-DPG is bound to hemoglobin.[6,15] In the "free" state, 2,3-DPG at physiologic concentrations modulates properties of the red cell membrane.[8] It binds directly to band 3 and thereby interferes negatively in the interactions between protein 4.1, protein 4.2, ankyrin, and band 3.[16] 2,3-DPG also releases spectrin from the membrane skeleton, and interferes negatively in the interactions between spectrin–actin–protein

4.1 and the glycophorin C complex.[8,17,18] This decreases the number of connecting links between the cell membrane and the cytoskeleton, and increases lateral mobility of integral membrane proteins.[10,19] The rise and fall of 2,3-DGP concentrations with each pass through the circulatory system therefore result in repetitive destabilization and restabilization of the membrane–cytoskeleton architecture (Figure 9.2). "Free" 2,3-DPG increases cell flexibility by weakening the links between the membrane and the cytoskeleton and facilitates gas exchange by allowing the red cell to slip into narrow capillaries and splenic sinusoids. However, further experiments are needed to clarify the full physiologic implications of the interactions between 2,3-DPG, cell membrane proteins and the cytoskeleton.

The Pentose shunt (hexose monophosphate shunt)

Under normal, steady-state conditions, most glucose is metabolized in red cells by way of the glycolytic pathway, but there is another important metabolic pathway called the *pentose shunt* or *hexose monophosphate shunt* (Figure 9.3). Some of the glucose-6-phosphate (G-6-P) formed when glucose is phosphorylated in the hexokinase reaction enters this pathway. Glucose-6-phosphate dehydrogenase (G-6-PD) catalyzes the oxidation of G-6-P to 6-phosphogluconolactone, reducing nicotinamide adenine dinucleotide phosphate (NADP) to NADPH. After hydrolysis of the lactone to 6-phosphogluconic acid, another oxidative step reduces additional NADP to NADPH, and releases carbon dioxide from the six-carbon compound, forming the pentose sugar ribose-1-phosphate. After a series of rearrangements, two normal intermediates of the main glycolytic pathway, fructose-6-phosphate and glyceraldehyde-3-phosphate, are formed and rejoin the main metabolic stream.

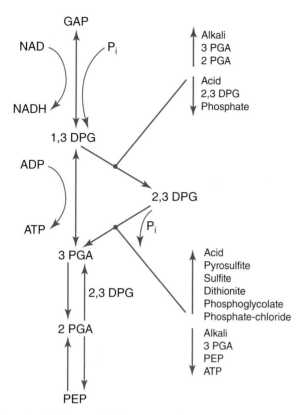

Figure 9.4 Regulation of the formation and breakdown of 2,3-DPG. The steady-state concentration of 2,3-DPG is governed by the rate of its formation from 1,3-DPG and by its breakdown to 3-phosphoglyceric acid. Both reactions are catalyzed by the same multifunctional enzyme modulated by a variety of substances. Depending on the reaction, the enzyme is abbreviated DPGM or DPGP in the figure. Abbreviations are as in Figure 9.3.

The pentose shunt is important to the red cell as a source of NADPH. It is this reduced nucleotide that maintains glutathione in its reduced form.[20] Reduced glutathione is important for the elimination of peroxide, protection of protein SH groups, limitation of lipid peroxidation, and detoxification processes. The pentose shunt also plays an important role for the red cell by providing ribose-5-phosphate needed for the production of phosphoribosyl pyrophosphate (PRPP), an essential substrate for the synthesis of adenine nucleotides required for continuing ATP synthesis (discussed further in this chapter).

Alternative substrates for red cell metabolism

Glucose is the natural substrate for human red cell energy metabolism, but red cells are also capable of metabolizing other sugars (i.e., fructose, mannose, galactose, and the three-carbon sugar dihydroxyacetone). However, none of these other sugars have proven to be useful in the design of blood preservatives.

The presence in red cells of the enzyme nucleoside phosphorylase makes it possible for red cells to use nucleosides such as inosine to support ATP synthesis:

$$Inosine + P_i \rightarrow Ribose - 1 - P + Hypoxanthine$$

In this reaction, ribose-1-phosphate is formed without the expenditure of ATP. Ribose-1-phosphate is then readily converted to fructose-6-phosphate by the pentose shunt, which feeds into

the glycolytic pathway leading to the generation of ATP. In the rejuvenation of red cells (see later in this chapter), inosine allows ATP-depleted red cells to prime their metabolic pump (the glycolytic pathway). It has not been possible to include inosine in blood preservatives because the product of its metabolism, hypoxanthine, is rapidly converted to uric acid in the body. Because many patients who receive blood transfusions have impaired liver function or may already have hyperuricemia because of hereditary or acquired factors, a blood product that increases plasma uric acid level cannot be considered safe.[21]

Regulation of energy metabolism
Glucose metabolism

In nucleate cells, metabolic regulation is dependent on protein synthesis, which in turn is regulated by increasing or decreasing the rate of DNA transcription or the translation of messenger RNA. Red cells do not have these options. Instead, the rate of glucose metabolism is regulated by feedback mechanisms acting on the glycolytic enzymes.[22] However, in spite of extensive studies, our understanding of the control of glucose metabolism by red cells is still incomplete.

The N-terminal cytoplasmic domain of the band 3 protein binds hemoglobin, cytoskeletal proteins, and glycolytic enzymes.[23] Based on current evidence, de Rosa et al.[8] point out that interaction between hemoglobin in the T state and band 3 causes a release by displacement of glycolytic enzymes, which results in increased activity of the main glycolytic pathway. On the contrary, hemoglobin in the R (highly oxygenated) state is associated with increased activity of the pentose shunt because the enzymes of the main glycolytic pathway show reduced activity when bound to band 3.[24]

The rate of glucose metabolism by red cells is influenced by many factors other than basal enzyme activity. Negative feedback mechanisms are involved in the control of the glycolytic pathway. Both hexokinase and phosphofructokinase are inhibited by hydrogen ions (low pH).[25] The principal reason that the rate of glycolysis slows markedly during red cell storage is the accumulation of lactic acid.

2,3-DPG concentration

The concentration of 2,3-DPG depends on the rate of its formation and degradation. Many effectors determine whether the mutase or the phosphatase activity of the diphosphoglycerate mustase–phosphatase predominates (Figure 9.4). The hydrogen ion concentration is the most important physiologic modulator.[26] At low pH, phosphatase activity is stimulated and mutase activity is inhibited. Thus, high pH favors 2,3-DPG maintenance and production during storage at the expense of ATP formation, whereas low pH leads to the rapid loss of 2,3-DPG with an increase in ATP production as long as DPG lasts. Modulation of red cell metabolism by elevating pH has been the principal means used to retard the decline of 2,3-DPG levels that occurs during liquid storage of red cells (see later in this chapter). After depletion of ATP during storage, 2,3-DPG levels in transfused red cells return to 50% of normal in 7 hours and almost to 95% at 72 hours.[27]

The pentose shunt activity

The rate of the pentose pathway is influenced by the availability of NADP and the concentration of NADPH. Under oxidative stress, NADPH is oxidized to NADP and the activity of the pentose pathway increases, which is consistent with the observation of increased pentose shunt activity when hemoglobin is in the R state.

Adenosine triphosphate

In the red cells, ATP is synthesized by the glycolytic pathway, but its regulation is complex. ATP is used in a number of different metabolic pathways, particularly by the kinases that phosphorylate sugars (i.e., hexokinase and phosphofructokinase) and proteins, and by ATPase-driven ion pumps (i.e., Na^+-K^+-ATPase, Mg^{2+}-ATPase, and Ca^{2+}-ATPase). Moreover, red cell membrane shape and rigidity are controlled by the ATP-dependent cytoskeleton.

$$ATP + AMP \leftrightarrow 2\,ADP$$

ATP is in equilibrium with ADP and adenosine monophosphate (AMP), as shown above. Production of ATP from ADP in glycolysis normally keeps AMP concentrations low. As the level of ADP increases when glycolysis slows, some is converted to AMP. AMP, in turn, is deaminated in the AMP-deaminase reaction and the total red cell pool of adenine decreases during storage, which leads to the depletion of ATP if adenine is not added to the anticoagulant and/or additive solution.

Guanine nucleotides

Red cells contain and turn over guanine nucleotides, which perform at least two functions in red cells. First, G proteins play a role in the signal transduction of membrane shear into secretion of the local vasodilators, cyclic AMP and ATP.[28] Second, high concentrations of GTP inhibit red cell transglutaminase, a primitive coagulation system that also interacts with the cytoplasmic domain of band 3 and with protein 4.1.[29] The GTP concentration is reduced when red cells age so that transglutaminase, which has a factor XIII–like activity, can facilitate the removal of senescent red cells by binding them to fibrin clots.

Synthetic processes

Red cells are only able to assemble a limited repertoire of important molecules from simpler precursors. They retain the capacity to synthesize nucleotides through a "salvage pathway" and to synthesize glutathione from its precursor amino acids. Adenine is able to enter the erythrocyte, and purine nucleotides are synthesized through the adenine phosphoribosyl transferase reaction:

$$Adenine + PRPP \rightarrow AMP + PP$$

This reaction is critical in blood storage. The beneficial effect of addition of adenine to stored blood depends on it. Phosphoribosyl pyrophosphate (PRPP), one of the substrates for the formation of AMP in this reaction, is synthesized from pentose–phosphate formed in the pentose shunt. Guanine nucleotides form in an analogous reaction and are catalyzed by a different enzyme, hypoxanthine–guanine phosphoribosyl transferase. Red cells also actively synthesize a number of other small molecules, including reduced glutathione, nicotinamide adenine dinucleotide (NAD), and S-adenosyl-L-methione.[13]

Membrane metabolism

The red cell membrane is composed of a phospholipid bilayer containing cholesterol molecules and membrane proteins.[30] The phospholipids are disposed with a predominance of phosphatidyl choline and sphingomyelin in the outer leaflet and phosphatidylinositol, phosphatidylethanolamine, and phosphatidylserine (PS) in the inner leaflet. Loss of phospholipid asymmetry results in exposure of PS, which is an important apoptopic marker on the red cell surface. Exposure of PS on the outer cell surface promotes red cell removal from the circulation, whereas the surface glycoprotein CD47, which decreases during storage, inhibits phagocytosis.[31] The phospholipid asymmetry is maintained by the ATP-dependent flippase (aminophospholipid translocase) activity. This activity counteracts phospholipid scrambling, which moves PS from the inner to the outer cell surface. Flippase activity decreases during storage but can be corrected by rejuvenation of the red cells.[32] Phospholipid scrambling is normally low during storage but can be enhanced by photodynamic treatment for pathogen inactivation.[33]

Maintaining the iron of hemoglobin in a reduced state is a prerequisite for effective oxygen transport. The enzyme involved is methemoglobin reductase, which is NADH driven and reduces Fe^{3+} to Fe^{2+}. Protection of the SH groups of hemoglobin and membrane proteins from oxidation is also a crucial function. This is accomplished by maintaining adequate amounts of reduced glutathione (GSH) by reduction of NADPH to NADP. The oxidation of GSH to GSSG catalyzed by peroxidase reduces H_2O_2 to H_2O and Fe^{3+} to Fe^{2+}. Adequate levels of ATP, NADH, NADPH, and 2,3-DPG for these metabolic functions are secured by the glycolytic pathway with its pentose and 2,3-DPG shunts. In addition, the synthesis of NAD and NADP from nicotinic acid must also occur.

Membrane proteins such as glycophorin and band 3 extend through the lipid membrane. Branches of carbohydrates anchored to membrane proteins protrude from the outer surface of the membrane. The inner surface of the membrane is lined by the cytoskeleton, which is anchored to the membrane through the N-terminal cytoplasmic domain of band 3. The tetrameric form of band 3 binds ankyrin and constitutes, with proteins 4.1 and 4.2, a major attachment site for spectrin. A second attachment site for spectrin involves actin and protein 4.1 in the glycophorin C complex. Both attachments (Figure 9.2) are weakened when the concentration of "free" (non-hemoglobin-bound) 2,3-DPG is increased; this appears to be of importance for cell flexibility and gas delivery.[8] Membrane shape and deformability are controlled by the ATP-driven cytoskeleton. Because some capillaries in the microcirculation have a diameter of only half that of a red cell, loss of flexibility and deformability is a serious storage lesion responsible for removal of rigid cells (Figure 9.1).

The red cell membrane also contains a number of transport proteins such as the glucose transporter, Ca^{2+}-ATPase, the Na^+-K^+-ATPase, the GSSG (oxidized glutathione) transport ATPases, and amino acid transporters, in addition to various other transport channels.

A prime metabolic activity of the red cell is maintaining osmotic stability through the activity of its membrane pumps, which are ATP driven. The Na^+-K^+-ATPase is highly sensitive to changes in temperature and scarcely functions at 4 °C. During storage in the cold, sodium diffuses into the cells and potassium leaks out until a new equilibrium is reached. The leakage of potassium is further increased by irradiation. Increased potassium content in plasma or in the additive solution of stored red blood cells (RBCs) presents a potential hazard to neonates, although under most other circumstances it can be ignored.[14] Citrate in plasma increases potassium toxicity, and reducing RBC supernatant volume results in less potassium leakage before equilibrium is reached. Studies performed over 30 years ago indicate that restoration of potassium after transfusion is slow and can take more than 6 days.[14] More recent studies in cells with better ATP concentrations show much faster restoration.

Although the macromolecules of the membrane are produced by red cell precursors, some of the components of the membrane are metabolically quite active. For example, cholesterol in the membrane exchanges readily with cholesterol in the plasma, phosphatidylinositol undergoes active phosphorylation, and some proteins are phosphorylated by protein kinases and dephosphorylated by phosphatases. These reactions may influence the functional status of membrane components, but their importance is not yet fully understood.

Eryptosis: programmed cell death in red cells

Although RBCs lack the nucleus and mitochondria associated with apoptosis in most cell populations, they undergo a unique form of programmed cell death called *eryptosis*, which is associated with low pH, increased cell calcium, or energy loss with low ATP concentrations.[34] The process is marked by irreversible shape change, loss of membrane by microvesiculation, and exposure of negatively charged phospholipids on their cell surface. Oxidative damage also appears to play an important role. Presumably, eryptosis marks RBCs at the end of their normal lifespan for removal from the vascular system by splenic or other macrophages.[35]

Eryptosis is critically limiting in RBC storage because falling pH and ATP concentrations are a concomitant of closed system storage with the accumulation of acid breakdown products of glycolysis and acidic inhibition of glycolysis.[36] The accumulation of hemoglobin-containing microvesicles in the supernatant appears to be a good marker of the process, as is increasing RBC calcium content with activation of calpain enzymes.

Summary

In the circulation, red cells metabolize glucose by the glycolytic pathway with its pentose and 2,3-DPG shunts. The energy gained provides ATP to maintain ion and glucose concentration gradients between the plasma and erythrocyte and to secure red cell deformability. It also secures NADH to keep hemoglobin in the reduced state and NADPH to protect SH groups on hemoglobin and membrane proteins. Finally, the production of 2,3-DPG is important for the optimal dissociation of oxygen from hemoglobin, whereas the rise and fall of non-hemoglobin-bound 2,3-DPG with each pass through the circulatory system induce repetitive changes in the membrane–cytoskeleton architecture, which could have implications for red cell flexibility and gas transport.

Red cell preservation in transfusion medicine

Liquid preservation
General considerations and principles

RBCs are the most commonly transfused blood components, and their use in a variety of physical circumstances and clinical conditions has shaped their development as products. As an example, the US military's need to reduce the weight and breakage of blood bottles during shipment led to the development and adoption of plastic blood bags.[37] This led to closed-system sterile component production and, fortuitously, exposing RBCs to the plasticizer diethylhexyl phthalate (DEHP), which reduced hemolysis during storage.[38] Arguments over the removal of plasma between blood bankers, who wanted the plasma to make albumin and coagulation factors, and surgeons, who wanted the blood to flow quickly in trauma patients, led to the development of additive solutions.[39] Again, there were unforeseen consequences, as removal of plasma led to better RBC storage and reduced transfusion reactions. Regulatory agencies have also played a role, as the US Food and

Drug Administration (FDA) recognizes that 4 million patients a year receive RBCs and that the product must be safe for all.[40] Ideas such as adding antibiotics to blood bags to prevent bacterial contamination, which kills approximately five patients a year in the country, would come at the risk of exposing millions to allergenic and toxic drugs with the probability of greater harm than good being achieved.

As a result of many competing forces, development and adoption of new RBC storage technology have been slow.[41] Five major improvements occurred in the last 60 years: (1) the addition of phosphate, (2) the use of plastic bags, (3) the addition of adenine, (4) the development of additive solutions, and (5) the use of leukoreduction, which reduces hemolysis. The reasons for this slow progress have had to do with the perception of little need for change, limited investment in change, lack of understanding of RBC storage lesions, poor developmental strategies, and conservative regulatory stances.[42] The major ongoing efforts, the development of advanced additive solutions and pathogen reduction methods, make slow progress for similar reasons.

For 60 years, it has been a societal goal that RBCs for transfusion should be available, safe, effective, and cheap.[37] Making red cells readily available requires both the ability to take liquid units out of the refrigerator and administer them immediately to critically ill or injured patients and the ability to find rare units in frozen national and international inventories. Storage systems contribute to blood safety by isolating individual units in closed systems and reducing product breakdown and bacterial growth through cold storage. A major goal of storage systems is to maintain effectiveness by preserving the lifespan and function of fresh RBCs to the greatest extent possible. Keeping blood cheap requires controlling per-unit costs and not increasing health risks that will make new demands on other parts of the system. At the present time, the unit costs of RBCs remain low, and controlling those costs has been one factor in limiting progress on storage systems.

A short history of RBC storage systems

Rous and Turner developed the first red cell storage solution in 1916, a simple mixture of citrate and glucose.[43] It was used initially to store rabbit RBCs for heterophil agglutination testing for syphilis, but when the cells appeared to be intact four weeks later, they were reinfused back into the donor rabbits, raising the hematocrit without increasing the reticulocyte count or bile in the urine, which suggested that the reinfused cells were circulating.[44] A year later, Rous's postdoctoral fellow, Oswald H. Robertson, used this Rous–Turner solution to build the first successful blood bank in the Harvard Medical Unit attached to the British Expeditionary Force in France.[45]

The major problem with the Rous–Turner solution was that it could not be heat sterilized, as the sugar caramelized, so there was a risk of bacterial contamination from the open mixing of the ingredients and adding the solution to the bottles. In 1943, Loutit and Mollison solved this problem by lowering the pH of the solution to 5.0 to make acid–citrate–dextrose (ACD) solution.[46] ACD solution could be autoclaved in sterile vacuum bottles and was used as the standard blood-collecting solution in the United States and Britain for many years. It was made first to be used in a 1:4 ratio with collected whole blood and later concentrated to be used at a 1:7 ratio, as is now standard, to reduce the dilution of the blood.

In exploring why RBCs seemed to do better in the lower volume of the anticoagulant solution, it became clear that the cells passively lose phosphate. This loss could be prevented by adding phosphate to the solution.[47] Citrate–phosphate–dextrose (CPD) in a 1:7 volume ratio, 63 ml for 450 ml of whole blood, stored red cells slightly better than the older ACD.[48] CPD became the standard anticoagulant in the United States, but ACD persisted in Europe, and both were used for 21-day storage with recovery of 70–80% of the RBC 24 hours after reinfusion of the stored cells back into their original donor.

At about the same time, Gabrio and her colleagues recognized that nucleotides were important for red cell metabolism, but almost a decade passed before researchers determined that adenine was the critical intermediate.[49–51] In 1968, Shields formulated a mixture of CPD and adenine, CPDA-1, and showed that it markedly improved whole blood storage.[52] However, during the subsequent 11 years that the FDA debated the safety of adenine, plastic bags revolutionized blood banking, and this excellent whole blood storage solution turned out to work less well with the packed RBCs left behind when plasma was removed.[53] Beutler and West showed that the higher the hematocrit of RBC in concentrates, the lower the red cell ATP concentrations and the in vivo recovery.[54] The obvious answer was to add back more volume and nutrients in the form of an "additive solution," but the initial attempt to do this with a solution of bicarbonate, adenine, glucose, and phosphate (BAGP) did not work.[55] CPDA-1 was finally licensed as a five-week storage solution in 1979, but only after Hogman had developed a simple additive solution of saline, adenine, and glucose (SAG) that also worked for five-week storage but without the adverse effects associated with the high pH.[56] SAG went on to immediate use in Sweden.

The use of SAG was associated with 1% hemolysis by the end of five weeks of storage, so mannitol was subsequently added (SAG-M) as a "membrane stabilizer."[57] This reduced the hemolysis by more than 50%. Drawing whole blood into CPD, making component products, and storing the RBC concentrate with an additional 100 ml of SAG-M (CPD/SAG-M) are the standard RBC storage system in Europe. Minimal variants of this basic solution, additive solution-1 (AS-1) and additive solution-5 (AS-5), are widely used in the United States. Also used is a more substantial variant using citrate and phosphate in the place of mannitol (AS-3 or SAG-CP). All of the variants appear to be equivalent and provide about 82% recovery with about 0.4% hemolysis after six weeks of storage.[58]

The most important limits of the first generation of additive solutions are the loss of membrane with resulting loss of deformability and viability that occur with prolonged storage. The progressive loss of 2,3-DPG may also be important in some situations, although the clinical impact is not well understood. More advanced additive solutions have been developed and licensed, but are not yet widely available.[39] They work by providing phosphate and buffering and are capable of 7–8 weeks storage. They are considered to be attractive more for their ability to improve recovery, reduce membrane loss, and improve 2,3-DGP and/or ATP concentrations for all stored RBC than for their ability to extend storage further.

Collection and separation procedures

The volume of whole blood removed for storage, processing, and transfusion was historically 450 ml, a pint, in Western countries. For some newer collection systems, this amount has been increased to 500 ml, a half-liter, to increase the collection with each donation and to offset the losses associated with filtration leukoreduction. Products derived from both collection volumes, whether leukoreduced or not, are considered one unit. The interdonor differences in hematocrit and platelet count are sufficiently great that the yields

of red cells, platelets, and plasma in components prepared from units of either whole blood collection volume show considerable overlap. Some have argued for a more standard definition of a unit, perhaps based on grams of hemoglobin, but it would make blood collection more difficult and wasteful.[59]

As noted above, the volume of anticoagulant–nutrient solution is normally one-seventh the volume of the collected blood, 63 ml for a 450 ml whole blood collection and 70 ml for 500 ml. This volume ratio has been a standard for more than 50 years and was used with the anticoagulant–nutrient solutions ACD-A, CPD, and CPDA-1. There has long been a question of whether the first few drops of blood to enter the collection system are injured by their sudden immersion in the acid anticoagulant, but the red cells seem to tolerate this process with minimal hemolysis or loss of viability.[60,61] At the end of collection, venous blood with a pH of about 7.35 has been mixed with anticoagulant–nutrient solution with a pH of 5.0–5.6, with a resulting pH of about 7.05 in the mixture. The high buffer capacity of the hemoglobin molecule limits the effects of the acidic primary collection solution.

Whole blood in anticoagulant–nutrient solution was licensed for storage for three or five weeks, but has now been largely replaced by separately stored blood components. Making components from whole blood not only serves more patients but also improves the storage of the individual blood elements. Red cells are best stored cold, platelets at room temperature, and plasma frozen. Removing the white blood cells (WBCs) also improves RBC storage by removing a cell population with high-energy requirements and potential for damaging red cells by released enzymes.[62]

Schemes for separating whole blood into components are based on centrifugation. The standard "platelet-rich plasma" method used in the United States involves performing a low-speed "soft" spin to sediment the red cells against the pole of the bag opposite the connections to the satellite bags and then squeezing off the supernatant platelet-rich plasma from the top of the bag into the first satellite bag with pressure applied to the sides of the base of the bag. Thus, typically, 500 ml of whole blood with a hematocrit (Hct) of 42%, consisting of 210 ml of red cells and 290 ml of plasma, is collected into 70 ml of anticoagulant–nutrient solution increasing the volume in the bag to 570 ml and reducing the Hct to 36%. Removing most of the supernatant plasma will increase the Hct in the bag to 80–90%, consisting of the original 210 ml of red cells and the remaining 22–45 ml of plasma/anticoagulant–nutrient solution mixture. Of the original 290 ml of plasma and 70 ml of anticoagulant–nutrient solution, about 90% is removed in this initial separation process. In Europe, an initial hard spin is generally preferred in order to harvest buffy coat for the production of platelets and increase the volume of the separated plasma. As noted above, the red cells do better if most of the plasma volume and anticoagulant–nutrient solution are replaced.

Recently, separation of whole blood into plasma and RBC by using a hollow-fiber filtration system has been described.[63] Red cell parameters were similar to those obtained when routine centrifugation methods were used, and the filter did not cause hemolysis. Levels of plasma factor VIII and factor XI were slightly reduced with this prototype; however, there was no evidence of activation of the coagulation or complement systems, and filters that do not interact with coagulation factors can be made.

Anticoagulant–nutrient solutions

Anticoagulant–nutrient solutions were developed from ACD to CPD to CPDA-1. This path is the result of the discovery of the

Table 9.1 Compositions and Properties of Some of the Common Acid Citrate Preservative Solutions

	ACD-A	ACD-B	CPD	CPDA-1	CP2D
Citric Acid	35	21	14	14	14
Sodium Citrate	97	58	116	117	117
Dextrose	136	81	141	142	284
Monosodium phosphate			15.8	16	16
Adenine				2	
pH	5.0		5.6	5.6	5.6
Volume ratio used (mL anticoagulant:mL blood)	1:7	1:4	1:7	1:7	1:7

ACD is acid–citrate–dextrose has two formulations (A and B); CPD is citrate–phosphate–dextrose; CPDA-1 is citrate-phosphate-dextrose, and adenine; a CPDA-2 was developed but never licensed. CP2D is CPD with double-dose dextrose. All concentrations are in mmoles/L.

Table 9.2 Compositions of the Common Licensed First-Generation RBC Additive Solutions

	SAG	SAG-M	AS-1	AS-3	AS-5
NaCL	150	150	154	70	154
Phosphate				23	
Adenine	1.25	1.25	2	2	2
Glucose	45	45	111	55	45
Mannitol		30	41.2		29
Citric Acid				2	
Na$_3$Citrate				30	

SAG is saline–adenine–glucose; SAG-M is saline–adenine–glucose–mannitol; AS-1 is a patented SAG-M variant formula sold as Adsol® by Fenwal; AS-3 is a patented formula sold as Nutracel® by Pall; and AS-5 is a patented SAG-M variant formula sold as Optisol® by Terumo, All concentrations are in mmoles/L.

critical nutrients for RBC during prolonged storage: dextrose, phosphate, and adenine. The recognition that RBC concentrates occasionally ran out of glucose led to development of CP2D, with twice the amount of glucose in CPD, and a never-licensed CPDA-2 with a third more glucose than CPDA-1.[64,65] The molar contents of the four licensed additive–nutrient solutions are shown in Table 9.1. Note that all of the anticoagulant–nutrient solutions are acidic, reducing the pH of the stored blood below 7.2 and leading to a burst of ATP production at the expense of the rapid depletion of 2,3-DPG as large amounts of 3-phosphoglycerate enter the glycolytic pathway.

The amounts of the nutrients in the additive nutrient solutions are critical depending on the intended storage times. There is enough glucose in whole blood to keep the red cells healthy for four days. Whole blood, stored in citrate alone for up to four days, was considered the safest form of storage before autoclavable solutions containing sugar were developed. The high glucose content of CP2D was necessary because it was first used with an additive solution that did not contain sufficient glucose, adenine–saline. Phosphate exists at 1–1.3 mmol/L in plasma, but it needs to be present at higher concentrations in the nutrient solution to prevent diffusive loss against the high concentrations in the red cells when 2,3-DPG breaks down. Adenine is only needed for storage beyond 3 weeks and is an ingredient of all of the additive solutions.

In emergencies in remote locations, it may be necessary to collect fresh whole blood before new supplies of fully tested components are available. Under these circumstances, drawing whole blood into the primary collection bag containing the anticoagulant–nutrient solution and holding the whole blood at room temperature for up to 24 hours is associated with good short-term preservation of function of the blood components.[66] The national blood services of Finland and Israel collect all of their whole blood on one day and process it on the next, holding it at 20 °C overnight in the anticoagulant–nutrient solution before separating it into components.[67,68] The Council of Europe Committee of Experts on Quality Assurance in Blood Transfusion Services has since 2005 advised that whole blood rapidly cooled after collection to 20–24 °C can keep at this temperature up to 24 hours after collection before separation into red blood cells, platelets, and plasma.[69] A large international study has examined the metabolic trade-offs involved in the warm overnight hold of whole blood before processing.[70] The warm hold did reduce the initial storage pH and lead to a burst of ATP synthesis, but the differences are lost in the larger individual donor differences by six weeks.

Additive solutions

First generation

The first widely used additive solution, SAG, represented an attempt to replace the volume and sugar lost with plasma removal and add the adenine necessary for storage beyond three weeks.[54] It was made with normal saline with 4.5% weight/volume glucose and 2 mmol/L of adenine. Stored RBC had good viability for five weeks but 1% hemolysis. In screening a large number of compounds for additives that would reduce the hemolysis, mannitol was identified as a compound that both reduced hemolysis and had an excellent safety record with intravenous (IV) infusion. The addition of 30 mmolar mannitol reduced hemolysis and increased the osmolarity of the solution further.[55] The solutions are made acidic to a pH of about 5.6 with hydrochloric acid to allow the glucose to be heat sterilized, but the solutions have essentially no buffer capacity so they do not make the RBC concentrates much more acidic than they were when separated from plasma. SAG-M and its close relatives, AS-1 and AS-5, are the most widely used additive solutions.

Other widely used first-generation additive solution systems include CP2D/AS-3 in the United States and CPD/MAP (mannitol, adenine, and phosphate) in Japan.[71] Table 9.2 provides a comparison of the ingredients and concentrations of the more common of these first-generation additive solutions.

Second generation

Second-generation additive solutions started with attempts to rebalance the final suspending solution and a search for additional nutrients for the packed RBC concentrates. BAGP was the result of the original attempt by Beutler to preserve both ATP and 2,3-DPG by raising the pH.[52] However, raising the pH substantially above 7.2 led to high concentrations of 2,3-DPG at the expense of ATP and no improvement in storage function. The composition of a representative group of second-generation additive solutions is shown in Table 9.3.

The pH of RBC during storage is very important. Above pH 7.2, the bifunctional enzyme diphosphoglycerate mutase–phosphatase converts almost all 1,3-DPG into 2,3-DPG, depriving the cell of new ATP.[27] Below a pH of about 6.4, the activities of the initial enzymes of glycolysis, hexosekinase and phosphofructokinase, are too low to support ATP production. In this narrow pH range between 7.2 and 6.4, hemoglobin, the mineral salts in the suspension, and bicarbonate all serve to buffer the protons produced by glycolysis. The approximately 60 g of hemoglobin present in a RBC can buffer about 8 mEq of protons in that pH range.[72] However, conventional

Table 9.3 Composition and Properties of Some of the Second-Generation RBC Additive Solutions

	BAGPM	PAGGS-M	PAGGG-M	ErythroSol-1	ErythroSol-2	AS-7
NaCL		72				
NaGluconate			72			
Bicarbonate	115					26
Phosphate	1	32	32	20	18	12
Adenine	1	2	2	1.5	1.3	2
Glucose	55	52	52	45	38	80
Mannitol	27	55	40	40	50	55
Guanosine		1.5	1.5			
Na$_3$Citrate				25	21	
pH of solution		6.3	6.3	7.4	8.8	8.4
pH of RBC suspension		6.9	6.9	7.2	7.3	7.2
Volume	100	110	110	114	150	110

BAGPM is bicarbonate–adenine–glucose–phosphate–mannitol, the original additive solution developed by Beutler; PAGGS-M, which is phosphate–adenine–glucose–guanosine–saline–mannitol, is licensed in Germany; PAGGG-M is phosphate–adenine–glucose–guanosine–(sodium) gluconate–mannitol, and it was developed by de Korte as a chloride-free variant of PAGGS-M; ErythroSol-1 and -2 were developed by Hogman; and AS-7 was developed by Hess and Greenwalt. All concentrations are in mmoles/L.

first-generation acidic additive solutions, which result in an initial pH of 7.0, fail to take advantage of a quarter of that pH range and buffer capacity. Adding 20 mmol/L of phosphate delivers 2 mmol in the 100 ml of additive solution and buffers about 1 mmol of additional protons. Adding 20 mmol/L of bicarbonate again delivers 2 mmol to the final RBC suspension, which will be protonated to make carbonic acid, converted to CO_2 and water by red cell carbonic anhydrase, and buffer 2 mmol of protons as the CO_2 diffuses out of the plastic bag. Attention to formulation and pH balance in the design of second-generation RBC additive solutions can almost double the amount of ATP energy available to stored red cells by depressing diphosphglycerate mutase activity while sustaining glycolysis.

Finding additional critical nutrients has been less successful. The only approved second-generation additive solutions are PAGGS-manitol and AS-7. In PAGGS-mannitol, the initials stand for phosphate, adenine, glucose, guanosine, and saline.[73] Guanosine was added because guanosine triphosphate was detected in red cells and known to decrease during storage. However, guanosine nucleotides play only a minimal role in critical events in RBC storage, inhibiting the primitive coagulation enzyme transglutaminase, and the solution worked only modestly better than first-generation additive solutions with a 74.6% 24-hour in vivo recovery after seven weeks in 10 units in the only published series.

As ingredients were added to advanced additive solutions, the salt concentration was generally reduced to maintain osmotic balance. Reducing the chloride concentration in the suspending solutions caused intracellular chloride to passively leave the red cells, but this can only occur if other anions countered the flow and phosphate, bicarbonate, and hydroxyl ions are the only available anions.[74] The influx of these anions initially increases the intracellular pH, but eventually the pH falls. PAGGG-M, in which the sodium chloride is replaced by sodium gluconate, is an example of an attempt to take advantage of the "chloride shift" phenomenon to maintain red cell 2,3-DPG.[75]

The ErythroSol solutions were developed based on the ideas of using the "chloride shift" to increase the intracellular pH while using a more alkaline final suspending solution and additional phosphate to simultaneously maintain ATP.[76] ErythroSol-1 used half-strength citrate (0.5 CPD) and had problems with incomplete anticoagulation in blood collected from donors with low (but acceptable) hematocrit levels. ErythroSol-2 used full-strength CPD and an alkaline additive solution made with disodium phosphate. In both systems, the glucose was placed in a separate bag from the

rest of the additive solution during manufacture and sterilization and only added at the time of RBC component production. The original description of ErythroSol-2 suggested that the optimal pH had been determined to preserve both ATP and 2,3-DPG.[77] However, subsequent work and evaluation of ErythroSol-4 as part of an international trial showed no differences in ATP and DPG content or hemolysis between it and SAG-M and PAGGG-M.[68]

The experimental additive solution-81 (EAS-81) has now been licensed in the United States and Europe as AS-7.[78] It was the end result of work that reexamined the use of bicarbonate as a buffer to prevent erythro-apoptosis by maintaining high concentrations of red cell ATP and limited hemolysis with mannitol and hypotonic conditions.[79] Formulating the solutions to get the starting pH as close as possible to 7.2 preserves the 2,3-DPG concentrations for two weeks.[80] The buffering provided by the bicarbonate allows RBC storage for at least eight weeks and excellent storage with recoveries of 88% at six weeks based on a very large study involving 54 recovery measurements (Figure 9.5).[81]

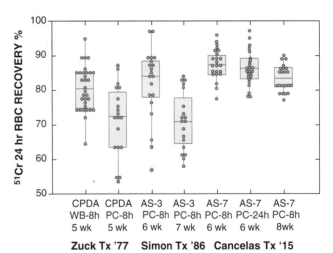

Figure 9.5 Chromium-51 autologous in vivo RBC recovery measures for RBC stored in successive generations of storage systems. CPDA-1 shows the decrease in mean recovery from whole blood stored at a hematocrit of 38% to packed cells with a hematocrit of 80%. AS-3 is a representative first-generation additive solution showing 84% mean recovery at 6 weeks but failure at 7 weeks. Bicarbonate buffered AS-7 allows better storage, storage for 8 weeks, and storage after warm overnight hold. See Refs.[53,64,80,81].

Finally, increasing the volume of these advanced additive solutions increases the buffering capacity and allows greater storage time. With 300 ml of additive solutions, Hess and his colleagues were able to achieve storage times of 10–12 weeks, but the higher volume and lower storage hematocrit probably make such solutions inappropriate for clinical use, especially in infants and massively transfused trauma patients.[82]

Additional factors influencing RBC quality

Temperature and time lapses during collection and component preparation

Whole blood is collected at body temperature and must be maintained at room temperature if platelets are to be prepared from the collection. By present US regulations, whole blood must be separated into its components in eight hours if platelets and fresh frozen plasma are to be manufactured. If only RBC and frozen plasma are to be made, the whole blood can be held on ice for up to 24 hours. The problems with holding blood at room temperature are twofold. Red cells metabolize glucose at higher rates when warm, producing more lactate and protons that reduce the pH and further slow metabolism[70] In addition, labile coagulation factors are lost. Attempts to validate the 24-hour warm hold for six-week RBC storage using first-generation additive solutions have not been successful, but in Israel and Finland, where this system is used, RBC are stored for only five weeks because of the efficiency of their national blood services and short supply lines.[83] AS-7 is now licensed in Europe for eight weeks of storage after an overnight hold.

As noted above, fresh whole blood is occasionally collected in emergencies on the battlefield or in isolated locations such as Pacific Island nations and stored at room temperature for short periods. Based on the above experience and experimental data, blood probably maintains reasonable functionality for 24–72 hours if maintained between 19 and 25 °C.[66] However, such use can only be recommended in the most urgent of situations.

Temperature and time lapses during storage

RBCs that have been allowed to rewarm to greater than 10 °C during storage are considered unfit for transfusion and are destroyed by FDA regulation. This has led to the wide use of the "30-minute rule," meaning that units are discarded if they have been off ice for more than 30 minutes. Experimental work has shown that glucose is metabolized about 10 times as fast at 25 °C as at 4 °C and that RBCs stored at 25 °C lose viability 10 times as fast so that a day of storage at room temperature would reduce the in vivo recovery equivalent to 10 days of 4 °C storage.[84,85] Thus, the regulation is very conservative with regard to temperature effects on metabolism, but it is also intended to prevent bacterial overgrowth in contaminated units.

Storage containers

Polyvinyl chloride (PVC) bags plasticized with DEHP are the standard RBC storage containers. The presence of DEHP reduces hemolysis by fourfold during storage by intercalating into the red cell membrane.[86] Other plasticizers, such as butyryl-n-trihexyl citrate, work almost as well, but they are more expensive (~5% more for a multibag set with leukocyte filter) and have an unusual smell when initially unwrapped.

Although questions about the safety of DEHP have been raised, they are based on very limited animal testing and must be balanced against the obvious safety value of being able to visually inspect the contents of blood bags and reduce RBC losses by extending shelf life. The general trend in Europe to avoid the slowly degradeable plasticizer, DEHP, has resulted in the introduction of butyryl-n-trihexyl citrate plasticized multibag systems in Sweden, Spain, and Norway, but the use of PVC bags with DEHP remains prevalent in Europe and almost universal in the rest of the world.

Leukocyte reduction

Leukocyte reduction improves RBC storage by removing a highly metabolically active blood component that would make the bag more acidic sooner. WBCs also secrete cytokines, and when they die after exposure to the cold, they release proteolytic, glycolytic, and lipolytic enzymes that damage the red cell surface. On the other hand, some red cells are damaged and many red cells are lost in the leukocyte reduction filters (typically, 15–35 ml of blood is lost in the filters depending on its size and whether whole blood or concentrated red cells are being leukoreduced). Red cells from donors with sickle cell trait may also clog filters. Leukocyte reduction improves the red cell 24-hour in vivo recovery by several percent according to the best estimates.[60] (See also Chapter 24.)

Washing

Washing RBC in saline to remove the plasma causes small losses of red cells in the bag transfers as well as loss of the supporting nutrients, glucose, phosphate, and adenine. Because the cells are used soon after washing, generally within 6–24 hours, only the glucose loss is physiologically important. There is still a small amount of glucose inside the washed RBCs, but it is metabolized quickly, especially if they are not promptly refrigerated. In the absence of glucose, metabolism stops and the cells are very susceptible to oxidative stress and erythro-apoptotic changes.

Irradiation

During storage at 4 °C, red cells lose potassium. This potassium collects in the supernatant fluid in the closed storage bag at a rate of about 1 mEq/day until equilibrium is reached between intra- and extracellular concentrations, usually at about 60–70 mEq/L depending on the storage hematocrit (Table 9.4). Gamma irradiation in doses of 2500 cGy, given to prevent graft-versus-host disease, damages the red cell membranes and increases this rate of potassium loss to approximately 1.5 mEq/day; however, the reinfused red cells have normal in vivo survival.[87] The current FDA regulation that irradiated RBC expire 28 days after irradiation limits the potential maximum potassium concentration by limiting the period of potassium loss. Nevertheless, care must be taken in all situations when large volumes of older, high-potassium RBC are used to prime cardiopulmonary bypass, dialysis, or apheresis circuits or infused into the central circulation and then administered at high flow rates.

Table 9.4 Effect of Storage Duration of Characteristics of RBC Concentrates in AS-1

	35-day	42-day	49-day	56-day
	(n = 25)	(n = 10)	(n = 10)	(n = 10)
% recovery	86	82	76	71
% hemolysis	0.28	0.32	0.51	0.68
ATP μM/g Hb	3.1	2.7	2.3	2.3
[K+] meq/L in plasma	45	50	52	60

Unpublished data obtained from the US FDA under the Freedom of Information Act.

Pathogen reduction

Pathogen reduction systems developed so far require additional manipulation of and stresses on the stored RBCs that are system specific. Examples from two such proposed systems are as follows. Diethyleneamine (DEA) was proposed as a red cell–permeable nucleic acid crosslinker with broad pathogen killing potential and minimal direct red cell toxicity. However, the system required exposure of the RBCs to DEA for 20 hours at room temperature and extensive secondary washing to reduce the remaining amounts of this carcinogenic chemical. When the time- and temperature-related decrease in RBC pH was added to the effects of washing the RBC with large volumes of acidic solutions and storing them in an acidic additive solution, red cell recovery suffered.[88] Riboflavin, a photoactive oxidizer, has also been proposed as a highly red cell–permeable molecule for pathogen reduction in conjunction with UV light. However, RBCs are so optically dense that the units must be diluted and transferred to large bags only a few millimeters thick for photo-treatment, and the photo-treatment must be done above a critical temperature. The bag transfers all involve losses of red cells, the choice of diluent fluid is important, and the hemoglobin and other optically active molecules in the red cells are also damaged by the light exposure. The red cells need additional energy to attempt to correct the damage. Finally, the reconcentrated treated RBCs need to be stored in an additive solution that is balanced to maximize their lifespan. (See also Chapter 56.)

Rejuvenation

Red cell loss of viability during storage is different than red cell senescence in the body. In the body, red cells undergo cumulative oxidative damage that leads to reduced enzyme activities and cross-linking of cytoskeletal components. These are essentially irreversible processes and are ultimately associated with macrophage clearance of old red cells possibly mediated by phosphatidyl serine exposure or neoantigen formation. The changes that lead to loss of viability during storage are largely reversible by a process called *rejuvenation*. Hogman showed that rejuvenating red cells at the end of six weeks of storage in SAG-M increased their 24-hour in vivo recovery from 77 to 89%.[89]

This rejuvenation is a strictly metabolic recharging of red cells at the end of their storage period. Such cells have a low pH as well as low ATP and 2,3-DPG concentrations. They can be rejuvenated by incubation in a high-pH solution of phosphate, inosine, pyruvate, and adenine (PIPA, Rejuvesol®, Cytosol Labs, Braintree, MA) for 2 hours. Such incubation increases their ATP and 2,3-DPG concentrations and increases their in vivo recovery, probably by allowing them to internalize negatively charged membrane phospholipids that would otherwise signal clearance by macrophages. Return of the normal distribution of phospholipids also prevents red cells from participating in plasma coagulation reactions. Rejuvenation does not reverse the oxidative damage to band 3 of the cell membrane, desialation of glycoproteins, or loss of membrane. However, the fact that RBCs can be rejuvenated at the end of storage by increasing their pH and ATP suggests that improved storage could be achieved by a method designed to maintain pH and ATP. This is the fundamental idea behind second-generation additive solutions.

Frozen storage of RBCs

RBCs can be frozen, and in the frozen state they are stable for long periods. Valeri has reported on RBCs stored for 37 years.[90] Four methods of freezing RBCs have been extensively tested, two

have been developed for practical use, and one remains in common use.[91]

During red cell freezing, water turns to ice and the salt concentration of the remaining intracellular water increases, drawing in more water and expanding the cell. Under normal circumstances, this leads to cell rupture. Rupture can be prevented by freezing the cells so rapidly that water does not have time to enter, or by diluting the total cellular water with a cryoprotectant so that not enough water enters to rupture the cell. Although several cryoprotectants can work, glycerol is the standard material used because of its cost and safety. The two systems for RBC cryopreservation that have been developed for clinical use both use glycerol. One system used a "low" glycerol concentration of about 20% and rapid cooling by plunge freezing in liquid nitrogen; the other uses a "high" glycerol concentration of about 40% and slow cooling in −80 °C freezers. The low-glycerol frozen RBCs must be maintained in the vapor phase of liquid nitrogen, whereas the high-glycerol frozen RBCs are stable at temperatures below −65 °C. The high cost of maintaining liquid nitrogen freezers and the difficulty of transporting products frozen in liquid nitrogen both limit the utility of the low-glycerol system. High-glycerol frozen RBCs can be transported on dry ice. When the RBCs are thawed, the glycerol must be removed promptly to prevent it from poisoning the red cell metabolism and to protect the recipient as the glycerol-loaded red cells would swell and rupture if placed directly into the bloodstream. Thus, once thawed, the RBCs must be deglycerolized by washing in a set of graded salt solutions. In the past, the glycerolization and deglycerolization of RBC for freezing were open manual processes, so the thawed RBCs had to be used within 24 hours or discarded.

The recent partial automation of a closed system for glycerolizing and deglycerolizing RBCs now allows them to be kept post thaw in the liquid state for two weeks.[75] RBCs collected in any of the standard licensed systems can be frozen up to six days after collection and stored for up to 10 years. The deglycerolized RBCs are then stored in AS-3. Net losses of red cells in the freeze–thaw–wash process are of the order of 5–15%, and the 24-hour in vivo recovery of infused red cells is about 78% after two weeks.[92] Frozen RBCs entail substantial costs for processing and storage, probably four times that of a standard liquid unit, so only for the rarest blood units is there an advantage for frozen inventory.

Other systems of freezing and freeze-drying have been demonstrated, but are associated with greater than 1% hemolysis and so would require a washing step before administration. This limitation prevents their use in emergency medicine, and they are too costly and labor intensive to compete with glycerol frozen RBCs.[90]

Oxygen delivery

RBCs have many functions, but the most important are bulk oxygen transport and microvascular perfusion for the delivery of oxygen and removal of CO_2. There is evidence that RBC metabolism and storage lesions affect both of these aspects of oxygen delivery. Bulk oxygen transport involves the loading of oxygen onto RBC hemoglobin in the lungs and its distribution to the arterioles of critical organs, including the heart, brain, liver, kidneys, gut, and skeletal muscle. Bulk oxygen transport also depends on RBCs being dense, flexible discs that flow in the middle of the bloodstream surrounded by poorly oxygen-soluble plasma that limits premature oxygen off-loading. Loss of RBC density through swelling, their flexibility through membrane loss, and their ability to slide smoothly back and forth over each other because of shape change have been discussed previously. Each of these storage lesions reduces the effectiveness of the laminar flow mechanism and increases the diffusive loss of arterial oxygen to nearby veins, creating *shunt*. The neural and endocrine mechanisms that maintain blood volume, pressure, and pulsatile flow are numerous and generally beyond the scope of this chapter. However, the heart is the critical organ first affected by limitation of bulk oxygen delivery. Oxygen extraction in the left ventricle is typically 70% at rest, twice that of the brain, making coronary artery vasodilation, increased heart muscle perfusion, and increased oxygen extraction the primary mechanisms by which the heart adapts to an increasing workload. The first two of these response mechanisms are primarily driven by adrenergic activity, and the RBCs have adrenergic receptors whose stimulation appears to reduce RBC aggregation and increase deformability.[93] These adrenergic pathways require ATP and GTP. Effects of RBC storage on RBC bulk viscosity have been described, and the restoration of stored RBC ATP content through "rejuvenation" largely restores bulk viscosity to prestorage levels.[94] All this suggests that maintaining RBC energetics during storage to maintain ATP and GTP concentrations to limit membrane loss and change will have the greatest effects on bulk oxygen transport.

Since the discovery of the effect of 2,3-DPG on the oxygen affinity of hemoglobin, it has been common to discuss the oxygen delivery functionality of stored RBCs in terms of their 2,3-DPG content. This is an oversimplification for several reasons. Firstly, although it is clear that low 2,3-DPG can reduce oxygen delivery in animal models by as much as 12% at the critical point where low hemoglobin concentrations make oxygen delivery flow dependent, these concentrations are well below standard transfusion triggers.[95] Secondly, 2,3-DPG works in red cells by binding and stabilizing deoxyhemoglobin. This moves the base of the oxy-hemoglobin dissociation curve to the right and increases the P50, but most oxygen transport occurs at the top of the binding curve and is relatively unaffected by DPG concentrations, as the arterial PO2 is much higher than the P50. However, 2,3-DPG plays an important role in red cell membrane oxygen transport and cytoskeleton architecture because of its interaction with attachment points between the cell membrane and the cytoskeleton, and the interaction of deoxyhemoglobin with band 3. These interactions, the critical importance of oxygen transport, and the retrospective data that suggest an association between adverse patient outcomes and increased storage time of banked RBCs drive continuing efforts to reduce 2,3-DPG depletion during storage with modern additive solutions. Until that is achieved, it has been recommended in Norway to use RBCs in SAGM, not older than 10 days, for the transfusion of intensive care ward patients.

However, the retrospective data suggesting that stored RBCs are dangerous are highly suspect. Such data are generally confounded by the common situations that sicker patients receive more transfused blood, sicker patients die at increased frequencies, and patients who receive more blood have a higher chance of receiving older blood.[96] Specifically, the study most frequently quoted to suggest that longer stored RBC units affect the outcome in cardiac surgery[97] is deeply flawed, with the excess numbers of patients receiving seven or more units in the arm receiving >14-day stored RBCs accounting for more than 60% of the excess mortality. There are now three large randomized trials, ARIPI, RECESS, and ABLE,[98] showing no effect of prolonged RBC storage on mortality in

neonates, repeat cardiac surgery patients, or critically injured patients, respectively. This is in spite of the fact that 15–25% of the old red cells are removed from the circulation by the reticuloenthelial system within 24 hours after transfusion. Cells age in storage, but the storage changes seem compensated in vivo by still poorly defined mechanisms.

At the microvascular level, oxygen delivery is maximized by increasing capillary density and perfusion and limiting shunting. These processes are controlled in large part by endothelial cells, and more than a dozen mechanisms are involved with intermediates as diverse as the respiratory gases O_2 and CO_2, nitric oxide, proteins like the endothelins, and lipid endoperoxides such as leukotrienes. Endothelial cells have the mitochondrial-derived energy, synthetic capability, and connections to provide the feedback between tissue oxygen tensions and end-arteriole sphincters that control capillary perfusion. Here, the connections between RBC deformability and secretory capacity appear most strongly connected to oxygen delivery. Probably most important for the microvascular flow of transfused RBCs is the loss of membrane, cell deformability, and ATP secretion that occurs with storage. Direct observation of the flow characteristics of fresh, stored, and stored rejuvenated RBCs suggests that ATP secretion in response to increased shear, by which red cells dilate small vessels to maintain their forward flow, is most important.[99] Membrane deformability, which is regulated by the ATP-modulated cytoskeleton, is also important for the passage of red cells through capillaries that are half their diameter. Maintaining high ATP concentrations is therefore again a critical function of modern additive solutions. Shear stress also regulates endothelial NO production, and increased shear stress by old rigid red cells could therefore have a positive influence on microvascular flow of old blood.

Validation of RBC quality and in vivo recovery

RBC storage systems have historically been validated by demonstrating that the stored cells do not hemolyze during storage and that they circulate normally after reinfusion. Measures of normal circulation have included increments in recipient hemoglobin, and determining the recovery and in vivo half life of the transfused red cells. Transfused red cells have been counted using differential agglutination, radioactive tracer labeling, and flow-cytometric differential counting.[100]

Chromium-51 labeling has been the standard method used in the United States for 50 years. There is a published standard method, but only a handful of laboratories perform the measurement, and a recent attempt to gather a decade's experience identified only 900 measurements.[56] Chromium-51 labeling persists in the United States because it is the only validated method compatible with autologous red cell reinfusion, and the infectious disease risks of allogeneic RBCs are considered unacceptable for storage system development work. The methods of red cell labeling have been the subject of an excellent review.[101]

When performing chromium-51 labeling, it is important to recognize that red cells from different donors may have very different 24-hour in vivo recovery values. In a typical study of a modern additive solution with an 84% mean recovery, individual units of donor RBCs have recoveries as high as 95% and as low as 65%.[62] These differences in viability correlate with differences in the red cell ATP concentrations, but poorly ($r^2 = .4$).

There have been attempts to measure the functionality of red cells, as opposed to their survival. Presumably, the functionality of red cells is related to their ability to deliver oxygen to tissues and to flow in the microcirculation. However, none of the red cells' rigidity or microcirculatory flow measures is widely available or validated. The level of 2,3-DPG is just a surrogate marker for red cell function and is limited by the difficulty of performing the test. In a recent shared sample exercise, 12 of the world's premier labs could not consistently measure 2,3-DPG.[102]

Finally, in countries that do not perform chromium-51 recovery measures, there has been a trend to using the ATP concentration as a red cell quality measure. Although the ATP is a poor surrogate for recovery in small clinical trials, its central role in the inhibition of erythro-apoptosis probably gives it special importance. Unfortunately, the measure is not very reproducible from laboratory to laboratory, so a wide margin of safety is required.[102]

Summary

RBC storage systems work remarkably well, making red cells for transfusion available, safe, effective, and cheap for the populations who can organize effective national blood systems. They are a product of slow and empiric development, and our present systems do not reflect our current understanding. They can be expected to improve in the future.

Key references

A full reference list for this chapter is available at: http://www.wiley.com/go/simon/transfusion

3 D'Alessandro A, Kriebardis AG, Rinalducci S, *et al*. An update on red blood cell storage lesions, as gleaned through biochemistry and omics technologies. *Transfusion* 2015;**55**:205–19.

8 De Rosa MC, Alinovi CC, Galtieri A, *et al*. The plasma membrane of erythrocytes plays a fundamental role in the transport of oxygen, carbon dioxide and nitric oxide and in the maintenance of the reduced state of the heme iron. *Gene* 2007;**398**:162–71.

9 Bruce LJ, Beckmann R, Ribeiro ML, *et al*. A band 3-based macrocomplex of intergral and peripheral proteins in the RBC membrane. *Blood* 2003; **101**:4180–8.

34 Lang F, Lang E, Föller M. Physiology and pathophysiology of eryptosis. *Transfus Med Hemother* 2012 Oct; **39**(5):308–14.

57 Hogman CF, Hedlund K, Sahlestrom Y. Red cell preservation in protein-poor media: III. Protection against in vitro hemolysis. *Vox Sang* 1981;**41**:274–81.

80 Cancelas JA, Dumont LJ, Maes LA, *et al*. Additive solution-7 (AS-7) reduces the red blood cell cold-storage lesion. *Transfusion* 2015 Mar; **55**(3):491–8.

81 Dumont LJ, Cancelas JA, Maes LA, *et al*. Overnight,room-temperature hold of whole blood followed by 42-day storage of RBCs in additive solution-7. *Transfusion* 2015 Mar; **55**(3):485–90.

91 Hess JR. RBC Freezing and its impact on the supply chain. *Transfusion Med* 2004;**14**:1–8.

93 Muravyov A, Tikhomirova I. Signaling pathways regulating red blood cell aggregation. *Biorheology* 2014;**51**:135–45.

99 Raat NJ, Hilarius PM, Johannes T, *et al*. Rejuvenation of stored human red blood cells reverses the renal microvascular oxygenation deficit in an isovolemic transfusion model in rats. *Transfusion* 2009 Mar; **49**:427–4.

102 Hess JR. Measures of stored red blood cell quality. *Vox Sang* 2014;**107**:1–6.

CHAPTER 10

Anemia and red blood cell transfusion

Jeffrey L. Carson[1] & Paul Hébert[2]

[1]Division of General Internal Medicine, Rutgers Robert Wood Johnson Medical School, Rutgers Biomedical Health Sciences, Rutgers University, New Brunswick, NJ, USA
[2]Centre Hospitalier de L'Université de Montréal (CHUM), University of Montreal, Montreal, Canada

Introduction

Red cell transfusion is an extremely common medical intervention. In the United States, more than 16 million red blood cell (RBC) units are transfused annually to 3.4 million patients.[1] Worldwide, 85 million units of blood are collected per year.[2] In Northern England, about 50% of units are given to medical patients, and 40% to surgical patients; hip replacement and coronary artery bypass graft (CABG) surgery were the most common surgical indications.[3] RBC units are also frequently administered to critically ill patients, as a supportive therapy to patients receiving chemotherapy and marrow transplants, and to patients with blood loss from medical conditions such as gastrointestinal bleeding.[4] Approximately 25% of all red cells transfused are given to patients with a primary diagnosis of cardiac disease,[5] and 8% of all cardiology admissions are transfused RBCs.[6] In recent years, blood use is declining as clinicians adopt a more restrictive approach to transfusion.[7] The latest estimates of the cost of a RBC unit range from $522 to $1183 (mean, $761 ± $294).[8]

This chapter reviews the current knowledge about red cell transfusion and the risk posed by anemia. This overview summarizes preclinical, observational data but emphasizes randomized clinical trials. Guidelines on transfusion practices are examined. The first three sections are based on systematic reviews of the literature. The fourth section describes an approach to decision making in red cell transfusion that is occasionally evidence based, but frequently based on the authors' views.

Adaptive mechanisms in anemia

In anemia, oxygen-carrying capacity decreases, but tissue oxygenation is preserved at hemoglobin levels well below 10 g/dL (Table 10.1). After the development of anemia, adaptive changes include a shift in the oxyhemoglobin dissociation curve, hemodynamic alterations, and microcirculatory alterations. The shift to the right of the oxyhemoglobin dissociation curve in anemia is primarily the result of increased synthesis of 2,3-diphosphoglycerate (2,3-DPG) in red cells.[9–11] This rightward shift enables more oxygen to be released to the tissues at a given PO_2, offsetting the effect of reduced oxygen-carrying capacity of the blood. In vitro studies have shown rightward shifts in the oxyhemoglobin dissociation curve with increases in temperature and decreases in pH.[12] Although clinically important shifts have been documented in a number of studies, hemoglobin oxygen saturation generally is measured in arterial specimens processed at standard temperature and pH. Therefore, current measurement techniques do not reflect oxygen-binding affinity or unloading conditions in the patient's microcirculatory environment, which may be affected by temperature, pH, and a number of disease processes. The shift in the oxyhemoglobin dissociation curve caused by decreases in pH (increase in hydrogen ion concentration) is the Bohr effect.[13] Because changes in pH rapidly affect the ability of hemoglobin to bind oxygen, this mechanism has been postulated to be an important early adaptive response to anemia.[14] However, the equations describing the physical process indicate that a very large change in pH is needed to modify the partial pressure of oxygen at which hemoglobin is 50% saturated with oxygen (P_{50}) by a clinically important amount (~10 mm Hg). As a result, the Bohr effect is unlikely to have significant clinical consequences.[12]

Several hemodynamic alterations occur after the development of anemia. The most important determinant of cardiovascular response is the patient's volume status, or more specifically left ventricular preload. The combined effect of hypovolemia and anemia often occurs as a result of acute blood loss. Acute anemia can cause tissue hypoxia or anoxia through both diminished cardiac output (stagnant hypoxia) and decreased oxygen-carrying capacity (anemic hypoxia).[15] The body primarily attempts to preserve oxygen delivery to vital organs by compensatory increases in myocardial contractility and heart rate as well as increased arterial and venous vascular tone mediated through increased sympathetic discharge. In addition, a variety of mechanisms redistribute organ blood flow. The adrenergic system plays an important role in altering blood flow to and within specific organs. The renin–angiotensin–aldosterone system is stimulated to retain both water and sodium. Losses ranging from 5% to 15% in blood volume result in variable increases in resting heart rate and diastolic blood pressure. Orthostatic hypotension often is a sensitive indicator of relatively small losses in blood volume not sufficient to cause a marked decrease in blood pressure. Larger losses result in progressive increases in heart rate and decreases in arterial blood pressure accompanied by evidence of organ hypoperfusion. The increased sympathetic tone diverts an ever decreasing global blood flow (cardiac output) away from the splanchnic, skeletal, and cutaneous circulation toward the coronary and cerebral circulation. Once vital organ systems such as the kidneys, the central nervous system, and the heart are affected, the patient is considered in hypovolemic shock. Although the American College of Surgeons Committee on Trauma[16] has categorized the cardiovascular and systemic response

Rossi's Principles of Transfusion Medicine, Fifth Edition. Edited by Toby L. Simon, Jeffrey McCullough, Edward L. Snyder, Bjarte G. Solheim, and Ronald G. Strauss.
© 2016 John Wiley & Sons, Ltd. Published 2016 by John Wiley & Sons, Ltd.

Table 10.1 Physiologic changes associated with normovolemic anemia

Oxyhemoglobin Dissociation Curve
- Oxyhemoglobin curve shifted to the right because of increased 2,3-biphosphoglycerate levels.
- Rightward shift in the oxyhemoglobin curve is not a result of the Bohr effect in patients.
- The shift in the oxyhemoglobin curve has been clearly established in many forms of anemia (excluding hemoglobinopathies).
- Shift in the oxyhemoglobin curve has been clearly established in a number of human diseases.

Hemodynamic Alteration
- Changes in blood viscosity result in many of the hemodynamic changes.
- Increased sympathetic activity.
- Increased myocardial contractility.
- Decrease in systemic vascular resistance.
- Redistribution of cardiac output toward the heart and brain and away from the splanchnic circulation.
- Maximal global oxygen delivery occurs at hemoglobin values of 10–11 g/dL.
- Global oxygen delivery declines above and below hemoglobin values of 10–16 g/dL.

Cardiac Output
- Cardiac output increases with increasing degrees of anemia.
- Increased cardiac output is a result of increased stroke volume.
- The contribution of increased heart rate to the increase in cardiac output is variable.

Coronary and Cerebral Blood Flow
- Coronary and cerebral blood flow is increased.
- Coronary artery disease in the presence of moderate degrees of anemia (hemoglobin values below 9 g/dL) results in impaired left ventricular contractility or ischemia.
- Moderate anemia does not aggravate cerebral ischemia in patients with cerebrovascular disease.

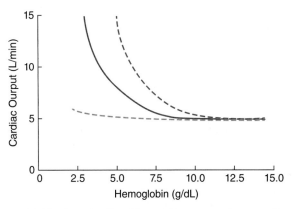

Figure 10.1 The theoretic effect of hemoglobin concentration on cardiac output. The curves illustrate how cardiac output increases as hemoglobin concentration decreases. The solid curve is meant to describe the increase in a healthy adult. The dashed line on the top shows how the cardiac output response can be accentuated in a young athlete, and the lower dashed line might correspond to someone with poor cardiovascular function.

to acute blood loss according to degree of blood loss, many of these responses are modified by the rapidity of blood loss and patient characteristics, such as age, coexisting illnesses, preexisting volume status, hemoglobin value, and the use of medications having cardiac effects (β-blockers) or peripheral vascular effects (antihypertensives).

The compensatory changes in cardiac output most thoroughly studied are the cardiovascular consequence of normovolemic anemia. When intravascular volume is stable or high after the development of anemia (as opposed to hypovolemic anemia and shock), increases in cardiac output have been consistently reported. Indeed, an inverse relationship between hemoglobin level (or hematocrit) and cardiac output has been clearly established in well-controlled laboratory studies (Figure 10.1).[17–19] Similar clinical observations have been made in the perioperative setting[20] and for chronic anemia.[18] Unfortunately, the strength of inferences from clinical studies is limited by confounding factors arising from major coexisting illnesses such as cardiac disease, a lack of appropriate control patients, and significant weaknesses in study design. Researchers have attempted to determine the level of anemia at which cardiac output begins to rise. Reported thresholds for this phenomenon identified in primary clinical and laboratory studies have ranged from 7 to 12 g/dL of hemoglobin.[18] Two major mechanisms are thought to be responsible for the physiologic processes underlying increased cardiac output during normovolemic anemia: (1) reduced blood viscosity and (2) increased sympathetic stimulation of the cardiovascular effectors.[21] Blood viscosity affects both preload and afterload, two major determinants of cardiac output,[21–23] whereas sympathetic stimulation primarily increases the two other determinants, heart rate and contractility. Unlike the situation for hypovolemic anemia, in this setting the effects of blood viscosity appear to predominate.[22,23]

Complex interactions exist among blood flow, blood viscosity, and cardiac output. In vessels, blood flow alters whole blood viscosity, and blood viscosity modulates cardiac output. Under experimental conditions in a rigid hollow cylinder, blood flow is directly related to the fourth power of the diameter and to driving pressure. It is inversely related to the length of the vessel and to blood viscosity (Poiseuille–Hagen law).[21,24] Also, blood viscosity increases as flow decreases because of increasing aggregation of red cells. Thus, viscosity is highest in postcapillary venules, where flow is the lowest, and viscosity is lowest in the aorta, where flow is the highest. In postcapillary venules, there is a disproportionate decrease in blood viscosity as anemia worsens, consequently augmenting venous return at a given venous pressure. If cardiac function is normal, the increase in venous return or left ventricular preload is the most important determinant of increased cardiac output during normovolemic anemia. The conclusion is based on experiments in which viscosity was maintained during anemia by means of high-viscosity colloidal solutions. In such studies, the cardiovascular effects of hemodilution were attenuated[22] compared with similar levels of hemodilution accompanied by reduced whole blood viscosity. Decreased left ventricular afterload, another cardiac consequence of decreased blood viscosity, also may be an important mechanism for the increase in cardiac output as anemia worsens.[22]

Sympathetic stimulation can result in increased cardiac output through enhanced myocardial contractility[25] and increased venomotor tone.[26,27] The effects of anemia on left ventricular contractility in isolation have not been clearly determined, given the complex changes in preload, afterload, and heart rate. Only one before-and-after hemodilution study was performed with load-independent measures to document increased left ventricular contractility.[25] Chapler and Cain[26] summarized several well-controlled animal studies indicating that venomotor tone increases as a result of stimulation of the aortic chemoreceptors. If sympathetic stimulation is significant in the specific clinical setting, contractility is increased from stimulation of the β-adrenergic receptors.[21,28]

The inverse relationship between cardiac output and hemoglobin level has led investigators to attempt to determine the hemoglobin level that maximizes oxygen transport. Richardson and Guyton[29] evaluated the effects of hematocrit on cardiac performance in a canine model. They established that optimal oxygen transport occurred between hematocrits of 40% and 60%. Others determined maximum oxygen delivery to be in the lower end of the range, at a hematocrit of 40–45% (hemoglobin 13–15 g/dL).[30,31] However, in one of the most widely quoted studies addressing this topic,[32] investigators found peak oxygen transport to occur at a hematocrit of 30% (hemoglobin concentration, 10 g/dL). Unfortunately, global indices of optimal oxygen delivery mask any differences in blood flow between specific organs.[33,34] In addition, attempting to identify a single optimal hemoglobin concentration that maximizes oxygen delivery neglects the large number of factors interfering with adaptive mechanisms during management of patients other than healthy, young patients with anemia.

Will the transfusion of allogeneic RBCs reverse any adaptive response to acute or chronic normovolemic anemia? Assuming that oxygen-carrying capacity is not impaired during storage and that hematocrit is restored after a transfusion, the cardiovascular consequences will be reversed. However, the storage process alters the properties of red cells. These alterations may impair flow and oxygen release from hemoglobin.[10]

Microcirculatory effects of anemia and red cell transfusion

At the level of the microcirculation, three putative adaptive mechanisms increase the amount of oxygen supplied to tissues by capillary networks. In a model of the microcirculation proposed by Krogh,[35] oxygen supply to the tissues is enhanced through recruitment of previously closed capillaries, increased capillary flow, and increased oxygen extraction from existing capillaries. The degree of anemia, the specific tissue bed, and a variety of disease processes affect microcirculatory blood flow and oxygen supply.[24,36] As the degree of hemodilution becomes more pronounced and hematocrit decreases, blood viscosity decreases disproportionately in capillary networks. This occurs because the hematocrit is highest in the capillary network; as a consequence, there is a larger decrease in capillary viscosity.

Stored red cells have properties that differ from those of their in vivo counterparts; many are related to the duration of storage (see Chapter 9). Characteristically, older RBC units have lower levels of 2,3-DPG. The result is a leftward shift in the oxyhemoglobin dissociation curve, which can impede delivery of oxygen to the tissues.[14] In addition, storage of red cells decreases the deformability of their membrane.[37] As a consequence, stored red cells may impede flow in the microcirculation[38] and may have limited ability to release oxygen to tissues. However, these storage lesions are reversible within 24–48 hours.[39]

There are reports[40] suggesting that disease processes such as sepsis impair red cell deformability. In conjunction with significant systemic microcirculatory dysfunction, the decrease in red cell deformability may dramatically affect tissue oxygen delivery in sepsis and septic shock.[40] This body of evidence suggests that RBC transfusions increase systemic oxygen delivery but may have adverse effects on microcirculatory flow.

Interaction between pathophysiologic processes and anemia

Several disease processes affecting either the entire body or specific organs potentially limit adaptive responses and make patients more vulnerable to the effects of anemia. Specifically, heart, lung, and cerebrovascular diseases have been proposed to increase the risk of adverse consequences of anemia. Age, severity of illness, and therapeutic interventions also may affect adaptive mechanisms.

The heart, specifically the left ventricle, is particularly prone to adverse consequences of anemia. This is because the myocardium consumes 60% to 75% (extraction ratio) of all oxygen delivered by the coronary circulation.[30,33,41] Such a high extraction ratio is unique to the coronary circulation. As a result, oxygen delivery to the myocardium can increase substantially only with an increase in blood flow.[42] In addition, most left ventricular perfusion is restricted to the diastolic period, because pressures inside the left ventricle are too high to allow adequate coronary blood flow during systole. Thus, any shortening of its duration (e.g., tachycardia) decreases blood flow. Laboratory studies have been performed to investigate the effects of normovolemic anemia on the coronary circulation.[31,41,43] There appear to be minimal consequences of anemia with hemoglobin levels in the range of 7 g/dL if the coronary circulation is normal.[19,25] However, myocardial dysfunction and ischemia either occur earlier or are greater in anemic animal models with moderate- to high-grade coronary stenosis compared with controls with normal hemoglobin values.[44]

Data from studies with human subjects are inconsistent. Several clinical studies involving patients with coronary artery disease undergoing normovolemic hemodilution have not shown any increase in cardiac complications or silent ischemia during electrocardiographic monitoring.[45] In addition, a retrospective analysis involving 224 patients undergoing CABG surgery did not show a significant association between hemoglobin level and coronary sinus lactate level (an indicator of myocardial ischemia).[46] However, in two recent cohort studies, moderate anemia was poorly tolerated by perioperative[47] and critically ill patients[48] with cardiovascular disease. Thus, retrospective studies seem to support preclinical reports. It is also plausible that anemia results in considerable increases in morbidity and mortality among patients with other cardiac diseases, including heart failure and valvular heart disease, presumably because of the greater burden of the adaptive increase in cardiac output.

During normovolemic anemia, cerebral blood flow increases as hemoglobin values decrease. Investigators have observed increases ranging from 50% to 500% of baseline value in laboratory studies[49] and in one study with human subjects.[50] Cerebral blood flow increases because of overall increases in cardiac output, which is preferentially diverted to the cerebral circulation. As oxygen delivery begins to decrease, cerebral tissues are able to increase the amount of oxygen extracted from blood. A number of factors, including degree of hemodilution, type of fluid used for volume expansion, volume status (preload), and extent of cerebrovascular disease, are capable of potentially modifying global or regional cerebral blood flow during anemia.[51] The increase in global cerebral blood flow combined with the potential for improved flow characteristics across areas of vascular stenosis (improved rheologic properties of blood because of decreased viscosity) prompted a number of laboratory and clinical[51–54] studies to investigate hemodilution as therapy for acute ischemic stroke.[52–54]

The results of laboratory studies suggest that moderate degrees of anemia alone should rarely result in or worsen cerebral ischemia. None of the randomized clinical trials demonstrated that hemodilution in acute ischemic stroke improved clinical outcomes in patients. Because of the variety of variables that affect clinical outcomes, the negative findings may not fully rule out the possibility that hemodilution offers therapeutic benefit. Thus, the currently available evidence indicates that cerebrovascular disease does not appear to predispose patients to serious morbidity from anemia.

Changes in oxygen delivery to the brain during normovolemic anemia (either increases or decreases in blood flow) do not uniformly affect various cerebral pathologic conditions. For example, patients with high intracranial pressure from traumatic brain injury may be adversely affected by increased cerebral blood flow. However, after subarachnoid hemorrhage, mild degrees of normovolemic or hypervolemic anemia may improve overall oxygen delivery, possibly by overcoming the effects of cerebral vasospasm and thereby improving cerebral blood flow through decreased viscosity.[55] However, the effects of moderate to severe anemia in subarachnoid hemorrhage have not been assessed in laboratory or clinical studies.

One of the major consequences of redistributing some of the available cardiac output toward the coronary and cerebral circulation during normovolemic anemia is the shunting of flow away from other organs, including the kidneys and intestines. Critically ill patients may be adversely affected by this redistribution,[56] which could result in increased intestinal ischemia, bacterial translocation, and multiple-system organ failure.[57] Critical illness also can tax many of the body's adaptive responses. Specifically, cardiac performance may be impaired[58] or may already be at maximal capacity in response to increased metabolic demands. Pathologic processes affecting the microcirculation, particularly prevalent among critically ill patients, also may affect the patient's response to anemia and transfusions.

Clinical outcomes of anemia and red cell transfusion

Every medical decision must weigh risk versus benefit. The decision to administer RBC units must consider the risks of blood transfusion (see Chapters 6 and [51 52 53 54 55 56 57 58 59 60 61 62]), the risk of anemia, and the level of anemia at which blood transfusion prevents the associated adverse outcomes.

Risk of anemia
Preclinical laboratory studies
The critical hemoglobin threshold is similar in different animals.[2] Results of studies suggest that healthy animals can tolerate hemoglobin levels between 3 and 5 g/dL after normovolemic hemodilution. Electrocardiographic changes consistent with ischemia occur at hemoglobin levels less than 5 g/dL, whereas lactate production, depressed ventricular function, and death have occurred at hemoglobin levels of 3 g/dL or less. Some animals survive with hemoglobin levels as low as 1–2 g/dL.[59] However, results of studies with animals suggest a decreased ability to tolerate anemia in the

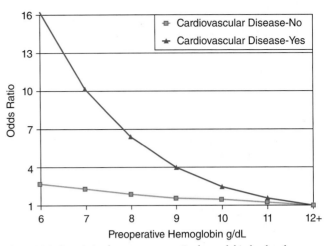

Figure 10.2 Association between preoperative hemoglobin level and mortality among patients with and without cardiovascular disease.[47] In a population of patients who refused blood transfusion, the risk of death was higher among patients with cardiovascular disease (top line) than among patients without cardiovascular disease (bottom line) for each preoperative hemoglobin level. (Source: Carson et al., 1996.[47] Reproduced with permission of Elsevier.)

presence of cardiac disease. In dogs with experimentally induced coronary stenosis varying from 50% to 80%, ST-segment changes or locally depressed cardiac function occurred at hemoglobin levels in the range of 7–10 g/dL.[60,61]

Human studies
Studies involving patients who refuse blood transfusion for religious reasons provide critical insight into the effect of anemia on humans. The largest study was performed with 1958 adult surgical patients who refused transfusion for religious reasons.[47] The mortality was greatest among patients with the lowest preoperative hemoglobin concentrations. Among patients with underlying cardiovascular disease, the risk of death was markedly greater than for patients without cardiovascular disease, especially in those patients with a hemoglobin concentration less than 10 g/dL. Among patients without underlying cardiovascular disease, the difference in mortality at hemoglobin levels greater than or less than 10 g/dL was not as great (Figure 10.2). These results, as well as data on animals and physiologic data, suggest that anemia is not tolerated as well in the presence of cardiovascular disease.

Two studies in patients who declined blood transfusion for religious reasons evaluated the mortality and morbidity associated with nadir postoperative hemoglobin concentrations less than 8 g/dL (Table 10.2).[62,63] Mortality was very low (0.9%) in patients with

Table 10.2 Unadjusted Rate of Death by 1 g/dL Decrements of the Nadir Postoperative Hb Level in the Two Series of Bloodless Surgery Patients[62,68]

Postoperative Hemoglobin	Carson et al. (2002)[68] N = 300		Shander et al. (2014)[62] N = 293		Totals N = 593	
	N	Mortality N (%)	N	Mortality N (%)	N	Mortality N (%)
1.1–2.0	7	7 (100%)	0	—	7	7 (100%)
2.1–3.0	24	13 (54.2%)	6	3 (50%)	30	16 (53.3%)
3.1–4.0	28	7 (25.0%)	16	3 (18.8%)	44	10 (22.7%)
4.1–5.0	32	11 (34.4%)	25	6 (19.4%)	57	17 (29.8%)
5.1–6.0	54	5 (9.3%)	49	7 (14.3%)	103	12 (11.7%)
6.1–7.0	56	5 (8.9%)	58	3 (5.2%)	114	8 (7.0%)
7.1–8.0	99	0 (0%)	133	2 (1.5%)	232	2 (0.9%)

hemoglobin concentrations between 7 and 8 g/dL but steadily rose with lower hemoglobin levels. The risk of death increased sharply below a hemoglobin concentration of 5 g/dL.

In a series of studies, the effect of anemia was evaluated among healthy volunteers who underwent isovolemic reduction of hemoglobin level to 5 g/dL. Transient and asymptomatic electrocardiographic changes were found in five of the 87 volunteers included in two studies.[64,65] These changes occurred when the hemoglobin level was between 5 and 7 g/dL and in patients with faster heart rates.[65] Changes in critical oxygen delivery were not measured. Subtle but reversible changes in cognition were identified in nine volunteers younger than 35 years at a hemoglobin level between 5 and 7 g/dL.[66] Self-rated fatigue was found in eight volunteers when the hemoglobin level decreased to 7 g/dL. Fatigue increased as hemoglobin levels decreased to 5 g/dL.[67] The results of these studies suggest that important clinical effects can be detected in young, healthy humans with hemoglobin levels between 5 and 7 g/dL.

It is uncertain how these results apply to older patients with comorbid factors who are also under stress from surgery or acute illness. An analysis of 31,000 patients 65 years of age or older undergoing major noncardiac surgery examined the association between preoperative hematocrit and mortality or cardiac morbidity (cardiac arrest or Q-wave myocardial infarction).[69] Mortality rose monotonically when the hematocrit was less than 36%. Cardiac events were more frequent when the hematocrit was less than 39%. These results, in contrast to experimental data, suggest that mild anemia is associated with increased mortality and morbidity. However, anemia may be only a marker of underlying disease, and studies are needed to demonstrate improved outcome if anemia is corrected by transfusion.

Efficacy of transfusion
Observational studies

There are many observational studies that evaluated the effect of RBC transfusion on clinical outcomes.[70] With few exceptions,[71–73] the studies found that transfusion was harmful. The validity of these studies is uncertain because the decision to transfuse often correlates with the illness burden of the patient. It is likely that comorbidity was not adequately adjusted for in these studies. Only randomized clinical trials can overcome this limitation.[74]

Clinical trials in adults

There have been 26 randomized clinical trials in adults that have contrasted the effects of different transfusion thresholds (Table 10.3).[75–100] The clinical settings varied, although each trial randomly assigned patients to transfusion on the basis of a restrictive (less transfusion) or a liberal strategy (more transfusion). In general, the restrictive triggers (specified hemoglobin concentrations that had to be attained) ranged from 7 to 9 g/dL, and liberal transfusion triggers from 9 to 10 g/dL, although there were other transfusion strategies used. There is overlap between the liberal and restrictive transfusion groups in these trials. Most of the trials are relatively small, with only one larger than 1000 patients. Overall, patients in the restrictive transfusion group received approximately 40% less transfusion than patients in the liberal transfusion group. We describe in detail four of the most important trials.

Most influential trials in adults
TRICC

The Transfusion Requirements in Critical Care (TRICC) trial was the first well-powered trial to evaluate clinically important outcome.[79,83] In the main study, the investigators randomly assigned 838 volume-resuscitated ICU patients to a restrictive strategy in which patients received allogeneic RBC transfusions at hemoglobin levels of 7 g/dL (and were maintained between 7 and 9 g/dL) or to a liberal strategy of receiving RBCs at 10 g/dL (and maintained between 10 and 12 g/dL). Average hemoglobin levels (8.5 vs. 10.7 g/dL) and RBC units transfused (2.6 vs. 5.6 units) were significantly lower in the restrictive as opposed to the liberal group. The 30-day mortality was slightly lower in the restrictive transfusion group (18.7% vs. 23.3%), although the finding was not statistically significant ($p = 0.11$). Mortality was lower in the restrictive transfusion group in patients less than 55 years of age ($p < 0.02$) and less ill patients defined by APACHE II scores less than 20 ($p < 0.02$). Furthermore, the restrictive transfusion group had fewer patients with myocardial infarction (0.07% vs. 2.9%; $p = 0.02$) and congestive heart failure (5.3% vs. 10.7%; $p < 0.01$).

FOCUS

Transfusion Trigger Trial for Functional Outcomes in Cardiovascular Patients Undergoing Surgical Hip Fracture Repair (FOCUS) enrolled 2016 patients undergoing surgical repair of hip fracture.[90] Patients had a history of cardiovascular disease (myocardial infarction, stroke or transient ischemic attack, congestive heart failure, or peripheral vascular disease) or cardiovascular risk factors (diabetes mellitus, hypertension, renal insufficiency, smoking, hypercholesteremia) and hemoglobin concentration less than 10 g/dL. The patients were randomly allocated to liberal transfusion trigger and blood was administered to maintain the hemoglobin above 10 g/dL, or restrictive transfusion and blood was administered when the hemoglobin concentration was less than 8 g/dL or for symptoms. The symptoms of anemia included chest pain thought to be cardiac in origin, congestive heart failure, or unexplained tachycardia or hypotension unresponsive to intravenous fluids. The primary outcome was inability to walk across the room without human assistance or death 60 days after randomization, which occurred in 35.2% in the liberal transfusion trigger and 34.7% in the restrictive-transfusion trigger (odds ratio in the liberal transfusion trigger, 1.01; 95% confidence interval [CI], 0.84 to 1.22). In-hospital acute coronary syndrome or death occurred in 4.3% in the liberal transfusion group and 5.2% in the restrictive transfusion group, respectively (absolute risk difference, −0.9%; 99% CI, −3.3 to 1.6). Mortality was similar between the groups at 30 days, 60 days, and a median of 3.1 years.[101] The causes of death were also similar.[101] The frequencies of other complications, including delirium,[102] were similar in the two groups.

Upper gastrointestinal bleeding

A total of 921 patients with severe upper gastrointestinal bleeding were enrolled in a trial comparing a liberal transfusion strategy (defined as a transfusion threshold of 9 g/dL) versus a restrictive transfusion threshold of 7 g/dL.[95] Patients were excluded if they had massive exsanguinating bleeding, acute coronary syndrome, symptomatic peripheral vascular disease, stroke or transient ischemic attack, high risk of further bleeding, recent history of trauma or surgery, and other reasons. All patients at the time of enrollment

Table 10.3 Randomized Controlled Trials in Adults

Study	Setting	Subjects: Eligibility and Comparability	Transfusion Strategy	Blood Usage Units/Pt Mean (SD)	Proportion Transfused % (n)	Hb/Hct Levels, Mean (SD)	30-Day Mortality % (n)	Length of Hospital Stay (Mean±SD^a)
Topley et al. (1956)[75]	Trauma (N=22)	>1 L blood loss; considered to be at no clinical risk in raising the blood volume ≥100% of normal, or allowing it to reach 30% below normal.	*Liberal:* Achieve red cell volume ≥100% of normal.	11.3 (6.9)	100% (10)	Lowest Hb: (15.6±2.0) g/dL	—	—
			Restrictive: Maintain red cell volume 70–80% of normal.	4.8 (6.7)	67% (8)	Lowest Hb: (11.3±0.7) g/dL	—	—
Blair et al. (1986)[76]	Gastrointestinal bleeding (N=50)	Acute severe upper gastrointestinal hemorrhage	*Liberal:* Patients received at least 2 units of PRBC immediately on admission to hospital.	4.6 (1.5)	100% (24)	Admission Hct: 28 (5.9)% Discharge Hct: 37.0 (7.8)%	8.3% (2)	—
			Restrictive: Patients were not transfused PRBC during the first 24 hours unless Hb < 8.0 g/dL or shock persisted after initial resuscitation with colloid.	2.6 (3.1)	19.2% (5)	Admission Hct: 29 (8.2)% Discharge Hct: 37.0 (7.1)%	0% (0)	—
Fortune et al. (1987)[77]	Trauma or acute hemorrhage (N=25)	Patients who had sustained a Class III or Class IV hemorrhage and had clinical signs of shock.	*Liberal:* Hct was brought up to 40% slowly over a period of several hours by the infusion of PRBC.	—	—	Average Hct for 3-day period: 38.4 (2.1)%	—	—
			Restrictive: Hct was kept close to 30% by the administration of PRBC.	—	—	Average Hct for 3-day period: 29.7 (1.9)%	—	—
Johnson et al. (1992)[78]	Cardiac surgery (N=38)	Patients undergoing elective coronary revascularization and able to donate at least three units of packed cells preoperatively.	*Liberal:* Patients received blood transfusion to achieve an Hct value of 32% as long as autologous blood was available.	2.05 (0.93)	100% (18)	Hct at 4 hours postop: 31.3%	—	7.6 (1.9) days
			Restrictive: Patients received transfusions only if the Hct value fell below 25%.	1.0 (0.86)	75% (15)	Hct at 4 hours postop: 28.7%	—	7.9 (4.3) days
Hebert et al. (1995)[79]	Critical care (N=69)	Critically ill patients admitted to 1 of 5 tertiary level intensive care units with normovolemia after initial treatment who had Hb concentrations <9.0 g/dL within 72 hours.	*Liberal:* Patients were transfused PRBC if their Hb 10.0–10.5 g/dL or less; Hb concentration maintained at 10.0–12.0 g/dL.	Mean units per patient: 4.8 Total units: 174	—	Admission Hb 93 (13)g/dL Average daily Hb 109g/L	25% (9)	Median (IQR) 31 (13–64)
			Restrictive: Patients were transfused PRBC only if their Hb 7.0–7.5 g/dL; Hb concentration maintained at 7.0–9.0 g/dL.	Mean units per patient: 2.5 Total units: 82	—	Admission Hb 97 (14)g/dL Average daily Hb 90 g/L	24% (8)	Median (IQR) 38 (25–62)
Bush et al. (1997)[80]	Vascular surgery (N=99)	Patients undergoing elective aortic and infrainguinal arterial reconstruction.	*Liberal:* Transfused with PRBC to maintain Hb> 10.0 g/dL.	Total units: 3.7 (3.5) Intraop: 2.4 (2.5)	88% (43)	Hb during 48 hr postop. period 11.0 (1.2) g/dL	8% (4)	11 (9)
			Restrictive: Transfused only if Hb level fell below 9.0 g/dL.	Total units: 2.8 (3.1) Intraop: 1.5 (1.7)	80% (40)	Hb during 48hr postop. period 9.8 (1.3) g/dL	8% (4)	10 (6)

(continued)

Table 10.3 (Continued)

Study	Setting	Subjects: Eligibility and Comparability	Transfusion Strategy	Blood Usage Units/Pt Mean (SD)	Proportion Transfused % (n)	Hb/Hct Levels, Mean (SD)	30-Day Mortality % (n)	Length of Hospital Stay (Mean±SD*)
Carson et al. (1998)[81]	Orthopaedic surgery (N = 84)	Hip fracture patients undergoing surgical repair who had postoperative Hb levels less than 10.0g/dL.	*Liberal:* Patients received 1 unit of PRBCs at the time of random assignment and then as needed to maintain Hb >10.0g/dL.	Total median 2 (1–2)	98.8% (83)	Lowest Hb: 9.4 (1.0)	2.4% (1)	6.3 (3.4)
			Restrictive: Transfusion was delayed until the patient developed symptoms or consequences of anaemia, or Hb value <8.0 g/dL in the absence of symptoms.	Total median 0 (0–2)	45.2% (38)	Lowest Hb: 8.8 (1.2)	2.4% (1)	6.4 (3.4)
Hebert et al. (1999)[83]	Critical care (N = 838)	Critically ill patients admitted to 1 of 22 tertiary level and 3 community intensive care units (ICU) with normovolemia after initial treatment who had Hb concentrations <9.0 g/dL within 72 hours.	*Liberal:* Patients were transfused with PRBC to maintain Hb concentration at 10.0–12.0 g/dL.	Total 5.6 (5.3)	100% (420)	Hb: (g/dL) (mean daily) 10.7 (0.7)	23.3% (98)	35.5 (19.4)
			Restrictive: Patients were transfused to maintain Hb concentration maintained between 7.0 and 9.0 g/dL.	Total 2.6 (4.1)	77% (280)	Hb: (g/dL) (mean daily) 8.5 (0.7)	18.7% (78)	34.8 (19.5)
Bracey et al. (1999)[82]	Cardiac surgery (N = 428)	Patients undergoing first-time elective coronary revascularization.	*Liberal:* Received RBC transfusions on the instructions of their individual physicians, who considered the clinical assessment of the patient and the institutional guidelines, which propose an Hb level <9.0 g/dL as the postoperative threshold for RBC transfusion.	Postop: 1.4 (1.8) Total: 2.5 (2.6)	Postop: 48%(104) Total: 64%(138)	Hb: (g/dL) mean net reduction in Hb (admission to discharge) 4.2 (1.9)	2.7% (6)	7.9 (4.9)
			Restrictive: Received an RBC transfusion in the postoperative period for an Hb level <8.0g/dL, unless the patient experienced blood loss >750 ml since the last transfusion, hypovolemia with hemodynamic instability and excessive acute blood loss, acute respiratory failure or inadequate cardiac output and oxygenation, or hemodynamic instability requiring vasopressors.	Postop: 0.9 (1.5) Total: 2.0 (2.2)	Postop: 35%(74) Total: 60%(127)	Hb: (g/dL) mean net reduction in Hb (admission to discharge) 4.2 (1.7)	1.4% (3)	7.5 (2.9)
Lotke et al. (1999)[84]	Orthopedic surgery (N = 127)	Patients undergoing primary total knee arthroplasty who were able to donate 2 units of autologous blood preoperatively	*Liberal:* Received their autologous blood (PAD) immediately after surgery, the first unit beginning in the recovery room and the second unit delivered on return to the ward.	—	Postop: 100%(65)	Mean Postop. Hb: (g/dL) Day 1 (11.4) Day 3 (10.7)	—	—
			Restrictive: Received all their autologous blood (PAD) if their Hb level had fallen below 9.0g/dL.	—	Postop: 26%(16)	Mean Postop. Hb: (g/dL) Day 1 (10.6) Day 3 (10.0)	—	—

Study	Setting	Intervention	Units transfused	% transfused (n)	Hb/Hct	Mortality	Length of stay, Median (range)
Grover et al. (2006)[85]	Orthopedic Surgery (N = 260)	*Liberal:* RBC transfusion for Hb < 10.0 g/dl; concentrations maintained between 10 and 12 g/dl.	(median, range) 0 (0–10)	43% (46)	Day 1: 11.0 (1.41); Day 3: 11.0 (1.26); Day 5 11/1 (0.93)	In-hospital (unsure of denominated) (1)	Median (range) 7.5 (5–13)
		Restrictive: RBC transfusion for Hb <8 g/dl; concentrations maintained between 8 and 9.5 g/dl.	(median, range) 0 (0–5)	34% (37)	Day 1: 9.7 (1.52); Day 3: 9.6 (1.36); Day 5 9.8 (1.23)	In-hospital (unsure of denominated) (0)	Median (range) 7.3 (5–11)
Foss et al. (2009)[86]	Orthopedic surgery (N = 120)	*Liberal:* RBC transfusion for Hb <10 g/dL.	Median (interquartile range) 2 (1–2)	74% (44)		0% (0)	18.4 (14.4)
		Restrictive: RBC transfusion for Hb 8 g/dL.	Median (interquartile range) 1 (1–2)	37% (22)		8% (5)	17.0 (12.9)
Zygun et al. (2009)[87]	Critical care (N = 30)	*Restrictive:* RBC transfusion for Hb 8 g/dL. *9 g/dL Threshold:* 2 units RBC transfused when Hb <9 g/dL. *8 g/dL Threshold:* 2 units RBC transfused when Hb <8 g/dL.	Median (interquartile range) 1 (1–2)	37% (22)		8% (5)	17.0 (12.9)
Hajjar et al. (2010)[88]	Cardiac surgery (N = 502)	*Liberal:* RBC transfusion to maintain Hct ≥30%.	Median (interquartile range) 2 (1–3)	78% (198)	10.5 g/dL	5 %	
		Restrictive: RBC transfusion to maintain Hct ≥24%.	Median (interquartile range) 0 (0–2)	47% (118)	9.1 g/dL	6 %	
Carson et al. (2011)[90]	Orthopedic surgery (N = 2016)	*Liberal:* Patients received 1 unit of PRBCs at the time of random assignment and then as needed to maintain Hb ≥10.0 g/dL.	Median (interquartile range) 2 (1–2)	97% (970)	Prior to transfusion: 9.2 (0.5)	5.2% (52)	(Randomization to discharge, censored at 30 days) United States Subjects: 3.67 (3.38); Canadian Subjects: 12.03 (9.31)
		Restrictive: Transfusion was delayed until the patient developed symptoms or consequences of anemia, or Hb value <8.0 g/dL in the absence of symptoms.	Median (interquartile range) 0 (0–1)	41% (413)	Prior to transfusion: 7.9 (0.6)	4.3% (43)	(Randomization to discharge, censored at 30 days) United States Subjects: 3.97 (3.89); Canadian Subjects: 12.70 (9.48)
Cooper et al. (2011)[91]	Acute myocardial infarction (N = 45)	*Liberal:* Patients received RBC transfusion when Hct <30% to maintain 30% to 33%.	2.5 (1.3)	100%	Average daily Hct: 30.6%	5% (1)	8.5 (5.6)
	Acute myocardial infarction and Hct ≤30% within 72 hours of symptoms	*Restrictive:* Patients received RBC transfusion when Hct <24% to maintain 24% to 27%.	1.6 (2.0)	54%	Average daily Hct: 27.9%	8% (2)	10.4 (7.2)

(continued)

Table 10.3 (Continued)

Study	Setting	Subjects: Eligibility and Comparability	Transfusion Strategy	Blood Usage Units/Pt Mean (SD)	Proportion Transfused % (n)	Hb/Hct Levels, Mean (SD)	30-Day Mortality % (n)	Length of Hospital Stay (Mean±SD*)
Shehata et al. (2012)[92]	Cardiac surgery (N = 50)	Elective cardiac surgery patients with a Cardiac Anesthesia Risk Score (CARE) of 3 or 4, or aged 80 and older	Liberal: RBC transfusion for Hb ≤9.5 g/dL intraoperatively (on cardiopulmonary bypass) or Hb ≤10 g/dL postoperatively.	99 units in 22 patients	88% (22)	Day 6: 10.7 g/dL	(In-hospital) 4% (1)	7 (4)
			Restrictive: RBC transfusion for Hb ≤7.0 g/dL intra operatively (on cardiopulmonary bypass) or Hb ≤7.5 g/dL postoperatively.	50 units in 13 patients	52% (13)	Day 6: 9.1 g/dL	(In-hospital) 16% (4)	9 (12)
Carson et al. (2013)[93]	Symptomatic coronary artery disease (N = 110)	Acute coronary syndrome or stable angina undergoing cardiac catheterization and Hb <10 g/dL	Liberal: RBC transfusion to maintain Hb ≥10g/dL.	1.58 (1.13)	94.5% (52)	Day 1: 10.3 (1.00); Day 2: 10.78 (0.78); Day 3: 10.64 (0.71)	1.8% (1)	
			Restrictive: RBC transfusion for symptoms or Hb <8.0g/dL.	0.49 (1.03)	27.3% (15)	Day 1: 9.03 (0.82); Day 2: 8.98 (0.80); Day 3: 9.12 (0.75)	13.0% (7)	
So-Osman et al. (2013)[94]	Orthopedic surgery (N = 603)	Elective hip/knee replacement surgery	Liberal: Hospital standard of care.	Median (interquartile range) 0 (0–2)	39.1% (119)	Day 1: 10.3 (1.4); Day 4: 10.5 (1.2); Dishcare: 11.4 (1.2)	(at 14 days) 1% (3)	9.6 (5.1)
			Restrictive: RBC transfusion determined by patient clinical risk (low, intermediate, high).	Median (interquartile range) 0 (0–1)	26.4% (79)	Day 1: 10.6 (1.6); Day 4: 10.5 (1.2); Discharge: 11.4 (1.3)	(at 14 days) 0% (0)	10.2 (7.4)
Villanueva et al. (2013)[95]	GI bleeding (N = 921)	Acute upper GI bleeding	Liberal: RBC transfusion for Hb <9 g/dL; target range for the posttransfusion hemoglobin level of 9–11 g/dL.	3.7 (3.8)	86% (384)	(discharge) 10.1 (1.0) g/dL	(at 45 days) 9% (41)	11.5 (12.8)
			Restrictive: RBC transfusion for Hb <7 g/dL; target range for the posttransfusion hemoglobin level of 7–9 g/dL.	1.5 (2.3)	49% (219)	Discharge: 9.2 (1.2) g/dL	(at 45 days) 5% (23)	9.6 (8.7)
Walsh et al. (2013)[96]	Critical care (N = 100)	Critically ill patients aged ≥ 55 years requiring ≥ 4 days mechanical ventilation with a Hb ≤ 9.0 g/dL	Liberal: RBC transfusion for Hb ≤9.0 g/dL; target Hb concentration of 9.1–11.0 g/dL.	Median (interquartile range) 3 (2–5)	100% (49)	During intervention: 9.6 (0.6) g/dL Last recorded: 9.8 (0.9)	32.7% (16)	Median (interquartile range) 31 (19–42)
			Restrictive: RBC transfusion for HB ≤7.0 g/dL; target Hb concentration of 7.1–9.0 g/dL.	Median (interquartile range) 2 (1–7)	78.4% (40)	During intervention 8.2 (0.5) g/dL Last recorded: 8.8 (1.2)	23.5% (12)	Median (interquartile range) 34 (13–64)
Prick et al. (2014)[99]	Postpartum (N = 521)	Women with acute anemia (Hb 4.8–7.9 g/dL) 12–24 hours postpartum	Liberal: RBC transfusion to achieve Hb ≥8.9 g/dL (minimum 1 unit RBC).	Median (interquartile range) 2 (2–2)	97% (252)	Discharge: median (interquartile range) 9.0 (8.5–9.5)		Median2
			Restrictive: No intervention.	Median (interquartile range) 0 (0–0)	13% (33)	Discharge: median (interquartile range) 7.4 (6.8–7.7)		Median2
Holst et al. (2014)[97]	Intensive care unit (ICU; N = 1000)	Septic shock and Hb ≤9 g/dL	Liberal: Received 1 unit RBC when Hb ≤9 g/dL.	Median (interquartile range) 4 (2–7)	98.8% (483)	Median (interquartile range) Lowest Hb Day 3: 9.3 (8.9–9.8)	(90-day Mortality) 45.0% (223)	
			Restrictive: Received 1 unit RBC when Hb ≤7 g/dL.	Median (interquartile range) 1 (0–3)	63.9% (312)	Median (interquartile range) Lowest Hb Day 3: 7.7 (7.1–8.2)	(90-day Mortality) 43.0% (216)	

Study	Population	Intervention					
Robertson et al. (2014)[100]	Traumatic brain injury	*Liberal:* IV erythropoietin/saline and RBC transfusion to maintain Hb 10 g/dL	7.1 (Range 1–21)	72.3% (73)	Day 9: Median (interquartile range) 11.4 (10.7–12.2)		
		Restrictive: Erythropoietin/saline and RBC transfusion to maintain Hb 7 g/dL	4.7 (Range 1–22)	52.5% (52)	Day 9: Median (interquartile range) 9.7 (8.6–10.9)		
Pinheiro de Almeida et al. (2015)[98]	Adult cancer patients admitted to the ICU post-major abdominal surgery	*Liberal:* RBC transfusion when Hb <9.0 g/dL while in ICU.	Median (interquartile range) 2 (1–3)	42.3%	Hb prior to transfusion: 7.9 (0.5)	8.2% (8)	Median (interquartile range) 13 (10–20)
		Restrictive: RBC transfusion when Hb <7.0 g/dL while in ICU.	Median (interquartile range) 1 (1–3)	20.8%	Hb prior to transfusion: 6.8 (0.5)	22.8% (23)	Median (interquartile range) 14 (10–22)
Murphy et al. 2015[103]	Cardiac surgery (N = 2003)	*Liberal:* RBC transfusion when Hg <9.0 g/dL.	Median (interquartile range) 2 (1–3)	94.9%	Approximately 1 g/dL higher than restrictive group	19 (1.9%)	Median (interquartile range) 7 (5–10)
		Restrictive: RBC transfusion when Hg 7.5 g/dL.	Median (interquartile range) 1 (0–2)	63.7%	Approximately 1 g/dL lower than liberal group	26 (2.6%)	Median (interquartile range) 7 (5–10)

Hb, hemoglobin level, PRBC, packed red blood cells.

were transfused one unit of red blood cells. Survival at six weeks was higher in the restrictive transfusion group (95%) compared to the liberal transfusion group (91%; 0.55; 95% CI, 0.33 to 0.92; $P = 0.02$). Recurrent bleeding occurred more frequently in the liberal transfusion group (16%) than the restrictive transfusion group (10%) ($P = 0.01$). In a subgroup of patients, portal pressures were higher in the liberal transfusion group than the restrictive transfusion group.

Septic shock

A total of 1005 patients with septic shock and a hemoglobin level less than 9 g/dL, and cared for in the intensive care unit, were enrolled in a trial comparing higher transfusion threshold (9 g/dL) to lower transfusion threshold (7 g/dL).[97] Few patients were excluded. The most common reasons were if they received transfusion prior to enrollment in the trial, had acute coronary syndrome, had life-threatening bleeding, and others. The primary outcome was death at 90 days. Secondary outcomes included use of life support, mechanical ventilation, renal replacement therapy, transfusion-associated acute lung injury, transfusion-associated circulatory overload, and number of ischemic events in ICU, which included cerebral ischemia, acute myocardial ischemia, intestinal ischemia, or limb ischemia. The median number of units transfused in the lower threshold group was one, and in the higher transfusion group was 4. Ninety-day mortality occurred in 43% of the lower transfusion group and 45.0% of the higher threshold group (relative risk, 0.94; 95% CI, 0.78 to 1.09; $P = 0.44$). Ischemic events occurred in 7.2% of the lower transfusion group and 8.0% of the higher transfusion group. Myocardial ischemic events occurred in 2.7% of the lower transfusion group and 1.2% of the higher transfusion group. No patients were classified as having transfusion-associated circulatory overload in this trial. There were no differences in other outcomes.

TITRe2

A total of 2003 patients undergoing cardiac surgery with hemoglobin concentration less than 9 g/dL were randomly allocated to a liberal transfusion threshold of 9 g/dL or a restrictive transfusion threshold of 7.5 g/dL.[103] The primary outcome was a composite of serious infection and ischemic event (stroke, myocardial infarction, gut infarction, or acute kidney injury) within 3 months of enrollment in the trial. The primary outcome occurred in a similar number of patients in both groups. However, there were more deaths at 90 days in the restrictive group (4.2%) than the liberal group (2.6%) (hazard ratio = 1.64; 95% CI, 1.00 to 2.67; $P = 0.045$). At 30 days, the differences in mortality was smaller and non-significant (2.6% for the restrictive group vs. 1.9% for the liberal group). There were no differences in infectious events, sepsis, or wound infections. The other clinical trials in cardiac surgery are described below.

Clinical settings of special interest

Acute coronary syndrome

There have been two small clinical trials evaluating transfusion thresholds in acute coronary syndrome. The first trial enrolled 45 patients with acute myocardial infarction with hematocrit less than 30% and was randomly allocated to liberal transfusion to administer blood transfusion to maintain hematocrit over 30% or restrictive transfusion to administer blood transfusion for hematocrit less than

24%.[91] All patients in the liberal transfusion group and 54% of the restrictive transfusion group, respectively, received transfusion. The primary outcome of in-hospital death, recurrent myocardial infarction, and new or worsening congestive heart failure occurred in eight patients (33%) in the liberal group and three patients (13%) in the restrictive group ($p = 0.046$). Most of the differences between the two groups were the result of increased risk of congestive heart failure in the liberal group.

The second trial enrolled 110 patients with acute myocardial infarction or coronary artery disease undergoing cardiac catherization with hemoglobin concentration less than 10 g/dL.[93] Patients were randomly allocated to a liberal transfusion strategy in which transfusion was administered to maintain a hemoglobin concentration greater than 10 g/dL or a restrictive transfusion strategy in which transfusion was administered if hemoglobin was less than 8 g/dL or for symptoms (definite angina requiring treatment with sublingual nitroglycerin or equivalent therapy, and unexplained tachycardia or hypotension). The primary outcome was composite of death, myocardial infarction, or unscheduled revascularization. This occurred in 6 patients (10.9%) in the liberal group and 14 (25.5%) in the restrictive group (risk difference= 15.0%; 95% CI of difference 0.7% to 29.3%; $p = 0.054$ and adjusted for age $p = 0.076$). Death at 30 days was less frequent in the liberal group ($n = 1$, 1.8%) compared to the restrictive group ($n = 7$, 13.0%; $p = 0.032$).

Cardiac surgery

There have been four published clinical trials in patients undergoing cardiac surgery that evaluated transfusion thresholds. The TITRe2 trial is described above. The first trial enrolled 428 patients undergoing cardiac bypass surgery and compared mortality, morbidity, and fatigue in those randomized to 8 g/dL threshold (restrictive) or 9 g/dL threshold (liberal).[82] There were no differences in mortality (3 [1.4%] of 215 restrictive patients and 6 [2.7%] of the 222 liberal patients), morbidity, or fatigue, although the difference in the transfusion thresholds was small. The second trial enrolled 502 patients undergoing cardiac bypass to hematocrit of 24% (restrictive) or 30% (liberal) from the start of surgery to hospital discharge.[88] The primary outcome was a composite of all-cause mortality, acute renal injury requiring dialysis, acute respiratory distress syndrome, or cardiogenic shock and occurred in 10% liberal and 11% restrictive (between-group difference, 1% [95% CI, −6% to 4%]; $P = 0.85$).

The third trial was a pilot study performed in 50 high-risk cardiac surgery patients.[92] The restrictive transfusion protocol administered transfusion if the hemoglobin level was ≤7 g/dL during the intraoperative time period and ≤7.5 g/dL during the postoperative time period. The liberal transfusion protocol administered transfusion if the hemoglobin level was ≤9.5 g/dL during the intraoperative time period and <10 g/dL during the postoperative time period. The trial was too small to reliably examine clinical outcomes; the larger TRICSIII trial is now underway.

Oncology patients

There are several clinical settings in oncology patients where transfusion is frequently administered. These include patients undergoing chemotherapy, stem cell transplantation, chronic anemia in patients with cancer, and surgery for cancer. Currently, there is only one published trial in cancer patients who underwent surgery.[98] 198 patients undergoing abdominal surgery at a cancer hospital and admitted to intensive care unit were randomly allocated to 9 g/dL threshold (liberal) or 7 g/dL threshold (restrictive).

The primary outcome was a composite outcome of major cardiovascular complications and eight secondary outcomes. Unexpectedly, the liberal transfusion group had superior outcomes to the restrictive transfusion group (liberal, 19.6%; restrictive, 35.6%; $P = 0.012$).

Children

Blood is frequently transfused in critically ill infants and children. In a recent survey, 14% of patients in pediatric ICUs received blood transfusion.[104] There have been four clinical trials evaluating liberal versus restrictive transfusion thresholds in this population[105] (see Table 10.4). One hundred hospitalized preterm infants with birthweights between 500 and 1300 g were randomly assigned to two transfusion levels.[106] The transfusion protocol adjusted the hematocrit level that led to transfusion depending on the respiratory status of the infant. A primary outcome was not designated among the 15 clinical events evaluated. Infants in the restrictive group received a median of two units less than the liberal group during the study, and the mean difference in hemoglobin concentration was ~2 g/dL. There were no differences between the liberal and restrictive transfusion groups for most outcomes, including survival, patent ductus arteriosus, retinopathy, or bronchopulmonary dysplasia. Infants assigned to the restrictive group had more apneic events and more neurologic events (combined parenchymal brain hemorrhage or periventricular leukomalacia). These differences in outcomes should be interpreted as hypothesis-generating because the composite neurologic outcomes were not designated a priori,[107] apnea was assessed by an unblinded nurse[107] and the differences were small, and the large number of outcomes increase the risk of false-positive results.

In the second study, 451 infants weighing less than 1000 g, whose gestational age was less than 31 weeks, and who were less than 48 hours old were randomly assigned to receive transfusion at either a low or high transfusion threshold.[108] The thresholds used varied by respiratory support using a prespecified transfusion algorithm. The primary composite outcome was in-hospital death, severe retinopathy, brochopulmonary dysplasia, or brain injury on cranial ultrasound. The mean hemoglobin concentration was ~1 g/dL different between groups, and the number of RBC transfusions were not significantly different. There was no difference in the composite outcomes (low threshold, 74.0%, vs. high threshold, 69.7%). This trial did not confirm the hypothesis that restrictive transfusion is associated with brain injury in preterm infants.

The largest study involved 637 children admitted to pediatric ICUs.[109] When a 7-g/dL threshold was compared to a 9.5-g/dL threshold, the mean hemoglobin concentration was ~2 g/dL lower in the restrictive group. RBC units were transfused to 46% of patients in the restrictive group and 98% in the liberal group. The frequency of new or progressive multi-organ dysfunction (primary outcome) was 12% in both groups, and there were no significant differences in any of the secondary outcomes including death, which occurred in 4% of both groups.

The fourth trial enrolled 107 children from 6 weeks to 6 years of age with noncyanotic congenital defects undergoing corrective cardiac surgery.[110] The patients were randomly allocated to liberal transfusion group for hemoglobin levels less than 10.8 g/dL and restrictive transfusion for hemoglobin level less than 8 g/dL. The length of stay was statistically significantly although only slightly shorter in the restrictive group (median = 8 [IQR 7–11]) versus liberal group (median = 9 [IQR 7–14] days; $p = 0.047$). There were no differences in other outcomes.

Meta-analysis

A meta-analysis combined data from published clinical trials as of 2012 in adults.[111,112] The restrictive transfusion threshold was associated with fewer red blood cell transfusions (mean difference, −1.19 units per patient; 95% CI, −1.85 to −0.53). The hemoglobin level of patients in the restrictive transfusion group was −1.48 g/dL lower than that of the liberal transfusion group. Length of hospital stay was not prolonged by restrictive transfusion strategy. The rates of cardiac events were inconsistent among the trials. Restrictive transfusion was not associated with an increase in mortality. Incorporating all trials published up to March 2015 (Figure 10.3), the risk ratio (RR) for 30-day all-cause mortality was 0.96 (95% CI, 0.78 to 1.16).

Animal models and in vivo data in humans consistently found evidence of immunosuppression after transfusion. Prior meta-analyses in 2012 found the rate of infections was decreased by 19% with the use of restrictive transfusion strategies, although the results are not significant (RR 0.81, 95% CI 0.66–1.00).[111] Five trials reported data for pneumonia. In contrast to overall infections, there was no significant difference between transfusion strategies (RR 0.93, 95% CI 0.76–1.15).[111]

However, a recent updated meta-analysis examined healthcare-associated infections.[113] This analysis included 17 trials with sufficient information for analysis. The overall risk of serious infections was not elevated (RR 0.92, 95% CI 0.82–1.04). However, restrictive strategy was associated with fewer serious infections (RR 0.84, 95% CI 0.73–0.96). These findings are likely not to be statistically significant when the results of the most recent trials are added to the analysis.[97,103]

Patients may be transfused with the expectation that it will improve the ability to walk and perform activities of daily living. The FOCUS trial evaluated liberal versus restrictive transfusion strategies on the ability to walk and a large number of other activities of daily living.[90] The liberal transfusion group did not improve any of the functional measures compared to restrictive transfusion strategy.

Most of the other published data examining the association between anemia and function were generated from clinical trials performed to evaluate the use of recombinant human erythropoietin in end-stage renal failure and patients undergoing cancer chemotherapy. These limited data suggest that increasing the hemoglobin level of patients with marked anemia (hemoglobin <10 g/dL) increases exercise tolerance.[114] The studies with negative findings[115] evaluated the effect of increasing hemoglobin level beyond the 10 g/dL threshold. A review of the use of erythropoietin in the care of patients with cancer-related anemia concluded that patients receiving erythropoietin had increased levels of energy and function.[115] Two clinical trials compared use of erythropoietin to achieve a high hemoglobin concentration (13–15 g/dL) versus a lower hemoglobin concentration (10.5–11.5 g/dL) in patients with chronic renal insufficiency.[116] Only one study found improvement in function and quality-of-life measures.[116] The US Food and Drug Administration has concluded that there is insufficient evidence to conclude that erythropoietin-stimulating agents alleviate fatigue or increase energy.

Transfusion guidelines

Since the National Institutes of Health Consensus Conference developed landmark guidelines for transfusion of blood components,[117] many organizations have issued guidelines with the intent of aiding clinical decisions. The administration of RBCs is based on

Table 10.4 Results of the Randomized Controlled Trials in Children

Study	Setting	Subjects: Eligibility and Comparability	Transfusion Strategy	Blood Usage Units/Pt Mean (SD)	Proportion Transfused % (n)	Hb/Hct Levels mean (SD)	Primary Outcome %	30-Day Mortality % (n)	Other Outcomes % (n)	Length of Hospital Stay (Mean±SD*)
Bell et al. (2005)[106]		100 preterm infants with birth weights of 500–1300 grams	Liberal: Algorithm of high transfusion thresholds	5.2 (4.5)	88%	Not reported	No outcome designated as primary among the 15 events evaluated	(In-hospital) 2% (1)	Patent ductus arterosis, 39%; intraventricular hemorrhage, 33%; periventricular leukomalacia, 0%; retinopathy, 60%; bronchopulmonary dysplasia, 38%	Median 74 (54–96)
			Restrictive: Algorithm of low transfusion thresholds	3.3 (2.9)	90%	Not reported		(In-hospital) 4% (2)	Patent ductus arterosis, 31%; intraventricular hemorrhage, 29%; periventricular leukomalacia, 14%; retinopathy, 51%; bronchopulmonary dysplasia, 35%	Median 73 (62–95)
Kirpalani et al. (2006)[108]	Neonatal intensive care units (N=451)	Infants weighing <1000 g, < gestational age, and to be < 48 hours old at the time of enrollment	Liberal: Algorithm of high transfusion thresholds	5.7 (5.0)	95%	Week 1: 14.9 (1.7); Week 2: 13.1 (1.3); Week 3 12.0 (1.5); Week 4 11.2 (1.3); Discharge 10.8 (1.6)	Combination of death or survival selected complications* = 69.7%	17.5%	—	—
			Restrictive: Algorithm of low transfusion thresholds	4.9 (4.2)	89%	Week 1: 14.3 (1.9); Week 2: 11.9; Week 3: 10.9 (1.5); Week 4 10.1 (1.2); Discharge 10.6 (1.8)	Combination of death or survival selected complications* = 74.0%	21.5%	—	—
Lacroix et al. (2007)[109]	Pediatric ICU (N=637)	Critically ill children with Hgb < 9.5 g/dL	Liberal: Threshold of 9.5 g/dL	0.9 (2.6)	98%	Lowest Hgb in ICU 10.8 g/dL	New or Progressive MODS**-12%	4% at 28 days	Nosocomial infections 25%	ICU Stay 9.9 (7.4) days
			Restrictive: Threshold of 7.0 g/dL	1.7 (2.2)	54%	Lowest Hgb in ICU 8.7 g/dL	New or Progressive MODS-12%	4% at 28 days	Nosocomial infections 20%	ICU Stay 9.5 (7.9) days
De Gast-Bakker et al. (2013)[110]	Pediatric cardiac surgery (N=107)	Children 6 weeks to 6 years of age with noncyanotic congenital cardiac defects undergoing corrective surgery with cardiopulmonary bypass	Liberal: RBC transfusion (10 ml/kg) for Hb <10.8 g/dL	258 ml (±87)	100% (54)	Pediatric ICU discharge 12.2 (1.2)	Length of stay in hospital median (interquartile range) 9 (7–14)		Length of stay in PICU 2 (1–5); duration of ventilation (hours) 16 (9–27)	Median (interquartile range) 8 (7–11)
			Restrictive: RBC transfusion (10 ml/kg) for Hb ≤8.0 g/dL	186 ml (±70)	100% (53)	Pediatric ICU discharge 10.2 (1.2)	Length of stay in hospital median (interquartile range) 8 (7–11)		length of stay in PICU 2 (1–4); duration of ventilation (hours) 20 (9–52)	Median (interquartile range) 9 (7–14)

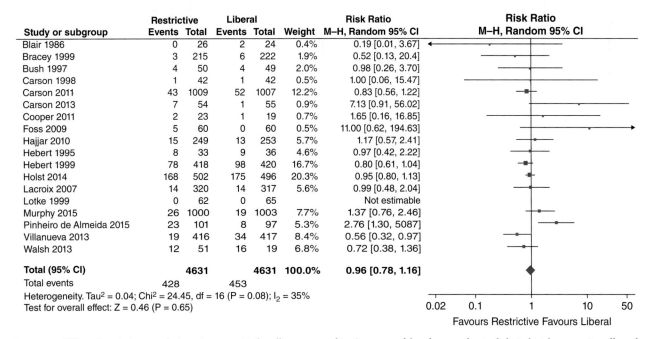

Study or subgroup	Restrictive Events	Total	Liberal Events	Total	Weight	Risk Ratio M–H, Random 95% CI
Blair 1986	0	26	2	24	0.4%	0.19 [0.01, 3.67]
Bracey 1999	3	215	6	222	1.9%	0.52 [0.13, 20.4]
Bush 1997	4	50	4	49	2.0%	0.98 [0.26, 3.70]
Carson 1998	1	42	1	42	0.5%	1.00 [0.06, 15.47]
Carson 2011	43	1009	52	1007	12.2%	0.83 [0.56, 1.22]
Carson 2013	7	54	1	55	0.9%	7.13 [0.91, 56.02]
Cooper 2011	2	23	1	19	0.7%	1.65 [0.16, 16.85]
Foss 2009	5	60	0	60	0.5%	11.00 [0.62, 194.63]
Hajjar 2010	15	249	13	253	5.7%	1.17 [0.57, 2.41]
Hebert 1995	8	33	9	36	4.6%	0.97 [0.42, 2.22]
Hebert 1999	78	418	98	420	16.7%	0.80 [0.61, 1.04]
Holst 2014	168	502	175	496	20.3%	0.95 [0.80, 1.13]
Lacroix 2007	14	320	14	317	5.6%	0.99 [0.48, 2.04]
Lotke 1999	0	62	0	65		Not estimable
Murphy 2015	26	1000	19	1003	7.7%	1.37 [0.76, 2.46]
Pinheiro de Almeida 2015	23	101	8	97	5.3%	2.76 [1.30, 5087]
Villanueva 2013	19	416	34	417	8.4%	0.56 [0.32, 0.97]
Walsh 2013	12	51	16	19	6.8%	0.72 [0.38, 1.36]
Total (95% CI)		**4631**		**4631**	**100.0%**	**0.96 [0.78, 1.16]**
Total events	428		453			

Heterogeneity. Tau^2 = 0.04; Chi^2 = 24.45, df = 16 (P = 0.08); I$_2$ = 35%
Test for overall effect: Z = 0.46 (P = 0.65)

Figure 10.3 Effect of restrictive transfusion triggers on 30-day all-cause mortality. Summary of data from randomized clinical trials comparing effect of restrictive versus liberal transfusion strategies on mortality in adults (expressed as relative risks). (Updated Cochrane Database of Systematic Reviews March 2015.)

the balance of benefits, risks, and costs. Physicians making transfusion decisions are faced with massive amounts of sometimes conflicting information. Since 1983, concerns about the transmission of human immunodeficiency virus and other viruses through blood components have significantly modified both real and perceived risks and benefits. Many organizations responded by issuing clinical practice guidelines advocating a more restrictive approach to the use of allogeneic RBC units and other components.[118] In recent years, there have been additional guidelines that benefit from accumulating clinical trial evidence.

Although some of the specific recommendations varied among the guidelines, most of the recommendations were similar.[119–128] Based on results of the TRICC trial and other evidence, all the guidelines published in the past few years recommended a 7 g/dL threshold in intensive care unit patients and often in other patient populations. Many guidelines suggested 8 g/dL threshold in patients with preexisting cardiac disease. Most of the guidelines also recommended that transfusion be guided by clinical judgment rather than hemoglobin level.

The AABB guideline recommendations (chaired by Dr. Carson) emphasized that the results of clinical trials should serve as the basis of all recommendations.[126] Furthermore, these guidelines addressed hemodynamically stable patients and provided recommendations when transfusion should be considered, but not necessarily given. There were four general recommendations: (1) adhering to a restrictive transfusion approach using a 7–8 g/dL threshold in hospitalized stable patients; (2) adhering to a restrictive transfusion approach in patients with preexisting cardiovascular disease using a 8 g/dL threshold; (3) no specific recommendation was provided for patients with acute coronary syndrome because there were no large clinical trials available to guide treatment; and (4) suggesting that the transfusion decision might be influenced by symptoms but emphasizing that there were not good trials documenting the efficacy of this approach.

Decision making in red cell transfusion
Approach to evaluating a bleeding patient
In the care of a bleeding patient, the physician must first determine the degree of blood loss and rate of bleeding. As part of the initial assessment, the healthcare team must rapidly address the patient's ABCs (airway, breathing, and circulation). Although blood loss usually leads to circulatory compromise, the severe form, termed *hemorrhagic shock*, often leads to airway and breathing concerns. Once airway and breathing have been assessed and cleared, assessment of the heart rate and blood pressure—in addition to a rapid scan of the scene and the patient—will reveal obvious threats such as dramatic blood loss. During the initial assessment, patients must be completely uncovered and rapidly examined to rule out rapidly bleeding wounds, obvious signs of massive bleeding such as a rapidly expanding abdomen in patients with a ruptured abdominal aortic aneurysm, or severe hematochezia in patients with severe lower gastrointestinal bleeding. The focus is on possible causes of bleeding and important comorbid conditions, such as cardiovascular disease that could exacerbate any injury. An emergency complete blood cell count, type and crossmatch, prothrombin time, and partial thromboplastin time should be obtained. From these data and the clinical examination, the source and rate of bleeding are estimated. A decision can be made about the rate of RBC unit transfusion as well as any curative and supportive measures. For patients with gastrointestinal bleeding, consultations may be requested from the gastroenterology and possibly surgery departments. In the care of patients with postoperative bleeding, measures such as angiography or exploratory surgery should be considered.

In patients with active bleeding, the hemodynamic status and need for emergency intervention must be determined. Crystalloid is administered to maintain intravascular volume. Red cell transfusions are administered rapidly to maintain adequate oxygen-carrying capacity. Clinical judgment is needed to (1) estimate how much more bleeding may occur and how much lower the hemoglobin level will decrease, and then (2) perform expectant transfusion. Vital signs are examined for a decrease in blood pressure and for tachycardia. The patient is asked about symptoms that can result from anemia, including cardiac ischemia (chest pain), congestive heart failure (dyspnea, paroxysmal nocturnal dyspnea, and edema), fatigue, dizziness, weakness, and orthostatic hypotension unresponsive to intravenous fluids. The hemoglobin level is measured at regular intervals.

It is important to determine the presence of coronary artery disease because results of studies with animals and with human subjects suggest that patients with coronary artery disease may be less tolerant of anemia. Review of the medical history for angina, myocardial infarction, and CABG surgery is essential. The electrocardiogram is examined for evidence of old myocardial infarction or ischemic changes. The chest radiograph is examined for cardiomegaly and other changes consistent with congestive heart failure. Patients with a history of peripheral or cerebral vascular disease are more likely also to have asymptomatic coronary artery disease.

In the care of patients with moderate to severe blood loss that has abated, there is more time for complete assessment of the source of bleeding, development of a course of management, and thorough evaluation of the patient. After bleeding has stopped and equilibration has occurred, the hemoglobin level stabilizes and the nadir hemoglobin level can be determined.

Surgical patient

Patients undergoing major surgical intervention often experience hemodynamic instability and frequently require RBC unit transfusion as a consequence of considerable blood loss. Various aspects of transfusion management for surgical patients are discussed in Chapters 48 and 49. One of the goals of resuscitation is to maintain oxygen delivery well beyond the anaerobic threshold. Hemoglobin concentration should be maintained above a value that maintains adequate DO_2 and minimizes exposure to allogeneic RBC transfusion. However, optimal intraoperative thresholds have not been established. Current methods of monitoring effective circulatory blood volume and utilization of oxygen at the tissue level have limitations. Therefore, maintenance of adequate hemoglobin level has been recommended.[129] Frequent measurement can assist the anesthesiologist in administering one RBC unit at a time when blood loss is predictable. Blood loss exceeding 20% of blood volume in a short time may necessitate transfusion of multiple RBC units as well as administration of plasma and platelets (the exact ratio is pending clinical trials). Reliable intraoperative measurements can be performed easily at the point of care with hemoglobin measurements obtained with standard blood gas analyzers. However, the accuracy of this measurement is influenced by the amount of intravenous fluid administered by the anesthesiologist and the fact that insufficient time has passed for equilibration to occur. Therefore, expert clinical judgment is required.

Standard anesthetic practice mandates intraoperative monitoring of cardiac function with measurement of continuous electrocardiographic and noninvasive or invasive blood pressure monitoring. Both monitoring techniques are essential but are insensitive to significant blood loss. This can delay recognition of significant anemia until late in the process. However, optimal intraoperative thresholds have not been established, and there are limitations to the current methods of monitoring effective circulatory blood volume and utilization of oxygen at the tissue level. A patient can have profound anemia without appreciable changes in either measurement. More sophisticated and invasive monitoring of cardiac function includes measurement of right- and left-sided ventricular filling pressure by means of central venous pressure and pulmonary artery catheters. Both techniques provide estimates of the effective circulating blood volume and are frequently used in high-risk surgery and in ICUs. Repeated measurement of central pressure and fluid challenges provide much more reliable assessment of effective circulating blood volume than does an isolated single measurement. Continuous monitoring of cardiac output with either pulmonary arterial catheters or esophageal Doppler techniques can be performed in many centers. Most of these techniques are reliable and frequently are used intraoperatively and during critical illness.[130] However, current monitoring techniques have a number of major limitations in guiding transfusion requirements. Careful clinical observation in conjunction with the physiologic data provide many of the necessary tools in the diagnosis and detection of clinically important anemia. The more difficult task is knowing how best to administer RBC units, intravenous solutions such as colloids and crystalloids, and vasoactive drugs.

Few data exist on whether invasive monitoring and different treatment strategies cause more harm than good. Most experienced anesthesiologists and critical care physicians have developed an approach to management of blood loss and hemodynamic instability. There is still enormous practice variation in selecting specific therapies. Randomized clinical trials are needed to assist in clinical decision making.

Chronic anemia

In chronic anemia, there is time for compensation to develop and for careful observation of the patient. Anemia is associated with an increase in blood flow resulting from decreased viscosity, greater release of oxygen caused by higher levels of 2,3-DPG, and an increase in cardiac output. There is time to determine whether these physiologic events are clinically important in the individual patient and carefully determine whether the patient has symptoms. Besides cardiac symptoms (angina, dyspnea), anemia can lead to nonspecific symptoms, such as fatigue, weakness, dizziness, reduced exercise tolerance, and impaired performance of activities of daily living. There also may be time to implement alternative treatments to correct anemia, depending on the cause. Iron, vitamin B_{12}, and folate can be replaced. Erythropoietin can be administered. It is important to correct preoperative anemia because the hemoglobin level strongly correlates with the probability of transfusion.[131]

Transfusion threshold

Recent clinical trials have assessed the optimal threshold for transfusion, and there are reliable data for many clinical settings. A 7 g/dL threshold should be used in critical care patients because several trials have confirmed that it is safe to withhold blood until the hemoglobin level decreases to less than 7 g/dL.[83,97] A 7 g/dL threshold should also be used in patients with acute gastrointestinal bleeding because one trial found a lower mortality than patients transfused at 9 g/dL.[95] However, it can be difficult to anticipate how low the hemoglobin level might fall in rapidly bleeding patients. Thus, blood pressure and pulse along with clinical judgment must be strongly considered in an actively bleeding patient. In postoperative surgical patients (orthopedic[90] and cardiac surgery[82,88]), an 8 g/dL threshold has been tested and proven to be as safe as a 10 g/dL threshold. It is possible that these patients would also tolerate a 7 g/dL threshold, but none of the currently published trials have tested the lower threshold. Patients with preexisting cardiovascular disease were included in the FOCUS trial that demonstrated the safety of an 8 g/dL threshold.[90] However, it is unclear what transfusion threshold is appropriate for patients with acute coronary syndrome or in those undergoing cardiac surgery. There have been only two small trials performed in patients with acute myocardial infarction, although one study of 110 patients provided a signal that these patients might benefit from the 10 g/dL threshold.[93] Similar results were found in the most recent trial in cardiac surgery. At this time we have no specific recommendation in these two groups of patients, and it is necessary to rely on clinical judgment. Patients with symptoms of anemia should be transfused as needed. No set of guidelines applies to every patient. In the end, careful clinical assessment of each patient with thoughtful consideration of risks and benefits should guide the transfusion decision.

Dose and administration

In patients who experience acute blood loss, the rate of administration of RBCs is guided by the rate of bleeding and hemodynamic compromise. In the treatment of rapidly bleeding patients, RBCs should be given at the rate necessary to maintain oxygen transport while definitive therapy is instituted. Rates may range from 5 to 10 units over 10–15 minutes in patients who are exsanguinating to rates in the range of one unit every 2–4 hours (1 mL/kg/hour) in patients with severe left ventricular dysfunction. When blood loss is predictable and not massive, RBC units should generally be administered one at a time. In the care of patients with chronic anemia, enough blood should be given to control symptoms. In most adult patients, 1 RBC unit increases the hemoglobin level approximately 1 g/dL and hematocrit approximately 3%. Ordinarily, 1 RBC unit is given over 1 to 2 hours. After transfusion of each RBC unit, measurement of hemoglobin level is repeated, and the patient reassessed.

Future

During the next decade, advances and risks may dramatically alter transfusion practice. Research is underway to develop safe red cell components. Further clinical trials should be performed to better describe the clinical effect of different transfusion strategies. Trials are especially needed in patients with acute coronary syndrome, neurological disorders, and acute and chronic hematological disorders. It is possible that within the next one or two decades, a cost-effective oxygen carrier will be developed that will reduce the use of allogeneic RBC units.

Summary

Red cell transfusion is an extremely common treatment throughout the world. Blood is administered to improve oxygen delivery. Patients compensate for anemia through increased cardiac output and through redistribution of blood flow to the cardiac and cerebral circulation. Particular attention must be paid to maintaining adequate oxygen delivery to the heart. The preponderance of evidence suggests that a hemoglobin level of 7 to 8 g/dL is a safe threshold for red cell transfusion. For patients with acute cardiovascular disease, a higher transfusion threshold should be considered. RBC units should usually be administered one at a time, and the patient and hemoglobin level reassessed after each transfusion. Transfusion decisions should consider the rate of bleeding, the presence of underlying medical problems, the hemodynamic status of the patient, the presence of symptoms, and whether anemia is acute or chronic.

Disclaimer

J.L. Carson has disclosed no financial relationship, and P. Hébert has disclosed no financial relationship.

Key references

A full reference list for this chapter is available at: http://www.wiley.com/go/simon/transfusion

47 Carson JL, Duff A, Poses RM, *et al.* Effect of anaemia and cardiovascular disease on surgical mortality and morbidity. *Lancet* 1996; **348** (9034): 1055–60.

83 Hebert PC, Wells G, Blajchman MA, *et al.* A multicenter, randomized, controlled clinical trial of transfusion requirements in critical care. Transfusion Requirements in Critical Care Investigators, Canadian Critical Care Trials Group. *New Engl J Med* 1999; **340** (6): 409–17.

90 Carson JL, Terrin ML, Noveck H, *et al.* Liberal or restrictive transfusion in high-risk patients after hip surgery. *N Engl J Med* 2011; **365** (26): 2453–62.

95 Villanueva C, Colomo A, Bosch A, *et al.* Transfusion strategies for acute upper gastrointestinal bleeding. *N Engl J Med* 2013; **368** (1): 11–21.

97 Holst LB, Haase N, Wetterslev J, *et al.* Lower versus higher hemoglobin threshold for transfusion in septic shock. *N Engl J Med* 2014; **371** (15): 1381–91.

103 Murphy GJ, Pike K, Rogers CA, *et al.* Liberal or restrictive transfusion after cardiac surgery. *N Engl J Med* 2015; **372** (11): 997–1008.

109 Lacroix J, Hebert PC, Hutchison JS, *et al.* Transfusion strategies for patients in pediatric intensive care units. *New Engl J Med* 2007; **356** (16): 1609–19.

126 Carson JL, Grossman BJ, Kleinman S, *et al.* Red blood cell transfusion: a clinical practice guideline from the AABB*. *Ann Intern Med* 2012; **157** (1): 49–58.

CHAPTER 11

Sickle cell anemia, thalassemia, and congenital hemolytic anemias

Keith Quirolo[1] & Elliott Vichinsky[1,2]

[1]Department of Hematology/Oncology, UCSF Benioff Children's Hospital Oakland, Oakland, CA, USA
[2]Department of Pediatrics, University of California San Francisco, San Francisco, CA, USA

Each year, an estimated 300,000 infants are born with either of the two most common hemoglobinopathies: the sickle cell diseases or the thalassemias. These inherited diseases are the most prevalent monogenetic disorders worldwide. Sickle cell disease makes up 85% of the total infants, and thalassemias the remaining 15%. It is increasingly apparent that sickle cell disease and thalassemia have become a major health challenge in emerging countries as more infants with hemoglobinopathies survive beyond infancy and into adulthood.

The prevalence of significant hemoglobin trait[1] (Hb S, Hb C, Hb E, Hb D, etc., and β thalassemia and α^0 thalassemia) varies from about 1% in all of Europe to as high as 18% in all of Africa; the prevalence in the American population is 3%. The presence of disease is 10.8/1000 in Africans, 0.6/1000 in Americans, and 0.2/1000 in all of Europe. Half of the people in the world with sickle cell disease live in three countries: Nigeria, Democratic Republic of Congo, and India. In West Africa, about 1,000 infants a day are born with sickle cell disease.

In the world's population, 1.5% are β thalassemia mutation carriers. Hemoglobin E–beta^0 thalassemia (Hb E/β^0 thalassemia) is the genotype responsible for approximately one-half of all severe β thalassemia worldwide. The distributions of the phenotype and genotype of North American thalassemia patients today—as well as their transfusion management—are dramatically different from those in the past decades.[2] The majority of patients, previously of Mediterranean descent, are now largely of Asian, Indian, and Middle Eastern origin.[2] In Thailand, about 3,000 affected children are born annually, with estimates of about 100,000 living patients. In southern China, the gene frequencies for β-thalassemia and for Hb E are over 4%, resulting in thousands of annual births of β thalassemia major and hemoglobin Hb E/β^0 thalassemia. Due to the diaspora occurring in the past and present, sickle cell disease and thalassemia can now be found in areas that are free of malaria.

Sickle hemoglobin is a structural variant causing severe disease in the homozygous state and when in combination with other hemoglobin variants. The α and β thalassemias are genetically diverse with more than 200 mutations accounting for decreased production of hemoglobin in those affected. The thalassemia phenotype varies from mild to severe states of anemia. The heterozygote is mildly protective against malaria with increased prevalence in some areas of the world. Red cell transfusions are indicated for both of these hemoglobinopathies. In sickle cell disease, transfusions prevent and/or treat complications and ameliorate anemia. In the thalassemias, transfusion prevents the anemia associated with decreased or absent hemoglobin production.

Malaria, blood groups, and hemoglobinopathy

Infections that are endemic and lethal in children are particularly effective for the selection of mutations that provide survival advantage. Malaria is a devastating parasitic disease with a very high mortality rate among children and pregnant women. Due to the high infection and mortality rates, malaria is an extremely strong force for selection. It is estimated that worldwide there are three billion people at risk for infection; there are 250 million clinical episodes of malaria and between one million and 500,000 deaths annually.[3] Ninety percent of deaths occur in sub-Saharan Africa, where many of the hemoglobin polymorphisms and blood group variants are found. Mutations providing even a slight survival advantage are numerous, primarily changing the red cell membrane and hemoglobin. Without the genetic pressure from malaria, human history and the practice of hematology and transfusion medicine would be much different than they are today. An understanding of malaria and the mutations it has caused lays a foundation for understanding sickle cell disease, thalassemia, and transfusion therapy of the hemoglobinopathies.

In Africa between 50,000 and 300,000 years ago, a genetically similar species to *Plasmodium falciparum* infecting western gorillas jumped species and infected humans.[4] It is thought that all of the *Plasmodium* species in sub-Saharan Africa jumped from chimpanzees, macaques, and gorillas to humans. However, the direction of transfer to New World monkeys cannot be determined for *Plasmodium malariae* or *Plasmodium vivax*; the parasite may have been transmitted from humans to monkeys.[5] Currently, there are four species of malaria parasites infecting humans: *P. falciparum*, *P. vivax*, *Plasmodium ovale*, and *P. malariae*. *P. falciparum* is the most common of these species, occurring in about 40% of infections. It is

Rossi's Principles of Transfusion Medicine, Fifth Edition. Edited by Toby L. Simon, Jeffrey McCullough, Edward L. Snyder, Bjarte G. Solheim, and Ronald G. Strauss.
© 2016 John Wiley & Sons, Ltd. Published 2016 by John Wiley & Sons, Ltd.

also the most lethal, accounting for the vast majority of deaths and severe disease. *P. vivax* may account for another 40% of cases, causing morbidity but not the mortality of *P. falciparum*.[6] The most recent jump[7] is the fifth species of *Plasmodium* to infect humans: *Plasmodium knowlesi*. Still considered a zoonosis, this *Plasmodium* sp. has macaque monkeys as a reservoir, and is known to infect human populations in Southeast Asia. *P. knowlesi* infections are reported to be as severe as those of *P. falciparum*.[8]

The association between hematological disease and malaria was first noted in the 1940s by Haldane[9] in the Mediterranean and Beet[10] in Africa. Six common diseases are associated with resistance to malaria:[11] thalassemia (both α and β thalassemia), glucose-6-phosphate dehydrogenase deficiency, hemoglobin C, Southeast Asian ovalocytosis, and hemoglobin S. There are six blood groups with mutations associated with malarial disease: the Duffy blood group, Gerbich blood group, MNS blood group, Knops blood group, and possibly ABO and Lewis blood groups.

Blood groups

The human blood groups are either receptors for the malaria parasite or are involved in the rosetting of red cells infected with the malarial parasite.

Duffy blood group

The Duffy blood group gene locus, DARC, is an acronym for *Duffy antigen receptor for chemokine*. The gene resides on the long arm of chromosome 1 (1q21-q22). The gene notation for the blood group is FY. Polymorphisms are responsible for the Fy^a and Fy^b antigens. These antigens differ in only one amino acid at position 42: Fy^a glycine, Fy^b aspartic acid. There are four common Duffy phenotypes. Within the Duffy blood group system, there are six separate antigens.[12] The Duffy antigen is the receptor for *P. vivax* and *P. knowlesi*. The Duffy antigen is also a nonspecific chemokine receptor. See Table 11.1.

The merozoite of *P. vivax* requires the Duffy-binding protein (PvDBP) in order to bind to the DARC on the red cell. *P. vivax* and *P. knowlesi* genes encode for only one binding protein; the absence of DARC on the red cell is protective against invasion by these parasites.

The Duffy negative allele in Africans is the result of a mutation in the erythroid-specific promoter at position 33 of the GATA-1 transcription factor region blocking the expression of the Duffy antigen on red cells. The mutation is in the Fy^b allele, designated erythroid silent: Fy^{Es}. The Duffy antigen remains present on somatic cells in the presence of the erythroid silent mutation.

Gerbich blood group[13]

The Gerbich blood group is expressed on glycophorin C and glycophorin D. There are 11 antigens in this group. The gene, GYPC, is located on chromosome 2, 2q14>2q21. Both glycophorins are encoded by this gene. There are two initiation codons; initiation at the first codon results in glycophorin C; initiation at the second codon results in glycophorin D. These glycophorins interact with the 4.1R protein, stabilizing the red cell membrane. A reduction of these antigens leads to hereditary elliptocytosis. Glycophorin C is one of the receptors of *P. falciparum* (EBA-140).[14] There have been reports of increased Gerbich negativity in the coastal areas of Papua New Guinea, an area where malaria is endemic. There is evidence that the Gerbich phenotype is associated with malaria infection.[14] There is no homology between this group and the glycophorins of the MNS system.

MNS blood group system

The MNS blood group system includes three red cell antigens on two glycophorins. M and N are found on glycophorin A, and S on glycophorin B. These two glycophorins carry two receptors for *P. falciparum*: EBA-175 on glycophorin A and EBA-1 on glycophorin B. The glycophorins are encoded on chromosome 4, 4q28>4q31 in sequence GYPA, GYPB, GYPE. These are homologous genes probably arising from GYPA. There is no evidence of a glycophorin on the red cell membrane arising from GYPE.[15] The MNS system is complex with unequal crossovers, deletions, gene conversions, and point mutations leading to 46 different antigens. It is second in complexity only to the Rh system. See Table 11.2.

Knops blood group[16]

The Knops blood group is found on the complement receptor 1 (CR1), a glycoprotein present on the red cell as well as other circulating blood cells. CR1 is one of a group of membrane proteins termed the *regulators of complement activation*; they include decay accelerating factor (DAF/CD55), membrane cofactor protein (CD46), and membrane inhibitor of reactive lysis (MIRL/CD59). CR1 also binds C4b/C3b immune complexes for transfer to the liver or spleen where the immune complexes are ingested by macrophages, returning the red cells to the circulation. CR1 has a binding site for *P. falciparum* entry into the host red cells. CR1 and a malaria red cell membrane protein are involved in red cell rosetting during cerebral malaria.

ABO, Lewis blood groups

There is evidence that *P. falciparum* influenced the distribution of the ABO blood groups to favor group O in areas where *P. falciparum* was present.[17] Group O decreases the adhesive properties of infected red cells relative to groups A and B.[18] Empirically, there are higher rosette levels, increased size, and increased adhesion in groups A and AB. Group B patients[19] have an intermediate

Table 11.1 Prevalence of Duffy Antigens

| Red Cell Phenotype | Prevalence % | | Allele |
	Caucasians	African Americans	
Fy (a+b−)	20**	10**	FY*01/Fy*01 or FY*A/FY*A
Fy (a−b+)	32	20	
Fy (a+b+)	48	3	
Fy (a−b−)	Rare	67%	

** 70–90% of Asians have this mutation; FYB^{ES} is the notation for the erythroid silent GATA mutation primarily seen in African Americans.

Table 11.2 Plasmodium Receptors

Plasmodium sp.	Parasite receptor	Red cell receptor
P. vivax	Duffy binding protein	Duffy A, Duffy B
P. falciparum	EBA-175	Glycophorin A (MN)
P. falciparum	EBA-140	Glycophorin C (Gerbich)
P. falciparum	EBA-1	Glycophorin B (Ss, U)

From: Jesse Qiao, MD, PowerPoint presentation, UT Health Science Center, January 28, 2013.

level of rosettes, with the lowest level of rosette formation being seen in group O individuals. It is proposed that the distribution of blood group O should be highest in areas of malaria and lowest in areas without malaria, and that group A should be lower in these areas, which is indeed the case. Blood group O is common in equatorial regions, and group A is more common in northern latitudes. Infections with severe malaria are more common in group A1 versus group O, even though group O is much more common in the populations studied. Inhibition of this effect can be demonstrated *in vitro* using soluble A and B antigen, blocking the PfEMP-1 receptor. This could also occur *in vivo* due to the effect of the Lewis gene transferase, which increases the levels of A and B antigen in the serum.[20] This would account for the increased Le (a−b−) seen in individuals with African ancestry.

Enzymopathy

Glucose-6-phosphate dehydrogenase (G6PD) deficiency

G6PD is expressed in all cells. It is the first enzyme in the pentose phosphate pathway and is responsible for the production of the NADPH needed for the regeneration of reduced glutathione. Reduced glutathione converts hydrogen peroxide (H_2O_2) to water. It is the only NADPH source in the red blood cell protecting it from oxidative damage. It is located on the X chromosome (Xq28). G6PD is the most common enzymopathy in humans. The disease affects males and females who are homozygotes; in some cases, G6PD can affect heterozygotes due to lyonization. The gene is polymorphic with 140 different variants. The normal allele is B. There are three alleles in Africa: B, A, A−. The two A alleles have 85% and 12% of normal activity; only the A− allele provides protection against malaria.[21] The A allele differs from B by one amino acid, and the A− from A by one amino acid. The A− is always on an A background, which may be required for malaria protection. The most severe form of G6PD is the *Mediterranean* allele, also a one-amino-acid substitution, producing only 3% activity. It is found in the Mediterranean, India, and Indonesia.

Thalassemia

Alpha thalassemia

Alpha thalassemia is the most common single-gene disease in the world. Four common mutations lead to α thalassemia, and all are α globin gene deletions. In Africa, the most common deletion is $-\alpha^{3.7}$. The deletion types have not been studied in terms of their protective effect against malaria. It is assumed they are equally effective. Homozygous α+ thalassemia ($-\alpha/-\alpha$) has been found to be protective against severe malaria. In some malarial areas, such as parts of India and Asia, the incidence of homozygous α thalassemia is 80%. In sub-Saharan Africa, the incidence is 50% or less in spite of endemic severe malaria. This is thought to be due to the negative effect (negative epistasis) of the combination of hemoglobin AS and α thalassemia.[22] In children with homozygous hemoglobin A, both the α thalassemia heterozygous[23] and homozygous[24] forms are protective. The protective effect is a decrease of disease progression from parasitemia to severe malaria. The actual biology of this effect has not been defined, but there is decreased rosette formation, increased phagocytosis,[25] and increased immune recognition in α thalassemia red cells.

Beta thalassemia

Although β thalassemia is prevalent in malarial areas, the evidence for β thalassemia being protective against malaria is less convincing, primarily due to the fact that the areas around the Mediterranean where β thalassemia has been prevalent are now free of the malaria parasite. In Africa there are few, if any, published studies of the effect of the sickle β thalassemia phenotypes on survival in patients with malaria. The majority of β mutations in Africans are β plus mutations (−88 C>T and −29 A>G). In African Americans, there are 14 β mutations.[26] The two most common β plus mutations are the same as noted. The most common β zero mutation is Codon 6 −A, also seen in Africans.

Membrane mutation

Southeast Asian ovalocytosis

Southeast Asian ovalocytosis does not occur in Africa, but hereditary elliptocytosis has a prevalence of up to 1.5% in some populations.[27] There is *in vitro* evidence that spectrin mutations may impede the entry of *P. falciparum* into red cells, but there is no published clinical evidence of an effect on survival.[28]

Structural hemoglobin mutations

Hemoglobin E

First described in 1954, hemoglobin E is a structural thalassemic mutation that is predominant in Southeast Asia. Hemoglobin E is the result of a point mutation at codon 26 of the β globin gene (Glu>Lys). Although this thalassemia is common in malarial areas, it is not clear how this mutation would protect against *P. falciparum* malaria. These red cells may be less susceptible to invasion.[29]

Hemoglobin C

Hemoglobin C occurs almost exclusively in West Africa, having a frequency of 50% in the Ivory Coast. Unlike hemoglobin S, where there is a disadvantage for the homozygote, there appears to be no selective disadvantage to the homozygote CC or the heterozygote AC. Hemoglobin C is not as effective in the prevention of severe malaria compared to hemoglobin S, which is probably why it is not more prevalent in sub-Saharan Africa. Both AC and CC are protective, with levels of protection differing depending upon reports.[30,31] Protection from severe malaria is due to a decreased parasite survival in CC cells and changes in the red cell surface in CC and AC red cells, particularly PfEMP1, leading to decreased cyto-adherence and an increase in acquired immunity.[32] This theory has been questioned[33] in a report that there was no increase in antibody response between AS and AC children infected with malaria. The presence of hemoglobin C in the erythrocyte alters the red cell membrane as well as hindering the development of *P. falciparum* within the cell.[34]

Hemoglobin S

Hemoglobin S (ß[6] Glu6Val, GAG>GTG) is common in West and Central Africa where malaria is endemic. The more prevalent the malaria, the more prevalent is this hemoglobin mutation. Hemoglobin S also occurs in North Africa, the Mediterranean, and India. It is estimated that the hemoglobin S mutation occurred as recently as 250–700 years or as long ago as 1750 years. The mutation for hemoglobin S occurred much more recently than the mutation for hemoglobin C, which is estimated to have occurred 3000 years ago. Hemoglobin S has become the dominant mutation due to superior protection against *P. falciparum* in the heterozygote.

Hemoglobin AS is highly protective against malaria.[35] A recent study[36] showed that hemoglobin AS was 90% effective in preventing malaria in 2591 children with severe malaria compared to a group of 2048 control children in Ghana. In this study, AC was only associated with a decrease in cerebral malaria. Although AS is clearly protective against severe malaria, it is not known how sickle hemoglobin provides this protection. There are several mechanisms that could account for the protection afforded by AS. Most of the research has been done in areas where *P. falciparum* is prevalent.

Red cells infected with *P. falciparum* have increased polymerization of hemoglobin and have an intracellular environment that decreases parasite growth. This could be due to high levels of potassium, elevated levels of hemoglobin, or microRNA that may reduce growth by inhibiting mRNA transcription in the parasite. There is also decreased rosetting of infected AS red cells in the circulation, likely due to a reduced expression of surface adherence proteins. The expression of these adherence proteins, such a *P. falciparum* membrane protein-1 (PFWMP1), leads to cycloadherence and increased endothelial activation in infected persons.

Recently,[37] a murine model has shown that heme oxygenase I induction by hemolysis with the production of CO creates tolerance to malaria and could be another mechanism of protection provided by hemoglobin AS. The expression of the heme oxygenase I gene, Hmox1, is increased by plasma free hemoglobin. Heme oxygenase I has been shown to be protective in inflammatory disease.[38] The protection against severe malaria is due to the effect of carbon monoxide on signal transduction by binding iron in the prosthetic groups' effector molecules and the inhibition of heme release from hemoglobin. There is no decrease in parasitemia, but there is tolerance induced by heme oxygenase I production of CO. This mechanism could also explain the decrease in malaria mortality in the thalassemias and in G6PD deficiency.

Hemoglobin SS pathophysiology

Unlike homozygous hemoglobin C, which results in the crystallization of hemoglobin at normal oxygen tension, homozygous hemoglobin S results in hemoglobin polymerization at low oxygen tension. Polymerization can also occur at low pH and with temperature elevation. Hemoglobin S polymerization distorts the red cell membrane, disrupting the asymmetry found in the normal red cell membrane. When the red cell membrane loses its asymmetry,[39] phosphatidylserine is exposed on the surface of the red cell. This exposure leads to a hypercoagulable[40] state and activates the cellular elements of the blood and vascular endothelium. The distortion also leads to rigidity of the membrane and hemolysis. Hemolysis increases plasma red cell arginase and plasma free hemoglobin, depleting nitric oxide[41] and decreasing cyclic guanosine monophosphate. Hemolysis and red cell membrane instability increases red cell membrane microparticles in the plasma. These changes in the red cell membrane and the activation of cellular elements and the vascular endothelium account for many of the clinical findings in sickle cell disease. Other modifiers of sickle cell disease[42] include proteins S and C deficiency, α thalassemia,[43] fetal hemoglobin production, nutritional factors, as well as others that influence the phenotypic expression of sickle cell disease.

Sickle cell disease is both a vasculopathy, with red cell adhesion to the vascular endothelium, and a hemolytic anemia with plasma free hemoglobin and microparticles. As each of these pathologies has a separate disease manifestation, there has been a proposed "phenotypic" model of sickle cell disease in which one or the other of these features predominates. See Figure 11.1.

Hemoglobin S can polymerize in the presence of other hemoglobin variants as well as hemoglobin A. These combinations are referred to as *sickle cell disease* if they cause clinical symptoms or have the potential to cause symptoms. Hemoglobin S combined with hemoglobin C, $D^{Los\ Angeles}$, β thalassemia, O^{Arab}, or CHORI cause symptomatic sickle cell disease. The only common hemoglobin-inhibiting polymerization is hemoglobin F. The sickle phenotype is affected by coinheritance of α thalassemia[43] and by the level of hemoglobin F.[44]

The most common sickle combinations are SS, SC, S β ^{0}, and S β+ thalassemia. $β^0$ refers to a thalassemia major mutation, and $β+$ refers to a mutation in which there is decreased hemoglobin A production, with S being the dominant hemoglobin. It would be expected that S β+ thalassemia would be a relatively benign combination, but this is not necessarily true. There are at least 14 β+ mutations commonly occurring in African Americans.[26] The mutations produce a wide range of hemoglobin A concentrations in the red cell, determining the phenotypic expression of this combination.

Even though the genotype of homozygous S is the same, the phenotype is not.[45] There are many variables that influence the phenotype,[46] the level of fetal (F) hemoglobin and an α gene deletion being the two most common. However, there are biomarkers that could potentially change the phenotypic presentation of sickle cell disease. Biomarkers in sickle cell disease have been reviewed, and although there are over one hundred variables considered as possible biomarkers of severity, only the most commonly used laboratory tests are clinically relevant: complete blood count with reticulocyte count, renal and hepatic function testing, and urine albumin–creatinine ratios are the most useful.[47] Initial steps have been taken in genome-wide surveys to find single nucleotide polymorphisms associated with severity, but clinical relevance has not been found to be associated with most of these single nucleotide polymorphisms.[48]

It is usually not possible to predict the severity of a child's course with sickle cell disease. In a review of the data from the Cooperative Study of Sickle Cell Disease, pain, persistent leukocytosis, and anemia in children under the age of 24 months were associated with poor outcome in the long term.[49] Other predictors of poor outcome in sickle cell disease are an abnormal transcranial Doppler (TCD) velocity (predicting stroke in children homozygous for hemoglobin S or with S β^0 thalassemia) or an elevated tricuspid jet velocity on an echocardiogram in adults.

Clinical review of sickle cell disease/transfusion indications

Red cell transfusion has been a therapy for sickle cell disease for decades, becoming more prevalent since the institution of nucleic acid amplification technology (NAT), leukoreduction, and routine red cell phenotyping for transfusion. There are numerous indications for transfusion in children and adults with sickle cell disease. Reviewed are the most common indications for transfusion and a brief description of each.

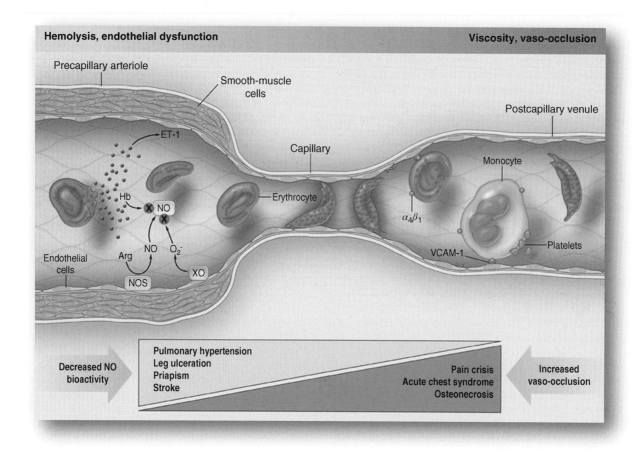

Figure 11.1 "Phenotypic" model of sickle cell disease.

Cerebrovascular disease (stroke)

Cerebral vascular disease is the most common indication for the transfusion of children with sickle cell disease. Stroke and cerebral vascular disease can be prevented by transfusion in children who have an abnormal transcranial Doppler. Children who have preexisting cerebral vascular disease at diagnosis will likely have progressive cerebral vascular disease. There is an increased risk of progressive hemorrhagic stroke in adults who are treated with chronic transfusion therapy for stroke.

Stroke prevention

Stroke risk for children with homozygous hemoglobin S is 200 times that for children without sickle cell anemia.[50] It is estimated that 10% of children will have a stroke before the age of 20 years. Stroke risk continues with age, with hemorrhagic stroke more common between the ages of 20 and 30 years.[51]

The STOP I study revealed that TCD screening beginning between two and three years of age in children with homozygous hemoglobin S or S β^0 thalassemia predicts increased risk of stroke. The institution of chronic red cell transfusion therapy for abnormal timed average mean maximum (TAMMv) can prevent brain injury.[52] Children with abnormal transcranial velocity (TAMMv >200 cm/sec) frequently have normal brain magnetic resonance imaging and angiography (MRI–MRA), but this does not indicate they are at decreased risk of stroke. The elevation of the TAMM velocity is proportional to the risk of stroke.[53] In the preliminary study leading to the STOP Study, there were strokes in children with TAMMv much less than 200 cm/sec.[54] It would be prudent to evaluate patients with MRI–MRA–Perfusion scans and treat patients with persistently elevated conditional TCD TAMMv with either hydroxyurea (no findings on MR study) or chronic red cell transfusion (findings on MR study). Patients with cerebral vascular pathology should be transfused for life. Children who have normal TCD studies cannot be considered at no risk for stroke as MRI–MRA studies have shown ischemia and cerebral vascular disease in these children as well.[55] See Table 11.3.

Once instituted, transfusion therapy should not be discontinued abruptly. The STOP II study was discontinued by the data safety monitoring board due to an increased rate of stroke and reversion to abnormal TCD in the non-transfused group.[56] The early events in

Table 11.3 Transcranial Doppler Screening

	TAMMv[1]	Treatment	Imaging
Normal	<170 cm/sec	Screen annually	Follow[2]
Conditional	≥170 cm/sec	Institute transfusion therapy	Brain MRI–MRA–perfusion scan
Abnormal	≥200 cm/sec	Institute transfusion therapy	Brain MRI–MRA–perfusion scan

[1] Timed average mean maximum velocity per STOP I study.
[2] Consider MRI–MRA at age five years to screen for occult ischemic or cerebral vascular disease per the SIT study.

this study may have been related to reticulocytosis following the discontinuation of transfusion, although this has not been documented.

Children who appear normal on physical examination and by history are at risk for so-called *silent stroke* or occult cerebral infarct.[57] Thirty percent of children with homozygous hemoglobin S will have evidence of occult infarct on MRI.[58] There is an undefined increased risk of stroke or increased occult infarcts in these children, even if they have a normal TCD. The risk of stroke in children with preexisting occult cerebral ischemia was studied in the SIT Study (Silent Cerebral Infarct Multi-Center Clinical Trial).[59] In this study, it was shown that the risk of a further increase in size (3 mm or more) of the initial area of ischemia, or of stroke, was reduced by 58% in the transfusion arm compared to the control arm. This would mean that 13 patients would have to be treated for three years to prevent one event. The optimum age and frequency for screening with MRI for occult ischemic injury are not known. By six years of age, the prevalence of brain ischemia is 27%. TCD as well as an MRI at MRI at age five years and further MRI–MRA–Perfusion scans if the child demonstrated soft neurologic signs or had decreased academic achievement at school.

A preliminary study indicated there was an association between mildly elevated blood pressures, anemia, and silent infarct.[60] Children who have abnormal sleep studies with obstructive or central apnea are at increased risk for stroke.[61] Overall, children with hemoglobin SS have a cumulative risk of cerebral vascular disease of 49.9% by the age of 14 years.[62]

Stroke risk is increased for at least two weeks following an episode of acute chest syndrome. Posterior leukoencephalopathy has been reported with acute chest syndrome[63] and is associated with blood transfusion, corticosteroid administration, and fluid overload with hypertension. Blood pressures for patients with sickle cell disease are lower than normal.[64] Blood pressure should be closely monitored in patients who are receiving blood transfusion for acute chest syndrome or another catastrophic event requiring red cell transfusion.

The STOP studies showed that stroke risk is decreased and acute strokes can be prevented by chronic red cell transfusion therapy. There is evidence that preexisting cerebral vascular disease is progressive in spite of appropriate chronic red cell transfusion therapy.[65,66] The TWiTCH Study revealed that, in selected patients, switching from transfusion to hydroxyurea did not lead to an increase in the TAMMv on transcranial Doppler compared to transfusion. The study did not show that there was equal protection from stroke with this change in therapy.

Secondary stroke prevention

Overt stroke has become less common in children and young adults since the institution of transcranial Doppler screening. Chronic transfusion therapy is not completely protective for progressive cerebral vascular disease and stroke[66] that is present when transfusion therapy is initiated. Children and adults who have severe brain injury following a completed stroke should be placed on transfusion for life. Red cell exchange can eliminate or decrease iron burden in patients with overt stroke on chronic transfusion.[67] It should be the preferred method for chronic transfusion therapy for secondary prevention of stroke. The SWITCH study would suggest that patients who have overt stroke or cerebral vascular disease are more likely to have a good outcome with transfusion and chelation versus hydroxyurea and phlebotomy.[68]

Transfusion

The goal of transfusion therapy is to decrease hemoglobin S by dilution in simple transfusion and by removal of affected cells and replacement in red cell exchange. For acute events, the *post*-transfusion percentage of hemoglobin S is optimally less than 30%. During chronic transfusion, the goal for the *pre*transfusion hemoglobin S is between 30 and 35%. The hemoglobin should not be above 11 g/dl with simple transfusion. With red cell exchange, the goal for hemoglobin should be 9 g/dl, which in some patients will lead to a reduction in iron overload. Red cell exchange is the preferred initial treatment for acute stroke.

Ophthalmologic complications

Transfusion is indicated for retinal arterial occlusion with visual loss, particularly if blindness is a possibility. Transfusion for invasive retinal surgery is indicated. Laser therapy for routine management of sickle cell vascular retinopathy does not require transfusion, although patients with severe sickle retinopathy with visual loss should be considered for transfusion. Hemoglobin SC patients would require red cell exchange transfusion.

The incidence of retinopathy is the greatest in hemoglobin SC disease (33%) and S β[0] thalassemia (13%), and lowest in homozygous S (3%).[69] Over the age of 30 years, 43% of SC patients and 13% of SS patients will have retinopathy. Hyphemia[70] is a medical emergency in both sickle cell disease and sickle cell trait causing glaucoma and blindness. Retinal artery occlusion,[71] suspected or confirmed, is an indication for transfusion.

Transfusion

Transfusion is initiated until a definitive diagnosis is determined and a long-term care plan made. Retinal arterial occlusion is an indication for chronic transfusion therapy. Patients with hemoglobin SC or SS with elevated hemoglobin are transfused by red cell exchange. The percentage of hemoglobin S should be less than 40%, and for SC it is convenient to use a goal of hemoglobin A greater than 60%.

Respiratory disease[72]

There is no indication for transfusion for obstructive or restrictive lung disease in patients with sickle cell disease. Severely anemic adults who have restrictive lung disease may benefit from transfusion to improve oxygenation. Obstructive or central sleep apnea are risk factors for stroke. Transfusion for central sleep apnea depends on the clinical assessment. Echocardiography should be performed to evaluate for pulmonary hypertension, and nighttime oxygen administration should be considered.

Children and adults with sickle cell disease are at increased risk for obstructive restrictive lung disease and asthma.[73] Asthma is a risk factor for acute chest syndrome and for stroke.[74] Children frequently present with both restrictive and obstructive disease[75] on pulmonary function testing without symptoms. Nitric oxide depletion occurs in both sickle cell disease and asthma.[76] Treatment for asthma is recommended for children with sickle cell disease who have a history of acute chest syndrome and abnormal pulmonary function testing.[72] Children and adults with respiratory disease would benefit from hydroxyurea therapy to reduce the incidence of acute chest syndrome.

Tonsillectomy and adenoidectomy for sleep apnea with hypoxia are considered high-risk surgeries, and preoperative transfusion is indicated.[77] A sleep study will determine whether nocturnal hypoxia is persistent in a patient who has had a tonsillectomy and adenoidectomy.[78] Nocturnal oxygen administration should be instituted, and the patient evaluated for pulmonary hypertension. In the absence of severe anemia, transfusion is not indicated for patients with abnormal pulmonary function testing.

Cardiopulmonary: pulmonary hypertension and acute chest syndrome

Transfusion for acute chest syndrome can be lifesaving. Transfusion for pulmonary hypertension may be indicated if treatment with sildenafil is considered, as there is an association between the use of sildenafil and increased pain in sickle cell disease. Transfusion alone may decrease pulmonary arterial pressure.

Pulmonary hypertension has been a known complication of sickle cell disease for over 30 years.[79] It is only recently[80] that pulmonary hypertension has become a major focus in the treatment of sickle cell disease. The interest has increased as the pathophysiology of pulmonary hypertension has become understood[81] and there are therapies for pulmonary hypertension that were not available previously. Screening by cardiac echocardiogram beginning at the age of 10–15 years is recommended. Adults who have pulmonary artery pressures estimated to be 25 mmHg (Trjet 2.5 m/sec.) have an increased risk of morbidity and mortality.[80] Patients with pulmonary artery pressures of 30 mmHg or higher should be considered for cardiac catheterization to determine true pulmonary hypertension.[82] If it is determined that a patient has elevated pulmonary pressures with increased pulmonary artery vascular resistance, they are considered for treatment. Sildenafil (a phosphodiesterase type 5 inhibitor) was shown to increase pain episodes in patients with sickle cell disease during the Walk PHaSST Study, which was terminated by the US National Institutes of Health. Treatment has not been studied beyond sildenafil alone. One study of bosentan showed that this therapy was well tolerated in sickle cell disease.[83]

A recent study[82] has shown that the incidence of cardiac catheterization-proven pulmonary hypertension is much less frequent than estimated by echocardiogram. In this study, those patients who were diagnosed as having pulmonary hypertension were older, had increased six-minute walk, increased N-terminal pro brain natriuretic peptide, and evidence of increased hemolysis. Only 1.5% of 398 patients had increased pulmonary arterial resistance, and only 24 had evidence of pulmonary hypertension by capillary wedge pressure. It is not known what significance elevated echocardiographic tricuspid-regurgitation jet velocity is in pediatric patients. In adult patients, it is a risk factor for morbidity and mortality.

Transfusion[84]

For documented pulmonary artery hypertension, transfusion alone has been successful in reducing pulmonary artery pressures in some cases.[85] Sildenafil could be added to transfusion if transfusion therapy was not effective. In pediatric patients, hydroxyurea has been found to be effective in a small study.[86] There is no consensus as to the optimal therapy for documented pulmonary hypertension. Aspirin has been recommended for splenectomized patients to prevent pulmonary hypertension due to platelet aggregation in the lungs. There have been no studies of the effectiveness of aspirin for this indication.

Acute chest syndrome

Acute chest syndrome[87] accounts for about 25% of hospital admissions and is a leading cause of death in sickle cell disease. Recurrent episodes of acute chest syndrome can cause lung scarring leading to restrictive lung disease in children and adults with sickle cell disease. Obstructive[75] pulmonary disease is common when pulmonary function is formally evaluated. Children and adolescents may not have symptoms of obstructive disease. Asthma is a risk factor for acute chest syndrome.[72] Acute chest syndrome is a risk factor for encephalopathy[88] and stroke.[89] Acute chest syndrome can develop within 72 hours of a painful event in adults. Elevated phospholipase A2, in conjunction with fever and respiratory symptoms, predicts acute chest syndrome, and expectant transfusion may arrest its development.[90,91]

The National Acute Chest Syndrome Study Group reviewed the common features and evaluation of acute chest syndrome in sickle cell disease.[87]

- Patients should be continuously monitored, and transfusion should be considered if there is a new infiltrate and oxygen saturation is less than 90–95%.
- Chest pain and low oxygen saturation, without infiltrate, should be the threshold for considering pulmonary emboli as a cause of these symptoms.

Transfusion

For patients who present with acute chest syndrome and severe anemia, simple transfusion may be sufficient to increase oxygenation and reduce risk of more severe disease. Hyperviscosity and hypervolemia can complicate simple transfusion.[92] Patients who present with an elevated hemoglobin (8 g/dl or higher) should receive an exchange transfusion as the initial therapy. Neurologic changes[63] during acute chest syndrome are more frequent in adults and are an indication for exchange transfusion as stroke risk is increased during, as well as following, an episode of acute chest syndrome. There is an association between blood transfusion, corticosteroid use, and stroke/posterior leukoencephalopathy, usually precipitated by hypertension.

Red cell exchange transfusion

Red cell exchange transfusion[93] is the safest and most effective method of transfusion for severe acute chest syndrome. It provides for isovolumetric red cell exchange without changes in viscosity. The end hematocrit and percentage of hemoglobin S are predictably obtained. The transfusion goal should be a reduction in the percentage of hemoglobin S to 30% or less with an end hematocrit of 9–10 g/dl. Ventilated patients should have an end hematocrit of 10 g/dl.

Chronic transfusion for six months following a severe episode of acute chest syndrome is reasonable therapy. Hydroxyurea should be considered for all patients who have had an episode of acute chest syndrome, particularly if they have obstructive lung disease.[72]

Immune dysfunction/sepsis risk

Children and adults who are septic frequently have a precipitous drop in their hemoglobin. Patients who appear septic should have a type and screen at presentation in the event they need an emergent transfusion.

Infection remains the most common cause of death at all ages in sickle cell disease.[94] Patients with sickle cell disease have decreased ability to opsonize bacteria,[95] and 95% of children homozygous for hemoglobin S develop functional asplenia[96] by the age of five years. Functional asplenia occurs in hemoglobin SC at an older age with much higher PITT counts.[97] The incidence of infection is greatest in infancy and early childhood, then decreases with age. The effect of pneumococcal vaccine[98] and penicillin prophylaxis[99] has decreased the incidence of death from overwhelming pneumococcal sepsis in sickle cell disease. Children with sickle cell disease are more likely to have bacteremia[100] with acute chest syndrome, they are at risk for pyelonephritis and urosepsis, and they have an increased incidence of osteomyelitis[101] with salmonella. Children with sickle cell disease can appear deceptively nontoxic with infections that prove fatal.

Transfusion

In the absence of multiorgan failure, simple transfusion to maintain the hemoglobin between 9 and 10 g/dl is recommended. Severe sepsis with multiorgan failure would be an indication for red cell exchange to decrease the percentage of hemoglobin S to 30% with an end hemoglobin of 9 to 10 g/dl.

Renal disease

Transfusion for renal disease would include patients with declining renal function and anemia and patients with a kidney transplant. Priapism has not been reported to respond to transfusion.

Renal disease is common in children and adults with sickle cell disease.[102] Total renal blood flow is increased in sickle cell disease due to anemia, with hyperfiltration present in infants by about one year of age. Microalbuminuria is present in about 30% of adolescents. The inability to concentrate urine (hyposthenuria) is extremely common in sickle cell disease, and it has been reported to be reversed in childhood with chronic transfusion therapy. Both proximal and distal tubular disease is present in patients with sickle cell disease. Distal tubule dysfunction causes a mild renal tubular acidosis. Proximal tubular disease causes an increase in tubular secretion making creatinine a poor indicator of glomerular filtration rate. Microscopic hematuria is common, frank bleeding can follow renal papillary necrosis. Blood loss from renal papillary necrosis may appear to be severe, but it generally does not require transfusion. An uncommon complication of papillary necrosis is hydronephrosis due to ureter obstruction.

Renal findings in sickle cell disease include:
- Decreased ability to concentrate urine;
- Decreased ability to excrete potassium;
- Inability to lower urine pH; and
- Hematuria/papillary necrosis.
  Risk factors for renal failure include:
- Anemia, proteinuria, and hematuria.

Acute renal failure can occur in sickle cell disease during episodes of sepsis and multiorgan failure. Rhabdomyolysis can occur with dehydration and has been described during acute painful episodes. Exchange transfusion and dialysis are lifesaving.

Priapism

Priapism is a common symptom in sickle cell disease.[103] It is estimated that as many as 40% of males will have an episode of priapism during childhood and adolescence, but the actual incidence is unknown. Priapism leads to permanent ischemic damage and impotence.[104] Severe priapism prognosticates a more severe course of sickle cell disease.[104] Priapism may be induced by hemolysis.[105] There are no reports of priapism in the setting of delayed hemolytic transfusion reactions (DHTRs) or other settings of hemolysis.

Transfusion

Transfusions, both simple and exchange, have not been shown to have an effect on acute priapism.[106] There have been reports of neurologic events when treating priapism with exchange transfusion[107] due to increased viscosity and fluid overload. Patients with a renal allograft should have either simple or exchange transfusion for graft protection. The hemoglobin should be kept between 9 and 10 g/dl with a percentage of hemoglobin S between 30 and 40%.[108]

Gastrointestinal

There is no indication for transfusion as nutritional support for patients who have growth or pubertal delay. Transfusion for children or adults who have hepatic disease may be indicated.

Common gastrointestinal complications in sickle cell disease are cholelithiasis, cholecystitis, choledocholithiasis, hepatic sequestration, and intestinal ischemia.[109] Surgical emergencies occur as frequently in sickle cell disease as in other populations.

Hepatic disease is relatively common in sickle cell disease.[110] The pathology includes viral hepatitis, hepatic sequestration, hepatic iron injury, and intrahepatic cholestasis.[111] During hepatic sequestration, the transaminases are elevated as well as the bilirubin, and the ALT (alanine aminotransferase) can remain elevated for several weeks. Overtransfusion in hepatic sequestration has led to hyperviscosity morbidity.[112] Intrahepatic cholestasis is a rare complication of sickle cell disease. Exchange transfusion has been successful in some cases.[113] Liver biopsy is contraindicated in the presence of hepatic congestion and coagulopathy. Elevation of bilirubin above 13 mg/dl with a predominantly direct component can be a sign of intrahepatic cholestasis, a sometimes fatal complication of sickle cell disease.[111] Bilirubin levels greater than 30 mg/dl or higher can lead to hepatorenal syndrome and death.

Transfusion

The most common surgical diagnosis in patients with sickle cell disease is cholelithiasis.[114] The complications of this surgery have been reported.[115] Red cell exchange transfusion may be effective for intrahepatic cholestasis.

Skeletal (avascular necrosis/osteomyelitis)

There is no indication for transfusion for avascular necrosis of bone. Hyperviscosity occurring during simple transfusion could, theoretically, contribute to avascular necrosis. Microparticle formation has been implicated in avascular necrosis.[116]

Bone in sickle cell[101] disease is a major area of pathology. Bone infarcts are perhaps the most common source of severe acute pain in patients with sickle cell disease. Infarcts can cause nerve compression,[117] digital shortening following dactylitis, and avascular necrosis of both the shoulders and the hips. Rib infarcts[118] are thought to contribute to acute chest syndrome, sternal infarcts are common, and the vertebral bodies [119] in sickle cell disease owe their peculiar shape to damage from necrosis.

Transfusion

Hip replacement is the most common orthopedic surgery in sickle cell disease.[120] Shoulder replacement is much less common.[121] Simple transfusion is recommended in the absence of elevated hemoglobin, in which case a red cell exchange could be considered.

Integument (skin ulcers)

Transfusion has been used to increase oxygenation for patients with chronic skin ulcers. There is better therapy for treatment, although transfusion following skin grafting could be helpful to decrease microvascular occlusion.

The most common problem of the skin in sickle cell disease is skin ulcers.[122] They are usually due to skin trauma, not recalled by the patient. There may be a relationship between skin ulceration and hydroxyurea in adult patients.[123]

Transfusion

Blood transfusion has been used in the treatment of skin ulceration. There are anecdotal reports of other therapies:[124] vascular flaps,[125] special dressings,[126] and arginine butyrate.[127]

Hematologic (severe anemia)

Children and adults with anemia and a low reticulocyte count due to infection or other cause may benefit from transfusion. Children with parvovirus infection require transfusion if they have severe anemia with an inadequate reticulocyte count. Splenic and hepatic sequestration require transfusion.

Sickle cell anemia and sickle β^0 thalassemia can have significant anemia. Patients with sickle β thalassemia have microcytosis, making the diagnosis of iron deficiency problematic.[128] A one or two α gene deletion (always *trans* in African Americans) will lead to microcytosis. Patients with severe anemia (hemoglobin of 5 g/dl or less) should be transfused to improve oxygen delivery and prevent complications of anemia. Chronic anemia results in a vascular overloaded state, and transfusion should be performed cautiously. Patients otherwise well with a brisk reticulocyte count and safe hemoglobin can be monitored. Other etiologies of anemia should be considered.

A child presenting with an enlarged spleen or liver is diagnostic of splenic or hepatic sequestration: Both are life-threatening. Parvovirus is the next most common etiology of acute anemia in children.

Overtransfusion can lead to hyperviscosity and morbidity when treating sequestration; blood may be released from the congested organ, increasing the hematocrit to dangerously high levels. Children who have life-threatening splenic sequestration should be transfused on a monthly basis to prevent recurrence and should have a laparoscopic splenectomy as soon as they have been fully immunized. There is significant morbidity in children who have hepatic sequestration. Hepatorenal syndrome should be entertained as a possible complication.[129]

Transfusion

Simple transfusion is indicated for anemia due to parvovirus aplastic anemia. Cautious transfusion for sequestration with a target hemoglobin of 8–9 g/dl is the safest approach to these patients.

Surgery

It has been shown in a prospective randomized trial that transfusion prior to surgery decreases morbidity and mortality.

Surgery is common in sickle cell disease.[114] Cholelithiasis and osteonecrosis are the most common indications for surgery. Patients with sickle cell disease have many risk factors for morbidity during surgery: Acute chest syndrome is the most common, and some patients may have stroke risk, although stroke as a complication of surgery is uncommon. Hyposthenuria can lead to dehydration in the sickle cell patients awaiting surgery. Rhabdomyolysis can occur due to dehydration and prolonged positioning during surgery. Pain management is not usually a problem following surgery. Transfusion is the standard of care for surgery with a prolonged anesthesia time. Surgery that has a long anesthesia time leads to atelectasis, increasing the risk of acute chest syndrome postoperatively.

Transfusion guidelines for surgery have been reported for the general patient with sickle cell disease, but not for patients who have comorbid conditions.[77,130,120] Surgical procedures can be classified as low, medium, and high risk.

- *Low (transfusion not indicated)*: Eyes (laser for retinopathy), skin (minor, biopsy), nose, ears (tympanostomy tubes), and dental (when anesthesia is less than one hour, or conscious sedation or local analgesia is used);
- *Medium to high*: Head and neck with possible airway edema (tonsillectomy-adenoidectomy), genitourinary system, and intraabdominal (laparoscopic) (when the general anesthesia is more than one hour); and
- *High*: intracranial, vertebral, cardiovascular, and intrathoracic, or the anesthesia is greater than four hours.

  Preoperative: Hydration when NPO (*nil per os*), transfusion, teaching the use of the incentive spirometer, and expectations for care following surgery.[131] Undiagnosed asthma is a common risk factor for perioperative complications. Therefore, screening for bronchoreactive lung disease and preventative use of bronchodilators is recommended. Blood transfusion to a hemoglobin of 10 g/dl is recommended for medium and high-risk surgeries to prevent complications.[132] For hemoglobin SC or other sickle cell disease patients with hemoglobin 10 g/dl or higher, exchange transfusion should be considered, particularly in patients with hemoglobin SS, S β0 thalassemia, and SC who are to have high-risk or prolonged procedures.
  Intraoperative:[133] Warm room, warm blood, and meticulous fluid management.
  Postoperatively: Pain management, fluid management, and evaluation of any respiratory or neurologic symptoms. Incentive spirometry every 2 hours, and oxygen therapy to maintain oxygen saturation over 95%. Common postoperative complications of surgery include:[134]
- Acute chest syndrome;
- Fluid overload;
- Alloimmunization;
- Rhabdomyolysis; and
- Neurologic complications.

Pain

Transfusion as an intervention for an acute, uncomplicated, pain episode has not been studied. For patients who have chronic pain, a trial of transfusion may allow patients to be pain free while they are withdrawn from pain medications and learning other coping skills. It is not recommended that patients be maintained on both transfusion and opioid medications for pain unless there is a physiologic indication such as avascular necrosis.

Pain is the pathognomonic symptom of sickle cell disease.[135] Pain in sickle cell disease is not necessarily sickle cell vaso-occlusive pain.

Acute pain that *is* sickle cell related includes:

- Acute painful episodes;
- Acute chest syndrome;
- Priapism;
- Cholecystitis (ascending cholangitis);
- Dactylitis;
- Left upper quadrant pain: splenic sequestration/infarct;
- Right upper quadrant pain: hepatic sequestration;
- Skin ulcer (even before skin breakdown);
- Pain with internal rotation of the hip: early avascular necrosis of hip; and
- Pain with arm extension: shoulder avascular necrosis.

Chronic pain that *is* sickle cell related includes:

- Avascular (osteo) necrosis (non-acute);
- Arthropathies (vertebral infarcts/collapse);
- Leg ulcers (chronic);
- Chronic osteomyelitis;
- Intractable chronic pain; and
- Neuropathic pain.

Transfusion

A fall in hemoglobin and hyperhemolysis can occur during painful events in patients with sickle cell disease.[136] Transfusion should be judicially used in the event of anemia occurring during a painful episode. Transfusion can be used during a period of weaning from chronic pain medication. It is not recommended to treat chronic pain with both transfusion and opioid.

Pregnancy[137]

There is controversy concerning transfusion during pregnancy. Studies have shown there is little to no benefit to the fetus, but that mothers have less painful events when transfused during the latter half of pregnancy compared to nontransfused women with sickle cell disease.[138] Pregnancy carries a high risk for the mother and fetus compared to normal women. Maternal complications occur even in the chronically transfused patient. Chronic transfusion should be considered for all women during pregnancy.

Some young women do relatively well with pregnancy,[139] but generally there is an increase in morbidity.[140] Pregnancy-related complications occur more frequently in women with hemoglobin SS. Transfusion has been offered to women in the last trimester of pregnancy, but should be offered early if there is any comorbidity. There is no indication that this improves fetal outcome, but it does decrease complications for the mother.[141–143] A recent study of partial exchange transfusions during pregnancy revealed that, even with transfusion, there is still an increase in morbidity for women with sickle cell disease during pregnancy.[144] Some studies have shown that red cell exchange transfusion significantly decreases morbidity and mortality during pregnancy.[138,145]

Transfusion

Transfusions for complications of pregnancy are indicated to prevent morbidity and mortality. Consider prophylactic simple red cell transfusion during pregnancy. Red cell exchange may provide an additional benefit. See Table 11.4.

Table 11.4 Sickle Cell Disease Indications for Transfusion

Cerebral Vascular Disease	
Stroke prevention	Transfusion by simple or red cell exchange for cerebral vascular disease, occult brain ischemia, abnormal TCD
Secondary stroke prevention	Transfusion by simple or red cell exchange for stroke
Ophthalmologic complications	Transfusion for arterial infarct
Respiratory disease	No indication for transfusion
Cardiopulmonary disease	
Pulmonary hypertension	Red cell exchange for catheterization proven pulmonary hypertension
Acute chest syndrome	Simple transfusion for low hemoglobin, red cell exchange if clinically severe or for elevated hemoglobin at presentation
Immune dysfunction sepsis	Simple transfusion for severe anemia
Renal disease	Consider transfusion for severe anemia
Priapism	Transfusion not proven effective
Skeletal	Transfusion not effective
Integument	Consider transfusion for severe anemia
Severe anemia	
Parvoviral infection	Simple transfusion for anemia
Splenic sequestration	Simple transfusion
Hyperhemolysis	Avoid transfusion if possible
Surgery	Transfusion to hemoglobin of 10 g/dl
Pain	Transfusion not proven to be effective
Pregnancy	Role for transfusion, red cell exchange may be beneficial

Thalassemia

The thalassemias are the most common monogenetic diseases worldwide.[146] These syndromes are classified according to whether the mutation causing the defect affects the α globin gene cluster or the β globin gene cluster. There is one β globin gene cluster on each chromosome 11 (β/β). Duplicated α gene clusters occur on chromosome 16 (αα/αα). Mutations in the globin genes reduce or eliminate the synthesis of the respective globin molecule. The majority of α gene mutations are deletional, although structural mutations occur. There are about 100 α gene mutations reported. β globin mutations are primarily point mutations leading to absent β globin synthesis (β^0 mutations) or decreased β globin synthesis (β^+ mutations). There are well over 200 β globin gene mutations. Structural variants of the globin genes can lead to thalassemic gene combinations. There are also deletions of β globin regulatory elements and of the other genes in the β globin cluster that lead to changes in expression of the gamma globin gene (HPFH). The β globin gene cluster is also regulated by genes on distant chromosomes such as BCL11A, KLF1, and others.

β Thalassemia[147]

β thalassemia presents with a diverse phenotype. Among this group are individuals who do not require regular transfusion but do require intermittent transfusion during illness, and individuals who require lifelong chronic transfusion therapy. The goal of transfusion is normal growth and development and the prevention of complications of ineffective erythropoiesis. Iron accumulation from transfusion and/or ineffective erythropoiesis is a major problem for patients with β thalassemia.

The major predictor of the β thalassemic phenotype is the α/β-globin chain imbalance with more severe disease in those genotypes with excess α globin and decreased β globin production. A β-gene heterozygote predicted not to require transfusion might require transfusions due to duplicated or triplicated α-genes leading to a greater α/β gene imbalance than expected.

The β thalassemias can be classified into four general categories: silent carrier, trait/thalassemia minor, thalassemia intermedia, and thalassemia major. β thalassemia carriers have no hematologic abnormalities, but do have elevated hemoglobin A2 on hemoglobin electrophoresis. Those with β thalassemia trait (β thalassemia minor) have elevated A2 as well as mild anemia and microcytosis. They do not require red cell transfusion. β thalassemia intermedia presents late with variable levels of anemia and is of the non-transfusion-dependent-thalassemia (NTDT) phenotype. Some mutations with this phenotype will go on to chronic transfusions due to the severity of their anemia or complications of their disease. β thalassemia major presents early and is transfusion dependent.

A common structural mutation occurring in combination with β^0 mutations is hemoglobin E.[148] Hemoglobin E is structurally abnormal, and the mutation causes abnormal RNA processing leading to decreased hemoglobin production. Hemoglobin E/β^0 thalassemia can be grouped into three types: severe with very low hemoglobin production (4–5 g/dl), moderate (hemoglobin 6–7 g/dl), and mild with hemoglobin levels in the 9–12 g/dl range. These phenotypes are influenced by the β^0 mutation, the production of fetal hemoglobin and α-genotype. Patients with the most severe phenotype require lifelong chronic transfusion.

Regularly transfused patients with thalassemia have complications that are primarily due to the increased absorption of iron from the gastrointestinal tract and iron derived from chronic transfusion.[149] The NTDT group has morbidity associated with ineffective erythropoiesis and splenectomy. The decision to begin transfusion should be considered after careful assessment of the genotype and the presentation over several months. Transfusion may not be necessary in some NTDT patients in childhood, but a transfusion requirement may develop in adulthood. Due to gastrointestinal absorption of iron, many NTDT patients will require chelation in the absence of transfusion.

Transfusion goals for β thalassemia

Even with identical genotypes, the baseline hemoglobin for the β thalassemia syndromes is not predictable. The baseline hemoglobin should be established for each child prior to the initiation of transfusion therapy. If the baseline is below 6 or 7 g/dl, chronic transfusion therapy should be initiated. The goal for transfusion-dependent β thalassemia is a pretransfusion hemoglobin of 9 to 10 g/dl, which requires transfusion every month in infants and young children, increasing to every three weeks in adults.[150] Patients who have an annual transfusion requirement of greater than 200 ml/kg/year should be evaluated to determine if their transfusion requirement can be reduced. If not splenectomized, they may have hypersplenism or be overtransfused to hemoglobin levels higher than necessary. Chelation becomes increasingly difficult with intensive transfusion therapy. (See Table 11.5.)

α Thalassemia[151]

The majority of patients with α thalassemia syndromes will not require chronic transfusion therapy. Exceptions are those patients with hemoglobin H constant spring and surviving infants with hydrops fetalis. Intermittent transfusions are more common in these diseases.

Table 11.5 Simple Transfusion versus Non-transfusion-Dependent Thalassemia (NTDT)[156] Complications

Chronic Transfusion	NTDT
Hypothyroidism	Silent cerebral infarct
Hypoparathyroidism	Pulmonary hypertension
Left heart failure: cardiac hemosiderosis	Hepatic fibrosis and cirrhosis
Hepatic failure	Hepatocellular carcinoma
Viral hepatitis	Splenomegaly
Diabetes mellitus	Thrombophilia
Hypogonadism	Extramedullary hematopoiesis
Osteoporosis	Osteoporosis
	Skin ulcers
Complications due to transfusion or dietary hemosiderosis and thrombophilia	

Single-gene deletions (−α/αα) are not detectable without α gene mapping. Alpha gene mutations that occur in *trans* (−α/−α) or *cis* (−−/αα) are indistinguishable hematologically and are frequently referred to as *α thalassemia traits*. Single mutations on the same gene are a$^+$ thalassemia mutations. Two common mutations are the 3.7 and 4.2 deletions. The case in which both genes are deleted on the same chromosome is the α^0 thalassemia mutations. A common α^0 thalassemia mutation is the SEA deletion, $--^{SEA}/\alpha\alpha$. Nondeletional mutations may occur as single mutations or in combination (−α/αNDα). These combinations can be detected on the complete blood count with microcytosis and occasionally mild anemia. The combinations by themselves do not require transfusion and are referred to as the *α thalassemia trait*.

Combinations of α^0 thalassemia and α^+ thalassemia can lead to a phenotype requiring red cell transfusions on an intermittent basis or chronically. Hemoglobin H disease (−α/−−) is the most common α^0 thalassemia-α^+ thalassemia combination.[152] It is rare that patients with hemoglobin H require transfusions, but transfusion may be needed during illness. Hemoglobin H disease manifests with a mild anemia and splenomegaly. In contrast, hemoglobin H constant spring ($--/\alpha^{CS}\alpha$) is a much more severe disease with anemia, requiring intermittent or chronic transfusion and occasionally occurring early in life. Most patients will develop hypersplenism and thrombophilia. Thrombosis following splenectomy is common in this nondeletional form of hemoglobin H disease. Later in life, cholelithiasis and skin ulcers can occur. Both hemoglobin H disease and H constant spring are in the NTDT group of thalassemias, although some H constant spring patients will require frequent or chronic transfusions later in life.[153]

The most severe form of α thalassemia is Bart's hydrops fetalis ($--^{SEA}/--^{SEA}$). The affected embryo develops severe hypoxia in the third trimester and will not survive without intrauterine transfusions or exchange transfusion at birth. Other a^0 thalassemia mutations may cause fetal demise earlier in gestation. These infants require chronic transfusion therapy or progenitor cell transplantation if they survive.

Monitoring during acute illness and simple red cell transfusion for severe anemia is needed in patients with hemoglobin H disease and hemoglobin H constant spring. For those patients requiring chronic transfusion, the goal should be a pretransfusion hemoglobin of between 9 and 10 g/dl. (See Table 11.6.)

Transfusion methods

Red cell product

A red cell antigen phenotype and/or genotype is obtained prior to transfusion with the purpose of identifying absent red cell antigens

Table 11.6 Clinical Severity Beta Thalassemia and Alpha Thalassemia

Phenotype	Genotype	Clinical Severity
Beta Thalassemia		
Silent carrier	β^0/β, β^+/β	Asymptomatic
Trait/thalassemia minor	β^0/β, β^+/β	Microcytosis
Intermedia	Combinations of β^0, β^+ alone or in combination with gene duplications, deletional forms of $\delta\beta$ thalassemia, increased γ production, or $\delta\beta$ thalassemia and HPFH and $E\beta^0$ thalassemia	Late presentation Mild to moderate anemia May be transfusion dependent or independent
Thalassemia major	β^0/β^0, β^0/β^+, β^+/β^+, β^+/β^0	Early presentation Severe Transfusion dependent
Alpha Thalassemia		
Silent carrier	$-\alpha/\alpha\alpha$	Asymptomatic
Trait/minor	$-\alpha/-\alpha$, $--/\alpha\alpha$	Microcytic, hypochromic
Hemoglobin H: deletional	$--/-\alpha$	Mild to moderate anemia Transfusion independent Variable severity Usually moderate severity
Hemoglobin H: nondeletional	$--/-\alpha^{ND}$	Moderate severity Transfusions possible
Major (Bart's hydrops fetalis)	$--/--$	Possibly nonviable Immediate transfusion Chronic transfusion

in order to provide antigen-negative red cells for transfusion; this is done as soon as possible before the first transfusion. Common antigens causing alloimmunization are: D, E, e, C, c, K, k, Jk^a, Jk^b, Fy^a, Fy^b, S, s, M, N, Le^a, and Le^b.[154] It is recommended these antigens be phenotyped at a minimum. Genotype is predetermined by the platform used. This information will guide investigations when an alloantibody is suspected. Using partially phenotypically matched red cells for Rh (D, C, c, E, e) and Kell antigen significantly decreases incidence of alloimmunization.[155] Alloimmunization is reduced in sickle cell disease from 30% to less than 3%. For thalassemia, the age of beginning transfusion influences the rate of alloimmunization, with children beginning transfusion before one year of age having less alloimmunization (11% vs. 30%).[2] An antigen common in the Chinese thalassemia population is Mi^a, accounting for 30% of alloimmunization in Chinese thalassemia patients.[2] Other less common antigens can be involved in DHTRs, particularly in patients with sickle cell disease.

Sickle cell trait-negative blood products are recommended for sickle cell disease, although a patient with a rare phenotype could receive sickle trait-positive units when necessary.[154] Genotyping for the GATA box mutation seen in Fy^b can somewhat simplify the provision of phenotypically matched blood products. Silencing will preclude the need to honor this antigen. There may be a higher risk of Rh alloimmunization if using only African-American donors for sickle cell patients.[156] The blood provider should confirm phenotypes for chronically transfused patients rather than relying on historically antigen-negative units. Confirmation of the partial phenotype at the blood bank prior to being issued for transfusion is optional.

Testing for HIV; hepatitis A, B, and C; and liver function provides baseline prior to initiation of transfusion, particularly in older children, adults, and patients who have been previously transfused. Transfusion-transmitted disease testing should be repeated annually. Hepatitis screening should be repeated if there is a rise in transaminases. Immunize patients who do not have serologic evidence of infection or immunity for hepatitis B and hepatitis A. Patients with positive serology for hepatitis B or C infections should be followed for hepatocellular carcinoma.[157]

Leukoreduced products are indicated for all sickle cell and thalassemia patients. Red cells do not require irradiation for either thalassemia or sickle cell disease. Radiation damages the red cell membrane and shortens red cell survival. The only indication for irradiation is for patients who are immune suppressed or who will possibly have a progenitor cell transplant.[158] Cytomegalovirus (CMV) infections should be prevented in CMV seronegative patients, particularly those likely to receive a progenitor cell transplant and women who are pregnant. Units that have been leukocyte-reduced by the blood supplier are widely accepted to be efficacious; there is no demonstrated need to combine with seronegative units shown to lack antibody. There are extremely rare cases of window-period CMV donations from newly infected donors that can transmit CMV infection.[159] Red cells are not required to be washed unless the recipient has had a urticarial or other transfusion reaction that could conceivably be ameliorated by washed units. Transfusion of CMV negative units is recommended for transfusion during pregnancy.[160] Patients considered for a progenitor cell transplant and who are CMV negative should receive CMV-negative red cells. When a referred patient is recommended for transfusion therapy and the indication for transfusion is unclear, reassess the need for chronic transfusion in both sickle cell disease and thalassemia patients. Sickle cell disease patients may be able to be weaned to hydroxyurea, and thalassemia patients may fit the category of NTDT.

HLA-type full siblings of patients with chronically transfused sickle cell anemia and transfusion-dependent thalassemia all are candidates for progenitor cell transplantation.[161]

Simple transfusion

Simple transfusion is the only method of transfusion in thalassemia. Simple transfusion can be performed with a minimal amount of infrastructure. The volume for simple transfusion should be calculated for pediatric patients, and transfusion should not be by whole units. A simple method of calculating red cell requirement is: the desired hemoglobin minus the current hemoglobin, multiplying by a "transfusion factor" of 3/hematocrit of transfused red cells (3/Hct), and then by the weight of the patient in kilograms:

$$(Hgb^d - Hgb^c)(3/Hct)(Wt. \text{ in } Kg)$$
$$= \text{milliliters of red cells to transfuse.}^{162}$$

Red cell units can be "split" by the blood bank to conserve the blood supply. Overtransfusion can lead to hyperviscosity in patients with thalassemia or sickle cell disease, and has led to morbidity in both. Simple transfusion in patients with anemia leads to a mild volume overload that is tolerated by most patients, but it can lead to cardiac overload in older patients or those with cardiomyopathy that requires monitoring.[163] Diuretics should be considered if the transfused volume is greater than 20 ml/kg. The pretransfusion goal for chronically transfused thalassemia and sickle cell patients should be a hemoglobin of 9–10 g/dl. The goal for simple transfusion should be a posttransfusion hemoglobin of 11 g/dl for sickle cell anemia and of 12–13 g/dl for thalassemia. In sickle cell disease, the pretransfusion hemoglobin S should be <30% for patients who have cerebral vascular disease and <40% if transfusion is for other indications. Thalassemia major patients may require monthly transfusions as infants and children, whereas adult patients usually require transfusions at three-week intervals. Patients with sickle cell disease should be transfused on a monthly basis.

Red cell exchange

Red cell exchange is the preferred method of transfusion for sickle cell disease for chronic transfusion as well as emergent situations in which the percentage of hemoglobin S must be reduced rapidly and the patient is not severely anemic. Exchange transfusion is isovolumetric to avoid fluid overload, and can decrease iron accumulation in some patients. Exchange can be performed manually as phlebotomy and infusion with red cells diluted to a predetermined hematocrit or as an automated procedure using erythrocytapheresis.

Erythrocytapheresis

Automated red cell exchange is the preferred method for transfusion where it is available.[164] The posttransfusion hematocrit and percentage of hemoglobin S can be predictably achieved, and the procedure provides for a continuous isovolumetric red cell transfusion. For emergent situations, the percentage of hemoglobin S should be 30% with a hemoglobin between 9 and 10 g/dl. The procedure is safe, and very few adverse events have been reported. The barriers to automated red cell exchange are the infrastructure required, intravenous access, and the expertise of the medical staff to perform the procedure. Alloimmunization has been shown to be equal to or less than that of simple transfusion. Hypocalcemia is a possible problem that is easily corrected with infusions of calcium gluconate.

Central intravenous access is necessary for acute procedures. Double lumen dialysis catheters are used and placed in either the femoral vein or the internal jugular vein. Intravenous access is the major barrier to chronic transfusion by automated red cell exchange. Young children generally do not have venous access for red cell exchange and are not developmentally able to tolerate the procedure. Most children who are five years of age or older are able to cooperate with the procedure, and many will have peripheral intravenous access. Access by angiocatheter is preferable with an 18 gauge for adults and a 22 gauge for children. The flow rates recommended by the manufacturer should be used for the procedure.

In the absence of peripheral access, an implantable dialysis catheter[165] is required for chronic transfusion. Currently, these catheters are not available in a size for pediatric patients until they weigh between 30 and 40 kg. The current catheter requires a large noncoring needle, and the placement should be done as a sterile/clean procedure to prevent infection. Ideally, the catheter should only be used by the apheresis staff for red cell exchange. It is recommended to use 1000 u/ml heparin for heparin lock and to use TPA if there are any problems related to flow during a procedure.

Hypocalcemia can be avoided with the use of calcium gluconate infusion. Calcium gluconate diluted to 50 mg/ml is infused at 0.25–0.5 mg/kg/minute. Ionized calcium monitoring is to provide the optimum infusion rate initially and less frequently once a rate is established. A bolus of calcium gluconate for symptomatic hypocalcemia can be given: 250 mg over five minutes for adults and 5 mg/kg for children over five minutes.

The transfusion goal for erythrocytapheresis should be an end hematocrit of 27%. This will reduce the iron burden of patients who come to transfusion with higher hematocrits. Many patients will not need chelation, and the postexchange transfusion hematocrit can eventually be equal to the pretransfusion hematocrit. This is a practical goal for chronic transfusion where whole units are used and end hematocrit is easily obtained.

Transfusion using percentage of hemoglobin S (fraction of cells remaining [FCR]) should be used in acute situations where the initial percentage of hemoglobin S is estimated to be close to 100% and the percentage of hemoglobin S is required to be a low level, such as 30%. Large-volume exchanges should be done with monitoring of the ionized calcium and replacement with calcium gluconate.

Manual exchange transfusion

There is no universal standard for the performance of manual exchange transfusions.[166] This method is used in developed, resource-rich countries as well as resource-poor countries. Partial exchange transfusions have used a predetermined phlebotomy followed with simple transfusion or successive aliquots of whole blood being removed and replaced by whole blood diluted to a desired hematocrit with albumin or normal saline. Hypocalcemia can be a problem due to the citrate in the red cell preservation solution. It is recommended that the exchange transfusion be accomplished by exchanging 25–50% total blood volume and repeating if necessary to reach the desired percentage of hemoglobin S and hematocrit.

Transfusion monitoring

Although alloimmunization is reduced in patients who are transfused with partially phenotypically matched blood products, alloimmunization is not prevented. Suspected transfusion reactions should be pursued to determine whether alloimmunization has occurred. Autoantibodies are relatively common and are not prevented by providing phenotypically matched products. Autoantibodies are known to mask alloantibodies.

For sickle cell disease, it has been shown that a dedicated pool of African-American donors for patients requiring chronic transfusion may increase the rate of Rh alloimmunization.[156] Both the donors and recipients are likely to have Rh variant genes leading to a high rate of Rh alloimmunization. Almost 60% of patients transfused from African-American donors were alloimmunized in a recent study. The rate of Rh alloimmunization in chronically transfused patients was 45% versus 12% in the episodically transfused patients. High-resolution genotyping of donors and recipients may resolve this problem.

The mean pretransfusion hemoglobin for chronically transfused sickle cell disease should ideally be 9–9.5 g/dl. The hemoglobin post transfusion should not exceed 12 g/dl. Hemoglobin levels higher than 12 g/dl increase blood viscosity with the potential for increased morbidity.[167] Sickle cell patients receiving simple transfusions should be transfused at four-week intervals with the goal of a hemoglobin S percentage as close to 30% as possible prior to transfusion for stroke or stroke risk.[168] The optimal hemoglobin S percentage for other complications is not defined, but a goal of less than 45% hemoglobin S would be reasonable. If the pretransfusion hemoglobin S is higher than the target hemoglobin S, the patient may need an increased frequency of transfusions or increased volume of transfusion, and this is more easily accomplished with erythrocytapheresis. The administration of hydroxyurea (25 mg/kg/d) to patients who are chronically transfused may increase fetal hemoglobin and reduce erythropoiesis, increasing control of the patient's hemoglobin S.[169]

During transfusing by erythrocytapheresis, the goal for the end hematocrit should be 27%. A higher end hematocrit will lead to increased iron accumulation. An end hematocrit of 27% will slow iron accumulation in some patients and can eliminate iron overload in others.[170] Increasing the numbers of units exchanged can reduce the hemoglobin S (FCR), although a large number of units will lead to removal of the donor red cells near the end of the red cell exchange with only minor decreases in the FCR. The use of an end hematocrit higher than the pretransfusion hematocrit cannot be avoided in all patients, such as those who have a high rate of hemolysis. The goal of exchange transfusion should not be marrow suppression but a low percentage of hemoglobin S with an adequate hematocrit in order to avoid iron overload. Patients who come to transfusion with a high hematocrit may benefit from a depletion exchange procedure. A depletion exchange is a two-stage exchange with a phlebotomy to a predetermined hematocrit in the first stage and an exchange transfusion to a higher hematocrit in the second stage. Depletion exchange can lead to less blood exposure in some patients. There may be a slightly higher incidence of adverse events, primarily hypocalcemia.

For sickle cell patients treated with simple transfusion, the goal should be the suppression of erythropoiesis by increasing the hemoglobin at the end of the transfusion to between 11 and 12 g/dl. During simple transfusion, evaluate total blood requirement every 12 months, and calculate all blood given to the patient (total volume) divided by an average weight over the past six months (cc/kg/year). If transfusion requirement is greater than 200 cc/kg/year, the cause for such a high transfusion requirement should be explored. There is a point at which chelation becomes difficult or impossible with high annual transfusion requirements.

The transfusion goal for thalassemia is higher than that for sickle cell disease. The pretransfusion hemoglobin should be between 9 and 10 g/dl. This may require monthly transfusion in infants and young children, with transfusions every three weeks in adolescent and adult patients. The posttransfusion hemoglobin should be 12–13 g/dl. Splenomegaly can lead to significant hypersplenism with an increase in blood requirement. Splenectomy should be considered if the annual blood requirement is over 200 ml/kg/year. Splenectomy can reduce the annual red cell requirement. Prior to splenectomy, patients should be fully immunized. Treatment with aspirin following splenectomy can decrease the risk of pulmonary hypertension.[171] Aspirin is not an effective treatment once pulmonary hypertension is established.[172] See Table 11.7.

Hyperviscosity

Overtransfusion should be avoided in the hemoglobinopathies. Hyperviscosity can lead to complications in patients with thalassemia as well as sickle cell disease. The level of hematocrit that may cause morbidity in thalassemia is higher than in sickle cell disease. A hematocrit of greater than 36% in sickle cell disease following a simple transfusion can lead to hypertension and posterior leukoencephalophy or stroke. Patients who have thalassemia can have morbidity with hematocrits of over 45%.

Transfusion to a hematocrit greater than 36% can lead to morbidity in sickle cell anemia, particularly if the percentage of hemoglobin S is not reduced to below 50%. Red cell transfusion to a hematocrit between 30% and 33% is adequate for all indications. Erythrocytapheresis[173] enables an isovolumetric transfusion, but

Table 11.7 Complications: Regular Transfusion versus Non-Transfusion-Dependent Thalassemia

Beta Thalassemia Major Chronic Transfusion: Hemosiderosis	Non-Transfusion-Dependent Thalassemia
Hypothyroidism	Silent cerebral infarct
Hypoparathyroidism	Pulmonary hypertension
Cardiac hemosiderosis, left-sided heart failure	Hepatic fibrosis, cirrhosis, hepatocellular carcinoma
Hepatic failure; viral hepatitis possible	Splenomegaly
Diabetes mellitus	Thrombophilia
Hypogonadism	Extramedullary hematopoiesis
Osteoporosis	Osteoporosis
	Skin ulcers

hyperviscosity[174] remains an issue if not carefully monitored by the apheresis physician. The goal for end hematocrit during erythrocytapheresis should reduce an elevated hematocrit to 33% to avoid the complications of hyperviscosity in some patients with sickle cell anemia and α thalassemia, those with SC disease, or others presenting with elevated hematocrit.[175] Transfusion to increase the hemoglobin to above 33% only can be detrimental.[176] Transfusion to a hematocrit greater than 38% has resulted in increases in blood pressure, congestive heart failure, stupor, coma, intracerebral infarct, or hemorrhage.[177]

At a hematocrit of 25%, patients with homozygous S have a blood viscosity slightly less than homozygous A with a hematocrit of 45%.[178] Above a hematocrit of 45%, hemoglobin A blood becomes more viscous and oxygen transport declines.[174] Oxygen delivery with hemoglobin S begins to decline with a hematocrit of 30–35%. During hypoxia, these effects are increased if the percent hemoglobin S is greater than 30%.[167]

Alloantibodies and autoantibodies

Autoimmunization[179] or alloimmunization[180] should be considered if the pretransfusion hemoglobin in a chronically transfused patient is less than 7.0–7.5 g/dl or is significantly less than usual following a transfusion. In sickle cell disease, it should be assumed that there is new antibody formation if the percentage of hemoglobin S and the reticulocyte count are both elevated. The indirect antiglobin test (IAT) and the direct antiglobin test (DAT) may be negative due to consumption of the antibody and antibody-coated red cells during hemolysis. An investigation for a new antibody should be undertaken prior to transfusion. Even micropositive IAT results should prompt a consideration of alloimmunization, as this could be the first indication of a new antibody. If an antibody is suspected after the initial screening, the specificity of the antibody must be determined by the blood bank reference laboratory or by a regional reference laboratory prior to transfusion.

Autoantibodies are known to obscure alloantibodies.[181] A high index of suspicion is needed to prevent severe delayed transfusion reactions in patients who have an autoantibody obscuring an alloantibody. The management of antibodies in patients who require chronic transfusions and develop alloimmunization is not straightforward.[182] If extended antigen typing is necessary, finding compatible units can be difficult or even impossible.

Autoantibodies are common in chronically transfused patients with sickle cell disease, and they may lead to increased transfusion requirements due to shortened red cell survival.[183] It is not clear why autoantibodies appear to be so prevalent in this group of patients.[184] Occasionally, the specificity of the autoantibody is an antigen occurring on the patient's red cells. Anti-e is the most common specificity in cases of autoimmunization when an antibody type can be identified. The term *least incompatible* is occasionally used by blood bank technicians, but has no meaning in transfusion medicine and is discouraged. When an autoantibody is detected, the patient's phenotype or genotype can be used to help determine if an underlying alloantibody exists. Safe blood can be provided if alloantibodies have been ruled out and the appropriate units are available for transfusion.[185]

The use of phenotypically or genotypically matched red cells for major antigens (D, C, c, E, e, and Kell) from the beginning of a chronic transfusion regimen can prevent alloimmunization to a significant degree.[186] Increased red cell exposure during erythrocytapheresis has been shown not to increase alloimmunization.[187] The safest units are those tested prior to transfusion for antigen negativity, rather than historically negative units.

Delayed hemolytic transfusion reaction

Acute hemolytic transfusion reactions are rare in sickle cell disease and thalassemia. DHTRs are much more common than would be expected for the general population. Some studies report up to 11% of patients will have DHTRs.[180] Many of these DHTRs will go unnoticed if they are not severe. A complete blood count with a reticulocyte count and a percentage of hemoglobin S prior to transfusion will be pathognomonic for a DHTR. The hemoglobin will be lower than baseline, the reticulocyte count will be higher, and the percentage of hemoglobin S will be higher than usual. The indirect antiglobin test may not be positive due to consumption of the offending antibody. The crossmatch may be compatible due to the absence of antibody in the recipient's plasma. With this presentation prior to a transfusion, the patient should not be transfused, and an investigation for the antibody should be undertaken.

Occasionally, patients will present 10–14 days following a transfusion with symptoms that can be mistaken for a vaso-occlusive episode. If they have hematuria, they may be suspected of having papillary necrosis. If fever is present, they may be suspected of having infection.[188] A complete blood count with a reticulocyte count will contribute to the diagnosis in a patient who has been recently transfused. Some patients will have hyperhemolysis with no red cell antibody found on investigation. The anemia can be severe, requiring immune suppression and support.

Hyperhemolysis[189]

Patients who have sickle cell disease can have dramatically decreased hemoglobin levels or other complications during vaso-occlusive episodes. These events have been termed *hyperhemolytic episodes*.[136,180,190] They may or may not be associated with a recent transfusion. They are not isolated to sickle cell disease.[191]

Hyperhemolytic transfusion reactions related to transfusion can be life-threatening and are similar to, but distinct from, other types of hyperhemolytic episodes. Continuing to transfuse in the face of falling hemoglobin during an immune-mediated hyperhemolytic transfusion reaction can exacerbate the hemolysis leading to life-threatening anemia. There have been no prospective studies to guide therapy. Immune suppression is often used with steroids, immunoglobulin, and rituximab, generally in that order. High-dose erythropoietin has also been recommended.[192] Transfusions should be reserved as a lifesaving measure. Apheresis has been used as an adjunct to treat hyperhemolysis with serial plasmapheresis followed by red cell exchange or by plasma to red cell exchange.[193] Frequently, no inciting antibody will be found, so patients can be successfully transfused once the event has resolved.

There is a relationship between transfusion, corticosteroid use, hypertension, intracranial hemorrhage, and stroke.[194] Patients should be monitored for hypertension and fluid overload when they are receiving intensive therapy for hyperhemolysis.

Iron overload and chelation therapy

Iron is regulated by absorption because there is no mechanism for excretion. Nonheme iron is absorbed from the intestinal lumen as ferrous iron (Fe^{2+}) by divalent metal transporter 1.[195] The iron can be stored in the enterocyte and returned to the villi surface or transported from the enterocyte to the circulation. The membrane transporter for iron entry to the circulation is ferroportin. Cellular expression of ferroportin is controlled by intracellular iron, iron-responsive elements, and heme. Ferroportin is regulated in a negative manner by hepcidin, a peptide hormone produced by the hepatocytes. Hepcidin is regulated by iron via elements of the bone morphogenetic protein pathway and in an unknown manner by erythropoiesis. Hepcidin is also regulated by inflammation, increasing production with increasing levels of IL6 and possibly other cytokines. The physiology and regulation of hepcidin are complex.[196]

Hepcidin regulation is partly responsible for the decreased effects of iron loading in sickle cell disease compared to thalassemia.[197] Most of the disparity between hemosiderosis in thalassemia versus sickle cell disease is due to the ineffective erythropoiesis of thalassemia, which significantly decreases hepcidin production in the liver, increasing iron absorption and increasing the release of iron from the enterocytes, as well as from macrophages and hepatocytes. Patients with sickle cell disease do not have the degree of ineffective erythropoiesis and have a chronic inflammatory state with the absorption of half as much iron from the diet compared to patients with thalassemia.[198] Due to decreased iron absorption and effective erythropoiesis, there are less transferrin saturation and less non-transferrin-bound iron (NTBI) in sickle cell disease compared to thalassemia. Increases in NTBI are associated with tissue damage, particularly in the endocrine organs. Increases in cardiac iron from NTBI are associated with cardiac disease in thalassemia.[199] Morbidity and mortality from other causes are amplified in adult patients with transfusion-induced hemosiderosis.[200]

Monitoring iron overload[201]

Serum ferritin is a routinely available laboratory test, but it results in inaccurate determination of iron loading when used alone.[202] Serial trends are more important than single results. The chronic pro-inflammatory state of sickle cell disease makes serum ferritin levels a suboptimal method in making major iron chelator dose adjustments.[202] Measurement of hepatic iron by liver biopsy has been replaced by noninvasive, reliable imaging techniques such as the superconducting quantum interference device (SQUID, or ferritometry) or MRI.[203] Specialized software is needed for MRI iron determination. In addition to evaluation of hepatic hemosiderosis, which reflects total body iron stores, $T2^*$ cardiac MRI[204] quantitates cardiac iron.[205] Due to differences in iron loading, $T2^*$ MRI rarely shows cardiac dysfunction in patients with sickle cell disease who have been transfused for less than 10 consecutive years.[206] Cardiac iron is much more significant for patients with thalassemia.[207] In thalassemia, there is a relationship between iron, pancreatic function,[208] and pituitary function.[209]

Initiation of chelation

Chelation should be considered after 1–2 years of transfusion therapy, when the serum ferritin is approximately 1500 ng/ml, or when the hepatic iron is greater than 7 mg/gram dry weight.[210] Optimal iron chelation should maintain serum ferritin between 500 and 1000 ng/ml. Because ferritin underestimates iron in sickle cell disease, it is important to have a quantitative measurement as a baseline for future evaluation. Compliance with chelation therapy is probably the most important factor in reducing the morbidity of chronic transfusion therapy.[211] Frequent evaluation of compliance and counseling is necessary in most patients for effective therapy.

Treatment with deferoxamine (desferal)

Iron is removed much more efficiently when deferoxamine is infused over a long period at a relatively low dose. The dose depends upon the age of the patient and the degree of iron overload. Side effects of deferoxamine are greater with lower levels of iron and in children under 2–3 years of age.

Subcutaneous deferoxamine should be administered at 30–50 mg/kg. Eight to 12 hours, 5–7 days per week is the standard dose for home therapy. Starting at fewer days per week may help the family adapt to and accept the new therapy. Ascorbic acid (vitamin C) 2-mg/kg/day (100–250 mg maximum) orally after infusion has been initiated increases iron excretion, but without deferoxamine, it will increase oral iron absorption.[212]

Oral iron chelators

Ferriprox (L-1, deferiprone)

Deferiprone has been used in Europe and in other countries and found to be relatively safe and effective in removing iron. Deferiprone has a short half-life requiring three-times-a-day dosing. The daily dose is 75 mg/kg per day. It may be used as a monotherapy, but it is the novel effect of this drug to remove cardiac iron that has made it attractive in combination chemotherapy in patients with cardiac hemosiderosis. One of the side effects, agranulocytosis (1.7%), is serious. This is a rare complication that requires monitoring of the leukocyte count while this drug is being administered. Neutropenia (6.2%) can precede agranulocytosis; neutrophil counts are monitored weekly. Some patients also experience joint swelling and pain during therapy with this chelator.

Exjade (deferasirox)

Deferasirox is the most recently developed iron chelators and has been extensively studied.[213] It is an oral iron chelator with a relatively long half-life. This allows for once- daily dosing. It has become the most-used iron chelator in the United States. The starting dose is 20 mg/kg/per day. It generally maintains a negative iron balance when used at 30 mg/kg. A tablet is available. Renal function should be closely monitored.

Patients with significant iron overload

Deferoxamine combined with deferasirox or deferiprone is an effective chelation approach for severe hemosiderosis.[214] A physician familiar with the toxicity of these drugs should oversee their administration.

Assessment and monitoring of iron overload

Annual assessment of endocrine function including thyroid, parathyroid, pancreas, adrenal, pituitary gland, and bone density should be performed.

Evaluate serum ferritin level quarterly. Ferritin levels greater than 3000 ng/ml (in the absence of hepatitis or other inflammatory process) and hepatic iron greater than 7 mg/gm dry liver weight are considered evidence of iron burden in thalassemia. Signs of elevated iron should prompt an evaluation of compliance, the chelation protocol, the annual and semiannual transfusion requirement, as well as hepatitis status and liver function.

Assessment of side effects and toxicity of iron chelators

Patients require ongoing monitoring for chelator toxicity. All patients should have hearing and vision screening, and monitoring of growth, renal, and liver functions. Patients treated with deferasirox require monthly renal function testing. Deferiprone use requires weekly monitoring of white cell count.

Congenital hemolytic anemia (see Table 11.8)

Red cell enzymopathies
Glucose-6-phosphate dehydrogenase deficiency

Glucose-6-phosphate dehydrogenase deficiency (G6PD) is the most common enzymopathy in humans.[215] G6PD is the first enzyme in the pentose phosphate pathway providing reducing power for the red cell. Without mitochrondia, the pentose phosphate pathway is the only source of NADPH available to the red cell, which provides for a high level of reduced glutathione. In the absence of NADPH production, there is no protection against cellular oxidative damage through the regeneration of reduced glutathione by glutathione reductase. Without this reduction potential in the red cell, oxidative membrane damage and hemolysis occur when the cells are presented with excessive oxidative stress.

G6PD has classical X-linked inheritance with the deficiency primarily affecting males, although females homozygous for the deletion or heterozygous with lyonization can be symptomatic with the disease. There are over 160 mutations leading to inactivation of the G6PD enzyme; most are single base mutations leading to amino acid substitutions and inactivation.[216]

The G6PD mutation has been most common in areas were malaria is prevalent as there is restricted parasite growth in the affected red cells.[217] As would be expected, the highest prevalence is in Africa, the Mediterranean, the Middle East, Southeast Asia, and the Pacific Islands. Although there are numerous mutations leading to the inactivation of G6PD, two common mutations are found: one in African and in areas of the African Diaspora, and one in the countries surrounding the Mediterranean, Israel, India, and Indonesia. The African variant is G6PDA-, the other second most common variant is G6PD Mediterranean. In the absence of oxidative stress, these mutations do not cause hemolysis. The presence of the mutation does not appear to have an effect on growth, development, or life expectancy.[218] There is evidence that there may be a reduction in coronary artery disease in males with this deficiency.[219]

Infection is the most common cause of acute hemolysis in G6PD deficiency. Viral hepatitis can be complicated by renal failure. The severity of the hemolysis depends on the type of infection and other compounding factors, but it can be severe. Numerous drugs have been implicated with hemolysis in G6PD deficiency; the degree of

Table 11.8 Inherited Hemolytic Disorders

	Membrane Defects			
	Mutation	Inheritance	Prevalence in disease population	Severity
Spherocytosis (HS) prevalence: 1/2000–3000	Ankyrin-1	AD, AR, *de novo*	60% in the HS population	Mild to Moderate
Spherocytosis (severe)	α spectrin	AR (Homozygote)	<5% in HS population	Severe
Elliptocytosis (HE) Prevalence: 3–5/10,000 (US)	α, β spectrin	AD		Mild anemia
Severe HE	α, β spectrin	AR (Homozygote)		Severe
Pyropoikilocytosis	α, β spectrin	AR (Homozygote)	African descent predominates	Severe in childhood
SEA ovalocytosis	Band 3	AD	Southeast Asian descent	Mild
Stomatocytosis overhydrated (DHSt)	RhAG Mutation	AD	Rare	Severe
Stomatocytosis dehydrated (DHSt)	PIEZO1 (North America)	AD	Rare	Less severe
Enzymopathy				
G6PD deficiency prevalence: common in African descent, Sardinian, Greek, others	X chromosome: numerous variants Class I,II,III	X-linked recessive	Common	Mild to severe with exposure to oxidants
Pyruvate kinase deficiency prevalence: rare	47 mutations leading to deficiency	AR	Most common of the related glycolytic enzymopathies	Moderate to severe

AD, Autosomal dominant; AR, autosomal recessive.

hemolysis can vary between individuals and with re-exposure in the same individual.[220] Favism is thought to be associated with the Mediterranean mutation and leading to severe hemolysis, particularly if fresh fava beans are ingested.

Pyruvate kinase deficiency

Pyruvate kinase deficiency (PKD) is much less common than G6PD, but is the most common cause of hemolytic anemia due to an enzyme abnormality of the glycolytic pathway. It is a more common cause of nonspherocytic hemolytic anemia than Class I G6PD. There are four isoenzymes (M_1, M_2, L, and R) found on two chromosomes: the gene for the L and R isoenzymes (PK-LR) on chromosome 1 (1q21) using different promoters to produce the two isoenzymes. The gene for M_1 and M_2 isoenzymes (PK-M) on chromosome 15 (15q22) with alternate splicing of RNA produces these two isoenzymes.[222] The R isoenzyme is expressed exclusively in red cells. The deficiency is autosomal recessive. The prevalence is unknown, but mutations have been reported in European and Asian populations.[223] One hundred and fifty-eight mutations are known to cause nonspherocytic hemolytic anemia.

Congenital nonspherocytic hemolytic anemia

Congenital nonspherocytic hemolytic anemia includes Class I variants of G6PH and PKD. There are 61 Class I variants of G6PD that lead to a severe chronic hemolytic anemia.[221] These patients present younger, at a median age of 4 years versus 22.5 years for other mutations. There are three mutations that seem to be the most common worldwide: G6PD Guadalajara 1159 C>T, G6PD Beverly Hills 1160 G>A, and G6PD Nashville 1178 G>A. These patients present with neonatal hyperbilirubinemia, chronic hemolytic anemia,

Table 11.9 Classes of G6PD Deficiency

WHO Classification	
Class 1	Severely deficient; chronic nonspherocytic hemolytic anemia
Class II	Severely deficient: (1–10% activity) acute hemolytic episodes
Class III	Moderately deficient: (10–60%) mild
Class IV	Normal activity (60–150%) normal
Class V	Increased activity (>150%)

jaundice, hyperbilirubinemia, moderate splenomegaly and reticulocytosis, and cholelithiasis. They require chronic red cell transfusion and may not respond to splenectomy. (See Table 11.9.)

Red cells are dependent on glycolysis for the production of adenosine triphosphate (ATP). Pyruvate kinase catalyzes two steps in the production of ATP. Deficiency results in ATP depletion and loss of red cell integrity. Upstream intermediates are increased in the red cell, including 2,3-diphosphoglycerate, which inhibits hexokinase, exacerbating the defect in the enzyme pathway. Due to this increase in 2,3 DPG, transfusion should not be determined by the hemoglobin, but by clinical symptoms of hypoxia.

The degree of anemia can be predicted by the neonatal jaundice and the need for exchange transfusion. Most of these infants will go on to require chronic red cell transfusions during infancy until they have had a splenectomy. The effect of splenectomy cannot be predicted, but it can raise the hemoglobin 2–3 g/dl, alleviating the need for transfusion.

Two missense mutations are associated with severe PKD (994A and 1529A). The most severe disease is found in "null" mutations with intrauterine growth retardation, severe anemia at birth requiring exchange transfusion, and transfusion dependence until splenectomy. Death has occurred in the neonatal period in infants with this severe genotype.[224] Hemosiderosis may occur without transfusion therapy or as a complication of chronic transfusion therapy in these patients. The transfusion requirement can decrease with age.

Disorders of the red cell membrane

The red cell membrane has a unique structure that is elastic, deformable without fragmentation, and rapidly responsive to changes in stress.[225] These properties are due to the structure of the lipid bilayer membrane and the underlying cytoskeleton. The lipid bilayer has an asymmetric distribution of phospholipids with phosphatidylserine (PS) localized to the inner layer. Both PS and internally located phosphoinositides interact with the spectrin and protein 4.1R anchoring the membrane to the cytoskeleton. Loss of this asymmetry, with PS translocated to the outer membrane, leads to phagocytosis and the membrane destruction seen in sickle cell disease and thalassemia. Key components of the membrane include band 3, glycophrin C, RhAG, α and β spectrin, actin, and ankyrin.

Hereditary spherocytosis

This membrane disorder occurs in all racial groups, but it is particularly common in northern Europeans where the prevalence is one in 3000. The inheritance is dominant in 75% and recessive in 25%. Sphereocytosis is recognized as mild with compensated hemolysis in about 6% of cases, although many patients may go unrecognized; moderate in 60% with hemoglobin of 8–10 g/dl and reticulocytosis of >8%; moderately severe (10% of total patients) with hemoglobin in the range of 6–8 g/dl, higher reticulocyte counts, splenomegaly, and intermittent transfusion requirement; and a small number (<5% of total patients) who have severe disease and a transfusion requirement. The most severe cases have autosomal recessive inheritance.

Loss of membrane determines the severity of this disease, leading to sequestration of defective red cells in the spleen. The most common defects are inherited abnormalities in ankyrin (50%), spectrin (20%), and band 3 (15–20%). Splenectomy will significantly decrease the severity of anemia in this disease. Rh-deficient cells or Rh-null cells have decreased or absent RhAG leading to stomatocytosis; this is less than 1% of the total cases.[226]

Hereditary elliptocytosis

Hereditary elliptocytosis (HE) has a worldwide distribution, but it is more common in malarial areas. The majority of mutations are related to α-spectrin, occurring in about 65% of cases. In 30% of cases, the mutation is β-spectrin; homozygotes have severe anemia. A small number, 5%, of mutations are in the 4.1R protein. Most mutations are missense mutations; notable is Arg28His, which is seen in African Americans and leads to severe hemolytic anemia. Hereditary pyropoikilocytosis is not a distinct membrane disorder; it is a HE variant that is either homozygous or a compound heterozygote for a spectrin mutation.[227]

Hereditary ovalocytosis

Hereditary ovalocytosis is common in malarial regions of Southeast Asia and the Philippines. The inheritance is autosomal dominant; only heterozygotes have been seen, with the assumption that homozygosity is incompatible with life. Only one mutation has been identified, a 27 base pair deletion of band 3. This membrane disorder is relatively benign with no or minimal hemolysis.

Hereditary stomatocytoses

These disorders lead to overhydrated hereditary stomatocytosis (OHSt) or dehydrated stomatocytosis (DHSt). Southeast Asian ovalocytosis is included in this group, a benign disorder.[228] DHSt may occur with pseudohyperkalemia, with perinatal fluid effusions, or as a single finding. DHSt is dominantly inherited. The precise mutation causing DHSt is not known. There is a compensated mild to moderate hemolytic anemia. OHSt has been characterized as having dominant inheritance of mutations in the RHAG gene in some cases. Other mutations have not been characterized. Hemolytic anemia can be mild to moderate. There have been case reports of thromboembolic events following splenectomy for hemolytic anemia in stomatocytosis.[229]

The congenital hemolytic anemias are a diverse group of blood diseases that generally do not require red cell transfusion. In the few severe presentations, patients will require red cell transfusions on a chronic basis or intermittently with viral illness and fever. In the case of G6PD deficiency, acute anemia due to exposure to inciting drugs, foods, or chemicals can require emergent transfusion.

Key references

A full reference list for this chapter is available at: http://www.wiley.com/go/simon/transfusion

2 Vichinsky E, Neumayr L, Trimble S, et al. Transfusion complications in thalassemia patients: a report from the Centers for Disease Control and Prevention (CME). *Transfusion* 2014;**54**:972–81, quiz 1.

3 Lopez C, Saravia C, Gomez A, Hoebeke J, Patarroyo MA. Mechanisms of genetically-based resistance to malaria. *Gene* 2010;**467**:1–12.

18 Cserti-Gazdewich CM, Dhabangi A, Musoke C, et al. Cytoadherence in paediatric malaria: ABO blood group, CD36, and ICAM1 expression and severe *Plasmodium falciparum* infection. *Brit J Haematol* 2012;**159**:223–36.

45 Powars DR, Chan LS, Hiti A, Ramicone E, Johnson C. Outcome of sickle cell anemia: a 4-decade observational study of 1056 patients. *Medicine (Baltimore)* 2005;**84**:363–76.

47 Rees DC, Gibson JS. Biomarkers in sickle cell disease. *Brit J Haematol* 2012;**156**:433–45.

51 Gueguen A, Mahevas M, Nzouakou R, et al. Sickle-cell disease stroke throughout life: A retrospective study in an adult referral center. *Amer J Hematol* 2014;**89**:267–72.

56 Abboud MR, Yim E, Musallam KM, Adams RJ. Discontinuing prophylactic transfusions increases the risk of silent brain infarction in children with sickle cell disease: data from STOP II. *Blood* 2011;**118**:894–8.

59 DeBaun MR, Gordon M, McKinstry RC, et al. Controlled trial of transfusions for silent cerebral infarcts in sickle cell anemia. *N Engl J Med* 2014;**371**:699–710.

68 Ware RE, Helms RW. Stroke with transfusions changing to hydroxyurea (SWiTCH). *Blood* 2012;**119** (17): 3925–32.

146 Weatherall DJ. The inherited diseases of hemoglobin are an emerging global health burden. *Blood* 2010;**115**:4331–6.

CHAPTER 12

Autoimmune hemolytic anemias and paroxysmal nocturnal hemoglobinuria

Andrea M. McGonigle,[1,2] Paul M. Ness,[1] & Karen E. King[1]

[1]Transfusion Medicine Division, Department of Pathology, The Johns Hopkins Medical Institutions, Baltimore, MD, USA
[2]Division of Transfusion Medicine, Department of Pathology and Lab Medicine, David Geffen School of Medicine at UCLA, Los Angeles, CA, USA

The hallmark of the autoimmune hemolytic anemias (AIHAs) and paroxysmal nocturnal hemoglobinuria (PNH) is shortened red blood cell survival. Although AIHA and PNH share the critical feature of shortened red cell survival, the mechanisms underlying this characteristic differ significantly between the two diseases. In the case of AIHA, autoantibodies directed against the patient's own red blood cells lead to accelerated red cell destruction. In PNH, lack of surface complement-regulatory proteins as well as the loss of other surface proteins, leads to exquisite sensitivity of the red cells to complement-mediated lysis.

The AIHAs are classified by characteristics of the responsible autoantibodies and their clinical settings (Table 12.1). Serologic differences in optimal temperature of reactivity allow for the differentiation of warm AIHA from cold AIHA; these broad divisions correlate with responsiveness to specific therapy and prognosis. Both warm and cold AIHAs can be further characterized as either a primary, idiopathic autoimmune phenomenon or a secondary process associated with an underlying clinical condition; this information also provides guidance on the most appropriate therapeutic approach. In contrast, PNH occurs in the context of a somatic gene mutation and some component of bone marrow dysfunction. This somatic mutation, which results in decreased glycosylphosphotidylinositol anchored proteins, ultimately leads to increased sensitivity to complement with effects of intravascular hemolysis and increased risk of thrombosis.

Autoimmune hemolytic anemias

Classification

The AIHAs are categorized into three broad subtypes: warm AIHA, cold AIHA, and drug-induced immune hemolytic anemia (Table 12.1). The distinction between warm and cold AIHAs is based on the causative antibody's optimal temperature of reactivity in vitro. Warm AIHA is due to autoantibodies which optimally react at 37 °C. Cold AIHA is associated with autoantibodies that optimally react at 0 °C,[1] but are also able to react at higher temperatures in cases with higher thermal amplitudes. Cold AIHA is further subdivided into the more common cold agglutinin disease (CAD) and the infrequent paroxysmal cold hemoglobinuria (PCH), based on serologic and clinical properties.

Because temperature of optimal reactivity and mechanism of action are known to vary amongst immunoglobulin classes, it is not surprising that warm and cold AIHA differ with respect to the most common immunoglobulin class of the causative autoantibody. Warm AIHA is typically due to an immunoglobulin G (IgG) autoantibody. CAD is usually associated with IgM autoantibodies. PCH is due to a unique type of IgG autoantibody called the Donath–Landsteiner antibody, which is also known as a biphasic cold hemolysin. This type of IgG can bind to red cells at low temperatures, activate complement, and subsequently lead to hemolysis at 37 °C.

The AIHAs, both warm and cold, can be further characterized by their clinical associations. Primary AIHA is idiopathic. Secondary AIHA is associated with an underlying disorder, such as an autoimmune disease, an infection, or a malignancy, most commonly of the lymphoproliferative type. The underlying disorders most frequently associated with AIHAs vary between the warm and cold autoantibody types. The AIHAs also demonstrate variability in severity of clinical presentation, related to the rate of hemolysis and the time course of the development of anemia. Clinically, AIHAs may have an acute presentation with a sudden development of severe anemia. Alternatively, they may present as a chronic phenomenon with a gradual decrease in hemoglobin and hematocrit over a prolonged period of time. The AIHAs may also be transient, most often seen when associated with an infectious etiology.

In drug-induced immune hemolytic anemia, autoantibodies are not categorized by temperature of optimal reactivity or immunoglobulin type, but instead by their proposed pathophysiologic mechanisms, which include the drug adsorption mechanism, the immune complex mechanism, and the autoimmune induction mechanism. The antibodies in drug-induced immune hemolytic anemia frequently demonstrate reactivity at warm temperatures, and consequently, patients may present with symptoms that are indistinguishable from those of warm AIHA.

Warm autoimmune hemolytic anemia

Epidemiology and risk factors

The incidence of AIHA is approximately 1–3 cases in 100,000 individuals per year.[2–4] Warm AIHA is the most common type, accounting for about 80% of all AIHAs.[5] Individuals of all ages,

Rossi's Principles of Transfusion Medicine, Fifth Edition. Edited by Toby L. Simon, Jeffrey McCullough, Edward L. Snyder, Bjarte G. Solheim, and Ronald G. Strauss.

Table 12.1 Classification of the Autoimmune Hemolytic Anemias

Warm Autoimmune Hemolytic Anemia
- Autoantibodies with optimal reactivity at 37 °C
- Usually an IgG (sometimes due to IgA) autoantibody
- Etiologies
  1. Primary: idiopathic
  2. Secondary
     a. Malignancies: leukemia, lymphoma, ovarian tumors
     b. Autoimmune/connective tissue disorders: systemic lupus erythematosus
     c. Immunodeficiency states
     d. Infectious diseases: HIV

Cold Autoimmune Hemolytic Anemia
I. **Cold Agglutinin Disease**
- Autoantibodies with optimal reactivity at 0 °C, with higher thermal amplitudes in clinically significant disease
- Usually an IgM autoantibody
- Etiologies
  1. Primary: idiopathic
  2. Secondary: B-cell neoplasms, *Mycoplasma pneumoniae*, and infectious mononucleosis

II. **Paroxysmal Cold Hemoglobinuria**
- Autoantibodies with biphasic reactivity: binding of antibody at cold temperatures and hemolysis at 37 °C
- A particular IgG autoantibody called Donath–Landsteiner or biphasic hemolysin
- Etiologies
  1. Primary: idiopathic
  2. Secondary: tertiary syphilis, upper respiratory tract infection of viral origin

Drug-Induced Immune Hemolytic Anemia
- Autoantibodies usually reactive at warm temperatures
- Pathophysiologic mechanism
  1. Drug adsorption mechanism
  2. Immune complex mechanism
  3. Autoimmune induction mechanism

from 1 month to the elderly, can be affected by AIHA.[6] Most patients with primary or idiopathic disease are women[7–9] aged 40–50 years.[2,10] The mean age of idiopathic warm AIHA is 49 years.[7] Secondary causes of warm AIHA include malignancies (such as leukemia, lymphoma, and ovarian tumors), autoimmune and connective tissue disorders (such as systemic lupus erythematosus [SLE]), immunodeficiency states, and infectious diseases.[11] Women also have a higher incidence of secondary AIHA, often associated with SLE or other autoimmune disorders.[10] The age distribution of secondary AIHA is expected to correspond to the age distribution of the underlying disease; leukemia and lymphoma are more common causes in older individuals, and SLE is a more common cause in younger patients. Warm AIHA may also occur in association with thrombocytopenia, a combination known as Evans syndrome. The thrombocytopenia in this syndrome is a form of autoimmune-mediated idiopathic thrombocytopenic purpura.[12]

Pathophysiology

There are two distinct mechanisms of immune-mediated red cell destruction: extravascular hemolysis and intravascular hemolysis.[9] Macrophages located in reticular tissue of the spleen and liver (known as the mononuclear phagocyte system or reticulo-endothelial system) are responsible for extravascular hemolysis. The spleen is the most common site of extravascular hemolysis,[13] because there is increased interaction between antibody-coated red cells and macrophages created by the movement of red blood cells from the cords of Billroth through tiny gaps in sinusoidal walls to gain entry to the sinusoids.[14] However, the liver also participates in

extravascular hemolysis when large amounts of IgG coat the red cells.[13]

The hemolysis of warm AIHA usually proceeds via the extravascular hemolysis mechanism.[9] As previously discussed, warm autoantibodies are typically IgG autoantibodies that are optimally reactive at 37 °C.[9] Consequently, IgG autoantibodies bind to red blood cells at normal body temperature. The antibody-coated red cells then circulate to the spleen and liver where macrophages adhere[9] to the Fc portion of the IgG bound to the red cells.[13] Once bound to macrophages, the antibody-coated red cells are then subjected to either complete or partial phagocytosis by the macrophage. Complete phagocytosis results in removal of the antibody-coated red cells from circulation. Partial phagocytosis, which is more common,[15] results in removal of a portion of the red cell membrane and the formation of spherocytes.[9] Spherocytes are released back into the circulation but have a decreased life span.[15] After a brief period of circulation, they pass back through the spleen where they become lodged in tiny gaps in sinusoidal walls as they attempt to reach the sinusoids, and they are destroyed.[16]

The degree of extravascular hemolysis depends on the subclass of IgG, quantity of bound IgG, and antibody specificity. There are four subclasses of IgG: IgG1, IgG2, IgG3, and IgG4. Macrophage Fc receptors have the highest affinity for IgG1 and IgG3 subclasses.[17,18] Macrophages have variable affinity for IgG2, but they have the lowest affinity for IgG4. Not surprisingly, the most common subclasses of IgG found in warm AIHA are IgG1 and IgG3, followed by IgG2. Subjects with IgG4-coated red cells are not expected to demonstrate hemolysis.[1] Based on macrophage affinity, one might suspect that the greatest degree of extravascular hemolysis would be observed when red cells are coated by IgG1 and IgG3 subtypes. Although this is partly true, in the case of IgG1, the quantity of immunoglobulin coating each red cell also plays a role in the degree of hemolysis. Studies suggest that at least 1200 IgG1 molecules[17,18] must coat each red cell before macrophages can effectively bind and subsequently phagocytose them. Consequently, there is a demonstrated relationship between the quantity of IgG1 sensitizing the red cells and the severity of AIHA.[19] In contrast, IgG3 is associated with hemolysis even when the quantity coating the red cells is too low to be detected by a direct antiglobulin test (DAT),[1] which is an average of 335 +/− 72 molecules.[20,21] In the case of IgG2, the situation is more complex. The gene that encodes the Fc receptor for IgG2 on macrophages has two alleles, resulting in differences in affinity. As a result, some people have macrophages with an Fc receptor that has a low-affinity for IgG2, and some are endowed with a receptor that has high affinity. Those individuals with high-affinity receptors for IgG2 have the capacity to destroy IgG2 coated red cells. However, in the case of IgG2 antibodies, destruction of red cells is also influenced by antigen specificity. For example, studies have shown that IgG2 alloantibodies against blood group A antigen lead to hemolysis, while hemolysis will not be seen due to IgG2 antibodies directed against Rh antigens.[22] Despite the findings of differing Fc receptor affinity and IgG2 alloantibody reactivity, the role of IgG2 autoantibodies in autoimmune hemolysis remains unclear. Practically speaking, in AIHA, red cell destruction due to IgG antibodies is primarily observed when the subclass of bound IgG is either IgG1 or IgG3.[1]

Although warm AIHA usually proceeds via the extravascular hemolysis mechanism, in some individuals presenting with severe hemolysis there may also be evidence of intravascular hemolysis,[9] which occurs when antibody-coated red cells are capable of activating complement. Red cell destruction occurs by the classical complement pathway, with formation of a membrane attack complex (MAC), forming pores in the red cell membrane leading to cell swelling and lysis. The ability of antibody-coated red cells to activate complement depends on many things, including the subclass and quantity of IgG coating the red cells. Subclasses IgG1 and IgG3 are the most commonly implicated in intravascular hemolysis, as they are thought to be more efficient at activating complement than other IgG subclasses.[23] In addition, studies have demonstrated that a high density of cell-bound IgG is required for efficient binding and activation of complement,[24] likely due to the need for two IgG molecules to be in close proximity to allow for binding and activation of the complement system. Since a high number of IgG molecules are required to coat the red cells before, by chance, two are in close proximity, the overall density would be expected to correlate with complement activation.[13,25]

Despite attempts to divide hemolysis discretely into extravascular and intravascular mechanisms for the purpose of understanding the pathophysiology of these disorders, they do not always occur discretely in clinical situations. Many cases of warm AIHA demonstrate both mechanisms of hemolysis. There may be a predominance of one type over another, but laboratory and clinical findings may ultimately overlap.[9]

Clinical features

Warm AIHA has a variable clinical presentation. Severe anemia as a result of hemolysis can present with varying degrees of fatigue, fever, dizziness, angina, shortness of breath (with exertion or even at rest), and flank pain. The severity of symptoms depends largely on the rate of hemolysis and the rate of decrease in hematocrit and hemoglobin. In chronic hemolytic anemia, the pace of the disease may allow for physiologic compensation and, therefore, less severe symptomatology. In addition, the presence of underlying conditions, such as cardiopulmonary disease, affects the ability to compensate for anemia, even when the hemolytic pace is slow. Patients may also develop jaundice, pallor, or dark urine consistent with hemoglobinuria. Hepatosplenomegaly is present in approximately half of all warm AIHA cases.[7,26] Patients with idiopathic AIHA have been shown to be at increased risk for venous thromboembolism.[7,27–29] It is important to note that approximately half of warm AIHA cases are due to secondary causes, and the clinical presentation of the underlying cause may predominate.

Diagnosis

The diagnosis of warm AIHA is based on laboratory findings indicative of shortened red cell survival and serologic evidence of autoantibody directed against red cell antigens, optimally reactive at 37 °C.

Laboratory findings

Complete blood counts will demonstrate typical features of anemia, with hemoglobin and hematocrit as low as 5 g/dL and 15%, respectively.[30] The anemia is typically macrocytic, due to concomitant bone marrow compensation and marked reticulocytosis, related to decreased red cell survival.[31] However, reticulocytopenia may also be seen in as many as one-third of cases. Reticulocytopenia should be treated as a hematologic emergency as it is often associated with the development of life-threatening anemia.[31] In the case of Evan's syndrome (warm AIHA associated with autoimmune thrombocytopenia), the platelet count is also low.[12] Other findings include hemoglobinemia, hemoglobinuria, elevated lactate dehydrogenase and indirect bilirubin, and decreased haptoglobin.[2,10]

The peripheral blood smear typically shows evidence of extravascular hemolysis, demonstrable by the presence of spherocytes.[32] Due to the relatively short lifespan of spherocytes, their presence in the peripheral blood should be taken as evidence for ongoing extravascular hemolysis.[16] Indirect evidence of bone marrow compensation, in the form of polychromatophilic macrocytes (which are suggestive of reticulocytes) or even nucleated red blood cells (when the rate of hemolysis is brisk), may also be seen in the peripheral blood smear.

Serology

Serologic evaluation reveals that the hemolytic process is immune mediated. DATs using polyspecific reagents, including both anti-IgG and anti-C3 (C3d), are typically positive in patients with warm AIHA.[33–35] IgG alone is demonstrated by DAT in 20–66% of warm AIHA,[36,37] and IgG in combination with C3 coat the red cells in 24–64% of cases. Complement alone is found in only 7–14% of warm AIHA[36,37] (Table 12.2). When the DAT demonstrates IgG, eluates of the antibody coating the red cells confirm the finding of IgG. Indirect antiglobulin tests, using either untreated or enzyme-treated red blood cells at 20 °C or 37 °C, typically demonstrate IgG antibody in the serum. Indirect antiglobulin tests may be negative if the antibody is adsorbed onto the patient's red cells; when the amount of autoantibody exceeds the binding capacity of the patient's red cells, the antibody will be detectable in the patient's serum. Although 97–99% of patients with warm AIHA will have a positive DAT, 50–90% of patients will have a positive indirect antiglobulin test, depending on the testing methodology.[2]

The IgG eluted from the red cells frequently demonstrates panagglutination when tested against a panel of commercially available red cells. Likewise, the serum typically demonstrates panagglutination. Occasionally, the autoantibody may demonstrate apparent specificity; these specificities are more often and more clearly seen in the serum as compared to the eluate. Specificity is most frequently seen as broad reactivity with antigens of the Rh system. Less commonly, specificity is toward a single Rh antigen.

Table 12.2 Typical Serologic Features of Autoimmune Hemolytic Anemia

	Warm Autoimmune Hemolytic Anemia	Cold Agglutinin Disease	Paroxysmal Cold Hemoglobinuria
Direct antiglobulin test	IgG only or IgG and C3; less commonly, C3 only	C3 only	C3 only
Immunoglobulin class	IgG, rarely IgA	IgM	IgG biphasic hemolysin
Eluate	IgG	Nonreactive	Nonreactive
Serum	IgG agglutinating red cells at the antihuman globulin phase, panagglutination	IgM agglutinating antibody, often with titers >1000, reacting at 30 °C in albumin	IgG biphasic hemolysin or Donath–Landsteiner antibody
Antibody specificity	Rh	I, i	P

Alternatively, the autoantibody may demonstrate relative specificity for glycophorin A.[38] On occasion, autoantibodies may demonstrate apparent specificity that appears consistent with an alloantibody. In these cases, there is transient decreased expression of the corresponding antigen. Following resolution of the AIHA, expression of that antigen will increase, returning to normal levels. Subsequent testing of the patient's convalescent red cells with retained serum will confirm the nature of the antibody as an autoantibody.

DAT-negative warm AIHA

In 1–3% of patients with warm AIHA, the DAT is negative[33–35,39] indicating that the quantity of bound IgG is too low to be detected by a DAT, or that the bound autoantibody is not of the IgG immunoglobulin class. As few as 230 molecules of IgG3 can result in hemolysis, yet this number is insufficient to produce a positive DAT.[40] Although IgG is the most common immunoglobulin class associated with warm AIHA, other immunoglobulin classes have been shown to cause AIHA, including IgA and IgM; these immunoglobulin classes are not detectable by routine antihuman globulin reagents. In 14% of warm AIHA cases, IgA was found coating the red cells.[41] It should be noted that cases solely attributable to IgA autoantibody are rare (less than 1%) and often IgG and/or IgM are found in combination with IgA.[42] Note that there are no anti-IgA or anti-IgM reagents that are currently licensed for serologic testing. In patients presenting with clinical features highly suggestive of warm AIHA, extended testing to identify DAT-negative cases should be performed, because DAT-negative cases often respond to typical therapy for warm AIHA.

Differential diagnosis

Other causes of anemia, such as hemorrhage or bone marrow failure, should also be considered. Other hemolytic disorders such as thrombotic thrombocytopenic purpura and the microangiopathic hemolytic anemias should be ruled out. Drug-induced immune hemolytic anemia produces a clinical syndrome with serology virtually indistinguishable from that of warm AIHA. The patient's clinical history should be reviewed for all recent medications. Although there are extensive lists of drugs that have been associated with drug-induced IHA in hematology texts, a suggestive drug history should be evaluated and suspected drugs discontinued even if they have not been previously reported.

Positive DAT results in patients without hemolytic anemia

Confirmation of the immune-mediated cause of a suspected warm AIHA should be sought and serology performed to determine the type of autoantibody coating the red cells. However, it is worth bearing in mind that disproportionate weight should not be placed on the results of the DAT. Up to 0.1% of healthy donors and 8% of hospitalized patients were found to demonstrate a positive DAT in the absence of signs of hemolysis.[43] Although a positive DAT can provide supportive evidence for warm AIHA in a patient with hemolysis, it is not independently indicative of the disease. The solitary finding of a positive DAT is not diagnostic of warm AIHA. Note that a negative DAT does not exclude the possibility of warm AIHA, because an IgA-mediated warm AIHA can present with a negative DAT and signs and symptoms of immune-mediated hemolysis.

Treatment

Treatment in warm AIHA is aimed at relieving clinical symptoms and transfusion dependence.[44]

Corticosteroids

The primary initial treatment for warm AIHA is corticosteroids. A standard therapeutic approach for adults includes prednisone 1.0 to 1.5 mg/kg per day or 60 to 100 mg/day for 1–3 weeks. A clinical response may be evident within several days to one week. Response rates of up to 80% within 3 weeks of treatment have been achieved with this therapy.[11] Most hematologists recommend continuation of higher corticosteroid doses for the first two weeks of therapy. Following initial response with improvement of hemoglobin and stabilization of hematologic parameters, the corticosteroid dose may be reduced.[45] Sudden decreases in dosage or rapidly progressive tapers may lead to relapse. If clinical relapse does occur, the prednisone dose should be increased. Maintenance doses of prednisone greater than 15 mg per day to maintain a hematocrit of at least 30% are considered therapeutic failures.

The adverse effects of corticosteroid therapy are well established. Initial complications include insomnia, increased appetite, weight gain, and emotional lability. Diabetes and hypertension may worsen. Long-term corticosteroid use is associated with the development of a cushingoid habitus, osteoporosis, avascular necrosis, posterior subcapsular cataracts, and glaucoma. Steroid use is associated with an increased risk of infection. Because of these serious adverse effects, steroids must be used judiciously and doses should be tapered as quickly as possible. Giving steroids every other day may reduce the complication rate.

The efficacy of corticosteroid therapy is likely related to several factors. Steroids have been shown to have an early effect on tissue macrophages, leading to less efficient clearance of IgG- and C3-coated red blood cells within the first eight days of therapy.[46] Steroids also affect antibody avidity and ultimately lead to a decrease in antibody production.[47] Following corticosteroid therapy, permanent remission is uncommon; it is seen in only 20–35% of adult patients.[48,49] When clinical response cannot be maintained despite high doses of corticosteroids, other therapies, such as splenectomy, rituximab, and cytotoxic therapy, are employed.[45] Although splenectomy has traditionally been the therapeutic approach following corticosteroid failure, rituximab is being used as a second-line approach with greater frequency. If a patient does not respond to rituximab, the selection of the next most appropriate therapeutic intervention should be based on evaluation of the specific patient and the severity of hemolysis.

Splenectomy

Splenectomy should be reserved for patients who show no initial response to steroids or who require large maintenance doses. It is nearly as clinically effective as steroids[45] and approximately 60–70% respond within two weeks.[50,51] In about 50% of patients who clinically respond to splenectomy, steroid therapy is still required, but at much lower doses than required preoperatively.[52] Despite an initial response, late clinical relapses are still seen in some patients. These relapses are thought to be due to enhanced antibody production as well as increased clearance of antibody-coated red cells by the liver.[7,49]

It should be remembered that postsplenectomy patients are particularly vulnerable to infection by encapsulated bacteria. When these infections occur, patients can rapidly progress to bacteremic shock due to an inability to efficiently clear the bacteria by phagocytosis. Overwhelming postsplenectomy sepsis syndrome represents a medical emergency with a risk of 3.2% in postsplenectomy patients and a mortality rate of 1.4%.[53] Pneumococcal and meningococcal vaccines are strongly recommended to prevent infection and mortality in these patients. Some clinicians advocate the use of prophylactic antibiotic regimens; commonly, prophylactic penicillin (250 mg twice a day) is given. Others prefer regimens of amoxicillin or bactrim. Febrile illness in splenectomized patients should be treated promptly with expeditious administration of antibiotics.

Rituximab and other monoclonal antibodies

Rituximab is a genetically engineered monoclonal antibody against CD20. It targets B-cell precursors and mature B cells. Plasma cells are not directly targeted as they do not carry the CD20 antigen. Most commonly, it has been reserved for cases of warm AIHA requiring large maintenance doses of steroids, for patients who cannot tolerate prednisone, and for patients who cannot undergo splenectomy. More recently, rituximab is being used as a second-line therapeutic approach following corticosteroid therapy, instead of the traditional secondary approach of splenectomy.[54] Typical dosing in warm AIHA is 375 mg/m² weekly for 2–4 weeks and possibly longer for some patients. Its use as a single-agent therapy has been shown by several case studies and retrospective reports to be efficacious in both adults and children with warm AIHA resistant to therapy, including some patients with Evans syndrome.[55–64] The combination of rituximab plus glucocorticoids has been evaluated in two small studies with promising initial results. Patients demonstrated higher initial clinical response rates and relapse-free survival over a three-year time period, when compared to glucocorticoid therapy alone. However, rituximab is expensive and can cause infusion-related reactions. Therefore, studies with longer term follow-up are needed before rituximab can be routinely recommended.

Alemtuzumab, a monoclonal anti-CD52 antibody, has been used as single-agent therapy and in combination with rituximab. Its use has only been studied in a handful of papers, with side effects including marked immunosuppression and infections.[65–67]

Immunosuppressive and cytotoxic therapy

Treatment with azathioprine or cyclophosphamide has demonstrated efficacy in reducing autoantibody formation and increasing hemoglobin levels.[45,68,69] Immunosuppressive agents should generally be reserved for cases of warm AIHA requiring large maintenance doses of steroids, or for patients who cannot tolerate prednisone[45] and cannot undergo splenectomy. Azathioprine takes at least one month to demonstrate an effect, and treatment failure is considered when there is no response after four months. Cyclophosphamide may be more effective than azathioprine[45,68] but has many side effects, including nephrotoxicity, that require careful monitoring. Although it has shown efficacy in treating warm AIHA in many trials,[70,71] it has also failed to demonstrate efficacy in others.[72] In select cases of refractory, severe warm AIHA, high-dose cyclophosphamide (50 mg/kg/day × 4 days) has been used with success as measured by induction of durable remission.[73] This intensive therapy has also been successfully used in other autoimmune diseases, including aplastic anemia.

Cyclosporine in combination with mycophenolate mofetil has been used with good results in some patients who are resistant to standard therapy. This combination has also demonstrated efficacy in patients with Evans syndrome and resistant disease.[70,74,75]

Other therapies

Danazol, an attenuated androgen, has been used in some cases of warm AIHA,[76,77] following the failure of steroid therapy either due to refractoriness or relapse.[77,78] The mechanism of action is unknown, but it appears to be most effective when used in initial treatment courses in combination with glucocorticoids.

Intravenous immunoglobulin (IVIG) shows neither clear efficacy nor failure; only 40% of patients respond to therapy,[79] and the response is typically only sustained if IVIG infusions are continued every three weeks.[80]

Therapeutic plasma exchange may be used as a temporizing measure. However, it is neither effective nor practical for long-term treatment. Severe warm AIHA is considered a Category III indication for plasma exchange therapy by the American Society for Apheresis, suggesting that the optimal role of apheresis has not been established for this disease with only case reports and case series demonstrating variable efficacy.[81]

Transfusion management

Support of patients with warm AIHA often requires red blood cell transfusion for severe and life-threatening anemia. Due to the broad reactivity of autoantibodies in this disease, serologic evaluation to select appropriate red cells for transfusion is often complex and time-consuming. Sometimes transfusion is clinically required before the serologic workup is complete. Frequently, even after completion of the serologic workup, red blood cells selected for transfusion are still incompatible with the patient's plasma. This finding should not be surprising given that the antibody found in the patient's serum is often broadly reactive with a variety of commercial red blood cells and it is actively attaching to the patient's own red blood cells. Transfusion of blood to a patient in true clinical need should not be delayed due to inability to find compatible red blood cell units. Most patients with AIHA show no adverse response to transfusion of serologically incompatible blood,[82–84] and the survival of transfused incompatible units is comparable to that expected for the patient's own red blood cells.

When assessing the need for transfusion, it is helpful to recall that patients with chronic anemia have a long history of physiologic compensation. They may appear hemodynamically stable even with life-threatening anemia. The onset of confusion in a patient with worsening anemia and/or reticulocytopenia should warrant immediate transfusion. Even young adults and children with gradual onset of anemia should be transfused to maintain a hemoglobin level above 4 mg/dL; higher hemoglobin levels are needed for older patients and patients with cardiovascular disease.[85]

Selection of blood for transfusion

ABO discrepancies and difficulty with Rh typing can arise in association with warm autoantibodies. When ABO discrepancy occurs, accurate ABO typing cannot proceed until the IgG autoantibody coating the red cells is removed. Rh typing may also be problematic, although use of low-protein, monoclonal reagents may improve results in the setting of immunoglobulin-coated red cells. When transfusion is urgent, recall that group O red cell components can be issued and administered, even if ABO typing is incomplete.

In many patients with autoantibodies, their history of transfusion or pregnancy allows for the possibility of an alloantibody in addition to their autoantibodies. Underlying alloantibodies have been seen in 32–40% of patients with AIHA.[86,87] Thus, identification of alloantibodies that may be obscured by the presence of a panreactive autoantibody is of great importance. The use of adsorption techniques is required for the removal of panagglutinating autoantibody from the patient's serum so that any underlying alloantibodies can be tested against commercially available red cells for identification.

Autologous adsorption, utilizing the patient's own red cells to draw off autoantibody, is a useful technique in patients who have not been transfused in the last three months.[88] If the patient has been recently transfused, allogeneic adsorptions may be required.[89,90] Adsorption techniques, particularly allogeneic adsorptions, are complex, labor-intensive, and time consuming.[86] Therefore, they may be incomplete when a transfusion is clinically necessary.

Identifying the patient's phenotype aids in the provision of appropriate blood for transfusion by focusing the alloantibody evaluation only on those alloantibody specificities the patient is capable of making. Phenotypically matched blood should be safe for transfusion even when the alloantibody workup is unenlightening.[87] In addition, provision of phenotype-matched blood may prevent the formation of alloantibodies.[91,92]

The practice of finding "least incompatible blood" is not suggested. This practice includes selection of red cell units based on crossmatch results having the lowest strength of agglutination. This practice is used by some when all crossmatches are incompatible. However, use of "least incompatible blood" has not been shown to improve safety of transfusion for recipients.[93] In addition, this practice is expected to lead to increased delays in the provision of blood due to time spent performing multiple crossmatches to compare the strength of agglutination.

Prognosis

Historically, the outcome of warm AIHA was poor, with a 38% mortality rate in the 1950s and 1960s.[26] More recent data indicate 91% survival at 1 year and up to 73% survival at 10 years.[94] The prognosis for children is excellent,[95–97] with most experiencing self-limited disease.[98,99]

Cold autoimmune hemolytic anemia

The autoantibodies responsible for cold AIHA optimally react at 0 °C.[1] When they react at warmer temperatures, demonstrating broader thermal amplitude, clinically significant hemolysis may ensue. Cold AIHAs are further subdivided into the more common CAD and the less common PCH, based on serologic and clinical properties. CAD is typically due to IgM autoantibodies.

Cold agglutinin disease
Epidemiology and risk factors

CAD accounts for 15–25% of cases of AIHA.[36,100] The classic patient is a female in her 70s.[3] In the largest study of patients with CAD to date, 61% of patients were female, and the median age at diagnosis was 72 years.[101] CAD following viral infections is more typically seen in children with transient disease.

Acute, transient CAD is most often due to *Mycoplasma pneumoniae* infection in adults and infectious mononucleosis in children. Chronic disease is typically associated with hematologic malignancies in older patients. In adults with chronic CAD and no obvious hematologic malignancy, flow cytometry can often detect an abnormal clone that may be responsible for the hemolysis and treatable by chemotherapy. Chronic disease does not usually occur in children.[9]

Pathophysiology

The red blood cells in CAD are typically coated with IgM. IgM binds to red cells at low temperatures, due to either the environmental cold or the relative decrease in temperature observed in the extremities. Once bound, IgM activates the classical pathway of complement, leading to the generation and binding of C3 to the red cell. If a critical amount of C3 is generated by complement activation, formation of the MAC may proceed, leading to red cell lysis and intravascular hemolysis. Hemolysis generally occurs if IgM is capable of remaining bound to the red cell and is immunologically active at both cool and warm temperatures, displaying broad thermal amplitude. If, on the other hand, the IgM has a narrow range of activity (or thermal amplitude), it has a smaller range of temperatures over which it can remain bound and activate complement. In this case, C3 will be formed and bound at cooler temperatures, and the amount of C3 generated may very well be below the amount needed to form the MAC.[102,103] In that case, the C3-coated red cells circulate to the spleen and liver where macrophages recognize and bind C3, and they phagocytose the red cells via extravascular hemolysis. Simultaneously, complement regulatory proteins work to inactivate C3 bound to red cells. Those red cells whose bound complement has been inactivated will still circulate through the spleen and liver, although the spleen will not recognize the inactive bound complement. The liver will recognize the inactive bound complement and sequester these red cells, frequently allowing them to return to the circulation after a period of time. Thus, when hemolysis in CAD occurs by way of the reticuloendothelial system, it is generally at a decreased pace and lesser degree, as compared to intravascular hemolysis. Extravascular hemolysis is the more common pathway in CAD. Unlike extravascular hemolysis in warm AIHA, in CAD, it more commonly occurs in the liver.[10]

Although the pathways of intravascular and extravascular hemolysis in IgM-mediated CAD are discussed as discrete entities for the purpose of understanding, these pathways are often not discrete. The percentage of hemolysis accounted for by each mechanism will depend on the titer of IgM, thermal amplitude of reactivity, and resultant number of red cells with sufficient complement activation for MAC formation.

Clinical features

As with other types of AIHA, patients with CAD present with symptoms of progressive anemia.[104] Given the pathophysiology, it is not surprising that there is an association between the thermal amplitude of the IgM autoantibody and severity of symptoms. Those patients having autoantibodies with a high thermal amplitude, immunologically reactive at higher temperatures, are more likely to have severe symptoms of hemolysis.[105] Those with low thermal amplitude, the more common occurrence, typically demonstrate an indolent course with a slower hemolytic rate than warm AIHA.[105] In either case, the anemia can be exacerbated by exposure to cold temperatures, such as during the winter or in a cold operating room, with acute hemolytic crises accompanied by frank hemoglobinuria. In addition, as with warm AIHA, the quantity of IgM, as measured by titration, is associated with the degree of hemolysis and observable symptoms. A higher titer autoantibody is more likely to be clinically significant.

On physical examination, these patients demonstrate pallor and jaundice, consistent with chronic anemia. Acrocyanosis of the tip of the nose, ears, fingers, and toes is common[101] and is resolved with warming.[104] Unlike, warm AIHA, hepatosplenomegaly is not a major feature.[101] In patients with secondary CAD due to an underlying process, whether it be a hematopoietic malignancy or infection, the symptoms associated with the underlying disease may predominate.

Diagnosis

Laboratory features

The first noticeable laboratory finding may actually be observed at the time of collection of a blood sample. The blood sample will demonstrate progressive agglutination as it cools from body to room temperature. The agglutination is reversible by warming the sample. On the wards, this phenomenon can be observed by holding the sample in your hands for a period of time. If the specimen cools prior to receipt in the lab or throughout the process of automated testing, spurious results such as macrocytosis may be encountered.[106] These spurious results frequently provide the first suggestion of this diagnosis. In order to avoid preanalytical testing problems, it is often necessary to maintain blood samples at 37 °C, most simply achieved by expeditiously collecting the blood sample and promptly placing it in a warm location (such as the transporter's axilla) for transport to the laboratory. Routine hematologic evaluation will reveal anemia with decreased hemoglobin and hematocrit. The peripheral blood smear will show agglutination with formation of irregular aggregates or clumps of red cells.

Serology

In CAD, a cold reactive, IgM antibody will be demonstrated by serology. The DAT will be negative with monospecific IgG reagent, but will be positive with C3 reagent (Table 12.2). Eluate studies are typically not performed, as they are not indicated in the setting of negative DAT results with anti-IgG. Instead, the IgM antibodies are further investigated by performing cold agglutinin titers and thermal amplitude measurement. Thermal amplitude measurement is often done in the presence of 30% bovine albumin as this medium enhances agglutination. These tests are important because higher titers and thermal amplitude are more likely to be associated with clinically apparent disease. Clinical CAD is most commonly seen in patients with cold autoantibodies having a titer >1000 and/or serum studies using 30% bovine albumin showing reactivity at 30 °C.[107] Because healthy individuals may often have low-titer cold autoantibodies, it is important to avoid misidentifying a patient with another cause for anemia as CAD based upon low-titer antibodies.

Cold panels, testing the patient's serum against cord blood cells, which mainly demonstrate the i antigen, and adult red blood cells, which mainly demonstrate I antigen, can be used to determine if the autoantibody demonstrates specificity. The most frequent antibody specificities are anti-i or anti-I.[108] The finding of anti-i is often associated with infectious mononucleosis, whereas anti-I is typically associated with *Mycoplasma pneumoniae* infections. Other antigen specificities such as Pr have also been demonstrated, albeit rarely.[109]

Differential diagnosis

As with warm AIHA, other etiologies of anemia should be considered and excluded. Nonimmune causes of hemolysis, such as microangiopathic hemolysis and mechanical hemolysis, should also be excluded. Once an immune-mediated process for the hemolysis has been established, alloimmune antibodies (especially in the recently transfused patient) must be ruled out. For an autoimmune process, serologic evaluation will determine the immunoglobulin class of the causative antibody, the temperature of optimal activity, and the thermal amplitude and titer in an effort to determine if the autoantibodies are capable of causing clinically significant disease.

Positive cold agglutinins in patients without hemolytic anemia

Cold reactive autoantibodies are commonly found in normal individuals. As with warm AIHA, the serologic findings in suspected CAD should always be correlated with clinical presentation, so as not to overstate their importance. Cold reactive autoantibodies in the absence of hemolysis are not diagnostic of CAD.

Treatment

Avoidance of cold

The mainstay of therapy for CAD is avoidance of the cold. Many patients with mild, chronic anemia are able to use this simple tactic to avoid transfusions for prolonged periods of time. Warming techniques during hypothermic surgeries should also be considered.[110]

Rituximab

Rituximab has been used with encouraging results in patients without an underlying hematologic malignancy.[111] Response rates as high as 79–83% have been demonstrated, although response rates in warm AIHA are still better. The role of prednisone in conjunction with rituximab is unclear at this time.[101,112–118]

Cytotoxic agents

Chlorambucil has been used with some success, but is associated with the side effect of bone marrow suppression.[68] Chemotherapeutic agents may be useful even in idiopathic cases where a malignant clone can be identified by hematologic analyses.

Other therapies

Therapeutic plasma exchange may be used as a temporizing measure, such as prior to surgery or during severe hemolysis, but the body temperature must be maintained at 37 °C and the use of an in-line blood warmer is recommended. The IgM antibodies in CAD have a larger intravascular volume and are more efficiently removed by apheresis than the IgG antibodies causing warm AIHA. Based predominantly on evidence from case reports, the American Society for Apheresis has deemed severe CAD as a category II indication for plasma exchange, indicating that apheresis is an acceptable second-line therapy.[81]

Other treatments such as IVIG,[39] interferon alpha,[119] erythropoietin, splenectomy, and glucocorticoids[103] are rarely useful in patients with CAD.

Transfusion management

Supportive care of patients with CAD occasionally includes transfusion. Transfusion may be episodic for those with well-controlled, mild, chronic disease. It may be urgent for those presenting with an acute exacerbation due to cold exposure.

As with warm AIHA, the serology and therefore provision of appropriate blood products may be complex. ABO typing in patients with CAD can be difficult. This test relies on the appearance of red cell agglutination as a positive result. Because the blood from patients with this disease agglutinates as the temperature declines and sometimes even at room temperature, the cold agglutinins can interfere with interpretation of this test. Warm washing of the red cells to remove the IgM autoantibody may be utilized to facilitate accurate ABO typing. Group O red cells can be transfused if ABO typing cannot be determined. For patients with a positive antibody screen, the distinction between a cold agglutinin reactive at room temperature and possible underlying alloantibodies must be made. Use of a prewarming technique, where the patient sample is warmed before being tested against an antibody panel of commercially available red cells, may prove useful. One can attempt to determine the specificity of the autoantibody; often, the antibody has specificity against the I antigen. It is not considered necessary to transfuse blood that is negative for the I antigen.[1] Transfusion with the use of a blood warmer is typically recommended, although not proven to be required.

Prognosis

The prognosis for CAD is better than for warm AIHA. The majority of patients have CAD as a transient problem following a viral infection and subsequently recover without recurrences. Other patients have a chronic, indolent course. There are rare reports of severe and even fatal CAD in the historic literature.[120,121] Although these cases did demonstrate an IgM autoantibody, the autoantibodies in these cases had unusually high thermal amplitudes.

Paroxysmal cold hemoglobinuria
Epidemiology and risk factors

PCH is uncommon, accounting for 2% of the AIHAs.[36] It is most commonly seen in children. When syphilis was more common, PCH was also seen in adults. Historically, PCH was seen in association with tertiary syphilis infection. As the incidence of syphilis declined, so too did the incidence of PCH. At present, PCH occurs most often in association with viral infections; the prototypical presentation is a child with a recent upper respiratory infection.

Pathophysiology

In PCH, the responsible autoantibody is an unusual IgG, called a *biphasic hemolysin* or *Donath–Landsteiner antibody*. This antibody binds red cells at cool temperatures and in the process irreversibly binds complement. At warmer temperatures, the antibody no longer stays bound. However, complement remains bound and becomes activated, leading to formation of the MAC resulting in intravascular hemolysis.

Clinical features

The typical presentation is a child with a recent history of upper respiratory tract infection. They may present with the dramatic appearance of hemoglobin in the urine. In addition to hemoglobinuria, jaundice, pallor, and fever may also be seen.[104] Hepatosplenomegaly is not a prominent feature. A history of cold exposure is usually not obtained.

Diagnosis

Laboratory findings

PCH often presents with laboratory evidence of anemia, which may be quite severe due to intravascular hemolysis.[122,123] Reticulocytosis may or may not be present.

The peripheral blood smear can demonstrate dramatic findings associated with complement binding and intravascular hemolysis, including spherocytes as well as fragmented red blood cell forms. Anisocytosis and poikilocytosis may be present. Polychromatophilic red cells may or may not be seen and are indirectly indicative of reticulocytosis. Erthyrophagocytosis by neutrophils may also be seen.

Serology

In patients with PCH, DATs are positive with anti-C3 complement reagent. They are negative with anti-IgG reagent, and eluate studies are therefore also negative. Antibody panels usually demonstrate specificity for the P antigen (Table 12.2). A special test, called the *Donath–Landsteiner test*, must be undertaken to demonstrate the biphasic nature of this antibody. In this test, the patient's serum is combined with normal serum as a fresh source of complement. Test red cells expressing the P antigen are then combined with the patient's serum. The mixture is subjected to the cold and then subsequently warmed to 37 °C. If hemolysis occurs, the test is positive, indicating the diagnosis of PCH.

Differential diagnosis

Given the rather dramatic presentation of intravascular hemolysis, the differential diagnosis should focus on excluding other causes of severe, acute intravascular hemolysis.

Treatment

Although the presentation is dramatic, the majority of cases of PCH are self-limited following a viral infection. Therefore, patients require supportive care during their acute illness, including blood transfusion. Corticosteroids are frequently used; however, their utility has not been established.

Transfusion management

Since the disease is typically self-limited, transfusion is commonly only required in the acute phase. Selection of blood appropriate for transfusion is aided by the fact that the causative biphasic autoantibody does not interfere with compatibility testing. The antibody itself does not bind red cells at temperatures above 4 °C and is therefore unable to exert its effects during routine testing.

Because the autoantibody usually demonstrates specificity for the P antigen, some advocate the use of red cell components negative for this antigen. However, donors with the p phenotype are uncommon and, consequently, these units are typically only available through rare donor registries. The provision of units with p phenotype is unlikely under urgent circumstances. Furthermore, it is more important to replace blood expeditiously in these patients than to obtain P antigen–negative blood. We recommend the selection of leukoreduced red cells to prevent febrile, nonhemolytic transfusion reactions, because these reactions would complicate an already complex clinical situation. It is unclear if the use of a blood warmer for transfusion is necessary, as the causative antibody is not reactive in compatibility testing greater than 4 °C. However, their use may be reassuring, especially for clinicians dealing with life-threatening anemia in a child.

Prognosis

The prognosis is excellent, with the disease typically following a self-limited course over a few days to weeks. The greatest risk to patients is in the acute phase when they may present with severe anemia and require urgent transfusion and supportive treatment.

Other types of autoimmune hemolytic anemias
Autoimmune hemolytic anemia due to warm IgM antibodies

Epidemiology and risk factors

AIHA due to warm IgM antibodies is rare. Most reported cases occur in adults.[124,125] However, a few cases in children have been reported.[126,127]

Pathophysiology

The causative autoantibody is an IgM antibody capable of coating red cells at body temperature. IgM is efficient at activating complement and causing intravascular hemolysis, via formation of the MAC. In addition, IgM may simultaneously bind to several red cells, causing them to link. These agglutinates of red cells linked by antibody may cause sludging and reduce perfusion to organs, leading to end-organ ischemia and tissue necrosis.

Clinical features

The classic presentation of AIHA due to warm IgM antibodies is intravascular hemolysis accompanied by tissue ischemia and/or infarcts. Cutaneous infarcts are manifested by visible gangrene. Ischemic infarcts elsewhere are frequently discovered by radiologic studies. Ischemia can be widespread, involving the brain, heart, and kidneys. These severely ill patients can therefore develop multi-organ failure.

Diagnosis

Laboratory findings

Laboratory results are often spurious due to the agglutination of samples caused by in vitro red cell linkage. When laboratory evaluations are possible, findings include anemia, hyperbilirubemia, elevated lactate dehydrogenase, hemoglobinemia, hemoglobinuria, and decreased haptoglobin.

Serology

Serologic studies demonstrate spontaneous agglutination that cannot be resolved with warming of the sample. Even repeated warm washes will not disperse the agglutination. The diagnostic finding is an IgM autoantibody with high thermal amplitude. Treatment with dithiothreitol (DTT) or 2-mercaptoethanol (2-ME) may be used to disrupt the IgM autoagglutinin in order to perform further serologic testing.

Treatment

The goal of therapy is to decrease in vivo red cell agglutination by the rapid reduction of antibody. Whole blood and plasma exchange have been used successfully as temporizing measures. Despite immunosuppressive drugs, cytotoxic agents, and exchange protocols, successful long-term treatment approaches have not been identified and the mortality rate is high.

Prognosis

Autoimmune hemolytic anemia due to IgM autoantibodies is virtually universally fatal.[124]

Warm and cold, or mixed AIHA

In addition to the outlined distinct cases of warm versus cold AIHA, some patients present with elements of both types of AIHA. There may be a predominance of one type over another, but laboratory and clinical findings ultimately overlap. Mixed AIHA comprises approximately 7% of all cases of idiopathic AIHA.[128] Of note, this entity typically responds to treatments appropriate for warm AIHA; these patients frequently have a rapid response to corticosteroid therapy. Consequently, it is of the utmost importance to identify the warm autoantibody component; misclassification of mixed AIHA as CAD could delay appropriate therapy.

Drug-induced immune hemolytic anemia
Epidemiology and risk factors

Drug-induced immune hemolytic anemia can occur in any age group; it may occur in association with a wide variety of medications, including prescription drugs, over-the-counter medications, and toxin exposures. The most commonly implicated drug class in current practice is the cephalosporins.[129] In the largest series of drug-induced immune hemolytic anemias, the odds ratio for developing immune hemolytic anemia was significantly increased with cotrimoxazole (trimethoprim/sulfamethoxazole), fludarabine, lorazepam, and diclofenac.[130]

Pathophysiology

Three different mechanisms have been proposed for drug-induced immune hemolytic anemia, including the drug adsorption mechanism, immune complex mechanism, and autoimmune induction mechanism.

In the drug adsorption mechanism, the drug attaches to the surface of the red blood cell. The resultant antibody formed is directed against the drug. The antibody binds to the drug, which remains bound to the red cell. The antibody–drug coated red cell is removed, typically via extravascular hemolysis. The prototypic drug associated with this mechanism is penicillin, particularly with very high doses.

In the immune complex mechanism, circulating drug stimulates the immune system to produce antibody directed against the drug. The antibody binds to the circulating drug, and the resulting immune complex can then bind to a red cell. It is unknown whether binding to the red cell is specific or nonspecific. The red cells, coated by antibody–drug complexes, are typically removed via brisk, intravascular hemolysis. The prototypic drug for this mechanism is quinidine.

In the autoimmune induction mechanism, the drug induces autoantibody formation. The resulting immune-mediated hemolytic anemia is serologically and clinically indistinguishable from warm AIHA. The autoantibody may persist even long after the offending drug has been discontinued. The prototypic drug demonstrating this mechanism of immune hemolytic anemia is α-methyldopa, a medication commonly used to treat hypertension in the past.

Although explanation of these mechanisms as discrete entities is helpful to understand the many ways in which drugs, antibodies, and red cells can interact, there is little laboratory evidence of these purported mechanisms. In addition, some patients have laboratory findings that overlap with more than one mechanism. A unifying theory was therefore proposed by Garratty, which argues that the antibodies against the drug itself, against the red cell membrane or components of both, could be present simultaneously (Figure 12.1). The specificity of the formed antibodies depends on the site of interaction between the drug and red cell. The unifying theory explains how patients may present with clinical evidence of multiple simultaneous pathophysiologies of drug-induced immune hemolytic anemia.[129,131]

Clinical features

The clinical presentation of drug-induced immune hemolytic anemia can be broad, ranging from mild anemia to severe hemolysis with life-threatening anemia. There may be hemoglobinemia and hemoglobinuria as well as renal failure. As previously described, the hemolysis produced is frequently indistinguishable from warm AIHA.

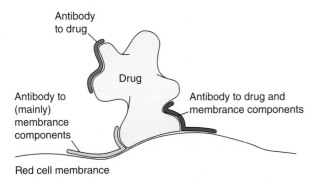

Figure 12.1 Proposed unifying theory of drug-induced antibody reactions. The thick lines represent antigen-binding sites of the drug-induced antibody. Antibodies may be made to the drug (producing in vitro reactions typical of a drug adsorption [penicillin-type] reaction); the membrane components or mainly membrane components (producing in vitro reactions typical of an autoantibody); or part-drug, part-membrane components (producing and in vitro reaction typical of the immune-complex mechanism).[129] This unifying theory was proposed by George Garratty, PhD. (1935–2014), who made significant contributions to the study of drug-induced immune hemolytic anemias. (Source: Garratty (2004).[129] Reproduced with permission of American Red Cross.)

Diagnosis

Serology

As with pathophysiology, the serologic findings can be divided into three categories. Warm reactive IgG antibodies are seen in cases of extravascular hemolysis associated with drug exposure and presumed to be due to the drug adsorption mechanism. The DAT is positive in these patients, revealing coating of red cells by IgG. The DAT may or may not show complement coating of the red cells. The indirect antiglobulin test (patient serum combined with reagent red blood cells) is positive only if the red cells are pretreated with the specific drug, such as penicillin.[132]

In cases of intravascular hemolysis presumed to be due to the immune complex drug mechanism, IgG, IgM, or both are found in association with complement. The DAT is usually positive for complement coating of the red cells as demonstrated by positivity with anti-C3 reagent. The indirect antiglobulin test is positive only if the drug is added to the reaction.

In cases demonstrating evidence of the autoimmune induction mechanism, the serologic findings are almost indistinguishable from those of warm AIHA, with a DAT positive for IgG but not C3 and panreactivity in serum studies. The antibodies may even show broad specificity for Rh antigens and may persist after the drug is discontinued.[133–135]

Specific drugs or drug metabolites can be utilized in additional serologic testing to demonstrate the connection between the antibody and presence of the drug. If testing is positive specifically in the presence of a drug, the association is confirmed. However, this testing is complex and typically only available through a reference laboratory.

Differential diagnosis

The differential diagnosis for drug-induced immune hemolytic anemia includes all causes of hemolytic anemia. Attempts should be made to determine the patient's drug history, including prescription medications, over-the-counter drugs, and chemical exposures. Although long lists of causative drugs have been compiled, it

should be kept in mind that the majority of these drugs are implicated in case reports. A convincing clinical picture should prompt discontinuation of the drug, even if it has not previously been associated with hemolytic anemia.

Treatment

Treatment is aimed mainly at discontinuing the causative drug. Corticosteroids are frequently given, although there are only empirical data to support their use.

Transfusion management

Transfusion support may be necessary for patients presenting with massive intravascular hemolysis. The hemolysis may be so great as to cause renal failure, requiring supportive therapies. This severe presentation is typically associated with patients demonstrating IgG, IgM, or a combination of the two and complement on their red cells, presumed secondary to the immune complex mechanism of drug-induced immune hemolytic anemia. In the case of hemolysis persisting even after discontinuation of the offending drug, as is presumed to be due to the autoimmune induction mechanism, a prolonged period of transfusion support may be required.[9]

Prognosis

The prognosis is excellent for this form of AIHA; full resolution of hemolysis is expected. The offending drug or toxin must be avoided indefinitely.

Paroxysmal nocturnal hemoglobinuria

Paroxysmal nocturnal hemoglobinuria (PNH) is a rare type of hemolytic anemia that can present with thrombosis and bone marrow dysfunction.[136] It is a clonal disorder of hematopoietic stem cells with its biochemical pathogenesis based in a somatic gene mutation.[137] The somatic mutation ultimately decreases availability of an enzyme required for synthesis of the anchor molecule, glycosylphosphatidylinositol (GPI), responsible for binding numerous proteins to the external surface of red blood cells. Two of the affected proteins, which are responsible for the majority of symptoms seen in PNH, are the complement-regulatory proteins CD55 and CD59. Without GPI binding of CD55 and CD59 to the cell surface, the red cells lack their normal defenses against random complement activation and have increased sensitivity to complement-mediated lysis.

Epidemiology and risk factors

PNH is rare, occurring at a rate of approximately 1–10 cases per million people.[138,139] It has been diagnosed in patients of all ages.[140,141] The median age at diagnosis is early thirties.[141–143] Pediatric cases account for only 10% of reported cases of PNH.[144,145] No apparent gender predilection has been identified.[142]

Although PNH can occur de novo, virtually all patients demonstrate some degree of bone marrow failure.[136] Likewise, red cells or granulocytes deficient in GPI-linked molecules, such as CD55 and CD59, are identified in a large number of patients with bone marrow disorders such as aplastic anemia and, to a lesser extent, low-risk myelodysplastic syndrome (MDS).[142,146] The leading hypothesis for this close association is that there is a selective growth advantage for PNH clones in these disorders; however, the exact etiology of PNH clones in these patients remains unclear.[146–149] Additionally, the finding of PNH clones may not always be clinically significant. In aplastic anemia and MDS, PNH clones are so commonly found that screening for undetected clones is recommended in patients with these disorders.[150,151] In most cases, the percentage of abnormal cells is so small that clinical symptoms are not observed and therapy for PNH is not indicated.[146] Furthermore, the stem cell mutations underlying PNH can be found at a low frequency in healthy controls.[152,153] Therefore, many questions remain unanswered, including what leads to multipotent stem cell mutations, why the clones sometimes expand to a high enough percentage to cause clinical disease, and why bone marrow failure exists in virtually all cases.

Although paroxysms of hemolysis may occur without preceding risk factors, it is generally agreed that factors leading to complement activation can trigger hemolytic episodes. Infection, trauma, pregnancy, and surgery are examples of known triggers of complement activation that may form the background upon which a PNH paroxysm occurs.[154]

Pathophysiology

PNH is a clonal disorder of multipotent hematopoietic stem cells that ultimately causes increased sensitivity to complement in its progeny cells. In virtually all cases, a somatic mutation in the X-linked phosphatidylinositol glycan class A (PIG-A) gene underlies the disorder. The PIG-A gene encodes for the PIG-A enzyme, which is needed in the first step of biosynthesis of the GPI anchor molecule.[137] GPI anchor molecules are needed to bind numerous proteins to the external surface of hematopoietic cells.[137] The majority of symptoms seen in PNH are due to the lack of binding of two of the affected proteins, CD55 and CD59. These complement-regulatory proteins are normally needed on the external surface in order to neutralize complement activation. CD55 accelerates the destruction of C3 convertase, reducing the activation of complement component C3 and its effect of leading to extravascular hemolysis by macrophages in the spleen and liver.[155] CD59 prevents the MAC from completing its action of pore production in the lipid bilayer of the cell and its effect of cell lysis through hypertonic cell swelling.[156] In brief, the PIG-A mutation leads to decreased or absent GPI molecules,[137] which, in turn, results in decreased or absent binding of proteins such as CD55 and CD59[136] to the cell surface and, ultimately, increased cell sensitivity to complement.

Two conditions must be met in order for the mutation to cause clinical symptoms: it must occur in a multipotent hematopoietic stem cell, and the stem cell carrying the mutation must undergo clonal expansion.[152,157] Evidence for the former requirement is that rare, circulating blood cells with PNH mutations can be seen in healthy blood donors[152,153] and low-frequency PNH clones in MDS rarely, if ever, lead to clinical disease.[136,158] Mutations in these cases appear to arise in hematopoietic cells without self-renewal capacity. If the mutation occurs in a multipotent hematopoietic stem cell, it will result in hematopoietic progeny (red cells, platelets, and white blood cells) that also harbor the mutation.[136] Patients with aplastic anemia, unlike those with MDS, more commonly develop PNH because mutations in these patients arise from multipotent hematopoietic stem cells.[136] Yet it is not enough that the mutations occur in a cell capable of creating progeny in all hematopoietic lineages. Low-frequency mutations do not cause clinical disease.[146] On the contrary, patients with greater than 20–25% of their neutrophils and greater than 3–5% of their red cells lacking CD55 and CD59 surface

proteins are more likely to demonstrate clinical signs of hemolysis and require specific treatment than those with lower values.[146] Likewise, patients with a higher proportion of PNH neutrophils (and monocytes) are more likely to demonstrate thrombosis,[159] with neutrophil clone sizes greater than 50% being highly predictive of thrombotic risk.[160] Although there are several purported hypotheses,[153,161–166] the mechanism by which PNH cells can achieve clonal expansion remains unknown.

The ultimate clinical effect of having a sizeable PNH cell population depends on the type of surface protein and cell affected. Affected red blood cells show decreased or absent CD59 and, as a result, are exquisitely sensitive to intravascular hemolysis from random complement activation. They also show decreased or absent CD55, causing them to be incapable of reducing C3 activation and making them vulnerable to extravascular hemolysis in the spleen and liver. On the other hand, the increased sensitivity to complement resulting from lack of CD55 and CD59 in platelets results in their inappropriate activation and an increased risk of thrombosis.[167] In affected leukocytes, absence of a receptor for urokinase-type plasminogen activator reduces the potential of these cells to convert plasminogen to plasmin.[168] The decreased formation of plasmin, which has a significant role in fibrinolysis, may also lead to increased risk of thrombosis.[169,170] Although all patients with PNH are at risk for thrombosis, there is increased risk with larger PNH clone size.[142] When thrombosis occurs in PNH patients, it often does so in atypical locations such as the portal circulation, although the reason is unclear.[136]

Secondary effects of sizeable PNH clonal populations are also seen. Increased intravascular hemolysis leads to large amounts of free hemoglobin, which overwhelm the normal mechanisms of clearance, such as binding by haptoglobin.[171,172] The circulating free hemoglobin in plasma then scavenges and reacts with nitric oxide.[172,173] The depletion of nitric oxide is thought by some to contribute to arterial constriction, decreased blood flow to organs, kidney damage, and pulmonary hypertension.[174] However, others believe that chronic kidney disease is due to tubular damage caused by microvascular thrombosis[175–177] and iron deposition from hemolysis.[136] Microthrombi may also contribute to pulmonary hypertension.[136] Decreased nitric oxide may also lead to smooth muscle dystonia manifested as chronic dysphagia, abdominal pain, and erectile dysfunction.[178]

In patients with PNH clones and clinical hemolysis, the hemolysis typically occurs at a chronic baseline rate punctuated by episodic periods of an increased hemolytic rate. The pathophysiology of these episodic exacerbations of hemolysis is thought to be due to enhanced complement activation in certain situations; infection, trauma, pregnancy, surgery, strenuous physical activity, and alcohol use are examples of known triggers.[154,179] Additionally, repletion of iron in a deficient patient is a known trigger of PNH exacerbations; it is thought to cause increased hemolysis by increasing the number of PNH clones.[180] Both enhanced complement activation and increased PNH clone size may form the background upon which a PNH paroxysm occurs.

Finally, although the PIG-A mutation described is prototypical for and present in the vast majority of PNH cases, other mutations have been described.[181,182]

Clinical features

PNH classically presents with the triad of hemolytic anemia, thrombosis, and bone marrow dysfunction.[136] Because the clinical findings are variable, three clinical categories of PNH have been described. In classical PNH, patients frequently have >50% PNH granulocytes, and episodic hemolytic anemia accounts for the majority of the clinical picture. These patients may present with fatigue, jaundice, and a history of dark urine, consistent with hemoglobinuria. The hemoglobinuria may be nocturnal, as implied by the disease's moniker; however, it may also occur at other times. These patients are also the most likely to develop thrombosis.[136] The second clinical category of PNH is clinically apparent disease occurring in the context of bone marrow disorders, most frequently aplastic anemia. In the context of an underlying bone marrow disorder, patients with PNH also present with symptoms of anemia, which is more likely due to bone marrow failure; they are less likely to demonstrate symptoms of hemolysis (jaundice, dark urine). They often have low platelet counts and a lower risk of thrombosis. The third category is subclinical PNH. By definition, these patients are asymptomatic[136] and typically have less than 10% PNH red blood cells or granulocytes in their peripheral blood.[136,150] The discrete definition of this disease into three clinical categories may be useful for understanding the variable clinical presentations, but it is not perfect. A particular point of confusion not addressed by these categories is that some element of bone marrow failure underlies virtually all PNH cases.

As mentioned above, patients with PNH clones and clinical hemolysis experience a chronic baseline rate of hemolysis punctuated by episodes of increased hemolysis. Infection, trauma, pregnancy, surgery, strenuous physical activity, alcohol use, and iron replacement in deficient patients are known triggers[154,179] of hemolytic paroxysms in PNH.

Thrombosis is rarely the presenting symptom of PNH,[183] but it is common over the course of the disease and occurs in up to 40% of patients.[179] Additionally, thrombi are the most common life-threatening complication in PNH.[159,177] The thromboses in PNH patients are often in atypical locations, most commonly affecting abdominal and cerebral vasculature, with veins more often affected than arteries. Commonly affected abdominal veins include the hepatic, portal, mesenteric, and splenic veins. The sagittal and cavernous sinuses are the most frequently affected cerebral vasculature. Overall, the most common site of thrombosis in these patients is the hepatic veins;[136] thrombi in this location cause a decrease in the normal flow of blood out of the liver, a process termed *Budd–Chiari syndrome*.[184,185] Despite frequently presenting in these atypical locations, thrombosis may occur in any site, and deep venous thrombosis, pulmonary emboli, and dermal thrombi are relatively common.[136] When thrombosis does occur, it tends to be progressive despite anticoagulant therapy.[159,177]

Patients with PNH may also present with symptoms of increased smooth muscle tone, manifested by chronic dysphagia, abdominal pain, and erectile dysfunction.[178] Over time, these patients may develop renal insufficiency and pulmonary hypertension. There is greater than a sixfold increase in risk of developing chronic kidney disease in PNH patients.[175] Although clinically significant pulmonary hypertension in PNH is rare, testing for terminal pro-brain natriuretic peptide[186] and transthoracic Doppler echocardiography[187] indicates that pulmonary hypertension is present in approximately half of these patients.

Most patients have a chronic illness that persists without therapy; interestingly, a small subset of patients may achieve spontaneous, long-term remission. A recent study found that 15% of patients had a spontaneous, sustained remission.[140]

Diagnosis

Laboratory findings

With the variable clinical presentation of PNH, the associated laboratory findings vary as well. In classical PNH, which includes patients with intravascular hemolysis and the highest risk of thrombosis, one can expect to find anemia, reticulocytosis, elevated lactate dehydrogenase,[137] elevated bilirubin, and decreased haptoglobin. Bone marrow evaluation demonstrates an overall hypercellular marrow with erythroid hyperplasia but no karyotypic abnormalities.[150,188] Patients with PNH in the context of an underlying bone marrow disorder also have anemia, but their laboratory results are predominated by the effects of bone marrow failure more so than intravascular hemolysis. These patients have severe thrombocytopenia, normal or only mildly elevated lactate dehydrogenase,[136] normal or only mildly elevated bilirubin,[189] and lower levels of reticulocytes than patients with classical PNH.[136] Patients with subclinical PNH have normal or only modestly aberrant blood counts.[136]

Peripheral blood smear findings are variable and include a broad array of anisocytosis and poikilocytosis.[190]

Serology

In PNH, the DAT is classically negative.[189] Patients undergoing eculizumab therapy may have a positive DAT; this therapy prevents formation of the MAC and intravascular lysis, but it does not prevent C3 coating of the red cells.[191–193]

Confirmatory tests
Acidified serum test (HAM test)

The earliest confirmatory test for PNH was the acidified serum test, or HAM test (named after its developer, Thomas Ham).[194] In this assay, red cells are combined with acidified serum. PNH red cells are more sensitive to complement and more likely to undergo lysis in the presence of acid. Spectrophotometry is utilized to quantify the presence of free hemoglobin liberated from hemolysis. This test is easy to perform, inexpensive, and reliable, but it cannot quantify the number of PNH cells present.[195] A positive test is not specific for PNH and may be seen in other disorders leading to enhanced sensitivity to complement (such as congenital dyserythropoietic anemia type II [HEMPAS] where hemolysis is enacted by an anti-HEMPAS antibody that binds complement).

Flow cytometry

Because of the sensitivity and specificity of flow cytometry for detection of PNH cells, it has become the gold standard. Classically, flow cytometry of the peripheral blood is aimed at detecting the marked reduction or absence of the GPI-anchored proteins, CD55 and CD59, on red cell or granulocyte surfaces. Monoclonal antibodies that bind each of these GPI-anchored proteins are tagged with a fluorescent label and combined with a patient sample, allowing the detection of cells capable of binding the antibody. This analysis provides useful information regarding the quantity of cells lacking or deficient in CD55 and CD59 as well as the strength of expression of these proteins on the cell surface.[195] In normal patients, all red cells and granulocytes demonstrate strong expression of CD55 and CD59. In patients with PNH, a variable proportion of red cells and/or granulocytes lacking CD55 and CD59 will be demonstrated in addition to a population of cells with strong expression of these surface proteins.[195] Flow cytometry of monocytes and granulocytes may be more accurate, as their numbers are not affected by recent red blood cell transfusions or hemolysis. Lymphocytes show variable expression of GPI-anchored proteins and are therefore undesirable for use in PNH diagnosis.[195] Ideally, PNH should be confirmed with findings of decreased or absent GPI-anchor proteins in two or more cell lines.[188,196]

The newest flow cytometry test, called fluorescent aerolysin (FLAER), is also aimed at detecting a marked reduction or absence of GPI-anchored proteins. The concept underlying FLAER is that GPI-anchored proteins bind a bacterial toxin called aerolysin. PNH cells lack GPI-anchored proteins and therefore lack the ability to bind the aerolysin toxin. By tagging the aerolysin toxin with a fluorescent label, the amount of cells capable of binding the toxin and the strength of binding can be quantified.[197] The sensitivity of FLAER is much higher than that achieved with a CD55- and CD59-based assay.[198] The detection rate is further improved when the FLAER reagent is combined with fluorescent labeled antibodies for GPI-anchored proteins on granulocytes and monocytes.[195] Red cells are not commonly included in analysis with a FLAER assay as they express glycophorin, which is capable to weakly binding aerolysin and thus affecting assay accuracy.[179] Peripheral blood flow cytometric analysis is preferred to that of bone marrow for routine analysis; it shows no diagnostic disadvantage and represents an analysis of cells that are more homogeneous with respect to stage of maturation and expression of GPI-anchor proteins.[195]

Differential diagnosis

The differential diagnosis includes consideration of other causes of anemia. If hemoglobinuria or other signs of intravascular hemolysis are present, other causes of hemolytic anemia must be ruled out, such as G6PD deficiency and PCH.

Treatment

In treating PNH, the choice of therapy (or therapies) depends on the type of symptoms the patient is experiencing (hemolysis versus thrombosis) as well as the degree of anemia. Indeed, therapy does not need to be initiated in an asymptomatic patient found to have PNH clones; these patients can be actively monitored for development of symptoms.

Anticoagulants and thrombolytic agents

Historically, anticoagulants represented one of the mainstays of therapy in PNH. Use of prophylactic anticoagulants in patients with PNH neutrophil clones greater than 50%, in the absence of contraindications, has been recommended.[199,200] However, this recommendation has been called into question,[201] particularly in the current era of eculizumab therapy. Problems with anticoagulant therapy include their lack of complete efficacy in preventing thrombotic events; in fact, the risk of thromboemboli remains high even with prophylaxis.[177,202] Additionally, anticoagulants increase the risk of bleeding, which may be compounded when patients also have thrombocytopenia.[201] Some experts recommend against routine prophylactic use of anticoagulants;[201] they are currently used in only 25% of patients with no history of thrombosis.[142] On the contrary, patients with other underlying risks for thrombosis such as pregnant patients or patients undergoing a recent surgery should still be considered for prophylactic anticoagulation.[201] Even in patients with a history of thrombosis,

anticoagulants have lacked success.[150,188] In patients receiving eculizumab, thrombotic event rates decline independent of prior or concurrent anticoagulant therapy,[203] making eculizumab the recommended therapy for the majority of patients with PNH and thrombosis. Despite these data, the discontinuation of anticoagulants in patients undergoing eculizumab is controversial,[201] and anticoagulants are still used in 70% of patients with PNH and a history of thrombotic event.[142]

Particular attention should be paid to clone size and symptoms of abdominal or chest pain. The risk of thrombotic events has been shown to correspond with clone size. In addition, patients with abdominal or chest pain have a greater risk of thrombosis.[142] Thrombolytic therapy with tissue plasminogen activator may be life-saving in severe thrombus formation, such as Budd–Chiari syndrome.[203]

Eculizumab

Eculizumab is a monoclonal IgG antibody that binds to the C5 complement protein, thereby inhibiting formation of the MAC[204–206] and reducing intravascular hemolysis of red blood cells in patients with PNH.[188] It was approved by the FDA for use in reduction of hemolysis in PNH in 2007.[207] It has been shown to be efficacious in reducing red cell transfusions,[176,204,207,208] thrombotic events,[176,177,204,209] lactate dehydrogenase levels,[204,207] nitric oxide depletion,[191] abdominal pain,[208] pulmonary hypertension,[186] and surgery-triggered hemolysis.[210] Eculizumab also leads to improvement in time-dependent renal function[204] and quality-of-life scores.[186,205,206] Survival rates are significantly increased both in the short term and long term.[176,204] The reduction of lactate dehydrogenase level is sustained over the course of treatment.[204] The drug is not curative,[211] and therapy must be continued for life.[137] Specific guidelines for use are still being determined. Some suggest eculizumab for patients with symptoms of hemolysis that are not managed by transfusion alone;[212] others use eculizumab in patients with fatigue that affects quality of life, transfusion dependence, thrombosis, frequent symptoms associated with smooth muscle dystonia (dysphagia, abdominal pain, or erectile dysfunction), renal insufficiency, or end-organ disease complications.[188] Its use may be particularly indicated in the perioperative period[210,213] or pregnant patient.[214–217] See the "Special Clinical Situations" section.

Despite its successes, not all patients respond to eculizumab therapy, and some have persistent symptoms and chronic need for red cell transfusion.[211] Some patients who fail to respond were found to have specific mutations of C5.[218] Other patients experience continued extravascular hemolysis, due to continued accumulation of C3 on the surface of red blood cells.[191,192,219] Further support of this mechanism is the observation of positive DATs with anti-C3 reagent in patients undergoing eculizumab treatment.[211] Eculizumab does not treat underlying bone marrow failure.[211]

Overall, eculizumab is well tolerated,[171,175,177,186,204–206,220] with the occurrence of adverse events decreasing over time. There is no evidence for cumulative toxicity.[204] Its use is associated with an increased risk of infection, particularly serious meningococcal infections. Meningococcal vaccine must be administered two weeks prior to treatment, patients' vaccination status should be kept up to date per current medical guidelines, and they should be followed for signs of infection to expedite prompt antibiotic treatment.[207] The most detrimental side effect of eculizumab is its extreme cost, averaging over $400,000 per year of treatment.[211]

Hematopoietic cell transplantation

The only potentially curative therapy for PNH is hematopoietic cell transplantation. However, transplantation using either bone marrow or peripheral blood stem cells as the graft source,[221] is associated with substantial morbidity and mortality[222–224] including high rates of rejection, side effects from the preparative regimen, and graft-versus-host disease.[221] Hematopoietic cell transplantation is considered for patients with severe clinical symptoms who are unresponsive to eculizumab therapy or for whom eculizumab therapy is not an option due to cost or lack of availability.[136] Using bone marrow as a source of stem cells may lead to a lower incidence of graft-versus-host disease, as compared to using peripheral blood.[224] Nonmyeloablative conditioning regimens show promise for improved outcomes and reduced morbidity and mortality.[221,225–228]

Hematopoietic cell transplantation may also be indicated for treatment of the patient's underlying bone marrow disorder, independent of PNH.

Immunosuppressive therapy

Patients with underlying bone marrow disorders, such as aplastic anemia, are more likely to receive immunosuppressive therapy with cyclosporine and/or antithymocyte globulin[142] than other PNH patients. Immunosuppressive, but not bone marrow–suppressive, therapy is likely the most effective therapy in patients with underlying bone marrow disorders. Corticosteroids may reduce hemolysis and improve anemia in some patients, but they carry an added risk of long-term toxicity.[188] In addition, others have reported little success with corticosteroid use in treating patients with underlying bone marrow disorders,[150] and their use is therefore becoming less common.

Other therapies

Given that eculizumab is successful in most PNH patients but that some continue to have extravascular hemolysis due to C3 deposition, novel therapies targeting C3 and other components of the complement activation pathway are being tested in vitro and in animal models, with promising results.[229–232]

In patients with marked hemolysis, replacement of iron (for iron-deficient patients), B_{12}, and folate to support production of new red blood cells may be indicated.

Special clinical situations

Complement activation is triggered by infection, trauma, pregnancy, and surgery.[154,210] Therefore, the use of eculizumab may be particularly indicated in the perioperative period[210,213] or for pregnant patients.[214–217]

Pregnancy

As previously discussed, pregnant patients with PNH frequently experience thrombosis. The risk of thrombosis in the setting of PNH is exacerbated by the hypercoagulability of pregnancy. Anticoagulant therapy may be an appropriate strategy to reduce morbidity and mortality during pregnancy. Eculizumab may also be useful and safe in pregnancy. The molecule is a hybrid IgG2 and IgG4, and IgG2 does not cross the placenta well.[233] Only a handful of case reports on the use of eculizumab in pregnant PNH patients exist, and there is great heterogeneity in the use of therapy prior to pregnancy, time of discontinuation (either during or following pregnancy), and concomitant use of anticoagulant therapy.

Teratogenic effects of eculizumab have not been observed.[214–216] Fetal outcomes to date have been good.[214–217]

Elective surgery

Few reports of perioperative eculizumab use suggest it may be helpful in preventing hemolytic paroxysms. One group reported successful cardiopulmonary bypass surgery in a PNH patient on maintenance therapy,[213] whereas another reported prevention of hemolysis using perisurgical induction with eculizumab for distal gastrectomy.[210]

Underlying bone marrow disorders

Asymptomatic patients with PNH clones do not need to be treated for PNH. Many of these patients have underlying bone marrow disorders, such as aplastic anemia or MDS, and therapy should be targeted toward those conditions instead of PNH.[188,214]

Children

PNH in children is rare; reports on their treatment are therefore also rare. Studies on the use of eculizumab in children have suggested its use is safe and effective.[234]

Transfusion management

Historically, blood transfusions have been a mainstay of therapy for PNH patients with moderate to severe hemolysis and anemia. They are still recommended for patients with severe, symptomatic anemia. Unlike with the warm and cold AIHAs, special testing and selection of specific red cells for transfusion are not required in PNH unless the patients develop a positive antibody screen. The red cell components do not typically need special modifications, such as washing or irradiation. However, leukoreduced red cell components should be selected to prevent febrile nonhemolytic transfusion reactions and alloimmunization, as would be indicated for any patient receiving chronic transfusions. Previous reports of the need to wash red cells have been discredited, because the hemolysis reported with unwashed cells was most likely due to minor incompatibilities. Platelet transfusion may also be given for a variety of clinical indications, including treatment of sequelae in patients with thrombocytopenia undergoing anticoagulant and/or thrombolytic therapy. Although not required based on the sole indication of PNH, blood product modifications may be necessary because of the patient's associated conditions or therapy, such as hematopoietic cell transplantation.

Prognosis

The 10-year survival rate for PNH patients between 1940 and 1970 was 50%.[140,143,176] More recently, the 10-year survival rate for PNH was 75%.[235] A small subset of patients may achieve long-term remission. A recent study found that 15% of patients had a spontaneous, sustained remission.[140]

Key references

A full reference list for this chapter is available at: http://www.wiley.com/go/simon/transfusion

2 Petz LD, Garratty G. *Immune hemolytic anemias*. 2nd ed. Philadelphia: Churchill Livingstone/Elsevier Science, 2004.

44 King KE. Review: pharmacologic treatment of warm autoimmune hemolytic anemia. *Immunohematology/Amer Red Cross* 2007; **23** (3): 120–9.

52 Petz LD. Treatment of autoimmune hemolytic anemias. *Curr Opin Hematol* 2001; **8** (6): 411–6.

85 Ness PM. How do I encourage clinicians to transfuse mismatched blood to patients with autoimmune hemolytic anemia in urgent situations? *Transfusion* 2006; **46** (11): 1859–62.

87 Shirey RS, Boyd JS, Parwani AV, Tanz WS, Ness PM, King KE. Prophylactic antigen-matched donor blood for patients with warm autoantibodies: an algorithm for transfusion management. *Transfusion* 2002; **42** (11): 1435–41.

112 Berentsen S. How I manage cold agglutinin disease. *Brit J Haematol* 2011; **153** (3): 309–17.

129 Garratty G. Review: drug-induced immune hemolytic anemia—the last decade. *Immunohematol/American Red Cross* 2004; **20** (3): 138–46.

136 Brodsky RA. Paroxysmal nocturnal hemoglobinuria. *Blood* 2014; **124** (18): 2804–11.

205 Hillmen P, Young NS, Schubert J, *et al.* The complement inhibitor eculizumab in paroxysmal nocturnal hemoglobinuria. *New Engl J Med* 2006; **355** (12): 1233–43.

CHAPTER 13

Carbohydrate blood groups

Laura Cooling

Department of Pathology, University of Michigan, Ann Arbor, MI, USA

Blood group antigens of the H, ABO, Lewis, and historical "P" blood groups are defined by small carbohydrate epitopes expressed as posttranslational modifications on glycoproteins, mucins, and glycolipids. Their synthesis is complex and dependent on several distinct glycosyltransferases and interrelated biosynthetic pathways. In many cases, carbohydrate antigens share features of more than one blood group (e.g., ABO and Lewis).

ABO system

Discovered in 1900 by Karl Landsteiner, the ABO blood group system remains the most important blood group system for blood transfusion and transplantation. ABO antigens are widely expressed on human tissues and fluids, leading to their designation as *histo-blood group* antigens.[1] ABO antigens are differentially expressed during cellular development and can be detected as early as human embryonic stem cells.[2] This can be observed in bone marrow, where hematopoietic progenitor cells strongly express H-antigens (H, Le^Y), but not A/B antigens, which are restricted to developing erythroblasts and megakaryocytes.[3,4] ABO can also be detected on vascular endothelium, skin, and tissues arising from embryonic endoderm and mesoderm, including epithelial cells of the respiratory, gastrointestinal, and genitourinary tracts.[1]

Chemistry and biosynthesis

The ABO system (ISBT 001) contains two structurally related carbohydrate antigens, A and B. The O or H antigen is the biosynthetic precursor of A and B antigens and is listed under a separate blood group system (ISBT 018). All three antigens consist of 2–3 terminal oligosaccharides on glycoproteins and glycolipids. As shown in Figure 13.1, the minimum A-antigen epitope is a trisaccharide composed of a subterminal β-galactose (Gal) bearing both an α1 → 2fucose and α1 → 3 n-acetylgalactosamine (GalNAc). The B antigen resembles the A antigen except for the presence of an α1 → 3Gal. Not surprisingly, group A red cells can be converted to group B-active cells through loss of the acetyl group. Clinically, this is observed in the acquired B phenotype, in which group A patients transiently type as group B due to infection by deacetylase-producing bacteria.[5]

In red cells, synthesis of H and A/B antigens proceeds in a stepwise fashion from a type 2 chain or lactosamine (Galβ1-4GlcNAc-R) precursor (Figure 13.1). Initially, the H-enzyme, FUT1, adds an α1 → 2 fucose to the terminal galactose to make type 2 H-antigen. H-antigen can then serve as a substrate for A and B synthesis. In group A individuals, A-transferase (GTA) recognizes UDP-GalNAc to transfer an α1 → 3GalNAc to H-antigen. Likewise, B-transferase (GTB) recognizes UDP-Gal to transfer an α1 → 3Gal to synthesize group B antigen. Group AB, in which both A and B antigens are expressed, reflects co-inheritance of GTA and GTB. The group O phenotype, on the other hand, reflects the complete absence of ABO enzyme activity due to ABO-null alleles. As a result, these individuals only express the H-antigen precursor. Because A/ B expression is dependent on H-antigen synthesis, the absence of FUT1 activity due to mutations (e.g., Bombay phenotype) or transcriptional repression is also associated with absent A/B expression.

On red cells, it is estimated that 65–75% of ABH antigens are expressed as N-linked glycans on glycoproteins, especially Band 3 (Diego blood group, AE1).[6] At one million copies, Band 3 is the major glycoprotein on red cells and accounts for 50% of all ABH antigens.[7] The remaining ABH antigens are present on O-linked glycans (10%), glycosphingolipids (GSL, 5%), and polyglycosylceramides (10–15%), also known as *erythroglycans*.[6] The latter are massive, branched, multivalent type 2 chain glycolipids composed of 40 or more oligosaccharides and potentially 4–6 ABH epitopes.[8]

ABH antigens can be expressed on different oligosaccharide scaffolds, which often demonstrate developmental and tissue specificity (Table 13.1). Furthermore, the oligosaccharide backbone can influence ABH valency and spatial presentation, as well as contribute to the immune epitope. On red cells, platelets, and endothelium, ABH is primarily expressed on type 2 chain or lactosamine-based structures. Genitourinary and gastrointestinal tissues, on the other hand, are rich in type 1 chain ABH antigens.[1] Type 1 chains are structurally similar to type 2 chains except for linkage of the galactose residue (Galβ1 → 3GlcNAc-R). In addition, the synthesis of type 1 chain H-antigen is dependent on *Secretor* or *FUT2*, a related α1,2-fucosyltransferase. Secretor-positive (*Se*) individuals also secrete type 1 ABH antigens in body fluids, including saliva and plasma.

Type 3 and type 4 chain structures share a terminal Galβ1 → 3 GalNAc-R (Table 13.1). Type 3 chain A, also known as *mucinous A*, is a polymer of repeating A motifs. Type 4 chain ABH, or *globo-ABH*, is a GSL-specific antigen related to the GLOB blood group system (see the "P Blood Group System" section). Although both type 3 and 4 ABH antigens are found in trace amounts on red cells, their synthesis is relatively tissue-restricted to gastrointestinal and/

Rossi's Principles of Transfusion Medicine, Fifth Edition. Edited by Toby L. Simon, Jeffrey McCullough, Edward L. Snyder, Bjarte G. Solheim, and Ronald G. Strauss.

© 2016 John Wiley & Sons, Ltd. Published 2016 by John Wiley & Sons, Ltd.

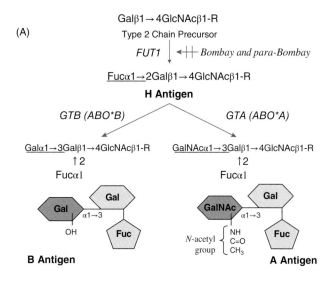

Table 13.1 Group A structures in humans

Name	Structure
Type 1 A (A-1)	GalNAcα1 → 3Galβ1 → 3GlcNAc → R[b] ↑ 2 Fucα1
Type 1, ALe[b]	GalNAcα1 → 3Galβ1 → 3GlcNAc → R ↑ 2 ↑ 4 Fucα1 Fucα1
Type 2 A (A-2)	GalNAcα1 → 3Galβ1 → 4GlcNAc → R ↑ 2 Fucα1
Type 3 A	(mucinous A) GalNAcα1 → 3Galβ1 → 3GalNAcβ1 → 3Galβ1 → R ↑ 2 ↑ 2 Fucα 1Fucα1
Type 4 A (globo-A, A₁)	GalNAcα1 → 3Galβ1 → 3GalNAcβ1 → 3Galα1 → 4Galβ1 → 4Glc → Cer ↑ 2 Fucα1

Cer, ceramide; Fuc, fucose; Gal, galactose; GalNAc, n-acetylgalactosamine; Glc, glucose; GlcNAc, n-acetylglucosamine.

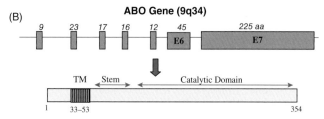

Figure 13.1 (A) Synthesis of group A and group B antigen. (B) Structure of the *ABO* gene and ABO glycosyltransferase.

or genitourinary epithelium.[1] There is evidence that both FUT1 and FUT2 are able to recognize type 3 and type 4 chain substrates;[9] however, it is believed that FUT2 is primarily responsible for type 3 and type 4 ABH synthesis in epithelial tissues.[10]

ABH antibodies

The ABH system is unique for the presence of naturally occurring antibodies against missing ABH antigens (Table 13.2). Specifically, a group A individual will possess anti-B, whereas anti-A will be produced by group B individuals. These antibodies are not present at birth but gradually develop after 4–6 months of age, with adult titers reached by 5–10 years of age.[11] Bacteria in the diet and the gastrointestinal microbiome appear to be the primary immune stimulus for the development of anti-A and anti-B: Many bacterial species express ABH-like structures on lipopolysaccharide that can crossreact with ABH antibodies and lectins.[12]

Antibodies against ABH and other carbohydrate antigens are considered to occur via a thymic-independent mechanism.[13] Specifically, carbohydrates presented as multivalent, repetitive epitopes can directly stimulate B-cells, independent of accessory T-cells, with the production of IgM antibodies. More recent studies in mice also implicate invariant natural killer cells (iNKTs) in ABH antibody formation.[14] Finally, the absence of ABH antibodies against self-antigens may occur through antigen–antibody complexes with specific deletion of antibody-producing B splenocytes.[15]

Serology of the ABO system

The ABO system contains four major phenotypes, based on the inheritance of A and B antigens: A, B, AB, and O (or none).[11] ABO is unique among all other blood groups in that both red cells and plasma/serum testing are required (Table 13.2). The forward-type or red cell grouping is performed by directly testing red cells for the expression of A and B antigens with commercial antisera. The back-type or serum grouping involves testing plasma or serum against commercial A₁ and B red cells for the presence of anti-A and anti-B. Both the forward and back type must agree for a valid ABO phenotype.[11]

Weak ABO subtypes

The ABO system contains several weak subtypes. All are characterized by decreased A/B and a parallel increase in H-antigen expression. Weak subtypes can be associated with ABO typing

Table 13.2 ABO serology

ABO Type	GT Genes*		RBC Grouping (Forward or Antigen Type)			Serum Grouping (Back Type)		
	FUT1	ABO	Anti-A	Anti-B	UEA-1†	A₁ RBC	B RBC	O RBC
A₁	+	+	++	0	0	0	+	0
A₂	+	+	+	0	+	+/0	+	0
B	+	+	0	++	0	+	0	0
O	+	0	0	0	++	+	+	0
Oₕ (Bombay)	0 (hh)	+	0	0	0	+	+	+

*Inheritance of at least one functional *FUT1* or *ABO* gene.
†Testing for H-antigen with lectin *Ulex europeaus* (UEA-1). Not routinely performed except to resolve ABO typing discrepancies.

discrepancies during serum grouping due to the presence of unexpected anti-A or anti-B activity. In some instances, A/B expression is so weak that red cells can forward type as group O.

The most common ABO subtype encountered is A_2, which occurs in 20% of group A donors in the United States and Europe. A_2 red cells have 75% less A antigen than A_1 cells and can possess an anti-A_1. Because of the inefficiency of the A_2-glycosyltransferase (GTA), A_2 red cells also differ in the type of A antigen synthesized. Specifically, A_2 red cells lack globo-A.[16] These differences are more pronounced in other tissues such as platelets and endothelium, where there is little or no A-antigen.[17,18] Studies in A_{weak} subtypes confirm a profound decrease in the array and complexity of A-antigens synthesized with weak GTA activity.[19] A_2 and A_{weak} red cell subtypes are serologically distinquished from A_1 red cells by their lack of reactivity with the lectin *Dolichos bifloris* (DBA).[11] Weak A/B subtypes have increased reactivity with *Ulex europeaus (UEA)*, an anti-H lectin.

Bombay and *para*-bombay

Bombay and *para*-Bombay are autosomal-recessive, H-deficient phenotypes due to homozygous inheritance of amorph *FUT1* alleles (*hh*). As a result, these individuals are unable to synthesize type 2H antigen, the precursor of A and B antigens. Serologically, red cells are negative for H, A, and B antigens, accompanied by the presence of naturally occurring anti-A, anti-B, *and* anti-H in plasma. In routine testing, these individuals may initially type as an apparent group O but will have a strong positive antibody screen due to allo-anti-H, which recognizes group O screening cells.

The Bombay and *para*-Bombay phenotypes are distinguished by the presence or absence of soluble type 1 ABH substance, which is under the control of *FUT2/Secretor*. The classic Bombay phenotype is an H-deficient nonsecretor (*hh, se/se*), with an absence of both type 1 and type 2 chain ABH antigens. As nonsecretors, these individuals will also type as Le(b-) (see the "Lewis Blood Group" section). In contrast, *para*-Bombay individuals are typically H-deficient secretors (*hh, Se/Se,* or *Se/se*) and retain synthesis of type 1 H antigen on mucosa and in secretions. Unlike Bombay cells, *para*-Bombay red cells may have trace amounts of ABH antigen on red cells due to adsorption of soluble type 1 ABH from plasma. There are also examples of *para*-Bombay arising from

an H-deficient, weak Secretor (*hh* and Se^W/se) as well as an H-weak nonsecretor (H^W/h and *se/se*).[20]

Molecular biology
ABO gene

The ABO system contains two autosomal, co-dominant consensus alleles, A^1 (*ABO*A1*) and *B* (*ABO*B*), responsible for GTA and GTB, respectively. The active enzyme is encoded over seven exons, spread over a 19 kb region on chromosome 9q34.1.[20,21] This is in stark contrast to most blood group–related glycosyltransferases (H, Secretor, Lewis, P1PK, and GLOB), in which the active enzyme is located within a single exon. Most mutations effecting ABO activity arise within exons 6 and 7, which account for 75% of the active enzyme. Exon 6, which encodes the stem region, is a hot spot for recombination. *ABO*A1* is generally considered the ancestral gene, with *ABO*B* and *ABO*O* alleles arising through convergent evolution.[22] A more recent study, however, suggests that ABO is an ancient balanced polymorphism originating early in hominid history and maintained in multiple primate lineages.[23]

ABO belongs to the GT6 family of glycosyltransferases, a large family (184) of animal and bacterial α-galactose/α-galactosaminyltransferases that includes the enzymes for Forssman antigen and linear B—two histo-blood group antigens found in animals. The enzyme is a 354-amino-acid, type II transmembrane glycoprotein with a short amino-terminal cytosolic (amino acids 1–32) and transmembrane (33–53) domains, followed by a "stem region" and a large, globular catalytic domain (64–354).[21] The enzyme has a single N-glycan site (Asn[113]), five cysteines, and a DxD motif (Asp[211]–Val[212]–Asp[213]). DxD motifs are found in many glycosyltransferases that require Mn^{2+} or other cations for catalysis.[24] Crystallography of the ABO protein shows it has a complex secondary and tertiary structure, composed of two functional domains separated by a catalytic cleft that contains the DxD motif and a highly conserved Glu[303].[25] The H-antigen acceptor binds to the carboxy-terminal half, whereas the UDP-nucleotide sugar donor binds to the more amino-terminal half of the enzyme. Initial binding of the UDP-nucleotide sugar leads to conformational changes in the enzyme necessary for H-antigen acceptor binding and catalysis.[25,26]

A comparison of GTA and GTB enzymes shows they are virtually identical, differing by only four amino acids at 176, 235, 266, and 268 (Table 13.3).[21] Using recombinant enzymes, Yamamoto *et al.*

Table 13.3 Examples of *ABO* alleles

Allele Name	RBC Type	88	176	234	235	266	268	Gene Type
		\multicolumn{6}{Amino Acid Position}		
ABO*A.01	A1	Thr	Arg	Pro	Gly	Leu	Gly	AAA
ABO*AW.08	A_{weak}	Thr	Arg	Pro	Gly	Leu	**Arg**	AAX
ABO*B.01	B	Thr	**Gly**	Pro	**Ser**	**Met**	**Ala**	BBB
ABO*BW.18	B_{weak}	Thr	**Gly**	Pro	**Ser**	**Met**	**Thr**	BBX
ABO*cisAB.01	cisAB	Thr	Arg	Pro	Gly	Leu	**Ala**	AAB
ABO*cisAB.02	cisAB	Thr	**Gly**	Pro	**Ser**	Leu	**Ala**	BAB
ABO*cisAB.03	cisAB	Thr	**Gly**	**Ser**	**Ser**	**Met**	**Ala**	BBB
ABO*cisAB.04	cisAB	Thr	**Gly**	Pro	Gly	**Met**	Gly	ABA
ABO*cisAB.05	cisAB	Thr	**Gly**	Pro	**Ser**	**Met**	Gly	BBA
ABO*BA.02	B(A)	Thr	**Gly**	**Ala**	**Ser**	**Met**	**Ala**	BBB
ABO*BA.03	B(A)	Thr	**Gly**	Pro	Gly	**Met**	**Ala**	ABB
ABO*O.01	O	fs118stop	—	—	—	—	—	
ABO*O.02	O	Thr	**Gly**	Pro	Gly	Leu	**Arg**	AAX
GWA Studies								
Ref SNP ID (rs)			8176719		8176743	1876746	8176747	

* *Gene type* refers to amino acid positions 235, 266, and 268. These three positions strongly influence substrate specificity and differ between A (AAA) and B (BBB) alleles. Amino acids that differ from the *ABO*A.01* consensus allele are highlighted in bold.

†Deletion mutant (261ΔG) leading to a frameshift and premature stop codon.

demonstrated that only three polymorphisms define whether the enzyme has GTA or GTB activity: Gly235Ser, Leu266Met, and Gly268Ala.[21] Because both GTA and GTB recognize and transfer a sugar to H-antigen, any differences in the two proteins must reflect binding of the nucleotide sugar donor. The factors determining how these three amino acids determine whether the enzyme will utilize UDP-Gal or UDP-GalNAc appear to be the size and geometry of the UDP-binding pocket. In general, the amino acids associated with GTA are biochemically "smaller" than those in GTB and are thus able to accommodate the larger UDP-GalNAc donor.[25] Evidence to support the latter includes crystallography studies, where Leu[266] in GTA directly interacts with the GalNAc acetoamido group, whereas no binding or interaction is observed with Met[266,25]. The adjacent Gly268Ala polymorphism is also believed to be critical for UDP-donor preference;[21] however, this has been challenged. Crystallographic data show both Ala[268] and Gly[268] interacting with galactose hydroxyl groups of the H-antigen acceptor regardless of UDP-donor specificity.[25] Other amino acids interacting with the H-antigen acceptor include Tyr[126], Glu[303], and amino acids 233–245, which includes the Gly235Ser polymorphism. The DxD motif near the nucleotide binding pocket binds Mn^{2+}, which helps coordinate the UDP-phosphate group.[25]

Mutations in *ABO* are responsible for weak ABO phenotypes. To date, over 100 *ABO* weak alleles have been identified.[20] Most weak alleles possess missense mutations affecting enzyme activity; however, mutations affecting transcription, mRNA processing, translation, and Golgi trafficking are also known.[20,27–30] The most common mutant allele is *ABO*A2.01* associated with the A_2 phenotype.[20] *ABO*A2.01* has a single nucleotide deletion (1061ΔC) near the carboxy terminus that leads to a frameshift and translation of an additional 20 amino acids. Some alleles contain mutations within or proximal to the DxD motif (Val212Met, Met214Arg, and Phe216Ile) and highly conserved Glu[303] (Asp302Gly, *ABO*AW.42*, and *BW.27*). A few alleles contain mutations affecting amino acids directly interacting with the H-antigen acceptor (amino acids 233–245: Arg241Trp, *ABO*AW.04, AW.11*, and *AW.23*), including mutations at amino acid 268 (*ABO*AW.08* and *BW.18*; Table 13.3). *ABO*AW.08* is a common cause of ABO discrepancies due to extremely weak GTA activity.[31]

The ABO system also contains hybrid *ABO* alleles able to synthesize both A and B antigens. The *cis*AB phenotype was initially identified following apparent anomalous inheritance of both A and B antigens. These individuals typically type as A_2B with unusually weak B expression, often accompanied by an allo-anti-B.[32] For many years, it was assumed that *cis*AB was the result of unequal crossover events, leading to a hybrid A–B gene. It is now clear that *cis*AB is a consequence of polymorphisms at or near key amino acids (234, 235, 266, and 268) necessary for UDP-donor and H-antigen acceptor binding.[20,21] As shown in Table 13.3, *cis*AB alleles share features of both GTA and GTB enzymes. Similar features are observed in *ABO*BA* alleles responsible for the B(A) phenotype. The B(A) phenotype is observed in rare group B individuals who have small amounts of A antigen when tested with certain anti-A monoclonal antibodies.

Group O, on the other hand, is an autosomal-recessive phenotype due to inheritance of amorph *ABO* alleles. There are several group *ABO*O* alleles documented, but most can be classified as belonging to either the O^1 (*ABO*O.01*) or O^2 (*ABO*O.02, O03*) families (Table 13.3).[20] O^1 accounts for 95% of group O alleles and is characterized by a nucleotide deletion (261ΔG, fs88stop118), leading to a nonfunctional truncated protein. O^2 alleles share a missense

mutation at amino acid 268 (Arg[268]), which profoundly impacts enzyme activity. As noted, this same mutation is present in two weak A and B alleles. In general, heterozygous inheritance of an *ABO*O* allele (ex. A^1/O) does not impact expression on red cells but may be associated with weaker ABO expression on other tissues.[33]

Given the complexity and number of allelic variants, molecular typing is not used for routine donor or recipient ABO typing. Molecular testing is used, however, in genome-wide association (GWA) testing. For these studies, 3–4 single nucleotide polymorphisms (SNPs) are used as a surrogate for ABO typing (Table 13.3). The most common SNPs cover the three amino acid polymorphisms that distinguish GTA from GTB (235, 266 and 268) plus the O^1 allele (261ΔG). Any O^2 alleles should also be identified using this scheme. SNP rs8176704 is sometimes added to screen for the common A_2 allele.

Finally, *ABO* mRNA expression shows evidence of tissue-specific regulation. Like many genes, the ABO 5′UTR is CpG rich (82%) and is highly susceptible to transcriptional regulation by methylation.[34] In fact, loss of A/B expression in leukemia patients is frequently attributed to hypermethylation of the *ABO* promoter region.[35] Methylation patterns are heterogeneous between different tissues; however, methylation of a basal promoter region (−117 to +31) strongly suppresses *ABO* transcription in both epithelial and erythroid cell lines.[34,36] This proximal promoter contains sites for SP1, which is required for transcription, as well as other transcription factor binding proteins.[36,37] In erythroid cells, transcription is enhanced by two GATA sites located within intron 1 (+5819 and +5890).[30] The proximal promoter region can be repressed via an adjacent N-box site at −196 to −191.[38] The latter is a potential binding site for Hes-1, a member of the bHLH family of transcription regulators.[36]

Additional promoter and enhancer elements have been identified upstream of the CpG-rich proximal promoter. A minor distal transcription initiation site was located at −678 near several GATA transcription factor binding sites.[36] A CBF/NF-Y minisatellite enhancer region composed of 1–4 copies of a 43-bp sequence is located at −3800.[39] In some tissues, there is a correlation between the number of tandem repeats, ABO type, and transcriptional activity.[29,39]

H gene

The *H* gene or *FUT1* resides on chromosome 19q13 in conjunction with the *Secretor* gene and *Sec1*, a pseudogene.[20] *FUT1* contains four exons with the active enzyme located within exon 4. *FUT1* is highly specific for type 2 chain polylactosamine substrates and is solely responsible for H antigen synthesis on red cells.[40] In hematopoietic lines, *FUT1* is expressed by stem cells and erythroid-megakaryocytic progenitors but is classically absent from lymphoid and myeloid cells.[3,41] *FUT1* mRNA is commonly expressed in epithelial tissues and other tissues.[42] *FUT1* is not expressed by salivary and parotid glands, which exclusively utilize *FUT2/Secretor*.[42] This is the basis for testing saliva for *secretor* status.

The H enzyme is a 365-amino-acid glycoprotein composed primarily of a large 240-amino-acid catalytic domain containing two conserved N-glycans, two cysteines, and three α-fucosyltransferase motifs.[40,43] Motif I resides at amino acids 214–224 and is likely involved in recognition of the GDP-fucose donor. Motifs II and III may be involved in recognition of the galactose acceptor and are located at 256–269 and 309–318, respectively. The enzyme shares 80% homology with FUT2/Secretor, especially along the catalytic domain.[44]

Loss of FUT1 activity and ABH expression is associated with the Bombay and *para*-Bombay phenotypes.[20] The International Society for Blood Transfusion (ISBT) currently lists 19 null alleles (*h*) and 23 weak-H alleles (H^W) due to missense, frameshift, and nonsense mutations. Several mutations occur at conserved fucosyltransferase and N-glycan motifs or introduce new cysteine residues with the potential for aberrant folding (Table 13.4). Nearly all missense mutations involve amino acids conserved between *FUT1* and *FUT2*.[44] In several instances, mutations in the same homologous amino acids in *FUT2* are associated with weak and null *FUT2* alleles.

Although widely expressed, *FUT1* is transcriptionally regulated with evidence of tissue-specific promoters and alternate splicing. In erythroid cell lines, up to four different mRNA transcripts can be identified from two different, developmentally regulated transcription initiation start sites.[3,41,45] In undifferentiated K562 cells, an early pleuripotent hematopoietic cell line, *FUT1* is transcribed primarily from exon 1A. In bone marrow and more differentiated erythroblastic cell lines (HEL, TF1), however, transcription proceeds from exon 2. Several transcription factor binding sites are located immediately upstream of exon 2 (AP-2, Sp1, Ets-1, c-Rel, and Elk), including a retroviral long-terminal repeat sequence that lies within the basal promoter region.[45] Retroviral-type sequences have been shown to regulate other glycosyltransferases and may be susceptible to methylation.[46]

FUT1 transcription has also been studied in other cell lines and cancer. In general, *FUT1* transcription occurs from exon 1A in epithelial cells, whereas vascular endothelium starts at exon 3.[45] In colon carcinoma, there is upregulation of *FUT1* mRNA and Le^Y expression due to Elk-1, which promotes transcription from the E1A start site.[47] In ovarian cancer lines, *FUT1* is upregulated by c-jun, a member of the AP-1 transcription factor activator protein complex.[48]

Table 13.4 Weak and null *FUT1* alleles

Allele Name	Phenotype	Activity	Nucleotide Change	Amino Acid Change	Conserved in FUT2	Comments
Single-Point Mutations (SNPs)						
FUT1*01W.21	H^W	Weak	235G>C	Gly79Arg	Y (Gly51)	
FUT1*02W.01	H^W	Weak	269G>T	Gly90Val	Y (Gly62)	
FUT1*01W.01	H^W	Weak	293C>T	Thr98Met	Y (Met70)	
FUT1*01W.02	H^W	Weak	328G>A	Ala110Thr	Y (Ala82)	*FUT2* analog se^{244}
FUT1*01W.03	H^W	Weak	349G>T	His117Tyr	Y (Ala89)	
FUT1*02W.02	H^W	Weak	371T>G	Phe124Cys	Y (Phe96)	New cysteine
FUT1*01N.02	h	Absent	422G>A	Trp141Stop	Y (Trp113)	Truncated protein
FUT1*01W.04	H^W	Weak	442G>T	Asp148Tyr	Y (Asp120)	
FUT1*01W.05/06	H^W	Weak	460T>C	Tyr154His	Y (Tyr126)	
FUT1*01N.02	h	Absent	461A>G	Tyr154Cys	Y (Tyr126)	New cysteine
FUT1*01N.03	h	Absent	462C>A	Tyr154Stop	Y (Tyr 126)	Truncated protein
FUT1*01W.07	H^W	Weak	491T>A	Leu164His	N	
FUT1*01N.04	h	Absent	513G>C	Trp171Cys	Y (Trp142)	New cysteine
FUT1*01W.08	H^W	Weak	522C>A	Phe174Leu	N	
FUT1*01N.05	h	Absent	538C>T	Gln180Stop	N	Truncated protein
FUT1*01N.06	h	Absent	586C>T	Gln196Stop	Y (Gln168)	Truncated protein
FUT1*01W.09	H^W	Weak	658C>T	Arg220Cys	Y (Arg190)	Motif I
FUT1*01W.10	H^W	Weak	659G>A	Arg220His	Y (Arg190)	*FUT2* analog se^{569}
FUT1*01W.11	H^W	Weak	661C>T	Arg221Cys	Y (Arg191)	Motif I
FUT1*01W.24	H^W	Weak	649G>T	Val217Phe	Y (Val187)	Motif I
FUT1*01W.29	H^W	Weak	655G>C	Val219Leu	Y (Val189)	Motif I
FUT1*01W.12	H^W	Weak	682A>G	Met228Val	Y (Met198)	
FUT1*01N.18	h	Absent	684G>A	Met228Ile	Y (Met198)	Also FUT1*02W.03
FUT1*01W.13	H^W	Weak	689A>C	Gln230Pro	N	
FUT1*01N.08	h	Absent	695G>A	Trp232Stop	Y (Trp202)	Truncated protein
FUT1*01N.19	h	Absent	694T>C	Trp232Pro	Y (Trp202)	
FUT1*01W.14	H^W	Weak	721T>C	Tyr241His	Y (Tyr211)	
FUT1*01N.09	h	Absent	725T>G	Leu242Arg	Y (Leu212)	
FUT1*01N.10	h	Absent	776T>A	Val259Glu	Y (Val229)	Motif II
FUT1*01N.11	h	Absent	785G>A, 786C>A	Ser262Lys	Y (Ser232)	Motif II
FUT1*01W.15	H^W	Weak	801G>C	Trp267Cys	Y (Trp237)	Motif II
FUT1*01W.16	H^W	Weak	801G>T	Trp267Cys	Y (Trp237)	New cysteine
FUT1*01N.12	h	Absent	826C>T	Gln276Stop	N	Truncated protein
FUT1*01W.17	H^W	Weak	832G>A	Asp278Asn	Y (Asp248)	
FUT1*01W.19	H^W	Weak	917C>T	Thr306Ile	Y (Thr276)	Adjacent Motif III
FUT1*01N.14	h	Absent	944C>T	Ala315Val	Y (Ala285)	Motif III FUT2 analog Se^{W285}
FUT1*01N.16	h	Absent	980A>C	Asn327Thr	Y (Asn297)	Loss of conserved N-glycan site
FUT1*01N.15	h	Absent	948C>G	Tyr316Stop	Y (Tyr286)	Truncated protein
FUT1*01N.17	h	Absent	1047G>C	Trp349Cys	Y (Trp319)	New cysteine
Frameshift, Other						
FUT1*01N.06	h	Absent	547_548ΔAG	183fs		
FUT1*01N.20	h	Absent	764_768ΔC	256fs		
FUT1*01N.13	h	Absent	880_881ΔTT	294fs333Stop		
FUT1*01W.20	H^W	Weak	990ΔG	330fs336Stop		

Transfusion and transplantation

Transfusion

Anti-A, anti-B, and anti-A,B are clinically significant IgM antibodies, capable of fixing complement and causing intravascular hemolysis.[11] In contrast, anti-H is typically a low-titer, clinically insignificant cold autoantibody in most individuals. On occasion, group A_1 and B individuals possess an allo-anti-HI that can react with group O red cells at 37 °C. In contrast, the allo-anti-H observed in Bombay and *para*-Bombay individuals is always significant, and requires the transfusion of rare H-negative red cells. In cold autoimmune hemolytic anemia, autoantibodies with I and ABH activity are not uncommon (e.g., auto-HI and auto-sialyl-A).

For transfusion, red cells and plasma must be ABO compatible with the recipient to avoid acute hemolytic transfusion reactions.[11] Patients whose ABO type is unknown or cannot be resolved due to typing difficulties should receive group O red cells. In emergent situations requiring plasma transfusion support, patients without a valid ABO type should receive group AB or, possibly, group A plasma. Thawed group A plasma is increasingly used as the initial plasma replacement in the military and large trauma centers due to the scarcity of group AB plasma.[49]

ABO compatibility is not required for platelet and cryoprecipitate transfusion, although most transfusion services attempt to dispense ABO type-specific and ABO-compatible, if possible. Transfusion of ABO-incompatible platelets can adversely affect the posttransfusion increment, especially in group O recipients.[50] Two studies have shown that A_2 platelets are group O compatible and are as effective as type-specific platelets when transfused to either group A or O patients.[51,52]

Hemolytic disease of the fetus and newborn (HDFN)

ABO major incompatibility between the mother and fetus is not uncommon given the incidence of blood groups O and A in the population.[53] Severe HDFN due to ABO incompatibility, however, is relatively rare, with a reported incidence of 0.04%.[53] One reason is the inability of IgM antibodies to cross the placenta. In addition, A/B antigens are poorly expressed on fetal red cells and may not efficiently support complement fixation by maternal immunoglobulin G (IgG) antibodies. HDFN due to ABO incompatibility is most commonly observed in group O mothers, especially with a history of a prior, non-O pregnancy and immune-stimulated, anti-A/B IgG antibodies.

Transplantation

Solid organ transplantation

In general, organs selected for allotransplantation are ABO compatible with the recipient. Transplants of ABO-incompatible organs are at risk for acute and hyperacute rejection due to immune recognition of A/B antigens on endothelium and epithelial tissues. To improve the availability of organs, group A organ donors are now screened to identify non-A_1 (A_2, A_{weak}) donors.[54] Because of the relative absence of A-antigen on endothelium and epithelium, these organs can be transplanted successfully into group O and B recipients.[54]

Protocols have been developed to permit transplantation of ABO incompatible organs in selected patient populations. Due to their naïve immune state, infants and neonates can be transplanted with ABO incompatible hearts with good outcomes, minimal risk of acute rejection, and a decreased incidence of HLA antibodies.[55] Unlike adults, neonates lack preformed ABO antibodies and memory B cells, eliminating the need for splenectomy and aggressive immunosuppression. Over time, infants appear to develop a broad donor-specific tolerance to ABO and other antigens.[55] Likewise, there is evidence of equivalent outcomes for ABO-incompatible liver transplantation in infants and young pediatric patients.[56]

Unlike infants, ABO incompatibility is a significant barrier in adult transplantation. Several protocols have been developed for ABO-incompatible kidney transplantation. Recipients often undergo a series of pre-surgery plasma exchanges, coupled with immune suppression that may include steroids, ATG, rituximab, basiliximab, daclizumab, ecluzimab, or alemtuzumab.[57] ABO-incompatible liver transplantation is usually reserved for emergent situations in which an ABO-compatible organ is unavailable. Historically, ABO-incompatible liver transplants were associated with high rates (50%) of graft failure and retransplantion. More recent studies using aggressive immunosuppression have reported improved graft survival, although the risks of venous thrombosis and graft loss are still higher than with ABO-compatible transplants.[56]

Stem cell transplantation

Unlike solid organ transplantation, human progenitor or stem cell transplants are frequently ABO incompatible. It is estimated that 30–50% of all allotransplants are ABO mismatched.[58] ABO incompatibility has no impact on white cell engraftment but can lead to hemolysis, delayed red cell engraftment, pure red cell aplasia, and increased transfusion requirements.[58] There are also reports linking ABO mismatched transplants with an increased incidence of venous occlusive disease, severe graft-versus-host disease, and transplant-related mortality.

Several variables influence the impact of ABO incompatibility in stem cell transplantation, including the type of stem cell product, whether the donor is ABO major or minor incompatible, the conditioning regimen (myeloablative versus reduced conditioning), and the type of posttransplant immunosuppression.[58,59] In general, ABO major-incompatible marrow transplants have more significant delays in red cell engraftment and pure red cell aplasia than peripheral blood stem cell transplants.[59] Loss of recipient ABO antibodies and donor red cell engraftment is often faster in matched unrelated donors, especially in the presence of graft-versus-host disease and increased transfusion requirements.[59] It is hypothesized that loss of ABO antibodies may reflect a graft-versus-plasma cell effect and passive infusion of soluble ABH antigen, which could both adsorb recipient ABO antibodies and promote selective B-cell depletion.[15,59,60] Finally, ABO minor-incompatible transplants may be complicated by hemolysis due to donor lymphocyte syndrome.[58]

Biological role

ABO, cancer, and possible biological role

The biological role of ABH antigens is still unclear; however, the influence of ABH antigens in cancer biology may provide some insight. It is well known that loss of A and B expression in lung, esophageal, and bladder cancers is associated with a poorer prognosis.[61–64] In immortalized colon carcinoma cell lines, the absence of A or B is associated with increased chemotactic and haptotactic cell migration in vitro, which can be blocked by transfecting cells with GTA or GTB transferases.[65] Because integrins are sensitive to changes in glycosylation, it is hypothesized that A/B antigens on α- and β-integrins sterically interfere with heterodimer formation, integrin-mediated adhesion, and/or cell signaling.[65,66] In addition,

ABH is a terminal glycan modification and competes with sialyltransferase for reactive nonreducing β-galactosyl residues on glycoproteins. As a result, ABH has the potential to modulate cellular interactions with galactins, siglecs (sialic acid-binding lectin glycoproteins), cadherins, and growth factors.[67]

ABH may also influence cell sensitivity to apoptosis and immune regulation. Increases in H-antigen and α1,2fucosyltransferase activity are associated with decreased overall survival in colon cancer.[68] Furthermore, induction of H-activity can increase resistance to apoptosis by heat shock and serum deprivation.[64] Finally, H-antigen neoexpression may make tumors less antigenic, allowing tumors to escaped immune surveillance.[64]

There are associations between specific blood types and the incidence of cancer. The incidence of gastric and pancreatic cancer is higher among group A individuals, where A>B, AB>O.[69,70] When examined by A subtypes, the risk of pancreatic cancer is higher among A_1 individuals whereas no increase is observed for A_2.[70] In lung cancer, blood group O has a higher mortality.[62] There is some evidence that many of these associations reflect differences in the upregulation of inflammatory mediators.[62,69]

ABO and coagulation

There is a strong association between non–group O and thrombosis risk. Two recent systematic reviews and meta-analysis calculated that non–group O individuals have a twofold higher risk of thrombotic events than group O.[71] In European studies, non–group O was the single most important population risk factor for venous thrombosis, including both deep venous thrombosis and pulmonary embolism. Non–group O also has an increased risk of coronary heart disease, increased LDL, and total cholesterol.[71]

The observed linkage between ABO and thrombotic events appears to be multifactorial. GWA studies have found associations between ABO and serum levels of ICAM1, TNFα, P-selectin, E-selectin, LDL, and cholesterol levels.[71] More importantly, there is a clear correlation between vWF levels and ABO type, where $AB>A,B>A_2>O>O_h$ (Bombay).[71] The lower vWF levels in O individuals reflect accelerated vWF clearance relative to non-O individuals. Group O vWF is more susceptible to proteolysis by ADAMTS13. In addition, there is evidence of accelerated vWF uptake by macrophages.

ABO and malaria

ABO is considered a major host susceptibility factor in malaria.[72,73] In fact, there is evidence that selection pressure by *Plasmodium falciparum* may underlie the high prevalence of blood group O in malaria-endemic populations located along the equator.[72] Why blood group O provides a survival and reproductive advantage against malaria is multifactorial and a subject of ongoing intensive investigation. Studies in Africa suggest that blood group O may protect against placental malaria with higher fetal birth weights and hemoglobins.[73] One critical benefit is protection against red cell rosetting by some *P. falciparum* species.[74] The ability to rosette red cells is a major virulence factor associated with severe malaria, microvascular ischemia, thrombosis, and cerebral malaria.[72–74] The increased thrombotic risk in non–group O may also contribute to excess morbidity and mortality (see above). Finally, group O may provide an advantage in parasite clearance. Infected group O red cells appear more susceptible to oxidative damage as evidenced by carbonylation of cytoskeletal proteins, hemichrome formation, and Band 3 clustering.[75,76] These senescent changes may facilitate phagocytosis and clearance of infected red cells, thereby decreasing the level and severity of parasitemia.

ABO, cholera, and other enteric infections

Group O is a host risk factor for the development of severe cholera by *Vibrio* strains carrying the El Tor and Bengal cholera toxin subtypes.[73] These two strains have been shown to bind difucosylated H antigen (Le^Y) but not ABH-modified structures (BLe^Y).[78] It is hypothesized that Le^Y captures and concentrates cholera toxin, bringing it within close proximity to ganglioside GM1, the physiologic toxin receptor on small intestine epithelium. The result is increased cellular toxicity and secretory diarrhea in group O individuals. ABO has no impact on classical O1 cholera toxin infections.

Several other enteric pathogens also recognize ABH epitopes on intestinal epithelium. *Campylobacter jejuni* recognizes type 2 chain H and Le^Y antigens on jejunal epithelium.[79] Norovirus and rotavirus, two highly infectious nonenveloped viruses, recognize type 1 ABH and/or Lewis antigens in the upper small intestine.[73] Norovirus G1 strains prefer type 1 H antigens, whereas GII strains are more promiscuous, recognizing a host of fucosylated structures.[73,80] Individuals lacking type 1 antigens (nonsecretors) are resistant to most norovirus infections.[81,82] Most human rotavirus strains (P4, P6, P8) also recognize type 1 H and Le^b;[83] however, a few strains belonging to the PIII family (P9, P14, P25) have evolved to recognize the GalNAcα1 → 3 Gal epitope present on group A antigen.[84]

ABH antibodies and innate immunity

ABH antibodies, particularly anti-B, may play a role in the innate host defense against bacterial infection. As discussed in this chapter, ABH-like glycoconjugates are found on the LPS of many enteric bacteria.[12] In animal and in vitro studies, anti-B have been shown to bind bacteria with complement activation and increased phagocytosis.[73] Clinically, the absence of anti-B in group B and AB individuals has been linked to increased incidence of infection by *Escherichia coli* and *Salmonella*.[85,86]

ABH antibodies are also implicated in the susceptibility to infection by enveloped viruses and schistosomiasis.[73] Both HIV and the SARS-CoV virus express host ABH antigens on viral glycoproteins and lipid envelope. HIV and SARS-CoV can be blocked by monoclonal and/or human ABH antibodies in vitro, suggesting that ABO incompatibility at time of primary viral exposure could offer some protection.[87,88] This has been observed clinically with the SARS-CoV virus during a large hospital outbreak in China.[89] Most infections (68%) occurred among non–group O health care workers, whereas group O individuals were relatively resistant (OR=0.18). Finally, group B and O individuals may have an increased resistance to shistosoma infections due to anti-A.[73] Anti-A is hypothesized to bind and block GalNAc epitopes on female flukes necessary for fluke chemoattraction and mating.[90]

Lewis blood group

The Lewis blood group system was discovered shortly after World War II (1946–1948) and currently contains six antigens.[20] Serologically, Lewis status is defined by the expression of two main antigens, Le^a (LE1) and Le^b (LE2). Four additional antigens—Le^{ab} (LE3), Le^{bH} (LE4), ALe^b (LE5), and BLe^b (LE6)—reflect the biosynthetic and immunologic interaction of Le^a, Le^b, and ABO antigens. Unlike ABH, Lewis antigens are not of erythroid origin but are passively adsorbed onto red cells from a pool of Lewis-active GSL present in plasma. Adsorbed Lewis antigen is also found on platelets, lymphocytes, and endothelium. Cells synthesizing Lewis

Table 13.5 Lewis serology and genetics

	Incidence		Genes*			Secreted Antigens†		
Lewis Type	White	Black	*FUT2*	*FUT3*	ABH Secretor†	Le^a	Le^b	ABO
Le (a+b−)	22%	23%	se/se	Le	N	+	0	0
Le (a−b+)	72%	55%	Se	Le	Y	+	+	+
Le (a+b+^{w})	Rare	Rare	Se^w	Le	Y	+	↓	↓
Le (a−b−)	6%	22%	Se	le/le	Y	0	0	+
			se/se	le/le	N	0	0	0

* Inherited at least one functional allele of FUT3/Lewis (*Le*) and FUT2/Secretor (*Se*). Lewis-null and nonsecretors are homozygous for FUT3 (*le/le*) and FUT2 (*se/se*) amorph alleles, respectively.

† Presence of secreted ABH substances in saliva and body fluids.

antigens are typically of endodermal origin and include gastro-intestinal, urogenital and respiratory epithelium. Soluble Lewis antigen can be found in plasma, saliva, breast milk, and urine.

Serology

There are four possible Lewis phenotypes, although only three are commonly encountered in adults (Table 13.5): Le(a+b−), Le(a−−b+), and Le(a−b−). The Le(a+b+) is unusual but can be observed in neonates and up to 20% of Japanese, Chinese, and Polynesians.[20] There are racial and geographic differences in the distribution of Lewis phenotypes and alleles. Because Lewis antigens are adsorbed and not synthesized on red cells, Lewis phenotype is sensitive to changes in red cell turnover and plasma volume.[32] Lewis antigens can be transiently decreased in chronic hemolysis. Pregnancy, cirrhosis, and chronic renal failure can lead to decreased Lewis expression due to an expanded blood volume and changes in circulating lipid concentration.

Synthesis and biochemistry

Le^a and Le^b are fucosylated type 1 chain antigens and reflect the interaction of two autosomal-dominant fucosyltransferases: Lewis (FUT3) and Secretor (FUT2). As discussed earlier in this chapter, FUT2 is an H-type α1,2 fucosyltransferase specific for type 1 chain substrates, whereas FUT3 is considered an α1,3/1,4 fucosyltransferase, able to utilize both type 1 and type 2 chain substrates. As a result, FUT3 can synthesize type I Lewis antigens as well as type II chain Le^X and Le^Y antigens (Figure 13.2). This is observed in gastrointestinal mucosa, where deep glandular epithelial stem cells express FUT3 and type 2 chain precursor with synthesis of Le^X and Le^Y, but switch to type 1 chain synthesis upon further differentiation, with expression of Le^a and Le^b structures on villus epithelium.[1,73]

Synthesis of Le^a and Le^b proceeds from type 1 chain precursor, historically known as Le^C, along two different pathways. Le^a is a monofucosylated antigen and requires only FUT3, whereas Le^b, a difucosylated antigen, requires the action of both FUT3 and FUT2 for its synthesis. To synthesize Le^a, FUT3 transfers an α1 → 4 fucose to the subterminal n-acetylglucosamine (GlcNAc) of type 1 precursor. To synthesize Le^b, type 1 precursor is initially fucosylated by FUT2 to form type 1 H (Le^D), which then serves as a substrate for FUT3 to form Le^b. Le^b cannot be synthesized directly from Le^a due to steric blocking by the subterminal fucose. Once formed, Le^b can be further modified by ABO to form ALe^b (LE5) and BLe^b (LE6). In A$_1$ individuals, ALe^b is the predominant Lewis- and A-active GSL in plasma.[91] Because Le^b requires FUT2 for synthesis, it is accompanied by the synthesis and secretion of type 1 chain ABH antigens.

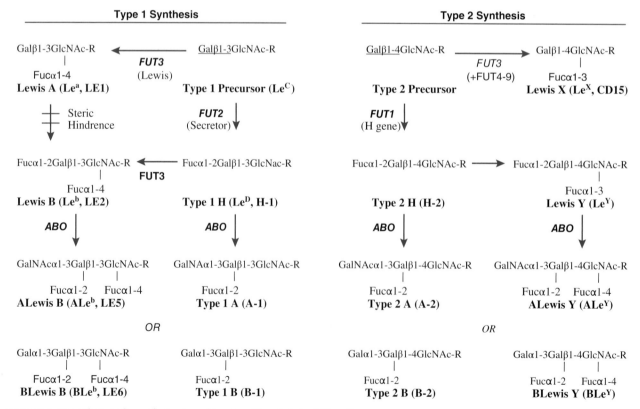

Figure 13.2 Biosynthetic pathways for Lewis, and type 1 and type 2 chain ABO, antigens.

It is now clear how FUT2 and FUT3 determine Lewis phenotype (Table 13.5). The Le(a+b−) phenotype reflects inheritance of at least one functional *FUT3* gene and homozygosity for *FUT2*-null alleles (*se/se*). As a result, Le(a+b−) individuals also fail to express type 1 chain ABH and are considered ABH "nonsecretors." Only type 1 chain precursor (Le[C]) and Le[a] are found in saliva and secretions.

The Le(a−b+) phenotype has inherited at least one functional *FUT3/Lewis* and *FUT2/Se* allele with secretion of Le[a], Le[b], and type 1 ABH antigens. The apparent absence of Le[a] on red cells is deceptive because both Le[a] and Le[b] are synthesized. It appears that FUT2 outcompetes FUT3 for type 1 precursor, leading to predominantly Le[b] synthesis.

Decreases in FUT2 activity account for the Le(a+b+) phenotype. In neonates, it is believed that there is a developmental delay in *FUT2* expression in gastrointestinal mucosa. In contrast, mutations leading to weak FUT2 activity underlie the Le(a+b+[w]) phenotype commonly encountered in Japanese, Chinese, and Polynesians.[20] Weak FUT2 activity permits FUT3 to successfully compete for type I precursor, tipping the balance toward Le[a] synthesis.

The Le(a−b−) phenotype is a *FUT3/Lewis*-null phenotype. Le (a−b−) may be either ABH nonsecretor or secretors, depending on the inheritance of *FUT2*. Le(a−b−) does not secrete Lewis-active substances.

Molecular biology of Lewis and secretor genes
Lewis gene (*FUT3*)
FUT3 is located on chromosome 19p13.3 as a tandem cluster of three homologous glycosyltransferases: FUT5−FUT3−FUT6.[20] All three genes belong to the GT10 family of α1,3 fucosyltransferase, which is widely conserved in vertebrates and bacteria.[43] The gene consists of three exons, although only exon 3 encodes the active enzyme. The translated protein is a 361-amino-acid, type II glycoprotein with five cysteines and two N-glycan sites.[92] Detailed analysis indicates that the globular catalytic domain starts around residue 86 and extends through the carboxy-terminus of the enzyme. *FUT3* shares two highly conserved α-fucosyltransferase motifs in the GDP-nucleotide donor (motif I, amino acid 152–171) and acceptor domains (motif II, amino acids 239–272) of the enzyme, respectively.[43] Motif I includes an N-glycan site and the DxD motif that interacts with divalent cations (Mn2+). The region immediately adjacent to motif I has been identified as critical for transferring fucose to type I substrates (amino acids 105–151).[93] This region contains two highly conserved cyteines (Cys[81],Cys[91]) that are believed to form disulfide bridges with formation of a small loop structure necessary for enzyme activity.[94] An additional conserved disulfide bond pair is located toward the carboxy-terminus (Cys[338],C[341]). The enzyme is believed to reside in the *trans*-Golgi.

FUT3 is tissue-restricted and correlates fairly well with *FUT2* expression.[42] The strongest *FUT3* expression is observed in trachea, intestine, bladder, and lower female reproductive tract.[42] Depending on tissue, up to four different mRNA transcripts can be produced due to differential splicing.[95] A basal promoter in the 5′UTR that is active in intestinal mucosa was located −636 to −674 bp upstream of exon 1 and contains AP-1 and c/EBPβ transcription binding sites. The 5′UTR also contains multiple c-Myc sites that can upregulate *FUT3* and an enhancer region (−674 to −854).[95,96] Gene suppression can occur by methylation and a negative regulatory region located between −855 and −1220.[95,97]

The blood group antigen gene mutation database lists 37 *FUT3* null (*le*) alleles associated with a Le(a−b−) phenotype. A majority of alleles (89%) have at least two mutations, and many alleles contain four or more SNPs. Several null alleles show distinct geographic and ethnic distributions. In whites, alleles containing T202C (Trp68Arg) and C314T (Thr105Met) are common (*le*[202,314]), whereas *le*[59], *le*[59,508], and *le*[59,1067] predominate in Japan, China, Korea, Northern India, Asia, and Brazilian Amazon.[73] In African and US black populations, several additional mutations have been identified, including G13A (Gly5Ser), G484A (Asp162Asn), G667A (Gly223Arg), and A808G (Val270Met). Of note, the G484>A affects the DXD site in Motif I, whereas A808>G mutates a highly conserved valine in Motif II.[43] In blacks, the most common alleles are *le*[13,484,667], *le* [484,667], and *le* [59,308].

Some mutations have an apparently greater effect on Lewis-GSL expression, leading to Lewis-type discrepancies between saliva, tissues, and red cells. A mutation in the transmembrane domain (Leu20Arg; *le* [59]) is associated with marked loss in Lewis-GSL synthesis but retains Lewis expression on intestinal glycoproteins.[98,99] It is believed this mutation leads to mislocalization and trafficking of the enzyme within the Golgi.[98] FUT3 also displays gene dosage with reduced enzyme activity in heterozygous individuals (*Le/le*).[100] Heterozygous individuals can red cell type as Le (a−b−) but retain Lewis expression on gastrointestinal and other tissues.[99,100]

Secretor gene (*FUT2*)
Like *FUT1*, FUT2/Se is a galactoside-2-alpha-L-fucosyltransferase, catalyzing the addition of an α1 → 2 linked fucose to a terminal galactose. Unlike FUT1, which is specific for type 2 chain precursors, FUT2 recognizes type 1 chain substrate with synthesis of type 1 chain ABH and Le[b] antigens. FUT2 is primarily responsible for the synthesis of type 3 and type 4 ABH antigens, which also share a terminal Galβ1 → 3HexNAc acceptor.[9,10] *FUT2* resides on chromosome 19q13.3 as part of a 100-kb gene cluster that includes *FUT1* and *Sec1*, an inactive *FUT2*-like pseudogene.[44] The *FUT2* gene contains two exons, with exon 2 encoding the active enzyme.[20,44] The translated protein is 343 amino acids long *FUT2* and shares 68% sequence homology with *FUT1*.[44] It shares three motifs common to eukaryotic and prokaryotic α1,2 fucosyltransferases at amino acids 184–204 (motif I), 226–239 (motif II), and 278–288 (motif III).[43] The *Sec1-FUT2-FUT1* gene cluster is susceptible to mutation and genetic recombination due to the high homology of the three genes and their proximity to several *Alu* sequences, including nine *Alu* repeats in exon 1.[101]

FUT2 is highly expressed in trachea, parotid, salivary gland, gastric and intestinal mucosa, uroepithelium (bladder and kidney), and female reproductive tract (vagina, cervix, and ovary): Little or no *FUT2* mRNA is observed in placenta, bone marrow, or spleen which uses *FUT1* almost exclusively.[42] Intestinal *FUT2* expression can be induced by commensal bacteria that utilize fucose as a nutrient[102] and could theoretically account for the developmental delay in Le[b] expression observed in newborns. Babies slowly acquire *FUT2*-inducing bacteria through ingestion of breast milk and other foods, only achieving a normal "adult-type" intestinal microbiome by 1 year of age.[103]

The minimal basal promoter for *FUT2* is located at −109 to −56 and includes several GC-rich regions. Multiple transcription factor binding sites are present, including those for CDX2 (8 sites), GATA, Sp1, AP2 (5 sites), and E2A.[96,101] CDX2 binding appears critical for *FUT2* expression in intestinal cell lines.[96] A SNP located at approximately −190 is associated with decreased transcription in colon cell lines and is unique to African populations.[104] Finally, *FUT2* mRNA

Table 13.6 FUT2 alleles associated with weak or absent expression

Allele Name	Phenotype	Activity	Nucleotide Change	Amino Acid Change	Conserved in FUT1	Comments
Single-Point Mutations (SNPs)						
FUT2*01N.01	se	Absent	244G>A, 385A>T	Ala82Thr	Y (Ala110)	See FUT2*01W.02
				Ile129Phe	N	FUT1 analog H^{W293}
FUT2*01W.01	Se^W	Weak	278C>T	Ala93Val	Y (Ala131)	
FUT2*01N.15	se	Absent	3012C>T	Pro101Leu	Y (Pro129)	
FUT2*01W.02	Se^W	Weak	385A>T	Ile129Phe	N	Common Se^W allele
FUT2*01N.17	se	Absent	412G>A	Gly138Ser	Y (Gly176)	
FUT2*01N.02	se	Absent	428G>A	Trp143Stop	Y (Trp171)	Truncated protein
						FUT1 analog h^{171}
FUT2*01N.03	se	Absent	569G>A	Arg190His	Y (Arg220)	Motif I,
						FUT1 H^{W65T} H^{W658A}
FUT2*01N.04	se	Absent	571C>T	Arg191Stop	Y (Arg221)	Motif I
						Truncated protein
						FUT1 H^{W659}
FUT2*01N.05	se	Absent	628C>T	Arg210Stop	N	Truncated protein
FUT2*01N.06	se	Absent	658C>T	Arg220Stop	Y (Arg250)	Truncated protein
FUT2*01N.07	se	Absent	664C>T	Arg222Cys	Y (Arg252)	New cysteine
FUT2*01N.10	se	Absent	400G>A, 760G>A	Val134Ile	N	
				Asp254Asn	Y (Asp285)	
FUT2*01N.16	se	Absent	960A>G	Gly247Ser	Y (Gly277)	Adjacent Motif III
FUT2*01N.12	se	Absent	849G>A	Trp283Stop	Y (Trp313)	Truncated protein
						Motif III
FUT2*01W.03	Se^W	Weak	853G>A	Ala285Thr	Y (Ala315)	Motif III
						FUT1 analog h^{994}
FUT2*01N.13	se	Absent	868G>A	Gly290Arg	Y (Gly320)	
FUT2*01N.14	se	Absent	950C>T	Pro317Leu	Y (Pro347)	
FUT2*01N.18	se	Absent	818C>A	Thr273Asn	Y (Thr303)	Loss of N-glycan
						FUT1 weak analog
						FUT1.01W.18
Frameshift, Other						
FUT2*01N.01	se	Absent	Gene deletion			
FUT2*01N.02	se	Absent	Deletion			
FUT2*01N.03	se^{fus}	Absent	FUT2-Sec1 gene fusion			
FUT2*01N.05	se^{fus}	Absent	FUT2-Sec1 gene fusion			
FUT2*01N.08	se	Absent	685_686ΔGT	230fs234Stop		
FUT2*01N.09	se	Absent	688_690ΔGTC	del230Val		
FUT2*01N.11	se	Absent	778ΔC	259fs275Stop		

has a long 3′ UTR that can form a large stem–loop structure, which could affect mRNA stability and translation.[101]

Individuals homozygous for two *FUT2*-null alleles (*se/se*) are considered nonsecretors and express only Le^a and/or type 1 precursor substance (Le^C) in their secretions and tissues (Table 13.5). ISBT currently lists 29 *FUT2* null alleles, many with distinct geographic and ethnic distributions (www.isbtweb.org). Most null alleles are the result of nonsense mutations leading to synthesis of a truncated protein (Table 13.6).[20] The most common null mutation is se^{428} (Trp143stop, *FUT2*01N.02*), an ancient mutation that arose nearly 3 million years ago. The se^{428} allele is the most frequent nonsecretor allele in whites and is common among Africans, Iranians, and Turks. As a consequence, it is frequently included in genetic studies (G428A, rs601338). Unusual *se* alleles due to *Alu*-mediated deletion and recombination have also been identified in India and Asia (Table 13.6; *FUT2*0N.01-.04*).[20] Of six missense mutations, two occur within or adjacent to conserved motifs (G569A, Arg190His; G868A, Gly290Arg), whereas a third introduces a new cysteine residue within the catalytic domain (C664T, Arg222Cys). All six SNPs occur among amino acids conserved in both *FUT1* and *FUT2*. In *FUT1*, SNPs in the homologous amino acids can be associated with weak H activity (H^w; Table 13.4).[20]

FUT2 variants with weak activity (Se^W) are common in Asia and tend to be missense mutations. In China and neighboring Asian countries, Se^{385} (Ile129Phe; *FUT2*01W.02*) is the predominate Se^W allele.[105] Missense mutations in conserved amino acids within the stem region (Ala93Val) and motif III regions (Ala285Thr, FUT2*01W.03) can also lead to weak activity.[20] Interestingly, the same missense mutation in *FUT1* (Ala315Val, *FUT1*01N.1*, h^{994}) leads to a complete loss of enzyme activity. Se^W/Se^W and Se^W/se individuals can type as Le(a+b^W), Le(a+b−), or Le(a−b−). Individuals with a Se^W/se genotype are particularly at risk for phenotyping as nonsecretors.[105]

Blood transfusion and transplantation

Lewis antibodies are generally low-titer, IgM saline agglutinins and are clinically insignificant.[11] Lewis antibodies can display ABO reactivity, reacting stronger with group O (anti-Le^{bH}), A (anti-ALe^b), or B (anti-BLe^b) red cells. With rare exceptions, they are not associated with HDFN or hemolytic transfusion reactions. There is a single small report linking a Le(a−b−) phenotype with an increased risk of rejection in kidney transplantation.[106]

Biological roles
Cancer

Sialyl-Le^a (sLe^a) is a receptor for E-selectin and important adhesion in cancer biology.[107] Epithelial tumors with high sLe^a (or sLe^x) expression have increased metastatic potential and a poorer clinical prognosis. Upregulation of *FUT3*, coupled with downregulation of *FUT2*, is an early step in the epithelial-mesenchymal transition during malignant transformation.[96] In cancer cell lines, FUT3 silencing by siRNA inhibits E-selectin binding and adhesion to endothelial cells, as well as reduces cellular proliferation.[107]

Atherosclerosis

A Le(a−b−) phenotype has been linked to a twofold increased risk of atherosclerotic disease and coronary death.[108] Although the basis for the observation is unknown, Le(a−b−) individuals did demonstrate lower triglyceride levels, which could potentially alter plasma Lewis-GSL concentrations. Molecular typing of 1735 individuals in the Framingham offspring study subsequently showed a 57% increased risk of atherothrombotic disease in confirmed *le/le* individuals.[109] Of three common *FUT3* mutations studied, the *le*[59] mutation had the strongest association with atherosclerotic disease.

Necrotizing enterocolitis and other inflammatory bowel disorders

Necrotizing enterocolitis occurs in 7–10% of premature infants and carries a high mortality rate (20–30%).[110] It is characterized by bowel inflammation and necrosis with evidence of a disturbed intestinal microbiota. Recently, a correlation between NEC, salivary H antigen, and *FUT2* genotype was identified.[111] Infants with low salivary H had a significantly higher risk of death from NEC and sepsis ($p < 0.001$). When examined by genotype, survival was highest among *Se/Se* homozygotes (98%) and *Se/se* heterozygotes (95%) when compared to *se/se* nonsecretors (87%).

From animal and human studies, there is evidence that fucosylation protects against infectious and inflammatory insults to the gastrointestinal tract. In adults, there is a direct spatial relationship between bacterial density and fucosylation, with highest density of bacteria and fucosylation in the colon and rectum.[112,113] As noted earlier, commensal bacteria that utilize fucose as a nutrient can specifically induce *FUT2* in intestinal tissue—a demonstration of a mutually beneficial symbiotic relationship.[102] In mice, inflammatory insults rapidly upregulate *FUT2*, leading to the shedding of fucosylated glycoproteins that promote commensal bacterial growth, while suppressing expression of bacterial virulence genes.[114] In addition, fucosylation protects against tissue injury with more rapid tissue recovery.[113] In contrast, nonsecretor animals are susceptible to chronic colitis, diarrhea, and weight loss.[114,115] Not surprisingly, nonsecretor has also been linked with Crohn's disease and is implicated in intestinal graft-versus-host disease, inflammatory bowel disorder, and altered microflora.[116,117]

Helicobacter pylori and other infections

H. pylori is a flagellated, Gram-negative pathogen of the stomach associated with chronic gastritis, gastroduodenal ulcers, and gastric cancer.[73] A major colonization and virulence factor is BabA, a 78 kD lectin that recognizes type 1 H and Le[b] structures. Surveys of BabA-positive strains from around the world show that most are "generalists," capable of binding Le[b], ALe[b], BLe[b], and type 1 H antigen. Le[b], however, is the preferred ligand in binding assays.[118] The ability to recognize ABH-modified-Le[b] structures may explain the lack of clear correlation between ABO type and *H. pylori* infection, despite older studies showing a linkage between group O and duodenal ulcers.[73] The correlation between *H. pylori* and secretor status is equally unclear, with some studies showing higher colonization rates and worse inflammation among nonsecretors.[119,120]

There is some evidence to suggest that a nonsecretor phenotype may increase the risk of cholera toxin and the related enterotoxigenic *E. coli*, which secretes a cholera-like toxin. Two studies have found an increased incidence of nonsecretor among cholera patients.[121,122] In the largest study of 522 subjects, infected symptomatic individuals were twice as likely to be Le(a+b−) nonsecretors.[122] Likewise, a nonsecretor phenotype may increase the risk of *E. coli* infection in young children. Le(a+b−) children were more likely to have symptomatic infections (71% vs. 29%), especially by strains expressing the CFA I adhesin.[123]

Secretor status is also considered a host susceptibility factor in several viral infections. As noted earlier, norovirus and rotaviruses recognize type 1 ABH structures. In most outbreaks, nonsecretors are relatively resistant to infection.[81,82] Nonsecretor may also provide mild protection against heterosexual HIV transmission, with HIV infection rates 14–30% lower than *Se*+ individuals.[124,125] One older study also showed a higher rate of influenza infection among *Se*+.[126]

I blood group

The I blood group (ISBT 027) was initially described in 1956 in a patient with a potent cold agglutinin and episodes of profound hemolysis characteristic of cold agglutinin disease.[127] Serologic studies showed a panagglutinin reactive with more than 22,000 donors, family members, and several animal species. After extensive testing, five compatible donors were identified, leading investigators to designate her antibody as an anti-I in order to "emphasize the high degree of individuality" of rare I-negative (i+) donors.[127] Dr. Lawrence Marsh later confirmed the inverse serologic relationship between I and i antigens after identification of an anti-i. This antibody was reactive with i[adult] and cord red cells but not adult, I+ red cells.[128]

I/i expression

The I antigen is a widely distributed, developmentally regulated antigen. At birth, cord red cells are I−i+, presumably as protection against HDFN due to ABO incompatibility (see later). After three months of age, I antigen progressively increases, accompanied by decreased i antigen, with a normal adult-type I+i− phenotype by 18–24 months.[128] I antigen on adult red cells can vary from 32,000 to 130,000/cell due to differences in the fine specificity of anti-I antibodies.[120] Estimates of i antigen on untreated cord and adult red cells are 25,000–75,000/cord and 1000–30,000/adult cell, respectively.[129] The i antigen is elevated on reticulocytes and can be increased on mature red cells as a sign of stressed erythropoiesis, dyserythropoiesis, and disordered Golgi trafficking.[129] Conditions associated with elevated i antigen include erythroleukemia, megaloblastic anemia, chronic hemolytic disorders, and hereditary erythroblastic multinuclearity with a positive acidified serum lysis test (HEMPAS).

I-null (i[adult])

An I−i+ phenotype is characteristic of i[adult] red cells, a rare autosomal-recessive phenotype due to mutations in the I gene (*GCNT2, IGnT*) with an estimated incidence of 1:4400 to 1:17,000.[128,130] Heterozygous family members can have an intermediate I+i+ phenotype consistent with gene dosage. Individuals with i[adult] can make an allo-anti-I reactive with normal adult red cells.

There are two clinical i[adult] phenotypes based on the presence or absence of congenital cataracts.[131,132] In non-Asians, there is an isolated deficiency of I antigen on red cells only. Conversely, many Asian i[adult] kindreds show a global loss of I antigen on all tissues, including human lens, accompanied by congenital cataracts.

(A)

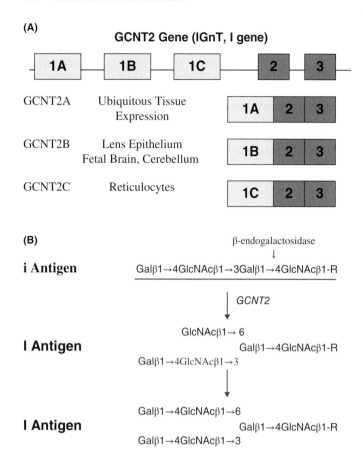

GCNT2 Gene (IGnT, I gene)

GCNT2A — Ubiquitous Tissue Expression

GCNT2B — Lens Epithelium Fetal Brain, Cerebellum

GCNT2C — Reticulocytes

(B)

β-endogalactosidase
↓

i Antigen   Galβ1→4GlcNAcβ1→3Galβ1→4GlcNAcβ1-R

↓ *GCNT2*

GlcNAcβ1→6

I Antigen   Galβ1→4GlcNAcβ1-R

Galβ1→4GlcNAcβ1→3

↓

Galβ1→4GlcNAcβ1→6

I Antigen   Galβ1→4GlcNAcβ1-R

Galβ1→4GlcNAcβ1→3

Figure 13.3 (A) Structure of the I gene (*GCNT2*) and three mRNA isoforms. (B) Synthesis of I antigen from i-active polylactosamine precursor.

Biochemistry

I and i antigens are biosynthetically and structurally related oligosaccharides, composed of repeating units of n-acetyllactosamine (LacNAc, $[Gal\beta \rightarrow 4GlcNAc]_n$). The mininum i antigen epitope is defined as a linear, unbranched type 2 chain oligosaccharide bearing at least two successive LacNAc units (Figure 13.3B).[133] The i antigen is sensitive to the enzyme β endo-galactosidase.

The I antigen is a branched, polylactosamine derivative of i antigen. The I gene (*GCNT2, IGnT*) encodes a β1-6 n-acetylgalactosaminyltransferase that transfers a β1 → 6 GlcNAc to a subterminal β1 → 3Gal.[131,132] Extensive studies with purified oligosaccharides indicate that the enzyme recognizes a four-sugar donor acceptor composed of two successive LacNac units.[134] This is consistent with isolated erythroid glycans, which show at least two LacNAc motifs between branch points.[8] The enzyme can form branches on both distal and centrally places β1 → 3Gal residues, but will not recognize LacNAc residues modified by fucose or neuraminic acid.[134] As a result, sialylation and fucosylation (ABH, Le^X, Le^Y) are regulators of I and i antigens, blocking both polylactosamine elongation and branching. Anti-I antibodies can recognize a variety of glycans but require a [−GlcNAcβ1 → 6 (GlcNAcβ1 → 3)Galβ1−] as part of the immune epitope (Figure 13.3B).[129,133]

Molecular biology and genetics

The I gene, *GCNT2* (IGnT), is located in an *Alu*-rich region on chromosome 6p24.2.[135] The gene consists of five exons, including three tissue-specific exon 1s (E1A, E1B, E1C; Figure 13.3A).[131,132] As a result, three different isoforms of the enzyme are produced depending on which exon 1 is utilized. *GCNT2A* (*IGnTA, IGnT2*) is expressed by most humans' tissues and is derived from exon E1A. *GCNT2B* uses exon E1B and is the only mRNA transcript identified in human lens. *GCNT2C* (*IGnTC*) is an erythroid-specific enzyme that is responsible for I antigen expression on red cells. *GCNT2* is highly homologous to *C2GnT*, a β1 → 6 n-acetylglucosaminyltransferase responsible for I-type structures on core 2 and core 3 O-glycans.[136]

The enzyme is 400–402 amino acids and, unlike most glycosyltransferases, does not require a metal ion for enzyme activity.[132] The enzyme retains nine highly conserved cysteines necessary for enzyme folding and five N-glycans but lacks the classic DXD motif found in metal-dependent transferases. Exon 1 encodes 77% of the translated protein, including the transmembrane domain, stem region, and UDP-nucleotide binding domain (UDP-GlcNAc).[129,132] The acceptor domain is primarily encoded by exons E2 and E3. Due to sequence differences in exon 1, the three *GCNT2* isoforms share only 66–73% homology and subtly differ in enzyme activity. In enzyme assays, the erythroid-specific GCNT2C isoform shows nearly twofold higher enzyme activity.[132]

GCNT2C is transcriptionally regulated in red cells.[137] Studies have identified a promoter sequence approximately 250 base pairs (−318 to −251) upstream of the E1C translation initiation site that contains transcription factor binding sites for Oct-2, Sp1, and C/EBPα. All three transcription factors bind the *GCNT2C* promoter region; however, only C/EBPα is absolutely critical for *GCNT2C* transcription. Interestingly, C/EBPα binding and transcriptional activation require dephosphorylation of a specific serine (Ser-21) on C/EBPα, possibly via ERK or p38 MAP kinase pathways.[137]

Table 13.7 *GCNT2* mutations associated with i_{adult} phenotype

	Mutation		Phenotype	
Exon	Nucleotide	Amino acid	i_{adult} RBC	Cataracts
E1C	243T>A	N81L	+	−
E1C	505G>A	A169T	+	−
E1C	683G>A	R228Q	+	−
E1C	651delA	V244X	+	−
E2	978G>A	W328X	+	+
E2	816G>C	E272D	+	+
E2	1006G>A	G336R	+	+
E3	1043G>A	G348E	+	+
E3	1148G>A	R383H	+	+
Deletion	Δ70 kb	E1B->E3	+	+
Deletion	Δ93 kb	E1B->E3	+	+

Phosphoserine residues are known to regulate C/EBPα function in early hematopoiesis and myeloid differentiation.[129]

The molecular basis for i_{adult}

Mutations in *GCNT2* are responsible for the i_{adult} phenotype.[131,132,135,138,139] Individuals with mutations in E1C, which is responsible for the erythroid-specific *GCNT2C*, show an isolated loss of I antigen expression in red cells only: I expression is retained in other tissues via *GCNT2A* and *GCNT2B*. These individuals are not at an increase for congenital cataracts (Table 13.7).

The i_{adult} with congenital cataracts is the result of mutations affecting all three *GCNT2* isoforms, leading to a tissue-wide loss of all enzyme activity.[132] To date, six point mutations have been identified in E2 and E3, which are shared by all three enzyme isoforms. In three unrelated kindreds, large deletions (70–93 kb) encompassing most of *GCNT2* (exons E1B, E1C, E2, and E3) were identified.[135] Because *GCNT2* resides in an *Alu*-rich region, it may be particularly susceptible to *Alu*-mediated deletion and genomic rearrangements.[135]

It is presumed that the absence of branched N-glycans in human lens underlies the development of congenital cataracts. This has not been substantiated in a *GCNT2*-null mouse model.[140] *GCNT2*-null mice had no apparent increase in either the incidence or onset of cataracts. This conundrum may reflect species-specific differences in glycan expression. Indirect evidence for the latter is the early development of cataracts in A3GALT-null mice, which are unable to synthesize oligosaccharides containing Galα1 → 3Gal (linear B) epitopes.[141]

Transfusion

Anti-I is a common, low-titer, IgM cold agglutinin in normal human sera.[129] Anti-I can demonstrate significant crossreactivity with i epitopes and can show a preference for polylactosamines bearing sialic acid or ABH epitopes. Anti-i, by contrast, is less frequent. Anti-i is commonly associated with infectious mononucleosis, Burkitt's lymphoma, and cirrhosis.[11,129] Many anti-i are sialoagglutinins with a preference for linear structures bearing a terminal sialic acid.[129]

An increase in anti-I/i titers and/or thermal amplitude is not uncommon following infection and in certain lymphoproliferative disorders. B cell malignancies, in particular, can secrete high-titer, monoclonal autoantibodies capable of inducing hemolysis and cold agglutinin disease. Monoclonal antibodies classically bear the V_H4–34 IgM heavy gene, which has inherent anti-I/i specificity due to hydrophobic sequences in the terminal FR1 domain of the

molecule.[142] Fine specificity (anti-I vs. anti-i) may be influenced by heavy (CDR_H3) and light chain ($V_\kappa CDR_L1$, $V_\lambda CDR_L3$) variable regions, which line the antigen-binding pocket.[143] In contrast, anti-I/i coincident with infection are polyclonal and reflect a global increase in IgM antibody.[129]

In general, antibodies against anti-I/i are clinically insignificant.[11] Blood typing difficulties and hemolysis can be observed in patients with high-titer antibodies, particularly if there is strong reactivity above 30–32 °C. These patients may require use of a blood warmer for transfusion. There are rare cases of hemolytic transfusion reactions with warm-acting anti-IH following transfusion of group O or A_2 red cells.[144]

Biological roles
Hemolytic disease of the fetus and newborn

There is a theory that the absence of I antigen on cord red cells is protective against HDFN due to ABO incompatibility. There is a parallel increase in both I and A/B antigens in the first few months of life, consistent with increasing erythroid *GCNT2C* activity.[129] Supporting evidence for the key role of branching in ABH expression can be found on the bi-attennary N-glycan of Band 3/Diego. On cord cells, the N-glycan is relatively simple and unbranched, with few ABH epitopes on the long, linear α1,6 mannosyl arm.[129,145] In contrast, adult red cells display a massive N-glycan with extensive β1–6 branching along both α1,6 and α1,3 arms, allowing display of multiple ABH epitopes per N-glycan.[7,129]

Galectins

Galectins are a family of small, soluble, lectin-type proteins that share a common β-galactoside binding motif.[146] One of the most widely studied galectins is galectin-3, which recognizes and binds polylactosamines bearing at least two successive LacNAc motifs.[146] Galectin-3 is abundantly expressed and secreted by macrophages and is implicated in giant cell formation, dendritic cells, fibrosis, and chronic inflammation.[147] Galactin-3 also binds and directly activates human neutrophils, promoting neutrophil recruitment, adhesion, and respiratory burst.

Embryonic development

I/i antigens are differentially expressed during embryonic development and are considered oncofetal antigens.[129] Recently, the i antigen was identified as a marker of human mesenchymal stem cells and might serve as a ligand for galactin-3.[148] Galactin-3 is hypothesized to play a role in the immunosuppressive properties of mesenchymal stem cells.

Breast and other cancers

GCNT2 is overexpressed in highly metastatic and basal-like breast cancer cells and was recently identified as a possible disease modifier in BRAC2 breast cancer.[149] A GWA study identified a polymorphism (rs9348512) located on chromosome 6p24, within 1 MB of *GCNT2*. Homozygosity for the minor "A" allele was associated with a 15% decreased risk of developing breast cancer and correlated with *GCNT2* mRNA levels. An increase in polylactosamines is also reported in colon and other epithelial cancers.[129]

P blood group system

The system historically known as the *P blood group* was initially discovered in 1927 by Landesteiner and Levine after immunizing rabbits with human red cells.[150] The resulting antibody recognized

Table 13.8 GSL structures related to globo, P1, and PX2 synthesis

GSL	Alias	Structure
GlcCer	CMH	Glc-Cer
LacCer	CDH	Galβ1-4Glc-Cer
GM3		NeuAcα2-3Galβ1-4Glc-Cer
Globo GSL		
Gb3	Pᵏ, CD77	Galα1-4Galβ1-4Glc-Cer
Gb4	P, globoside	GalNAcβ1-3Galα1-4Galβ1-4Glc-Cer
αGal-Gb4	NOR1	Galα1-4GalNAcβ1-3Galα1-4Galβ1-4Glc-Cer
Forssman	Forssman	GalNAcα1-3GalNAcβ1-3Galα1-4Galβ1-4Glc-Cer
Gb5	SSEA3	Galβ1-3GalNAcβ1-3Galα1-4Galβ1-4Glc-Cer
Fuc-Gb5	Globo H	Fucα1-2Galβ1-3GalNAcβ1-3Galα1-4Galβ1-4Glc-Cer
MSGG	LKE, SSEA4	NeuAcα2-3Galβ1-3GalNAcβ1-3Galα1-4Galβ1-4Glc-Cer
αGal-Gb5	"Band 0.03"	Galα1-4Galβ1-3GalNAcβ1-3Galα1-4Galβ1-4Glc-Cer
neolacto GSL		
Lc3		GlcNAcβ1-3Galβ1-4Glc-Cer
nLc4	Paragloboside	Galβ1-4GlcNAcβ1-3Galβ1-4Glc-Cer
αGal-nLc4	P1	Galα1-4Galβ1-4GlcNAcβ1-3Galβ1-4Glc-Cer
GalNc-nLc4	PX2	GalNAcβ1-3Galβ1-4GlcNAcβ1-3Galβ1-4Glc-Cer
NeuAc-nLc4	SPG	NeuAcα2-3Galβ1-4GlcNAcβ1-3Galβ1-4Glc-Cer

Cer, ceramide; Fuc, fucose; Gal, galactose; GalNAc, n-acetylgalactosamine; Glc, glucose; GlcNAc, n-acetylglucosamine; NeuAc, n-acetylneuraminic acid.

the P_1 antigen, which is variably expressed on most, but not all, human red cells. The P^k and P antigens were added to the system after the discovery of rare null phenotypes. The historical P system has now expanded into three blood group systems and six serologic antigens, which are assigned based on the last glycosyltransferase necessary for their synthesis.[151] The P1PK system (ISBT 003) encompasses P^k, P_1, and NOR antigens, which all share a terminal $\alpha1 \rightarrow 4$Gal epitope. GLOB (ISBT 028) contains the P and PX2 antigens, which terminate in a $\beta1 \rightarrow 3$GalNAc. FORS (ISBT 031) contains a single antigen, Forssman—a xenoantigen expressed by many animals and rare A_{pae} red cells. *Luke antigen on erythrocytes* (LKE) is a high-incidence antigen that is still classified under the GLOB collection 209. Other related antigens include galactosygloboside, globo-H, and globo-A antigens. Globo-A is a target for anti-A_1, whereas globo-H, galactosylgloboside, and LKE are oncofetal antigens found on stem cells and many epithelial cells.

Biochemistry and synthesis

Unlike ABH, Ii, and Lewis antigens, the antigens of the P system are exclusively expressed on glycospingolipids (GSLs). Chemically, GSLs consist of a carbohydrate head covalently linked to a ceramide lipid tail (*N*-aceylsphingosine), which anchors the molecule in the membrane. Most members of the P-system belong to the globo-series of GSLs and share a $Gal\alpha1 \rightarrow 4Gal\beta1 \rightarrow 4Glc$-Ceramide or Gb3 core (Table 13.8). Exceptions are P_1 and PX2, which are type 2 chain, neolacto GSLs derived from paragloboside.

Lactosylceramide (LacCer) is the precursor of both globo- and type 2 chain GSLs (Figure 13.4). Globo-family GSLs proceed from the addition of an $\alpha1 \rightarrow 4Gal$ to LacCer by A4GALT1 to form globotriaosylceramide (Gb3, P^k), the first globo-family GSL. Gb3/P^k may then serve as a substrate for B3GALNT1, which adds a terminal $\beta1 \rightarrow 3GalNAc$ to form globoside (Gb4, P antigen). In animals and rare A_{pae} cells, globoside/P antigen is further modified by the

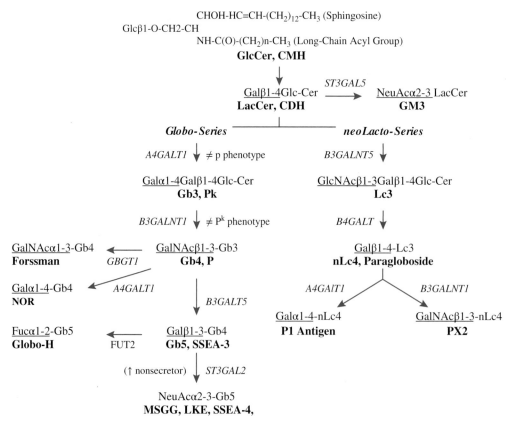

Figure 13.4 Synthesis of P blood group and related glycosphingolipid antigens.

addition of an $\alpha1 \rightarrow 3$GalNAc to form Forssman antigen.[151] The rare NOR antigen shares features of both P^k and P antigens, with an $\alpha1 \rightarrow 4$Gal terminus on a Gb4/P antigen core.[152]

Synthesis of LKE and extended globo-family antigens requires B3GALT5, which adds a terminal $\beta1 \rightarrow 3$Gal to form galactosylgloboside or Gb5.[153] B3GALT5 is a rate-limiting enzyme for both Gb5 and type 1 chain synthesis and shows developmental and tissue-specific expression.[154] Once formed, Gb5 can serve as a substrate for H-active fucosyltransferases to form globo-H.[9,10] In A_1 individuals, globo-H is converted to globo-A: Expression of globo-A is believed responsible for antigenic differences between A_1 and A_2 red cells.[16]

Gb5 can also be sialylated by the $\alpha2,3$sialyltransferase ST3GAL2 to form LKE antigen (MSGG, SSEA-4).[155] In genitourinary tissue, there is competition between FUT2 and ST3GAL2 for Gb5, leading to decreased LKE/MSGG synthesis on epithelial cells of secretors (Se+).[156] In some tissues, including red cells, LKE is further sialylated to form disialogalactosylgloboside (DSGG).[157,158] In human platelets, a minor GSL with a Gb5 core and terminal $\alpha1 \rightarrow 4$Gal was identified in 10–20% of donors.[159]

A4GALT1, the enzyme responsible for P^k synthesis, is also capable of recognizing paragloboside to form P_1 antigen. Unlike P^k, P_1 is a minor red cell GSL with variable expression. Paragloboside can also serve as an alternate substrate for β3GALNT1 to form PX2, a P-active GSL recognized by some allo-anti-P.[151] Synthesis of PX2 is limited to rare p null phenotypes, which lack Gb3/P^k (see the "Serology" section).

Serology

P_1/P_2: The classic P system contains two main phenotypes, P_1, and P_2. P_1 and P_2 have normal expression of globo-series antigens and only differ in the expression of P_1 antigen (Table 13.9). P_1 is the predominant phenotype in most populations and can vary in strength between individuals. The P_2 (P_1-negative) phenotype ranges from 6% in Blacks to 75–80% in some Asian populations (China and Vietnam).[20,73] The P_1 antigen is absent on p cells (see below). P_2 individuals can make a naturally occurring anti-P_1.

P^k: P^k is a rare autosomal-recessive phenotype due to homozygous inheritance of null B3GALNT1 alleles. P^k can occur on either a P_1 or P_2 background, giving rise to P_1^k or P_2^k phenotype, respectively (Table 13.9). P^k red cells lack Gb4/P and all subsequent globo-series GSLs (LKE, globo-H), accompanied by increased expression of P^k/Gb3, LacCer, and type 2 chain GSLs (paragloboside,

sialylparagloboside).[151,160] P^k variants, with increased P^k/Gb3 and decreased Gb4/P, have been described and may reflect decreased B3GALNT1 activity. P^k individuals make a potent, clinically significant allo-anti-P that is reactive with all red cells except rare P^k and p cells. Anti-P can contain reactivity against PX2 as well as other globo-GSLs (Gb5, LKE).[151,160]

p null: The p phenotype is a true globo-null phenotype due to homozygosity for amorph A4GALT1 alleles.[151] Red cells and other tissues lack P_1 and all globo-GSL (Figure 13.4). Red cells show a compensatory increase in type 2 chain GSLs, including paragloboside and PX2. Heterozygous individuals (A4GALT1+/−) show normal globo-GSL expression with no evidence of gene dosage. Sera from p individuals contain a mix of naturally occurring IgM agglutinins cross-reactive with P_1, P, and P^k cells (allo-anti-PP$_1$P^k). In solid phase testing, anti-P^k and anti-P are the predominant specificities.[160]

LKE: LKE, also known as Luke, is a minor, high-incidence ganglioside on red cells. There are three recognized LKE phenotypes: LKE-strong positive (LKE^S), LKE-weak positive (LKE^W), and LKE-negative (LKE^N).[161] LKE^N red cells often show a P^k variant-like phenotype, with increased P^k/Gb3 and decreased Gb4 expression.[161] LKE^N can also occur in weak P red cells, which have marked decrease in Gb3 and Gb4 expression.[160] In P_1 and P_2 individuals, LKE^N is associated with trace LKE/MSGG (10% normal) on red cells: True LKE-null is only observed in p and P^k phenotypes.[160] LKE/MSGG is also known as stage-specific embryonic antigen-4 (SSEA4) and is a marker of embryonic, mesenchymal, and cancer stem cells.[9,162–164]

NOR: NOR is a rare polyagglutinable phenotype that appears to have arisen in a Polish kindred.[151,152] NOR red cells express unusual penta- and hepatoglycosylglobo-GSLs that bear a Gal$\alpha1 \rightarrow 4$GalNAc terminus (Table 13.8). Normal human sera contain two classes of naturally occurring antibodies reactive with NOR, with slightly different specifities: type 1, anti-P^k+NOR and type 2, anti-NOR. NOR is not recognized by anti-P_1.

Genetics and molecular biology

P1PK synthase (A4GALT1)

A4GALT1 encodes an $\alpha1,4$ galactosyltransferase responsible for P^k, P_1 and NOR antigen synthesis.[151,165] A4GALT1 resides on chromosome 22q13 and is organized into three exons, with the active enzyme localized within exon 3. A4GALT1 belongs to the GT32

Table 13.9 P blood group serology

Type	Incidence	GT Genes*		Antigens on RBC†					Antibodies
		A4GALT1	B3GALNT1	P^k	P	LKE	P_1	Other	
P_1	80%†	+	+	+	+	+	+		
P_2	20%	+	+	+	+	+	0		Anti-P_1
LKE^S	80–90%	+	+	+	+	+	+/0		
LKE^W	10–20%	+	+	+	+	↓	+/0		
LKE^N	1–2%	+	+	+	+	tr‡	+/0		Anti-LKE
P_1^k	Rare	+	0	+	0	0	+		Anti-P
P_2^k	Rare	+	0	+	0	0	0		Anti-P, P_1
p	Rare	0	+	0	0	0	0	PX2	Anti-PP$_1$P^k
NOR	Rare	+	+	+	+	na	+/0	NOR	

*Inheritance of at least one functional glycosyltransferase (GT) gene (+).

†Incidence in US whites.

‡Trace antigen, not detected by hemagglutination.

family of glycosyltransferases and shares 43% homology with *A4GNT*, an α1,4 galactosyltransferase involved in gastric mucin synthesis.[165] *A4GALT1* mRNA is ubiquitously expressed in most human tissues.[42]

The predominant enzyme in P[1] and P[2] individuals is a 353-amino-acid type II glycoprotein containing two N-glycosylation sites, five cysteine residues, and a classic DXD motif.[165] There is evidence that A4GALT1 resides in the *trans*-Golgi network, possibly in a heterodimeric complex with LacCer synthase.[166] Synthesis of Gb3 and other globo-GSLs can be suppressed or disrupted by competing glycosylation pathways, altered Golgi trafficking, and lysosomal degradation.[166–168]

The basis of the P[1]/P[2] phenotype is still under investigation. In Japan, the P[2] phenotype was initially linked to polymorphisms in the promoter region (−551insC, −160A) that reportedly decreased *A4GALT1* transcription.[169] These findings were not consistently found, however, in a study of European donors.[170] Subsequently, Thursson *et al.* identified a minor *A4GALT1* mRNA transcript utilizing an alternate exon (exon 2a) that contained a SNP (42C>T) in P[2] individuals.[171] In addition, P[2] individuals had less *A4GALT1* mRNA than P[1] donors. More recently, a large systemic study that included several different ethnic groups identified 11 distinct SNPs within intron 1, including eight SNPs that showed linkage with the P[1]/P[2] phenotype.[172] An eloquent series of experiments using luciferase constructs bearing different combinations of SNPs showed that one SNP (3084G>T; rs4741348) was associated with P[2] and decreased *A4GALT1* transcription. It is hypothesized that this new SNP may involve binding by transcription factor binding proteins. *A4GALT1* does show evidence of gene dosage, where *A4GALT1* levels are highest in $P^1/P^1 > P^1/P^2 > P^2/P^2$.[171,172]

The NOR phenotype is the result of a missense mutation (Gln211>Glu) in the catalytic domain of the enzyme.[173] A comparison of *A4GALT1* sequences from humans, gorilla, pig, cattle, rat, and mouse indicates that Q211 is a conserved amino acid. Likewise, a homologous sequence motif (QxSRYxxNG) containing a Gln211 analog is present in the related *A4GNT*. It is hypothesized that the polymorphism broadens acceptor substrate specificity, allowing the enzyme to recognize either a β-Gal or β-GalNAc acceptor.[173] The p phenotype can arise from a variety of missense, frameshift, nonsense, and deletion mutations. Approximately 30 amorph *A4GALT1* alleles are described to date.[20,151]

P synthase (*B3GALNT1*)

B3GALNT1 is located on chromosome 3q26 and encodes a β1 → 3 n-acetylgalactosaminyltransferase responsible for P and PX2 antigen synthesis.[20,151] Originally named *B3GALT3*, *B3GALNT1* is a member of the GT31 family of glycosyltransferases and is ubiquitously expressed in most human tissues.[42,174] *B3GALNT1* is highly homologous to the β1,3-galactosyltransferase family, likely arising late in evolution from *B3GALT5*.[175] The gene contains five exons with the open reading frame located in exon 5. The translated enzyme is 331 amino acids with three β1,3 galactosyltransferase motifs, five potential N-glycans, and six cysteines, including four cysteines conserved among other β1,3 galactosyltransferases.[174,175] Seven null alleles associated with the P[k] phenotype are reported to date.[20]

Forssman synthase (*GBGT1*)

GBGT1 encodes an α1 → 3galactosaminyltransferase belonging to the GT6 family of α1,3-Gal/GalNAc transferases and is responsible for Forssman synthesis.[176] Members of the GT6 family arose from a common ancestral gene and include the *ABO* gene, isogloboside synthase (*A3GALT2*), and the enzyme necessary for linear B synthesis (*GGTA1*).

GBGT1 is located on chromosome 9q34 as a pseudogene.[176] Like the *ABO* gene, the open reading frame is spread over several exons. Surprisingly, *GBGT1* mRNA can be detected in a wide host of human tissues despite the absence of Forssman expression. The absence of Forssman antigen in humans and apes is the consequence of two inactivating mutations (Gly230Ser; Gln296Arg) that arose late in primate evolution. Using recombinant enzyme constructs, Yamamato and colleagues were able to restore enzyme activity in human GBGT1, where Gly230+Gln296 > Gly230 > Gln296.[176] Gly230 is homologous to Gly235 in the human ABO gene, which is crucial for UDP-GalNAc and H-antigen acceptor recognition. Forssman expression on rare A[pae] red cells is due to an Arg296>Gln mutation that restores partial enzyme activity. It is hypothesized that de novo Forssman expression reported in some cancers could reflect a similar process.[176]

Transfusion medicine

P[2] individuals can make a naturally occurring anti-P[1], a low-titered, IgM agglutinin.[11] Anti-P[1] is generally clinically insignificant, although rare acute hemolytic transfusion reactions have been reported. High-titer anti-P[1] can be observed in bird fanciers and certain Helminth infections due to the presence of P[k]- and P[1]-like substances in bird droppings and parasites.[11,73] Although there is no evidence that anti-P[1] is advantageous against Helminth infections, it is interesting that the highest incidence of P[2] occurs in regions with a high incidence of *Echinococcus* infection.[73]

Unlike anti-P[1], the allo-anti-PP[1]P[k] and allo-anti-P present in p and P[k] individuals are always clinically significant antibodies, capable of causing acute hemolytic transfusion reactions and spontaneous abortion.[11] A hemolytic auto-anti-P is also seen in paroxysmal cold hemoglobinuria. The antibody is a biphasic, IgG hemolysin and is identified using the Donath–Landsteiner test.

Anti-LKE is rare, with only six known cases.[160] Most examples of anti-LKE were low-titer, IgM antibodies and clinically insignificant. There is one report of a hemolytic transfusion reaction associated with a high-titer anti-LKE in a patient with newly diagnosed lymphoma.[160]

Biological role
Development and cancer

Globo-GSLs are expressed on embryonic stem cells, where they may play a role in development. Two extended globo-GSLs, Gb5 (SSEA-3) and LKE/MSGG (SSEA-4), are markers of embryonic stem cells, embryonic carcinoma, and teratocinomas.[162] In vitro studies with human embryonal carcinoma cell lines have shown homotypic cell–cell adhesion and signaling mediated by Gb4–Gb5 interactions.[177] In murine embryos, LKE/MSGG-enriched lipid rafts participate in cytokinesis, localizing along the cleavage furrows in cooperation with actin and E-cadherin.[178] In mice, deletion of *B3GALNT1*, with loss of Gb4, Gb5, and MSGG, is embryonic lethal.[179]

Several globo-GSLs are increased in malignancy and serve as cancer markers. Gb3 is elevated in Burkitt's lymphoma and is a marker of apoptotic germinal center B cells.[151] Globo-H, Gb5, and MSGG are expressed by breast cancer and cancer stem cells.[9,164,180] In breast cancer, MSGG-enriched lipid rafts contribute to tumor invasion through their interaction with integrins, cSrc, and FAK.[180] A MSGG-binding protein FKBP4 was recently identified in breast cancer cells.[181] Finally, MSGG and/or disialosylgalactosylgloboside

(DSGG) are elevated on renal cell carcinoma.[158,182] DSGG binds siglec-7 and is associated with pulmonary metastasis and inhibition of NK cells.[182,183]

Immune response

Gb3 is expressed on B-cells and may serve as a stimulatory glycolipid antigen for iNKT cells.[184] In addition, Gb4 was identified as an endogenous ligand for toll-like receptors (TLRs), a member of the innate immune system expressed on monocytes, spleen, and phagocytic cells.[185] In Gram-negative sepsis, the TLR4–MD2 complex binds bacterial LPS via the lipid A tail, triggering an intense inflammatory response. In *A4GALT1*-knockout mice, exogenous Gb4 administration can reduce LPS-induced inflammation and mortality by binding TLR4-MD2 and blocking LPS binding. In wild-type mice, LPS upregulates *A4GALT1* transcription with upregulation of Gb4 synthesis, coupled with recruitment of TLR4-MD2 into Gb4-enriched lipid rafts.

Parvovirus B19 and HIV

P antigen is a receptor for parvovirus B19, the causative agent of erythema infectiosum or fifth disease.[73] B19 is an erythrovirus, preferentially infecting marrow erythroblasts, resulting in reticulocytopenia, anemia, and, on occasion, aplastic crisis and pure red cell aplasia. Erythroblasts may be particularly susceptible to B19 due to their high concentration of Gb4.[73] Although Gb4 is necessary for infection, it is not sufficient—suggesting a possible co-receptor. Current research suggests that infection requires a two-step process, in which B19 initially binds Gb4, leading to a conformational change in the viral capsid.[186] The modified B19 can then bind a secondary receptor probably localized within a Gb4-enriched lipid domain. Once bound, the B19–receptor–lipid complex undergoes clathrin-mediated endocytosis.[186]

GSL-enriched lipid rafts play an important role in HIV fusion, endocytosis, and HIV budding.[187] In human lymphoid cells, there is an inverse relationship between Gb3 and HIV infection. Lymphocytes from p individuals are hypersusceptible to HIV in vitro, whereas lymphocytes from P^k donors, or patients with Fabry disease, are HIV resistant.[188,189] Other investigators, on the other hand, have identified Gb3 as a co-receptor, facilitating the interaction between HIV, CD4, and CXCR4.[190]

Shigella, E. coli, and *Streptococcus suis*

Shigella dysenteriae and enterohemorrhagic *E. coli* express shiga toxins (Stx) that recognize GSLs bearing a terminal Galα1 → 4Gal epitope, including P_1, Gb_3, and "band 0.03."[73] Gb3, however, is the physiologic receptor in infection and development of hemolytic uremic syndrome (HUS). Gb3-enriched lipid rafts are necessary for toxin binding, Stx-mediated cell signaling, and endocytosis. Six studies have examined the correlation between P_1/P_2 phenotype, HUS, and clinical outcomes with mixed results.[73] A study from the *E. coli* O157:H7 network, however, found a fourfold increased risk of HUS in P_1^{strong} individuals.[191] Gb3 is also a receptor for *S. suis*, a pathogen of pigs that can cause life-threatening infections in humans.[73]

Globo-GSLs are also receptors for P-fimbriated, uropathogenic *E. coli* strains. P-fimbria recognize all globo-GSLs, although LKE/ MSGG is the preferred receptor in solid phase testing. The ability of *FUT2* to decrease MSGG synthesis is likely responsible for the 3.4 to 26-fold higher incidence of UTI in nonsecretors.[192,193] The impact of the P_1/P_2 phenotype on *E. coli* UTI is less clear. Early pediatric studies showed a slight increase in UTI and recurrent pyelonephritis in P_1 children.[73] In contrast, studies in adults have found little or no association between UTI and P_1 phenotype.[192]

Key references

A full reference list for this chapter is available at: http://www.wiley.com/go/simon/transfusion

20 Reid ME, Lomas-Francis C, Olsson ML. *Blood group antigen FACTs Book*. 3rd ed. Waltham, MA: Academic Press, 2012.

21 Yamamoto F. Review: ABO blood group system—ABH oligosaccharide antigens, anti-A and anti-B, A and B glycosyltransferases and ABO genes. *Immunohematology* 2004; **20**: 3–22.

25 Brockhausen I. Crossroads between bacterial and mammalian glycosyltransferases. *Front Immunology* 2014; **5**: 492:1–21. doi: 10.3389/fimmu.2014.00492

32 Issitt PD, Anstee DJ. *Applied blood group serology*. Durham, NC: Montgomery Scientific, 1998.

43 Breton C, Oriol R, Imberty R. Conserved structural features in eukaryotic and prokaryotic fucosyltransferases. *Glycobiology* 1998; **8**: 87–94.

73 Cooling L. Blood groups in infection and host susceptibility. *Clin Micro Rev* 2015 Jul; **28** (3): 801–70.

129 Cooling L. Polylactosamines, there's more than meets the "Ii": a review of the I system. *Immunohematology* 2010; **26**: 133–55.

132 Yu L-C, Twu Y-C, Chou M-L, *et al.* The molecular genetics of the human *I* locus and molecular background explain the partial association of the adult i phenotype with congenital cataracts. *Blood* 2003; **101**: 2081–8.

151 Kaczmarek R, Buczkowska A, Mikolajewicz, Krotkiewski H, Czerwinski M. P1PK, GLOB FORS blood group systems and GLOB collection: biochemical and clinical aspects. Do we understand all yet? *Transf Med Rev* 2014; **28**: 126–36.

CHAPTER 14

Rh and LW blood group antigens

Connie M. Westhoff[1,2] & Don L. Siegel[2]

[1]Laboratory of Immunohematology and Genomics, New York Blood Center, New York, NY, USA
[2]Division of Transfusion Medicine and Therapeutic Pathology, Department of Pathology and Laboratory Medicine, Perelman School of Medicine at the University of Pennsylvania, Philadelphia, PA, USA

Summary

Although the Rh and LW antigens are carried on entirely different proteins, they are incorporated together in this chapter on the basis of a historic serologic connection (and confusion) and evidence that they are physically associated within the red cell membrane.

Rh blood group system

History and nomenclature

The Rh system is second only to the ABO system in importance in transfusion medicine because Rh antigens, especially D, are highly immunogenic and cause hemolytic disease of the fetus and newborn (HDFN) and hemolytic transfusion reactions (HTRs). HDFN was first described by a French midwife in 1609 in a set of twins, one of whom was hydropic and stillborn, whereas the other was jaundiced and died of kernicterus.[1] That a wide range of observed clinical scenarios involving red cell hemolysis were related—from severely hydropic stillborn fetuses to infants with mild or significant levels of jaundice and kernicterus—was not realized until 1932.[2] The cause of red cell hemolysis remained elusive until 1939, when Levine and Stetson described a woman who delivered a stillborn fetus and also suffered a severe hemolytic reaction when transfused with blood from her husband. Levine and Stetson correctly surmised that the mother had been immunized by a fetal red cell antigen inherited from the father and suggested that the cause of the erythroblastosis fetalis was maternal antibody in the fetal circulation.[3] They did not give the target blood group antigen a name. Meanwhile Landsteiner and Wiener, in an effort to discover new blood groups, injected rabbits and guinea pigs with rhesus monkey red cells. The antiserum they obtained agglutinated not only rhesus monkey red cells but also the red cells of 85% of White subjects, whom they called "Rh positive"; the remaining 15% of individuals studied were termed "Rh negative."[4(p182)] The "anti-Rhesus" serum seemed to be reacting similarly to the maternal antibody in serologic testing, hence the blood group system responsible for HDFN came to be known as "Rh." The anti-Rhesus serum, in actual fact, was detecting the LW antigen (subsequently named for Landsteiner and Wiener), which is present in greater amounts on D-positive than on D-negative red cells.[4(p394)] Years of debate followed concerning whether the human

antibodies and the Rhesus antibodies were detecting the same antigen and extended long after serologic profiles suggested they were reacting with different structures. Landsteiner and Wiener never accepted the LW terminology, because doing so would imply that they had not discovered the cause of HDFN.[5]

It was soon obvious that Rh was not a simple, single-antigen system. In 1941, Fisher named the C and c antigens (A and B had been used for ABO), and used the next letters of the alphabet, D and E, to define antigens recognized by additional antibodies. In 1945, the e antigen was identified.[4(p182)]

It is important for transfusion medicine specialists to appreciate that the often confusing nomenclature used to describe Rh antigens results from the difference in opinion that existed concerning the number of genes that were involved in their expression. The Fisher–Race nomenclature suggested that three closely linked genes (C/c, E/e, and D) were responsible, whereas the Wiener nomenclature (Rh-Hr) was based on his belief that a single gene encoded one "agglutinogen" that carried several blood group factors. Even though neither theory was correct (there are two genes—*RHD* and *RHCE*—correctly proposed by Tippett[6]), for written communication the Fisher–Race designation (DCE) for haplotypes is preferred, and for spoken communication a modified version of Wiener's nomenclature is preferred (Table 14.1). The "R" indicates that D is present, and use of a lowercase "r" (or "little r") indicates that it is not. The C or c and E or e Rh antigens carried with D are represented by subscripts: 1 for Ce (R_1), 2 for cE (R_2), 0 for ce (R_0), and Z for CE (R_z). The CcEe antigens present without D are represented by superscript symbols: "prime" for Ce (r′), "double-prime" for cE (r″), and "y" for CE (r^y). The "R" versus "r" terminology allows one to convey the common Rh antigens present on one chromosomal haplotype in a single term (a phenotype).

The major Rh antigens are D, C, c, E, and e, but the Rh blood group system is one of the most complex because of the number of additional antigens that have been reported (Table 14.2). These additional antigens include compound antigens in *cis* (e.g., f [ce], Ce, and CE), low-incidence antigens arising from partial-D hybrid proteins (e.g., D^w, Go^a, and Evans), and antigens arising from various point mutations in the RhCE protein (e.g., C^w, C^x, and VS). Table 14.2 also includes the numeric designations for Rh antigens.[7] With a few exceptions (RH17 and RH29), the numeric designations are not widely used in the clinical laboratory.

Rossi's Principles of Transfusion Medicine, Fifth Edition. Edited by Toby L. Simon, Jeffrey McCullough, Edward L. Snyder, Bjarte G. Solheim, and Ronald G. Strauss.
© 2016 John Wiley & Sons, Ltd. Published 2016 by John Wiley & Sons, Ltd.

Table 14.1 Nomenclature and prevalence of Rh haplotypes

Haplotype-Based Antigens (Fisher–Race)	Shorthand for Haplotype (Modified Wiener)	Occurrence (%)		
		Whites	Blacks	Asians
DCe	R_1	42	17	70
DcE	R_2	14	11	21
Dce	R_0	4	44	3
DCE	R_z	<0.01	<0.01	1
ce	r	37	26	3
Ce	r'	2	2	2
cE	r''	1	<0.01	<0.01
CE	r^y	<0.01	<0.01	<0.01

Table 14.2 International society for blood transfusion (ISBT) numerical terminology and symbols for Rh antigens

Numeric	Symbol	Numeric	Symbol	Numeric	Symbol
RH1	D	RH27	cE	RH48	JAL
RH2	C	RH28	hr^H	RH49	STEM
RH3	E	RH29	"total"	RH50	FPTT
RH4	c	RH30	Go^a	RH51	MAR
RH5	e	RH31	hr^B	RH52	BARC
RH6	ce or f	RH32	Rh32†	RH53	JAHK
RH7	Ce	RH33	Rh33‡	RH54	DAK
RH8	C^w	RH34	Hr^B	RH55	LOCR
RH9	C^x	RH35	Rh35§	RH56	CENR
RH10	V	RH36	Be^a	RH57	CEST
RH11	E^w	RH37	Evans	RH58	CELO
RH12	G	RH39	C-like	RH59	CEAG
RH17	Hr_0*	RH40	Tar	RH60	PARG
RH18	Hr	RH41	Ce-like	RH61	CEVF
RH19	hr^s	RH42	Ce^s		
RH20	VS	RH43	Crawford		
RH21	C^G	RH44	Nou		
RH22	CE	RH45	Riv		
RH23	D^w	RH46	Sec		
RH26	c-like	RH47	Dav		

Note: Rh13 through 16, 24, and 25 are obsolete.
* High-frequency antigen. The antibody is made by D- -/D- - and similar phenotypes.
† Low-incidence antigen expressed by R^N and DBT phenotypes.
‡ Original described on R_0Har phenotype.
§ Low-frequency antigen on RhCeMA.

Genes and their expressed proteins

Two genes designated *RHD* and *RHCE* encode the Rh proteins.[8] They are 97% identical, each has 10 exons, and they are the result of a gene duplication on chromosome 1p34–36.[9] Rh-positive individuals have both genes, whereas most Rh-negative individuals have only the *RHCE* gene (see below).

RhD and RhCE are 417-amino-acid, nonglycosylated proteins. One protein carries the D antigen, and the other carries various combinations of the CE antigens (ce, cE, Ce, or CE). RhD differs from RhCE by 32–35 amino acids, depending on which form of RhCE is present (Figure 14.1).[10–13] This relatively large degree of difference explains why D is the most immunogenic of all the blood group proteins, because most other blood group antigen polymorphisms result from only single amino acid changes in the respective protein. The Rh proteins migrate in sodium dodecyl sulfate polyacrylamide gels with an approximate M_r of 30–32 kD and hence were sometimes referred to as the *Rh30 proteins*. They are predicted to span the membrane 12 times and are covalently linked to fatty acids (palmitate) in the lipid bilayer (Figure 14.1).[14]

Basis for antigen expression

D antigen

Rh-positive and *Rh-negative* refer to the presence or absence of the D antigen, respectively. The Rh-negative phenotype occurs in 15–17% of Whites, but is not as common in other ethnic populations and is very rare in Asia.[4(p182)] The absence of D on the red cells of people of European ancestry was caused by a complete deletion of the *RHD* gene[15] and occurred on a Dce (R_o) haplotype because the allele most often carried with the deletion is RHCE*ce. Deletion of the *RHD* gene is associated with being "Rh-negative" in all populations, but inactive or silenced *RHD* is also a cause of D-negative phenotypes in Asians or Africans. D-negative phenotypes in Asians occur with a frequency of <1%,[4(p182)] and most carry mutations in *RHD* genes associated with *RHCE*Ce*, indicating that they probably originated on a DCe (R_1) haplotype. Only 3–7% of South African blacks are D-negative, but 66% have *RHD* genes that contain a 37-bp internal duplication, which results in a premature stop codon. Additionally, 15% of D-negative phenotypes in Africans result from a hybrid *RHD IIIa-CE-D* gene that does not encode D epitopes. This is important when designing polymerase chain reaction (PCR)-based methods to predict the D status of the fetus and the possibility of HDFN. The population being tested, and the different molecular events responsible for D-negative phenotypes (i.e., gene deletion or gene mutation) must be considered. Even among D-negative whites, cases of a *RHD* gene that is not expressed because of mutation or nucleotide insertions have been reported.[16]

Weak D

An estimated 0.2–1% of whites (and a greater percentage of blacks) have reduced expression of the D antigen,[4(p195)] which is characterized by weaker than expected reactivity with anti-D typing reagents or, alternatively, as failure of such red cells to agglutinate directly with anti-D reagents, requiring the use of an indirect antiglobulin test for detection. The basis of weak expression of D is heterogeneous, but is primarily associated with the presence of point mutations in *RHD*. The mutations encode amino acid changes most often predicted to be intracellular or in the transmembrane regions of RhD rather than on the outer surface of the red cell (Figure 14.2).[17] These mutations primarily affect the efficiency of insertion and, therefore, the quantity of protein in the membrane, and they may not affect the expression of D epitopes. This explains why most individuals with a weak-D phenotype can safely receive D-positive blood and do not make anti-D. There are over 80 different mutations known to cause weak-D expression (Type 1 through Type 84). The long history of transfusing patients who have weak-D red cells with D-positive blood suggests that weak-D Types 1, 2, and 3 (which represent the majority of whites with weak D) are unlikely to make anti-D. Predicting which mutations alter D epitopes based on structural analysis can be helpful,[18,19] but documenting the RHD genotype of patients whose red blood cells (RBCs) type as D-positive but who make anti-D following stimulation with D-positive RBCs is definitive evidence of which mutations are associated with changes in D epitopes.

It is important that donor center typing procedures detect and label weak-D RBC units as D-positive, because they can stimulate the formation of anti-D in D-negative recipients. However, testing for weak expression of D antigen by indirect antiglobulin testing (IAT) is not required for transfusion recipients, who would then receive D-negative units without untoward effects. When weaker than expected reactivity with anti-D is seen when typing females of child bearing potential, *RHD* genotyping should be considered to guide transfusion therapy to conserve D-negative donor units,

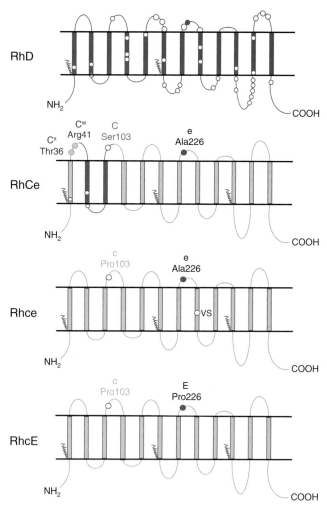

Figure 14.1 Predicted membrane topology of RhD and the major RhCE proteins. The amino and carboxy termini are cytoplasmic, and the proteins are predicted to transverse the membrane 12 times. The locations of the amino acid residues that differ between D and CE are represented by open circles, only nine of which are predicted to be extracellular. The C/c (Ser103Pro) polymorphism located on the second extracellular loop and the e/E (Ala226Pro) polymorphism on the fourth extracellular loop are shown. The shared region of RhD and RhCe responsible for expression of the G antigen is shown in dark blue. Amino acid changes responsible for C^x and C^w are located on the first extracellular loop; and the VS antigen, common in blacks, is located in the eighth transmembrane domain of Rhce. The zigzag lines represent covalent linkage to fatty acid in the lipid bilayer.

always in short supply, and to determine candidates for Rh immune globulin. Patients with weak-D types 1, 2, and 3 are not at risk for anti-D and can safely receive D-positive blood and females are not candidates for Rh immune globulin.[20]

A very weak form of D expression (D_{el}), which cannot be detected by routine serology methods but can be demonstrated by adsorbing and eluting anti-D, is relatively common in Asians (10–30% of apparent D-negative). Red cells with very low levels of D are primarily of concern for donor testing, because they have stimulated anti-D in D-negative recipients.[21]

Partial D

The D antigen has long been described as a "mosaic" because of the observation that some Rh-positive individuals produce anti-D when

exposed to D antigen. It was hypothesized that the red cells of these individuals lack some part of D and that they can produce antibodies to the missing portion. Molecular genetic analysis has shown that the missing portions of *RHD* are replaced by corresponding portions of *RHCE* in the great majority of cases (Figure 14.3).[16,19] The novel sequences of amino acids and the conformational changes that result from segments of RhD joined to segments of RhCE can generate new antigens (e.g., BARC, D^w, FPTT, DAK, Go^a, Evans, and Rh32) (Figure 14.3 and Table 14.2). The replacements are the result of gene conversion, the hallmark being that the donor gene is unchanged. Gene conversions involve single or multiple exons, whereas others involve short stretches of amino acids (Figure 14.3). Some also result from only single-amino-acid changes (e.g., DMH, DFW, and DII) (Figure 14.2). In contrast to the single-amino-acid changes that cause weak D (above), which are predicted to be cytoplasmic or transmembrane in location, those that cause partial-D phenotypes are often predicted to be located on the extracellular loops of the protein (Figure 14.2).

From a clinical standpoint, individuals with partial-D antigens are at risk for anti-D, and ideally females of childbearing potential with partial D should receive D-negative blood and, if they become pregnant, are candidates for Rh immune globulin. Some RBCs with partial D react weaker than expected with anti-D reagents, but they cannot be distinguished from weak-D RBCs, which are not at risk for anti-D. RHD genotyping can guide clinical decision making for Rh immune globulin prophylaxis and transfusion.[20] In practice, many individuals with partial-D phenotypes will type strongly D-positive and will be recognized only after they have made anti-D following a transfusion with D-positive cells or pregnancy with a D-positive fetus. Routine *RHD* genotyping would overcome the limitations of serologic D typing of these individuals.

Elevated D

Several rare phenotypes, including D−−, Dc−, and DC^w−, have enhanced expression of D antigen and no, weak, or variant CE antigens, respectively.[4(p205)] These phenotypes are analogous to the partial-D rearrangements described in the "Partial D" subsection, only they involve the opposite situation—that is, replacement of portions of *RHCE* by *RHD*. The additional *RHD* sequences in *RHCE* along with a normal *RHD* explain the enhanced D and account for the reduced or missing CE antigens. Although these represent altered *RHCE* genes (see below), they are included here because of their elevated D phenotype. Individuals with such altered CE phenotypes can make anti-Rh17 when immunized. Anti-Rh17 reacts with all cells that have conventional Rhce, RhCe, or RhcE protein, and only RBCs with the D−− phenotype (or those expressing the same Rhce variant) are compatible.

C/c and E/e antigens

The four major forms of the *RHCE* gene encode four different proteins: RhCe, −ce, −cE, and −CE (Figure 14.1).[12] C and c differ by four amino acids: Cys16Trp encoded by exon 1, and Ile60Leu, Ser68Asn, and Ser103Pro encoded by exon 2 (Figure 14.1, open circles on RhCe). Of those four amino acids, only the residue at 103 is predicted to be extracellular and is located on the second loop. All the amino acids encoded by exon 2 of *RHCE*Ce are identical to those encoded by exon 2 of *RHD* (Figure 14.1, dark blue on RhCe). This suggests that *RHCE*Ce arose from the transfer of exon 2 from *RHD* into an *RHCE*ce gene, respectively. The sharing of exon 2 encoded amino acids by RhD, RhCe, and RhCE accounts for the expression of the G antigen on red cells that are D or C positive.

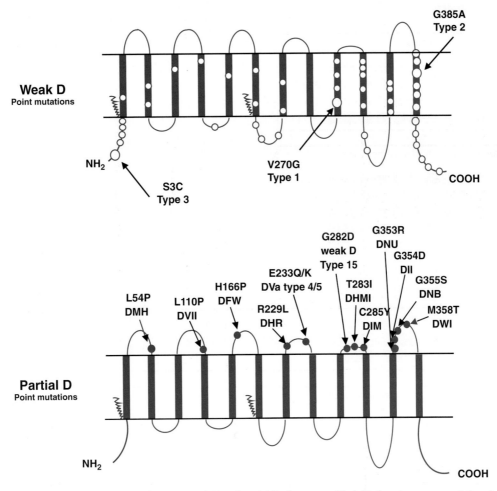

Figure 14.2 Predicted location of point mutations that cause weak-D and partial-D phenotypes. Weak-D phenotypes carry mutations in *RHD* that primarily cause amino acid changes predicted to be intracellular or in the transmembrane regions of D (upper panel). The specific amino acid mutation and the location in the protein are indicated. The partial-D phenotypes that carry mutations in *RHD* are predicted to be located on extracellular loops of RhD (lower panel). The specific amino acid mutation and location in the protein, as well as the common name for each, are indicated.

Individuals who lack D and C can make anti-G, which can be distinguished from a combination of anti-D and anti-C by absorption and elution studies.[5] The presence of anti-G can explain why a D-negative person who was transfused with D-negative/C-positive red cells (or exposed to such cells through pregnancy) can subsequently appear to have made anti-D. The identification of anti-G is generally of academic interest only because transfusion requirements for such an individual would be the same (i.e., RBCs that are both D and C negative). However, in the case of a pregnancy, it is important to identify individuals with anti-G only, as Rh immune globulin prophylaxis would be indicated. E and e differ by one amino acid, Pro226Ala, predicted to reside on the fourth extracellular loop of the protein (Figure 14.1, solid circle). The E antigen arose from a single point mutation that occurred in exon 5 of a *RHCE*ce* gene, giving rise to *RHCE*cE*.

Altered CE

C[w] and C[x] are low-incidence antigens that result from single-amino-acid changes (Gln41Arg and Ala36Thr, respectively) predicted to be located on the first extracellular loop of RhCE (Figure 14.1, light blue circles).[22] These antigens are more common in Finns (4%) and are most often present on RhCe. C[w] is also associated with the deletion phenotype DC[w]− (Figure 14.3).

V and VS antigens, which are expressed on RBCs of more than 30% of blacks, result from a Leu245Val substitution located in the predicted eighth transmembrane segment of Rhce (Figure 14.1).[23] The V−VS+ phenotype results from a Gly336Cys change on the 245Val background.[24] V+ and VS+ are associated with weak and altered expression of e, indicating that Leu245Val causes a local conformation change on the fourth extracellular loop where the e-specific amino acid resides.

Most individuals have e-positive red cells, but the e antigen is considered to be second in complexity to D because variant expression has frequently been observed.[25] The e antigen is altered on many red cells from African blacks, and some of the alleles encoding altered expression are shown (Figure 14.3). Extensive discussion is beyond the scope of this chapter, but these alleles are prevalent in patients with sickle cell disease (SCD),[26,27] who not infrequently produce anti-e following transfusion, despite having an e-positive red cell phenotype. RH genotyping of the patient can help to determine if the anti-e is allo- or auto-antibody and to inform selection of blood for transfusion.[28]

E variants are not common and include EI, EII, and EIII, which result from a point mutation (EI) or gene conversion replacement of RhcE amino acids with RhD residues (EII and EIII) with concurrent loss of some E epitope expression. Category EIV red cells, which

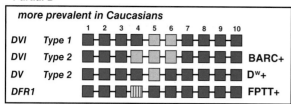

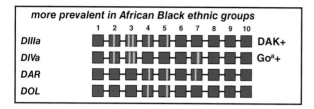

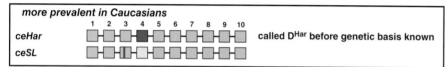

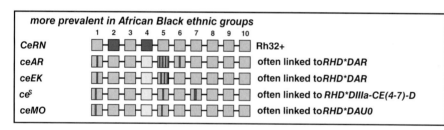

Figure 14.3 Gene conversion events between *RHCE* and *RHD* produce chimeric Rh proteins and new antigens (shown on right-hand side). Dark blue (*RHD*) and light blue (*RHCE*) boxes represent the 10 exons that encode Rh proteins. Gene conversion events involve amino acid changes (vertical bars) or whole exons (filled boxes). Replacement of portions of *RHD* by *RHCE* (upper set of panels) causes many of the partial-D phenotypes, some of which are shown here. Replacement of portions of *RHCE* by *RHD* causes altered RhCE expression (lower set of panels).

have an amino acid substitution in an intracellular domain, do not lack E epitopes but have reduced E expression.[28]

Variants of c are infrequent. The very rare RH:-26 results from a Gly96Ser transmembrane amino acid change that abolishes Rh26 and weakens c expression.[29] The lack of c antigen variants in humans compared to the other Rh antigens, and the preservation of expression of c on the red cells of nonhuman primates, suggest that the two proline residues involved form a stable structure that is resistant to perturbations and changes in Rhce.[30]

In summary, point mutations and genetic exchange, mainly involving gene conversion events between *RHD* and *RHCE*, are primarily responsible for the large number of Rh antigens. Additional complexity results because many of the Rh epitopes are highly conformational, and single-amino-acid changes in one part of the protein, including changes within the transmembrane regions, can affect the expression of cell-surface-exposed antigen epitopes.

RH genotyping

DNA-based testing methods were introduced to the blood bank and transfusion medicine community over two decades ago. Assays for blood group antigens encoded by single nucleotide polymorphisms (SNPs) are highly reproducible and correlate with red cell phenotype. Semi-automated testing platforms are now being used for routine antigen typing.[31] Genotyping for the two most important blood group systems, ABO and Rh, are more challenging because of the many different mutations that cause weak expression of A and

B, and inactive O, and because of the numerous variant Rh antigens and hybrid *RH* alleles. Multiple regions of the genes must be sampled, and hybrid genes are problematic for analysis. RH genotyping is performed principally in a reference laboratory setting at the present time.

RHD zygosity testing

Serologic testing for red cell expression of D, C/c, and E/e can only predict the likelihood that a sample is homozygous (D/D) or heterozygous (D/−) for *RHD*. Genotyping enables zygosity to be determined by assaying for the presence of a recessive D-negative allele. In prenatal practice, paternal *RHD* zygosity testing is important to predict the fetal D status when the mother has anti-D. Several different genetic events cause a D-negative phenotype, and multiple assays must be performed to accurately determine zygosity. If the father is *RHD* homozygous, the fetus will be D-positive, and monitoring of the pregnancy will be required. If the father is heterozygous, the D type of the fetus can then be determined to prevent invasive and unnecessary testing.

Fetal typing

Genotyping is important in the prenatal setting to determine whether the fetus has inherited the paternal antigen to which the mother has a clinically significant antibody. Fetal DNA can be isolated from cells obtained by amniocentesis. The discovery that cell-free, fetal-derived DNA is present in maternal plasma or serum by approximately five weeks gestation allows maternal plasma to be used as a source of fetal DNA.[32] Fetal DNA in maternal plasma is derived from apoptotic syncytiotrophoblasts, increases in concentration with gestational age, and is rapidly cleared following delivery.[33] The small quantity of cell-free fetal DNA present relative to maternal DNA requires positive controls for isolation of sufficient fetal DNA to validate negative results. Isolation of fetal DNA from maternal plasma has become routine in several European countries to determine fetal D status prior to administration of Rh immune globulin.[34] This has been most successful for D typing because the D-negative phenotype in the majority of samples is caused by the lack of *RHD*. Testing for the presence or absence of a gene is less demanding than testing for a single gene polymorphism or SNP. Testing the maternal plasma for the presence of a fetal *RHD* eliminates the unnecessary administration of antepartum Rh immune globulin (RhIG) to the approximately 40% of D-negative women who are carrying a D-negative fetus. RhIG is not entirely risk free as it is a human blood product, and this approach is cost-effective for some healthcare systems.[35] Noninvasive testing for fetal K and HPA-1a status has also been reported.[36]

Distinction between weak D and partial D

As indicated above, altered expression of D antigen is not uncommon. Weak-D phenotypes have amino acid changes that primarily affect the quantity of RhD in the membrane. Partial-D phenotypes have amino acid changes that alter D epitopes, or often are hybrid proteins with portions of RhD joined to portions of RhCE. The distinction between weak-D and partial-D phenotypes is of clinical importance because the latter make anti-D. Routine serologic typing reagents cannot distinguish between these red cells; however, *RHD* genotyping strategies can discriminate between weak D and partial D.

Detecting patients at risk for production of antibodies to high-incidence antigens

Alloimmunization is a serious complication of chronic transfusion, particularly in patients with SCD requiring long-term transfusion support. Many transfusion programs attempt to prevent or reduce the risk and incidence of alloantibody production in patients with SCD by transfusing RBC units that are antigen matched for D, C, E, and K. Although this approach reduces the incidence of alloimmunization, variant *RHD* and *RHCE*ce* genes are common in African blacks and individuals of mixed ethnic backgrounds. The prevalence of *RH* alleles that encode altered D, C, and e antigens in this patient group explains why some SCD patients become immunized to Rh, despite Rh antigen matching for D, C, and E.[26,37] These antibodies often have complex, high-incidence Rh specificities, and it can be difficult or impossible to find compatible units. *RH* genotyping can identify those patients who are homozygous for variant *RH* alleles and at risk for production of alloantibodies to high-incidence Rh antigens, and can identify compatible donors for transfusion.

Rh_{null} phenotype

Rh_{null} individuals lack expression of all Rh antigens. They suffer from a compensated hemolytic anemia, and they have variable degrees of spherocytosis, stomatocytosis, and increased red cell osmotic fragility.[38] The phenotype is rare and occurs on two different genetic backgrounds: the "regulator" type, caused by mutation in the *RHAG* gene at an unlinked locus, and the "amorph" type, which maps to the *RH* locus.[5] In the more common regulator

type of Rh_{null}, the suppression of Rh antigens is caused by a lack of, or a mutant, Rh-associated glycoprotein (RhAG) protein.[39] RhAG is a 409-amino-acid glycosylated protein that co-immunoprecipitates with RhD and RhCE.[40] It shares 37% amino acid identity with the RhD–RhCE proteins and has the same predicted membrane topology. RhAG is not as polymorphic as RhCE and RhD, and only four antigens have been identified;[41] however, it is important for targeting the Rh proteins to the membrane during erythroid maturation. RhAG has one N-glycan chain that carries ABO and Ii specificities.[42]

The amorph type of Rh_{null} results from mutations in *RHCE* on a D-negative background.[43] Amorph-type red cells express no Rh protein and have reduced amounts (∼20%) of RhAG.

Rh membrane complex

Additional complication in Rh protein structures arises because they exist in the red cell membrane as complexes with several other proteins. Rh and RhAG are associated in the membrane as a core complex.[44] The fact that several other proteins interact with the Rh core complex is based on observations of Rh_{null} cells. These red cells have reduced expression of CD47, an integrin-associated protein (IAP) that has wide tissue distribution, binds β_3 integrins, and is required for integrin-regulated Ca^{2+} entry into endothelial cells. Its function on the red cells is unknown; however, a role in red cell senescence has been suggested.[45] Rh_{null} cells also have reduced glycophorin B (GPB), a sialoglycoprotein that carries S or s and U antigens. GPB appears to aid RhAG trafficking to the membrane, because the RhAG protein in GPB-deficient cells has increased glycosylation, reflecting longer dwell time in the endoplastic reticulum. Rh_{null} cells also lack LW, a glycoprotein of unknown function that belongs to the family of intercellular adhesion molecules (ICAM-4). Band 3 (the anion exchanger) enhances the expression of the Rh antigens in transfected cells, suggesting that band 3 may also be associated with the Rh core complex.[46] The Rh core complex is linked to the membrane skeleton through interactions between CD47 and protein 4.2[47] and through a novel Rh/RhAG–ankyrin cytoskeleton connection.[48]

Rh function
Rh glycoproteins (RhAG, RhBG, and RhCG)

The Rh blood group proteins are well known because of their importance in blood transfusion. However, the mammalian family of Rh proteins also includes RhAG in erythrocytes, and the related proteins, RhBG and RhCG, in other tissues.

Protein sequences with similarities to the mammalian Rh proteins were first found in *Caenorhabditis elegans*, and these homologs, in turn, showed similarity to the ammonia transporters from bacteria, yeast (MEP), and plants (AMT).[49] The relationship of the Rh glycoproteins to the AMT and MEP ammonia transporters from these other organisms has been substantiated by functional transport data[50–52] and structural modeling.[53,54] The Rh proteins reveal the power of comparative genomics and proteomics, in which sequence analysis and homology modeling can give important insight into mammalian protein function.

The non-erythroid Rh glycoproteins, RhBG and RhCG, are present in the kidney, liver, brain, and skin where ammonia production and elimination occur. In the kidney collecting segment and collecting duct, RhBG and RhCG are found on the basolateral and apical membranes, respectively, of the intercalated cells where they mediate transepithelial movement of ammonia from the interstitium to the lumen.[55] In the liver, RhBG is found on the basolateral membrane of perivenous hepatocytes, where it may function in ammonia uptake. RhCG is also present in bile duct epithelial cells, where it is positioned to contribute to ammonia secretion into the bile fluid.[56]

The mechanism of ammonia transport by Rh glycoproteins is an electroneutral process that is driven by the NH_4^+ concentration and the transmembrane H^+ gradient.[57,58] Functional studies of the kidney, liver, and brain Rh homologs, along with the erythrocyte RhAG/Rh proteins, promise to lead to development of a unifying hypothesis of ammonia transport in mammals by the Rh family of proteins.

RhCE and RhD

The more recently evolved erythrocyte blood group proteins, RhCE and RhD, when expressed in heterologous systems do not transport ammonia.[59] RhCE and RhD lack the highly conserved histidine residues located in the membrane pore that are critical for ammonia transport. RhCE and RhD may be evolving a new function in the red cell membrane as phylogenetic analysis indicates the RhCE/D proteins are rapidly evolving.

Clinical relevance of Rh protein expression in RBCs

Lack of Rh expression (i.e., Rh-null RBCs) most often results from absence or mutations in RhAG. RhAG is important for ion balance in RBCs.[60,61] Mutations in the RhAG ammonia conductance channel are associated with altered ion transport. Hereditary overhydrated stomatocytosis (OHSt), an autosomal dominant macrocytic hemolytic anemia, is caused by a Phe65Ser mutation in RhAG. OHSt red cells exhibit cation leak with elevated Na^+ and reduced K^+ content, and loss of ammonia conductance.

Immune response to Rh
Medical aspects

Human red cells can express more than 400 different blood group antigens. Typing patient and donor cells for every known antigen with the intention of providing perfectly matched blood would not be practical or feasible. Fortunately, such extensive testing is not required for a number of reasons, the most important of which is that exposure to the majority of foreign red cell antigens through transfusion does not lead to the production of clinically significant alloantibodies. D is one notable exception. As many as 80% of D-negative patients on deliberate immunization with D-positive red cells may develop high-titer, high-affinity, D IgG antibodies that may persist for the rest of their lives even if they are never exposed to the antigen again. The antibodies can cause HTRs and can cross the placenta, causing HDFN when present in a D-negative female carrying a D-positive fetus. Therefore, because of its extraordinary immunogenicity and clinical significance, the D antigen is currently the primary blood group antigen in the United States for which it is routine to prophylactically match blood before transfusion for all patients so as to avoid immunization. Although other Rh antibodies to C, c, E, and e can cause HTRs and HDFN, they are much less immunogenic than D (~1% rate of sensitization), and the use of RBCs lacking one or more of those antigens is indicated for patients only after sensitization has occurred (management of patients on chronic transfusion, including those with sickle cell anemia and thalassemia, differ as described in the preceding section).

In practice, D-positive patients can be transfused with either D-positive or D-negative RBCs—the absence of D will cause no harm—but it is deemed prudent to reserve the rarer units of D-negative blood (~15% of donor units) for D-negative individuals who must receive them. In cases of trauma and/or massive transfusion in which the patient's D status is unknown, efforts are made to provide D-negative blood, especially for females of childbearing potential, until the appropriate testing can be completed. When D-negative blood is in short or critical supply, it may be necessary to transfuse D-negative patients with D-positive units. In such scenarios, D-negative units are reserved for females of childbearing potential and for patients whose serum contains anti-D from a previous sensitization.

Unlike ABO blood group antigens, which are expressed by all transfused blood cells including platelets, the D antigen is present only on red cells. Theoretically, the selection of platelet units for transfusion should be independent of the D status of the donor. However, a transfusion of pooled platelet concentrates may introduce as much as 5 mL of donor red cells, which may be sufficient to alloimmunize a D-negative patient. Therefore, the standard of care is to avoid transfusing D-negative patients, particularly females of childbearing potential, with platelet units derived from D-positive donors. If such units are unavailable and platelet transfusion must be undertaken, the administration of RhIG can be considered. A standard 300-μg dose of RhIG, which may inhibit the immunizing potential of up to 15 mL of D-positive red cells, would neutralize the effects of D-positive red cells from several mismatched platelet transfusions. If mismatched platelet transfusions are repeatedly given over time and their content of D-positive red cells is not expected to exceed the volume of red cells for which a standard dose of RhIG is indicated, then a single dose of the drug should be sufficient for at least 2–4 weeks of prophylaxis given the 3-week half-life of IgG.[62] With respect to the transfusion of plasma products, the D status of the donor is not an issue because plasma products do not contain cellular or soluble material capable of inducing anti-D immune responses.

Serologic aspects

The immune response to Rh, like that to other peptide antigens, is typically thymus-dependent, requiring T-cell help. Upon exposure to a foreign Rh antigen, an IgM response may develop, but this is quickly followed by the production of IgG antibodies. Consequently, nearly all examples of Rh antibodies are IgG molecules (mostly IgG1 and IgG3), which bind optimally to red cells at 37 °C and require the addition of an antiglobulin reagent to produce hemagglutination. Although IgG1 and IgG3 subclasses classically initiate complement activation, the vast majority of anti-Rh-containing sera do not do so. The usual explanation for this cites the relatively low copy number of Rh antigens per red cell, which results in Rh molecules situated too far apart on the cell surface to permit the simultaneous binding of C1q by multiple Rh IgG antibodies. Therefore, hemolysis from the transfusion of Rh-incompatible RBCs is generally extravascular because of the phagocytosis of IgG-coated erythrocytes by cells of the reticuloendothelial system.

After anti-D, the Rh antibodies most commonly found in the sera of alloimmunized individuals are anti-E > anti-c > anti-e > anti-C. In approximately 50% of cases of warm-type autoimmune hemolytic anemia (WAIHA), autoantibodies are believed to be directed to Rh antigens by virtue of their "pan-reactivity" with all red cell phenotypes except Rh_{null} cells. However, direct binding of autoantibodies to putative epitopes common to D and C/E polypeptides or to other components of the Rh membrane complex (RhAG, CD47, etc.) has yet to be demonstrated in WAIHA. The difficulties in approaching this problem are largely technical in nature and relate to both the inability to produce workable quantities of pure patient autoantibody in vitro (i.e., clone the autoantibody-producing B lymphocytes) and the inability to purify Rh proteins in a way that retains their native, conformationally dependent epitopes.

Molecular aspects

The characterization of Rh antibodies on a molecular level, particularly that of anti-D, has been the focus of much study not only because of their clinical significance, but also because of the need to develop suitable in vitro methods for their production.[63] Ironically, because of better transfusion practice and the use of RhIG, alloimmunization of antigen-negative individuals is significantly less common (as are sera donors willing to be purposely hyperimmunized), so that supplies of Rh antibodies for use as typing reagents and for the preparation of RhIG are dwindling. To better understand the molecular makeup of Rh antibodies, investigations have focused on analyzing their variable regions in order to determine whether there are commonly shared genetic and/or structural features among Rh antibodies made by different individuals.

Early work using rabbit antisera specific for different human heavy-chain variable region gene products suggested a restriction in the use of certain heavy-chain gene families by the anti-D contained in polyclonal sera from several dozen anti-D donors.[64] Subsequent studies with rodent idiotypic antibodies demonstrated cross-reactive idiotypes among polyclonal anti-D preparations[64,65] and among different examples of human monoclonal anti-C, -c, -D, -E, -e, and -G produced by transformed B cells.[66] A more direct approach using nucleotide sequencing to examine immunoglobulin gene diversity examined a cohort of four IgM and 10 IgG monoclonal anti-D variable regions.[67] A restricted use of the human heavy-chain variable region genes V_H3–33 and V_H4–34 was found with a shift in repertoire usage toward V_H3–33 for anti-D that had isotype switched to the more clinically relevant IgG. The restriction of anti-D heavy chains to the use of these and other highly related V_H genes has been confirmed and extended through the analysis of many additional examples of anti-D produced through both tissue culture and recombinant means.[68–73] The use of molecular approaches such as site-directed mutagenesis,[74] complementarity-determining region (CDR) sequence randomization,[75] and heavy-chain/light-chain "shuffling"[76] has demonstrated the genetic relatedness among anti-D molecules directed against different D epitopes as well as among antibodies with D and E specificity. These studies and others[77,78] have supported the hypothesis that a restricted "Rh footprint" for D alloantibodies and a process termed "epitope migration"[68] play a role in the molding of the anti-Rh immune repertoire.[79]

Although the precise significance of immunoglobulin germline gene restriction by Rh antibodies is not fully understood, it may have practical significance for the preparation of anti-D for both therapeutic and diagnostic use. For example, the V_H genes used to encode anti-D are among the most cationic of the human germline V_H genes[80] and may account for the relatively high pI of polyclonal anti-D-containing antisera originally noted over 50 years ago.[81] Although the cationic nature of the antibodies may be important for binding to D, it has also been suggested that a constitutive net-positive charge may be necessary to permeate the highly negative red cell zeta potential, thus permitting antibody to contact antigen.[82] Secondly, although IgM D monoclonal antibodies are well suited for antigen typing because they may serve as direct agglutinins, the fact that they are most often encoded by V_H4–34 (the germline gene to which cold agglutinins are also restricted)[83,84] may explain why many IgM monoclonal anti-D typing reagents falsely

agglutinate D-negative cells when used at cooler than recommended temperatures. This phenomenon may also explain the body of literature claiming that the D antigen was present on numerous nonerythroid cells. Using IgM anti-D, these investigators may have been detecting antigens of the I/i blood group system.

With respect to the development of recombinant formulations of RhIG that would function as effectively as naturally derived anti-D, attention has shifted from an initial focus on the variable regions of the antibodies that make contact with the D antigen to the effector functionality of the anti-D, particularly the role that Fc glycosylation may play in inducing immune prophylaxis.[63,85,86]

LW blood group system

History and nomenclature

The LW antigens are the "true" Rhesus antigens shared by humans and the rhesus monkey. As discussed earlier, the confusion occurred because LW antigens are more abundant on D-positive than on D-negative red cells. When the situation was clarified, the term *Rh* remained associated with the human antigen, so the real Rhesus antigen was renamed *LW* in honor of Landsteiner and Wiener.[5] The confusion can be understood today in the transfusion service when a weak example of anti-LW^a often appears initially to be anti-D. The LW system has undergone additional terminology revisions. The historical terminology of LW$_1$, LW$_2$, LW$_3$, LW$_4$, and LW$_0$ to describe phenotypes was based on both the LW and the D status of the red cells but is now obsolete.[5] The phenotypes are LW(a+b−), LW(a−b+), LW(a+b+), and the rare LW(a−b−); the antigens are designated LW^a, LW^b, and LW^ab.

Genes and their expressed proteins

LW is encoded by a single gene located on chromosome 19. The 42-kD LW glycoprotein is a member of the family of ICAMs and has been renamed ICAM-4 (CD242). LW passes through the red cell membrane once, and the N-terminal extracellular region is organized into two immunoglobulin superfamily (IgSF) domains.[87]

Basis for antigen expression

LW^b is the common antigen, whereas LW^b has an incidence of less than 1% in most Europeans.[4(p393)] The LW^a/LW^b polymorphism is caused by a single amino acid substitution, Gln70Arg, on the LW glycoprotein.[88] An increased frequency of the uncommon LW^b antigen in Latvians and Lithuanians (6%), Estonians (4%), Finns (3%), and Poles (2%) suggests that the LW^b mutation originated in the people of the Baltic region. The LW^ab antigen was originally defined by an alloantibody made by the only known (genetically verified) LW(a−b−) person, who lacks expression of all LW antigens.[5] Rh antigen expression was not altered, and there was no clinical evidence of an associated pathology. The *LW* gene in this rare LW(a−b−) individual has a 10-bp deletion and a premature stop codon in the first exon.[89] Rh$_{null}$ red cells also lack LW antigens but do not have defective *LW* genes. Rh proteins appear to be required for LW to traffic to the membrane, and association with RhD is preferred.

LW antigens require divalent cations (e.g., Mg^{2+}) for expression and have intramolecular disulfide bonds that are sensitive to dithiothreitol (DTT) treatment.[5] This is helpful to differentiate anti-LW from anti-D, because the D antigen is resistant to DTT. DTT-treated and untreated D-positive red cells can be prepared and tested for reaction with patient serum.[90] Also helpful in identifying anti-LW is the fact that LW antigens are expressed equally well on group O D-positive and D-negative cord blood red cells.[4(p395)]

Transient loss of LW antigens has been described in pregnancy and patients with diseases, particularly Hodgkin's disease, lymphoma, leukemia, sarcoma, and other forms of malignancy, in the absence of any overt associated RBC abnormality. Transient loss of LW antigens is associated with the production of autoanti-LW that can appear to be alloantibody.[4(p395)]

LW function

LW glycoprotein, ICAM-4, is a ligand with broad specificity for a number of β1, β2, β3, and β5 integrins, including $\alpha_L\beta_2$ (LFA-1), $\alpha_M\beta_2$ (Mac-1), $\alpha_4\beta_1$ (VLA-4), $\alpha_V\beta_1$, $\alpha_V\beta_5$, as well as platelet integrin $\alpha_{2b}\beta_3$.[87,91–94] In addition, LW binds to the I domains of CD11a/CD18 and CD11b/CD18 on leukocytes.[87,95] The function of LW glycoprotein on mature red cells is not known, but LW may have a role in erythroblastic island formation through interaction with macrophage integrins.[96,97] LW appears to play a pathophysiologic role in the development of vaso-occlusion in SCD mediated by endothelial cell integrins[98,99] and of thrombosis mediated by activated integrins on platelets.[94]

Summary

The molecular basis for the Rh antigens has now been elucidated. A gene deletion or silent *RHD* gene explains the absence of the D antigen in many Rh-negative individuals. The large number of amino acid differences between the RhD and RhCE proteins explains why exposure in an individual lacking D often results in a vigorous immune response characterized by a very heterogeneous population of antibodies. The proximity of *RHD* and *RHCE*, duplicated genes on the same chromosome, has resulted in numerous exchanges by gene conversion between them. This has generated new polymorphisms and explains the many antigens observed in this blood group system. Rh antigen expression is affected not only by changes in extracellular amino acids but also by intracellular changes, highlighting the conformational nature of these blood group antigens and complicating attempts to map the epitopes to specific amino acid residues.

RH genotyping can be used to determine paternal *RHD* zygosity to predict HDFN, and the fetus can be typed from amniocytes or from the maternal plasma. *RH* genotyping can also identify patients facing long-term transfusion therapy who are homozygous for variant *RH* alleles and at risk for production of alloantibodies to high-incidence Rh antigens. When partnered with *RH* genotyping of donors, this approach promises to have a positive impact on transfusion therapy outcomes by reducing alloimmunization, especially in patients with SCD.

Rh antibodies show restriction in their use of particular variable-region immunoglobulin germline genes. Antibodies to serologically distinct epitopes may be genetically related, and epitope migration may be an important process that helps shape the composition of the anti-Rh immune repertoire. Questions remain concerning the function of the Rh proteins. The discovery that Rh protein homologs also exist in the liver and kidney indicates that the Rh blood group antigens belong to a conserved family of proteins that function in ammonia transport. Similarly, the function of LW on the mature red cell is not entirely clear, but its ability to interact as an adhesion molecule with a broad range of integrin-binding specificity suggests an important role in both normal red cell development as well as disease-associated processes such as vaso-occlusion and thrombosis.

Key references

A full reference list for this chapter is available at: http://www.wiley.com/go/simon/transfusion

1   Bowman JM. RhD hemolytic disease of the newborn. *New Engl J Med* 1998; **339**: 1775–7.

4   Daniels G. *Human blood groups*. Wilmington, DE: Wiley-Blackwell, 2013.

19 Westhoff CM. The structure and function of the Rh antigen complex. *Semin Hematol* 2007; **44** (1): 42–50.

20 Sandler S, Flegel W, Westhoff C, et al. It's time to phase in RHD genotyping for patients with a serologic weak D phenotype. *Transfusion* 2015; **55**: 680–9.

31 Casas J, Friedman DF, Jackson T, et al. Changing practice: red blood cell typing by molecular methods for patients with sickle cell disease. *Transfusion* 2015 **55** (6 Pt. 2): 1388–93.

36 Avent ND. Prenatal testing for hemolytic disease of the newborn and fetal neonatal alloimmune thrombocytopenia: current status. *Expert Rev Hematol* 2014; **7** (6): 741–5.

51 Westhoff CM, Ferreri-Jacobia M, Mak DO, et al. Identification of the erythrocyte Rh blood group glycoprotein as a mammalian ammonium transporter. *J Biol Chem* 2002; **277** (15): 12499–502.

63 Kumpel BM. Efficacy of RhD monoclonal antibodies in clinical trials as replacement therapy for prophylactic anti-D immunoglobulin: more questions than answers. *Vox Sang* 2007; **93** (2): 99–111.

68 Chang TY, Siegel DL. Genetic and immunological properties of phage-displayed human anti-Rh(D) antibodies: implications for Rh(D) epitope topology. *Blood* 1998; **91** (8): 3066–78.

87 Bailly P, Tontti E, Hermand P, et al. The red cell LW blood group protein is an intercellular adhesion molecule which binds to CD11/CD18 leukocyte integrins. *Eur J Immunol* 1995; **25** (12): 3316–20.

CHAPTER 15

Other protein blood groups

Jill R. Storry

Blood Group Immunology, Clinical Immunology and Transfusion Medicine, University and Regional Laboratories Region Skåne, Lund University Hospital, and Division of Hematology and Transfusion Medicine, Department of Laboratory Medicine, Lund University, Lund, Sweden

Of the 35 currently known blood group systems, seven are carbohydrate in nature and are discussed in Chapter 13. Antigens of the remaining 28 blood group systems are carried by (glyco)proteins. Three of these 28 systems—Rh (ISBT 004), RhAG (ISBT 030), and the closely associated LW (ISBT 016)—are discussed in detail in Chapter 14. The remaining blood group systems are summarized in Table 15.1 and will be discussed here.

Many of the proteins carrying blood group antigens are functionally important; however, antibodies in only a few blood group systems represent a problem for the transfusion service, in that they may cause decreased survival/hemolysis of transfused antigen-positive red blood cells (RBCs) in patients with the antibody, or hemolytic disease of the fetus and newborn (HDFN) in a mother with antibodies directed at paternally inherited antigens on her baby's erythrocytes. In addition, the presence of such antibodies may delay availability of compatible units of RBCs for transfusion and, occasionally, may make transfusion of incompatible RBCs unavoidable, particularly in urgent settings or with antibodies to high-incidence antigens. This chapter addresses only those antigens that elicit formation of clinically significant antibodies and briefly comments on the other blood group systems. Further details may be found in review articles[1,2] and comprehensive textbooks.[3–5]

MNS blood group system (ISBT 002)

Structure and function of glycophorins A and B
Antigens of the MNS blood group system are carried by glycophorin A (GPA) and glycophorin B (GPB). Both molecules are present in a very high copy number in the plasma membrane: $0.5–1.0 \times 10^6$ copies of GPA and $1–3 \times 10^5$ molecules of GPB.[6] GPA and GPB are encoded by homologous genes at chromosome 4q28-q31 that undoubtedly arose by gene duplication. Both glycoproteins are integral membrane proteins with a single transmembrane α-helical segment and with the N-termini located extracellularly (Figure 15.3). GPA was the first protein whose primary structure was determined by amino acid sequencing.[7]

GPA carries the M and N antigens at its N-terminus. Although two amino acid substitutions underlie antigen specificity, an important requirement for recognition of these antigens by human antibodies is the presence of O-glycans attached to terminal serine and threonine residues.

GPB is homologous with GPA. Although the genes are greater than 95% identical, *GYPB* encodes a shorter protein because a point mutation at the 5′ splicing site of the third intron prevents incorporation of exon 3 into the translated mRNA. Because *GYPB* arose by duplication of the *N* allele of *GYPA*, *GYPA*N*, and the first 26 amino acids of GPB are therefore identical to those of GPA with N specificity, GPB expresses an N-like antigen designated as *N* (Figure 15.1).

The S and s isoforms of GPB differ at amino acid position 48. The S allele encodes methionine and the s allele, threonine. GPB also carries the U antigen whose epitope is adjacent to the point where GPB enters into the lipid bilayer[8] (Figure 15.1), although the molecular basis of this antigen is not known.

As is frequently the case with genes arising by duplication and located next to each other, unequal crossing over or gene conversion may easily occur. Consequently, numerous hybrid molecules containing portions of GPA and GPB have been described.[9] This phenomenon is responsible for many low-prevalence MNS antigens, which are carried by different hybrid proteins such as Mi[a], V[w], Hil, MUT, MINY, St[a], and DANE. GPA associates in the red cell membrane with the band 3 protein (SLC4A1). The epitope of the Wr[b] antigen from the Diego blood group system (see below) is formed by the association of GPA with band 3. This clearly demonstrates the intimate association of GPA and band 3 in the plasma membrane.[10]

MNS in transfusion medicine
The most commonly encountered antibodies are directed against the M, N, S, and s antigens. Anti-M is a common antibody and may be found in the sera of persons who have not been exposed to human erythrocytes. M antibodies are predominantly IgM with a thermal optimum below 30 °C; however, they frequently contain an IgG component, and occasionally are exclusively IgG. Nevertheless, anti-M is rarely clinically significant, and those examples of hemolytic anti-M are usually IgG and react at 37 °C. Selection of blood for transfusion can be made based on a negative cross-match irrespective of M antigen status. Similarly, anti-M is not considered to be an important antibody with regard to HDFN, although rare cases have been described.[11] Anti-N is rare, most likely because of the immune tolerance induced by the N antigen on GPB, and is usually a weak, cold-reactive antibody of no clinical significance. These should be distinguished from the strong and potentially clinically

Rossi's Principles of Transfusion Medicine, Fifth Edition. Edited by Toby L. Simon, Jeffrey McCullough, Edward L. Snyder, Bjarte G. Solheim, and Ronald G. Strauss.

Table 15.1 Overview of the protein blood group systems other than Rh, RhAG, and LW

ISBT Number	System Name	Gene Name ISBT	Gene Name HGNC	Erythrocyte Membrane Component	Number of Antigens	Examples of Antigens
002	MNS	*MNS*	GYPA, GYPB	Glycophorin A (CD235a), Glycophorin B (CD235b)	48	M, N, S, s, U
005	Lutheran	*LU*	LU	B-CAM (CD239)	21	Lu^a, Lu^b
006	Kell	*KEL*	KEL	Kell glycoprotein (CD258)	35	K, k, Js^a, Js^b, Kp^a, Kp^b
008	Duffy	*FY*	ACKR1	ACKR1 (CD234)	5	Fy^a, Fy^b
009	Kidd	*JK*	SLC14A1	SLC14A1	3	Jk^a, Jk^b
010	Diego	*DI*	SLC4A1	SLC4A1 (CD233)	22	Di^a, Di^b, Wr^a, Wr^b
011	Yt	*YT*	ACHE	Acetylcholinesterase	2	Yt^a, Yt^b
012	Xg	*XG*	XG,MIC2	Xg glycoprotein (CD99)	2	Xg^a
013	Scianna	*SC*	ERMAP	ERMAP	7	Sc1, Sc2, Sc3, Rd
014	Dombrock	*DO*	ART4	ART4	8	Do^a, Do^b
015	Colton	*CO*	AQP1	Aquaporin-1 (AQP1)	4	Co^a, Co^b
017	Chido/ Rodgers	*CH/RG*	C4A, C4B	Complement component C4A/C4B	9	Ch1, Ch2, Ch3, Rg1, Rg2
019	Kx	*XK*	XK	Xk glycoprotein	1	Kx
020	Gerbich	*GE*	GYPC	Glycophorin C (CD236), Glycophorin D	11	Ge2, Ge3, Ge4
021	Cromer	*CROM*	CD55	Decay accelerating factor (DAF, CD55)	18	Cr^a
022	Knops	*KN*	CR1	Complement receptor 1 (CR1,CD35)	9	Kn^a, McC^a, Sl^a
023	Indian	*IN*	CD44	CD44	4	In^a, In^b
024	OK	*OK*	BSG	Basigin (CD147)	3	Ok^a
025	RAPH	*RAPH*	MER2	CD151	1	MER2
026	JMH	*JMH*	SEMA7A	Semaphorin 7A (CD108)	6	JMH1
029	GIL	*GIL*	AQP3	Aquaporin 3 (AQP3)	1	GIL
032	JR	*ABCG2*	ABCG2	ABCG2	1	Jr^a
033	LAN	*ABCB6*	ABCB6	ABCB6	1	Lan
034	Vel	*SMIM1*	SMIM1	SMIM1	1	Vel
035	CD59	*CD59*	CD59	CD59	1	CD59.1

ISBT, International Society of Blood Transfusion; HGNC, Human Gene Nomenclature Committee.

significant antibodies observed in persons of the rare phenotype M+N–S–s–U– who do not express GPB (hence *N*), and for whom phenotypically similar, cross-match-compatible blood should be provided.

In contrast to anti-M and anti-N, antibodies to S, s, and U usually occur after exposure to allogeneic erythrocytes, and all should be considered to be clinically significant because all are capable of causing hemolytic transfusion reactions (HTRs) and HDFN. The appropriate antigen-negative, cross-match-compatible blood should be selected for transfusion.

Lastly, severe HDFN due to rare antibodies to low-prevalence MNS antigens has also been reported and should be suspected in a strongly DAT-positive or symptomatic newborn where alloantibodies cannot be detected by routine screening.

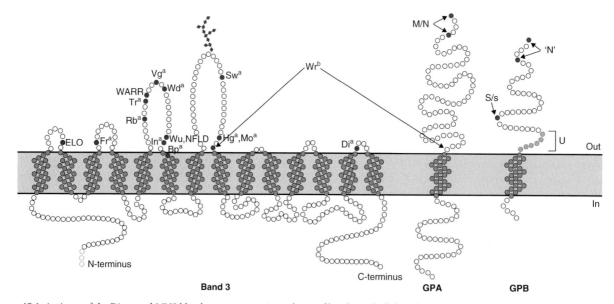

Figure 15.1 Antigens of the Diego and MNS blood group systems in a scheme of band 3 and of glycophorins A and B. The membrane domain of band 3 with 14 transmembrane segments is shown. Mutations underlying the Diego blood group antigens are located in the putative first, second, third, fourth, and seventh extracellular loops. Positions of the M and N antigens in GPA and of the 'N', S, s, and U antigens in GPB are indicated. Arrows point to the sites in band 3 and GPA that are involved in formation of the Wr^b epitope and, therefore, have to come into close contact in the membrane.

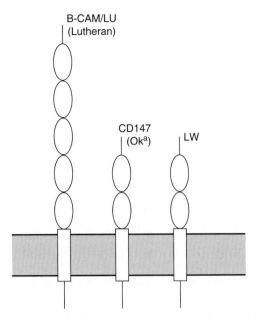

Figure 15.2 Members of the immunoglobulin superfamily carrying blood group antigens. B-CAM/LU contains five immunoglobulin domains and carries antigens of the Lutheran blood group system. CD147, or basigin, contains two Ig domains and carries the Ok^a antigen. CD147 is similar to the LW protein, which is discussed in Chapter 14.

Lutheran blood group system (ISBT 005)

Lutheran antigens reside on B-CAM/LU (Figure 15.2), a pair of spliceosomes (protein products arising from the same gene because of alternative splicing of hnRNA) that belong to the immunoglobulin superfamily (IgSF).[12,13] Basal cell adhesion molecule (B-CAM) is involved in adhesion of the basal surface of epithelial cells to the basement membrane. B-CAM/LU is a receptor for laminin.[14,15] Expression of B-CAM/LU is increased on erythrocytes from patients with sickle cell disease[14] and on a number of malignant epithelial tumors,[16] which also lose the polarity of B-CAM/LU expression found in normal tissues.

The Lutheran blood group system contains multiple antigens; however, clinically significant antibodies are rarely encountered. The most important antigens are Lu^a and Lu^b. The prevalence of Lu^a is less than 10% in most populations, whereas Lu^b is a high-prevalence antigen with an average occurrence of 99.8% in all populations. Lutheran antigens are poorly developed at birth and, not surprisingly, anti-Lu^a has been associated only rarely with mild cases of HDFN. It does not cause transfusion reactions. Lu^b is somewhat more immunogenic, and anti-Lu^b has caused mild or moderate HTRs and mild HDFN. Of historical note, Lu and Se (Chapter 13) were the first two loci for which an autosomal linkage in humans was demonstrated.

The null phenotype, Lu(a−b−), is rare but quite interesting. It may result from three different patterns of inheritance. A recessive pattern of inheritance is associated with exceedingly rare null alleles of the *LU* gene. In the most common dominant type (so-called *In (Lu)*), heterozygous inheritance of mutations in the gene encoding KLF1, a common erythroid transcription factor, results in marked suppression of not only the Lutheran glycoprotein but also P1, i, In^a and In^b, and AnWj (see the "Indian Blood Group System" section).[17,18] The third cause of the Lu(a−b−) phenotype was first hypothesized to be the consequence of an X-linked recessive

suppressor gene *XS2*.[19] Similar to In(Lu), the molecular basis has recently been identified as heterozygosity for a mutation in the *GATA-1* gene.[20] GATA-1 is an important transcription factor in the differentiation of erythrocytes and megakaryocytes, and mutations in *GATA-1* account for cases of dyserythropoeisis, thrombocytopenia, and anemia.[21] Interestingly, only P1 blood group antigen expression was decreased in addition to Lu antigens; however, the proband was thrombocytopenic, and macrothrombocytes were observed.

Kell and Kx blood group systems (ISBT 006 and 019)

Structure, function, and interaction of the Kell and XK proteins

Antigens of the Kell blood group system are carried by a 93-kD red cell membrane glycoprotein, which consists of a short cytoplasmic N-terminal portion, a single membrane-spanning α-helical segment, and a large, 665-amino-acid extracellular C-terminal portion held in a globular conformation by multiple disulfide bonds (Figure 15.3).[22] Kell antigens are inactivated by reducing agents such as dithiothreitol, suggesting that disulfide bonds are important in maintaining its antigenic conformation.

The Kell glycoprotein is a member of the neprilysin (M13) family of zinc metalloproteases. This family consists of Kell, neutral endopeptidase 24.11, two different endothelin-converting enzymes, the product of the *PEX* gene, and XCE.[23] Members of the M13 subfamily of membrane zinc endopeptidases have widely different roles, including processing of opioid peptides, Met- and Leu-enkephalin, oxytocin, bradykinin, angiotensin, endothelins, and parathyroid hormone. Kell protein has been shown to preferentially activate endothelin-3;[24] however, the in vivo physiologic role of Kell protein is probably complex, because K$_0$ (null) persons are apparently healthy.

Kell glycoprotein interacts in the erythrocyte membrane with the 37-kD protein XK, which plays an important role in the expression of Kell system antigens. In contrast to the Kell protein, XK is a multiple membrane-spanning protein with both of its N- and C-termini located intracellularly (Figure 15.3). The function of XK is not known; however, absence of XK results in McLeod neuroacanthocytosis syndrome, an X-linked, late-onset neuromuscular disorder.[25] Structurally, XK resembles the glutamate transporters, but it has very little amino acid sequence homology with this group of transport proteins. The Kell and XK proteins are covalently associated in the membrane by a disulfide link between cysteine 72 of Kell and cysteine 347 of XK (Figure 15.3).[26,27] The gene encoding the Kx antigen is located on the short arm of the X chromosome near the loci for X-linked chronic granulomatous disease (CGD) and Duchenne muscular dystrophy (DMD).[28]

Kell in transfusion medicine

The Kell blood group system is the second most important protein blood group system in transfusion medicine after Rh, because the antibodies can cause HTRs and HDFN. The most important antigens in this system are K (KEL1) and the antithetical k (KEL2). K and k are codominant autosomal alleles; and, although approximately 9% of whites and 2% of blacks are K-positive (i.e., K+k− or K+k+), the majority are K-negative (i.e., K−k+). Antigens of the Kell blood group system are highly immunogenic and, excluding ABO, K is second only to RhD in its potential to elicit production of alloantibodies.

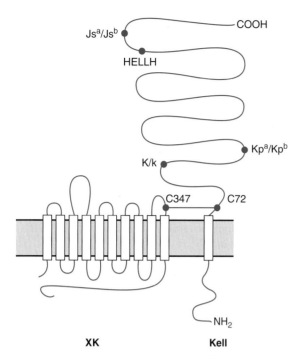

Figure 15.3 Schematic representation of the Kell/XK complex in the red cell membrane. The XK protein is a multipass membrane protein, while Kell has only one transmembrane domain, most of which is exposed on the extracellular side. Due to multiple disulfide bonds, the extracellular portion of Kell is a globular structure; however, it is represented here schematically so that the positions of the main antigens can be shown. A disulfide bond between Cys72 of Kell and Cys347 of XK connects the two proteins. The position of the pentameric sequence HELLH is shown. Sequences HEXXH are involved in zinc binding and catalytic activity of zinc endopeptidases. The K/k polymorphism at amino acid 193 changes the consensus sequence for N-glycosylation at Asn191, which is not glycosylated in K. This difference in glycosylation may be important for the marked antigenicity of K. Positions of two additional sets of antithetical antigens Kp^a/Kp^b and Js^a/Js^b at amino acids 281 and 597 are indicated.

Anti-K is commonly found. Fortunately, because more than 90% of donor units are K negative, it is easy to obtain blood for transfusion to individuals with anti-K. In contrast, although anti-k is relatively rare, it is also of clinical significance and only 1 in 500 random donor units is antigen-negative. The other two sets of antithetical antigens to which antibodies are often found are Kp^a/Kp^b and Js^a/Js^b (Figure 15.3), although there are many other rare polymorphisms.

Mothers with anti-K are relatively rare, but since the introduction of Rh prophylaxis, anti-K accounts for nearly 10% of cases of severe HDFN. In contrast to RhD, anti-K titers are not good predictors of fetal anemia. In addition, affected Kell-alloimmunized infants have lower reticulocyte counts and amniotic fluid bilirubin concentrations than RhD-sensitized infants. Because Kell glycoprotein is synthesized early in erythropoiesis, anti-K has been hypothesized to suppress erythropoiesis at the progenitor cell level.[29,30] In rare cases, administration of recombinant erythropoietin (rHuEPO) to the newborn has been tried with some success in cases where the mother has a Kell blood group system antibody causing prolonged anemia in a newborn whose RBCs and their progenitors express the cognate antigen in question.[31,32]

It is important to determine if a fetus is at risk when the mother has anti-K. The putative father should be typed and if he carries the K antigen, genotyping from amniocentesis or cell-free fetal DNA (cffDNA) in the mother's plasma can be performed using molecular techniques.

Null phenotypes

There are two rare but clinically interesting null phenotypes. Rare individuals have erythrocytes that completely lack the Kell glycoprotein. Although these cells exhibit the null phenotype (K$_0$), they are morphologically normal and survive normally in vivo. In contrast, individuals lacking the XK protein, and thus Kx antigen, exhibit depressed levels of the Kell glycoprotein.[22] This phenotype, known as the McLeod neuroacanthocytosis syndrome, is associated with acanthocytic erythrocytes and a mild chronic hemolytic anemia.[25] It is associated with late onset of neuromuscular symptoms that include muscle weakness or atrophy, cognitive alterations, and psychiatric symptoms. Association of the McLeod phenotype with other rare syndromes, most frequently with CGD and DMD or Becker muscular dystrophy (BMD), is caused by large gene deletions encompassing *XK* together with adjacent gene *CYBB* that encodes a large subunit of cytochrome b$_{558}$ and is associated with X-linked CGD, and *DMD* that encodes dystrophin.[33]

Duffy blood group system (ISBT 008)

Structure and function of the Duffy protein

The Duffy gene encodes a glycoprotein of 336 amino acids with a molecular weight of 36 kD. The Duffy glycoprotein has seven transmembrane α-helical domains and is homologous with proteins of the G-coupled protein receptor family.[34] The Fy^a and Fy^b antigens are carried on the extracellular N-terminus; the C-terminus is intracellular (see Figure 15.4). Duffy protein functions as a chemokine receptor and is also known as the Duffy antigen receptor for chemokines (ACKR1).[35] Duffy binds both CXC chemokines, such as interleukin-8 (IL8) and melanocyte growth-stimulating activity (MGSA), as well as CC chemokines, such as regulated on activation, normal T-cell expressed and secreted (RANTES) and macrophage chemoattractant protein-1 (MCP1).[34] It is currently not known why a red cell, with its limited metabolism and response to chemokine binding, would carry a significant number of chemokine receptors at its surface. One possible explanation is that the chemokine receptor acts as a scavenger for locally released chemokines. However, individuals who do not express the Duffy protein either on erythrocytes or in all tissues are phenotypically normal, suggesting that the Duffy protein is dispensable.

Duffy is the primary receptor for the human malarial parasite *Plasmodium vivax*, which infects the erythrocytes of Duffy-positive individuals.[36] The binding site for *P. vivax* is located in the N-terminal extracellular domain of Duffy. *P. vivax* merozoites invade primarily reticulocytes, although reticulocytes and mature erythrocytes do not substantially differ in Duffy expression. This suggests that an additional receptor has to play a role in erythrocyte invasion.

Duffy in transfusion medicine

The two main alleles of the Duffy blood group system are the antithetical codominant antigens Fy^a and Fy^b whose genetic determinant is a Gly/Asp polymorphism in position 44 (Figure 15.4).[37] These two alleles occur with similar frequencies in persons of European ancestry, Fy^a being somewhat more common. The Fy (a−b−) phenotype is extremely rare among whites, but approximately two-thirds of African Americans and more than 90% of

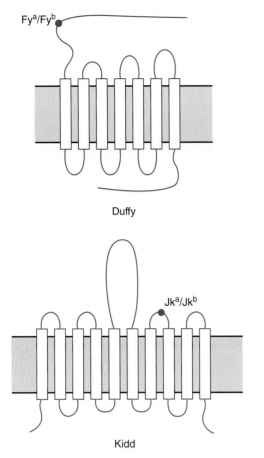

Fy^a/Fy^b

Duffy

Jk^a/Jk^b

Kidd

Figure 15.4 Schematic depiction of proteins carrying the Duffy and Kidd blood group antigens. The Duffy antigen receptor for chemokines (DARC) consists of seven transmembrane segments. The N-terminus is located extracellularly, functions as both the chemokine and *P. vivax* attachment site, and carries the Fy^a/Fy^b polymorphism. The Kidd protein has 10 transmembrane segments, both N- and C-termini are intracellular, and the amino acid determining the Jk^a/Jk^b polymorphism is located in the fourth extracellular loop.

native West Africans are Fy(a−b−). This is most likely caused by the genetic adaptation for resistance to *P. vivax* malaria. However, it is not clear why this genetic advantage would lead almost to fixation of the Fy(a−b−) phenotype in the indigenous population of West Africa. In contrast to the other malarial parasites, *P. vivax* causes a relatively mild form of malaria.[34] Furthermore, despite the high prevalence of Duffy-negative individuals in West Africa, the Duffy protein has recently been shown to be a co-factor in platelet factor 4 (PF4)-dependent killing of *P. falciparum* parasites, suggesting that it has a protective role in this disease.[38]

A long-standing conundrum of immunohematology has been the well-known fact that transfused Fy(a−b−) people of African ancestry never develop anti-Fy^b. This mystery was solved by the characterization of the mutation causing the Fy(a−b−) phenotype in native West Africans. The underlying mutation is a T → C substitution in the GATA site of the promoter region.[39] This substitution prevents binding of the erythroid transcription factor GATA1 and abolishes transcription of the gene in the erythroid cells, while leaving the transcription of the *FY* gene in other tissues unaffected. Because the mutation occurred in the *FY*B* allele, the Fy^b antigen remains expressed in certain endothelial, epithelial, and brain cells,

and, consequently, the transfusion recipient does not form antibodies against Fy^b. The GATA-1 mutation has been found on the *FY*A* allele in individuals from Papua New Guinea.[40]

Fy^a antibodies are found relatively frequently, constituting 6–10% of the clinically significant antibodies identified by immunohematology laboratories. For reasons not well understood, Fy^b is a relatively poor immunogen and, consequently, anti-Fy^b is considerably less common. Both immediate and delayed HTRs caused by Fy^a incompatibility have been described, ranging from mild to severe hemolysis. HDFN is usually mild; only a few cases of severe HDFN have been reported. In contrast, anti-Fy^b is associated only rarely with cases of mild HDFN and is usually found in delayed HTRs, although on rare occasions it has caused severe acute hemolysis.

Kidd blood group system (ISBT 009)

Kidd is an integral protein with 10 transmembrane domains and both N- and C-termini located intracellularly (Figure 15.4). Of the five extracellular loops, the longest, third loop is N-glycosylated, and the relatively short fourth loop carries an Asp280Asn polymorphism corresponding to the Jk^a/Jk^b antigens.[41] Kidd protein is expressed not only on the red cell surface but also on neutrophils and in the kidney.

The two main antigens of the Kidd blood group system, Jk^a and Jk^b, are found with almost identical frequencies in white populations. Jk^a is a better immunogen, and anti-Jk^a is found more frequently than anti-Jk^b. Anti-Jk^a may cause severe immediate or delayed HTRs and, occasionally, HDFN. It is one of the most dangerous immune antibodies because of its tendency to decrease to undetectable levels in between transfusions and its relatively low affinity for Jk(a+) erythrocytes. For these reasons, it accounts for a large proportion of delayed HTRs. Anti-Jk^b may also cause immediate or delayed HTRs, albeit less severe than those caused by anti-Jk^a (see http://www.shotuk.org/shot-reports/ for more information). Several cases of mild HDFN caused by anti-Jk^b have been reported.

The finding that cells of the Jk(a−b−) phenotype are resistant to lysis by 2M urea led to the discovery of the function of the glycoprotein carrying the Kidd antigens. Based on this finding and on in vitro expression of the cloned Kidd cDNA,[42–44] it is now known that the protein is the primary erythrocyte urea transporter (SLC14A1), although the importance of urea transport for red blood cells is not completely understood. Its presence or absence may not be critical for red cell structure and function, because carriers of the Jk(a−b−) phenotype have erythrocytes indistinguishable from those of controls. While individuals with the Jk(null) phenotype lack SLC14A1 completely, weakly expressed forms of the protein have been found, in which the Jk^a and/or Jk^b antigens may be barely detectable.[45–47]

Diego blood group system (ISBT 010)

Antigens of the Diego blood group system are carried by band 3 (SLC4A1, anion exchanger 1), the most abundant integral protein of the red cell membrane together with GPA (see above). Band 3 is also one of the most important proteins for the structure and function of the membrane because it maintains red cell integrity by linking the red cell membrane to the underlying spectrin-based membrane skeleton. It also mediates exchange of chloride and bicarbonate anions across the plasma membrane, thereby significantly increasing the carrying capacity of blood for carbon dioxide.

Band 3 consists of a cytoplasmic and a membrane domain. The membrane domain contains 14 transmembrane helices connected by ecto- and endoplasmic loops (Figure 15.1).[48,49] The fourth loop of band 3 is N-glycosylated, and the attached carbohydrate chain carries over half of the red cell ABO blood group epitopes.[50] Several disorders of red cell structure and function have been associated with mutations in the band 3 gene, including Southeast Asian ovalocytosis,[51] autosomal dominant spherocytosis, and distal renal tubular acidosis.[52]

Despite being the most abundant protein of the red cell membrane, it was only in 1992 that Spring *et al.*[53] reported that the Memphis II variant of erythroid band 3 protein carries the Di[a] blood group antigen. Di[a] was originally described in South American Indians by Layrisse *et al.* in 1955.[54] The antithetical antigen Di[b] was reported by Thompson *et al.* in 1967.[55] Di[a] and Di[b] represent co-dominantly expressed gene products. Di[a] is a low-prevalence blood group antigen in persons of European ancestry who carry the antithetical high-prevalence antigen Di[b]. Prevalence of Di[a] is as high as 8% in certain areas of Southeast Asia and reaches up to 40% in some groups of South American Indians. Di[a] was used as one of the original markers for studying migration of people from Southeast Asia across the Bering Strait and southward through the American continents.[56] Cloning and sequencing of *SLC4A1* identified the substitution 854 Pro→Leu in the last extracellular loop of band 3 as the molecular basis of the Di[a] antigen. Di[b] corresponds to the wild-type band 3 with proline in position 854.[57]

Subsequently, the low-prevalence blood group antigen Wr[a] was mapped to the fourth extracellular loop.[10] The antithetical Wr[b] antigen is observed only when both GPA and band 3 protein are expressed in the erythrocyte membrane; thus, erythrocytes that lack GPA (so-called En(a−) phenotype) but have normal band 3 are also Wr(b−) (Figure 15.1). Numerous additional low-prevalence antigens are associated with single point mutations on band 3 and included in the Diego system.[58-60] Positions of the amino acid polymorphisms in the band 3 molecule are shown in Figure 15.1, which also indicates the regions of band 3 and GPA that interact in the membrane and are involved in formation of the Wr[b] antigen.

Some antigens of the Diego blood group system have been localized to the regions of band 3 protein that have been implicated in the adhesion of abnormal erythrocytes, such as sickle cells or malaria-infected erythrocytes, to vascular endothelium.[61,62] Erythrocytes from carriers of low-prevalence blood group antigens in band 3 may serve as a model for evaluation of the sequence requirements for adhesion. The so-called *senescent* or *aging red cell antigen* may also be located in the extracellular loops of band 3.[63]

Xg blood group system (ISBT 012)

The Xg system contains two antigens, Xg[a] and CD99, carried by glycoproteins of 180 and 185 amino acids, respectively.[64] The function of Xg glycoprotein in erythrocytes is not known, although it is 48% homologous to CD99, an adhesion molecule. Xg[a] was described in 1962 as the first sex-linked blood group antigen,[65] and the antigen-positive incidence was shown to be significantly different in men (62%) than women (89%).[66] The *XG* gene is located in the pseudoautosomal region of the X chromosome,[64] and consequently escapes lyonization (X-inactivation). Xg[a] antibodies are clinically insignificant.

Scianna blood group system (ISBT 013)

The seven antigens of the Scianna blood group system are carried by the erythrocyte membrane-associated protein (ERMAP), potentially a receptor/signal transduction molecule specific for erythroid cells.[67] Mild HDFN and mild postransfusion hemolysis caused by anti-Sc-2 and anti-Sc-3 antibodies have been reported.

Colton and GIL blood group systems (ISBT 015 and 029)

Antigens of these two blood group systems are carried by members of the large aquaporin family. Antibodies against the two antigens of the Colton blood group system, the high-prevalence Co[a] and the less common, antithetical Co[b], are rare and have only rarely been associated with mild HTRs and mild HDFN. These two antigens, together with the high-prevalence Co3 and Co4 antigens present on all erythrocytes except those of the very rare null phenotype Co (a−b−), are carried by aquaporin-1 (AQP1),[68] a member of a large family of water channels.[69] It is present in the membrane as a tetramer. Expression of AQP1 in *Xenopus* oocytes is associated with dramatic swelling and lysis of the cell;[70] however, the Co(a−b−) phenotype is associated with only slightly abnormal erythrocytes and with normal kidney function despite the fact that AQP1 is the major water channel of human kidney.[71] The GIL antigen is carried by aquaporin-3 (AQP3), which differs from AQP1 in that it transports glycerol, water, and urea.[72]

Chido/Rodgers blood group system (ISBT 017)

Antigens of the Chido/Rodgers blood group system are the only protein antigens that are not produced by erythrocytes but instead adhere to the red cell surface (Lewis antigens are glycolipids). They are carried by the complement component C4. Although antibodies against the nine known antigens of the system are generally benign, a severe anaphylactic reaction following a transfusion of platelets to a patient with anti-Ch3 has been described.[73]

Gerbich blood group system (ISBT 020)

As in the MNS system, antigens of the Gerbich system are located on glycophorins C and D (GPC, GPD). The glycophorin terminology is in fact the only common feature of these two classes of glycophorins. There is otherwise no homology between the Gerbich and MNS genes. GPC and GPD are the products of a single gene, *GYPC*, and are the products of alternative splicing. GPC is produced by a full-length gene transcript, whereas the less abundant GPD is produced from a second initiation methionine that encodes a protein that is 21 amino acids shorter. Although present in much smaller copy numbers than GPA and GPB, GPC plays an important role in the structural integrity of the red cell membrane.[74] In the Leach phenotype, deletions of exons 3 and 4 or a frameshift mutation leads to complete absence of glycophorins C and D from the plasma membrane.[75] The affected individuals have moderate elliptocytosis and decreased red cell deformability and mechanical stability. Antibodies in the Gerbich system, to both the high- and low-prevalence antigens, are rare and, in the vast majority of cases, clinically insignificant.

Knops blood group system (ISBT 022)

Antigens are located on the C3b/C4b complement receptor 1 (CR1, CD35). CR1 protects erythrocytes from autohemolysis by inhibiting the classical and alternative complement pathways through cleavage of C4b and C3b. CR1 is a large 190- to 280-kD molecule. It contains 30 complement control protein domains (CCPDs) of about 60 amino acids. Seven CCPDs form a long homologous repeat (LHR) of about 450 amino acids. Various forms of CR1 contain up to six LHRs.[76] Erythrocyte CR1 binds immune complexes and carries them to the liver and spleen for removal. Expression of CR1 on erythrocytes varies widely from 20 to 1500 molecules and is decreased in hemolytic anemias, AIDS, systemic lupus erythematosus, and other autoimmune disorders. *Plasmodium falciparum*–infected erythrocytes deficient in CR1 have greatly reduced rosetting capacity, indicating an essential role for CR1 in rosette formation and raising the possibility that CR1 polymorphisms in Africans that influence the interaction between erythrocytes and parasite-encoded protein PfEMP1 may protect against severe malaria.[77] CR1 could therefore be a potential target for future therapeutic interventions to treat severe malaria.

Indian blood group system (ISBT 023)

The four antigens of this system, In[a], In[b], INFI, and INJA, reside on CD44, an adhesion molecule expressed in leukocytes, fibroblasts, epithelial cells, and other tissues. CD44 is an important lymphocyte marker that functions as a hyaluronan receptor[78] and a lymphocyte homing receptor (Figure 15.2). Transfection of nonadherent cell lines with CD44 cDNA confers an adherent phenotype.[79] As with the Lutheran antigens, expression of In[a] and In[b] is suppressed by *In (Lu)*. The high prevalence antigen, AnWj, is also associated with CD44 and is a receptor for *Haemophilus influenzae*.[80] Antibodies to Indian blood group system antigens are rare and of limited clinical significance. Anti-AnWj is extremely rare.

Blood group antigens on glycosylphosphatidylinositol-linked proteins: Cartwright (ISBT 011), Dombrock (ISBT 014), Cromer (ISBT 021), JMH (ISBT 026), and CD59 (ISBT 035)

The common denominator of antigens in these blood group systems is the linkage of the carrier protein to the glycosylphosphatidylinositol (GPI) anchor (Figure 15.5). The Cartwright (Yt) blood group system consists of two antigens, Yt[a] and Yt[b], which are located on red cell acetylcholinesterase. The function of acetylcholinesterase on erythrocytes is not understood, although it appears to play a role in vascular signaling.[81] Most examples of anti-Yt[a] are benign.

The eight antigens of the Dombrock system are located on ART-4, a member of the adenosine 5′-diphosphate (ADP)-ribosyltransferase ectoenzyme gene family.[82] Dombrock expression is developmentally regulated during erythroid differentiation and occurs at highest levels in the fetal liver. Do[a] and Do[b] antigens differ in a single amino acid substitution within the RGD motif of the molecule.[83]

The Cromer blood group system contains 18 antigens located on decay-accelerating factor (DAF, CD55), a complement regulatory protein. Extraordinarily, much of the polymorphism appears restricted to one ethnic group or another, making it a very interesting blood group system.[84] Antibodies to Cromer blood group antigens are of limited clinical importance, and due to the expression of DAF on the placenta, antibodies disappear over the course of pregnancy and pose no threat to the fetus.[85] Although DAF was the first complement regulatory protein identified, it plays only a minor role in complement-mediated lysis, the more important being CD59 (MIRL). This was clearly demonstrated in the case of the null phenotype, Inab, which is associated with lack of DAF expression on all circulating cells but not with increased hemolysis.[86]

The six high-prevalence antigens of the JMH blood group system reside on a GPI-linked protein, semaphorin 7A (CD108), which is part of a plasma membrane complex associated with intracellular protein kinases.[87] CD108 is expressed in multiple tissues and may play a role in signal transduction. Anti-JMH is generally a weak, clinically benign antibody found in older people.

CD59 was recently assigned blood group system status following the report of an antibody produced in response to transfusion in a CD59-deficient girl.[88] The clinical significance of the antibody is not known, although the absence of CD59 in this and other patients has severe clinical consequences.

Antibodies in these blood group systems have been associated only occasionally with mild HTRs or HDFN. Not surprisingly, expression of all GPI-linked antigens is decreased in paroxysmal nocturnal hemoglobinuria (PNH), a multisymptomatic disorder caused by defects in the X-linked phosphatidylinositol glycan class A (*PIG-A*) gene, which participates in an early step of GPI anchor synthesis.[89] The pathophysiology of PNH is due almost exclusively to the absence of CD55 and CD59, which are important regulators of the complement system: CD55 accelerates the rate of destruction of membrane-bound C3 convertase and thus limits C3 activation; and CD59 reduces the amount of the membrane attack complex (MAC) formed by preventing C9 accumulating and thus lytic pore formation. Anemia, due to both hemolysis and bone marrow

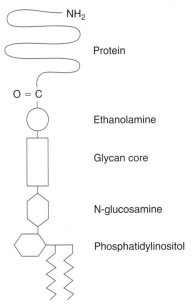

Figure 15.5 Schematic representation of a GPI-anchored protein. The membrane anchor is provided by phosphatidylinositol. The inositol moiety binds to a glycan core via a molecule of N-glucosamine. The glycan core is attached via ethanolamine to the C-terminus of the protein.

failure, and thrombosis are also common in PNH patients.[89] See Chapter 12 for a complete discussion of PNH.

Other minor blood group systems: OK (ISBT 024), RAPH (ISBT 025), JR (ISBT 032), LAN (ISBT 033), and VEL (ISBT 034)

The three high-prevalence antigens of the OK blood group system are carried on basigin (CD147), a widely distributed IgSF molecule.[90] Rare Ok(a−) individuals have so far been reported only in Japan, and absence of the high-prevalence antigens OK2 and OK3 has been described in single families.[91] As with LW, its extracellular domain contains two immunoglobulin domains. The function of the Ok glycoprotein in erythrocytes is not known, but it has recently been described as a novel receptor of *P. falciparum*.[92]

MER2 is the only antigen of the RAPH system carried on CD151.[93] CD151 is a tetraspannin that is expressed not only on erythrocytes but also on basement membranes, where in the kidney and in skin it is thought to facilitate binding of integrins to the extracellular matrix to maintain integrity.[1]

Two proteins in the ABC transporter family were recently found to carry blood group antigens and thus solved the molecular whereabouts of two previously uncharacterized high-prevalence antigens. The Jr[a] antigen was localized to ABCG2, where the Jr(a−) phenotype represented the null phenotype.[94,95] ABCG2 is a well-characterized protein that confers multidrug resistance (e.g., in breast cancer), and is also important in porphyrin homeostasis. It has a high affinity for urate, and Japanese Jr(a−) individuals have a higher incidence of gout. Anti-Jr[a] is not usually considered clinically important; however, it has caused severe HDFN.[96]

The high-prevalence Lan antigen is carried on ABCB6, a mitochondrial porphyrin transporter considered essential for heme synthesis.[97] Like Jr(a−), Lan− individuals represent the null phenotype and lack the protein. ABCB6 is highly expressed during erythropoiesis. Anti-Lan is not generally considered clinically important, and antigen expression is variable.[98]

Expression of the clinically important Vel antigen has been shown to be dependent on SMIM1, a small transmembrane protein of unknown function.[99–101] Intriguingly, the protein is well-conserved across species, suggesting that it is an important protein, and GWA studies suggest that it might play a role in iron metabolism.[102]

Anti-Vel is considered clinically significant and has caused severe hemolytic transfusion reactions.

Summary

The century-long history of modern transfusion medicine and immunohematology practice led to the characterization of an enormous number of blood group antigens with often confusing terminology. These antigens have been arranged into a complex framework of blood group systems, collections, and low- and high-prevalence antigens.[103] Advances in biochemical and molecular biology techniques in the past two decades led to a detailed structural characterization of most proteins carrying blood group antigens and to a better understanding of the relation between gene variations, amino acid polymorphisms, protein structure, and immunogenicity of individual antigens. Better understanding of the molecular biology, biochemistry, and immunogenicity of proteins carrying blood group antigens will undoubtedly contribute to accurate compatibility testing and to safe transfusion of erythrocytes.

Disclaimer

The author has disclosed no conflicts of interest.

Key references

A full reference list for this chapter is available at: http://www.wiley.com/go/simon/transfusion

2 Reid ME, Mohandas N. Red blood cell blood group antigens: structure and function. *Semin Hematol* 2004; **41**: 93–117.

4 Daniels G. *Human blood groups*. 3rd ed. Oxford: Wiley-Blackwell, 2013.

7 Tomita M, Furthmayr H, Marchesi VT. Primary structure of human erythrocyte glycophorin A. Isolation and characterization of peptides and complete amino acid sequence. *Biochemistry* 1978; **17**: 4756–70.

23 Turner AJ, Isaac RE, Coates D. The neprilysin (NEP) family of zinc metalloendopeptidases: genomics and function. *Bioessays* 2001; **23**: 261–9.

35 Horuk R, Martin A, Hesselgesser J, *et al.* The Duffy antigen receptor for chemokines: structural analysis and expression in the brain. *J Leukocyte Biol* 1996; **59**: 29–38.

76 Krych-Goldberg M, Atkinson JP. Structure–function relationships of complement receptor type 1. *Immunol Rev* 2001; **180**: 112–22.

CHAPTER 16

Red cell immunology and compatibility testing

Connie M. Westhoff

Laboratory of Immunohematology and Genomics, New York Blood Center, New York, NY, USA

Introduction

Immunohematology is the study of the immune response to blood cells. This chapter reviews the basic concepts of immunity as they apply to production of antibodies to red blood cells (RBCs), also called atypical *allo*antibodies. Antibodies to platelets and neutrophils, as well as *auto*antibodies and drug-induced antibodies, are discussed elsewhere.

The relevance of immunohematology to transfusion medicine is addressed through discussion of the principles of serologic and DNA-based testing and the application to blood transfusion and donor–recipient compatibility. Identification of the blood group specificity of alloantibodies (antibody identification) is performed by testing plasma or serum against red cells of known phenotypes. Importantly, modern immunohematology uses knowledge of the blood group antigen profile of the patient to aid and inform the process of antibody identification and selection of units for transfusion. This is feasible with the use of DNA-based testing, which provides an extended RBC antigen profile performed as a single assay. The chapter also includes a discussion of the steps and requirements for pretransfusion compatibility testing and release of blood components for transfusion, as well as efforts to track adverse transfusion events through biovigilance programs and to reduce alloimmunization by extended antigen matching.

Red cell immunology

The immune response

Immune responses can be divided into two categories: humoral immunity and cell-mediated events. Humoral immunity is B-cell mediated and results in the production of antibody. Cell-mediated immunity involves the activation of T cells, which regulate the immune response through the production of cytokines and direct interactions with other elements and cells of the immune system.[1] Beginning during fetal development and continuing after birth, B and T cells produce receptors that enable lymphocytes to recognize foreign antigens from self.

Antigen receptors on T cells and B cells

The antigen receptors of both T and B cells consist of two polypeptide chains synthesized under the direction of two different chromosomal loci. In the early stages of lymphocyte development, the genetic material at each of these loci undergoes a process of rearrangement, known as *somatic recombination*, which is unique to each cell.[1] The loci consist of gene segments, grouped into families on the basis of sequence similarity, and the gene rearrangement process entails selection and joining of the segments for each portion of the immunoglobulin molecule (Figure 16.1) and elimination of unused genetic material.

Each B-cell and T-cell receptor chain consists of a constant region, and a variable region associated with antigen binding and peptide–MHC (major histocompatibility complex) recognition. For B cell receptors, which are immunoglobulin molecules, the amino acid sequences of the constant regions determine the isotype, and amino acid sequences of the variable region determine the idiotype and antigenic specificity. For both receptors, one chain contains three gene segments (V, D, and J), whereas the other chain contains rearrangements of V and J segments. The human immunoglobulin loci are polymorphic between individuals as far as the number of genomic V, D, and J segments, but the heavy chain locus has at least 51 V gene segments, 6 J region gene segments, and 27 D region gene segments, and the number of possible combinations for different antibody binding regions is over 8000. At the light chain loci, there are at least 71 V gene segments and 9 J gene segments. Further amino acid sequence variation is introduced by imprecise splicing of the gene segments and addition of extra nucleotides (called *N nucleotides*), which are not encoded in the genome, to V–D and D–J joints in the heavy chain variable region. Given all these mechanisms and assuming the combination of gene segments is random, the number of different antibody variable regions is virtually unlimited.[1]

Exposure to foreign protein antigens

If foreign protein antigens enter the host, antigen-presenting cells (APCs) process the antigen and display antigen-derived peptides in association with host Class II MHC molecules on the cell surfaces. This peptide–MHC complex is recognized as foreign by the T-cell antigen receptor on T lymphocytes. In contrast, B-cell receptor antibody molecules on B lymphocytes recognize foreign epitopes on the protein. Cytokines produced by the activated T cells cause antigen-specific B cells to develop into immunoglobulin-secreting plasma cells. Plasma cells have a short but active life of antibody production. Some antigen-specific B cells develop into memory cells that persist in the circulation long after their initial activation.[1]

Rossi's Principles of Transfusion Medicine, Fifth Edition. Edited by Toby L. Simon, Jeffrey McCullough, Edward L. Snyder, Bjarte G. Solheim, and Ronald G. Strauss.
© 2016 John Wiley & Sons, Ltd. Published 2016 by John Wiley & Sons, Ltd.

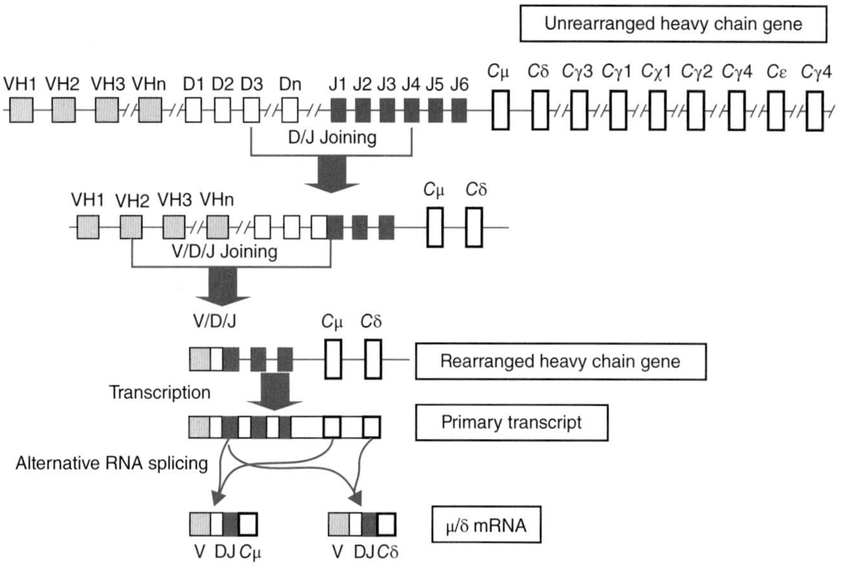

Figure 16.1 Diagram of gene rearrangement generating antibody diversity at the immunoglobulin heavy chain locus on chromosome 14. The un-rearranged locus (top) shows the V, D, and J gene segments on the left and the constant region segments to the right. Gene rearrangement occurs by selection and joining of one D and one J segment (exon) to form a D/J unit. This is then joined by one V exon. The V/D/J unit, via alternative splicing, is joined to Cμ or Cδ heavy chain gene segments. In later generations, clonal progeny can undergo isotype switching in which the same variable region V/D/J is joined to other sequences from the constant region.

Primary response

The first immunoglobulin class to appear in the bloodstream is immunoglobulin M (IgM); the lag phase (time between antigen exposure and appearance of antibody) can vary from days to weeks. Shortly after the appearance of IgM antibody, IgG antibody of the same specificity usually becomes detectable. The IgM component disappears over time, whereas the IgG component persists indefinitely but can drop in titer to undetectable levels. Cytokines from activated T cells are essential for this immunoglobulin class switching and for generation of memory B cells.

Secondary (anamnestic) response

On re-exposure to a foreign antigen, a memory response is activated within a few hours or days, resulting in a sharp rise in the level of IgG antibody, higher than was produced in the primary response.

T-cell independent response

Antibodies produced in response to foreign carbohydrate antigens are primarily IgM. This is because B-cell antigen receptors can be activated by direct binding to repeating polysaccharide epitopes, such as the blood group A or B antigens. Structures that have multiple identical repeat carbohydrate chains can initiate B-cell proliferation and antibody secretion without T-cell help. In the absence of T-cell help, isotype switching from IgM to other isotypes does not occur.[1,2]

Affinity maturation

The affinity of IgG antibody for specific antigen increases progressively during the immune response, particularly after stimulation with low doses of antigen. Affinity maturation is most pronounced after secondary challenge with antigen and involves somatic mutation and clonal selection of B cells with higher affinity antibody receptors for the antigen. These two interrelated processes occur in the germinal centers of the secondary lymphoid organs:

1 *Somatic hypermutation:* Mutations in the variable, antigen-binding coding sequences (known as complementarity-determining regions [CDRs]) of the immunoglobulin genes. The mutation rate is up to 1,000,000 times higher than normal. Although the exact mechanism is not known, a major role for the activation-induced (cytidine) deaminase has been discussed. The increased mutation rate results in 1–2 mutations per CDR per cell generation, and these mutations alter the binding specificities and affinities of the resultant antibodies.[2]

2 *Clonal selection:* B cells that have undergone somatic hypermutation must compete for antigen binding to survive. The follicular dendritic cells (FDCs) in the germinal centers present antigen to the B cells, and only those with the highest affinities for antigen will survive. B-cell progeny that have undergone somatic hypermutation but bind antigen with lower affinity or not at all will be deleted by programmed cell death or apoptosis. Over several rounds of selection, the resultant secreted antibodies produced will have effectively increased affinities for antigen.[2]

Clonality

Only antigen-activated B cells proliferate and mature into antibody-secreting plasma cells. The number of progenitor B cells that are initially activated will determine the heterogeneity of the immune response. A polyclonal response occurs when many different B cells are activated simultaneously, best exemplified by anti-D made in D-negative individuals who lack the RhD protein, which carries many foreign epitopes. A more restricted oligoclonal (pauciclonal) response occurs when the antibody-producing cells originate from a few B cells, exemplified by anti-Fy[a] produced by a Fy(b+) individual, which represents a single amino acid change. Monoclonal antibodies, which are commonly used as reagents in the laboratory, are specific for a single epitope. Antigen-specific monoclonal antibody responses are rarely found in vivo and are usually associated with some leukemias and multiple myeloma. Rather, monoclonal antibodies are isolated in vitro from polyclonal responses using hybridoma technology.

Immunoglobulin molecules

Figure 16.2 portrays the basic structure of an antibody molecule, which consists of four polypeptide chains: two identical light chains of 211–217 amino acids, and two identical heavy chains of 440 or more amino acids. Antigenic specificity is conferred by the first half of the N-terminal amino acids of the light chains and the first quarter of the N-terminal amino acids of the heavy chains; these are described as *variable regions*. The remaining portions of both chains are referred to as *constant regions*.[1]

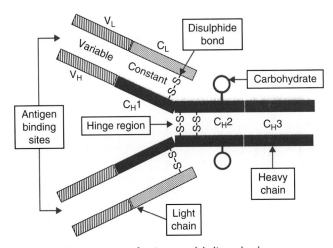

Figure 16.2 Basic structure of an immunoglobulin molecule.

Table 16.1 Characteristics of blood group antibodies

Immunoglobulin Characteristic	IgM	IgG	IgA
H-chain isotype	μ	γ	A
Subclasses	2	4	1
L-chain types	κλ	κλ	Κλ
Sedimentation constant	19 S	7 S	11 S
Molecular weight	900–1000 kD	150 kD	180–500 kD
Electrophoretic mobility	Between β and γ	γ	Γ
Serum concentration (mg/dL)	85–205	1000–1500	200–350
Antigen binding sites	10 (5)	2	4
Fixes complement	Often	Some	No
Placental transfer	No	Yes	No
Direct agglutinin	Yes	Usually not	Usually not
Hemolytic in vitro	Often	Usually not	No
Example	Anti-A, anti-B	Anti-D	Anti-Lu^a

Light chains

The constant region of the light chains can have one of two different amino acid sequences, designated kappa (κ) and lambda (λ). A single B cell will synthesize an immunoglobulin molecule containing either κ or λ chains, but never both.

Heavy chains

The constant region of heavy chains, designated by the Greek letters α (alpha), δ (delta), ε (epsilon), γ (gamma), and μ (mu), gives rise to five types of immunoglobulin classes, or isotypes, termed IgA, IgD, IgE, IgG, and IgM, respectively. A single B cell will synthesize an immunoglobulin molecule containing only one type of heavy chain.

Blood group antibodies

Blood group antibodies are immunoglobulins that bind to antigens on the surface of red cells, platelets, and neutrophils. The focus of this chapter is primarily on antigens expressed on the RBC. The antibodies can be acquired either "naturally," meaning from exposure to common environmental stimuli, or through exposure to foreign red cells via pregnancy or transfusion. Most blood group antibodies are either IgG or IgM; only occasionally are they IgA.[3] The IgD and IgE immunoglobulins have not been implicated as blood group antibodies.

Physical properties

The physical properties and serologic characteristics of the three immunoglobulin antibody classes with blood group specificity are summarized in Table 16.1. IgM antibodies are pentameric and have 10 antigen binding sites, are direct agglutinating, and often fix complement to the red cells. Antibodies to A and B antigens are predominantly IgM; they are found in persons whose red cells lack the corresponding antigen. They are stimulated by antigens present in the environment, including plants and bacteria that carry blood group A- and B-like polysaccharides. In adults with a normal immune system, these antibodies are almost always present when the corresponding antigens are absent on the red cells.

In contrast to anti-A and anti-B, most other blood group antibodies are immune in origin and do not appear in plasma/serum unless the host is exposed to foreign red cell antigens through blood transfusion or pregnancy. The majority are IgG,

which have two sites for antigen binding (Figure 16.2). Most IgG antibodies do not activate complement, but this depends on both the subclass of IgG and the number and nature of the antigen on the cells.

Antibodies to red cell antigens, other than naturally occurring anti-A and anti-B, are considered "unexpected" alloantibodies, and are directed to antigens absent on the RBCs of the individual. Antibodies in the recipient can cause accelerated destruction of antigen-positive transfused red cells, and some potent antibodies in donor plasma may destroy recipient RBCs. In pregnant women, IgG antibodies may cross the placenta and cause hemolytic disease of the fetus and newborn.[3]

There are more than 300 different blood group antigens described.[4] The immunoglobulin class and clinical relevance of some of the antibodies encountered are shown in Table 16.2.

Red cell antigen–antibody interactions

Red cells normally repel one another. The force of repulsion (zeta potential) at the surface depends not only on the electronegative surface charge, but also on the ionic cloud that surrounds it. The electronegative charge is imparted primarily by the carboxyl (COO^-) group of N-acetyl-neuraminic acid, which is a constituent of alkali-labile tetrasaccharides that are attached to MN and Ss sialoglycoproteins (glycophorins A and B, respectively). The magnitude of this charge is modified by the formation of an ionic cloud of positively charged (+) sodium ions and negatively charged (−) chloride ions at the red cell membrane surface (Figure 16.3). The net effect of this ionic cloud is to decrease the electrostatic repulsion between cells.[5]

For in vivo enhancement of the interaction of red cell antigens with blood group antibodies, three variables are considered: the surface charge of the red cells, the dielectric constant of the medium, and the mutual attraction between antigen and antibody. The latter involves electrostatic (Coulombic) and hydrogen bonds, and van der Waals interactions, and there must be structural complementarity between the antigen and its binding site on antibody molecules.

There are two phases of red cell antigen–antibody agglutination interactions; these often occur simultaneously. The first phase is one of association, involving binding of antibody to antigens on the red cell membrane. The second phase involves the formation of an agglutination lattice of antibody-coated cells. For the latter to occur,

Table 16.2 Blood group antibody, class, clinical significance, and % antigen-negative (compatible) donors[7]

Antibody	Ig Class[†]	C3-Binding	Effect of Ficin	HDFN[‡]	HTR[§]	%Compatible Whites	Blacks	Comments
A	M, G	Yes	↑	Moderate	Yes	57	73	No dosage
A₁	M	rare	↑	No	Rare	66	81	Present in 1% A₂, 25% A₂B
At^a	G	No		No	Yes	Rare	Many	1 case mild HDFN
B	M, G	Yes	↑	Moderate	Yes	91	80	No dosage
Bg	G	No		No	No	99	99	To HLA[‖]
C	G, M	No	↑	Mild	Yes	32	73	
c	G, M	No	↑	Yes	Yes	20	4	Often with anti-E
Ch	G	No	↓	No	No[#]	4	4	antibody to C4d[#]
C^w	G, M	No	↑	Yes	Yes	98	99	
Co^a	G	No		Mild	Mild	Rare	Rare	
Co^b	G	Rare		Mild	Yes	90	90	
Cr^a	G	No		No	Mild	None	Rare	
Cs^a	G	No		No	No	2	4	
D	G, M	No	↑	Yes	Yes	15	8	
Di^a	G	No		Yes	Yes	>99	>99	64% American Indians
Di^b	G	No		Mild	Yes	Rare	Rare	4% American Indians
Do^a	G	Yes	↑	No	Yes	33	45	
Do^b	G	Yes	↑	No	Yes	18	11	
E	G, M	No	↑	Mild	Yes	71	78	Often with anti-c
e	G, M	No	↑	Rare	Yes	2	2	
f (ce)	G, M	No	↑	Mild	Mild	35	8	Compatible with c−
Fy^a	G	Rare	↓	Yes	Yes	34	90	
Fy^b	G	Rare	↓	Mild	Yes	17	77	
Ge	G, M	Yes	↓Some	No	Yes	Rare	Rare	
H	M, G	Yes	↑	No	Yes	Rare	Rare	In O$_h$ blood
Hy	G	No		No	Mild	Rare	Rare	In Blacks
I	M, G	Yes	↑	No	Yes	Rare	Rare	In i adults
Jk^a	G	Yes	↑	Yes	Yes	23	8	
Jk^b	G	Yes	↑	Mild	Yes	26	51	
JMH	G	No	↓	No	No	Rare	Rare	HTLA[¶]
Js^a	G	No		Yes	Yes	>99	80	
Js^b	G	No		Yes	Yes	Rare	1	
K	G, M	Rare		Yes	Yes	91	98	
k	G	No		Yes	Yes	Rare	Rare	
Kn^a	G	No	↓	No	No	2	1	
Kp^a	G	No		Yes	Mild	98	>99	
Kp^b	G	No		Mild	Mild	Rare	Rare	
Lan	G	Some		Mild	Yes	Rare	Rare	
Le^a	M	Yes	↑	No	Rare	78	77	
Le^b	M	Yes	↑	No	No	28	45	
Lu^a	G, A	Rare		Rare	No	92	95	
Lu^b	G, A	Rare		Mild	Mild	Rare	Rare	
M	M, G	Rare	↓	Rare	Rare	22	26	
McC^a	G	No	↓	No	No	2	6	HTLA[¶]
N	M, G	No	↓	Rare	Rare	28	25	Potent in N–U–
P₁	M	Some	↑	No	Rare	21	6	
P+P₁+P^k	M, G	Yes	↑	Yes	Yes	Rare	Rare	
Rg	G	No	↓	No[#]	Rare	2	2	Antibody to C4d[#]
S	G	Some	↓	Yes	Yes	45	69	
s	G	Rare	↓	Yes	Yes	11	7	
Sc1	G	No		No	No	Rare	Rare	
Sc2	G	No		Yes	No	99	99	
Sl^a	G	No	↓	No	No	2	55	
U	G	No		Yes	Yes	Rare	1	
V	G	No	↑	No	Yes	>99	70	
Vel	M, G	Yes	↑	Yes	Yes	Rare	Rare	
Wr^a	M, G	No		Yes	Yes	>99	>99	
Xg^a	G	No	↓	No	No	23	23	
Yk^a	G	No	↓	No	No	8	2	HTLA[¶]
Yt^a	G	No	↓Some	No	Some	Rare	Rare	

[†] Predominant immunoglobulin class shown first.

[‡] HDFN = reported to cause hemolytic disease of the fetus and newborn.

[‖] HLA = antibody to antigen present on white blood cells that is variably expressed on red cells.

[¶] HTLA = antibody, usually of high titer, to antigen of low site density on RBC. Incorrectly called high-titer, low-avidity antibody.

[#] C4d = antibody to epitopes found on the fourth component of human complement (C4). Hives and anaphylaxis reported with plasma containing products.

[§] Hemolytic Transfusion Reaction.

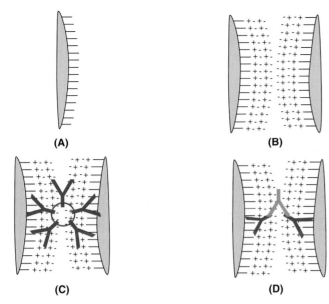

Figure 16.3 (A) Red cells carry a strong negative electric charge, imparted primarily by the carboxyl (COO⁻) group of N-acetyl-neuraminic acid. (B) When suspended in saline, red cells are kept apart by virtue of their negative surface charge. The magnitude of this charge is modified by the formation of an ionic cloud of positively charged (+) sodium ions and negatively charged (−) chloride ions at the red cell membrane surface. The force of repulsion that exists between red cells in suspension is referred to as the *zeta potential*. (C) In order for antibody molecules to cause agglutination of adjacent red cells, they must be able to span the intercellular distance. Pentameric IgM antibody molecules can readily bridge the distance between adjacent red cells causing agglutination. (D) IgG molecules (black) cannot readily cause direct agglutination. The bound IgG antibody can be detected by antihuman IgG antibody (e.g., rabbit antihuman IgG), depicted here in gray, causing agglutination.

antibody molecules must be able to span the distance between adjacent red cells.

Interaction between red cells and blood group antibodies can be observed either directly by examination of red cell and antibody mixtures for agglutination (clumping) and/or hemolysis, or indirectly by use of an antihuman globulin reagent in the antiglobulin test. These two serologic techniques are summarized in Table 16.3.

Table 16.3 Types of red cell serologic tests

Direct Tests	Indirect Tests
Mix serum and red cells.[†] Centrifuge. Examine for agglutination and hemolysis.	Mix serum and red cells.[*] Incubate (37 °C). Centrifuge. Examine for agglutination and hemolysis.[†] Wash, to remove unbound globulins. Add antihuman globulin reagent. Centrifuge. Examine for agglutination.[‡]

[†] Can incubate at room temperature.
[*] An enhancement reagent, to promote antibody uptake, may be incorporated here.
[‡] Confirm negative test results with IgG-coated red cells.

Agglutination reactions

IgM antibody molecules can cause direct agglutination of RBCs carrying the corresponding antigen. Examination for agglutination may be performed either macroscopically or microscopically, but the latter may detect nonspecific reactivity and is not routinely performed. The strength of the observed reactions are graded, and numerical values are assigned based on a scoring system.[6]

Hemolysis

IgM antibodies, in particular anti-A and anti-B, can also cause direct lysis of antigen-positive red cells in the presence of complement. Hemolysis results from the action of complement, a series of α and β globulins that act in sequence as enzymes (e.g., esterases) to form a complex (membrane attack complex) that causes rupture of the red cell membrane through which intracellular hemoglobin can escape (see Figure 16.4). For initiation of the complement cascade, the Fc portions of two immunoglobulin heavy chains must be in close proximity on the red cell surface. Initiation of the complement cascade readily occurs when a single pentameric IgM antibody molecule is bound; for it to occur with IgG antibodies, there must be closely adjacent heavy chain regions of two IgG molecules at the cell surface. Furthermore, not all IgM antibodies bind complement to red cells, and complement binding does not always proceed to complete red cell lysis (intravascular hemolysis). Rather, activated C3b may be cleaved to C3d, which remains bound to red cells and may be detected by the antiglobulin test (see the "Antiglobulin Test" section).[6]

Red cells coated with C3b are also removed by cells of the reticuloendothelial system (extravascular hemolysis).

Antiglobulin test

IgG antibodies do not readily cause direct agglutination of red cells, although some IgG antibodies will cause direct agglutination if the red cell zeta potential is reduced, or if there are a large number of antigens on the RBC, for example the M antigen carried on glycophorin A. Zeta potential can be decreased by raising the dielectric constant of the red cell suspending medium by the addition of colloids such as bovine serum albumin, or by treating the cells with proteolytic enzymes such as papain or ficin, which cleave the proteins that carry the negatively charged neuraminic acid residues.

IgG antibodies, as well as complement components bound to red cells by either IgM or IgG antibodies, are detected by the antiglobulin test. This test, once called the Coombs' test, entails the use of antibodies raised in animals (usually rabbit), or prepared by hybridoma technology, to detect human IgG and complement bound to red cells. Antihuman globulin (AHG) will react with human globulins, either bound to red cells or free in plasma or serum. Red cells must be washed free of unbound globulins before testing with AHG to avoid false-negative tests caused by neutralization of AHG by unbound globulins.

Direct antiglobuin test

The direct antiglobulin test (DAT) is used to detect antibodies bound to red cells in vivo; such antibodies may be seen in patients with autoimmune hemolytic anemia, infants with hemolytic disease of the fetus and newborn, and patients manifesting an alloimmune response to a recent transfusion.[6]

Indirect antiglobulin test

An indirect antiglobulin test (IAT) is used to detect and identify unexpected antibodies in the serum or plasma. These antibodies

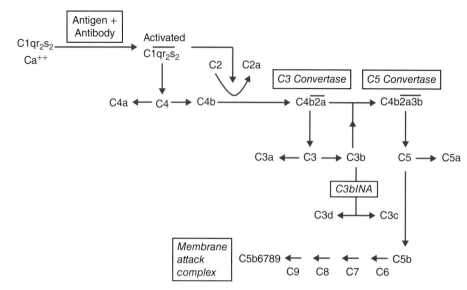

Figure 16.4 Classical pathway for complement activation.

may be seen in blood donors, transfusion recipients, and prenatal patients who have been previously transfused or pregnant.[6]

Compatibility testing

Compatibility testing comprises pretransfusion procedures and laboratory tests with the goal to provide blood for transfusion that will have the optimal clinical effect. The elements of pretransfusion testing can be placed into one of three categories: those related to donor unit testing and processing, those related to patient sample collection and testing, and those that serve as a final check between the donor unit and intended recipient (Table 16.4). Proper performance of each element will enable the right unit of blood to be transfused to the right patient. The most important part of the process is proper identification of the patient, both at sample collection and at administration of the blood product. The most common cause of morbidity and mortality following blood transfusion is ABO incompatibility due to mislabeling of the sample, wrong blood in tube (WBIT), or misidentification and transfusion to the wrong patient.[8,9]

Donor testing
Collection facility

ABO, Rh, and antibody detection tests on donor blood, tests for infectious diseases, and labeling of donor units are functions often carried out by a regional donor center; however, some hospital-based transfusion services continue to procure a portion of their blood needs. Donations come from the population at large (allogeneic donors), but may also be collected from patients for their own use in elective surgical procedures (autologous donors); or, rarely, some patients request that they receive blood from relatives or friends (directed donations), but this practice is discouraged with the implementation of extensive tests for infectious disease and the safety of the blood supply (Chapter 62).

The volume of tests performed at donor centers necessitates use of automated equipment. ABO grouping entails testing both donor red cells and serum/plasma, and the results must be concordant for the unit to be labeled. Red cells are tested with anti-A and anti-B; and the serum/plasma is tested against A_1 and B red cells. Anti-A,B

Table 16.4 Elements of pretransfusion testing[10]

Element	Requirement
Patient Consent	Blood bank or transfusion service medical director to participate in development of policies and processes
Patient Sample Collection	
Identification	Positive identification of intended recipient and blood sample at time of collection
	Mechanism to identify phlebotomist
Label	Two independent identifiers (e.g., first and last names, patient unique number)
	Date of collection
	Affixed to sample before leaving side of intended recipient
Timing	Within 3 days of red cell transfusion if patient was transfused or pregnant within previous 3 months, or if patient history is uncertain or unavailable
Donor Unit Confirmatory	
	Testing from an attached segment, after the label has been affixed
ABO and Rh	Anti-A and anti-B on RBCs of units labeled group A or group B
	Anti-A,B on units labeled group O
	Direct tests with anti-D for units labeled as Rh-negative
Patient Sample Testing	
ABO and Rh	Anti-A and anti-B on RBCs; serum or plasma with A_1 and B red cells; concordance between red cell and serum results
	Test with anti-D; test for weak expression optional
	To reduce risk of misidentification of the sample, perform ABO/Rh on second sample collected at a separate phlebotomy, or compare with previous records, or electronic identification verification
Unexpected antibodies	Method that will demonstrate clinically significant antibodies using reagent red cells that are not pooled
	Comparison of current ABO, Rh, and antibody screen with historical records
Donor/Patient Testing	
Crossmatch	Antiglobulin test if clinically significant antibodies detected, currently or in the past
	Tests for ABO incompatibility only if no clinically significant antibodies detected, currently or in the past
Electronic	Computer system validated to ensure only ABO-compatible blood is selected may be used to detect ABO incompatibility

and/or A$_2$ red cells are often also used to detect subgroups of A that may be nonreactive in direct tests with anti-A alone.

Rh typing for the D antigen on blood donor samples must be performed by a method that will detect weak expression of the D antigen as D is highly immunogenic[8] and weak expression of the antigen can evoke an immune response. Donor red cells that initially type as Rh-negative in direct agglutination tests can be tested further for weak D by an IAT, or more commonly at donor centers enzyme treatment of the RBCs is a used in automated tests to enhance reactivity of weak D antigen. All D-positive and weak D-positive blood is considered Rh-positive.[6,10] Some RBCs that express very weak D antigens, including those only detected by adsorption/elution of anti-D (termed Del), are not detected as Rh-positive.[6] This is a shortcoming of serologic methods as the units are labeled as Rh-negative. Hence, production of anti-D in a patient receiving RBCs labeled as Rh-negative should be reported to the donor center for follow-up testing of the blood donor.

Transfusing facility

The ABO group of units of whole blood or RBCs, and the Rh type of those labeled Rh-negative, must be confirmed by the transfusion facility on a segment from the unit before transfusion.[10(p35)] This "retyping" for confirmation of ABO only requires testing of the RBCs with anti-A and anti-B, and units labeled group O can be tested with anti-A,B alone.[6] For confirmation of the D type of units labeled Rh-negative, only direct testing with anti-D is necessary; testing for weak expression of D is not required, nor is repeat testing for unexpected antibodies or for markers of infectious diseases.[6] For transfusion facilities that also collect blood, confirmatory testing for first-time donors must be performed after the original ABO and Rh label has been affixed using a sample from a segment attached to the donor unit.

Patient testing
Sample collection

The major cause of fatal, hemolytic transfusion reactions is ABO-incompatible transfusion resulting from patient and/or sample misidentification somewhere in the process from specimen collection to transfusion. Facilities must have validated processes and procedures that define each step in the process. Some considerations include:

1 *Requisition.* Forms requesting blood and blood components must contain two independent patient identifiers, usually the first and last names and a unique numerical identifier such as a hospital registration number.[10(p34)] The name of the requesting physician, gender and date of birth of the patient, clinical diagnosis, and previous transfusion or pregnancy history are additional useful pieces of information.

2 *Patient identity.* The collection of a properly labeled blood sample for pretransfusion testing from the correct patient is critical to safe blood transfusion. The person collecting the sample must positively identify the patient from the wristband containing two unique patient identifiers (generally patient's full name and unique hospital registration number) that remains attached to the patient throughout the hospitalization and blood transfusion. The information on the requisition form must be compared with that on the wristband; blood samples should never be collected if there is a discrepancy.[10(p35)]

In the absence of a wristband, the nursing staff should follow hospital procedure for identifying and attaching a wristband to the patient before any samples are drawn. In an emergency, a temporary identification number should be used, and cross-referenced with the patient's name and hospital identification number once they are known.

3 *Labeling.* Blood samples must be clearly labeled at the bedside with the patient's unique identifiers. There must be a mechanism to identify the date of sample collection and the individual who collected the sample. Conventionally, the phlebotomist signs or initials the tube and signs or initials the requisition form so that there is a permanent record of the phlebotomist.[10(p35)]

4 *Confirmation of sample identity.* Prior to testing, the information on the blood sample label must be compared with that on the requisition. A new sample must be obtained whenever there are discrepancies or if there is any doubt about the identity of the sample. It is unacceptable to correct a mislabeled sample.[10(p35)]

5 *Type of sample.* Either serum or plasma may be used for pretransfusion testing. Anticoagulated (plasma) samples are more commonly used and are required if testing is automated. Some technologists prefer to use serum rather than plasma for compatibility testing to facilitate detection of antibodies that primarily coat red cells with the C3d component of complement. Bound C3d will not cause lysis but can be detected with AHG reagents containing anti-C3d. EDTA, citrate, and other commonly used anticoagulants chelate calcium ions that are essential for complement activation.

6 *Age of specimen.* To ensure that the specimen used for compatibility testing is representative of a patient's current immune status, serologic studies must be performed using blood collected no more than three days in advance of the transfusion when the patient has been transfused or pregnant within the preceding three months, or when such information is uncertain or unavailable.[10(p36)] From a practical standpoint, it is often simpler to stipulate that all pretransfusion samples must be collected within three days before red cell transfusions, rather than ascertain whether or not each patient has been recently transfused or pregnant.

7 *Storage.* Blood samples used for compatibility testing, including donor red cells, must be stored at refrigerated temperatures for at least seven days after transfusion.[10(p35)] This ensures that appropriate samples are available for investigational purposes should adverse responses occur.

ABO typing

Reagent antisera and red cells for ABO typing are available commercially. Anti-A and anti-B are monoclonal antibodies prepared by hybridoma technology. Reagent red cells are usually suspended in a preservative medium containing EDTA, to prevent lysis of the red cells by complement-binding anti-A and anti-B. ABO grouping is performed using a direct agglutination technique (Table 16.3). Red cells are tested with anti-A and anti-B, and the serum or plasma with A1 and B red cells. Use of anti-A,B and A2 red cells is optional, but it is generally considered unnecessary when routinely ABO typing potential transfusion recipients.[6]

The expected findings for each of the four ABO phenotypes are shown in Table 16.5. When interpreting the results of ABO grouping tests, the reciprocal relationship that exists between the absence of A and/or B antigens on red cells and the presence of anti-A and/or anti-B in the serum is considered. If there is conflict between cell and serum ABO tests, group O blood can be provided for transfusion until the discrepancy is resolved and reliable conclusions of the patient's ABO type can be made.

Table 16.5 The Expected Reactions of the Four Common ABO Phenotypes: Results of Blood Typing Tests

Blood Type	Anti-A	Anti-B	A₁ Red Cells	B Red Cells
O	0	0	4+	4+
A	4+	0	0	4+
B	0	4+	4+	0
AB	4+	4+	0	0

O = no agglutination; 4+ = strong agglutination.

Rh typing

In the United States, anti-D for testing patient samples is a blend of monoclonal IgM and monoclonal/polyclonal human IgG. With blended anti-D reagents, the IgM component causes direct agglutination of D-positive red cells and the IgG component permits detection of the weak expression of D by application of the antiglobulin test.[14]

Only direct tests with blended anti-D reagents are required on patient samples; the test for weak D is not required. To avoid incorrect designation of a D-negative recipient as D-positive because of autoantibodies or abnormal serum proteins, a control system appropriate to the anti-D reagent is required.[6] A negative test with anti-A and/or anti-B is considered an appropriate control system, but apparent Group AB, D-positive samples require an Rh control reagent.

Tests for unexpected antibodies

Table 16.2 lists the majority of blood group alloantibodies encountered and provides the approximate percentage of compatible units that are likely to be encountered in Caucasian and black donor populations.

Methods for testing samples for unexpected antibodies in the serum or plasma of prospective transfusion recipients must be those that detect clinically significant antibodies.[10(p36)] An IAT after 37 °C incubation of patient serum or plasma with reagent red cells is required. A number of options exist regarding the selection of methods for pretransfusion antibody detection (Table 16.6). Decisions relative to these options are within the purview of the blood bank medical director. They should be made based on the type of patients served, the causes and frequency of previous significant antibody-mediated transfusion reactions, and the availability of resources, with the realization that no one method will detect all clinically significant antibodies.

Tube test methods

A variety of red cell suspending media or additives are used either to enhance antibody uptake or to potentiate the agglutination phase of antibody–antigen interactions (Table 16.6). Low-ionic-strength saline (LISS) solution, normal saline, or red cell preservatives (modified Alsever's solution) are used as red cell suspending media. In contrast, bovine serum albumin (22% or 30% w/v), LISS additives, or polyethylene glycol (PEG) are commonly added directly to serum–red cell mixtures.[11]

Antibody uptake is accelerated when red cells are suspended in LISS or PEG. The magnitude of the ionic cloud (Figure 16.3) surrounding negatively charged red cells suspended in LISS (approximately 0.03 M) is lower than that surrounding red cells suspended in normal saline (0.15 M NaCl). The ionic cloud, imparted by negatively charged carboxyl groups, hinders association between antibody and antigen; thus, reducing the magnitude of the ionic cloud promotes antibody association and also causes an increase in attraction between the negatively charged red cell membrane and positive charges on the antigen-binding sites of antibody molecules. The net effect of additives is that more antibody can be bound in a shorter period of time using LISS or PEG as opposed to saline. Consequently, incubation times can be reduced to 10–15 minutes for LISS, or 15–30 minutes for PEG, compared to 30–60 minutes for saline.[11]

In contrast, albumin promotes the second stage of antigen–antibody interactions, namely, the agglutination of antibody-coated red cells. Albumin can promote the direct agglutination of IgG-coated red cells; however, albumin is not used in the United States in a manner that promotes direct agglutination of antibody-coated red cells. Rather, the enhancing effect of albumin on red cell–antigen interactions can be attributed to its formulation as a low-ionic solution.[11]

It is common practice to examine saline, albumin, and LISS tests for direct agglutination before subjecting them to an IAT. These examinations can be made immediately after mixing cells and serum followed by centrifugation (immediate-spin tests) and again after incubation at 37 °C. For antiglobulin testing, either anti-IgG or polyspecific AHG (containing anti-IgG and anti-C3) may be used. However, use of polyspecific AHG may lead to the detection of a number of unwanted positives. PEG tests should not be examined for direct agglutination, and antiglobulin reagent containing anti-C3 is not routinely used.[11]

Gel column testing

A gel test for detecting red cell antigen–antibody interactions was first described in 1990 by Lapierre and colleagues.[12] Cards consisting of six microcolumns, each containing agarose gel suspended in anti-IgG, are commercially available. Atop each card is an incubation chamber in which reagent red cells and test plasma are dispensed. The cards are incubated at 37 °C and then

Table 16.6 Methods for Pretransfusion Antibody Detection

	Serum	Red Cells	Incubation	AHG*
Saline	2–3 drops	1 drop, 3–5%	30–60 min; 37 °C	IgG/PS
Albumin	2–3 drops	1 drop, 3–5%	15–30 min; 37 °C	IgG/PS
Low-ionic-strength saline (solution)	2 drops*	2 drops, 2%*	10–15 min; 37 °C	IgG/PS
Gel	25 µL†	50 µL, 0.8%	15 min; 37 °C	IgG
Polyethylene glycol (PEG)	2 drops†	1 drop	15–30 min; 37 °C	IgG
Solid-phase adherence	1 drop	‡	10–15 min; 37 °C	IgG

* Drop volumes should be equal.
† Plus 4 volumes of 20% polyethylene glycol.
‡ Predetermined by reagent supplier.
AHG, antihuman globulin; PS, polyspecific AHG; RT, room temperature.

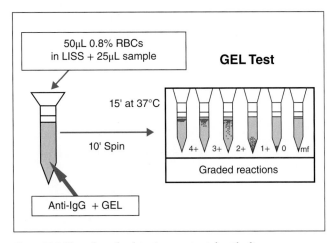

Figure 16.5 The gel test for detecting unexpected antibodies.

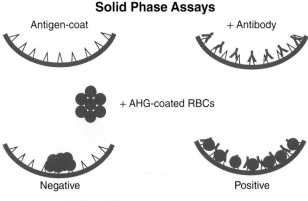

Figure 16.6 Solid-phase adherence assays.

centrifuged. As the red cells pass through the gel, they are separated from the serum/plasma and come into contact with anti-IgG. If the red cells become coated with antibody during incubation, they will be agglutinated by anti-IgG. The agglutinated red cells become trapped in the gel; unagglutinated red cells pellet to the bottom of the microcolumn (Figure 16.5).

Column technologies offer several advantages over test tube procedures. When compared to tube tests, the time savings are reflected in no centrifugation/reading for direct agglutination after incubation, no addition of antiglobulin reagent, and no need to validate negative tests using IgG-coated red cells. Reproducibility is increased through use of measured volumes of reactants, elimination of the washing process, and less subjective reading of tests. The stability of reactions facilitates validation and review of results by a second technologist. Testing can be automated, or semiautomated using liquid sample handling devices.

Solid-phase adherence methods
Two forms of solid-phase adherence assays are available for red cell serologic testing. For direct tests, antibody is fixed to wells of a microplate (e.g., anti-A and anti-B for donor/recipient ABO typing), and red cells are added. Following centrifugation, red cells expressing the corresponding antigen will efface across the well; red cells lacking the antigen will pellet to the bottom of the well.

For indirect tests (e.g., for detecting unexpected antibodies), red cell membranes are affixed to microplate wells; test serum or plasma are added, and the plates washed to remove unbound globulins. Indicator red cells, which are coated with anti-IgG, are then added, and the plates are centrifuged. The indicator red cells efface across the well in a positive test, and pellet to the center of the well in a negative test (Figure 16.6).

Automated pretransfusion testing
Automated systems for pretransfusion testing are particularly suited for large hospital-based transfusion services, and include:
1 Gel column technology;
2 Solid-phase adherence technologies; and
3 Liquid microplates or microplates containing dried antisera for ABO/Rh typing, and modified solid-phase methods for antibody detection.

Automated systems perform sample and reagent pipetting and analysis of agglutination reactions. Standard features include

positive sample identification, process control through automated documentation of reagent lot numbers and expiration dates, batch and random access operating modes, STAT sample interrupt, and image analysis. The test results can be transmitted via an interface into the laboratory computer system.

The benefits of automation include technologist time savings, positive sample identification, standardized testing (compliance with current good manufacturing practice), and increased workload capacity.

Reagent red cells for antibody screening
The FDA mandates that sets of reagent red cell samples licensed for use in pretransfusion antibody detection tests carry the C, c, D, E, e, Fy^a, Fy^b, Jk^a, Jk^b, K, k, Le^a, Le^b, P^1 M, N, S, and s antigens. Reagent red cells for antibody detection are available commercially as sets of either two or three samples. The Rh phenotypes present in two-sample sets are R^1R^1 (D+C+c−E−e+) and R^2R^2 (D+C−c+E+e−). In three-sample sets, an rr (D−C−c+E−e+) sample is also provided. Use of three red cell samples facilitates the identification of anti-D and enables inclusion of red cells from individuals homozygous for particular blood group genes. Such red cells often have a stronger expression of an antigen when compared to red cells from individuals heterozygous for the same gene; this phenomenon is known as *dosage*.

The principles of antibody identification
When unexpected antibodies are present, as indicated by positive antibody screening tests, they must be identified. This involves testing the patient's serum or plasma against a panel of fully phenotyped reagent red cell samples and the patient's own cells. A typical panel is shown in Table 16.7, which illustrates the results of antibody identification tests with a sample containing both anti-M and anti-K. Tests performed in this example include a reading for direct agglutination after room temperature incubation and after incubation at 37 °C. Results of testing with LISS additive and tests with ficin-treated red cells are displayed.

A typical approach follows:
1 The reactions with the patient's own red cells (AC) are examined. If the AC is positive, autoantibodies may be present and the patient may have a positive DAT. Therapy with certain drugs can also cause the AC and DAT to be positive.[6,11] Alternatively, the AC may react because alloantibodies have formed to recently transfused red cells that are still circulating in the recipient. The AC is negative in the case shown, so autoantibodies likely are not present.

Table 16.7 Results of tests between a panel of reagent red cells and a serum containing anti-M and anti-K

Panel		RH							MNS				P1	LE		KEL				JK		FY		XG		LISS			FICIN	
	D	C	c	C^w	E	e	f	M	N	S	s	P_1	Le^a	Le^b	K	k	Kp^a	Js^a	Jk^a	Jk^b	Fy^a	Fy^b	Xg^a		RT	37	IAT	37	IAT
1 r'r	0	+	+	0	0	+	+	+	+	+	0	0	0	+	0	+	0	0	+	+	0	+	+	1	3+	1+	0	0	0
2 R_1R_1	+	+	0	0	0	+	0	0	+	+	+	+	+	0	0	+	0	0	+	+	+	+	+	2	0	0	0	0	0
3 R_1R_1	+	+	0	+	0	+	0	+	0	0	+	+	0	+	+	+	0	0	+	+	+	0	+	3	4+	3+	3+	0	3+
4 R_2R_2	+	0	+	0	+	0	0	0	+	0	+	+	0	+	0	+	0	0	0	+	+	+	+	4	0	0	0	0	0
5 r''r	0	0	+	0	+	+	+	+	0	+	0	+	0	+	0	+	0	0	+	+	0	+	+	5	4+	3+	3+	0	0
6 rrV	0	0	+	0	0	+	+	+	+	0	+	+	0	0	0	+	0	0	0	+	0	+	+	6	3+	1+	0	0	0
7 rr	0	0	+	0	0	+	+	0	+	0	+	+	0	+	+	0	0	0	0	+	+	0	0	7	0	0	4+	0	4+
8 rr	0	0	+	0	0	+	+	+	+	+	+	+	+	0	0	+	0	0	+	0	+	+	0	8	3+	1+	0	0	0
9 rr	0	0	+	0	0	+	+	+	0	+	0	+	0	+	0	+	0	0	+	0	0	+	+	9	4+	3+	3+	0	3+
10 rr	0	0	+	0	0	+	+	+	+	+	+	0	+	0	+	+	0	0	+	+	+	0	+	10	3+	1+	3+	0	3+
11 Ror	+	0	+	0	0	+	+	+	+	0	0	+	0	+	0	+	0	+	+	+	0	0	0	11	3+	1+	0	0	0
PATIENT																								AC	0	0	0		

2 The graded reaction strengths are examined. Variability in reaction strength may be an indication of dosage, that is, the antibody reacts stronger with red cells from homozygotes (double-dose) than with red cells from heterozygotes (single-dose). Given the varying degrees of reactivity of positive red cell samples in Table 16.7, more than one antibody appears to be present, and M+N− red cells react significantly stronger than M+N+ red cells.

3 A process of "ruling out" is undertaken by evaluating the non-reactive cells and the antigens present on the nonreactive cells. Only reagent red cell samples 2 and 4 are nonreactive. The presence of antibodies to antigens present on these two cells (D, C, c, E, e, N, S, s, P_1, Le^a, Le^b, Jk^a, Jk^b, Fy^a, Fy^b, and Xg^a) can be eliminated from initial consideration. This leaves the possibility of antibodies to M, K, C^w, f, Kp^a, and Js^a. However, C^w, Kp^a, and Js^a are low-prevalence antigens not present on the reagent red cells used for antibody detection, and f antigen will not be present on a two-sample screening set of R^1R^1 and R^2R^2 cells, so these specificities are not responsible for the positive antibody screen. Thus, the results suggest the presence of anti-M and anti-K.

4 The test phase at which reactivity is observed is evaluated. Antibodies that are often IgM (Table 16.2), such as anti-M, -N, -Le^a, and -P_1, react as direct agglutinins at room temperature. Antibodies that are usually IgG (e.g., anti-Rh, -K, -Fy, -Jk, and -S) react preferentially by an IAT, although during the early stages of the immune response, IgM antibodies of these specificities can be encountered.

With the example here, the anti-M appears to react best at room temperature, and the anti-K reacts best by IAT. This is consistent with the anti-M being IgM, although many examples of anti-M do have an IgG component,[3,7] whereas the anti-K is most likely IgG (Table 16.2). Anti-f does not appear to be present because f-positive cell samples 1, 6, 8, and 11 are nonreactive by IAT.

5 The results of tests with enzyme-treated red cells, if performed, are evaluated. Knowledge of the anticipated behavior of certain antibodies with enzyme-treated red cells can be very helpful when identifying antibodies—especially when dealing with sera containing mixtures of alloantibodies. Antigens of the MNS, FY, and XG systems are cleaved by treatment of red cells with proteolytic enzymes such as papain or ficin, and negative or weak reactions are observed when antibodies to these antigens are tested with ficin- or papain-treated red cells. In contrast, treatment of red cells with proteolytic enzymes enhances reactivity with Rh antibodies, as well as antibodies such as anti-Le^a, -P_1, and -Jk^a. The double-dose M-positive red cell samples (3, 5, and 9) react in LISS tests at 37 °C and by IAT. These cells are nonreactive when pretreated with ficin, as expected. In contrast, K antigen is not affected by ficin treatment, so there is no difference in the reactions of ficin and LISS tests with cell samples 3, 7, and 10. Anti-f can now be completely eliminated because, if present, it should have reacted with all the K-negative ficin-treated cells from donors with r (ce) haplotype.

6 There must be sufficient negative test results with red cells that lack the corresponding antigen and sufficient positive test results with red cells that carry that antigen. To obtain a confidence level of >95% ($p = 0.05$), there should be at least three nonreactive antigen-negative red cell samples and at least three reactive antigen-positive red cells. This requirement has been met for both the anti-M and the anti-K.

7 The red cells from the patient are tested with anti-M and anti-K, and should lack both M and K antigens. There are exceptions of alloantibody formation when the corresponding antigen appears to be present on the autologous red cells. Most notably, this is seen in the Rh system in individuals with partial antigens who make antibody to the portions of antigen that are absent from their red cells.

The above illustration represents a basic approach to antibody identification. More complex cases involving autoantibodies, multiple alloantibodies, mixtures of both auto- and alloantibodies, and antibodies to high-prevalence antigens often will require the resources of an immunohematology reference laboratory.

Blood group DNA-based typing in pretransfusion testing

Blood group antigens other than ABO and RhD are often referred to as *minor blood group antigens*. Testing for antigens beyond the ABO and RhD groups is referred to as performing an *extended phenotype*. For pretransfusion testing, knowing which common clinically significant antigens are expressed on the patient's RBCs and which antigens the patient lacks, and hence may have the corresponding antibody in the serum or plasma, is very useful for antibody identification. In the past, this information has not been readily available because performing extended typing for multiple minor RBC antigens by manual serologic methods is time consuming and costly. In contrast, with DNA-based testing, an extensive antigen profile on the patient (and blood donor) can be obtained in a single assay. This enables antigen matching of patients with donors for transfusion, especially for patients who are chronic transfused and have multiple blood group antibodies, or patients with auto-antibodies reactive with all red cells when compatibility cannot be demonstrated by routine serologic methods.[13,14]

Donor–recipient testing
Recipient prior records check
As part of blood transfusion safety and quality assurance, the results of current ABO, Rh, antibody detection, and compatibility tests must be checked against records of any previous tests [10(p36–37)], if performed. This must be accomplished before blood is released for transfusion, preferably when a sample is first received for pretransfusion testing. The records must be reviewed for ABO and Rh, difficulties in typing, clinically significant antibodies, severe adverse events related to transfusion, and any special transfusion requirements. Discrepancies between past and present ABO and Rh typing results must be thoroughly investigated. Importantly, previously identified clinically significant antibodies must be taken into consideration when selecting and crossmatching blood for present and future transfusions to avoid delayed transfusion reactions, as a majority of clinically significant antibodies drop to serologically undetectable levels.[15]

Selection of blood for transfusion
ABO and Rh
RBCs or whole blood selected for transfusion must be compatible with the serum of the intended recipient. To avoid the hemolytic and often fatal consequences of an ABO-mismatched transfusion, red cells carrying A and/or B antigens should not be transfused to a patient unless the patient's red cells also carry those antigens. Group O individuals should receive group O red cells, but AB individuals can receive red cells of any ABO type. Rh-negative individuals, particularly females of childbearing potential, should receive Rh-negative blood.

Unexpected antibodies
When the identified antibodies, or those previously identified and not now reacting, are known to cause accelerated destruction of transfused incompatible red cells, blood selected for transfusion must be tested with FDA-licensed methods and reagents, if available, and shown to lack the corresponding antigen or antigens.[10(p37)] Examples of potential significant antibodies include those directed toward antigens of the RH, JK, KEL, and FY systems, and the S and s antigens of the MNS system, as well as some other antibodies active at 37 °C and/or by an IAT as indicated in Table 16.2. Antigen testing performed by the donor center and included on the product label or tie tag does not require repeat testing.[10(p35)] When antibodies with specificities directed toward M, N, P_1, and Lewis antigens are present, particularly when the antibodies react best at or below room temperature, blood selected for transfusion need only be shown to be compatible by IAT following 37 °C incubation; demonstrating that compatible units lack the relevant antigen(s) is optional and not required. When autoantibodies are present, it must be determined that the autoantibody is not masking a concomitant, clinically significant alloantibody.[6,11]

Crossmatch
Before issue of RBCs or whole blood, a sample of the recipient's serum or plasma must be tested against the donor cells from an integrally attached segment, with the exception of emergency

release. The method used should be capable of detecting ABO incompatibility and demonstrate clinically significant antibodies, including an IAT. However, if no clinically significant antibodies were detected in the antibody screening and there is no history of alloantibodies, only testing to detect ABO incompatibility is required.[10(p38)]

Serologic detection of ABO incompatibility
Detection of ABO incompatibility can be done serologically by performing an immediate-spin crossmatch between the prospective recipient's serum or plasma and donor red cells. Use of EDTA–saline to prevent false-negative results from prozone by complement-fixing high-titer anti-A and anti-B has been suggested.[11]

Computer detection of ABO incompatibility
Computer software may be designed and used to detect ABO incompatibility between the sample submitted for pretransfusion testing and the donor unit selected for transfusion.[10(p38)] This has been termed an *electronic crossmatch* (EXM) and replaces the immediate-spin test for detecting ABO incompatibility.

There are a number of requirements, including validation of the system on site, and that the system recognize and correlate antibody detection results, comparison of previous records, concordant ABO on the recipient from at least two determinations, donor component and unit number and ABO/Rh retype results, as well as logic to alert the user to discrepancies between donor unit labeling and confirmatory test interpretation, and to ABO incompatibilities between the recipient and the donor unit. FDA guidance on requirements is available.[16] The advantages of implementing an EXM include technologist time savings, reduced sample handling, avoidance of "false"-positive test results on immediate-spin crossmatch due to cold agglutinins or rouleaux, and decreased turnaround time.

Antiglobulin crossmatch
When clinically significant unexpected antibodies are present, or a patient's records indicate that such antibodies have been detected previously, blood selected for transfusion must be tested with the patient's serum or plasma by an IAT. Any of the methods described in this chapter for antibody detection can be used.

An antiglobulin crossmatch can also be performed routinely on recipients with nonreactive screening tests for unexpected antibodies. However, the predictive value of a positive IAT crossmatch following nonreactive screening tests for unexpected antibodies is sufficiently low that many large hospital transfusion services do not perform an IAT crossmatch except as required above. Those that choose to perform an optional IAT crossmatch aim to detect ABO incompatibility, detect unexpected antibodies to low-incidence antigens that are missed in pretransfusion screening tests, detect antibodies manifesting dosage, and consider this testing as a second safety check for antibodies potentially missed in screening tests due to technical error.

Extended antigen matching by DNA-based typing
When a patient has a positive DAT due to autoantibodies with serum autoantibody reactive with all cells on the antibody panel and donor red cells, time- and resource-consuming differential allogeneic absorptions will be required to determine the presence or absence of alloantibodies underlying the autoantibody.[6,11] Establishing the patient's most probable extended red cell antigen phenotype can be performed on samples with a positive DAT by

DNA-based assays. This approach also allows for matching the antigen profile of the absorbing RBCs to that of the patient, thereby reducing the number of cell types required for absorption. Most importantly, it also allows for matching the antigen profile of the donor to that of the patient for the most clinically significant, common antigens (e.g., C, c, E, e, Fy^a, Fy^b, Jk^a, Jk^b, and S, s) when transfusion is required. This avoids the use of "least incompatible" blood for transfusion, and allows transfusion of units "antigen-matched for clinically significant blood group antigens" to mitigate delayed transfusion reactions and to circumvent additional alloimmunization.

Labeling

Before blood is released for transfusion, the container shall have an affixed label or tie tag indicating the recipient's two independent identifiers (usually first and last names and hospital identification number), the donor unit number, and the interpretation of compatibility tests, if performed.[10(p41)]

Issue

At the time that blood and blood components are issued, there must be a final check of transfusion service records to include the recipient's two independent identifiers, ABO group and Rh type; the donor unit number (or pool number for platelets and cryoprecipitate) and ABO group and Rh of the donor, if required; the expiration date and time, if applicable; the interpretation of crossmatch tests, if performed; and the date and time of issue.[10(p42)] The unit must be inspected visually before release; if any abnormality in color or appearance is noted, the unit should not be issued. A record must be made of this inspection.

Emergency release

When a patient's ABO group is not known, group O RBCs are issued.[10(p43)] For female patients of childbearing potential, these should also be Rh-negative. If the ABO group and Rh type have been determined on a current sample, type-specific or ABO-compatible RBCs may be issued. The container label or tie tag should conspicuously indicate that compatibility testing was not completed at the time the unit was released. Testing should be completed expeditiously, and the records should contain a signed statement from the requesting physician indicating the need for transfusion before completion of compatibility (or any other testing, including infectious disease) testing.

Administration of blood and blood components

The blood bank or transfusion service director should participate in the development of recipient consent for transfusion, as well as protocols for administration of blood and components, including the use of infusion devices and the identification, evaluation, and reporting of adverse events related to transfusion.[10(p43–44)]

The physician's written order must be reviewed, and after issue and immediately before transfusion all information must be verified bedside, including: the recipient's two independent identifiers and ABO/Rh, donation number and donor ABO/Rh, interpretation of tests, and special transfusion requirements, and that the unit is satisfactory in appearance and has not expired.

The patient's medical records must include the transfusion order, documentation of patient consent, name of component, donation number, date and time of transfusion, pre- and posttransfusion vital signs, amount transfused, and identification of the transfusionist and any adverse events.

Biovigilance

Blood transfusion is not without risks, ranging in severity from febrile nonhemolytic reactions to red cell alloimmunization, disease transmission, and death from bacterial contamination or transfusion of incompatible blood.

Biovigilance systems and networks have been established to track adverse reactions and incidents associated with blood collection and transfusion. These programs have been established in many countries to gather and analyze data to identify trends and risks and to recommend best practices and interventions with the goal of providing improved patient care and safety, while reducing overall costs. The program provides benchmarking internally and against national averages, consistent definitions for adverse reactions, and analysis by experts for the purpose of recommending nationwide health and safety enhancements, for risk mitigation, and to facilitate better understanding of reactions.[17,18]

Adverse event reporting of patient outcomes in the United States is focused through a patient safety organization (PSO) dedicated to confidentially analyzing data on adverse reactions and incidents associated with blood transfusion to communicate best practices and to design interventions to improve patient safety.

Conclusion

Compatibility testing is designed to detect serologic incompatibility between the donor unit and the intended recipient, and to prevent both clerical and technical errors that may have serious if not fatal consequences. Most importantly, there can be no substitute for proper patient identification, proper sample labeling, and proper performance of serologic tests.

Although considerable resources have been spent to reduce infectious disease transmission following blood transfusion, the elimination of process errors in transfusion deserves serious attention and resource allocation. These include WBIT, resulting from misidentification of the patient at time of sample collection or mislabeling of the collection tube; inappropriate transfusion, which exposes patients to the hazards of transfusions that they did not need; and mis-transfusion with transfusion of the wrong unit or transfusion to the wrong patient.

Use of DNA-based testing (genomics) in transfusion medicine

DNA-based testing for blood group antigens was introduced more than a decade ago following cloning of the blood group genes. Most blood group antigens result from single nucleotide gene polymorphisms (SNPs) inherited in a Mendelian manner, making assay design and interpretation fairly straightforward. Current methods for testing include amplification of target gene sequences by polymerase chain reaction (PCR), followed by manual or automated downstream analysis. Semi-automated systems enable large-scale typing of patients and donors for multiple antigens.[14]

There is nearly complete concordance between DNA (genotype) and serology (phenotype). Discrepancies are most often due to gene mutations that weaken or silence expression of the antigen, or in many cases they are due to errors in the manual process associated with serologic testing and recording of results.[19] ABO and RhD typing is more complex and requires a higher resolution approach than is required for minor antigen typing.

DNA-based typing is very useful in a number of clinical situations encountered in transfusion medicine (Table 16.8). These include typing of patients who are multiply transfused, who have

Table 16.8 DNA-based typing for patient and donor testing

Transfusion Recipients	Prenatal Practice	Blood Donors
Type RBCs of patients who have been recently transfused	To determine gene copy number (zygosity) of paternal sample	Large-scale typing to locate donors negative for multiple antigens
Type RBCs of patients whose RBCs are coated with IgG (+DAT)	Type amniocytes to identify a fetus at risk for anemia or hemolytic disease	To detect weak D antigen expression to confirm D-negative typing of donors
To distinguish alloantibody from autoantibody	RHD genotyping of maternal sample for weak D or partial D	To detect weak expression of antigens (Fy^b, e, etc.)
To determine antigen profile in patient who has received an allogeneic stem cell transplant		To determine zygosity of reagent panel cells: D, S, and Fy
Type RBCs when no serologic reagents available: Do^a, Do^b; Js^a, Js^b; V/VS, etc.		
To resolve serologic typing discrepancies		

a positive DAT (with or without serum autoantibody), and who are receiving chronic transfusion therapy, and for locating antigen-negative blood, especially when no serologic reagent is available. Applications in prenatal medicine include assessment of risk for hemolytic disease when the mother has a blood group antibody, and accurate determination of the RhD status of a mother to guide Rh immune globulin prophylaxis.[20,21]

Disclaimer

The author has disclosed no conflicts of interest.

Key references

A full reference list for this chapter is available at: http://www.wiley.com/go/simon/transfusion

1 Kuby TJ, Kindt T, Osborne B, Goldsby R, Eds *Immunology*. 6th ed. New York: W.H. Freeman, 2006.

3 Daniels G. *Human blood groups*. 2nd ed. Cambridge, MA: Blackwell Science, 2002.

7 Reid ME, Lomas-Frances C, Olsson ML. *The blood group antigen FACTS book*. 3rd ed. Amsterdam: Elsevier, 2012.

8 FDA. Fatalities reported to the FDA following blood collection and transfusion. 2014. http://www.fda.gov/BiologicsBloodVaccines/SafetyAvailability/ReportaProblem/TransfusionDonationFatalities/ucm346639.htm

10 AABB. *Standards for blood banks and transfusion services*. Bethesda, MD: AABB, 2014.

CHAPTER 17

Platelet production and kinetics

Christopher A. Tormey[1,2] & Henry M. Rinder[2,3,4]

[1]Transfusion Medicine, Veterans Affairs Medical Center, West Haven, CT, USA
[2]Department of Laboratory Medicine, Yale School of Medicine, Yale University, New Haven, CT, USA
[3]Hematology Laboratories, Yale-New Haven Hospital, New Haven, CT, USA
[4]Department of Internal Medicine, Yale School of Medicine, Yale University, New Haven, CT, USA

Platelet production

Platelets are essential for normal hemostasis. In adult humans, a normal circulating concentration of $150–450 \times 10^6$ platelets per mL is maintained by the marrow's production and release into blood of at least 75–100 billion platelets per day.[1] This chapter will use the term *megakaryopoiesis* as synonymous with either *megakaryocytopoiesis* or *thrombopoiesis* to denote the complete pathway of cell production from earliest progenitor to the terminal circulating platelet. *Platelet biogenesis* will refer to the final physical stages of megakaryopoiesis that result in circulating platelets.

Early megakaryopoiesis: proliferation of megakaryocytes

In mammalian physiology, circulating platelets in the blood are anucleate cells derived from their bone marrow precursors, megakaryocytes (MKs).[2] Megakaryopoiesis, under homeostatic conditions, is under the overall control of two primary growth factors: thrombopoietin (TPO) and stem cell factor (SCF).[3,4] Thus, any mutation that renders the TPO receptor, cMPL, unresponsive (human congenital amegakaryocytic thrombocytopenia) or genetic deletions in mice of TPO or SCF will result in severe thrombocytopenia.[5,6]

MK development can be considered to include three stages: (1) proliferating progenitors with DNA content of 2N, (2) MKs undergoing endomitosis, and (3) cytoplasmic maturation of MKs preceding release of platelets. However, 2N MKs can mature and make platelets; studies have demonstrated that neonatal MK progenitors are hyperproliferative. Low-ploidy neonatal MKs are generated at a much higher rate than their adult counterparts, likely mediated by upregulated thrombopoietin signaling. It is likely that the fetal/neonatal rapidly expanding bone marrow is the impetus for this developmental difference in megakaryopoiesis.[7]

MK development does not occur in a single marrow location; instead, developing MKs move in a directed manner across distinct marrow spaces (Figure 17.1). The earliest MK progenitors proliferate near the cortical bone (i.e., in the osteoblastic or endosteal niche), where TPO acts in a synergistic fashion with other cytokines to promote MK evolution from stem cell precursors and subsequent proliferation of MKs.[8]

Hematopoietic stem cells (HSCs) give rise to a common myeloid progenitor cell. Biphenotypic megakaryocyte–erythroid precursors (MEPs) are then derived from this common myeloid precursor; TPO and other hematopoietic mediators, such as erythropoietin, SCF, and interleukin-11,[9] function synergistically to cause the bipotential precursor to differentiate toward the MK lineage and become promegakaryoblasts.[8] Promegakaryoblasts undergo endomitosis in order to increase their ploidy content (polyploidization), a process that is probably necessary for normal maturation into MKs in the adult marrow, but, as noted above,[7] is not required for cord blood–derived MKs and platelet production in utero. Still, both of these platelet production mechanisms, fetal and adult, are under the general control of TPO.[10,11]

Two major transcription factors involved in differentiation of the common myeloid precursor (CMP) are PU.1, which regulates granulocyte–monocyte precursors, and GATA1, which drives differentiation of the MEPs.[12] The downregulation of PU.1 expression in the CMP is the first event associated with the restriction of precursor differentiation to erythroid and MK lineages.[13] In response to TPO, SCF, and other cytokines and chemokines, the bipotential MEP can develop into the highly proliferative, early MK burst-forming unit (BFU-MK), or the smaller, more mature CFU-MK, both of which express CD34.[14] GATA1 is thought to have a specific effect on fetal megakaryopoiesis; GATA1 mutations occur in trisomy 21–associated transient myeloproliferative disorder, which generally resolves spontaneously following the newborn period.

The endomitotic cell cycle in MKs consists of G1, DNA replication in S, and then G2 phase but an aborted M phase. In the 2N to 4N transition, MKs fail to complete anaphase B, telophase, and cytokinesis. After the 4N stage, M phase is generally aborted prior to cytokinesis, and the cells demonstrate multiple pole spindles, then enter a Gap-phase that enables reentry into the subsequent S-phase, which occurs repeatedly to form multilobulated nuclei that may reach ploidy levels as high as 128N. The mechanism of

Rossi's Principles of Transfusion Medicine, Fifth Edition. Edited by Toby L. Simon, Jeffrey McCullough, Edward L. Snyder, Bjarte G. Solheim, and Ronald G. Strauss.
© 2016 John Wiley & Sons, Ltd. Published 2016 by John Wiley & Sons, Ltd.

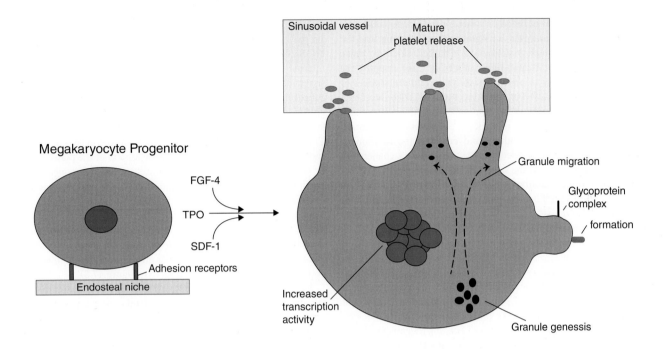

Terminal Megakaryocyte Maturation

Figure 17.1 The model of megakaryocyte terminal maturation in marrow sinusoidal niche. Megakaryocyte progenitors in the osteoblastic (or endosteal) niche mature under the influence of, among other cytokines, thrombopoietin (TPO), stromal cell–derived factor (SDF)-1, and fibroblast growth factor (FGF)-4. Once the maturing megakaryocyte has moved away from the cortical bone and into the vascular niche, adjacent to sinusoidal blood vessels, there is now increased transcription of proteins that will eventually appear as platelet membrane components (e.g., gpIb/IIIa) or are packaged within platelet granules (e.g., von Willebrand factor). Alpha and dense granules migrate along with the extension of membrane processes and eventually into the tips of these pro-platelet processes, which form the pre-platelet terminal ends. As these terminal ends extend into the sinusoidal vessels, shear causes release of the pre-platelets into the blood circulation; mature terminal platelets are then derived from the pre-platelets within the blood.

polyploidization is complex. Cyclin D3 is overexpressed (partly under the influence of TPO) in the G1-phase of maturing cells, which helps to overcome the normal block to polyploidization.[15] Aurora-B kinase (AIM-1 kinase), which mediates late anaphase and cytokinesis, had been hypothesized to be deficient during MK prophase and early anaphase, but others have found this critical kinase to be normally localized and completely functional in endomitotic MKs.[16] Other pathways mediating polyploidization include MKL1-induced downregulation of ARH-GEF2 (discussed later in this section), which is critical for late cytokinesis.[17]

Ploidy classes in MKs are identified as multiples starting with the diploid 2N baseline (i.e., 4N, 8N, etc.). The ploidy distribution obtained by flow cytometry in both fractionated and unfractionated normal human marrow demonstrates a ploidy value of 16N in 50% of the total MK population, with the remainder of MKs equally split between cells having 8N ploidy or lower and MKs of ploidy 32N or higher.[18] Mature MKs eventually give rise to circulating platelets by the acquisition of cytoplasmic structural changes necessary for platelet formation and release into the circulation.[19,20] MKs reach cell sizes of 50–100 microns in 128N.[21,22]

As the MK matures, the polyploid nucleus becomes eccentrically located within the cell, and the cytoplasm expands as it accommodates the formation of an extensive demarcation membrane system (DMS).[23] This mass of DMS is the reserve membrane supply that will subsequently form pro-platelet projections once the MK has migrated to its perivascular niche; release of pro-platelets into

sinusoidal blood vessels will then give rise to circulating pre-platelets, sometimes termed *reticulated platelets*.[24]

Control of megakaryopoiesis

Research into the regulation and ordering of megakaryopoiesis has expanded significantly in the past few years, aided by relevant murine models, as well as unilineage differentiation cultures. Upregulation of the chemokine receptor CXCR4 (whose ligand is CXCL12) is associated with MK maturation and differentiation.[25] Although CXCL12 by itself cannot stimulate MK growth and differentiation, this finding has importance for non-homeostatic regulatory mechanisms of platelet production because CXCL12 acts synergistically with TPO both in vitro and in vivo.[26–28] Inflammation is a significant and frequent cause of thrombocytosis perhaps as a compensatory process to promote angiogenesis and wound healing. The proinflammatory VEGFR1-mediated pathway has now been shown to stimulate further upregulation of CXCR4 on MKs in a murine model,[29] and the VEGFR1 pathway additionally stimulates MK endomitosis. CXCL12 also affects late megakaryopoiesis by stimulating MKs to migrate from the endosteal environs to the vascular niche; as noted in the "Late Megakaryopoiesis" section, MKs in the vascular niche can interact with sinusoidal blood vessels to release pro-platelets. Hence, inflammation mediated by VEGFR1 enhances platelet production at multiple levels via the chemokine CXCR4.[29]

It is important to understand megakaryopoiesis not only for in vivo production, but also because of potential ex vivo implications. Donation of blood or apheresis for platelet units that are eventually to be transfused is a significant undertaking, and the short shelf life of donor platelets (see Chapter 19) is a major impediment to medical care. Hence, there is some impetus for developing alternatives to platelet products or artificial sources of actual platelet products.[30] For the latter, human CD34+ stem cell populations have been described that can generate ex vivo functional MKs with ploidy levels up to 32N.[31–33] However, generating sufficient MK numbers in culture and ensuring the subsequent production of adequate platelets per MK are still very challenging aspects to this strategy. At the same time, though, such studies also improve our understanding of the physical environment of the marrow,[34–36] the specific niche requirements of MK differentiation and pro-platelet release,[37] and the requisite physical and cellular interactions needed for optimized megakaryopoiesis.[38–40]

Thrombopoietin

As noted above, megakaryopoiesis is the process of differentiation of HSCs that leads to platelet production characterized by an initial phase of proliferation of MK progenitors, followed by subsequent differentiation of maturing MKs that do not proliferate. Because both processes are mediated largely by TPO, this suggests that there is a physiologic balance in TPO's ability to both enhance and inhibit proliferation.[41] Regulation of this balance is important for timing and adequacy of platelet production. TPO has been shown to act via mitogen-activated protein kinase (MAPK) signaling to halt MK proliferation and induce the same MKs to undergo differentiation.[42] Besides MAPK, work on cell lines has shown that this balance of TPO-induced proliferation versus differentiation is also dependent upon JAK2 and MPL protein levels.[41] When either one of the JAK2 or MPL proteins is expressed at relatively lower levels, TPO exposure will induce preferential MK proliferation via weak MAPK signaling; by contrast, when both proteins are highly expressed and MAPK signaling is strongly activated, MK cell cycle arrest occurs,[20–22] which is accompanied by MK differentiation.[43,44]

Steady-state megakaryopoiesis supplies about 10^{11} platelets every day into the circulation. MKs will respond to changes in platelet lifespan, increasing by 10-fold with destructive thrombocytopenic conditions,[45,46] and the proportion of higher ploidy MKs also increases.[47] Compensatory responses of marrow MKs are evident within 24–48 hours after inducing thrombocytopenia; in response to thrombocytapheresis and in thrombocytopenia caused by immune destruction, there is a marked increase in MK number and size.[22,48] Reciprocal decreases in MK size, ploidy, and volume occur with experimentally induced thrombocytosis.[49,50] These alterations, found in both experimental animals and human subjects, are primarily mediated by TPO.[45]

TPO is the most potent cytokine for stimulating the proliferation and maturation of MK progenitor cells into their terminally differentiated form. TPO stimulates MKs to increase cell size and ploidy and to form pro-platelet processes.[45] TPO can also act in synergy with other hematopoietic cytokines and has been used to expand human HSCs and MK progenitor cells in vitro.[51–54]

Human thrombopoietin is encoded by the *THPO* gene, located on chromosome 3q26.3-3q27, which yields a 30 kDa, 353-amino-acid precursor protein. The mature molecule, composed of 332 amino acids, is acidic and heavily glycosylated. TPO shares high homology with erythropoietin (EPO) at its N-terminus. TPO binds to the c-Mpl receptor on platelets and MKs and selectively initiates proliferation, maturation, and cytoplasmic delivery of platelets into the circulation.[55,56] A large percentage (perhaps 50% or more) of

circulating TPO is produced constitutively by the liver, and its levels are partly regulated by the extent of TPO binding to c-Mpl receptors on circulating platelets and marrow MKs, which results in the internal elimination of TPO–c-Mpl complexes.[56,57] However, recent data suggest that hepatic secretion of TPO is only partially constitutive, and a significant regulation of TPO production occurs via the senescent platelet mass interacting with hepatocyte receptors (see the "Platelet Kinetics" section).[58] Blood and marrow levels of TPO are usually inversely related to marrow MK mass and peripheral platelet counts;[45] hence, regulatory aspects of the platelet mass by circulating TPO levels are sometimes termed the *sponge model*. High-affinity Mpl on platelets binds TPO, which is then internalized and degraded, allowing the circulating platelet mass to affect, at least in part, the amount of TPO available to marrow MKs for stimulation (see Figure 17.2); low platelet counts allow more available TPO to induce megakaryopoiesis. In the sponge model of TPO regulation, as long as constitutive liver production of TPO occurs, total platelet mass is preserved (Figure 17.2).

The sponge model does well to explain why plasma levels of TPO are increased by several orders of magnitude in patients with hypoproductive thrombocytopenia, and why TPO levels decline after recovery of hematopoiesis.[56,59] However, when severe platelet destruction via FcγR binding causes thrombocytopenia, such as in immune thrombocytopenic purpura (ITP), TPO levels are not as escalated as might be expected from the degree of thrombocytopenia. This was thought to be due to the markedly increased platelet turnover rate,[60] but data on platelet clearance via hepatic interaction suggest otherwise: that ITP bypasses normal senescent mechanisms of platelet loss that are partly responsible for upregulating TPO production.[58] Thus, megakaryopoiesis appears to be regulated by plasma levels of unbound TPO, which reflects the balance between constitutive TPO production, the rate of platelet and MK binding dictated by overall platelet levels, and TPO production regulation by senescent platelet clearance by the liver.

The TPO receptor (c-Mpl) is constitutively expressed on most hematopoietic progenitors, MKs, and terminal platelets but can be modulated by TPO binding and receptor internalization. Mpl binding to TPO induces conformational change in the receptor, which stimulates JAK2 and starts downstream signaling. TPO avidly binds to and activates the c-Mpl receptors on MK, which then initiate signal transduction via the JAK family of kinases constitutively bound to the membrane-proximal cytoplasmic domains of c-Mpl. Elimination of a functional c-Mpl gene (located on chromosome 1p34), or its congenital absence, results in severe thrombocytopenia accompanied by decreased HSCs and lineage-committed progenitor cells.[45]

Genetic regulation of megakaryopoiesis

Other critical regulators of megakaryopoiesis have recently been elucidated, and, as noted above with JAK2/MPL, these pathways affect both early MK proliferation and the later stages of MK differentiation and pro-platelet release. Studies of acute megakaryoblastic leukemia (AMKL) have found that two of the three myocardin family of genes (i.e., MKL1 and MKL2) may be important for megakaryopoiesis, and mutation of the MKL1 gene is part of the t(1;22) translocation found in some infantile AMKLs, where the *MKL1* gene is fused to the *RBM15* (RNA binding motif protein 15) gene.[61] MKL1 is known to act as a cofactor for serum response factor (SRF) to induce muscle differentiation.[62,63] Although SRF is a transcription factor widely expressed in hematopoietic cells, until recently it was not considered active in megakaryopoiesis. However,

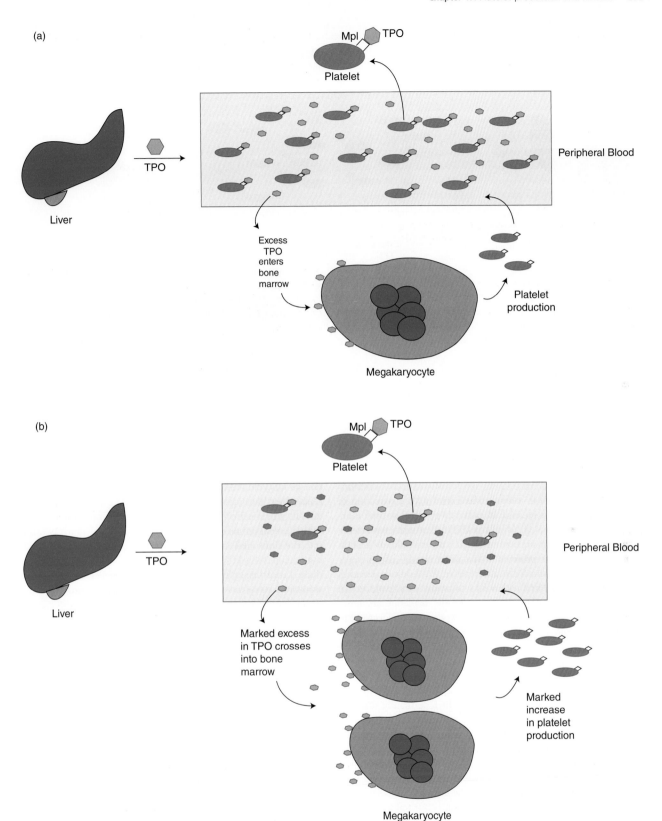

Figure 17.2 The "sponge" model of megakaryopoiesis. The liver constitutively secretes thrombopoietin (TPO) into the blood; Mpl receptors on platelets bind, internalize, and degrade TPO. In this model, the platelet mass determines the amount of free TPO in the circulation. During homeostasis (A), the normal platelet count reflects balanced platelet production and destruction; free TPO in blood moves to the marrow to stimulate steady-state megakaryopoiesis and normal ploidy (e.g., 8N) distribution. When destructive thrombocytopenia occurs, free TPO is increased (B) because there are too few platelets available for binding; a larger amount of TPO is available to the marrow, which results in an increased number of megakaryocytes with higher average ploidy (e.g., 16N). In contrast, reactive thrombocytosis (e.g., with chronic inflammation) results in less free TPO (C) available to transit to the marrow; decreased megakaryopoiesis results in fewer megakaryocytes with lower average ploidy (e.g., 2N) levels.

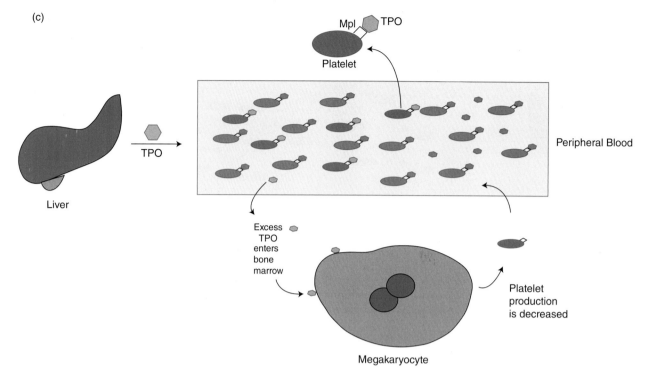

Figure 17.2 *Continued*

SRF can regulate cytoskeletal genes critical for MK differentiation, and it has a role in the actin cytoskeleton development of stem cells.[64] SRF, in association with cofactors other than MKL1, is also a downstream target for MAPK signaling.[65–69]

In murine models, hematopoietic-specific SRF knockouts demonstrated decreased platelet counts, concomitant with a reduction in polyploid MKs and an increase in early MKs with abnormal morphology.[61] The morphologic dysplasia and macrothrombocytopenia induced by SRF deletion are accompanied by downregulation of actin cytoskeletal regulatory proteins in the MKs, clearly disruptive of essential MK mechanisms for megakaryopoiesis.[70] Additional studies found that SRF is required with MKL1 to produce polyploidization during MK differentiation. The effects of SRF depletion are more extreme than those of MKL1 deletion, which also causes a decrease in platelet counts and an increase in MK progenitors in the bone marrow. These findings suggest: (1) SRF transcription is critical for terminal MK processes that lead to pro-platelet formation and platelet release; and (2) there are additional factors besides MKL1 that promote SRF-mediated megakaryopoiesis.[61,71] The authors suggested that MKL2 expressed in MKs might redundantly function with MKL1 in murine MK maturation.[71]

When both MKL1 and MKL2 are absent, the arrest of MK maturation (the majority of MKs with ploidy of 4N or less) is more dramatic than with absence of either alone. Expression of the guanine nucleotide exchange factor GEFH1, which promotes RhoA activity to complete cytokinesis,[72] may be linked to MKL1 regulation of MK maturation. GEFH1 expression is normally decreased early in MK endomitosis and subsequently rises with maturation, and SRF is known to bind to the GEFH1 promoter in hematopoietic cells.[73] By contrast, GEFH1 is increased when MKL1 is absent, and GEFH1 is not downregulated at any point during megakaryopoiesis. Hence, MKL1 regulation of SRF-influenced transcription is probably most relevant to early MK maturation. RUNX1 also plays a role in early MK maturation because it silences the nonmuscle myosin

IIB heavy chain, MYH10, a required event for the transition from mitosis to endomitosis.[74]

Late megakaryopoiesis: differentiation of megakaryocytes

Once they have completed the proliferative phase, MKs subsequently migrate from the peri-cortex, partly under the control of matrix metalloproteinases (MMPs), through the marrow stroma into the sinusoidal area (i.e., the vascular niche). It is here that the nonproliferating MKs form extensive pro-platelet processes; when these processes extend through the endothelial cells lining the sinusoidal blood vessels, pro-platelets are released into the circulation (Figure 17.1).

Differentiated polyploid MKs are responsible for terminal platelet production; as MKs differentiate, a central invaginated membrane branching system, often termed the *demarcation membrane system* (DMS), forms that is contiguous with the plasma membrane.[75] This is similar to the open canalicular system (OCS) of the platelets and possibly the precursor for the OCS. The DMS, which begins in earlier MKs, will eventually provide the membranes needed for pro-platelet production and release into the circulation.

MKs synthesize some of their α-granule constituents (e.g., von Willebrand factor), while other granule contents (e.g., fibrinogen) are incorporated into the granules by endocytosis and/or pinocytosis of plasma proteins. There is growing evidence that α granules are not identical and are actually quite heterogeneous in their content; moreover, they have the capacity for differential release with activation.[76]

Physical MK changes that lead to platelet production and release

The terminology of platelet production is still defined by individual studies, but in this chapter, we will affirm that the differentiated pro-platelet-producing MK is the result of the extension of multiple branched membrane evaginations. The elongated branching projections will be called *pro-platelets*, and the platelet-sized end swellings are termed *pre-platelets*. It appears that the DMS of the differentiated MK is particularly adapted to production of platelets via continuous directed remodeling of its underlying cytoskeletal structure; investigations into this dynamic process have focused on the roles of actin, microtubular rearrangements, and the surface integrin proteins.

Platelet biogenesis from MKs starts with (1) microtubule reorganization into pseudopod structures, (2) followed by spreading of these structures and their eventual development into pro-platelet processes, accompanied by (3) organelle inclusion within the processes such that the organelles are eventually concentrated at the tips of the pro-platelet branches, and, finally, (4) actin-dependent branching to extensively amplify pro-platelet processes, with the DMS serving as the membrane reservoir for this expansion.

Ultrastructural studies of the differentiated MKs demonstrate that late-stage MKs are characterized by peripheralization of the DMS membranes. This is accomplished by the membranes thinning out (evagination), such that they produce branching processes, termed *pro-platelets*, which finally extend into sinusoidal blood vessels. These processes have platelet-sized swellings all along their structure, but most importantly, the swellings at the branch tips appear to be the source of pro-platelets. Pro-platelets appear in the blood after vascular shear forces interact with the projections that extend through the extracellular matrix; shear causes the pro-platelet tips to separate and enter the sinusoidal vessels on their way into the peripheral blood circulation.[75]

Microtubules are critical for pro-platelet membrane process elongation.[61] Repeated rounds of microtubule extension (bundling) and bending to form pro-platelet processes can be characterized by physical forces such that, on balance, final platelet size can indeed be correctly predicted to be in the micron radius range.[77,78] The subsequent branching of these processes is the end result of multiple rounds of fission at both the midbody and the ends of the projections; these fission events are the result of actin-dependent bending and branching that amplify the pro-platelet ends, thereby resulting in an increased potential number of platelets to be released once membrane projections penetrate the sinusoidal vasculature.[79] Live-cell imaging has been used to examine the related MK-specific mechanisms of drug-induced thrombocytopenia. Trastuzumab emtansine is known to result in thrombocytopenia; the drug is taken up by mouse MKs and has been shown to inhibit MK differentiation and to disrupt pro-platelet formation. This inhibitory effect of trastuzumab emtansine is mediated by its induction of abnormal tubule organization within MKs, resulting in abnormal tubule thickness and fewer branching processes.[80]

Like platelet activation, there is a role for shear forces in megakaryopoiesis, specifically relative to both MK maturation and platelet release.[81] DNA synthesis can be enhanced by shear stress in immature MKs, and similarly, both MK fragmentation and generation of pro-platelets are increased.[81] The penetration of pro-platelet extensions into sinusoidal vessels is the precursor to release of platelet precursors and whole/partial MK fragments into blood; both processes will give rise to terminal circulating platelets.[37,82–84] High shear stress is known to promote higher pro-platelet formation via cytoskeletal remodeling.[37] It is possible that shear forces act physiologically because hemodynamic stress in humans (e.g., exercise) has been shown to elevate platelet counts.[85,86]

The end tips of the pro-platelets are released, as noted in this chapter, when they are exposed to shear forces; based on

ultrastructural images, barbell-shaped pro-platelets and circular pre-platelets are released from the differentiated MK into the blood. Thus, current studies suggest that terminal platelet formation actually occurs within the blood[77] and, to some unknown extent, within the pulmonary bed as well.[84,87] The circular pre-platelets may be identical to reticulated platelets and/or to the large platelets that are present in several of the defined macrothrombocytopenia syndromes. In studies of hemostasis in human ITP, reticulated platelets (RPs) have been found to contain twice as much α-granule content as older circulating platelets.[88] RPs also have an increased density of membrane receptors compared to older platelet cohorts, bolstering evidence that the RP subset may represent the circular pre-platelets or released pro-platelets.[89]

Data also suggest that circular pre-platelets can revert to a barbell pro-platelet form. When barbell pro-platelets divide, they form two platelets that are larger (i.e., have a demonstrably higher median MPV) when compared with older circulating platelets. However, these intermediate stages of terminal platelet formation after pro-platelet excision are relatively dynamic, and the exact sequence of platelet maturation has not been confirmed by independent studies.

There is also evidence that a small fraction of in vivo circulating platelets, which are thought to be terminally differentiated, may duplicate in the bloodstream under the stimulation of thrombocytopenia;[75] the latter physiology may perhaps be analogous to circular pre-platelets reverting to the barbell pro-platelet form, which subsequently is able to divide and form two distinct terminal platelets. Such young pre-platelets should be differentiated from the majority of circulating platelets that can neither divide nor revert to a barbell shape. It is also likely that such younger platelets have greater ability for continued protein translation, and there is imaging evidence for higher content of ribosomes, hence the possibility that these platelets also possibly represent the reticulated platelets, as defined by elevated RNA content, in comparison to the majority of circulating, older platelets.

Insights into platelet production and sizing

The physical forces that regulate pro-platelet extension and their release and final differentiation to a specific number and size of mature circulating platelets appear to be governed by conservation of mass.[90,91] Some defects in platelet receptors and/or skeletal proteins (e.g., actin, tubulin, and the spectrin proteins) have helped to elucidate these physical influences and shed light on normal terminal production of platelets from the differentiated MK.

In the macrothrombocytopenia syndromes, there appears to be a defect in terminal platelet production (i.e., regulation of pro-platelet formation, release, and/or maturation to circular pre-platelets). There is evidence that the β3 integrin plays a role in pro-platelet formation and platelet size. In Glanzmann's thrombocytopenia, where there is a β3 integrin defect producing larger platelets in some instances, there appears to be inability to constrict the ends of the pro-platelets.[92,93]

Pro-platelet extension is driven by extension and bending of microtubules that, in turn, are dependent on actin motility and actin filament turnover. Filamin A anchors receptors (β3 integrin, gpIb) to the cytoskeleton,[79,94,95] and human defects in Filamin A result in macrothrombocytopenia.[96] Although MKs are normal in number in Bernard Soulier syndrome (BSS), there is a disordered central membrane invagination system that appears to be dependent on the normal expression of gpIbα.[97,98] Knockout mice lacking gpIbα, but not gpV, have the identical macrothrombocytopenia phenotype as

BSS, making this a possible pathway defect for terminal platelet production.

Another macrothrombocytopenia syndrome, May–Hegglin anomaly, appears to have defective microtubule extension based on abnormal thickness of the packed microtubule layers;[75] this defect results in larger pro-platelet formation and release, but there is evidence that microtubule band thinning, and therefore normal extension, may also be inhibited through a distinct nontubule pathway. The May–Hegglin anomaly is caused by the MYH9 mutational defect in nonmuscle myosin IIA heavy chain[99] and produces an autosomal dominant macrothrombocytopenia in humans. Similar macrothrombocytopenia syndromes, but with varying associated phenotypes (e.g., Fechtner syndrome, Sebastian platelet syndrome, and Epstein's syndrome), are also thought to involve MYH9 defects.[100,101] The MYH9 defect has been shown to have normal MK ultrastructure by EM, that is, there is no early differentiation defect that affects the central membranes (DMS), nor is there disruption of internal granule structure.[102]

In vivo actin filament turnover is critical for the terminal processes of MK pro-platelet formation and subsequent normal platelet sizing; actin filament turnover does not appear to have an effect on MK maturation.[103] Actin depolymerizing factor (ADF)/cofilin severing proteins regulate actin turnover. Using murine knockouts, cofilin, but not ADF, was shown to be essential for normal platelet size and shape. Yet, if both proteins are knocked out, platelet formation is nearly absent; the latter is characterized by severe disruption of the MK central membrane system and disorganization and diminution of pro-platelet processes. Thus, actin has a major role in pro-platelet formation and pre-platelet conversion to the terminal platelet with normal maturation/sizing.

MK migration from the endosteal location to the vascular environs, and subsequent pro-platelet budding, clearly require dynamic rearrangement of the actin cytoskeleton, and podosomes are similarly dynamic contacts of the MK with the extracellular matrix (ECM).[104] Podosomes are actin-rich cores with an associated integrin ring structure. MK from Wiskott–Aldrich syndrome (WAS) cannot form podosomes, and WAS MKs prematurely release pro-platelets into the marrow, not blood.[105] MK podosomes have a role in degrading ECM to enhance MK motility to the vascular niche, and subsequently promote extension of pro-platelet processes into sinusoidal vessels. Normal MK formation of podosomes and their associated actin-rich protrusions across the sinusoidal basement membrane have been shown to be dependent on MMP function; both of these abilities are lost in WAS.[104]

Platelet kinetics

Platelet production as a component of platelet survival in the circulation

The kinetics of normal platelet production have been measured indirectly by determining the turnover rate of circulating platelets (platelet count divided by platelet survival corrected for recovery). The median overall rate of platelet production under steady-state conditions (platelet removal is equivalent to platelet production when the platelet count is constant) in healthy humans ranges from 35,000 to 44,000 platelets/μL/day.[106–109] The reliability of platelet turnover estimates depends on the accuracy with which each of the three variables used in calculating platelet turnover can be determined—mean platelet lifespan, recovery of platelets in the circulation, and blood platelet count. The summation error may be

considerable, as occurs among patients with severely enhanced platelet destruction (e.g., ITP).[108]

Platelet lifespan and its regulation

The human platelet lifespan is 9.5 ± 0.6 days,[106] and platelet disappearance is generally linear, hence thought to reflect platelet senescence.[109] With consumptive thrombocytopenia, the platelet lifespan is shortened, with exponential, likely random, platelet removal from circulation.[110] Platelet survival time has also been shown to shorten progressively as the platelet count decreases to <100,000/μL.[109,111] Therefore, a shortened platelet survival time in patients with thrombocytopenia does not necessarily indicate a destructive process.

Hanson and Slichter proposed a model for platelet removal that predicted shortening of platelet lifespan in relation to the level of thrombocytopenia.[109] The analysis indicated that 82% of normal platelet turnover is caused by platelet senescence; only 18% of platelet removal is due to the requirement of platelets to support vascular integrity. In this model, healthy hemostatic platelet loss represents about 7000–10,000 platelets/μL/day. Because there is evidence that clearance of platelets via hemostatic integrity is a fixed absolute requirement, thrombocytopenia caused by marrow hypoplasia causes the daily proportion of platelets removed by hemostatic consumption to rise significantly.[112] Hemostatic clearance in patients with megakaryocytic hypoplasia can actually be predicted by the platelet count (15.1–28.0% of overall platelet turnover).[112]

Kinetic modeling of platelet lifespan using labeling in murine populations suggests that, at steady state, circulating platelet senescence is internally programmed.[113] Because platelets contain the key components (Bcl-2 proteins, Bak and Bcl-x_L) of a critical apoptotic pathway that regulates lifespan,[114] it may well be that platelet lifespan and the induction of senescent platelet death are regulated by internal, programmed functions rather than external injuries or "hits."

When platelets become senescent, the physiology of their removal is postulated to include irreversible changes in membrane glycoproteins; increased platelet-associated immunoglobulin, as in ITP (with subsequent clearance of those high-immunoglobulin-expressing platelets by splenic macrophages); increased exposure of the negatively charged procoagulant lipid, phosphatidylserine, on the external platelet membrane; and decreased levels of surface sialic acid.[115] Mechanisms of platelet clearance have been examined in many studies, most with particular relevance to platelet storage (see Chapter 19), but such studies may shed light on in vivo platelet circulation. For example, desialylation of platelet receptors occurs when platelets are warmed after cold exposure;[116] warming activates sialidases in plasma that target the sialic acid residues on platelet glycoproteins. Cold exposure also primes MMP cleavage of gpIbα, and the end result of both pathways is increased platelet clearance by the liver.

This latter aspect (loss of sialic acid) of platelet senescence has recently reinforced the possibility that platelets themselves act directly on TPO mRNA expression[117–121] rather than MPL uptake of TPO as the exclusive model for regulation of hepatic production.[122–126] As platelets age in the circulation, they lose $\alpha 2,3$ sialic acid from surface glycoproteins; these desialylated platelets can then be cleared by binding to the hepatocyte Ashwell–Morell receptor (AMR), a heteromeric complex of asialoglycoprotein receptors 1 and 2.[58] Binding of platelets to the AMR induces hepatocyte TPO mRNA via JAK2–STAT3 signaling, and this may partly explain why TPO levels are higher than expected in essential thrombocythemia

Peripheral Blood

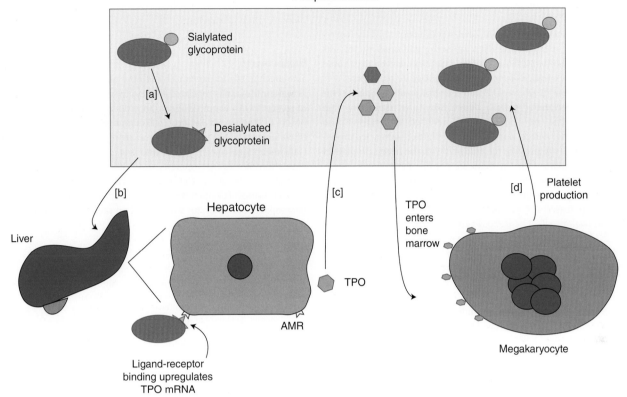

Figure 17.3 The *platelet feedback* model of megakarypoiesis. Liver secretion of thrombopoietin (TPO) into the blood is regulated by platelet-hepatocyte binding. Circulating platelets have α2,3 sialic acid on their surface glycoproteins; over time in the circulation, platelet desialylation (a) occurs. When aged desialylated platelets transit the liver (b), the desialylated platelet glycoproteins bind to their receptor, the hepatocyte Ashwell–Morell receptor (AMR). This ligand–receptor event upregulates hepatocyte TPO mRNA levels and increases TPO production. TPO secreted from the liver into the blood (c) can either bind to platelet Mpl or remain free in the circulation. Free TPO is then able to transit to the marrow (d), where it is available to stimulate megakaryopoiesis; fully sialylated platelets are then released from the marrow into the blood.

(ET) and lower than expected in ITP. In ET, where platelet lifespan is unchanged, one would expect a higher daily number of senescent platelets to be cleared by the liver, thereby inducing more TPO; by contrast, because platelets in ITP are primarily cleared by macrophage FcγR binding and would bypass the hepatocyte AMR, lower TPO production would be the result. In this model (Figure 17.3), senescent platelet regulation of TPO production accounted for up to 50% of secretion, suggesting that this pathway may even be equivalent to constitutive TPO production for regulation of platelet mass. It is unclear if the apoptotic pathway intrinsic to platelets initiates these sialylation changes, but the apoptotic mechanism does affect platelet survival,[114,127,128] including pro-apoptotic platelet clearance via the liver.[129]

As noted in the "Platelet Production" section, neonatal and adult MKs differ in their maturational abilities, and similarly, studies of neonatal platelets suggest kinetic differences from their adult counterparts. Murine studies that have examined platelet lifespan suggest that platelets survive one day longer in neonatal mice when compared to platelets in the circulation of adult mice of the same genotype.[130] The anti-apoptotic protein Bcl-2 was much higher in neonatal platelets compared with adult platelets, suggesting relatively increased resistance to apoptosis.[114,129] These findings additionally support the concept of programmed cellular senescence via

apoptosis, but they do not rule out additional processes governing nonhemostatic platelet clearance.

Newly released RPs are identified by their increased RNA content;[131] murine studies have directly confirmed that RPs are the platelet subset most recently released from MKs into the blood.[132,133] The RP% in humans correlates with thrombopoietic activity.[134] Analogous to red cell reticulocytes, RPs increase in response to destructive thrombocytopenia and decrease when MK hypoproliferation occurs with chemotherapy or intrinsic marrow aplasia.[135] The absolute RP count in humans with normal platelet counts ranges from 15,000 to 48,000/μL; this average platelet production agrees with isotopic labeling studies.

The RP% has proven valuable for detecting changes in overall platelet turnover. The RP% has been applied for predicting thrombopoietic recovery, transfusion independence, and thrombotic risk. An increase in the RP% was associated with subsequent graft-versus-host disease after allogeneic HSC transplantation.[136] Similarly, an asymptomatic increase in the RP%, with no change in platelet counts, from the first to second trimester in pregnancy, was associated with subsequent preeclampsia.[137] Asymptomatic patients with steady-state thrombocytosis and an elevated RP% or absolute RP count were at increased risk for subsequent thrombosis, and their relative risk was higher than the risk associated with a high platelet count alone.[138] The RP% and absolute RP count in thrombocytosis decrease with either successful aspirin therapy or hydroxyurea.[139,140]

A compensatory increase in platelet production and the corresponding rise in circulating RP% are well established in patients with ITP, in whom antibodies targeting platelet membrane epitopes cause platelet clearance via splenic macrophage Fc receptors.[141,142] Platelet lifespan in severe ITP can be shortened to hours. This increase in peripheral platelet destruction is so significant that platelet lifespans are shorter than predicted by Hanson and Slichter's model. Hence, posttransfusion platelet counts are probably the only way to provide the clinician with the necessary platelet survival information for the management of such patients.

Although the marrow can increase MK mass by 10-fold, this response is insufficient to maintain a normal platelet count with ITP; the increased RP% confirms the compensatory marrow production response.[143] The RP% is very sensitive to MK production, and RP changes may precede changes in platelet counts; in fact, the RP% has been shown to decline about 24 hours before platelet count recovery in ITP[88] and to similarly rebound prior to marrow recovery from chemotherapy-induced hypoplasia.[144] The RP% in both situations will eventually decrease as the platelet count approaches the normal range, indicating that restoration of a normal platelet lifespan rapidly downregulates MK platelet release.

Platelet sequestration

Approximately two-thirds of human platelets circulate while the remaining 30% of platelets are reversibly sequestered, primarily in the spleen.[145] Massive splenomegaly can cause severe thrombocytopenia (counts <50,000/μL) when as much as 90% of total-body platelet mass is sequestered in the spleen.[108,145]

Platelet accumulation in the spleen reaches 90% of maximum activity within 12.5 minutes after injection of labeled platelets.[145] Splenic pooling of platelets is reversible; intravenous epinephrine, which reduces blood flow to the spleen and causes the organ to empty passively into the circulation, will cause the platelet level to increase by 30–50%, but epinephrine does not affect platelet count in asplenic individuals.[146]

Splenectomy in humans may or may not affect platelet survival.[147] However, an animal model has demonstrated a significant (>40%) increase in platelet lifespan after splenectomy.[148] Patients with moderate splenomegaly, such as seen with cirrhosis and portal hypertension, have platelet counts in the range of 60,000–100,000/μL. Hepatic pooling of platelets probably accounts for 10% of total-body platelets, but this fraction may increase after splenectomy.[107,108]

Summary

The mechanistic understanding of how platelets are produced and how their lifespan is regulated are keys to improving the clinical care of patients with acquired thrombocytopenia and hematologic disorders that affect platelet production and survival. The possibilities of enhancing platelet storage or improving the outcome of platelet transfusion are certainly tied into the genetic and biochemical regulation of megakaryopoiesis and both the innate and environmental aspects of platelet kinetics. The following chapters on platelet storage (Chapter 19) and platelet transfusion and thrombocytopenia (Chapter 20) will expand on these critically important topics.

Key references

A full reference list for this chapter is available at: http://www.wiley.com/go/simon/transfusion

41 Besancenot R, Roos-Weil D, Tonetti C, *et al.* JAK2 and MPL protein levels determine TPO-induced megakaryocyte proliferation vs differentiation. *Blood* 2014; **124**: 2104–15.

58 Grozovsky R, Begonja AJ, Liu K, *et al.* The Ashwell-Morell receptor regulates hepatic thrombopoietin production via JAK2-STAT3 signaling. *Nature Med* 2015; **21**: 47–54.

71 Smith EC, Thon JN, Devine MT, *et al.* MKL1 and MKL2 play redundant and crucial roles in megakaryocyte maturation and platelet formation. *Blood* 2012; **120**: 2317–29.

75 Thon JN, Italiano JE, Jr. Does size matter in platelet production? *Blood* 2012; **120**: 1552–61.

81 Jiang J, Woulfe DS, Papoutsakis ET. Shear enhances thrombopoiesis and formation of microparticles that induce megakaryocytic differentiation of stem cells. *Blood* 2014; **124**: 2094–103.

91 Gieger C, Radhakrishnan A, Cvejic A, *et al.* New gene functions in megakaryopoiesis and platelet formation. *Nature* 2011; **480**: 201–8.

121 McIntosh B, Kauskansky K. Transcriptional regulation of bone marrow thrombopoietin by platelet proteins. *Exp Hematol* 2008; 799–806.

128 Debrincat MA. Mcl-1 and Bcl-xL co-ordinately regulate megakaryocyte survival. *Blood* 2012; **119**: 5850–8.

130 Liu ZJ, Hoffmeister KM, Hu Z, *et al.* Expansion of the neonatal platelet mass is achieved via an extension of platelet lifespan. *Blood* 2014; **123**: 3381–9.

144 Wang C, Smith BR, Ault KA, Rinder HM. Reticulated platelets predict platelet count recovery following chemotherapy. *Transfusion* 2002; **42**: 368–74.

CHAPTER 18

Platelet immunology and alloimmunization

Janice G. McFarland

Platelet and Neutrophil Immunology Laboratory, Blood Center of Wisconsin; and Department of Medicine, Medical College of Wisconsin, Milwaukee, WI, USA

Platelets express a variety of immunogenic markers on the cell surface. Some of these antigens are shared with other cell types as in the case of HLA antigens, which are shared with virtually all nucleated cells in the body, whereas others are observed to be essentially platelet specific. This chapter reviews the antigens expressed on platelets, the various patterns of alloimmunization to these antigens, and their impact on platelet transfusion responses. Strategies to treat and prevent alloimmunization are summarized.

Antigens on the platelet surface

Antigens shared with other tissues
HLA antigens

HLA class I, but not HLA class II, molecules are expressed on platelets. Class I A, B, and C antigens are all expressed on the platelet membrane, and in particular the A and B antigens are important targets for antibodies implicated in platelet transfusion refractoriness.[1] In fact, platelets are the major source of HLA class I antigens present in blood. Human platelets are reported to express on average about 20,000 molecules of HLA class I per platelet.[2] However, platelet expression of HLA antigens varies amongst individuals.[2–4]

Although platelets ultimately derive from nucleated precursors (the megakaryocytes) and hence might be anticipated to acquire their HLA antigens through mechanisms in common with other nucleated cells, early studies[5,6] demonstrated that, in vitro, platelets absorb and express soluble HLA antigens after incubation in plasma. These studies, as well as others purporting to show that HLA class I antigens could be stripped from the platelet membrane by chloroquine treatment,[7,8] suggested that HLA absorbed from plasma contributed significantly to the total HLA class I present on platelets. However, it is now recognized that low pH treatment of platelets does not "strip" the HLA class I heavy chain from the cell membrane of platelets. Rather, this treatment of platelets actually disrupts the trimolecular complex of HLA class I heavy chain, peptide, and β_2-microglobulin, destroying antigenic epitopes and preventing the binding of specific HLA antibodies.[9]

It is now clear that most HLA class I molecules on platelets are integral membrane proteins persisting from the megakaryocyte stage of development. Evidence for this includes studies of phorbol ester stimulation of platelets that resulted in phosphorylation of their HLA molecules,[10] and mRNA from platelets that is capable of producing small amounts of HLA class I,[11] both of which are consistent with HLA molecules being an integral part of the platelet membrane. In addition, peptides presented by HLA-A2 molecules on human platelets have been isolated, sequenced, and shown to be identical to those commonly expressed by HLA-A2 on nucleated cells.[9] One ubiquitously expressed peptide is derived from the megakaryocyte-platelet-specific glycoprotein (GP) IX. Detectable HLA class I surface molecules that were removed by either incubation at 37 °C or treatment with pH 3.0 citrate could be almost completely restored after addition of exogenous β_2-microglobulin and peptide ligand. This indicates (1) that platelets themselves are not able to load HLA molecules with endogenous peptides, but that this occurs during HLA protein synthesis at the megakaryocyte stage; and (2) although B2-microglobulin and peptide become unstable and dissociate from the platelet surface either when platelets are incubated at 37 °C or when treated with low pH, the class I heavy chain remains embedded in the membrane. The above evidence suggests, then, that the vast majority of HLA class I molecules on platelets are intrinsic transmembrane proteins synthesized and acquired at the megakaryocyte stage before platelets become cytoplasmic fragments.

ABH blood group antigens

Platelets express low levels of the blood group antigens I,[12] P,[12] and ABO(H),[13,14] but with the exception of ABH, antibodies against these antigens do not appear to have clinical relevance to transfused platelet recovery or survival. The A, B, and H antigens are expressed on the carbohydrate moieties attached to virtually all platelet glycoproteins.[13,15] The endothelial cell adhesion molecule PECAM-1 (CD31) accounts for the majority of these antigens per platelet while GPIa/IIa expresses the highest levels of ABH per molecule.[13] Several studies have demonstrated that levels of A and B antigens on platelets vary between individuals, with levels of A_1 antigens between individuals calculated to range from 2100 to 16,000 molecules per platelet.[13] Variability of expression also exists within an individual's own platelet population,[13,14,16] although not all groups have found this to be significant.[17] The variable expression of ABH on an individual's platelets, to the extent it occurs, may explain why early studies showed a rapid destruction of a subset of transfused ABO-incompatible platelets followed by near-normal survival of the remaining cells.[18,19] Notably, individuals of the A_2 subtype express no A antigens on their platelets and therefore these platelets can be successfully substituted for group O platelets for transfusion.[13,20] About 4–7% of non–group O individuals express

---

Rossi's Principles of Transfusion Medicine, Fifth Edition. Edited by Toby L. Simon, Jeffrey McCullough, Edward L. Snyder, Bjarte G. Solheim, and Ronald G. Strauss.

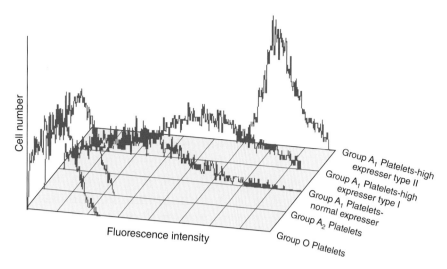

Figure 18.1 Fluorescence histograms of platelets after incubation with a fluorescent-labeled monoclonal antibody specific for the blood group A antigen and immunofluorescence detection by flow cytometry. Group A_2 platelets are not distinguishable from group O platelets—no A antigens are detected. Normal group A_1 platelets (middle histogram) show great variation in A antigen expression—broad histogram. Platelets from a Type 1 high expresser, like the normal expresser, give a broad histogram but have overall higher levels (histogram shifted to the right) of A antigen. Type II high expressers have much higher levels and show a more homogeneous (narrow histogram at top) expression of A antigens per platelet.

elevated levels of A and/or B antigens on their platelets.[13,14] A subset of these "high expressers," termed *type II high expressers*, have about 20-fold normal levels. ABO antibodies reacting with high expresser platelets have been implicated in both fetal/neonatal alloimmune thrombocytopenia (FNAIT)[21] and platelet transfusion refractoriness (PTR) (Figure 18.1).[14]

Similar to the controversy regarding the source of class I HLA antigens on platelets, the origin of ABH antigens on platelets has been debated with conflicting evidence suggesting that they were either absorbed from the plasma or integral to the platelet membrane. Group O platelets incubated in group A or group B plasma could be shown to acquire soluble A or B substance detectable with anti-A or anti-B typing reagents in agglutination tests.[22] However, more recent studies show that a great majority of blood group A, B, and H antigens on platelets are not passively absorbed from the plasma, but are expressed on many of the integral platelet membrane glycoproteins, including GPIIb, GPIIIa, GPIV, GPV, PECAM-1, GPIb/IX, GPIa/IIa, and CD109.[14,15,23–25] It is now believed that as in red cell development, A- and B-UDP sugars are attached in the Golgi apparatus of the megakaryocyte to the Type II H precursor chains present on these platelet glycoproteins. Studies by several groups using monoclonal probes specific for Type II H chains confirm that this membrane-intrinsic form of H substance is present on platelets and detectable in varying quantities according to the ABO group of the individual (greatest in group O and A_2 platelets; less in groups B, A_1, and A_1B; and least in O_h [Bombay]).[13,14,22,23] Although it is likely that a small amount of ABH on platelets is acquired by absorption of glycolipids expressing these antigens from the surrounding plasma, the majority, as for HLA, is intrinsically derived at the megakaryocyte stage.

Other antigens on platelets

Platelet GP IV or CD36 is expressed on various human cells, including platelets, monocytes and macrophages, capillary endothelium, erythroblasts, and adipocytes.[26,27] Some apparently normal individuals lack CD36 on their platelets (Type II deficiency) or platelets and monocytes (Type I deficiency).[28] CD36 deficiency is common in Asian (3–11%)[29] and African (3–6%),[30,31] populations but is extremely rare in European populations (0.1%).[30,32] It is interesting that the most common gene mutations responsible for CD36 deficiency in those of Asian and African ethnicity are different—a $C \rightarrow T_{478}$ point mutation in exon 4 (Asians[28,33]) and $T \rightarrow G_{1264}$ stop mutation in exon 10 (Africans[34]). The higher

frequency of CD36 deficiency in these groups is thought to be related to their living in regions of the world where malaria is endemic. CD36 is a known receptor for red cells infected with *Plasmodium falciparum*; thus, it is believed that CD36 deficiency may afford partial resistance to malaria infection. However, one report suggests CD36 deficiency may actually be a risk factor for more severe forms of malaria infection.[34] Type I CD36-deficient individuals can become sensitized from transfusion or pregnancy, producing antibodies directed at CD36 that have been implicated in cases of platelet transfusion refractoriness,[29,35] postransfusion purpura (PTP),[36,37] and FNAIT.[32,37,38] Successful transfusion responses can be achieved using CD36-deficient platelets in patients immunized against CD36.[32,35,38]

CD109 is a 175-kD glycoprotein found on cultured endothelial cells, activated T cells, several tumor cell lines, and platelets.[39] Two alloantigens, human platelet antigen-15b (HPA-15b) (Gov[a]) and HPA-15a (Gov[b]), have been identified on platelet CD109,[40] and unlike most platelet-specific alloantigens, both alleles are highly expressed: 77% (HPA-15a) and 65% (HPA-15b) in those of European ethnicity (Table 18.1). CD109 is a member of the α_2-macroglobulin/complement gene family,[41] and a single nucleotide polymorphism $A \rightarrow C_{2108}$ resulting in a Tyr:Ser$_{703}$ change in the protein defines the HPA-15a/b alloantigens.[42] The number of CD109 molecules expressed on platelets is small (<2000/platelet), and the HPA-15 antigens are labile in storage, making detection of HPA-15 antibodies difficult using currently available serologic methods, suggesting that alloimmunization to these antigens may be underreported. Results from several studies show that antibodies to HPA-15a or HPA-15b are uncommonly detected (0.2–1.0%) in sera collected from women who have given birth to infants affected with FNAIT, but are more frequently seen in sera from patients with PTP (2%) and platelet transfusion refractoriness (3–4%).[43–44] This suggests that HPA-15 may be as immunogenic as the HPA-5 antigen system, which is second only to the highly immunogenic HPA-1a (Pl[A1]) platelet antigen system.

Platelet-specific antigens

Antibodies recognizing platelet-specific antigens have been discovered in three clinical situations: mothers who give birth to infants with FNAIT, patients who develop dramatic thrombocytopenia after blood transfusion (PTP), and patients who have received multiple transfusions. To date, 33 HPAs expressed on six different platelet glycoproteins—GP IIb (CD41), GP IIIa (CD61), GP Ibα

Table 18.1 Human Platelet Alloantigens[46,47,50]*

Alloantigens	Other Names	Phenotypic Frequency (Caucasian)	Glycoprotein Location/ Amino Acid Substitution	Encoding Gene/ Nucleotide Change
HPA1a	PlA, Zw	72% a/a	GPIIIa	*ITGB3*
HPA1b		26% a/b	L33P	T176C
HPA-1c		2% b/b	L33V	C175G
		< 1 % a/c		
HPA2a	Ko, Sib	85% a/a	GPIb-alpha	*GPIBA*
HPA2b		14% a/b	T145M	C482T
		1% b/b		
HPA3a	Bak, Lek	37% a/a	GPIIb	*ITGA2B*
HPA3b		48% a/b	I843S	T2621G
		15% b/b		
HPA4a	Pen,	>99.9% a/a	GPIIIa	*ITGB3*
HPA4b	Yuk	<0.1% a/b	R143Q	G506A
		<0.1% b/b		
HPA-5a (Brb)	Br, Hc,	80% a/a	GPIa	*ITGA2*
HPA-5b (Bra)	Zav	19% a/b	E505K	G1600A
		1% b/b		
HPA-6bw	Caa, Tu	<1%	GPIIIa R489Q	*ITGB3* G1544A
HPA-7bw	Mob	<1%	GPIIa P407A	*ITGB3* C1297G
HPA-8bw	Sra	<0.1%	GPIIIa R636C	*ITGB3* C1984T
HPA-9bw	Maxa	<1%	GPIIb V837M	*ITGA2B* G2602A
HPA-10bw	Laa	1%	GPIIIa R62Q	*ITGB3* G263A
HPA-11bw	Groa	<0.5%	GPIIIa R633H	*ITGB3* G1976A
HPA-12bw	Iya	1%	GPIb-beta G15E	*GPIBB* G119A
HPA-13bw	Sita	<1%	GPIa T799M	*ITGA2* C2483T
HPA-14bw	Oea	1%	GPIIIa K611del	*ITGB3* 1909_1911delAAG
HPA-15a	Gov	35% a/a	CD109	*CD109*
HPA-15b		42% a/b	S682Y	C2108A
		23% b/b		
HPA-16bw	Duva	<1%	GPIIIa T140I	*ITGB3* C497T
HPA-17bw	Vaa	<1%	GPIIIa T195M	*ITGB3* C662T
HPA-18bw		<1%	GPIa Q716H	*ITGA2* G2235T
HPA-19bw		<1%	GPIIIa K137Q	*ITGB3* A487C
HPA-20bw		<1%	GPIIb T619M	*ITGA2B* C1949T
HPA-21bw		<1%	GPIIIa E628K	*ITGB3* G1960A
HPA-22bw		<1%	GPIIb K164T	*ITGA2B* A584C
HPA-23bw		<1%	GPIIIa R622W	*ITGB3* C1942T
HPA-24bw		<1%	GPIIb S472N	*ITGA2B* G1508A
HPA-25bw		<1%	GPIa T1087M	*ITGA2* C3347T
HPA-26bw		<1%	GPIIIa K580N	*ITGB3* G1818T
HPA-27bw		<1%	GPIIb L841M	*ITGA2B* C2614A
HPA-28bw		<1%	GPIIb V740L	*ITGA2B* G2311T

*Phenotypic frequencies for the antigens shown are for the white population only. Significant differences in gene frequencies may be found in African and Asian populations.

(CD42b), GPIbβ (CD42c), GPIa (CD49b), and CD109—have been described, including localization to platelet surface GPs, quantification of their density on the platelet surface, and determination of DNA polymorphisms in genes encoding for them (see Table 18.1).[46,47] (For a current list, see http://www.ebi.ac.uk/ipd/hpa/table1.html and http://www.ebi.ac.uk/ipd/hpa/table2.html.)[46] Thirteen antigens are clustered into one triallelic[48] (HPA-1) and five biallelic groups (HPA-2, HPA-3, HPA-4, HPA-5, and HPA-15). HPAs for which antibodies against only one of the alleles have been detected are labeled with a "w" for workshop (e.g., HPA-8bw). To date, 20 such low-frequency single-allele HPAs have been discovered, essentially all involved in FNAIT cases.[49]

Although the frequencies of HPA have been most extensively studied in Caucasian populations, it should be noted that they have been determined for other racial and ethnic groups as well and in some cases vary significantly from Caucasian frequencies. For example, HPA-lb is expressed on the platelets of approximately 15% of persons of European ancestry but of less than 1% of persons of Asian ancestry. (For more information regarding HPA frequencies in different populations, readers are directed to: http://www.ebi.ac.uk/ipd/hpa/freqs_1.html.)[46]

Alloimmunization to platelet antigens

Immunization to HLA antigens

Pregnancy and transfusion account for the development of HLA alloimmunization, with exposure to leukocyte-containing blood components resulting in high rates of antibody formation in patients receiving multiple transfusions over time. Antibodies to class I and not class II HLA antigens can significantly affect the recovery and survival of transfused platelets because the former and not the latter are expressed on the platelet surface. Among the class I antigens, the HLA-A and -B markers are most important.[1] HLA-C antigens are also present and reported to be expressed at approximately the same density as A antigens,[51] but with rare exceptions,[52] antibodies to HLA-C antigens do not appear to significantly affect transfused platelets.

The natural history of HLA sensitization in patients receiving platelet transfusions for hematologic diseases was studied in 1978,[53] before the advent of widespread use of leukocyte-reduced blood components. By actuarial analysis, 60% of patients who were not positive for lymphocytotoxic antibodies at the beginning of the study were projected to develop them as early as 10 days after primary exposure or four days after secondary exposure if they had been transfused or pregnant in the past. The number of transfusions was not related to the likelihood of immunization, an observation that was confirmed in a later study.[54] Patients who were alloimmunized at the beginning of the study had the poorest responses to transfused platelets, those who did not develop HLA antibodies had the best responses, and those whose antibodies developed during the period of observation had intermediate responses.[53] A later study of platelet preparation methods to reduce alloimmunization in newly diagnosed acute myelogenous leukemia (AML) patients found a similarly high HLA sensitization rate of 45% in the control group (131 patients) who received unmodified, pooled, whole blood–derived platelet transfusions over an eight-week period.[55] Rates of alloimmunization in other studies involving hematology–oncology patients receiving non-leukocyte-reduced blood components range to up to 70% (Table 18.2).

Table 18.2 Platelet Alloimmunization in Multitransfused Patients Receiving Non-Leukocyte-Reduced Blood Components*

Study	Number of Patients	Anti-HLA[†]	Anti-PSA[‡]	Loss/Decrease in Antibody
Seftel et al. (2004)[61]	315	61/315 (19%)		
TRAP (1997)[55]	131	59/131 (45%)	11/131 (8%)	
Atlas et al. (1993)[62]	134	95/134 (71%)		43/95 (38%)
Meenaghan et al. (1993)[63]	106	37/106 (35%)	45/106 (42%)	29/45 (64%)
Godeau et al. (1992)[64]	50	13/50 (26%)	4/50 (8%)	
Pamphilon et al. (1989)[56]	49	20/49 (41%)	11/49 (22%)	12/20 (59%)
Murphy et al. (1987)[65]	154	55/154 (36%)	5/154 (3%)	30/55 (54%)

*Frequency of HLA antibody and platelet-specific antibody formation in studies of patients with hematologic and oncologic diagnoses requiring repeated platelet transfusion. The final column contains frequencies of antibody loss or decline in these studies.

[†]HLA antibodies determined by lymphocytotoxicity testing.

[‡]Platelet-specific antibodies determined by a variety of methods.

The risk of HLA alloimmunization is influenced by several patient and blood component factors. Transfused patients who were exposed previously to allogeneic HLA via transfusion or pregnancy developed HLA antibodies sooner—and, in many studies, more often—than patients who were not exposed previously.[55–58] In the Trial to Reduce Alloimmunization to Platelets (TRAP) study,[55] 62% of previously pregnant women with AML receiving untreated blood components (control product) developed lymphocytotoxic antibodies compared with 33% of those who had not been pregnant or transfused previously. There is general agreement that primary alloimmunization to HLA antigens is unlikely to occur before 3–4 weeks after the first transfusion in patients receiving multiple transfusions, and that HLA antibodies detected sooner than this most likely represent secondary immune responses in patients with remote histories of transfusion or pregnancy.

The underlying disease for which patients require platelet transfusion also influences the rate of HLA alloimmunization. In one study, patients undergoing induction chemotherapy for AML were more likely to become alloimmunized than were patients being treated for acute lymphoblastic leukemia (ALL).[59] Although both groups of patients received similarly intensive chemotherapy and required roughly the same level of transfusion support, HLA antibodies developed in 44% of the AML group, compared with 18% of the patients with ALL ($p = 0.00002$). The authors postulated that the difference may be attributable to either an additional immunosuppressive effect of the high-dose corticosteroids given in ALL or to a decreased immune responsiveness in patients with ALL caused by their underlying disease. Others have corroborated this finding and have noted, moreover, that alloimmunization seems to occur sooner in patients with AML than in those with ALL.[56,60]

Except for prospective solid organ transplant recipients, there have been limited studies of HLA alloimmunization in patients without malignant hematologic-oncologic disorders who received transfusions of red blood cells (RBCs) or whole blood units, but interest in sensitization rates in such patients has increased, particularly with the advent of stem cell transplantation for hemoglobinopathies such as sickle cell disease. Sensitization to HLA can inhibit platelet transfusion responses (discussed further in this chapter), increasing the risk of thrombocytopenic hemorrhage in patients undergoing stem cell transplantation who require multiple platelet transfusions. One study of chronically transfused sickle cell disease patients determined that 85% of those with at least 50 past red cell transfusions had evidence of platelet-reactive antibodies, predominately anti-HLA, whereas 48% of those with fewer than 50 past exposures were sensitized. HLA antibodies were not detected in

those patients who had no past exposure to transfusion.[66] A second study of 60 thalassemia patients examined the development of HLA antibodies and found that 32 (53%) were positive for HLA antibodies at baseline and seven more became sensitized in the follow-up period of 1 year, for a total HLA sensitization rate of 65%.[67] The type of blood components used for these two groups of patients may have contributed to these significant rates of alloimmunization. Details about the type of RBC transfusions given in the first study were not provided in the report, but there did not appear to be any systematic attempts to give leukocyte-reduced units. Washed RBCs were routinely used in the second study, and these were estimated to have residual leukocyte content of $>5 \times 10^6$ per unit. Therefore, neither study used RBC units that were leukocyte reduced to the extent that HLA sensitization would be lessened (also discussed further in this chapter). A more recent report of β thalassemia patients from Middle Eastern countries coming to stem cell transplant also noted a high rate of HLA alloimmunization, presumably due to their being heavily transfused in the past.[68]

Still other investigators have sought to document the rates of HLA alloimmunization in nonhematologic conditions requiring shorter periods of transfusion support. In a study of 117 cardiac surgery patients who were exposed to a single episode of RBC transfusion, 18% became sensitized.[69] In contrast, in a second study of 40 more seriously ill patients requiring placement of left ventricular assist devices as a bridge to cardiac transplant, 45% formed Class I HLA antibodies after a course of support that included a number of platelet as well as RBC transfusions. By actuarial analysis, 63% of those who received more than six transfusions of pooled whole blood–derived platelets were projected to become HLA immunized.[70] This rate was strikingly similar to that of the patients with hematologic malignancies followed in the earlier study noted above who received non-leukoreduced blood.[53]

These studies documenting HLA alloimmunization in patients with non-hematologic-oncologic conditions suggest that, apart from patients with ALL, most patients who require repeated red cell and/or platelet transfusions for treatment of their hematologic-oncologic condition are at risk of becoming sensitized to HLA at a rate similar to that of patients who would be assumed to have normally functioning immune systems.

Both the number and type of platelet products also affect the sensitization rate. There is some disagreement in the literature regarding the importance of a dose–response relationship between platelet transfusions from different donors and the risk of alloimmunization. One study[54] failed to note such a relationship in a group of patients with AML receiving induction therapy. However, most of the patients in this study were exposed to more than 20 different platelet donors. Indeed, animal data[71] and human transfusion trials[72] suggest that, with fewer donor exposures (i.e., less than 20), there is a dose–response relationship between the number of exposures and the rate of alloimmunization. Fewer donor exposures can be achieved using apheresis platelets, which provide adequate doses of platelets from a single donor rather than pooled platelet concentrates. Alloimmunization can be delayed and perhaps reduced using this type of platelet product.[72]

Despite the established correlation between HLA antibodies and refractoriness to platelet transfusions (discussed in this chapter),[73,74] HLA antibodies are frequently a transient complication in patients with hematologic-oncologic diagnoses requiring repeated platelet transfusions. Studies document that 17% to 67% of patients demonstrating these antibodies eventually lose them (Table 18.2).[56,59,61,62,65,75,76] The loss of these antibodies may be related to discontinuance of the antigenic exposure after marrow recovery or to switching of platelet transfusion support to HLA-matched platelets; however, it can occur despite continued exposure to whole blood–derived platelet transfusions.[59,65,75,77] One interesting report[62] found that two-thirds of patients with decreasing anti-HLA reactivity despite continued exposure had developed anti-idiotypic antibodies that reacted with the V region of anti-HLA IgG. In 36% of these patients, the serum actually inhibited binding of the patient's own prior anti-HLA to appropriate lymphocyte targets. A history of pregnancy did not affect the ability to produce these anti-idiotypic antibodies. In contrast, those patients with persistently detectable anti-HLA did not develop anti-idiotypic reactivity. HLA antibodies that are detected before the onset of transfusion therapy (i.e., because of remote transfusion or pregnancy) tend to persist, whereas those antibodies that develop de novo during a transfusion support episode are more likely to be transient and to decrease in strength or disappear altogether despite continued exposure to allogeneic blood and platelets.[65]

The major route of primary HLA immunization to transfused platelets involves the *donor leukocytes*, and not the platelets, per se. In vitro experiments showed that highly purified HLA-A2+ platelets could not induce allo-cytotoxicity in HLA-A2-negative peripheral blood mononuclear cells (PBMCs)—not even in the presence of helper HLA-A2-negative PBMCs.[9] Studies in humans show that when leukocyte reduced platelets are transfused, primary immunization to HLA is very much delayed or does not occur at all,[78–81] whereas unmodified platelet concentrates are associated with a rate of HLA immunization ranging from 19% to 71% (Table 18.2). These observations implicate the leukocytes in both platelet and red cell transfusions as the source of primary immunization.

Early animal studies suggested that the production of major histocompatibility complex (MHC) antibodies requires recognition of class II MHC molecules on *donor* antigen-presenting cells (APCs) by *recipient* T cells.[82] Later work found that although the majority of MHC (or, in humans, HLA) sensitization in a platelet transfusion model was due to this direct pathway, by significant prestorage leukocyte reduction of platelets (i.e., to $<10^6$ WBC/μL) the majority of such antibody production could be inhibited; but exhaustively leukoreduced SCID mouse platelets (<0.05 WBC/μL) with very low levels of MHC class II–bearing WBCs were even more immunogenic than platelets that had had class II MHC WBCs added back to them. The results suggested that donor MHC class II–positive APCs must have a dual function in modulating their sensitization to MHC class I–bearing platelets. At normal concentrations, they are the dominant pathway through which antigen is presented to the recipient's immune system, whereas at levels lower than that required for this direct pathway, they actually inhibit the indirect pathway of recipient sensitization that requires recipient APCs presenting antigens to recipient T cells. Finally, removal of almost all donor APCs results in an uninhibited indirect pathway of alloimmunization and restored MHC antibody production.[1]

Immunization to platelet-specific antigens

The importance of HPAs in the clinical syndromes FNAIT and PTP is undisputed; however, their relevance to platelet transfusion practice is controversial.

One kind of evidence implicating HPA or platelet-specific antibodies in the destruction of transfused platelets is the failure of some transfusions of HLA-matched platelet concentrates given to patients who are refractory to random whole blood–derived platelets.[79] The poor responses to these platelet transfusions, despite HLA matching, indicate that other antigens, perhaps platelet-specific markers, are involved. The other kind of evidence involves the demonstration of platelet-reactive antibodies in the absence of anti-HLA activity. The conclusion drawn is that antibodies directed at platelet-specific antigens cause these reactions.[77,79] In contrast to antibodies to HLA antigens, the majority of platelet-specific antibodies identified using these strategies do not seem to be associated with poor transfused platelet recovery or survival, however.

With the advent of Phase III platelet antibody assays that detect platelet glycoprotein (GP)-specific reactions, it is now possible to assay directly the sera from multitransfused patients for platelet-specific antibodies. Using one such method, the monoclonal antibody-specific immobilization of platelet antigens (MAIPA) assay, one group documented that among 252 patients with hematologic-oncologic diagnoses receiving platelet transfusions, 20 (8%) developed platelet-specific antibodies with clear-cut specificities. The most common specificity in these patients was for HPA-5b in 10 of the 20; followed by HPA-1b in four; HPA-5a in two; and one each with HPA-2b, HPA-1a, HPA-1b plus HPA-5b, and HPA-1b plus HPA-2b.[83] This study confirmed earlier findings in the TRAP study where 8% of the 530 patients in the trial formed platelet-specific antibodies, the most common being anti-HPA-1b.[55]

These two studies confirm the finding that many of the best-documented platelet-specific antibodies detected in patients who receive transfusions are directed against platelet antigens, the phenotypic frequencies of which are less than 30% in the blood donor population.[55,69,83] Therefore, it is difficult to attribute refractory responses to whole blood–derived and/or HLA-matched platelet transfusions to these antibodies alone. Indeed, the majority of refractory patients with platelet-specific antibodies also have HLA antibodies.[84] Alloimmunization to high-frequency platelet-specific antigens would be expected to present a major challenge in finding compatible platelets to support a patient requiring multiple platelet transfusions. Fortunately, these cases are extremely rare.[69,85,86] Although platelet-specific antibodies directed at defined platelet alloantigens (HPAs) can result in transfusion failures,[87–89] most platelet glycoprotein reactivity lacking definite specificity does not seem to influence transfusion responses.[55,64,90]

There have been several reports of platelet transfusion refractoriness caused by antibodies to GPIV (CD36) in patients who are GPIV deficient.[29,31] These patients are difficult to support because virtually all platelet products available for transfusion would be incompatible (GPIV positive). In some cases, GPIV-negative platelets were obtained by large-scale screening of donor populations with a higher frequency of GPIV deficiency (African), and transfusion of those platelets resulted in good platelet increments for the patients.[91]

Immunization to blood group antigens

Several studies have documented the effect of ABO incompatibility on platelet transfusion therapy. In an early report of 91 alloimmunized thrombocytopenic patients receiving 389 transfusions, 24-hour transfused platelet recovery was reduced by 23% in ABO-incompatible donor–recipient pairs (donor-group A, B, or AB; recipient-group O, B, or A).[92] In the aggregate, patients receiving multiple platelet transfusions have been thought to demonstrate a statistically significant but clinically unimportant decrease in platelet recovery after transfusion of ABO-incompatible platelets (especially group A). In a subset, however, as many as 20% of group O patients could develop severe refractoriness to group A platelets.[14,20,93] Failure to respond to HLA-matched platelet transfusions in the absence of nonimmune clinical factors should prompt the clinician to examine the ABO group of the recipient and of the donors to determine whether ABO incompatibility might be responsible for the unexpected poor responses.

One report from Japan described a group O patient who failed to respond to two of 12 ABO-incompatible HLA-matched platelet transfusions.[14] Further evaluation determined that the platelets in the two unsuccessful transfusions were from donors who expressed unusually high amounts of group B substance on their platelets (high expressers), up to 20 times that found on group B, HLA-matched platelets that were successfully transfused in this patient.

Heal *et al.*[93] have examined the importance of ABO blood groups in platelet transfusion therapy. Forty patients with hematologic diseases receiving platelet transfusions were randomly assigned to receive either ABO-identical or ABO-unmatched platelets. The responses in the group of patients receiving ABO-unmatched transfusions (i.e., when either the recipient would be expected to have isoagglutinins to the ABH antigens on the transfused platelets, or the donor had such antibodies directed at the recipient's blood type) were significantly worse than those observed in patients receiving ABO-identical platelet transfusions. Analysis of the first 25 transfusions in each group showed a significantly better response in the ABO-identical arm (mean corrected count increment [CCI], 6600 vs. 5200; $p < 0.01$). This effect was most important in the first 10 transfusion episodes and tended to predict subsequent alloimmunization and refractoriness to platelet transfusions.[94] This finding seemed to be in conflict with earlier reports in which a minor, clinically insignificant impact of ABO mismatching was observed. The newer data were then reanalyzed using the earlier definitions of ABO *compatibility* (the patient lacks isoagglutinins to recipient ABO antigens) and *incompatibility* (the patient has isoagglutinins that are reactive with donor ABO antigens). In the reanalysis, no benefits of ABO compatibility were detected,[95] suggesting that there is a significant negative impact of *both* major and minor ABO incompatibility in platelet transfusions. An increased frequency of refractoriness in patients receiving ABO-unmatched platelet transfusions was also observed in a study of 26 patients (69% vs. 58%; $p = 0.001$).[96]

The mechanism for platelet destruction in platelet ABO-incompatible transfusions (the recipient has isoagglutinins against donor ABH) is not difficult to ascertain. Presumably, IgM and IgG anti-A or anti-B in the recipient interact with A and B substances on the transfused platelets, resulting in their destruction. Explanations offered for the biphasic survival curves of ABO-incompatible

platelets include (1) the elution of a portion of group A substance from the platelet surface; (2) the nonhomogeneous distribution of group A substance on donor platelets, with resultant rapid destruction of the subpopulation with highest expression; and (3) secondary injury to a subset of transfused platelets caused by the reaction between anti-A isoagglutinins and A red cells in the platelet concentrate.[13,18]

The suboptimal response of the *plasma*-incompatible transfusions (the donor has isoagglutinins against recipient ABH) is more difficult to explain. One report postulates that immune complexes involving soluble recipient ABH substance and donor A or B antibodies form. These immune complexes secondarily interact with the transfused platelets via the FcγRIIα receptor, or the complement receptors cC1q-R and gC1q-R, and mediate their destruction.[97] Some experimental evidence supports this theory, in that anti-A has been detected in an immune complex fraction of group A recipient plasma after transfusion with group O platelets, and these immune complexes bind to IgG FcγRIIα and the cC1q-R and gC1q-R receptors on group O platelets.[97] Indeed, in at least one study, plasma-incompatible platelet transfusions were even less effective than platelet-incompatible transfusions.[94] Immune complexes involving other plasma proteins such as C2, C4, albumin, and fibrinogen likewise have been implicated in refractory responses to platelet transfusion.[97,98]

Adverse effects of ABO-incompatible platelet transfusions may extend beyond reducing platelet transfusion increments and stimulating alloimmunization. In one retrospective cohort study of cardiac surgery patients, those patients who received mismatched ABO platelets were compared with those who received ABO-identical platelets. The mismatched group experienced significantly longer hospital stays, more days of fever, increased healthcare costs, and more red cell transfusions. Other negative outcomes including mortality and time in the intensive care unit were also increased in the mismatched group, but these differences failed to reach statistical significance. The authors postulated that the negative effects of ABO-mismatched platelet transfusions were again related to immune complexes that stimulated inflammatory pathways, leading to increased postoperative morbidity in these patients.[99] Although intriguing, these findings have yet to be confirmed by other groups. In fact, a later retrospective study involving more cardiac surgery patients failed to identify negative effects of ABO-mismatched platelet transfusions.[100]

An indisputable risk of ABO plasma-incompatible transfusions, particularly those involving group O donors and non–group O recipients, is acute hemolytic transfusion reaction caused by high-titer isoagglutinins in the donor plasma. With the marked shift from pooled whole blood–derived platelet concentrates to apheresis platelets, the risk of transfusing large volumes of ABO-incompatible plasma with potent ABO isoagglutinins is increased. Many blood providers have taken steps to alleviate this risk by reducing the volume of incompatible plasma or screening group O donors for high-titer isoagglutinins.[101]

Transfusion refractoriness

Alloimmunization is an immune response in a recipient stimulated by foreign donor antigens. In the platelet transfusion setting, these responses involve the production of antibodies directed at donor platelets. *Platelet refractoriness* describes a clinical condition in which patients do not achieve the anticipated platelet count increment from a platelet transfusion. It is possible to be alloimmunized to platelet antigens without being refractory to platelet transfusions, and also to be refractory to platelet transfusions without being alloimmunized. *Alloimmune refractoriness* occurs when the level of alloimmunization, as measured by the breadth of antibody response to platelet antigens, is sufficient to affect the majority of randomly selected platelet products.

The detection of alloimmunization is straightforward using standard laboratory techniques to detect antibodies in the patient's serum that are reactive with HLA or platelet-specific antigens. In contrast, the definition of the refractory state is less precise.[1,102] A standard dose of platelets (six units of pooled whole blood–derived platelet concentrates or one apheresis platelet unit) generally increases the platelet count by about 5000–7000 platelets/μL/unit in a 70-kg adult. This would result in a post-transfusion increment of about 30,000–40,000 platelets/μL 1 hour after platelet transfusion.[102] The TRAP study defined the refractory state as a corrected count increment (CCI) which normalizes transfusion responses for patient blood volume estimated using body surface area and platelet dose, of <5000 after two sequential ABO-compatible platelet transfusions.[55] Another measure of platelet transfusion response is the percent platelet recovery (PPR). Similar to the CCI, the PPR uses platelet dose and patient blood volume; the latter is estimated using the patient's body weight in kilograms rather than body surface area. Studies in normal autologous platelet donors show an average 1 hour PPR of approximately 66%.[74] Recovery less than 20–30% at 1 hour after the transfusion indicates a refractory response.[103]

The PPR and CCI have been criticized as measures of post-transfusion platelet response because both calculations, which correct for patient size and dose of platelets, fail to provide information about the impact of these two variables on the post-transfusion platelet count increment.[104] For example, a small dose of platelets given to a large patient might result in an acceptable PPR or CCI but a poor absolute platelet count increment. In order to better examine the impact of patient size and platelet dose, as well as other factors that affect the quality of the platelets (storage time, postcollection manipulations, etc.), regression analysis of post-transfusion platelet increments is suggested. It is also recommended by the same authors that because both the CCI and PPR calculations are biased in favor of platelet preparation techniques that provide fewer platelets, neither should be used to define platelet refractoriness. Regardless of which method is used, the actual platelet increment in patients who are highly refractory because of alloimmunization is extremely small to negligible.

It is important to recognize that refractoriness does not necessarily imply alloimmunization. Indeed, only about 30% of refractory responses to platelet transfusion is attributable to alloimmunization, the remainder being due to nonimmune factors that result in shortened platelet survival and/or markedly decreased platelet recoveries in patients who receive transfusions.[74,105,106] Multiple linear regression analysis has been used to demonstrate a number of factors related to clinical refractoriness, including HLA alloimmunization as well as splenomegaly, amphotericin therapy, disseminated intravascular coagulation, or recent allogeneic marrow transplantation.[107] Other studies have also demonstrated factors with negative effects on transfused platelets such as sepsis, fever, and drugs.[108,109] Individual patients may have significantly different responses to the same nonimmune causes of refractoriness, with some patients experiencing minimal impact and others having markedly impaired response to platelet transfusions. Some patients, particularly those with multiple clinical complications (e.g., sepsis

and fever), appear to respond poorly to platelets that are approaching the end of the recommended storage interval (five days). Such patients may experience an improvement in their platelet response after receiving "fresh platelets"—platelets that were collected less than 48 hours earlier.[102,110]

A cause of non-alloimmune refractoriness that can be overlooked in the infected, neutropenic, hematology–oncology patient is development of drug-dependent platelet-reactive antibodies. Vancomycin, a drug often used to treat serious Gram-positive bacterial infections in such patients, has been implicated. Drug-dependent platelet-reactive antibodies should be suspected in refractory patients when there is no evidence of alloimmunization or they fail to respond to HLA-selected platelets, and the refractory responses are temporally related to therapy with a drug.[111]

Treatment of the refractory alloimmunized patient

In the modern era wherein universal leukocyte reduction of blood products for patients receiving multiple platelet transfusions has become standard practice, the rate of alloimmunization (primarily to HLA class I antigens) remains about 20%,[55,106] and the rate of refractoriness due to alloimmunity is about half that rate. The refractoriness, if related to HLA immunization, can be transient or persistent. Several approaches can be considered to provide such patients with adequate platelet support—including provision of HLA-matched platelets or platelets selected by crossmatch tests.

Platelet selection

HLA-selected platelet transfusions

A standard approach to supporting a patient who is refractory to whole blood–derived platelet transfusions is to supply HLA-matched apheresis platelet concentrates. Because the primary cause of immune refractoriness to platelet transfusion is alloimmunization to class I HLA antigens, it follows that avoidance of incompatible HLA specificities should result in a more successful platelet transfusion response. In practice, up to 90% of alloimmune refractory patients benefit from an HLA-matched product. This was first demonstrated in a study that showed that patients who were refractory to platelets from unselected donors could be successfully supported by HLA-matched family member platelet transfusions.[112]

Certain "private" HLA antigens can be segregated into so-called cross-reactive groups (CREGs), defined by antibodies directed against shared "public" determinants.[113] Indeed, these shared determinants are the basis for the cross-reactivity and are different from the private determinants, which account for the highly polymorphic HLA system. Selection of platelet donors with antigens in the same CREGs as the antigens in the patient, so-called cross-reactive antigens, was demonstrated to be nearly as successful in supporting alloimmune platelet refractory patients as HLA-identical transfusions.[114] This appeared to be due to the relative inability of the patient's immune system to recognize these cross-reactive antigens as different, thereby greatly increasing the number of potentially successful platelet donors in a given pool.[115]

A disadvantage of relying on HLA-matched platelets, even when using selective mismatching with CREG associations, is that a pool of 1000–3000 or more HLA-typed potential apheresis donors is generally necessary to find sufficient HLA-compatible matches to support a typical patient.[116] Moreover, donor selection on the basis

Table 18.3 Classification of Donor/Recipient Pairs on the Basis of HLA Match

A	All four antigens in donor are identical to those in recipient.
B1U	Only three antigens are detected in donor; all are present and identical in recipient.
B1X	Three donor antigens are identical to recipient; the fourth antigen is cross-reactive with recipient.
B2U	Only two antigens are detected in donor; both are present and identical in recipient.
B2UX	Only three antigens are detected in donor; two are identical with recipient, and the third is cross-reactive.
B2X	Two donor antigens are identical to recipient; the third and fourth antigens are cross-reactive with recipient.
C	One antigen of donor is not present in recipient and non-cross-reactive with recipient.
D	Two antigens of donor are not present in recipient and non-cross-reactive with recipient.

of HLA type can lead to the exclusion of donors whose HLA types, although different from that of the recipient, may still be effective.

In alloimmune refractory patients, the best increases in CCI occur with the subset of grade A and B1U or B2U HLA-matched platelets, but platelets mismatched for some antigens (e.g., B44 and B45) that are poorly expressed on platelets can also be successful.[117] Although alloimmunized patients with high panel-reactive (HLA) antibody (PRA) values benefit only from platelet products that lack any incompatible class I antigens (match grades A, B1U, B1X, B2U, and B2UX; see Table 18.3), patients with lesser degrees of sensitization can sometimes benefit from less well-matched platelets. In one study, 73% of HLA single-antigen mismatched platelet transfusions (grade C match) were successful when provided to patients with PRA values less than 60%.[118] On the basis of these data, some experts suggest extending donor searches for alloimmunized patients to include single-antigen mismatches (grade C matches), particularly if the PRA is less than 60%.

Even with the additional donors that the above-cited studies may make available, HLA-matched platelets are frequently unavailable for many refractory patients. Use of the patient's HLA antibody specificity as an additional basis for selection of platelet products has been demonstrated to increase the numbers of potentially compatible donors. Antibody specificity prediction (ASP) allows procurement of platelet products from donors who lack HLA antigens to which the patient has raised an antibody. Such platelet donors often have frank mismatches for some or all of the class I antigens in the refractory patient. One study compared ASP platelets to those selected by standard HLA matching criteria and by platelet crossmatching. HLA-matched, crossmatched, and ASP-selected platelet transfusions were found to have similar platelet recoveries, whereas randomly selected control platelets had significantly lower PPR. For 29 alloimmunized patients, the mean number of potential donors found in a file of 7247 HLA-typed donors was only six when grade A HLA matches were required and 39 when BU matches were added. However, 1426 potential donors (20% of total) were identified by the ASP method. The authors suggest that careful HLA antibody specificity identification could greatly enhance the number of potential donors by identifying nonmatched products that lack these HLA antigens.[119] Other investigators using a computerized analysis of the lymphocytotoxicity (LCT) assay for private and public HLA class I epitopes in platelet recipients confirmed that there is value in carefully identifying HLA antibody specificities, allowing selection of many more donors by simply avoiding the

HLA antigens against which the antibodies are directed.[120] Current sensitive techniques for detecting and identifying class I HLA antibodies using flow cytometry or Luminex provide a precise way of determining the relative strength of multiple HLA antibodies that may be present in patient sera.[121–123]

Regardless of the method planned to select HLA-compatible platelets for alloimmune refractory patients, the HLA type of the patient should be determined before myeloablative therapy, and HLA antibody screening should be obtained periodically (preferably weekly) so that HLA-selected platelets can be provided when and if alloimmune refractoriness is diagnosed.

In a small number of patients who fail to respond to HLA-matched platelets and for whom no other nonimmune explanation can be found for refractoriness, platelet-specific alloantibodies may be the cause of the poor platelet increments. Approximately 8% of platelet multitransfused patients develop platelet-specific antibodies.[55] Many of these patients are also alloimmunized against HLA. One report described six patients who were highly alloimmunized to HLA but also had human platelet alloantibodies to HPA-1b or HPA-5b.[124] These patients were successfully supported with a pool of HLA-matched platelets that were typed for the HPA antigens.

Platelet crossmatching

Although the use of HLA-matched, selectively HLA-mismatched, and ASP-selected donors provides support for the majority of patients who are alloimmune refractory, there are limitations to these strategies. As many as 20–25% of refractory patients fail to respond adequately to HLA-matched platelets. In the absence of nonimmunologic clinical factors that can decrease platelet transfusion recovery and survival, these failures might be explained by ABO incompatibility, platelet-specific antibodies, and undetected HLA incompatibility.[125] These immune causes of transfusion failure cannot be addressed with HLA matching alone. In addition, many facilities do not have access to adequately sized HLA-typed donor files, so alternative methods of selecting compatible platelets for alloimmune refractory patients must be considered.

Many platelet and leukocyte antibody detection methods have been assessed as platelet compatibility tests. One method that has gained wide acceptance is the commercially available solid-phase red cell adherence (SPRCA) assay. The test is rapid and sensitive, particularly for the detection of HLA antibodies, and is therefore suitable for routine platelet crossmatching.[126,127] Good correlation between test results and posttransfusion platelet counts has been achieved with the SPRCA assay.[127,128]

To date, few studies have compared the efficacy of HLA matching to that of platelet crossmatching for supporting alloimmune refractory patients. One multicenter study[129] compared HLA selection and platelet crossmatching using three different techniques—the indirect immunofluorescence test for platelets, an enzyme-linked immunosorbent assay (ELISA), and a radioimmunoassay were used to test apheresis platelet concentrates. At least one pair of apheresis platelet components was transfused to each patient. One unit was selected by HLA matching, and the other by crossmatching. The results of the two donor selection methods were compared. Although the difference between 1-hour posttransfusion recoveries was not statistically significant, after 24 hours the HLA-selected transfusions were significantly more successful. This was even more apparent when only A and BU matches were considered. The authors concluded that when HLA-typed donors are available, A or BU matches were preferable to randomly chosen products selected by any of the crossmatch methods used in their study.

The quality of the HLA match is paramount to the transfusion success rate as shown in a study in which HLA matching apparently did not improve on the success rate of crossmatch-selected platelets.[128] Here, however, the HLA-selected platelets were seldom of A or BU match grade with the recipients.

The degree to which a patient is alloimmunized has an impact on the success of platelet transfusions selected by crossmatching assays. Using platelet concentrates from whole blood units and a radio-labeled antiglobulin technique, one study found that 70% of transfusions selected by the test were successful in supporting moderately alloimmunized patients.[130] In contrast, others found that only 41% of transfusions selected by either an ELISA or the SPRCA test were successful in a highly alloimmunized group of leukemia patients.[131] Moreover, only 15–24% of platelet concentrate segments tested were negative in these tests, indicating that many whole blood–derived platelet concentrates had to be screened in order to identify sufficient compatible platelets to pool for the transfusions. In the latter study, the most compatible platelet products selected by crossmatching were less successful in supporting the refractory patients than were HLA-matched platelets.

A report of an automated version of the SPRCA assay demonstrated how large numbers of platelet concentrates could be routinely tested to identify compatible pools of whole blood–derived platelets for refractory patients. In this study, a daily inventory of 100–120 whole blood–derived buffy coats were assessed to provide platelet support for 40 consecutive alloimmune refractory patients.[132] Platelets collected from routinely obtained donor samples, rather than from the concentrates themselves, were tested with patient serum. Using this system, up to 94 different platelet samples could be tested for each patient. Buffy coat platelets from five or six donors whose platelets yielded negative results were then pooled and transfused to the patient. The authors were able to demonstrate significant improvement in both 1-hour and 18- to 24-hour increments with the crossmatch-negative pools compared with random pools given in the month before the patients met the criteria for refractoriness in the study (two consecutive 1-hour posttransfusion CCIs <5000).

The cost of the kits for achieving each "successful" platelet increment (posttransfusion platelet count >10,000/µL) was about 450 euros. This did not include any costs for labor or administration of the crossmatching program. The authors noted that although the automated crossmatching strategy allowed rapid identification of compatible platelet pools from available inventories, a larger study, preferably a randomized controlled trial of this method versus HLA matching, would be necessary to confirm the value of this approach and more accurately capture the costs involved.

Experience using both the LCT assay and the SPRCA for analyzing antibodies to HLA and platelet antigens has been reported to aid in identifying patients who will benefit from either HLA-selected or crossmatch-selected platelets.[133] With the LCT assay, investigators found that if the PRA was <70%, adequate transfusion responses were seen in approximately 80% of transfusions that were selected simply by HLA criteria (ASP and CREGs). However, when the PRA was >70%, only about 25% of patients did well. When analyzing the results using crossmatching, patients with PRAs <80% did well with crossmatch-selected platelets; but when the PRA was 80–100%, there were many failures with the crossmatch-compatible products. It was suggested that at high levels of alloimmunization, crossmatching misses significant antibodies. One report compares the MAIPA assay to the LCT test for the detection of HLA antibodies. This study showed the MAIPA assay to be more

sensitive, detecting apparent HLA antibodies missed by the LCT assay. Moreover, these MAIPA-positive, LCT-negative HLA antibodies may be clinically relevant and affect the posttransfusion platelet count increment.[134] The advent of more sensitive methods for screening patients for HLA antibodies, when used to identify patients who are alloimmune refractory to platelet transfusions, may prove to be superior to the LCT assay for this purpose.[122,123,135]

With the considerable effort and expense entailed in their procurement, HLA- or crossmatch-selected platelet products should be reserved for those refractory patients who have definite evidence of alloimmunization by either HLA or platelet antibody testing. In the latter case, alloimmunity can be established in the context of performing a platelet crossmatch test if at least some of the platelet products tested with patient serum are reactive in the assay. In practice, when refractoriness is first recognized during use of random donor platelets, provision of a few HLA-selected products may be warranted before the results of definitive testing to document alloimmunization are available. In the event that such testing fails to document alloimmunity (i.e., no HLA- or platelet-reactive antibodies are identified), then support with randomly selected platelet products should resume.

Although the incidence of platelet-specific antibodies causing patients to be refractory to most or all attempted platelet transfusions is very small, this possibility should be investigated when most of the attempted crossmatches are positive or when HLA-matched transfusions fail. If platelet-specific antibodies are present, donors of known platelet antigen phenotype or family members, who may be more likely to share the patient's phenotype, should be tested.

Despite the effort and expense involved in providing platelets selected by crossmatching to refractory patients, as is the case with platelets selected by HLA matching, a positive impact on patient outcomes has not been demonstrated. A recent review of platelet crossmatching studies reported from the past four decades concluded that none provided adequate evidence that either mortality or morbidity related to bleeding could be reduced by using crossmatch-compatible platelets in refractory patients, regardless of the method chosen.[136]

Overcoming established alloimmunization

Strategies attempting to reverse established alloimmunity to HLA antigens have met with only limited success to date. Previously attempted methods include (1) methods to temporarily block the immune-mediated destruction of platelets, (2) suppression of the immune response to decrease the production of relevant antibodies, and (3) provision of modified platelets or alternative (nonplatelet) hemostatic compounds.

Blocking immune destruction of platelets

Several studies investigated the utility of high-dose intravenous immunoglobulin (IVIG) to increase the platelet count in association with transfusion in refractory patients. The results of these studies have been highly variable.[137–139] Initial uncontrolled trials were conducted with very small numbers of patients using whole blood–derived platelet transfusions. Studies using somewhat larger numbers of patients have been inconclusive. One study treated 11 refractory patients with 0.4 g/kg/day for 5 days with no benefit in the 1-hour posttransfusion recoveries.[137] Another found a modest beneficial effect of IVIG in a randomized placebo-controlled trial with 12 alloimmunized thrombocytopenic patients.[138] The same donor platelets were used before and after treatment with IVIG.

The posttreatment 1-hour CCIs in the IVIG group (seven patients) were significantly greater than in the five patients receiving placebo treatment—8413 and 1050, respectively. However, by 24 hours after the transfusion, there was no residual benefit of IVIG. The authors concluded that the use of IVIG could not replace HLA-matched platelet transfusions in supporting alloimmunized refractory patients.

Using very high-dose (6 g/kg) IVIG, other investigators could reverse the refractory response in some patients who failed to respond to HLA-selected LCT-compatible platelet transfusions.[139] Before treatment with IVIG, the patients had been refractory to HLA-matched platelet products. Following therapy, 13 of 19 patients responded with improvement in 1-hour posttransfusion platelet count increment using HLA-matched platelets. Those patients with PRAs <85% responded better than those who were more highly alloimmunized.

After initial reports of success with IVIG to improve platelet responses in immune refractory patients, other investigators examined the role of Rh immune globulin (RhIG) infusions in preventing refractory responses from developing. In this randomized control trial, patients treated with weekly intravenous RhIG infusions had rates of refractoriness similar to those treated with placebo, indicating that this form of reticuloendothelial system blockade was not helpful in preventing refractory responses.[140]

Suppression of the immune response to decrease antibody production

Other strategies evaluated to overcome the platelet refractory state include use of vinblastine-loaded platelet transfusions,[141] treatment with cyclosporin A,[142] immunoabsorption using staphylococcal protein A columns, and plasmapheresis.[143,144] A more recent report describes the coincident improvement in platelet response in a patient treated with bortezomib for multiple myeloma,[145] and a second one describes a patient whose alloimmune refractoriness resolved after conditioning for allogeneic stem cell transplantation.[146] Each strategy has had some limited success, and none can be recommended for routine use in this situation.

Provision of modified platelets or alternative (nonplatelet) hemostatic compounds

A novel approach has been developed involving transfusion with acid-treated whole blood–derived platelets. Treatment of platelets with citric acid modifies HLA class I antigens on the platelet surface, making them less recognizable to the immune system.[8,147] A small number of patients have been treated with such products but with very limited success. Several potential platelet substitutes are currently being investigated. These include lyophilized platelets, infusible platelet membranes, thromboerythrocytes, and thrombospheres. Whether these will have clinical relevancy remains to be determined by future investigation.[148,149]

The role of platelet growth factors in the treatment of patients who have undergone highly myeloablative therapy is not totally defined. Studies support the use of both interleukin-11 (IL11)[150] and recombinant human thrombopoietin in shortening the duration and blunting the severity of thrombocytopenia after chemotherapy. However, toxicity and the development of thrombopoietin-neutralizing antibodies have halted trials using the latter agent.[151] Less success has been demonstrated with these agents in the setting of myeloablation with stem cell transplantation. These drugs may play more of a role in preventing rather than managing platelet refractoriness because responsive patients would require

fewer platelet transfusions. Currently, only one product, recombinant human IL11 (Neumega, Genetics Institute, Cambridge, MA), is licensed in the United States for the prevention of severe thrombocytopenia and the reduction of the need for platelet transfusion following myelosuppressive but not myeloablative chemotherapy in patients with nonmyeloid malignancies.[152,153] There have been only limited case reports and no formal trials of the newer thrombopoietin mimetic agents romiplostim or eltrombopag for refractory patients.[154]

Prevention of alloimmunity

Alloimmunization to HLA antigens appears to be transient in some patients; however, for most patients, once the alloimmune refractory state is established, it is very difficult to reverse. Therapy for the refractory state is expensive and frequently requires more transfusions than therapy for patients who are not refractory.[155] Therefore, attention has turned to prevention of alloimmunization as a more practical way to ensure continued successful platelet support. Figure 18.2 represents an approach to managing platelet transfusions that encompasses both prevention of and platelet selection for refractoriness to platelet transfusions.

Several strategies have been used to prevent alloimmunization to platelet products. Antigenic exposure can be limited by the use of apheresis platelet transfusions. Both animal studies and trials involving humans have shown that HLA alloimmunization can at least be delayed (if not reduced) by the provision of apheresis platelets. Apheresis platelet products provide adequate platelet doses for adults from single donors rather than pools of whole blood–derived platelet concentrates, which typically expose patients to 5–8 different donors.[72] Indeed, the majority of platelet transfusions in the United States are now provided from apheresis collections, partly in order to reduce the rates of alloimmunization and refractoriness.[156]

A second promising method is treatment of blood components with ultraviolet B (UVB) irradiation.[157] UVB irradiation prevents the interaction of donor dendritic cells with recipient T lymphocytes, which is the major route of primary HLA alloimmunization to platelet transfusions. Additional studies have provided evidence that the inability of donor and recipient immune cells to interact following UVB irradiation may indicate a state of immunologic tolerance to a blood transfusion. Preliminary studies with UVB-treated platelets in thrombocytopenic patients with cancer demonstrated a reduced rate of HLA antibody formation. The TRAP study found that UVB irradiation could reduce the incidence of alloimmunization and platelet refractoriness.[55] Despite its effectiveness in reducing alloimmunization, UVB irradiation of platelet products is currently not approved for use in the United States.

Because the major pathway of primary alloimmunization against HLA class I involves antigen presentation in the context of HLA class II molecules on donor APCs,[1] significant work has centered on removing leukocytes from the donor blood components as a means of preventing alloimmunization. Clinical trials have demonstrated that reduction of leukocytes to a level $<5 \times 10^6$ in blood components is sufficient to reduce the risk of HLA alloimmunization.[55,79] Removal of leukocytes is most often accomplished by passing the components through third-generation leukocyte reduction filters. These filters remove the leukocytes by a combination of adhesion and pore size and are capable of producing a three- to four-log reduction in leukocytes. This process results in products that easily meet the US Food and Drug Administration's requirement for leukocyte-reduced blood components ($<5 \times 10^6$ total

Algorithm for Managing Platelet Support

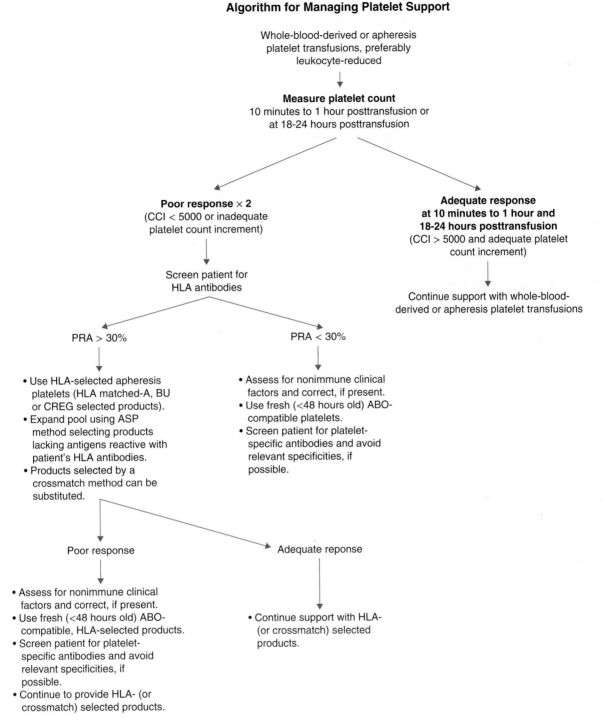

Figure 18.2 Algorithm for managing platelet support.

leukocytes). Although such filters can be used at the bedside, the preferred method is prestorage leukocyte reduction in the laboratory. The latter allows leukocyte-reduced blood components to be manufactured according to good manufacturing practice regulations with well-defined quality control. It also prevents leukocyte fragments, shown to be capable of passing through filters and sensitizing recipients in animal studies, from accumulating in stored blood components.[158] Leukocyte reduction of platelet products can be accomplished by using either of two techniques. With apheresis technology (by which the equivalent of six whole blood–derived platelet concentrates can be obtained from a single donor), the product is leukocyte reduced as it is collected. Alternatively, pools of whole blood–derived platelet concentrates can be filtered before a five-day storage period.

The majority of trials to date support the use of leukocyte reduction to reduce alloimmunization to blood components. In 1998, 18 clinical trials (some randomized controlled and some nonrandomized) using leukocyte-reduced red cells and platelets to prevent alloimmunization were reviewed.[159] Fourteen of the trials showed positive results using leukocyte-reduced blood to prevent HLA alloimmunization and platelet refractoriness, whereas three of the trials showed no benefit. In addition, a recent meta-analysis of eight randomized controlled trials demonstrated a clear, protective effect of white cell reduction in the prevention of HLA alloimmunization and platelet refractoriness.[160]

The most definitive clinical trial demonstrating the importance of leukocyte reduction in the prevention of alloimmunization and refractoriness to platelet transfusion was the TRAP study.[55] This trial compared four groups of patients: (1) patients receiving pooled platelet concentrates (control); (2) patients receiving leukocyte-reduced (filtered), pooled platelet concentrates; (3) patients receiving UVB-irradiated pooled platelet concentrates; and (4) patients receiving filtered platelets obtained by apheresis. All patients received leukocyte-reduced red cell components. Evidence of alloimmunization (by LCT assay) developed in 45% of the control group compared with 17–21% in the treated groups ($p \leq 0.0001$ for each treated group as compared with controls). There were no differences among the treated groups in rates of alloimmunization. In the control group, 13% of patients became refractory compared to 3–5% in the treated groups ($p \leq 0.03$ for each treated group as compared with controls). Individual treatments did not differ.

Several other important findings were noted in the TRAP study: (1) Clinical outcomes were similar in all four groups of the study, with no significant difference in the incidence of deaths caused by hemorrhage; (2) the incidence of refractoriness to platelet transfusions was low in the control group relative to previous reported studies; (3) patients who had never been pregnant had a lower risk of developing refractoriness than those who had previous pregnancies; (4) only about 8% of the patients in the study developed platelet-specific antibodies, and the treatment groups had no impact on this type of immunization; (5) the presence of platelet-specific antibodies did not correlate with refractoriness; and (6) a small percentage of patients in all groups were refractory to platelet transfusions yet did not have lymphocytotoxic antibodies—most likely, these patients had either clinical factors or drug-related causes of refractoriness.

Another large, single-institution, retrospective study was reported from Canada, where universal leukocyte reduction (ULR) of blood components was instituted between 1997 and 1999.[61] The study examined rates of alloimmunization and refractoriness in cohorts of patients undergoing chemotherapy for acute leukemia or stem cell transplantation before and after the introduction of ULR. Investigators found that alloimmunization to HLA, alloimmune refractoriness, and the need for HLA-matched platelets were all significantly reduced in the ULR cohort. Even taking into account the lower numbers of platelet transfusions given to the ULR patients, which likely resulted, in part, from changing the platelet transfusion trigger from 20,000/μL to 10,000/μL, leukocyte-reduced transfusions remained a significant independent variable driving the lower rates of alloimmunization and refractoriness in this patient population.

From the studies cited above, it is clear that both leukocyte reduction and UVB irradiation are capable of reducing the incidence of alloimmunization and platelet refractoriness. At the present time, leukocyte reduction of blood components is the most practical means of reducing the incidence of alloimmune platelet refractoriness and should be recommended for all patients at risk.

The identification and characterization of platelet antigens together with increased understanding of immunologic responses to these markers have been crucial in developing optimal platelet transfusion practices. Our understanding of the causes and mechanisms of both the immunologic and nonimmunologic aspects of the refractory response allows for improved strategies in the care of the potentially refractory patient.

Summary

Platelets express a variety of immunogenic markers on the cell surface. Some of these antigens are shared with other cell types as in the case of HLA antigens, which are shared with virtually all nucleated cells in the body. Other antigens are observed to be essentially platelet specific. This chapter has reviewed the antigens expressed on the platelet, the various patterns of alloimmunization to these antigens, and the impact on platelet transfusion responses. Strategies to treat and prevent alloimmunization were also summarized.

Disclaimer

The author has disclosed no conflicts of interest.

Key references

A full reference list for this chapter is available at: http://www.wiley.com/go/simon/transfusion

1 Pavenski K, Freedman J, Semple JW. HLA alloimmunization against platelet transfusions: pathophysiology, significance, prevention and management. *Tissue Antigens* 2012; **79**: 237–45. doi: 10.1111/j.1399-0039.2012.01852.x

47 Curtis BR, McFarland JG. Human platelet antigens—2013. *Vox Sang* 2013; **106**: 93–102. doi: 10.1111/vox.12085

55 Leukocyte reduction and ultraviolet B irradiation of platelets to prevent alloimmunization and refractoriness to platelet transfusions. The Trial to Reduce Alloimmunization to Platelets Study Group. *N Engl J Med* 1997; **337**: 1861–9.

101 Cooling L. ABO and platelet transfusion therapy. *Immunohematology* 2007; **23**: 20–33.

102 Slichter SJ. Algorithm for managing the platelet refractory patient. *J Clin Apher* 1997; **12**: 4–9.

119 Petz LD, Garratty G, Calhoun L, *et al.* Selecting donors of platelets for refractory patients on the basis of HLA antibody specificity. *Transfusion* 2000; **40**: 1446–56.

129 Moroff G, Garratty G, Heal JM, *et al.* Selection of platelets for refractory patients by HLA matching and prospective crossmatching. *Transfusion* 1992; **32**: 633–40.

136 Vassallo RR, Fung M, Rebulla P, *et al.* Utility of cross-matched platelet transfusions in patients with hypoproliferative thrombocytopenia: a systematic review. *Transfusion* 2014; **54**: 1180–91. doi: 10.1111/trf.12395

CHAPTER 19

Preparation, preservation, and storage of platelet concentrates

Ralph R. Vassallo, Jr.

University of Pennsylvania School of Medicine, Philadelphia, PA, USA

Platelets may be obtained for transfusion by centrifugation of 450–500 mL of whole blood drawn in citrate-based anticoagulants or by various apheresis instruments that selectively collect platelets over 45–120 minutes. In the United States, platelets collected by either method are suspended in autologous plasma or a combination of plasma and a saline-based additive solution at an average concentration of 1500×10^9/L, six times the mean blood platelet concentration. Modern manufacturing techniques isolate 70–75% of the platelets from a whole blood donation ($0.6–1.2 \times 10^{11}$).[1] Pooling of 4–6 whole blood–derived (WBD) units provides a single therapeutic adult dose. Alternatively, high-efficiency apheresis separators are able to harvest 65–75% of platelets from the 2–6 L of blood cycled through the instrument ($3–14 \times 10^{11}$), resulting in as many as three adult doses.[2]

Apheresis units represented approximately 91% of the platelet concentrates (PCs) transfused in the United States in 2011.[3] This is because of both their convenience (preparation for immediate transfusion and bacterial contamination screening are performed at the blood center rather than the hospital) and the perceived advantage of fewer donor exposures. Although WBD units can be pooled before storage and also easily tested for bacteria, they remain relegated to a supplementary role when apheresis capacity is suboptimal, despite their somewhat lower cost.[4]

Preparation of platelets from whole blood: the platelet-rich plasma method

Until the late 1960s, whole blood donations were routinely refrigerated at 1–6 °C to prevent bacterial proliferation. Following the introduction of plastic containers in the late 1940s, platelets were transfused primarily as platelet-rich plasma (PRP), directly infused after soft centrifugation to separate unneeded red cells.[5] Further attempts to concentrate platelets from PRP resulted in an irreversibly clumped mass at the bottom of the refrigerated bag. Success at augmenting recipient platelet counts was limited both by volume constraints and because platelets separated and stored in the cold circulated poorly in recipients.[6] Mourad recognized that if PRP were allowed to come to room temperature before hard centrifugation, following supernatant plasma expression into another container, the platelet pellet could be gently resuspended in approximately 50 mL of residual plasma after a short resting period.[7] Building upon this finding, Murphy and Gardner revolutionized platelet therapy by demonstrating that platelets maintained at room temperature (20–24 °C) throughout their entire ex vivo interval were easily concentrated and circulated almost four times longer than refrigerated ones in recipients.[6]

Since the early 1970s, room temperature citrated whole blood has been transported from the collection site to a manufacturing facility and processed into red blood cells (RBCs), plasma, and room temperature PC components (Figure 19.1A). Small changes to this process have been introduced over the years (e.g., optimization of bag materials and centrifugation protocols, introduction of new anticoagulants, and integration of leukocyte reduction filters into collection sets), but production of PCs from a PRP intermediate remains the only US Food and Drug Administration (FDA)-licensed method of WBD platelet production in the United States today. Room temperature whole blood storage was initially limited to four hours after collection, but current guidelines allow an eight-hour period between venipuncture and platelet production.[8,9] There is increasing interest in extending this period for operational reasons. The overnight hold of whole blood donations eliminates the need for multiple transport runs from remote collection sites to the manufacturing facility and allows manufacturing on one rather than multiple shifts. Data exist to support the maintenance of PRP platelet quality after an overnight hold, but RBC quality and lack of interest in shouldering extensive product revalidation costs remain problematic.[10,11]

Platelets derived from whole blood are known as *Platelets* (colloquially, random-donor platelets [RDPs]). AABB and the FDA require that a unit of platelets contains at least 0.55×10^{11} platelets.[12] Modern concentrates actually contain an average of 0.9×10^{11} platelets with a relatively wide ($\sim 0.27 \times 10^{11}$) standard deviation.[1] This requires a pool of at least five concentrates to ensure that, after a 6–10% loss during pooling, 99% of pools contain a dose of 3×10^{11}, the AABB/FDA-stipulated minimum content of apheresis platelets.[12] Prestorage leukocyte reduction is increasingly accomplished routinely during manufacture (*Platelets Leukocytes Reduced*) with a loss of 4–5% of platelet content in the filter.[13] Leukocyte reduction results in a ≥3 log reduction in white blood cell (WBC) content to a level below AABB and FDA requirements for $<0.83 \times 10^6$ WBCs per PC (one-sixth of the $<5 \times 10^6$ threshold required for apheresis platelets).[12] PRP-PCs are suspended in

Rossi's Principles of Transfusion Medicine, Fifth Edition. Edited by Toby L. Simon, Jeffrey McCullough, Edward L. Snyder, Bjarte G. Solheim, and Ronald G. Strauss.

© 2016 John Wiley & Sons, Ltd. Published 2016 by John Wiley & Sons, Ltd.

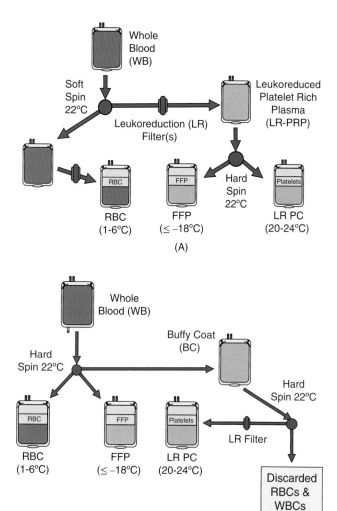

Figure 19.1 Platelet production methods. RBC, red blood cell; FPP, fresh frozen plasma; LR, leukocyte reduced; PC, platelet concentrate.

autologous plasma anticoagulated with citrate–phosphate–dextrose (CPD), or CPD with either twice the amount of dextrose (CP2D) or adenine (CPDA-1).

Platelets and *Platelets Leukocytes Reduced* platelets are frequently pooled into a licensed container specifically validated for prestorage pooling. This pool, produced by blood suppliers, has a five-day outdate (midnight of the fifth day following collection). This is substantially more flexible than the four-hour outdate for *Platelets* or *Platelets Leukocytes Reduced* platelets that are pooled after storage. Diversion of 8–10 mL for bacterial culture of these 40–70 mL products results in significant platelet loss. The cost and inconvenience of required bacterial contamination screening with point-of-issue tests have dramatically reduced the use of poststorage pooling.[14] *Platelets* and *Platelets Leukocytes Reduced* platelets are thus primarily used for neonatal transfusion for which one or two units constitutes a therapeutic dose.

Preparation of platelets from whole blood: the buffy coat method

In Europe, concern about WBC content in RBC components and the need for plasma derivatives resulted in a different method of component production.[15] Initial hard centrifugation results in the density-dependent partition of plasma, a platelet- and white-cell-containing buffy coat (BC), and red cells. Both manual and automated devices are available to express plasma and red cells into different containers, leaving the BC in the primary container. Four to six BCs are combined, resuspended in plasma from a male donor (in the United Kingdom) or in a platelet additive solution (PAS; continental Europe) and soft centrifuged to remove red cells and white cells (Figure 19.1B). The resultant product is passed through a leukocyte reduction filter to produce a prestorage pooled, leukocyte-reduced PC. This process results in lower initial white cell content, facilitating compliance with European standards for leukocyte reduction, which require $<1 \times 10^6$ WBCs in the resultant pooled product.[16] Compared with the PRP manufacturing process, the BC process yields an average platelet product with a nearly equivalent platelet content. In addition, the RBC component has about 20 mL fewer red cells and one log fewer white cells. There is also about 30–75 mL more recovered plasma.[17] In 2005, the Canadian Blood Services initiated a switch from PRP to BC production because of perceived advantages, the most important of these being logistical. BC production employs butanediol plates within transport containers to rapidly cool and hold whole blood at 20–24 °C for up to 24 hours before manufacturing. Automated pooling technology contributes to process control, making BC production even more economical.[18]

In Europe, 50% or more of transfusions are BC-WBD PCs.[19] Denmark, Germany, Spain, and the Netherlands prepare >85% of their concentrates from whole blood.[19] These countries demonstrate that a national platelet supply can be derived predominantly from collected whole blood rather than relying upon apheresis PC production when a 24-hour room temperature hold period is allowed before component separation.

In contrast to PRP-PCs centrifuged against the platelet container, BP-PCs are centrifuged against cellular elements of the whole blood unit. This may lead to less platelet activation during PC production relative to PRP-PCs.[20] Activation is one mechanism of platelet loss during storage.

Preparation of platelets by plateletpheresis

Support of HLA-alloimmunized platelet-refractory patients requires platelets from a single donor. Apheresis-derived platelets are known as *Apheresis Platelets* (colloquially, single-donor platelets [SDPs]). In the mid-1970s, automated instruments were developed to replace high-volume, dedicated-donor PC collections (serial whole blood donations alternating with red cell and plasma reinfusion). As these cell separators became more widely available, inevitably, the economics of supporting plateletpheresis programs drove collections beyond these niche needs, and apheresis-derived units were offered as a substitute for WBD units. Improved computer controls allowed apheresis technology to evolve beyond tedious automated cycles to continuous processing, which has significantly decreased procedure time and extracorporeal blood volumes. As the efficiency of apheresis separators improved and platelet yields increased well beyond the content of "standard" pools of six WBD-PCs, blood centers began to "split" apheresis units, providing therapeutic doses for two and sometimes three adults. In-process leukocyte reduction became possible with better separation controls, so *Apheresis Platelets Leukocytes Reduced* now routinely contain $<5 \times 10^6$ WBCs. Unlike WBD-PCs, red cell content in apheresis PCs is quite low in most units, often (but not always) below the dose of red cells associated with RhD alloimmunization.[21,22]

The various apheresis instruments collect platelets in slightly different ways, leading to subtle differences in platelet populations and postprocedure activation. (See Chapter 32 for more detail.) Several variations on the earliest models employed a disposable plastic centrifuge chamber from which a layer of concentrated platelets was siphoned into a collection bag. More commonly employed instruments use a spinning channel with two-stage plastic inlays to initially separate the red cells from the PRP, followed by plasma removal before collection of the final platelet product. Yet another technology uses an elutriation mechanism to move larger platelets away from the red cell layer, separates the PRP, and then hyperconcentrates platelets along a collection bag wall before plasma resuspension in a storage container. This heterogeneity of collection technologies means that apheresis products are not necessarily similar, nor will they always produce equivalent platelet increments in a given recipient.[23]

Alternative sources of platelets

Although not currently cost-effective, efforts to generate platelets ex vivo from CD34+ progenitor cells and embryonic or induced pluripotent stem cells may eventually be feasible.[24] These platelets appear morphologically normal and participate in thrombus formation, but so few can be produced that more extensive functional testing is difficult. Although bioreactors that simulate the marrow microenvironment may be the answer to yield insufficiency, this technology is unlikely to produce economical transfusable doses within the foreseeable future.

Storage conditions

Once the circulatory survival benefit of room temperature processing and storage was appreciated, platelets were kept for up to three days in the first generation of plastic containers. As improvements were made in platelet storage technology, shelf life was first increased to five days, and then to seven days. In 1986, the FDA mandated a return to a five-day shelf life because of increasing reports of bacterial sepsis associated with prolonged 20–24 °C storage.[25] Detection methods for bacterial contamination were required in 2004 (discussed in detail in Chapter 53), but reextension of storage has not been possible because of the poor sensitivity of available testing (29–40%).[14,26,27] Improvements in bacterial testing or the introduction of pathogen reduction technology, however, might once more allow seven-day platelet storage.

Platelets survive for approximately 9–10 days in the circulation and are removed by senescence, consumption during maintenance of vascular integrity (normally, $\sim 7.1 \times 10^9/L/day$),[28] or clot formation to control pathologic bleeding. Room temperature storage appears to slow platelet metabolic activity by almost 60% compared with in vivo activity at 37 °C.[29] This suggests that seven days of storage may lead to only three days' worth of in vivo senescent loss. Storage conditions that minimize platelet loss by inhibiting platelet activation, senescence (apoptosis), or metabolic exhaustion might, in theory, permit the extension of PC shelf life well beyond seven days. The critical variables affecting stored platelet health are (1) temperature, (2) metabolic fuel availability, and (3) respiratory capacity. The last is dependent on platelet content, gas diffusion through the plastic container, and agitation. Activation occurring during collection and processing appears to be somewhat reversible, but excessive activation may also lead to platelet loss.

Metabolic concerns during storage: temperature

When platelets are exposed to the cold, their plasma membranes undergo phase transitions that result in the coalescence of lipid rafts, in turn leading to platelet shape change and activation priming, clustering of neoepitope-expressing glycoprotein (GP)-Ibα domains with enhanced von Willebrand factor (vWF) binding capacity, and acceleration of platelet apoptosis.[28–32] This in vivo platelet cold sensitivity presumably facilitates activation at wound sites on the cooler body surface, while resulting in the removal of repetitively primed platelets to prevent core thrombosis.[30,31]

Membrane phase transitions begin at temperatures below 30 °C, bringing phosphoinositide-rich lipid rafts together.[31,33] Resultant phosphoinositide release results in an increase in intracellular calcium, which is associated with activation priming. Indeed, the immediate posttransfusion function of cold-stored platelets exceeds that of room temperature–stored platelets, prompting a call for reevaluation of the role of cold-stored platelets when immediate hemostasis is paramount (e.g., after trauma).[34] Hypothermic membrane changes also result in clustering of the principal vWF receptor, GP-Ib/IX/V.[31] Function of the receptor appears to be enhanced by clustering. However, lectin-binding domains of hepatic macrophage $\alpha_M \beta_2$ and hepatocyte asialoglycoprotein receptors recognize densely clustered GP-Ibα subunits that have lost or gained sugars during this process and rapidly remove these platelets. This explains the quite short circulation time of these potentially more hemostatically active chilled platelets.[34]

The reversibility of cold-induced platelet membrane changes is both time and temperature dependent. Figure 19.2 shows the effect of 18 hours of storage at various temperatures upon the half-life of radiolabeled autologous platelets after reinfusion into healthy volunteers. Temperatures above 20 °C resulted in normal platelet survival.[6] Holme et al.[35] reported that significant loss of platelet circulatory capacity occurred after 24 hours at 18 °C, 16 hours at 16 °C, 10 hours for 12 °C, and six hours at 4 °C. Storage above the 20–24 °C temperature described as optimal by Murphy and Gardner did not result in measurable damage, but was accompanied by increased metabolism compared with room temperature storage. The salutary metabolic effects of room temperature storage include decreased in vitro aging and slower accumulation of toxic metabolites within the platelet container. There is, however, a reversible loss

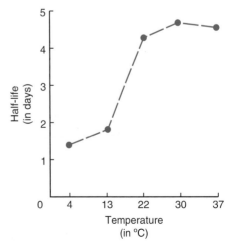

Figure 19.2 In vivo survival of radiolabeled autologous platelets stored at various temperatures for 18 hours.

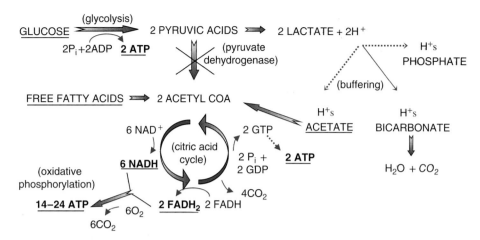

Figure 19.3 Pathways of platelet adenosine triphosphate (ATP) regeneration from inorganic phosphate (P_i) and adenosine diphosphate (ADP). Metabolic fuels are underlined. Energetic intermediates are underlined. Carbon dioxide (CO_2) is produced from hydrogen ion (H^+) buffering and oxidative metabolism of acetyl CoA. AMP, adenosine monophosphate; PPi, pyrophosphate; GDP/GTP, guanosine di-/triphosphate; NAD/NADH, nicotinamide adenine dinucleotide/reduced NAD; FADH/FADH$_2$, reduced flavin adenine dinucleotide forms.

of function that recovers only after a variable period of time in circulation.[34] The ability of room temperature–stored platelets to circulate for longer periods of time, despite transiently decreased activation capacity, is desirable in preventing spontaneous hemorrhage in chronically thrombocytopenic transfusion recipients.

Metabolic concerns during storage: metabolic fuel availability

Stored platelets must catabolize substances within their suspension medium to regenerate adenosine triphosphate (ATP), the principal "energy currency" of the cell spent in the maintenance of cellular integrity. Figure 19.3 shows the pathways for ATP regeneration.

Seminal studies of glucose consumption and lactate production in PRP-PCs revealed an approximately 1:2 ratio consistent with predominantly anaerobic metabolism of glucose.[36] Pyruvate dehydrogenase, which produces acetic acid for the aerobic citric acid cycle, appears to be downregulated in stored platelets. Glucose metabolism in platelets ends with the production of only 2 moles of ATP per mole of glucose consumed. Lactic acid is buffered primarily by plasma bicarbonate, which results in the production of CO_2.[37] This CO_2, a volatile acid, diffuses through the storage container wall. Progressive depletion of bicarbonate thus occurs through lactic acid buffering as well as slow spontaneous dissociation to CO_2 and water. Once bicarbonate is consumed, continued lactic acid production ultimately results in a deleterious decrease in product pH.

Aerobic metabolism through the citric acid cycle and oxidative phosphorylation is a far more efficient source of energy, yielding up to 13 moles of ATP per mole of acetic acid entering the cycle. Comparison of platelet oxygen consumption (approximately 6 moles of ATP produced per mole of O_2 consumed) with lactate production (1 mole of ATP per mole of lactate) suggests that approximately 85% of platelet energy is derived from aerobic metabolism in continuously agitated PCs.[36] Studies using radiolabeled palmitate identify free fatty acids derived from plasma triglycerides as the predominant metabolic fuel for platelets stored in plasma.[38] A small, rather insignificant component results from metabolism of the amino acid glutamine.[39] Efforts to identify plasma-sparing PASs led to the discovery that acetate could serve as an effective alternative fuel to plasma free fatty acids.[40] As described below, acetate also provides a valuable lactate-

buffering function through consumption of a hydrogen ion during its metabolism.

Under low oxygen conditions, glycolysis is upregulated six- to sevenfold, the so-called Pasteur effect.[41] Although this satisfies energy requirements in the absence of aerobic metabolism, it results in a considerable increase in lactic acid production, which can exacerbate plasma buffer exhaustion and produce deleterious declines in pH. Mechanical factors also affect platelet oxygenation. Mitochondrial oxygen starvation can occur with the interruption of agitation during shipping, accompanied by an expected increase in lactate generation and pH decrements.[42] Studies have shown that platelets begin to suffer deleterious effects below a pH of 6.5–6.8 at room temperature (22 °C) and are irreversibly damaged in the face of a sustained pH below 6.2 at 22 °C.[37,43] Efforts to extend platelet storage have been limited by the constitutive glycolytic production of lactate, even with maintenance of adequate oxygenation. Glycolysis can also be transiently upregulated by activation associated with platelet separation.[44] Attempts to develop glucose-free additive solutions to minimize the production of lactate have not been successful. Despite the presence of sufficient amounts of alternate fuels (e.g., acetate), once PCs exhaust their supply of glucose, they deplete their adenine nucleotides and a host of other metabolic intermediates, leading to cell death.[40,45] The reasons for this are poorly understood, but may be related to substrate depletion of the anti-oxidant pentose phosphate shunt and an as-yet-unexplained link between glucose metabolism and mitochondrial function. Adenine nucleotide depletion during storage has been characterized in PRP-PCs.[46] After seven days of storage, adenine nucleotide levels in PCs (in both metabolic and storage granular pools) decline to 70% of those initially present.[47] Although platelet ATP levels are not predictive of platelet quality except at extremely low levels, energy depletion is responsible for a host of deleterious effects that ultimately culminate in platelet senescence or necrosis.

Proteomic and metabolomic studies have shed additional light on platelet storage metabolism.[44,48,49] Regardless of the separation method, there appears to be a transition from active aerobic and glycolytic metabolism to a state of metabolic decay characterized by progressive depletion of intermediates. This is posited to occur as a result of mounting activation stimuli, both outside-in and inside-out, which reach an irreversible tipping point after three days of storage under current conditions. In vitro suppression of signaling proteins appears to delay the metabolic shift from maintenance to activation, but this laboratory approach has not resulted in an inhibitor suitable for clinical use.[44]

Metabolic concerns during storage: respiratory capacity

Maintenance of aerobic metabolism requires a PO_2 above 5–10 mmHg.[36] Because oxygen consumption is relatively constant per platelet, the presence of a high total platelet bag content stresses the oxygen permeability of the storage container. When PC consumption exceeds the ability of the container to transport oxygen, the PO_2 will decline to hypoxic levels over several days, leading to upregulation of glycolysis, lactic acid accumulation, and a deleterious decrease in pH. Gases diffuse across storage container walls driven by their gradients once the plastic is saturated. Each manufacturer's container has a different gas permeability related to wall thickness and the plastic's unique gas transport capacity. Oxygen delivery also depends upon the container's ratio of volume-to-surface area as well as continuous agitation, which promotes gas diffusion and helps maintain normal platelet oxygen consumption.

Kilkson et al.[36] demonstrated that across the CO_2 concentrations seen in PCs stored in the least permeable containers (10–100 mmHg), little pH change is attributable to the formation of carbonic acid from aqueous CO_2 and H_2O. Lactate concentration was shown to be the principal determinant of pH. Thus, high CO_2 permeability is not as critical as is good oxygen permeability. High CO_2 permeability, in fact, can lead to an early increase in pH as the PCO_2 falls from physiologic plasma levels, unbalanced by significant lactic acid accumulation. A pH >7.4 at 22 °C may result, which has been associated with cellular damage with earlier forms of agitation. Although European regulators have set 7.4 pH as the upper limit of acceptable end storage at 22 °C, a comprehensive study noted that with modern forms of agitation, a pH >6.3 at 22 °C had no predictive value for platelet viability (in PCs compliant with licensed maximum and minimum platelet contents and concentrations).[50]

From the foregoing discussion of metabolic fuel requirements, it is evident that high platelet content will increase constitutively produced levels of lactic acid and that high platelet concentrations also result in fewer plasma buffers per respiring platelet, both of which may lead to deleterious drops in pH. Less intuitive are the harmful effects of low platelet contents and concentrations. Adverse effects in these situations result from low CO_2 and lactate production, which initially result in an increase in PC pH. Why these products develop metabolic exhaustion and adenine nucleotide depletion is not entirely clear, but some forms of agitation further increase this effect at higher pH values.

The very first containers, made of polyvinyl chloride (PVC) plasticized with di-(2-ethylhexyl) phthalate (DEHP), were originally designed for freezing plasma. Serendipitously, they allowed enough oxygen and CO_2 diffusion across their walls to permit room temperature platelet storage of relatively lower content PCs for three days before the pH decreased to unacceptable levels. Containers were later specifically designed for improved gas permeability as trial and error revealed that PCs stored in more gas-permeable containers had lower rates of pH failure (pH <6.2 at 22 °C).[51] So-called second-generation containers appear to be able to store PRP-PCs for at least seven days without deleterious pH decrements. Because apheresis PCs and prestorage pooled PRP-PCs have such heterogeneous contents, each unit must be assayed to ensure that total platelet content and concentration limits validated by the container manufacturer are not exceeded. The platelet concentration of donor blood limits individual WBD-PC content to values below those accommodated by newer storage containers. Second-generation containers currently in use are manufactured from polyolefin, ethylene vinyl acetate (EVA), or PVC that is thinner or plasticized with different compounds such as triethyl hexyl trimellitate (TOTM) and butyryl-tri-hexyl citrate (BTHC).[52] These bags provide nearly twice the oxygen permeability of first-generation DEHP-plasticized PVC containers.[53]

The need for continuous agitation was also recognized as a means of facilitating oxygen utilization.[51,54] Several different types of platelet rotators have been used over the years. Ferris-wheel and elliptical rotators have given way to face-over-face tumblers (3–6 rpm) and flatbed platform shakers (50–70 cpm) because of inefficient maintenance of pH or damage to platelets at pH >7.4 at 22 °C.[37] Initially thought to promote the diffusion of oxygen throughout the PC, agitation appears to exert a more complex effect on platelet metabolism. Several groups have shown that PO_2 was maintained in unagitated PCs and that mixing of products even once a day could prevent injurious pH decrements in relatively lower content platelet products.[55,56] Agitation, therefore, may also facilitate oxygen utilization by platelet mitochondria or prevent settling and a platelet contact-mediated switch from oxidative to glycolytic metabolism.[57] In any case, even with relatively higher content PCs, agitation may be safely interrupted for 24 hours (as during shipping) without undue lactate accumulation and subsequent development of injuriously low pHs.[57,58]

The platelet storage lesion

Stored platelets experience a progressive decline in function accompanied by characteristic morphologic changes. Studies document up to 20% loss of platelet recovery through five days of storage.[59] In apheresis containers currently licensed in the United States, Day 7 recovery is approximately 83% of Day 5 recovery.[60,61] This progressive damage has been termed the *platelet storage lesion*.[62,63] Well-characterized changes are seen in common tests assessing platelet morphology, activation, cell metabolism and function, and apoptosis. Some, but not all, of these changes are reversible upon platelet transfusion.[64]

The gold standard for evaluating product efficacy remains post-transfusion bleeding assessments, but the large patient numbers required and related time and expense usually lead to the substitution of surrogate measurements such as patient adjusted count increments on the assumption that a circulating platelet is a functional one. An even less costly alternative involves the reinfusion of healthy volunteers with autologous stored platelets radiolabeled with chromium-51 or indium-111. (Cell kinetics is described in greater detail in Chapters 7, 18, and 22.) Percent recovery and survival may be calculated by serial assay of postinjection blood radioactivity. Platelet recovery is significantly affected by individual differences in splenic sequestration (usually ~33%) and blood volume estimation errors during calculations. In an effort to standardize interpretation, Murphy proposed that products be evaluated against concurrently injected fresh autologous platelets to establish a fixed, rather than floating, standard.[65] This facilitates comparison of interventions designed to ameliorate the storage lesion. Although in vitro tests have attempted to rapidly and economically predict the ability of transfused platelets to circulate, only extreme values have documented any correlation with outcomes.[66,67] Accordingly, batteries of tests are often examined to ensure product equivalency after minor changes, or as the first step in assessment of more substantive changes in storage methods.

Alterations from normal discoid morphology are observed during platelet storage. Kunicki described a scoring system that assigned 4 points to discs, 2 to spheres, 1 to dendritic forms, and none to ballooned platelets.[68] Multiplied by the percentage of each form seen under phase contrast microscopy, scores decline from a maximum of 400 as changes associated with the storage lesion progress. Others have advocated simply reporting the percentage of discoid forms. The extent of shape change assay uses aggregometry to measure the decrease in light transmission after adenosine diphosphate stimulation of stirred PRP in the presence of EDTA to prevent aggregation.[69] Because only discoid platelets can change shape and block more light, the assay provides a more objective measure of the percentage of discoid platelets. All three approaches appear to correlate somewhat with in vivo recovery and survival at high or low assay values, but predict less well for in-between values. Mean platelet volume decreases throughout storage when membrane loss from dendritic forms occurs or when activation or apoptosis result in microvesiculation.[70]

Platelet activation during processing and throughout storage is accompanied by surface expression of sequestered granular membrane proteins (P-selectin and CD63) and conformational changes of the fibrinogen receptor, GP-IIb/IIa. Release of specific granular contents into the supernatant (β-thromboglobulin, platelet factor 4, etc.) also occurs throughout platelet storage as a manifestation of activation. This may not be specific for activation, however, because granular content release also occurs with platelet lysis. Similarly, platelet procoagulant activity (surface expression of membrane phosphatidylserine) appears not only with activation but also during cellular apoptosis. None of these indicators of platelet activation appear to correlate reliably with platelet recovery and survival. Studies of storage medium supplementation with activation inhibitors, however, suggest that activation contributes in part to the platelet storage lesion.[71] As previously noted, use of activation inhibitors in storage media has not gained widespread acceptance because of inconsistent results, toxicity, and the expense of licensing novel storage systems.

The ability of stored platelets to function normally has been assessed in several ways, and only one functional assay—hypotonic shock response—has proven to be of value in assessing platelet viability. Measurements of platelet ATP levels do not consistently provide reliable information.[47] Aggregation studies similarly fail to predict platelet viability. Responsiveness to single agonists rapidly declines during storage, but can recover with plasma rescue or in vivo reinfusion.[44] Responses to agonist mixtures, although better preserved, are still not helpful in assessing viability.[72] The hypotonic shock response or osmotic reversal reaction exposes platelets to a hypotonic environment. Metabolically active platelets rapidly extrude water after initially swelling. Recovery of normal intracellular water content can be quantified using light transmittance. Significant changes in values for this assay have been shown to correlate with in vivo recovery and survival.

Markers associated with cellular apoptosis accumulate throughout platelet storage with evidence of caspase activation, structural protein degradation, and changes in mitochondrial membrane potential.[73,74] Apoptotic inhibitors, although ameliorating some of these changes, have not resulted in improvements in platelet viability, casting doubt upon cellular senescence as a significant contributor to the platelet storage lesion.

Platelet additive solutions (synthetic storage solutions)

In Europe, synthetic storage solutions, also called PASs, have been used routinely for two decades.[75] In the United States, PASs were approved for use in 2010. The use of PASs allows: (1) greater plasma recovery from whole blood donations for transfusion or fractionation; (2) minimization of the adverse effects mediated by plasma (e.g., allergic and febrile nonhemolytic transfusion reactions [FNHTRs] and possibly, reduction of ABO isoagglutinin-mediated hemolysis or antibody-mediated transfusion-related acute lung injury [TRALI]); (3) use of photochemical pathogen reduction technologies, because the presence of plasma may interfere with the technology system; and (4) potential improvements in platelet storage through engineered manipulation of the storage medium.[76,77]

Early studies demonstrated the feasibility of suspending PRP-PCs in a commercially available neutral intravenous crystalloid solution, Plasmalyte A.[78] The 10–20% plasma carried over in the storage medium provided the sole source of glucose and bicarbonate. In vitro results were quite encouraging, but although previous versions of this PAS containing additional glucose and citrate were shown to be promising in vivo, the solution was not successfully commercialized.[79] When Murphy tested another balanced salt solution, the in vivo results were disappointing.[80] In retrospect, the deletion of acetate from Murphy's so-called PSM-2 solution was likely responsible for the pH failures seen in vitro. Acetate can efficiently substitute in the citric acid cycle for free fatty acids, the primary in vivo substrate for oxidative metabolism (Figure 19.3), decreasing both the glycolytic rate and lactic acid generation.[81] Acetate must also be transformed to acetic acid to enter the cycle, removing hydrogen ions produced by the anaerobic metabolism of glucose. This bicarbonate-sparing buffering effect also helps preserve pH. From Murphy's experience and other studies, it appears likely that some glucose must be available throughout storage. Holme and Gulliksson both noted the association of glucose exhaustion (even in the presence of alternate fuels) with adenine nucleotide depletion and loss of platelet viability.[40] The addition of glucose to PAS, however, is technically difficult because glucose carmelizes upon heat sterilization at the neutral or slightly basic PAS pHs best suited to maintain PC pH. Accordingly, most commercially available PASs do not contain additional glucose and require 20–40% plasma carryover. Two as-yet FDA-unapproved solutions have gotten around this problem by adding bicarbonate to a separately sterilized glucose-containing low-pH base solution.[82,83] Table 19.1 lists the components of various solutions, including those currently FDA-approved and under investigation in the United States.

In addition to sparing bicarbonate, PAS contents have been designed to modulate the glycolytic rate and downregulate platelet activation. Citrate, important in maintaining anticoagulation, upregulates glycolysis and renders platelets more susceptible to activating stimuli. Consequently, use of the lowest possible concentrations of citrate in the medium appears desirable.[40] Phosphate similarly has both salutary and detrimental effects in PAS.[84] Phosphate serves as a buffer and in apheresis platelets suspended in acid–citrate–dextrose (ACD), instead of the CPD/CP2D used in PRP-PCs and BC-PCs, is important in maintaining adenine nucleotide levels. It also upregulates glycolysis and consequently mandates more plasma carryover or addition of glucose to PAS. Magnesium and potassium both appear to decrease platelet activation and may downregulate glycolysis as well.[40] Studies with a number of platelet activation inhibitors (e.g., prostaglandin E1 and theophylline)

Table 19.1 International council for commonality in blood banking automation (ICCBBA) designations for platelet additive solution products (with annotation of FDA-approved products and those under investigation in the United States)

	Citrate	Phosphate	Acetate	Magnesium	Potassium	Gluconate	Glucose
PAS-A	A	A			A		
PAS-B	B		B				
PAS-C[‡]	C	C	C				
PAS-D	D		D	D	D	D	
PAS-E	E	E	E	E	E		
PAS-F		[†]	F	F	F	F	
PAS-G	G	G	G	G	G		G*

‡ Fenwal's Intersol® is a PAS-C product.
† B. Braun's Isoplate®, a PAS-F product, includes PO_4.
* Haemonetics' "PAS-G" includes HCO_3^- and Fenwal's "PAS-5" includes HCO_3^- and Ca^{++}.

suggest that these substances may enhance PAS efficacy, but safety concerns related to routine transfusion in varied patient populations significantly hinder commercial applicability.[85]

Clinical studies comparing platelets stored in plasma with FDA-approved additive solutions have demonstrated that allergic reactions and FNHTRs were reduced by approximately two-thirds with a 65% PAS-C and 35% plasma apheresis platelet product.[86] Corrected count increments after transfusion, however, are approximately 25% lower with PAS platelets.[87,88] Once commercialized, additive solutions containing glucose and bicarbonate, which require 5% or less plasma carryover, may further reduce transfusion reaction rates, including antibody-mediated reactions like TRALI and ABO-mediated hemolysis.

Component modification

Several PC modifications are occasionally required for various subsets of patients. Cellular products containing viable lymphocytes must be irradiated before transfusion to patients who are susceptible to graft-versus-host disease. An irradiation dose of 25 Gy (15–50 Gy) has no significant effect on common in vitro parameters even after seven days of storage following irradiation as early as Day 1.[89] Similarly, little or no effect of irradiation was seen on in vitro storage parameters or in vivo recovery and survival after five days of storage of platelets irradiated with up to 30 Gy on Days 1 or 3.[90,91]

Patients with moderate to severe allergic reactions to plasma components or newborns with neonatal alloimmune thrombocytopenia receiving maternal platelets benefit from plasma removal by platelet washing. Some institutions also wash platelets to remove ABO-incompatible plasma.[92] Washing, however, leads to significant loss of platelets as well as a decrement in platelet function while also reducing the product shelf life to four hours. A standard saline wash procedure using the COBE 2991 instrument (TerumoBCT, Lakewood, CO) has been described.[93] Platelet losses range from 8% to 29%.[94,95] Functional impairment of saline-resuspended washed platelets resulted in a two-thirds loss of recovery versus an unwashed control in one study.[96] Other studies have reported better in vitro properties of washed platelets resuspended in additive solutions instead of the saline commonly used in the United States.[97] For IgA-deficient patients, saline alone may not remove as much IgA as citrate-buffered saline because of the low isoelectric point of IgA and its coprecipitation with platelets in an acidic saline wash fluid.[98]

For transfusions in utero or for volume-sensitive neonates, additional concentration of PCs can be achieved through volume reduction by centrifugation and plasma removal. This technique has also been used to minimize infusion of maternal antibodies or ABO-incompatible plasma, although washing is preferred when antibody removal is critical. Some have questioned the need for volume reduction for most neonates and have pointed out that nonmanipulated PCs are well tolerated in neonates not in extremis.[99] Procedures have been described for volume reduction that result in <15% loss of platelets and relatively preserved in vivo viability.[100] British standards call for a concentration in excess of 2000×10^9/L for in utero transfusion.[101] Volume-reduced PCs maintain acceptable in vitro properties in plastic syringes at room temperature or in neonatal incubators (at 37 °C).[102] PCs should be transfused as soon as possible after volume reduction in a closed system, employing sterile connection devices, and must be used within four hours if prepared in an open system, such as via spike entry.

Most apheresis platelets are leukocyte reduced during the separation process. Leukocyte reduction of WBD-PCs is usually accomplished by prestorage leukofiltration during separation or at prestorage pooling. Prestorage leukocyte reduction has resulted in a 75–90% reduction in FNHTRs after platelet transfusion.[103,104] Leukocyte reduction also reduces cytomegalovirus transmission and platelet alloimmunization.[105,106]

Novel storage techniques

The short shelf life and significant infrastructure needed to maintain room temperature, continuously agitated, liquid PCs have encouraged exploration of alternative storage approaches. Cold liquid storage clearly minimizes the impact of bacterial contamination and also promises to extend shelf life by further slowing platelet metabolism. The better functional status of these platelets compared with room temperature–stored platelets makes them an attractive alternative for trauma victims and bleeding surgical patients.[36] Whether the maintenance of a dual platelet inventory is necessary awaits clinical studies proving the superiority of cold-stored platelets in immediate hemostasis. Attempts to mask clustered GP-Ib/IX/V receptors with sugar moieties, a successful manipulation in mice transfused with briefly cold-stored platelets, have not reversed the rapid clearance of longer stored chilled platelets observed in humans.[107]

Cryopreserved platelets can be prepared and stored for up to 10 years, but cost, inconvenience, procedure-related platelet loss, and functional decrements remain barriers to wider implementation. There is, however, considerable military interest in frozen platelets because of their low volume, rapid availability, and less onerous transportation requirements. The most common method of freezing employs 5–6% dimethylsulfoxide (DMSO) as a cryo-protectant, and requires <−65 °C storage, with DMSO removal possible before freezing.[108,109] The use of cryopreserved platelets results in corrected count increments that are approximately half of the increments seen with liquid apheresis platelets.[109,110] Contemporary autologous reinfusion studies with modern cryopreserved platelets have observed a recovery of 52% and survival of 89% of fresh platelets. Controlled rate freezing appears superior to uncontrolled temperature reduction.[111,112] Nonmilitary use is generally limited to broadly alloimmunized patients refractory to allogeneic transfusion. Collected between successive rounds of high-dose chemotherapy, these units can support patients through short periods of severe thrombocytopenia.

Lyophilized platelets have been studied without great success in a resulting product. Animal studies in the 1950s showed no hemostatic effect of early preparations.[113,114] Bode and Read described a new technique using 1.8% paraformaldehyde to fix washed platelets, followed by freezing in 5% bovine albumin and lyophilization.[115] This preparation has been stored at −80 °C but may be stable at room temperature for shorter periods. Paraformaldehyde treatment appears to confer an additional benefit by killing bacteria and many viral pathogens. Although morphologically normal and able to support adhesion and thrombin generative functions, these platelets do not activate or aggregate. Observation of thrombosis, splenic accumulation, and short circulatory time in animal models has led to limited enthusiasm for the product.[116]

The role of platelet substitutes, including platelet microvesicles, liposome-based hemostatic agents, fibrinogen-coated albumin microspheres, and red cells coated with fibrinogen or RGD peptides, is beyond the scope of this chapter, and readers are referred to published reviews for additional information.[116–118]

Disclaimer

The author has disclosed a financial relationship with Fenwal, Inc.

Key references

A full reference list for this chapter is available at: http://www.wiley.com/go/simon/transfusion

4 Vassallo RR, Murphy S. A critical comparison of platelet preparation methods. *Curr Opin Heme* 2006;**13**:323–30.

6 Murphy S, Gardner FH. Platelet preservation. Effect of storage temperature on maintenance of platelet viability—deleterious effect of refrigerated storage. *N Engl J Med* 1969;**280**:1094–8.

10 Moroff G, AuBuchon J, Heaton A, Holme S. Preparation of components from units of whole blood held for 24 hours at 20–24 °C. *Vox Sang* 1994;**67**:48.

12 Levitt J, ed. *Standards for blood banks and transfusion services*. 29th ed. Bethesda, MD: AABB, 2014.

16 *Guide to the preparation, use and quality assurance of blood components*. 17th ed. Strasbourg: Council of Europe Publishing, 2013: 118.

CHAPTER 20

Thrombocytopenia and platelet transfusion

Michael F. Murphy, Simon J. Stanworth, & Lise Estcourt

NHS Blood & Transplant and National Institute of Health Research (NIHR) Oxford Biomedical Research Centre, Oxford University Hospitals University of Oxford, UK

Thrombocytopenia is caused by disorders impairing platelet production, causing platelet destruction or leading to platelet sequestration. In addition, there are both congenital and acquired disorders of platelet function. These latter conditions may lead to the functional equivalent of thrombocytopenia, often despite the presence of a normal platelet count. Platelet transfusion represents an important therapeutic option for most of these disorders. However, under certain circumstances, platelet transfusion is contraindicated. Therefore, correct diagnosis of the underlying etiology of thrombocytopenia is important.

Methods for the preparation of platelet products for transfusion include platelet pools derived from multiple whole blood donations and apheresis units from individual donors. These components may be further manipulated depending on the requirements of the recipient. Platelet refractoriness represents a significant problem that develops in some patients who require repeated platelet transfusions, and it is most frequently due to nonimmune platelet consumption. HLA alloimmunization is the most important immune cause, and it is managed by the provision of HLA-matched or crossmatched platelets. The development of platelet substitutes and the administration of thrombopoiesis-stimulating agents represent alternatives to platelet transfusion that are in various stages of clinical development and may ultimately reduce the need for donor-derived platelets.

Thrombocytopenia

Thrombocytopenia refers to any reduction in platelet number below the lower limit of the normal range, which is about 150,000/μL in most laboratories. In the absence of other factors, however, the risk of bleeding is considered to be relatively modest until the platelet count is less than 50,000/μL, and it is not considered to be severe until the platelet count is less than 25,000/μL.[1] However, congenital or acquired abnormalities in platelet function may be associated with bleeding even when the platelet count is in the normal range.[2,3] A systematic diagnostic approach facilitates the correct diagnosis and appropriate management of thrombocytopenia and platelet dysfunction. Careful assessment of the medical history is imperative, including a review of concomitant medications. The peripheral blood smear should be reviewed for morphologic abnormalities in any of the three lineages (myeloid, erythroid, and megakaryocytic),

which may provide important insight into the underlying diagnosis, be it congenital or acquired. The causes of thrombocytopenia are summarized in Table 20.1.

Impaired platelet production

Disorders of platelet production may be congenital or acquired. Congenital disorders are relatively rare, whereas acquired disorders are much more commonly encountered in clinical practice. In the absence of an apparent etiology, distinguishing decreased platelet production from increased platelet destruction or from splenic sequestration can sometimes be challenging. Decreased platelet production is generally characterized by normal platelet size on the peripheral blood smear and a normal mean platelet volume (MPV). In addition, the reticulated platelet count as measured by flow cytometry is low.[4] A bone marrow aspirate and biopsy may be required in order to determine the underlying disorder associated with thrombocytopenia.

Hematologic and nonhematologic malignancies, and myelofibrosis, are associated with replacement of the marrow space and a reduction in blood cell production and pancytopenia. However, sometimes reduction in the platelet count is the first indication of one of these abnormalities. Platelet transfusions may be used appropriately for supportive care as needed while the cause of the underlying disorder is identified.

Platelet sequestration

About one-third of the platelet mass is normally sequestered in the spleen.[5] Splenomegaly from any cause tends to increase splenic platelet pooling. Hematologic malignancies including the myeloproliferative disorders may result in marked splenomegaly. In particular, myelofibrosis may be associated with thrombocytopenia.[6] Portal hypertension from liver disease may also be associated with marked splenomegaly leading to thrombocytopenia or even pancytopenia. The thrombocytopenia associated with splenic sequestration alone is generally moderate enough so as not to be associated with bleeding. However, concomitant conditions, such as the coagulopathy of liver disease or dysfibrinogenemia, can exacerbate the tendency to bleed in this setting.[7] Individuals with alcoholic cirrhosis and portal hypertension who continue to consume alcohol may also have exacerbated thrombocytopenia resulting from suppression of platelet production.[8]

Rossi's Principles of Transfusion Medicine, Fifth Edition. Edited by Toby L. Simon, Jeffrey McCullough, Edward L. Snyder, Bjarte G. Solheim, and Ronald G. Strauss.
© 2016 John Wiley & Sons, Ltd. Published 2016 by John Wiley & Sons, Ltd.

Table 20.1 Causes of thrombocytopenia

Impaired Production
 Selective megakaryocyte depression:
  Rare congenital defects
  Drugs, chemicals, and viruses
 As part of general bone marrow failure:
  Cytotoxic drugs and chemicals
  Radiation
  Megaloblastic anemia
  Leukemia
  Infection
 Myelodysplastic syndromes
 Myeloma
 Myelofibrosis
 Solid tumors
 Aplastic anemia
Excessive Destruction or Increased Consumption
 Immune
 Autoimmune: ITP
 Drug induced (e.g., GP IIb/IIIa inhibitors, penicillins, and thiazides)
 Secondary immune (SLE, CLL, viruses, drugs, e.g., heparin and bivalirudin)
 Neonatal alloimmune thrombocytopenia
 Posttransfusion purpura
 Disseminated intravascular coagulation
 Thrombotic thrombocytopenic purpura
Sequestration
 Splenomegaly
 Hypersplenism
Dilutional
 Massive transfusion

Congenital platelet disorders

Hereditary disorders may affect platelet number, platelet function, or both. Some congenital disorders leading to severe thrombocytopenia or markedly abnormal platelet function are identified early in life, but others are identified only after excessive bleeding is encountered in adulthood at the time of trauma or surgery.[9] Although platelet transfusion is effective in the treatment of bleeding in congenital platelet disorders, it can lead to the production of platelet antibodies and thus should be reserved for serious bleeding episodes. ε-aminocaproic acid (EACA) or desmopressin (DDAVP) may be useful for minor bleeding or for perioperative management of minor procedures, depending on the severity of the underlying disorder. In the absence of any bleeding, patients should be counseled to avoid aspirin and nonsteroidal anti-inflammatory drugs (NSAIDs), and to take appropriate prophylactic measures before procedures (e.g., use of EACA before minor dental procedures).[9,10]

Acquired platelet disorders

Thrombocytopenia may be the primary manifestation of several different hematologic disorders. These include immune thrombocytopenic purpura (ITP) and the microangiopathic hemolytic anemias.

Immune thrombocytopenic purpura

ITP, covered in more detail in Chapter 21, is an acquired immune-mediated disorder characterized by isolated thrombocytopenia (platelet count $<100 \times 10^9$/l), in the absence of any obvious underlying cause.[11] In particular, red cell morphology is normal, and large platelets are often seen. In children, this condition is typically acute, is associated with an antecedent viral illness, and resolves spontaneously. However, in adults it often follows a chronic course and there are usually no precipitating factors. Signs and symptoms vary widely; some patients have little or no bleeding, whereas others can experience life-threatening hemorrhage.[11]

The standard initial treatment in adults is with corticosteroids (1 mg/kg/day). Individuals with moderate bleeding where a more rapid increase in the platelet count is required may be treated in addition with intravenous immunoglobulin at a dose of either 1 g/kg/day for one or two days or 0.4 g/day for up to five days.[12] In cases of severe or life-threatening bleeding, platelet transfusion is indicated. Although survival of transfused platelets is greatly reduced, they are likely to have some beneficial effect on active bleeding.[11]

Microangiopathic hemolytic anemia

Several different conditions can cause a similar appearance on the blood smear: thrombocytopenia and the presence of red cell fragmentation (schistocytes).[13] However, clinical distinction between thrombotic thrombocytopenic purpura (TTP)/hemolytic uremic syndrome (HUS) and disseminated intravascular coagulation (DIC) is critical. In addition, malignant hypertension and valvular hemolysis may result in a similarly appearing smear.

TTP represents a medical emergency.

TTP is a rare condition that has been characterized by a pentad of clinical findings:

- Microangiopathic hemolytic anemia (MAHA);
- Thrombocytopenia;
- Neurological deficits;
- Fever; and
- Renal abnormalities.

However, its onset is insidious and the classic pentad is rarely present at diagnosis. Early diagnosis and treatment are essential, and TTP is now often diagnosed and treated when only the first two clinical findings are present in the absence of any other known cause.[14] Coagulation tests are almost always normal. The pathophysiology of this disorder has become elucidated as resulting from reduction or inhibition in function of the von Willebrand factor (vWF)-cleaving protease ADAMTS13.[15]

Platelets are activated in TTP, leading to a hypercoagulable state. Therefore, transfusion with platelets should be reserved for individuals with thrombocytopenia and life-threatening hemorrhage. The therapy of choice is plasma exchange, although plasma infusion may be used as a temporizing measure.[16,17] Steroids are useful to suppress the autoantibodies inhibiting ADAMTS13 activity in severe ADAMTS13 deficiency.[16,17] Relapsing and refractory TTP have been treated successfully with the CD20 monoclonal antibody rituximab.[16,17]

HUS is characterized by the triad of thrombocytopenia, MAHA, and acute renal failure.[18,19] The most common form of HUS is associated with diarrheal illness with shiga-toxin-producing bacteria such as *Escherichia coli H:0157*.[18] Supportive care is usually all that is required, because spontaneous recovery is the rule. Atypical HUS (aHUS) has been used to classify any HUS not caused by shiga toxin. It has been associated with a variety of precipitating events including infections, drugs, autoimmune conditions, and pregnancy.[18-20] Until the beginning of the 2010s, plasma exchange was considered the gold standard for aHUS.[21,22] Eculizimab has now been shown to be highly effective in aHUS, with 85% of patients becoming disease free.[19]

DIC is most commonly associated with infection or malignancy, although it can also be observed in the setting of vascular lesions such as hemangiomas and intravascular dissections. In contrast to TTP and HUS, the consumptive coagulopathy that occurs is not exacerbated by the administration of platelets and other blood components.[23] Although primary therapy should address the underlying condition, transfusions of platelets and other blood components may be safely administered in the interim.

Malignancy

Thrombocytopenia is also a side effect of the cytotoxic chemotherapy administered for many different hematologic and nonhematologic malignancies. However, in addition, several hematologic malignancies are associated with inherent impairment in platelet function. Both the myelodysplastic and myeloproliferative syndromes are potentially associated with impaired platelet function out of proportion to any reduction in platelet number that is present.[24] In this setting, platelet dysfunction results from ultrastructural abnormalities and impaired signaling, and may be manifest in platelet aggregation assays.[25,26] Platelet transfusions are sometimes indicated in the bleeding patient despite apparently acceptable platelet numbers. It should be noted, however, that myeloproliferative syndromes are also associated in some situations with platelet activation and thrombosis. Because of the latter, agents such as EACA should be used cautiously in these disorders and reserved for situations with reduced platelet function or severe thrombocytopenia.

Uremia

Several nonmalignant acquired conditions are associated with platelet dysfunction. Of these, uremia is most commonly encountered in clinical practice. Elevated levels of metabolites, such as guanidinosuccinic acid, lead to impaired signaling from the surface receptors on the platelet through to cyclooxygenase.[27] Guanidinosuccinic acid also leads to inhibition of platelet aggregation by facilitating excess nitric oxide production.[28] Treatment of uremia with dialysis restores platelet function toward normal. For the patient with acute bleeding in the setting of uremia, several therapies have potential benefit.[29] DDAVP is administered to release additional vWF from endothelial stores and to try to restore platelet signaling. It is reasonably safe and effective in this setting. Alternatively, administration of cryoprecipitate facilitates the same end. Recombinant Factor VIIa has been used off label in a small number of patients with severe bleeding in this setting, but its safety and efficacy are not well documented.[30] For less acute bleeding, high doses of conjugated estrogens (several milligrams daily) may be effective. The mechanism of action is not well understood, and it usually takes several days to observe a beneficial effect.[29]

Dialysis

Although dialysis improves platelet function in uremia,[29] it is also associated with the development of thrombocytopenia. In particular, continuous venovenous dialysis or hemofiltration has been associated with a reduction in platelet number in some patients.[31] It is important to distinguish thrombocytopenia caused by the dialysis procedure from heparin-induced thrombocytopenia (see below), because patients are often treated with this anticoagulant in the intensive care setting.

Cardiac interventions

Cardiac procedures, use of ventricular assist devices, and cardiopulmonary bypass may all be associated with thrombocytopenia and/or defects in platelet function. Thrombocytopenia in cardiac catheterization is associated with the use of agents that inhibit GPIIb/IIIa function.[32] A hemorrhagic diathesis is exacerbated by the concomitant use of antiplatelet agents. Ventricular assist devices and cardiopulmonary bypass are also associated with platelet consumption.[33] As in the dialysis setting, the distinction of heparin-induced thrombocytopenia from other causes is critical. Platelet transfusion is indicated if simple platelet consumption is suspected, whereas it is relatively contraindicated when heparin-associated thrombocytopenia is present.

Heparin-induced thrombocytopenia

Heparin-induced thrombocytopenia is a special class of immune-mediated thrombocytopenia. It is a prothrombotic drug reaction caused by immunoglobulin G (IgG) antibodies to platelet factor 4 (PF4)/polyanion complexes that activate platelets.[34]

Although perhaps more commonly associated with unfractionated heparin, this syndrome is also associated with use of low-molecular-weight heparins. The diagnosis is suggested when the platelet count decreases by 50% or to less than 100×10^9/L in a patient receiving one of these drugs. Diagnosis requires a high clinical likelihood of the condition (e.g., 4Ts scoring system) plus the presence of platelet-activating antibodies.[34,35]

When heparin-induced thrombocytopenia is suspected, treatment consists of immediate discontinuation of any heparin-containing product and institution of an alternative anticoagulant, such as lepirudin or the direct thrombin inhibitor argatroban. Use of warfarin alone is contraindicated, because it decreases protein C levels and can lead to catastrophic thrombosis.[36] Platelet transfusion is contraindicated even in patients with low counts on anticoagulation, except in the circumstance of life-threatening bleeding.

Other medications and supplements

A number of medications, herbal remedies, and nutritional substances result in disorders of platelet function or number.[37,38] Aspirin and NSAIDs are among the most commonly used over-the-counter medications. In the case of aspirin, irreversible acetylation of cyclooxygenase in the platelet results in loss of function for the 5–7-day lifespan of the platelet. Conversely, NSAIDs are reversible inhibitors. This distinction is important in the bleeding patient. If a patient with life-threatening bleeding has consumed aspirin during the past several days, platelet transfusion may be indicated. However, in the case of NSAIDs, once at least four to five half-lives have elapsed, there is generally little utility in platelet transfusion unless a concomitant condition is present.

Immune-mediated thrombocytopenia (see Chapter 21) has been associated with the use of many different drugs. Most notably, quinine, quinidine, sulfonamides, sulfonamide derivatives such as furosemide, and vancomycin have been associated with autoantibody formation.[39,40] Although platelet transfusion may be necessary in patients with active bleeding, treatment consists primarily of discontinuation of the agent and observation. If necessary, treatment with intravenous immunoglobulin or corticosteroids may be initiated to hasten recovery of the platelet count.

Many other commonly encountered classes of drugs are associated with qualitative or quantitative changes in platelets. These include traditional anticonvulsants such as valproic acid, which has also been associated with immune-mediated thrombocytopenia, and more recently approved agents such as gabapentin.[41,42] Simple discontinuation of these agents is generally all that is required in order to facilitate resolution of the defects. Drugs that affect both platelet number and function include heparin (as mentioned).

Posttransfusion purpura

PTP is a rare but serious complication of blood transfusion, characterized by the sudden onset of severe thrombocytopenia (platelet count often less than 10×10^9/L) usually within 5–10 days of a blood transfusion.[43] It usually affects HPA-1a-negative women who have been previously alloimmunized by pregnancy. The transfusion precipitating PTP causes a secondary immune response, boosting the HPA-1a antibodies, although the mechanism of destruction of the patient's own HPA-1a-negative platelets remains uncertain. On average, 10 cases per year of PTP were reported to the UK hemovigilance scheme (SHOT) prior to the introduction of universal leukoreduction of blood components.[44–46] Since then, the number of cases of PTP reported has fallen progressively to an average of one case per year.[47]

Although the thrombocytopenia usually resolves spontaneously within a few weeks, there is a relatively high rate of bleeding associated with PTP, so that treatment should be considered. Platelet transfusions are usually ineffective in raising the platelet count.[48–50] Administration of immunoglobulin (0.4 g/kg for five days or the equivalent) has been shown to have some efficacy in this setting.[51]

Neonatal alloimmune thrombocytopenia

About 2% of women have platelets of the HPA-1b (Pl^{A2}) phenotype. When they become pregnant with a HPA-1a-positive fetus, about 10% develop HPA-1a antibodies. These antibodies cross the placenta and lead to fetal/neonatal thrombocytopenia even during the first pregnancy, unlike the situation with RhD-negative individuals in which prior sensitization is required. Neonatal alloimmune thrombocytopenia (NAIT) is most commonly manifest as skin and other minor bleeding after birth. However, it may cause intracranial hemorrhage either at the time of delivery or in utero usually after 30 weeks of gestation. The precise incidence of intracranial hemorrhage is unknown, but conservative estimates suggest that it is around 1 in 20,000 live births.[52]

For the management of an affected neonate, if the platelet count is $<30 \times 10^9$/L or if there are signs of bleeding with a low count, it is recommended that the neonate is transfused with donor platelets that are ideally both HPA-1a and -5b-negative, as these will be compatible with the maternal HPA alloantibody in $\geq$95% of cases. If HPA-1a-negative and -5b-negative platelets are not immediately available and there is an urgent clinical need for transfusion, then random, ABO- and RhD-compatible donor platelets should be used. The results of laboratory investigations should not delay immediate platelet transfusion, as full investigation may be time-consuming and the risk of intracranial hemorrhage is highest in the first 48 hours post delivery. In a typical case, the platelet count should recover to normal within a week, although a more protracted recovery can occur. Intravenous immunoglobulin is not recommended as first-line treatment, as it is only effective in about 75% of cases and there is a delay of 24–48 hours before a satisfactory count is achieved

For the antenatal management of women with a history of NAIT in a previous pregnancy, referral to specialists in fetal medicine and hematology is required. Treatment during the subsequent pregnancy involves the administration of immunoglobulin and steroids; the timing of the initiation of treatment and the doses depend on the history of hemorrhage and fetal/neonatal thrombocytopenia in previous pregnancies.[53]

Platelet transfusion

Platelet products

In the United States, whole blood–derived platelet units (also called random-donor units) are prepared as platelet-rich plasma (see Chapter 19).[54,55] Outside of the United States, the buffy coat method is often used for platelet preparation.[56] In this case, after centrifugation analogous to that used to separate plasma from the red cell pellet, the buffy coat layer atop the red cells is harvested. Both platelet preparation methods involve the pooling of four to six units and result in a similar quality product. Each unit contains at least 5.5×10^{10} platelets.[57] Apheresis platelets (often called single-donor platelets) are harvested from an individual through use of an apheresis device.[58] A six-unit pool or an apheresis unit contains around 3×10^{11} platelets, and this platelet dose generally leads to a platelet increment of 30 to 60×10^9/L in the platelet-naïve patient when measured one hour after administration. Although the products may be considered interchangeable in terms of efficacy and safety,[59] use of whole blood–derived platelets in some settings is preferred to use of apheresis platelets in the absence of special circumstances such as the need for HLA matching.[60]

Platelet storage and processing are described in detail in Chapter 19.

Platelet administration

Platelets contain ABO antigens on their surface. Transfusion of ABO-mismatched platelets, however, is not associated with a major reaction. Nonetheless, there are data to indicate that naturally occurring anti-A or anti-B in the recipient may lead to destruction of group A or B mismatched platelets and to poorer platelet increments.[61,62] When the supply allows, ABO-matched platelets should be transfused.

In contrast to ABO, Rh blood group antigens are not expressed on the surface of the platelet. However, red cells with these antigens are invariably contained in platelet products, albeit to a much lower extent in modern platelet products. Therefore, transfusion of platelets from RhD-positive donors to RhD-negative recipients can lead to RhD alloimmunization. Because of immune suppression, this is uncommonly encountered in patients with hematologic malignancies receiving RhD-mismatched platelets. However, it is recommended to administer RhD-negative platelets to RhD-negative recipients whenever available and to administer intravenous Rh immunoglobulin to female children and females of childbearing age who have hypoproliferative thrombocytopenia. A dose of 1500 IU will cover multiple platelet exposures.

Specific platelet transfusion products, such as for patients with acute leukemia, may be needed e.g., leukocyte-reduced, irradiated platelet products (see Chapters 16 and 54). Because of the potential reduction in the number of platelets, washing of platelets should be reserved for individuals with severe allergic reactions that cannot otherwise be overcome by appropriate medications.

Although acetaminophen 650 to 1000 mg and diphenhydramine 25 to 50 mg are frequently administered before platelet transfusion as primary prophylaxis against febrile and allergic reactions, few data exist to support this as routine practice.[63,64] However, once an allergic reaction has been observed (hives, wheezing, or dyspnea), diphenhydramine is the drug of choice to prevent additional reactions in the future. If a moderate allergic reaction recurs in an adult despite administration of these premedications, hydrocortisone 100 mg IV is often effective. Recurrence of severe allergic reactions despite premedication is an indication for the use of washed platelets.

Platelet concentrates must be administered to adults through a blood filter. This is generally a standard blood set with an infusion time of about 30 minutes.

Platelet transfusion is not without risk. Aside from the development of platelet refractoriness and allergic reactions that can be observed with any blood component, platelets are the component most commonly associated with the transmission of bacterial infection.[65] In the past, it has been estimated that about 1 in 5000 platelet units are contaminated with bacteria. Newer methods for bacterial testing have reduced the incidence of bacteremia associated with platelet transfusion. Nonetheless, there should be a heightened sense of awareness for the possibility of bacterial transmission in those receiving platelet transfusions, particularly if individuals are neutropenic and become febrile during or shortly after a platelet transfusion.

Prophylactic platelet transfusions

Prophylactic transfusion refers to maintenance of the platelet count above a certain threshold in patients who are neither bleeding nor actively consuming platelets because of immune destruction or infection. In patients with acute myeloid leukemia who have received 25 platelet transfusions, the mean one-hour platelet increment is reduced by about one-third and the 18- to 24-hour platelet increment is reduced by more than half in comparison to that observed after the first platelet transfusion.[66] Therefore, reduction in the number of unnecessary platelet transfusions is of significant benefit.

There have been several questions relating to the use of prophylactic platelet transfusions in patients with reversible bone marrow failure.

Should prophylactic platelet transfusions be given?

A systematic review identified three small randomized controlled trials (RCTs) that compared a prophylactic versus therapeutic platelet transfusion strategy.[67] All included studies were conducted at least 30 years ago and used outdated methods of platelet component production and patient supportive care.

Since this review, two large RCTS have addressed the question of whether prophylactic platelet transfusions should be used.[68,69] Both showed that prophylactic platelet transfusions reduced the risk of bleeding.[70] However, this effect was less marked in the prespecified subgroup of patients receiving autologous hematopoietic stem cell transplants (HSCTs). When considering these results as a *number needed to treat*, five patients receiving intensive chemotherapy or a stem cell transplant would need to receive prophylactic platelet transfusions over a 30-day period to prevent one patient from having clinically significant bleeding (WHO grade 2 or above) (95% CI, 3–18), whereas for autologous HSCT patients 43 patients would need to receive prophylactic platelet transfusions to prevent one patient from bleeding.[71]

What platelet transfusion threshold should be used?

A systematic review identified three RCTS that compared different platelet transfusion thresholds in patients with hematological malignancies.[67] Two compared a threshold of 20×10^9/L versus 10×10^9/L, whereas the third compared a threshold of 30×10^9/L versus 10×10^9/L. A fourth RCT excluded from the systematic review compared a threshold of 20×10^9/L versus 10×10^9/L.[72] A meta-analysis of all four studies (658 patients) showed no increase in the proportion of patients who bled and also showed a significant reduction in the number of platelet transfusions given.[73] However, this meta-analysis may not be sufficiently powered to detect an increased bleeding risk in the 10×10^9/L threshold arm of less than 50%. There has been a suggestion that platelet transfusion thresholds should be lowered, but automated haematology analysers are not yet accurate enough in counting very low platelet numbers.[74]

No randomized studies in adult patients have assessed the use of other transfusion thresholds, such as platelet mass, absolute immature platelet number, or immature platelet fraction.

For patients with chronic bone marrow failure, there is little evidence on which to base practice. A retrospective study considered platelet transfusion in outpatients with stable chronic severe aplastic anemia (AA).[75] Prophylactic platelets were given if the count was 5×10^9/l or less, or if the patient was unwell with fever (temperature $>38\,^{\circ}$C) or recent hemorrhage if the count was 10×10^9/l or less. Patients with significant bleeding or prior to minor surgery received platelets at counts $>10 \times 10^9$/l. In total, 55,239 patient days were reviewed with 18,706 days when the platelet count was 10×10^9/l or less. All deaths from hemorrhage were associated with alloimmunization or withdrawal from treatment. Three nonlethal major bleeding episodes occurred. The authors concluded that this restrictive policy, with a median transfusion interval of seven days, was feasible, safe, and economical.

Both national and international guidelines vary in their advice for platelet transfusion in stable nonbleeding patients with bone marrow failure resulting in chronic thrombocytopenia. Recommendations include a threshold of $<10 \times 10^9$/l, as used in patients with reversible bone marrow failure;[76] a threshold of 5×10^9/l or less;[77,78] or no prophylaxis.[79–81]

A recent RCT has assessed whether prophylactic platelet transfusions are beneficial in dengue hemorrhagic fever.[82] The study was small with only 87 patients enrolled. Platelet transfusion did not prevent progression to severe bleeding, nor did it appear to shorten time to cessation of bleeding. It was also associated with severe side effects; three patients showed severe anaphylactic reactions and hypotension, and one patient died due to transfusion-related lung injury (TRALI). Other studies have shown no correlation between the platelet count and risk of bleeding;[83,84] therefore, use of platelet transfusions in dengue fever should not be based solely on a platelet count.

National recommendations for adult intensive care patients are not based on RCTs.[85] For neonates, practive varies significantly between countries.[86] Several RCTs are in progress studying different platelet transfusion thresholds.[87–90]

What platelet transfusion dose should be used?

A systematic review identified six RCTS that compared different platelet transfusion doses in patients with hematological malignancies,[67] and one study that had not yet been published. No other studies have been identified within an ongoing review.[91] Four studies assessed clinically significant bleeding as an outcome measure (usually defined as WHO grade 2 or above). In this review, there was no evidence of a difference in the risk of bleeding between low-dose $(1.1 \times 10^{11}/m^2)$ and standard-dose $(2.2 \times 10^{11}/m^2)$ and between standard-dose and high-dose platelet transfusions $(4.4 \times 10^{11}/m^2)$. Low-dose transfusions decreased the total amount of platelets that patients received, but at the expense of a higher number of transfusion episodes. The UK dose for platelet transfusions is that at least 75% of units contain $>2.4 \times 10^{11}$ platelets per adult dose and should continue to be used as standard. Increasing the platelet dose from a standard- $(2.2 \times 10^{11}/m^2)$ to a high-dose $(4.4 \times 10^{11}/m^2)$ transfusion regimen does not increase the transfusion interval (a median of five days for both regimens).

Additional risk factors for bleeding

Numerous clinical factors have been associated with an increased risk of bleeding (Table 20.1). However, the majority of these postulated risk factors are based on low-level evidence, such as expert opinion or retrospective analysis of patient databases. Further studies are required to identify clearly which factors should prompt an increase in the transfusion threshold, and what this threshold should be. Inflammation has been shown to be associated with an increased risk of bleeding in mice.[92] Studies have differed in their opinion of whether fever increases the risk of bleeding in humans (Table 20.1). Currently, the platelet transfusion threshold is commonly raised to 20×10^9/L when patients have an infection or fever.[93]

Pre-procedure platelet transfusions
Bone marrow aspirates and trephines
According to the UK confidential registry of complications after bone marrow aspirates and trephines, the risk of significant bleeding is very low (less than 1:1,000), and the majority of patients had bleeding when they did not have a significant thrombocytopenia.[94–98]

Central venous catheters
Nineteen observational studies have reported bleeding outcomes in thrombocytopenic patients after insertion of central venous catheters (CVCs).[99–117] At least 1340 procedures were performed when the platelet count was $\leq 50 \times 10^9$/L. Only one case of severe bleeding (Hb drop >15 g/L) was reported throughout all of these studies.[116] Three of these studies looked at risk factors associated with bleeding. The two studies that did not perform the CVC procedure with ultrasound guidance found that the number of attempts, site of insertion (jugular vs. subclavian), and failed guidewire insertion significantly increased the risk of bleeding on multivariable analysis,[99,105] whereas the third study that used ultrasound guidance did not.[117] Systematic reviews of complications of CVC placement have found that ultrasound guidance significantly reduced failure and complication rates.[118,119] A small study in thrombocytopenic patients that compared ultrasound-guided versus landmark insertion techniques reiterated this finding.[115]

The Zeidler study[117] looked at risk of bleeding according to platelet count thresholds with multivariable analysis. The risk of bleeding only increased when the platelet count was less than 20×10^9/L (OR, 2.88; 95% CI, 1.23 to 6.75; $p = 0.015$); this analysis controlled for sex, type of leukemia, insertion site, and use of prophylactic platelet transfusions. All CVCs in this study were untunneled and inserted by experienced individuals.[117] In the large Haas study, no patient with thrombocytopenia had any bleeding that was not treated with simple pressure at the site of the tunneled CVC; their platelet count threshold for insertion was 25×10^9/L.[107]

One additional prospective study assessed insertion of peripherally inserted central catheters (PICCs) without prophylactic platelet transfusions. Of the 50 patients who had a line inserted with a platelet count less than 20×10^9/L, only one bleeding episode occurred (minor oozing).[120]

One prospective nonrandomized study has assessed the risk of bleeding after traction removal of tunneled cuffed CVCs in patients with abnormal platelet counts or international normalized ratio (INR).[121] Fourteen of the 179 patients enrolled in the study had a time to hemostasis of over five minutes, and only one of these patients had a platelet count $<100 \times 10^9$/L.

Lumbar punctures and epidural anesthesia
A wide-ranging review of the literature has been performed of the risk of spinal hematoma following lumbar puncture or neuraxial anesthesia.[122] We are aware of no new studies that have contributed

to the literature since this review. The authors' conclusions are based on case series, case reports, and expert opinion. The thresholds they recommend are that lumbar punctures can be performed safely when the platelet count is $\geq 40 \times 10^9$/L, and that epidural anesthesia can be performed safely when the platelet count is $\geq 80 \times 10^9$/L.

Liver biopsy
Percutaneous liver biopsies are considered safe when the platelet count is at least 50 to 60×10^9/L.[123,124] 2740 percutaneous liver biopsies were conducted in the HALT-C trial;[125] only 16 patients (0.6%) had a serious adverse event due to bleeding after the biopsy. Transjugular liver biopsy has been shown to be safe in patients with low platelet counts, and with more modern techniques it can produce comparable histological samples to percutaneous liver biopsies.[126–128]

Renal biopsy
Uncontrolled hypertension, high serum creatinine, anemia, older age, and female sex have all been shown to be risk factors for bleeding post renal biopsy as well as a prolonged bleeding time.[129–132] There have been no systematic studies that have assessed the effect of acutely lowering blood pressure prior to renal biopsy.[130] Dialysis may improve the bleeding tendency in patients with uremia.[29,133] DDAVP can be used successfully to prevent bleeding before invasive procedures.[29,134,135] Conjugated estrogens are a long-acting alternative to DDAVP, because they shorten the bleeding time with a more sustained effect.[29,136] Correcting anemia will decrease the bleeding time.[29] Transjugular renal biopsy has been used in patients in whom percutaneous renal biopsy has failed or been contraindicated, and gas produced a similar diagnostic yield and safety profile.[137] Avoid the use of platelet transfusions if possible because of the risk of allosensitization.[138]

Dental extraction
One recent small RCT (23 patients requiring 35 procedures and 84 teeth removed) has shown a low rate of bleeding complications with no blood products transfused, in patients prior to liver transplantation.[139] Patients had platelet counts $\geq 30 \times 10^9$/L and an INR ≤ 3.0, and they were randomized to the presence or absence of tranexamic acid on the gauze used to apply local pressure. A third of patients had a platelet count $<50 \times 10^9$/L. Only one patient in the control arm had postoperative bleeding, which was controlled with local pressure. This small study suggests that dental extractions can be performed safely with the use of local hemostatic measures alone, but more research is required before a recommendation can be made.

Surgery
There remains a lack of evidence to guide the prophylactic use of platelet transfusions before major surgery. Guidelines from around the world suggest a threshold of 50×10^9/l before major surgery,[79,140–142] and a threshold of 100×10^9/l prior to neurosurgery or ophthalmic surgery involving the posterior segment of the eye, because of the critical sites involved.[79,140–142] A platelet count increment after any platelet transfusion is desirable, but it may be limited by the circumstances.

Therapeutic platelet transfusions
The predominant usage of platelet transfusions is to prevent bleeding (up to 67%),[143] but therapeutic platelet transfusions are also needed to treat active bleeding from thrombocytopenia and/or

platelet dysfunction in a wide range of clinical scenarios. Although most clinical research of the use of platelet transfusions has been in the area of prophylactic transfusions in patients with hematologic malignancies, the management of the actively bleeding patient with severe thrombocytopenia and/or platelet dysfunction has received less attention and is arguably more challenging. The clinical scenario is often complex, and management depends on the nature and site of the bleeding, the severity of the thrombocytopenia, the presence or absence of other disorders of hemostasis, and the presence or absence of anemia, as well as the clinical condition of the patient.

Consensus guidelines have generally recommended a threshold for therapeutic platelet transfusions of at least 50×10^9/L if a patient is actively bleeding (Table 20.2). However, there are few definitive studies to substantiate these platelet transfusion triggers, and the level of evidence to support the recommendations is poor.

Platelet refractoriness

Platelet refractoriness is defined as the repeated failure to achieve satisfactory responses to platelet transfusions; this topic has been comprehensively reviewed recently.[144] The effectiveness of platelet transfusions can be assessed clinically in a bleeding patient through assessment of cessation of bleeding or not. However, where platelet transfusions have been given prophylactically, the response is assessed by measuring the posttransfusion platelet count increment. Various formulas have been devised to refine this assessment of the response to platelet transfusion.[79]

1 The percentage platelet recovery (R) is calculated from the platelet increment $\times 10^9$/L (PI), the blood volume (BV) in liters, and the platelet dose transfused $\times 10^9$ (PD):

$$R(\%) = PI \times BV \times PD^{-1} \times 100$$

2 The corrected count increment $\times 10^9$/l (CCI) is calculated from the platelet increment (PI), the body surface area of the patient in square meters (BSA), and the dose of platelets transfused $\times 10^{11}$ (PD):

$$CCI = PI \times BSA \times PD^{-1}$$

A platelet recovery of about 67% in a stable patient indicates a successful transfusion, but the minimum platelet recovery to define

a successful transfusion is considered as >30% at 1 hour post transfusion and >20% at 20–24 hours. A CCI of $>7.5 \times 10^9$/l at 1 hour and $>4.5 \times 10^9$/l at 20–24 hours is considered to be a successful transfusion. In practice, a 24-hour platelet increment of $<5 \times 10^9$/L following a platelet transfusion on two or more occasions is a good indicator of refractoriness to random donor platelets.

It is sometimes stated that the absence of a response one hour after transfusion indicates refractoriness from immunologic causes, and lack of a response at a later time following transfusion is caused by underlying clinical problems, but this rule is an unreliable way of determining the cause of platelet refractoriness.

There are many causes of platelet refractoriness, and they can be subdivided into immune and nonimmune. The main immune cause is HLA alloimmunization, which occurs predominantly in females with a history of pregnancy or in patients who have received multiple transfusions. Other immune causes include HPA alloimmunization, ABO incompatibility with high-titer ABO antibodies in the recipient, platelet autoantibodies, and drug-related platelet antibodies. On the other hand, a lack of response to platelet transfusion may be the result of an underlying acute illness, such as infection, or it may result from a more chronic condition, such as splenomegaly. Fever, sepsis, DIC, hemorrhage, and conditions associated with marrow transplantation such as veno-occlusive disease and graft-versus-host disease all contribute to platelet refractoriness.

Alloimmune platelet refractoriness is mainly caused by HLA antibodies, but its incidence has declined due to the implementation of leukocyte reduction of blood components and more aggressive treatment for patients with hematological malignancies and other cancers. The incidence of HLA alloimmunization varies with the type of blood components transfused, the patient's underlying condition, and the previous history of pregnancy and transfusion. For example, HLA alloimmunization is more frequent in patients with aplastic anemia than in patients with acute leukemia. The Trial to Reduce Alloimmunisation to Platelets found that in patients with acute myeloblastic leukemia receiving non-leukocyte-reduced blood components, the incidence of HLA alloimmunization was

Table 20.2 Platelet thresholds for therapeutic transfusion during active bleeding

Clinical Indication	Treatment Trigger	Level of Evidence*
Major bleeding and thrombocytopenia or massive hemorrhage	50 to 75	Grade C, level IV
Massive transfusion and multiple trauma or TBI	75 to 100	Grade C, level IV
Surgery	50 to 100	Grade B, level III, to Grade C, level IV
DIC	50	Grade C, level IV
DIC in neonates	100	Grade C, level IV
Intracerebral bleeding	100	Grade C, level IV
Platelet function defects	No threshold	Grade C, level IV

*Levels of evidence originate from the US Agency for Healthcare Research and Quality (www.ahrq.gov):

Statements of Evidence

Ia: Evidence obtained from meta-analysis of randomized controlled trials.

Ib: Evidence obtained from at least one randomized controlled trial.

IIa: Evidence obtained from at least one well-designed controlled study without randomization.

IIb: Evidence obtained from at least one other type of well-designed quasi-experimental study.

III: Evidence obtained from well-designed nonexperimental descriptive studies, such as comparative studies, correlation studies, and case studies.

IV: Evidence obtained from expert committee reports or opinions and/or clinical experiences of respected authorities.

Grades of Recommendations

A: Requires at least one randomized controlled trial as part of a body of literature of overall good quality and consistency addressing the specific recommendation. (Evidence levels Ia and Ib.)

B: Requires the availability of well-conducted clinical studies but no randomized clinical trials on the topic of recommendation. (Evidence levels IIa, IIb, and III.)

C: Requires evidence obtained from expert committee reports or opinions and/or clinical experiences of respected authorities. Indicates an absence of directly applicable clinical studies of good quality. (Evidence level IV.)

TBI, traumatic brain injury; DIC, disseminated intravascular coagulation.

33% in those who had never been pregnant, and 62% in those who had been pregnant; in patients receiving leukocyte-reduced blood components, it was 9% and 32%, respectively.[145]

The role of platelet-specific (or HPA) antibodies in platelet refractoriness is less clear. HPA antibodies have been detected at a frequency of 8%[69] to 20–25%[146] in various studies of multi-transfused hematology patients and are usually found in combination with HLA antibodies,[147] although they may occur in isolation. Most commonly, HPA alloimmunization is directed toward antigens with phenotypic frequencies below 30%. Some studies have suggested that there is no clear correlation between HPA antibodies and poor responses to platelet transfusions,[148,149] but others have found that matching for platelet-specific antigens in patients refractory to HLA-matched platelets may be beneficial.[150]

Platelet refractoriness is most commonly due to shortened platelet survival associated with nonimmune clinical factors, including DIC, splenomegaly, and intravenous antibiotics (especially antifungal drugs such as amphotericin B).[151,152] Fever has also been implicated in causing poor responses to platelet transfusions, although whether this is a reflection of sepsis, associated DIC, or antibiotic therapy rather than the temperature itself is unclear.[153]

The appropriate investigation and management of platelet refractoriness require consideration of information from a clinical assessment of the patient as well as laboratory investigations (Figure 20.1).[79]

The first step is a clinical evaluation for possible nonimmune clinical causes, and this step is all too frequently omitted.[154] Any significant clinical factors such as infection should be treated if possible, and prophylactic platelet transfusions from random donors continued as standard care. If poor responses to platelet transfusions persist, the patient should be tested for HLA antibodies, and, if present, platelet transfusions matched for the HLA-A and -B antigens of the patient should be used.

HLA matching of platelets uses databases of HLA-typed platelet donors who can then be asked to donate by apheresis. This requires logistic coordination, and may result in a time lag before the product is available. There are a number of ways to select HLA-matched platelet transfusions. Traditionally, recipient and donor are matched for HLA-A and –B antigens, as the most important antibodies in causing platelet refractoriness are directed against these antigens.[155] Refinements to HLA matching have been made, including grading of the quality of HLA match and its revision to include "permissive" mismatches,[156] the identification of the specificity of HLA antibodies and the issue of HLA-matched platelets based on their specificity,[157] and more recently the use of software tools such as *HLA matchmaker* to predict HLA compatibility by identifying immunogenic epitopes in antibody-accessible regions of HLA molecules.[158] A recent systematic review found that HLA-matched platelet transfusions improved one hour posttransfusion

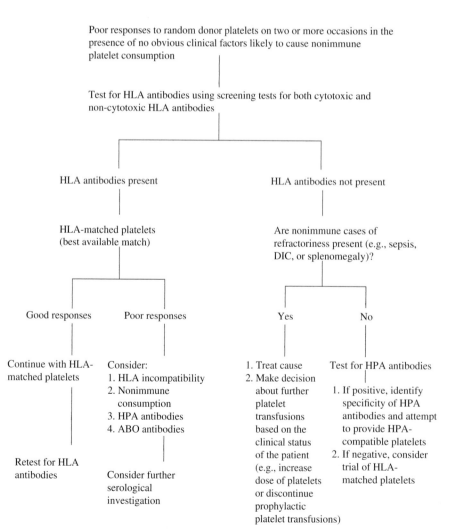

Figure 20.1 Algorithm for the investigation and management of patients refractory to platelet transfusions. Source: Phekoo *et al.*, 1997. Vox Sanguinis, 73, 81–86. Adapted with permission.

platelet increments but did not consistently improve the 24-hour increments, and failed to demonstrate any reduction in mortality or bleeding as the studies were inadequately powered for these outcomes.[159]

HPA antibodies are rare in the absence of HLA antibodies, and do not always cause platelet refractoriness. It is not necessary to test for HPA antibodies during the initial serological investigation of platelet refractoriness.

The use of HLA-matched platelet transfusions is also justified if there has not been time to carry out serological testing, particularly when platelet refractoriness is associated with bleeding. HLA-matched platelet transfusions are not indicated when full serological testing has failed to detect HLA antibodies. In this case, further consideration should be given to the identification of nonimmune clinical factors, and if they still appear to be absent, testing for HPA antibodies should be undertaken.

Responses to HLA-matched platelet transfusions should be carefully monitored, ideally with posttransfusion platelet counts both one hour and 20–24 hours post transfusion. If there are improved responses, HLA-matched platelet transfusions should continue to be used for further transfusions. If there are poor responses to HLA-matched platelet transfusions, the reasons should be sought, including HLA incompatibility, which is most likely to occur in patients with unusual HLA types with few well-matched donors; nonimmune platelet consumption; and HPA and ABO incompatibility. Further serological investigations including testing for HPA antibodies may be useful to differentiate between these possibilities. Depending on the results of these investigations, the appropriate management could be the use of ABO-identical or HPA-matched platelet concentrates if the specificity of the HPA antibodies can be identified.

Platelet crossmatching the patient's plasma against the lymphocytes and platelets of donors of HLA-matched platelet transfusions that have failed to produce satisfactory responses may be very helpful in identifying the cause of the poor responses.[160] Platelet crossmatching can also be used as an alternative approach to the management of refractory patients with HLA-matched platelet transfusions.[161–163] Typically, the patient's plasma is tested against platelet samples of ABO-compatible apheresis platelet donors. Donor platelets lacking reactivity are considered to be *crossmatch compatible*, and the associated platelet concentrates selected for transfusion in preference to those from random donors. An advantage of platelet crossmatching over a strategy of HLA-matched platelet transfusions is its timeliness when the HLA types of platelet-refractory patients are not yet known. A disadvantage is the need to carry out testing each time a platelet transfusion is required.

The management of patients with HLA and/or HPA alloimmunization with no compatible donors may be very difficult. There is no evidence that alloimmunized patients benefit from prophylactic transfusions of incompatible platelets that do not produce an increase in the platelet count, and prophylactic platelet support should be discontinued. If bleeding occurs, platelet transfusions from random donors or the best-matched donors, despite being incompatible, may reduce the severity of hemorrhage, although large doses of platelets may be required. Other management approaches for severe alloimmune refractoriness, such as the use of high-dose intravenous immunoglobulin, splenectomy, and plasma exchange, have not been shown to be effective.[81]

The management of patients with nonimmune platelet consumption is similarly problematic. Treatment of the underlying illness is indicated. Common practice is to continue with daily platelet transfusions as prophylactic platelet support, but it is not known whether this approach is effective, or whether platelet transfusions should be discontinued or the dose of platelets increased. Intravenous immunoglobulin is ineffective in this scenario. However, EACA and tranexamic acid may be useful in reducing bleeding in patients with severe thrombocytopenia (although tranexamic acid is not available in the United States). Even at relatively low doses of 1 g every six hours, EACA appears to be effective in this setting.

Leukocyte reduction of blood components has been shown to reduce the incidence of HLA alloimmunization and platelet refractoriness.[145]

Platelet substitutes and storage technologies

Platelet substitutes are in relatively early stages of development.[164] Among other approaches, ongoing efforts are being made to develop human platelet fragments that could be stored for lengthy periods and platelet cell surface molecules that are coupled to nanoparticles.[165–167]

The lesion that leads to the clearance of platelets that have been stored in the cold (below 12 °C) has been investigated extensively. In vitro, it appears that glycosylation (in particular, galactosylation) can prevent the clearance of refrigerated human platelets that are otherwise recognized by macrophage complement type 3 (CR3) receptors.[168,169] Whether modification of platelets in this manner will facilitate the effective transfusion of platelets in humans remains to be seen.

Thrombopoietin receptor agonists

Thrombopoietin is the primary regulator of megakaryocyte progenitor expansion and differentiation.[170] Its cloning in the mid-1990s led to the development of thrombopoietic drugs, and there was initial success in reducing the duration of thrombocytopenia with its use in cancer patients. However, trials were discontinued because healthy volunteers developed severe thrombocytopenia as a result of an immune response to the drug where antibodies cross-reacted with endogenous thrombopoietin. Focus shifted to the development of small-molecule peptide (romiplostim; Nplate marketed by Amgen) and nonpeptide thrombopoietin mimetics (eltrombopag; Promacta marketed by GlaxoSmithKline), and these have proved successful in the treatment of autoimmune thrombocytopenia. Efficacy in other settings of thrombocytopenia has not yet been demonstrated.

Summary

A variety of diverse congenital and acquired conditions are associated with thrombocytopenia or its functional equivalent. Congenital causes are rare, but acquired causes are relatively common. In particular, thrombocytopenia or platelet dysfunction associated with the administration of chemotherapy or with surgical procedures is a leading indication for platelet transfusion. The availability of a variety of platelet products for transfusion facilitates the supportive care of individuals receiving chemotherapy and the treatment of bleeding individuals with thrombocytopenia or its functional equivalent. Leukocyte-reduced whole blood–derived platelets and apheresis platelets are associated with similar rates of infection and alloimmunization, and they can be used interchangeably in most settings. A prophylactic platelet transfusion threshold of 10×10^9/L is generally acceptable for afebrile patients receiving cancer chemotherapy. Maintenance of a higher platelet count is indicated in a number of situations, including the settings of sepsis, DIC, hemorrhage, trauma, and surgery. Febrile and allergic reactions to platelet transfusion can often be managed conservatively with the administration of acetaminophen and diphenhydramine. Platelet refractoriness based on nonimmune and immune mechanisms remains a major issue when repeated transfusions are required. After platelet refractoriness following two transfusions has been documented, ABO matching, platelet crossmatching, and HLA matching may be used as initial strategies to address the situation. Because of the limitations of current storage techniques, research and development continue on platelet storage and substitutes. Thrombopoiesis-stimulating agents provide additional therapeutic alternatives for the management of thrombocytopenia in specific settings. However, much additional research and development will be necessary in order to establish their safety and efficacy in patients receiving cancer chemotherapy.

Disclaimer

The authors have disclosed no conflicts of interest.

Key references

A full reference list for this chapter is available at: http://www.wiley.com/go/simon/transfusion

9   Bolton-Maggs P, Chalmers E, Collins P, *et al.* A review of inherited platelet disorders with guidelines for their management on behalf of UKHCDO. *Br J Haematol* 2006;**135**: 603–33.

12   Neunert C, Lim W, Crowther M, Cohen A, Solberg L, Crowther MA. The American Society of Hematology 2011 evidence-based practice guideline for immune thrombocytopenia. *Blood* 2011;**117**: 4190–207.

16   Scully M, Hunt BJ, Benjamin S, *et al.* Guidelines on the diagnosis and management of thrombotic thrombocytopenic purpura and other thrombotic microangiopathies. *Br J Haematol* 2012;**158**: 323–35.

59   Heddle NM, Arnold DM, Boye D, Webert KE, Resz I, Dumont LJ. Comparing the efficacy and safety of apheresis and whole blood-derived platelet transfusions: a systematic review. *Transfusion* 2008;**48**: 1447–58.

64   Tobian A, King K, Ness P. Transfusion premedications: a growing practice not based on evidence. *Transfusion* 2007;**47**: 1089–96.

67   Estcourt L, Stanworth S, Doree C, *et al.* Prophylactic platelet transfusion for prevention of bleeding in patients with haematological disorders after chemotherapy and stem cell transplantation. *Cochrane Database Syst Rev* 2012: CD004269.

68   Stanworth SJ, Estcourt LJ, Powter G, *et al.* A no-prophylaxis platelet transfusion strategy for hematologic cancers. *N Engl J Med* 2013;**368**: 1771–80.

91   Estcourt L, Stanworth S, Doree C, *et al.* Different doses of prophylactic platelet transfusion for preventing bleeding in patients with haematological disorders after chemotherapy or stem cell transplantation. *Cochrane Database Syst Rev* 2014;**2014**: CD010984.

144   Murphy MF. Managing the platelet refractory patient. *ISBT Science Series* 2014;**9**: 234–8.

145   The Trial to Reduce Alloimmunization to Platelets Study Group. Leukocyte reduction and ultraviolet B irradiation of platelets to prevent alloimmunization and refractoriness to platelet transfusions. The Trial to Reduce Alloimmunization to Platelets Study Group. *N Engl J Med* 1997;**337**: 1861–9.

CHAPTER 21

Management of immune-mediated thrombocytopenia

Donald M. Arnold,[1] Ishac Nazi,[1] James W. Smith,[1] & Theodore E. Warkentin[1,2]

[1]Department of Medicine, Michael G. DeGroote School of Medicine, McMaster University, Hamilton, ON, Canada
[2]Department of Pathology and Molecular Medicine, Michael G. DeGroote School of Medicine, McMaster University, Hamilton, ON, Canada

Introduction

Thrombocytopenia, defined as a platelet count below the normal range, is one of the most common reasons for hematological consultation. Low circulating platelet numbers can be caused by platelet underproduction, sequestration, hemodilution, consumption, or destruction. This chapter explores the problem of immune-mediated thrombocytopenia, including autoimmune conditions (e.g., primary immune thrombocytopenic purpura [ITP]), secondary immune conditions (e.g., drug-induced immune thrombocytopenia [DITP] and heparin-induced thrombocytopenia [HIT]), and alloimmune conditions (e.g., neonatal alloimmune thrombocytopenia [NAIT]). Immune thrombocytopenia is characterized by a shortened platelet lifespan caused by platelet–antibody interactions and, in primary ITP, reduced platelet production likely because of immune-mediated alterations to bone marrow megakaryocytes. We begin with a review of routine and specialized laboratory testing used for the investigation of thrombocytopenic conditions, followed by a description of the most common immune-mediated thrombocytopenic syndromes and a review of current management.

Laboratory tests for the investigation of thrombocytopenia

Complete blood cell count and blood film

Platelets usually are quantitated during a complete blood cell count with a particle counter. A normal platelet count usually is 150,000–400,000/μL, although the reference range may be lower in Mediterranean populations (125,000–300,000/μL) that have larger sized platelets. The platelet count usually remains fairly stable throughout a normal human lifespan.[1] An exception occurs during pregnancy, when the platelet count decreases somewhat, perhaps the result of increased plasma volume (hemodilution). An elevated platelet count also is normal 10–14 days after a major surgical procedure (postoperative thrombocytosis, 250,000–1,000,000/μL) before return to preoperative baseline by three weeks after the operation.[2,3] Thus, a platelet count of only 170,000/μL 10 days after an operation in a patient with dyspnea who had received postoperative heparin prophylaxis could represent pulmonary embolism complicating HIT. A useful general rule is that isolated thrombocytopenia usually is caused by increased platelet consumption or destruction, whereas bicytopenia or pancytopenia usually is attributable to marrow dysfunction, hypersplenism, or hemodilution. Isolated, severe thrombocytopenia (platelet count less than 20,000/μL) often indicates platelet destruction by autoantibodies, alloantibodies, or drug-dependent immunoglobulin G (IgG) antibodies. Such severe thrombocytopenia occasionally occurs in patients with HIT[4] or septicemia, although platelet count nadirs are typically more than 20,000/μL in these two disorders characterized by in vivo platelet activation caused by heparin-dependent IgG antibodies or thrombin, respectively.

Examining the blood film is important to exclude pseudothrombocytopenia (spurious thrombocytopenia resulting from antibodies that cause ex vivo platelet agglutination) and to suggest various nonimmune causes of thrombocytopenia, such as toxic leukocytes indicating infection or fragmented red cells suggesting microangiopathic hemolysis. In contrast, primary immune thrombocytopenia is usually characterized by a reduction in platelet number with otherwise unremarkable morphologic features of all cell lines.

Platelet size and platelet RNA

A particle counter also is used to determine average platelet size, or mean platelet volume (MPV), which usually ranges from 7.0 to 10.5 fL. Disorders of increased platelet destruction usually are characterized by large platelets, and MPV ranges from 10 to 15 fL. Normal-sized or small platelets are common in disorders of underproduction or sequestration of platelets.

Young platelets contain residual amounts of RNA, which can be detected by means of flow cytometric analysis of platelets labeled with either thiazole orange or auramine-O. However, such quantitation of reticulated platelets (immature platelet count [IPC]) has not gained the acceptance that red cell reticulocyte assays have. Recent studies[5] have reported that elevated IPC is associated with greater risk of major adverse cardiovascular events (although a causal vs. confounded relationship remains uncertain[6]), and that reduced IPC may be used to identify subgroups of patients with ITP who have a marked defect in platelet production.[7]

Bone marrow examination

Disorders of increased platelet destruction are characterized by normal or increased numbers of megakaryocytes in the marrow.[8] Sometimes examination of the marrow yields enough information to determine the cause of the thrombocytopenia, such as myelodysplasia or megaloblastic anemia.

Rossi's Principles of Transfusion Medicine, Fifth Edition. Edited by Toby L. Simon, Jeffrey McCullough, Edward L. Snyder, Bjarte G. Solheim, and Ronald G. Strauss.
© 2016 John Wiley & Sons, Ltd. Published 2016 by John Wiley & Sons, Ltd.

Measurement of platelet life span

A platelet survival study is the definitive test for classifying the cause of thrombocytopenia. Indium-111 is the radiolabel of choice because of its higher labeling efficiency and efficient range of γ emissions. Indium-111 is not released from platelets by platelet autoantibodies. Three patterns of platelet survival can be observed: (1) normal platelet recovery (60% to 75%) and a normal survival time (7 to 10 days) characterize thrombocytopenia caused by underproduction; (2) markedly reduced platelet lifespan (hours) is found in patients with thrombocytopenia caused by increased platelet destruction; and (3) reduced platelet recovery (10% to 30%) with a normal or near-normal platelet survival time is consistent with platelet sequestration (hypersplenism). Platelet survival studies are rarely performed because these tests are complex and physicians usually infer the mechanism of the thrombocytopenia from the clinical situation.

Platelet–antibody assays

There are two broad categories of plateletantibody assays: (1) platelet-associated IgG assays, and (2) assays that identify the protein target of the antibody (direct binding assays). Measurement of platelet-associated IgG (PAIgG) has been widely available for many years. It can be used to detect either surface-associated immunoglobulin or complement using a labeled anti-immunoglobulin (and/or anticomplement) probe, or total PAIgG measured after platelet lysis. These assays have limited diagnostic usefulness, because a positive test result does not differentiate immune from nonimmune thrombocytopenia.[9]

Direct binding assays can quantify binding of a labeled anti-immunoglobulin probe to the platelet surface. The anti-immunoglobulin probe is labeled with a radioisotope, fluorescent marker, or enzyme. The labeled probe (e.g., anti-IgG, anti-IgM, or anticomplement) is incubated with washed test platelets, unbound probe is washed away, and the amount bound to the platelets is measured.[9] Although these assays are simple, a disadvantage is that platelet membranes nonspecifically adsorb proteins, including the labeled probe. Furthermore, even monoclonal anti-immunoglobulin probes may not differentiate immune from non-immune thrombocytopenic disorders.[9] Nevertheless, this type of assay can be diagnostically useful in special situations, such as detecting a drug-dependent increase in platelet surface-bound IgG in the presence of patient serum.[10]

Protein-specific platelet–antibody assays

The diagnostic usefulness of platelet–antibody assays has increased dramatically with the introduction of various protein-specific assays that help identify the platelet protein target of antibodies with either monoclonal antibodies or electrophoretic techniques. Current protein-specific antibody assays use detergents to extract the glycoprotein (GP) target from the membrane. This process increases the specificity of the test, but may affect antigenicity because the use of detergents and certain inhibitors (e.g., EDTA) may affect the structure of certain GP targets, such as the GPIIbIIIa complex, reducing the reactivity of some antibodies to HPA-1a.[11]

Various monoclonal antibody-based assays can be used to detect platelet antibodies. Perhaps most widely used is the monoclonal antibody immobilization of platelet antigen (MAIPA) assay. An improved modified MAIPA assay[12] is shown in Figure 21.1A. A technically simpler assay is the antigen capture enzyme immunoassay, in which platelet GP monoclonal antibodies interact with detergent-solubilized platelet samples (Figure 21.1B), rather than intact platelets.[10,13] Simplicity and improved specificity are advantages of these assays, especially the antigen capture assay. In addition to investigation of autoimmune thrombocytopenia, these assays can be adapted to study alloimmune disorders with a panel of platelet glycoproteins of known alloantigen phenotype, or drug-induced thrombocytopenia through demonstration of drug-dependent binding of antibody to specific platelet glycoproteins.[10] A disadvantage is that the identity of the target protein (and thus the monoclonal antibody to be used in the test) must be known in advance, and a number of different monoclonal antibodies are often needed. These assays also can give false-negative results if the patient antibody competes for the same epitope recognized by the monoclonal antibody. Some human sera contain antibodies that recognize murine IgG, which is why the modified MAIPA and antigen capture assays are preferred to the original MAIPA.[12]

Immunoprecipitation

Immunoprecipitation has the advantage of being able to identify novel protein targets of platelet antibodies and does not require the use of a known monoclonal antibody in advance. It is performed by incubating patient serum or plasma with platelets labeled with iodine-125 or tagged with nonradioactive biotin.[14] The proteins are then solubilized by the addition of detergent, and the antibody–protein complex is precipitated by addition of an anti-immunoglobulin bound to a solid phase (e.g., immobilized staphylococcal protein A). The labeled protein–antibody complexes are washed, and the platelet proteins are separated by denaturing gel electrophoresis and detected by autoradiography or use of enzyme-conjugated streptavidin. The target antigen is identified according to its electrophoretic mobility. Either the patient's platelets are used (direct immunoprecipitation), or patient serum or plasma is mixed with target platelets (indirect immunoprecipitation).

Immunoprecipitation offers advantages over immunoblotting because the antibody reacts with native, rather than denatured, platelet proteins. In particular, this technique has allowed detection of clinically significant antibodies against previously unrecognized platelet proteins, such as anti-HPA-15 (anti-Gov) on CD109, a 175-kD glycosylphosphatidylinositol (GPI)-anchored protein.[15] The main disadvantage of immunoprecipitation is technical difficulty. In addition, not all platelet proteins are optimally labeled (e.g., GPVI).

Immunoblotting (Western blotting)

In immunoblotting, patient serum is allowed to interact with platelet proteins that have been electrophoretically separated and then immobilized onto a solid phase (nitrocellulose). The test serum is added, and binding of patient antibody to specific protein bands is detected with labeled anti-immunoglobulin. Although immunoblotting offers the advantage of simplicity and the opportunity to store the immobilized proteins for long periods, a major disadvantage is that protein antigens are denatured in this method. This can destroy some platelet antigens (e.g., HPA-5 and -15) and may modify or expose epitopes to which normal sera can react (e.g., vinculin and talin), making interpretation difficult.[15,16]

Surface plasmon resonance (SPR)

A problem with many immunoassays is the requirement for wash steps. Even relatively gentle washes and dilutions can disrupt the binding of lower affinity antibodies to their glycoprotein targets. SPR was developed to investigate interactions between biomolecules in real time. The change in refractive index at the interface between

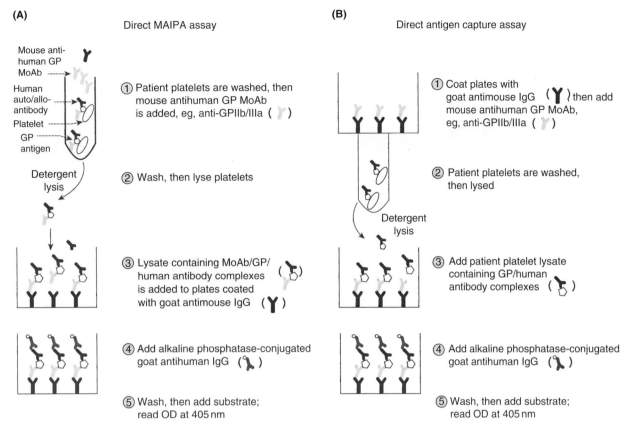

Figure 21.1 Modified monoclonal antibody immobilization of platelet antigen (MAIPA) assay and antigen capture assay. "Direct" versions of both assays are shown, that is, the patient's platelets are tested for the presence of platelet glycoprotein (GP)-bound autoantibodies. (In indirect assays, the patient's serum or plasma is added to target platelets to detect the presence of serum or plasma platelet glycoprotein antibodies.) (A) In the MAIPA assay, the antihuman GP monoclonal antibodies (MoAbs) are added to washed intact patient platelets before detergent lysis.[12] (B) In the antigen capture assay, the patient's platelets are washed, then lysed, and only later is GP MoAb added.[13] However, both assays resemble each other in the final stages (steps 4 and 5). A relative advantage of the antigen capture assay is that the platelet lysate can be stored and the assay performed later using any MoAb of choice, making this a technically simpler and more versatile assay. OD, optical density.

a gold surface and media can be measured as molecules in the fluid phase are passed over their targets bound to the surface. SPR has been used to investigate serum platelet antibodies, which may be low avidity and thus may escape detection by conventional protein binding assays. For example, SPR was used to confirm the diagnosis of NAIT in women who were suspected of having the disease but tested negative in other conventional immunoassays.[17,18] A disadvantage of SPR is the requirement for purified target protein to bind to the gold surface, limiting the method to abundant platelet glycoproteins that can be isolated efficiently. SPR has not yet been adopted into routine practice for platelet antibody investigations.

Tests for heparin-induced thrombocytopenia

Special tests are required to detect the antibodies that cause HIT. These assays are classified as platelet activation or platelet factor 4 (PF4)-dependent antigen assays.[19,20]

Platelet activation assays

Heparin-induced thrombocytopenia antibodies have potent heparin-dependent, platelet-activating properties. Aggregation of platelets (prepared as citrate-anticoagulated platelet-rich plasma) by patient plasma detected with conventional platelet aggregometry once was widely used for HIT; however, the sensitivity and specificity of this assay are relatively low for detecting HIT antibodies. In

contrast, assays performed with washed platelets that have been resuspended in calcium-containing buffer, such as the platelet serotonin release assay (SRA) or heparin-induced platelet activation assay (HIPA), are both sensitive and specific for detecting clinically significant HIT antibodies.[19,20] These assays are not widely available because they are technically demanding, require careful platelet donor selection, and require a panel of strong and weak positive serum controls. HIT antibodies have a characteristic activation profile: platelet activation at therapeutic, but not high, heparin concentrations and inhibition of activation by Fc receptor-blocking monoclonal antibodies. Strong serum-induced platelet activation that occurs in the absence of heparin is a feature of severe HIT, including "delayed-onset" and "spontaneous" HIT (discussed in this chapter).

PF4–heparin enzyme immunoassay

In 1992, Amiral *et al.*[21] identified PF4–heparin complexes as the antigen of HIT. Both commercial and in-house antigen assays based on enzyme immunoassay (EIA) methods have since become available. An intriguing feature of the HIT antigen is that certain polyanions other than heparin render PF4 antigenic. This is the basis of the PF4-polyvinylsulfonate EIA for PF4–heparin antibodies.[22]

Figure 21.2 compares the operating characteristics (sensitivity–specificity trade-offs) for three types of platelet–antibody assays.

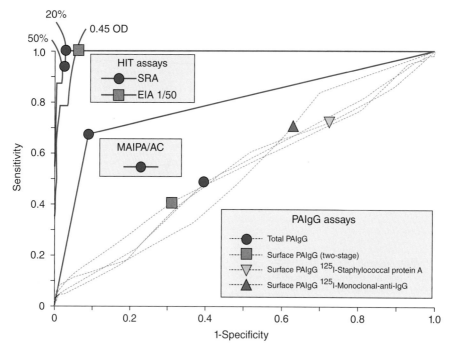

Figure 21.2 Operating characteristics of various platelet–antibody assays. The operating characteristics (sensitivity–specificity trade-offs at various diagnostic cutoffs between positive and negative results) show that assays for heparin-induced thrombocytopenia (HIT) are diagnostically useful (high sensitivity and specificity).[2,17,18] The data for the HIT assays show two diagnostic cutoffs (20% and 50% serotonin release) for the serotonin release assay (SRA), and one diagnostic cutoff (0.45 optical density unit) for the platelet factor 4/heparin enzyme immunoassay (EIA, performed with serum at 1/50 dilution). In contrast, the modified monoclonal antibody immobilization of platelet antigen (MAIPA) assay and antigen capture (AC) tests have moderate usefulness for diagnosis of autoimmune thrombocytopenia (high specificity but low to moderate sensitivity).[13] Conventional assays for platelet-associated immunoglobulin G (PAIgG) have minimal diagnostic value;[9] that is, sensitivity is similar to 1 − specificity. Open symbols are the diagnostic cutoff actually used for each assay. The data used for the MAIPA, AC, and PAIgG assays are from published sources.[9,13] Source: Warkentin (2001).[19] Reproduced with permission of Springer.

Classical PAIgG assays provide limited diagnostic information,[9] whereas the newer protein-specific platelet–antibody assays have moderate sensitivity and relatively high specificity for immune thrombocytopenia.[13] Both the antigen and washed-platelet activation assays are useful for diagnosis of HIT.[19,20]

Platelet genotyping

Serologic assays are generally reliable for detecting platelet alloantibodies. They also have been used to identify platelet antigens (platelet phenotyping). However, a disadvantage of antibody-based analysis is that there may not be sufficient platelets available from a patient with severe thrombocytopenia (e.g., posttransfusion purpura [PTP]) to allow determination of the reciprocal platelet alloantigen phenotype.[23] Secondly, specific phenotyping sera are available for only a few of the platelet antigens. Molecular techniques provide a reliable alternative to serologic phenotyping. Genomic DNA is used to determine the corresponding platelet alloantigen genotype and is readily available from a number of sources. Molecular techniques are useful in the evaluation of suspected NAIT. Analysis of fetal cells (obtained by amniocentesis, chorionic villus sampling, or sampling of fetal blood) can determine whether a fetus is at risk for this complication. Small amounts of tissue can be studied (e.g., 5–10 mL of amniotic fluid) because the technique of polymerase chain reaction (PCR) greatly amplifies the DNA. The possibility of significant maternal DNA contamination of a fetal sample can be assessed with the forensic technique of variable-number tandem repeat analysis of the sample.[24]

Polymerase chain reaction and restriction fragment length polymorphism

For all platelet alloantigen polymorphisms but one (HPA-4), the single-base substitution responsible for the change in the expressed amino acid is associated with a restriction endonuclease recognition site.[23] Accordingly, restriction fragment length polymorphism (RFLP) analysis was the first genotyping assay developed to identify platelet alloantigens. In the PCR–RFLP method, a section of DNA that encompasses the polymorphism is amplified using a pair of sense–antisense primers. The amplified product is subjected to restriction enzyme digestion, which cuts the amplified DNA into fragments depending on the nucleotide sequence. These are separated using agarose gel electrophoresis to identify the size and number of fragments, which indicate the platelet antigen genotype. One limitation is the possibility that another polymorphism within the amplified fragment could confound the genotyping by interfering with the restriction enzyme.[25] Phenotyping methods do not appear to be affected, suggesting that multiple methods for antigen typing may be warranted.[26]

Allele-specific polymerase chain reaction

Because PCR–RFLP is a comparatively labor-intensive technique, allele- or sequence-specific PCR (SSP-PCR) is commonly used. For this technique, one of the primers is specific for the particular allele to be amplified.[27] When the specific nucleotide corresponding to the allelic polymorphism is positioned at the 3′ end of the oligonucleotide primer, efficient amplification occurs only when the primer is 100% complementary to the genomic sequence. The advantage of this method is that the PCR product is visualized directly in agarose gels to determine the genotype. Appropriate controls must be included in the assay, including additional primers to amplify a ubiquitous gene (e.g., human growth hormone) to ensure that all assay constituents are working properly.

Real-time polymerase chain reaction
A modification of SSP-PCR is real-time PCR. Real-time PCR has improved both the speed and accuracy of genotyping.[28] The use of specifically designed hybridization probes tagged with fluorescent dyes for the PCR allows direct determination of the platelet genotype without gel electrophoresis or restriction enzymes in a single reaction. One hybridization probe, the donor, is tagged with a dye (fluorescein) and emits light at a specific wavelength when excited by a light source. The other probe, the acceptor, is tagged with a different dye. It straddles the single nucleotide polymorphism of interest and is 100% homologous to one of the platelet alleles. The acceptor probe usually is one nucleotide away from the donor probe in a head-to-tail arrangement, that is, the dyes are juxtaposed. The energy emitted by the dye of the donor probe is transferred to the adjacent dye of the acceptor probe, which emits light at a different wavelength. The intensity of the second light emitted is proportional to the amount of double-stranded DNA present. Unbound donor probe in the mixture can be excited but cannot transfer energy to the acceptor probe. On completion of the PCR, the platelet genotype is determined by means of melting curve analysis. Because the acceptor probe straddles the polymorphism and is 100% homologous to one of the alleles, the melting curve has a different temperature midpoint (T_m) depending on whether a mismatch is present. The acceptor probe can have as much as 5 °C to 8 °C difference in T_m between the two platelet alleles. In all, three melting curves are seen, one for each polymorphism and a composite melting curve when the heterozygous situation is present.[28] The advantage of fluorescence-based real-time PCR with melting curve analysis is that the PCR product is measured directly and no further manipulation is required. Any additional polymorphism in the region of the acceptor probe is detected in the melting curve analysis. Rapid thermal cycling and DNA extraction permit determination of a platelet genotype within two hours of specimen collection.

Immune-mediated thrombocytopenic syndromes
Immune thrombocytopenia results from antibody-mediated platelet destruction. The IgG-sensitized platelets are phagocytosed by monocytes and macrophages of the reticuloendothelial system. Reticuloendothelial cells are located throughout the body but are concentrated in the spleen, liver, lungs, and marrow. Pathogenic antibodies bind to platelets via their Fab termini, usually against specific autoantigen or alloantigen epitopes. Sometimes the target antigen is induced by a drug or drug metabolite. The result is a ternary complex that involves IgG, a drug, and a specific region on a platelet glycoprotein. Heparin-induced thrombocytopenia is an exception to these generalizations: Although HIT antibodies bind to PF4–heparin complexes via the Fab terminus, the Fc portion of IgG interacts with platelet FcγIIa receptors, resulting in platelet activation.[4]

The rate of platelet destruction is determined by the quantity and subclass distribution of IgG on the platelet, the amount of complement, and the efficiency of reticuloendothelial clearance.

The severity of thrombocytopenia reflects the balance between the rate of platelet destruction and the compensatory marrow thrombopoiesis.

Immune thrombocytopenia
Immune thrombocytopenia (ITP), previously known as primary idiopathic thrombocytopenic purpura, is a common disorder characterized by increased platelet destruction and impaired platelet production. It is a diagnosis of exclusion, defined by isolated thrombocytopenia with no other clinically apparent cause. Secondary ITP can occur in the setting of human immunodeficiency virus (HIV), hepatitis C, and *Helicobacter pylori* infections; systemic lupus erythematosus (SLE); drugs; and lymphoproliferative disorders. Causes of non-immune thrombocytopenia that are often confused with ITP include myelodysplasia, splenomegaly, and familial thrombocytopenia.[29] Although platelet–antibody assays allow for the detection of platelet GP-reactive autoantibodies in up to 75% of patients, the false-negative rate (at least 25%) gives this test a low sensitivity (e.g., a negative test does not exclude the diagnosis of ITP).[13,30]

Pathogenesis
Over 50 years ago, Harrington *et al.*[31] showed that ITP plasma infused into healthy volunteers caused acute severe thrombocytopenia. The platelet-destroying plasma factor was later shown to be IgG, although in some patients, IgM and IgA antibodies may be pathogenic. The immune target of the autoantibodies usually is one of the two major platelet glycoprotein complexes, with GPIIb/IIIa implicated more often than GPIb/IX.[32] Other less common autoantigen targets include GPIa/IIa and, possibly, nonprotein targets such as glycosphingolipids. The autoantibodies bind to platelets by way of their Fab terminus and cause premature platelet destruction via Fc receptor (FcγR)-mediated phagocytosis by macrophages in the spleen and other reticuloendothelial tissues. Platelet autoantibodies can also activate complement in vitro. Another proposed mechanism of platelet destruction is direct platelet lysis by cytotoxic T cells.[33]

Platelet production is also impaired in ITP. Platelet turnover is lower than expected, as shown by radiolabeled autologous platelet studies,[34] and some patients who respond to thrombopoietin (TPO)-based treatments have demonstrated an increase in the number of reticulated platelets, suggesting that this compensation was not maximal.[7] An increased megakaryocyte mass that has been observed in some patients[8] may account for the relative TPO deficiency, because these cells bind free TPO; conversely, platelet underproduction may result from megakaryocyte injury caused by autoantibodies.[35]

The cause of autoantibody formation in ITP is not known. Light-chain and immunoglobulin subclass restriction of platelet-reactive antibodies suggests an oligoclonal origin of autoantibodies in chronic ITP.[36] Furthermore, the autoepitopes involved may be fairly restricted in scope. Autoantibodies are produced by B lymphocytes, and the loss of T-cell tolerance to platelet proteins is a key feature.

Clinical and laboratory features
Stages of ITP have recently been defined by the international ITP Working Group: newly diagnosed ITP (within three months), persistent ITP (3–12 months), and chronic ITP (more than 12 months).[37] The prevalence of ITP has been estimated at 12.1 (95% confidence interval [CI], 11.1–13.0) per 100,000 adults.[38] If clinical

evaluation reveals weight loss, fever, lymphadenopathy, hepatomegaly, or splenomegaly, other diagnoses should be considered. Laboratory testing for patients with ITP should include testing for HIV, hepatitis C, and hepatitis B (in anticipation of possible rituximab treatment). Some guidelines recommend *H. pylori* testing, quantitative immunoglobulin levels, and thyroid screening (especially before splenectomy, because thyroid dysfunction may be associated).

Mucocutaneous bleeding is the hallmark of ITP and manifests as purpura (petechiae and ecchymosis), epistaxis, menorrhagia, oral mucosal bleeding, and gastrointestinal bleeding. Serious bleeding occurs in 9.6% of adults and 20.2% of children, and intracerebral hemorrhage occurs in 1.4% of adults and 0.4% of children.[39] Severe bleeding is highest among patients with chronic ITP, patients with previous bleeding, and patients over 60 years of age.[40] On the other hand, many patients even with severe thrombocytopenia have minimal or no bleeding, possibly because of the presence of small numbers of young, reticulated platelets with enhanced α-granule release to platelet agonists.[41] Often, morbidity is attributable to the treatments of ITP and less commonly to the disease itself.[42]

Treatment overview
Treatment strategies for ITP are based on the following principles:
1 Many patients do not bleed, even with low platelet counts ($<30 \times 10^9$/L), and may not need treatment.
2 The goal of treatment is to achieve a safe platelet count, not necessarily a normal count.
3 The urgency of treatment will dictate the type of therapy: Platelet transfusions may be useful when immediate (but transient) hemostasis is needed, intravenous immunoglobulin (IVIG) will start to increase the platelet count in most patients by 12–24 hours, and corticosteroids result in a platelet count response within 3–7 days.
4 Most adults have chronic ITP with low (but not infrequent) rates of spontaneous remission (up to 20%), whereas most children have acute ITP that improves spontaneously or with minimal treatment.[29]
5 Many adults will require treatment beyond first-line therapies, but the minimal amount of treatment should be used to maintain a hemostatic platelet count in patients with chronic ITP.
6 Drugs that interfere with platelet function—particularly aspirin, nonsteroidal anti-inflammatory agents, and alcohol—should be avoided.

First-line therapies

Corticosteroids
Corticosteroids, either prednisone (1 mg/kg/day tapered over 6–8 weeks) or high-dose dexamethasone (40 mg/day for four consecutive days, repeated monthly if necessary), are considered first-line treatments. Two prospective studies[43,44] compared conventional and lower dose prednisone therapy (1 mg/kg/day vs. 0.25 mg/kg/day in one trial; 1.5 mg/kg/day vs. 0.5 mg/kg/day in the other), and in neither study was there a significant difference in remission at 6-month follow-up evaluation. In the larger study,[44] however, the higher dose regimen showed a trend to a higher rate of complete remission (46% vs. 35%) as well as higher platelet counts at 14-day follow-up evaluation (77% vs. 51% having a platelet count greater than 50,000/μL).

High-dose dexamethasone has been used with success in patients with newly diagnosed ITP. In one study ($n = 125$), 84% of patients with acute ITP treated with a single course of high-dose dexamethasone (40 mg/day for four days) achieved a platelet count response (>50,000/μL), and of those, 50% had a response that lasted from 2 to 5 years.[45] In another study ($n = 37$), six courses of monthly high-dose dexamathosone resulted in an overall response rate of 83.8%, and a sustained response of 64.9% after two years.[46] However, repeated cycles of high-dose dexamethasone were often poorly tolerated, and these high rates of durable response have not been consistent in practice. In patients with chronic ITP, responses with high-dose dexamethasone are variable. In one study, all 10 treated patients achieved a response that lasted six months following six cycles of high-dose dexamethasone (40 mg/day for four days).[47] However, other subsequent studies were less encouraging. Using the same regimen, Stasi *et al.*[48] reported that 13 of 32 patients (40.6%) had transient responses only, and in the study by Warner *et al.*,[49] none of nine patients responded, and five could not tolerate the treatment. Overall, only approximately 20% of adult patients with ITP have a durable remission following corticosteroid therapy.

Adverse effects of corticosteroids include facial swelling, weight gain, and behavioral changes in up to 20% of patients.[29,50] Less common (1–5%) complications include infection, myopathy, hyperglycemia, psychosis, hypertension, hypokalemia, and osteoporosis. Osteonecrosis, most commonly involving the femoral head, occurs as a late side effect in approximately 5% of patients who undergo prolonged therapy, but it may occur even after intensive short-term exposure.[51]

Intravenous immunoglobulin
High-dose IVIG has been used to treat patients with ITP since 1981.[52,53] Reticuloendothelial blockade is the principal mechanism of action of IVIG, but many other mechanisms have been proposed, including the reduction of antibody synthesis, IgG molecules against the Fab regions of pathogenic autoantibodies ("anti-idiotypic antibodies"),[54] cytokine-induced pro- or anti-inflammatory effects,[55] up- or downregulation of various FcγRs, or the formation of soluble immune complexes. In a mouse model of ITP, the inhibitory IgG receptor, FcγRIIB, was required for IVIG to cause an elevation in platelet count,[56] and the transfer of IVIG-primed dendritic cells has been shown to recapitulate the effect of IVIG.[57]

The use of IVIG is indicated for patients with ITP with bleeding or for whom an invasive procedure is planned to raise the platelet count quickly. A French study of 122 adults with ITP showed that IVIG (0.7 g/kg/day for three days) raised the platelet count to over 50,000/μL within five days more frequently than did corticosteroids (methylprednisolone, 15 mg/kg/day for three days).[58]

The usual dose of IVIG is 1–2 g/kg, given either as 0.4 g/kg for five consecutive days or as 1 g/kg over two days. One trial showed no difference between one and two doses of 1 g/kg.[59] Thus, our approach is to give 1 g/kg as a single dose and to repeat the dose 1 or 2 days later if no significant platelet count increase has occurred.[60]

IVIG increases the platelet count to greater than 50,000/μL in approximately 80% of adult patients. Responses are usually transient, lasting 2–6 weeks. Tachyphylaxis after repeated courses may be observed in patients with severe ITP.

Common but mild side effects include headache in 10% of patients, backache, nausea, flushing, and fever.[61] Aseptic meningitis may occur rarely.[29] Chest pain, hypertension, hypotension, bronchospasm, and laryngeal edema have been reported. A boxed warning concerning the risk of thrombosis with IVIG was issued by the US Food and Drug Administration (FDA) in 2013 (http://www.

Table 21.1 Comparison of high-dose IVIG and intravenous RhIG for management of immune thrombocytopenic purpura

Characteristic	High-Dose IVIG	Intravenous RhIG
Side effects	Common: headache, hypertension, fever and chills	Common: mild hemolysis
	Rare: hemolysis, renal failure, myocardial infarction, stroke	Rare: severe hemolysis necessitating transfusion or hemodialysis, DIC
Response rate	~80%	~80%
Response duration	Usually transient	Usually transient
Pattern of platelet increase	Faster increase, higher peak, shorter duration of response	Slower increase, lower peak, longer duration of response
Influence of ABO, Rh type	No influence	Only D-positive patients respond
Influence of splenectomy	Unknown	Minimal response in patients without a spleen
Suitability for emergency management of ITP	Recommended	Not recommended

IVIG = intravenous immune globulin; RhIG = Rh immune globulin; DIC = disseminated intravascular coagulation; ITP = immune thrombocytopenic purpura.

fda.gov), because arterial and venous thrombosis have rarely been reported, particularly in elderly patients[62] (Table 21.1). Because IVIG is prepared from pooled plasma from thousands of donors, infection transmission is theoretically possible. Transfusion-related acute lung injury following IVIG also has been described.[63]

Intravenous Rh immune globulin

Like IVIG, the mechanism of action of intravenous Rh immune globulin (RhIg) is believed to be reticuloendothelial blockade, which occurs through occupancy of the reticuloendothelial cell FcγRs by IgG-sensitized red cells. The therapy is only effective in D-positive individuals.

Doses of 50–75 μg/kg of RhIg have been shown to produce a rapid increase in platelet count.[64] Hemolysis is an expected side effect, and rarely severe hemolysis with disseminated intravascular coagulation and renal failure has been reported with fatal outcomes.[65] Because of this, RhIg was voluntarily withdrawn from some European markets in 2009 (Table 21.1).

Second-line therapies

Splenectomy

Splenectomy is frequently successful, because the spleen is the major site of both autoantibody production and platelet destruction. Complete remission occurs in 70% of patients within 4–6 weeks.[66] In complete responders, normal platelet counts are reached within seven days in 90% and within six weeks in 98% of patients; spontaneous remission is encountered rarely thereafter. In a further 5–10% of patients, partial remission is achieved. In a systematic review of the efficacy of splenectomy for patients with ITP, younger age was an independent predictor of response to splenectomy;[66] however, other investigators have shown that response to IVIG[67–69] and splenic clearance of platelets (determined by radionuclide platelet imaging techniques)[70] are good predictors of response to splenectomy. The risk of relapse after a complete remission following splenectomy is low (approximately 10–15% at 10 years). Splenectomy is most often done using a laparascopic approach.

Perioperative management of splenectomy involves (1) optimization of the platelet count before surgery, (2) vaccination to minimize the risk of overwhelming postsplenectomy infection, and (3) prevention of thromboembolism. Adequate perioperative hemostasis usually can be achieved with preoperative high-dose IVIG or corticosteroids, and TPO receptor agonists may be a suitable alternative.[71] However, most patients do not have excessive bleeding; therefore, platelet transfusions should be reserved for the treatment of perioperative bleeding.

The presence of residual accessory spleen should be considered when splenectomy fails, or when patients relapse months or years after surgery.[72] Postsplenectomy blood film changes (e.g., Howell–Jolly bodies) do not necessarily eliminate the possibility of a residual accessory spleen. A durable platelet count response following accessory splenectomy performed because of postsplenectomy relapse of ITP is uncommon and can be expected in less than 50% of patients.

Perioperative morbidity after splenectomy is less than 10%. The most frequent complications are pleuropulmonary (pneumonia, subphrenic abscess, and pleural effusion) in 4% of patients, major bleeding in 1.5%, and thromboembolism in 1%. Morbidity is lower with a laparoscopic approach by an experienced surgeon. Overall mortality is approximately 1% following laparotomy and 0.2% following laparascopic splenectomy.[66]

Bacterial infection is the most feared complication of splenectomy. The risk of overwhelming postsplenectomy infection is approximately 1–3%. In a population-based Danish cohort study of 3812 patients who underwent splenectomy, the overall incidence rate of infection was 7.7 per 100 person-years (odds ratio compared to unsplenectomized patients with an indication for splenectomy, 1.7 [95% CI, 1.5–2.1] in the first 90 days).[73] In a review of the literature up to 1996, the frequency of infection was 2.1% and mortality was 1.2% among 484 patients who had splenectomy for ITP.[74] Life-threatening infections may occur many years after splenectomy, suggesting that the risk of severe infection may persist.[75] To reduce the risk of bacterial infection, all patients who undergo splenectomy should receive vaccinations against the encapsulated bacteria *Streptococcus pneumoniae*, *Haemophilia influenza* type B (HIB), and *Neisseria meningitidis*.

Postoperative thromboembolism is the most common cause of postoperative mortality; thus, for patients with delayed postoperative mobilization, prophylactic low-molecular-weight (LMW) heparin should be considered when the platelet count is recovering.

Rituximab

Rituximab is a chimeric monoclonal anti-CD20 currently indicated for the treatment of lymphoma and rheumatoid arthritis. The Fab portion binds to CD20 on B lymphocytes, which results in FcγR-mediated B-cell lysis by complement-dependent[76] and antibody-dependent pathways.[77–79] In ITP, rituximab depletes CD20-positive B cells, which are responsible for platelet autoantibody production. It can also correct T-cell dysfunction which has been associated with platelet count improvements after rituximab.[80] Rituximab may be a suitable alternative to splenectomy for some patients because of its association with lasting remissions in up to 20% of patients.[81]

A systematic review[82] of observational studies described outcomes in adults who had ITP for 1–360 months (half had splenectomy). A complete response to rituximab (platelet count greater than 150,000/μL) was seen in 43.6% of patients (95% CI, 29.5–57.7%) and an overall response (platelet count >50,000/μL) in 62.5% (95% CI, 52.6–72.5%). Responses lasted a median of 10 months. Data from randomized trials were less optimistic. In a recent meta-analysis, rituximab plus standard of care was more often associated with a complete platelet count response (platelets $>100 \times 10^9$/L without rescue treatment) compared with standard of care alone (46.8% vs. 32.5%; $p = 0.002$); however, responses were generally not sustained past 12 months.[83]

Results with rituximab in children are less encouraging. In a prospective single-arm study of 36 children with chronic ITP treated with rituximab, 11 (30.6%) achieved a platelet count of 50,000/μL or greater for four consecutive weeks.[84]

Toxicities of rituximab include infusional reactions, hepatitis B reactivation, and a possible association with progressive multifocal leukoencephalopathy.[85] Rituximab has been shown to impair vaccine responses for up to six months.[86]

Thrombopoietin receptor agonists

TPO receptor agonists are a releetively new class of medications indicated for the treatment of patients with chronic ITP. Romiplostim is administered by weekly subcutaneous injection, and eltrombopag is a daily pill. The clinical success of these medications has been one of the most important advances in ITP treatments since the discovery of IVIG. In phase III trials, each has been shown to be effective in increasing platelet counts compared with placebo or standard of care[87,88] in 60–80% of patients. Responses are sustained even after long-term follow-up.[89,90] The platelet count response is usually maintained as long as the medication is continued; however, once it is stopped, platelet counts typically drop to pretreatment levels, at which point patients may be at increased risk of bleeding.[91] However, some patients can successfully stop TPO receptor agonists and maintain durable platelet count responses.[92] Rare side effects include thrombosis and bone marrow reticulin formation;[93] however, the true risk of these complications remains uncertain. Potential long-term toxicities and high cost limit the prolonged use of these medications.[94]

TPO receptor agonists bind to and activate the c-Mpl receptor on hematopoietic stem cells and megakaryocytes, ultimately leading to increased platelet production. They do not resemble endogenous TPO, and thus cannot induce the formation of TPO-reactive autoantibodies, which was a problem with early formulations of pegylated recombinant human megakaryocyte growth and development factor (PEG-rHuMGDF).[95]

Where TPO receptor agonists should be positioned for the treatment of patients with ITP remains uncertain. They are good treatment options for patients who have failed second-line therapies, including splenectomy and rituximab. The use of these medications at an earlier stage of disease may improve short-term outcomes.[96]

Other treatments

Danazol

Danazol is an attenuated androgen with mild virilizing effects that can be used to treat men and nonpregnant women with ITP. Its mechanism of action is to decrease FcγR numbers and the rate of FcγR-mediated clearance of IgG-sensitized cells. Danazol decreases the number of monocyte IgG Fc receptors.[97] Usually, 400 to 800 mg is administered daily in divided doses, although some physicians use low doses (50 mg/day). A response usually occurs within two months, although when low doses are used, as long as six months may be needed.

Danazol appears to produce a sustained increase in platelet count in approximately 30–40% of treated patients. The response rate may be higher among patients with associated rheumatologic disorders.[98] Danazol must be continued to maintain the platelet count response, although attempts at dose reduction should be made. Danazol is generally well tolerated but may be associated with virilizing side effects in women, liver dysfunction, and rash.

Vinca alkaloids

Vinca alkaloids (vincristine and vinblastine) can produce generally short-lived increases in platelet count in approximately 65% of patients.[99] These drugs bind to platelet microtubules and so might work by being delivered to, and thereby inhibiting, reticuloendothelial macrophages. Repeated doses of vinca alkaloids are rarely used to treat patients with chronic ITP, mostly because of dose-dependent neuropathy.

Immunosuppressive agents

Cyclophosphamide, azathioprine, mycophenylate, and cyclosporine are immunosuppressive agents that have been used to treat patients with refractory ITP. Cyclophosphamide is an alkylating agent given in doses of 1–2 mg/kg/day, although high-dose cyclophosphamide has been used in combination with autologous stem cell transplantation.[100] Azathioprine and mycophenylate are purine antimetabolites that inhibit lymphocyte proliferation. Cyclosporine is a calcineurin inhibitor that selectively blocks T-cell-dependent biosynthesis of lymphokines, particularly interleukin-2, at the level of messenger RNA transcription.

These drugs, alone or in combination, have shown moderate success, with up to two-thirds of patients exhibiting a platelet count response.[101–103] However, only 20–30% have responses that persist after stopping the drug(s). Responses may occur as early as two weeks and as late as three months after initiation of treatment.

Azathioprine can have myelosuppressive effects on haematopoietic cells and may cause severe bone marrow toxicity in patients who lack activity of the enzyme thiopurine methyltransferase (TPMT) (1 in 300 individuals).[104] Mycophyenolate may also be associated with leukopenia. The concern over leukemic transformation has limited use of cyclophosphamide.[105] Animal studies suggest that intermittent cyclophosphamide may be less leukemogenic than daily administration. Cyclophosphamide also can cause hemorrhagic cystitis and hepatic toxicity. Cyclosporine is associated with hypertention and renal failure in some patients.

Special treatment situations

Emergency treatment of a bleeding patient

Any patient with ITP who has life-threatening bleeding needs immediate platelet transfusion. The patient then should receive IVIG (1 g/kg) over 4–6 hours to block the reticuloendothelial system, and corticosteroids should be considered for long-term disease control.

Preparation for invasive procedures

High-dose IVIG usually is the treatment of choice for severely thrombocytopenic patients with ITP who need urgent surgery or an invasive procedure. Prophylactic platelet transfusion should be administered only when maximal hemostasis is required, because transfusion-induced platelet count increments are usually transient. For situations in which at least 2 or 3 days are available before the planned procedure, less expensive and equally effective options include corticosteroids. TPO receptor agonists may be a reasonable alternative but must be started 2–3 weeks in advance.

Immune thrombocytopenia in pregnancy

Thrombocytopenia during pregnancy usually is not caused by ITP. Rather, a benign condition known as *gestational thrombocytopenia* is more common, occurring in approximately 5% of pregnancies at term. In this condition, maternal platelet counts do not fall below 70,000/μL.[106] Newborns of mothers with incidental thrombocytopenia are not at increased risk of neonatal thrombocytopenia.[107] The second most likely cause of thrombocytopenia is pregnancy-related disorders (e.g., preeclampsia and syndrome of hemolysis, elevated liver enzymes, and low platelet count [HELLP syndrome]). Preeclampsia occurs in approximately 10% of pregnancies and causes thrombocytopenia in one-fourth of affected mothers. Preeclampsia is associated with increased maternal and fetal morbidity and mortality. Secondary causes of immune thrombocytopenia that can occur in young women, such as SLE or HIV infection, should also be considered in the appropriate clinical context.

ITP in pregnancy is an important disorder because of the treatment implications for the mother and the possibility of fetal or neonatal thrombocytopenia caused by transplacental passage of IgG platelet autoantibodies. In the past, infants of mothers with ITP were delivered by cesarean section; however, today, this procedure is not routinely recommended for two reasons. Firstly, the frequency of severe fetal thrombocytopenia (platelet count less than 20,000/μL) is low (approximately 4%).[108] Secondly, there is no evidence that cesarean section leads to less intracranial bleeding compared with vaginal delivery.

Many pregnant women with ITP do not need specific treatment, unless the platelet count decreases below 20,000/μL or there is evidence of impaired hemostasis. The two preferred treatment options are intermittent high-dose IVIG and low-dose prednisone; however, IVIG is generally the treatment of choice (1 g/kg every 2–4 weeks) because side effects are more common with prednisone and include teratogenicity (first trimester) and preeclampsia (second and third trimesters). At delivery, thrombocytopenic patients should not be subjected to epidural analgesia. Platelet transfusions are almost never needed at delivery. In the largest cohort of infants born to mothers with ITP (119 pregnancies in 97 women), 10% of infants had a platelet count below 50,000/μL at birth, 15% required hemostatic treatments, and 1% died.[109]

There are no good predictors of fetal thrombocytopenia, not even the severity of maternal thrombocytopenia (indeed, women cured of ITP by splenectomy can bear infants with passive autoimmune thrombocytopenia).

If therapy for maternal thrombocytopenia is needed, IVIG is preferred. Splenectomy is rarely indicated for severe, refractory thrombocytopenia in pregnancy.[29] Cesarean section delivery should be reserved for obstetrical indications.

Immune thrombocytopenia in children

Acute ITP of childhood is a relatively common, generally self-limited, immune thrombocytopenic disorder with a peak incidence between 2 and 6 years of age. Boys and girls are equally affected, except for infants, in which males predominate.[110] Most children

(80–90%) with acute ITP recover completely within six months; the others have persistent thrombocytopenia. Acute ITP of childhood likely is a transient autoimmune disorder.[111]

The typical clinical manifestations are bleeding and bruising following a viral infection. The mortality is approximately 0.4%, and most deaths are caused by intracranial hemorrhage. Laboratory abnormalities include isolated thrombocytopenia and normal or increased MPV. A marrow examination usually is not performed on a child with typical clinical features of ITP, but is indicated for unexpected clinical or laboratory findings. Normal or increased numbers of megakaryocytes are observed. Sometimes, morphologically distinct lymphoid cells, called *hematogones*, constitute up to one-half of the marrow cells and may cause confusion with acute leukemia.[112] These nonneoplastic cells have the surface immunophenotypic profile of immature lymphocytes.

Acute ITP in children usually is a benign disease. Although rare, intracranial hemorrhage is the most feared complication. Clinical trials have focused on the time to increase the platelet count to safe levels as a surrogate endpoint for avoiding intracranial hemorrhage.

In a meta-analysis of six randomized trials ($n = 410$ children), IVIG was associated with a more rapid platelet count increase compared with corticosteroids.[113] On the basis of these results, high-dose IVIG is generally recommended for initial treatment of severe acute ITP in children. Oral prednisone or an additional dose of IVIG is added if the platelet count remains below 20,000/μL by 48 hours. It appears that lower doses of IVIG (e.g., 250–500 mg/kg/day for 2 days rather than the standard 1 g/kg/day) may also be effective.[114]

High-dose corticosteroid therapy (e.g., intravenous methylprednisolone at 30 mg/kg/day for 3 days; or oral methylprednisolone at 30–50 mg/kg/day for 7 days) also rapidly increases the platelet count in children with acute severe ITP.[115] Combined treatment with IVIG and pulse methylprednisolone may be indicated for those children felt to be at very high risk of intracranial hemorrhage.[116]

Approximately 10–20% of children with ITP eventually have chronic ITP, defined as a platelet count less than 100,000/μL for more than six months. As many as one-third of children who meet this definition can still enter late spontaneous remission, sometimes as long as 5–10 years after diagnosis. Chronic ITP in children resembles adult chronic ITP.

Some patients have no symptoms despite marked thrombocytopenia. These children generally do not need treatment. For children with symptoms, options include long-term or intermittent administration of corticosteroids, maintenance IVIG or RhIG, splenectomy, vinca alkaloids, and immunosuppressive agents.[117]

Intravenous immune globulin (2 g/kg over 2–5 days) increases the platelet count of most children with chronic ITP,[52,117] and repeated courses of IVIG have been used to defer or avoid splenectomy. This practice also appears to be cost-effective.[118] Unfortunately, approximately 25% of patients become refractory. Low-dose, alternate-day corticosteroid therapy may improve the results with maintenance IVIG.

Intravenous RhIG is effective in increasing the platelet count of most Rh-positive children with chronic ITP[119,120] and, at a dose of 75 μg/kg, appears to be as effective as IVIG.[121] The benefit is transient, and the median duration of benefit is approximately three weeks. RhIG can also be considered splenectomy-sparing in some patients.[120] However, RhIG is generally ineffective following splenectomy.[120]

Splenectomy is sometimes performed in children with chronic ITP who cannot be maintained on low-dose maintenance glucocorticoids, IVIG, or RhIG therapy. Because of the high probability of a cure (approximately 70%), some physicians perform splenectomy before instituting potentially toxic immunosuppressive therapy. However, in general, splenectomy is avoided in children, especially young children, because of the high risk of postsplenectomy sepsis, the possibility of late spontaneous remissions, and the efficacy of intermittent maintenance therapy with IVIG or RhIG. As with adults, children must receive vaccines for *S. pneumoniae*, *N. meningitides*, and *H. influenzae* type b at least two weeks before splenectomy.[122]

Results of use of immunosuppressive agents (azathioprine or cyclophosphamide) and vinca alkaloids to treat children with chronic ITP are variable and based on uncontrolled studies.[117] Pulse corticosteroids have been used in children, although few durable remissions occur. In one study, three of seven children achieved a platelet count above 50,000/μL six months after receiving high-dose dexamethasone. One child had a response that was maintained to one year.[123] Children with chronic ITP refractory to splenectomy occasionally obtain benefit from cyclosporine. Danazol can be tried in the adolescent patient. About one-third of pediatric patients with chronic ITP responded to rituximab in one study.[84]

Drug-induced immune thrombocytopenia

Drugs can produce several immune-mediated thrombocytopenic disorders[4,124–127] (Table 21.2). The most common is HIT (discussed separately), which paradoxically is associated with increased risk of thrombosis but not bleeding. In contrast, many other drugs in rare instances cause severe thrombocytopenia and bleeding, a syndrome called *drug-induced immune thrombocytopenic purpura* (DITP). Some drugs cause atypical clinical signs and symptoms (e.g., abciximab-induced thrombocytopenia) or trigger an illness that resembles thrombotic thrombocytopenic purpura (TTP) or HUS.

Typical drug-induced immune thrombocytopenia

The most common drugs that have been confirmed by laboratory testing to cause DITP are quinine, quinidine, trimethoprim/sulfamethoxazole, vancomycin, penicillin, rifampin, carbamazepine, and ceftriaxone.[128] The risk of DITP is approximately 1 case in 1000 for quinine and 1 in 25,000 for sulfamethoxazole–trimethoprim.[129] Quinine is present in certain beverages (e.g., tonic water), and consequently patients may not be aware of exposure.

Clinical criteria supporting a diagnosis of DITP are (1) thrombocytopenia occurs during drug treatment and is corrected completely after discontinuation of the drug; (2) the implicated drug was the only one used when thrombocytopenia occurred, or platelet count recovery occurred or persisted despite continuation or reintroduction of the other drugs used; (3) other causes of thrombocytopenia are excluded; and (4) reexposure to the implicated agent resulted in recurrent thrombocytopenia.[125] For reasons of patient safety, drug reexposure is rarely performed deliberately, but sometimes the outcome of unintentional reexposure can provide important diagnostic information (e.g., recurrent thrombocytopenia following ingestion of tonic water suggests quinine-induced thrombocytopenia). Meeting all four criteria provides definite evidence of causation, whereas meeting the first three criteria suggests a probable cause.[125]

Although many dozens of drugs have been suspected as causing DITP, laboratory evidence confirming the presence of drug-dependent platelet antibodies exists for relatively few drugs.[128] Supporting evidence for the drugs claimed to cause DITP is available (http://www.ouhsc.edu/platelets/).

Drug-induced immune-mediated thrombocytopenia typically begins abruptly and is severe; most patients have a platelet count less than 20,000/μL.[4,127,130] Although the interval between starting the drug and development of thrombocytopenia usually is 1 or 2 weeks, occasionally it can be several months or even longer after

Table 21.2 Drug-induced immune thrombocytopenic syndromes

Syndrome and Drug(s)	Comment
Heparin-induced thrombocytopenia	Prothrombotic reaction caused by heparin-dependent platelet-activating IgG antibodies that recognize platelet factor 4/heparin complexes; caused less often by low-molecular-weight heparin and fondaparinux than by unfractionated heparin
Drug-induced immune thrombocytopenic purpura (DITP)	Prohemorrhagic reaction caused by IgG antibodies that recognize drug (or drug metabolite) bound to platelet glycoprotein (GP); patients have severe thrombocytopenia and mucocutaneous bleeding.
• Quinine	Quinine-dependent anti-GPIIb/IIIa and GPIb/IX IgG implicated; drug is widely available (eg, tonic water)
• Quinidine	Antibodies usually distinct from quinine-dependent antibodies
• Rifampin	Rifampin-dependent anti-GPIIb/IIIa and GPIb/IX IgG implicated
• Sulfa antibiotics	Occurs in ~1 of 25,000 patients receiving trimethoprim-sulfamethoxazole
• Vancomycin	Vancomycin-dependent anti-GPIIb/IIIa IgG
• Iodinated contrast	Severe thrombocytopenia begins after radiologic procedure
• Acetaminophen	IgG recognizes metabolite of acetaminophen
• Many others	See published lists[153,154]
Atypical DITP	
• Abciximab	Abrupt onset of severe thrombocytopenia (platelet count nadir, 15,000 to 35,000/μL) perhaps by naturally occurring ligand-induced binding site antibodies
• Gold	Thrombocytopenia can persist for months after gold therapy is stopped
• MMR vaccine	Transient autoimmune thrombocytopenia (anti-GPIIb/IIIa) that occurs a few weeks after vaccination (resembles childhood acute ITP)
DITP: hapten mechanism	Indicates that IgG recognizes drug that remains bound to platelet surface even following platelet washing
• Penicillin	Not well-established
Drug-induced TTP/HUS	
• Ticlopidine	Estimated frequency, 1/2,000 to 1/5000
• Clopidogrel	Estimated frequency, 1/20,000
• Quinine	Quinine-dependent IgG against platelets and other cells found
• Cyclosporine	May be pathogenic factor in transplantation-associated TTP/HUS
• Others	See text

MMR = measles-mumps-rubella; ITP = immune thrombocytopenic purpura; TTP = thrombotic thrombocytopenic purpura; HUS = hemolytic uremic syndrome.

administration of the drug is started. Sometimes, thrombocytopenia persists for several weeks even after the drug is stopped, possibly because some of the IgG antibodies formed have drug-independent platelet reactivity.

The pathogenesis of DITP involves formation of a ternary complex involving a platelet glycoprotein (usually, the GPIIb/IIIa complex, less often GPIb/IX), drug (or drug metabolite), and the Fab terminus of IgG.[10,131,132] Such a mechanism has been invoked for quinine, quinidine, sulfonamide, rifampin, vancomycin,[131] and pentamidine, among others. Unlike the mechanism of HIT, platelet FcγRs are not involved. Furthermore, the drug does not function as a hapten; that is, drug-dependent IgG does not bind to platelets that have been washed after pretreatment with the implicated drug.[127] Limited evidence of a hapten mechanism of DITP has been suggested only for penicillin; that is, penicillin-dependent IgG binds to platelets that have been washed after pretreatment with penicillin. A proposed model suggests that drug-dependent antibodies are derived from a pool of naturally occurring antibodies with weak affinity for self antigens residing on platelet membrane glycoproteins; certain drugs are able to affect both antibody and antigen in such a way that their interaction is greatly enhanced, provided that B cells expressing such antibodies are induced to produce these.[127,133]

In a case of suspected DITP, as many drugs as possible should be discontinued. If further drug treatment is necessary, an immunologically non-cross-reactive substitute should be prescribed. Platelet transfusions should be given to patients with life-threatening bleeding or who are judged to be at high risk of bleeding (e.g., severe thrombocytopenia plus "wet purpura"). High-dose IVIG, 1 g/kg given over 6–8 hours for two consecutive days, may be of value, but can be ineffective if the relevant drug is not discontinued.[131] Corticosteroids are relatively ineffective in the management of this condition.[130]

Atypical drug-induced immune thrombocytopenia

Glycoprotein IIb/IIIa antagonist-induced thrombocytopenia

Thrombocytopenia is a relatively common side effect of the three approved GPIIb/IIIa antagonists—abciximab, tirofiban, and eptifibatide.[134] Often, the thrombocytopenia begins within hours of a first exposure; this is caused by naturally occurring antibodies.[135] In other patients, the thrombocytopenia begins about one week after initial—or abruptly upon repeat—drug administration; this clinical presentation reflects drug-induced antibody formation.[136]

Abciximab (ReoPro, Eli Lilly) is a humanized chimeric Fab fragment of a murine monoclonal antibody specific for an epitope on GPIIIa. It is used to prevent restenosis after coronary angioplasty. Approximately 0.5% of patients have moderate or severe thrombocytopenia within several hours of treatment with this drug.[134] Although approximately 20% of the normal population have antibodies that react against the papain cleavage site in abciximab, the remainder (1.6% overall) react against murine sequences incorporated into abciximab that confer specificity for GPIIb/IIIa. It is this latter group of antibodies that evinces pathogenicity. Perhaps surprisingly, given the degree of thrombocytopenia and use of a major platelet glycoprotein inhibitor, most patients do not have petechiae or bleeding[134] (although fatal bleeding episodes have been reported). Treatment with platelet transfusions and, perhaps, IVIG may benefit bleeding patients.

For approximately one-third of patients with apparent abciximab-associated thrombocytopenia, examination of the blood film shows platelet clumping. This finding suggests pseudothrombocytopenia

(ex vivo platelet clumping) caused by abciximab.[137] Such patients are not at risk for bleeding and do not need treatment.

Tirofiban and eptifibatide are synthetic compounds that mimic or contain the RGD (arg-gly-asp) peptide and bind tightly to the RGD recognition site in GPIIb/IIIa.[134] As with abciximab, the frequency of naturally occurring antibodies (approximately 1–2%) correlates roughly with their risk of inducing abrupt-onset thrombocytopenia upon first exposure. Delayed-onset thrombocytopenia beginning about one week after exposure has also been reported. For tirofiban, some drug-dependent antibodies produce platelet activation and increased risk of ischemic events.

Drug-induced autoimmune thrombocytopenia

Approximately 1–3% of patients treated with gold have thrombocytopenia that sometimes persists for weeks or months despite stopping the drug; thus, the disorder resembles chronic ITP.[138] It remains uncertain whether this is true drug-induced autoimmune thrombocytopenia or is caused by gold-dependent IgG antibodies that are slowly released from tissues. Procainamide, α-methyldopa, sulphonamide antibiotics, and interferons alfa and beta also may cause autoimmune thrombocytopenia.[127,139] In extremely rare instances, measles–mumps–rubella vaccination causes an acute ITP-like illness in which anti-GPIIb/IIIa IgG is formed.[140]

Drug-induced thrombotic microangiopathy

Drugs may cause a thrombotic microangiopathy (TMA) that closely resembles TTP or HUS.[141] Two general mechanisms for drug-induced TMA include immune (idiosyncratic, non-dose-dependent) and toxic (dose-dependent). Immune-mediated drug-induced TMA is caused by quinine,[142] with endothelium and other target cells affected by quinine-dependent antibodies. Paradoxically, immune-mediated TMA can even be caused by the antiplatelet agents ticlopidine[143] and clopidogrel.[144] Ticlopidine-induced TTP is estimated to occur in 1 in 2000–5000 patients who receive this drug after coronary stenting. The characteristic onset is between one and eight weeks after administration of the drug is started. Clopidogrel-induced TTP occurs in approximately 1 in 20,000 recipients, generally within the first two weeks of treatment. Autoantibodies to von Willebrand factor–cleaving metalloproteinase have been identified in these patients and may contribute to the pathogenesis.[145]

Other drugs that cause an illness that resembles HUS due to toxic effects include antineoplastic chemotherapy (e.g., gemcitabine, mitomycin C, cisplatin, and bleomycin) and immunosuppressive agents (e.g., cyclosporine and tacrolimus). Because some of the medical conditions leading to use of these drugs can be associated with microangiopathic blood film changes (neoplasia, organ rejection, graft-vs.-host disease, and vasculitis), causal relationships to the various drugs listed can be problematic.

The mortality of drug-induced TMA is high. Early recognition and discontinuation of the drug are essential. Response to plasma exchange has been observed. Many physicians would also give corticosteroids, although the efficacy remains unproven. Specific therapy for drug-induced HUS (dialysis, plasmapheresis, and corticosteroids) is individualized depending on the clinical situation. The prognosis is poor for drug-induced TTP in the setting of hematopoietic stem cell transplantation (HSCT).

Heparin-induced thrombocytopenia

Heparin-induced thrombocytopenia is a relatively common, IgG-mediated, adverse reaction to heparin that has a strong association with venous and arterial thrombosis.[2–4,146] Heparin-induced thrombocytopenia is a clinicopathologic syndrome; that is, the diagnosis is made most reliably on both clinical and serologic grounds.[147–149] Thus, HIT antibody formation without thrombocytopenia or other abnormalities is not HIT, whereas HIT antibody formation accompanied by an otherwise unexplained 50% or greater postoperative decrease in platelet count (even if the platelet count remains greater than 150,000/μL)[3] or complicated by necrotizing skin lesions at heparin injection sites[146] are examples of HIT syndrome. Indeed, the thrombocytopenia usually is much less severe in HIT[4] than in DITP[130] or GPIIb/IIIa antagonist-induced thrombocytopenia[134] (Figure 21.3). Another contrast from DITP is that even when severe thrombocytopenia occurs in HIT, petechiae and other types of bleeding typically are not observed.[146,150] Indeed, even the one characteristic hemorrhagic complication of HIT—bilateral adrenal hemorrhage—is caused by thrombosis (adrenal vein thrombosis leading to hemorrhagic necrosis).[146] HIT is an antibody-mediated disorder, and a minimum of five days is required for an immunizing exposure to heparin to generate sufficient levels of antibodies to cause thrombocytopenia.[146] Sometimes, onset of thrombocytopenia and thrombosis begins—or worsens—after all heparin has been stopped ("delayed-onset" or "autoimmune-like" HIT).[151–153] Some patients who have not previously been exposed to heparin will develop thrombocytopenia, thrombosis, and have detectable platelet-activating anti-PF4/heparin antibodies; such patients with "spontaneous HIT" have often had recent infection or surgery.[154]

The target antigen recognized by HIT antibodies consists of a multimolecular complex between PF4 (a platelet α-granule protein of the CXC family of chemokines) and heparin.[21] The HIT antibodies bind to one or more PF4 regions that have undergone conformational modification through binding to heparin. The formation of the antigen is somewhat nonspecific, because PF4 can be rendered antigenic by binding to certain other polyanions, such as pentosan polysulfate or polyvinylsulfonate.[22] At least 12–14 saccharide units are needed for heparin to form the antigen complex with PF4. This may explain why LMW heparin preparations are less immunogenic than unfractionated heparin and are less likely to

cause HIT.[2,3] Although LMW heparin sometimes causes HIT, it is likely that very small heparin preparations (e.g., fondaparinux, a synthetic anti-Factor Xa-binding pentasaccharide) or specially engineered heparins (e.g., highly sulfated heparin moieties bridged with nonsulfated spacer regions) only rarely cause HIT.[155,156]

Figure 21.4 illustrates several possible mechanisms to explain the intense thrombin generation that occurs in HIT.[157,158] These include the formation of procoagulant, platelet-derived microparticles[159] that result from cell signaling triggered by clustering of platelet FcγRIIa. Recent data suggest that in situ formation of IgG-PF4/heparin complexes on the platelet surface leads to platelet activation.[160] In vivo platelet activation is suggested by expression of P-selectin by circulating platelets in HIT as well as by increased levels of circulating microparticles. Tissue factor expression by endothelium[161] or monocytes[162] activated by HIT antibodies that recognize PF4 bound to surface glycosaminoglycans comprises other possible procoagulant events.

Marked in vivo thrombin generation helps explain several clinical features of HIT, including its association with venous and arterial thrombosis (hypercoagulable state), the occurrence of decompensated DIC with low fibrinogen levels and/or elevated prothrombin time in approximately 10–20% of patients, and the potential for deep vein thrombosis (DVT) to progress to venous limb gangrene, particularly in patients treated with warfarin.[158] This last syndrome results from impaired procoagulant–anticoagulant balance: Warfarin-induced protein C depletion leads to microvascular thrombosis caused by ongoing intense thrombin generation. Patients with warfarin-induced venous gangrene typically have a supratherapeutic international normalized ratio (INR), usually more than 3.5. The explanation is a concomitant severe decrease in factor VII that parallels the decrease in protein C. The importance of in vivo thrombin generation in HIT provides a rationale for consensus recommendations that an agent that reduces thrombin generation or directly inactivates thrombin be used for the management of this syndrome.[147,148,163]

The frequency of HIT varies among different patient populations. Medical patients appear to develop HIT less often than do surgical

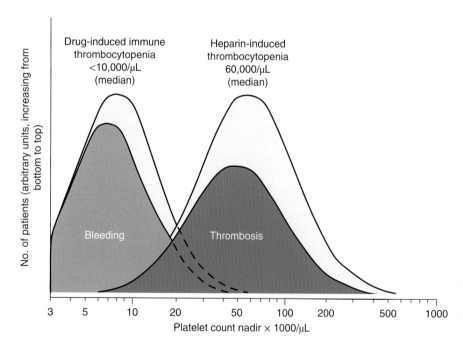

Figure 21.3 Platelet count nadirs ($\log_{10}$ scale) and clinical profile of classic drug-induced immune thrombocytopenic purpura (DITP) and heparin-induced thrombocytopenia (HIT). Classic DITP (e.g., caused by quinine, vancomycin, or glycoprotein IIb/IIIa antagonists, among many others) typically produces severe thrombocytopenia (platelet count nadir, ~10,000/μL) and associated mucocutaneous bleeding. In contrast, HIT typically results in mild to moderate thrombocytopenia (median platelet count nadir, ~60,000/μL) and associated venous or arterial thrombosis. Note that the relative heights of the two peaks are not drawn to scale; HIT is much more common than all other causes of DITP combined. Source: Warkentin (2007).[4] Reproduced with permission of Massachusetts Medical Society

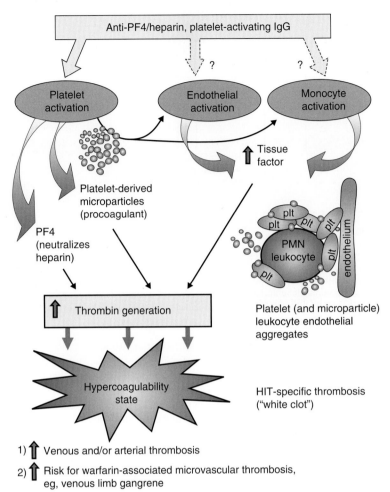

Figure 21.4 Pathogenesis of heparin-induced thrombocytopenia. Two explanations for thrombosis in HIT are presented. Activation of platelets by platelet factor 4 (PF4)–heparin IgG antibodies leads to formation of procoagulant, platelet-derived microparticles. Together with neutralization of heparin by PF4 released from activated platelets, there results a marked increase in thrombin generation. Such a "hypercoagulability state" is characterized by an increased risk of venous and arterial thrombosis, as well as predisposition to warfarin-associated microvascular thrombosis (e.g., venous limb gangrene). However, it is also possible that other unique pathogenetic mechanisms operative in HIT explain unusual thromboses, such as arterial "white clots." For example, HIT antibodies have been shown to activate endothelium and monocytes (leading to cell surface tissue factor expression), although this stimulation may be largely indirect through poorly defined mechanisms involving platelet activation and, possibly, formation of platelet-derived microparticles. Furthermore, aggregates of platelets and polymorphonuclear (PMN) leukocytes have been described in HIT. To what extent these cooperative interactions between platelets, microparticles, PMN leukocytes, monocytes, and endothelium lead to arterial or venous thrombotic events in HIT, either in large or small vessels, remains unclear. Source: Warkentin and Kelton (1996).[151] Reproduced with permission of American College of Physicians.

patients, and female gender is a minor risk factor for HIT.[164] The frequency of HIT can be as high as 5% when multiple risk factors are present (thromboprophylaxis with unfractionated heparin administered for two weeks to a female patient following major surgery), whereas the risk is very low or negligible in other settings (e.g., administration of LMW heparin during pregnancy).[2,3,165]

Iceberg model of HIT

Figure 21.5 illustrates the relation between clinical HIT and detectability of anti-PF4/heparin antibodies by either washed platelet activation assay or PF4-dependent EIA.[166] The key concept is that whereas both types of assay have high sensitivity for diagnosis of clinical HIT, the former assay has greater diagnostic specificity. It is estimated that substantial overdiagnosis (~50%) of HIT will result[167] if a positive EIA of any magnitude is considered diagnostic of HIT irrespective of the patient's clinical likelihood of HIT, as judged using a clinical scoring system (the 4Ts)[168] and the gold standard assay (platelet SRA).

Management of heparin-induced thrombocytopenia-associated thrombosis

Results of prospective and retrospective studies[3,4,150] indicate that approximately 50–75% of patients with HIT have new, progressive, or recurrent thrombosis. Thus, the need for an alternative anticoagulant is a common issue in the care of these patients.

Lepirudin is a direct thrombin inhibitor (DTI) derived from hirudin (leech anticoagulant protein) manufactured by means of recombinant technology. Although it is approved for treatment of HIT complicated by thrombosis, it was discontinued by the manufacturer in 2012.

Argatroban (Novastan, GlaxoSmithKline) is a small-molecule DTI approved in the United States for the management and prevention of HIT-associated thrombosis.[148,169] Features of argatroban include its short half-life (40–50 minutes) as well as its hepatic route of metabolism. No dose adjustments are needed for patients with moderate renal failure, although dose reduction is needed in the presence of hepatic insufficiency. Anticoagulant monitoring is usually performed using the aPTT; although simple, aPTT monitoring can result in systematic underdosing of argatroban in patients with baseline (pretreatment) elevation in aPTT, for example because of severe HIT-associated disseminated intravascular coagulation ("aPTT confounding").[170,171] Argatroban also prolongs the INR, which complicates the transition from argatroban to warfarin therapy. It is important to postpone introduction of warfarin until the thrombocytopenia has substantially recovered (platelet count at least 150,000/μL).[148]

Danaparoid sodium (Orgaran, Aspen Pharmacare) is a mixture of anticoagulant glycosaminoglycans with predominant anti–Factor Xa activity that decreases thrombin generation in patients with HIT.[172] A randomized trial showed a higher thrombosis resolution rate among patients treated with danaparoid and warfarin than among those treated with dextran and warfarin, especially for patients with severe thrombosis (92% vs. 33%; $p < 0.001$).[173] Although some HIT sera show in vitro cross-reactivity with

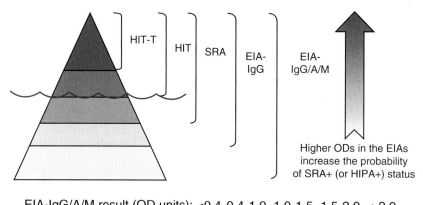

EIA-IgG/A/M result (OD units): <u><0.4</u> <u>0.4-1.0</u> <u>1.0-1.5</u> <u>1.5-2.0</u> <u>>2.0</u>
Probability of SRA+ status: ~0%   <5%   ~20%   ~50%   ~90%

Figure 21.5 "Iceberg model" of HIT. Clinical HIT, comprising HIT with (HIT-T) or without thrombosis (HIT), is represented by the portion of the iceberg above the waterline; the portion below the waterline represents subclinical anti-PF4/H seroconversion. Three types of assay are highly sensitive for the diagnosis of HIT: the washed platelet activation assay (e.g., the serotonin-release assay [SRA]), the IgG-specific PF4-dependent EIAs (EIA-IgG), and the polyspecific EIAs that detect anti-PF4/H antibodies of the three major immunoglobulin classes (EIA-IgG/A/M). In contrast, diagnostic specificity varies greatly among these assays, being the highest for the SRA and lowest for the EIA-IgG/A/M. The approximate probability of SRA+ status in relation to a given EIA result, expressed in OD units, was obtained from the literature. Modified with permission from Warkentin *et al.* (2000).[159]

danaparoid (i.e., enhanced platelet activation in the presence of danaparoid), this effect is usually weak; moreover, platelet-activating effects of many HIT sera are inhibited by danaparoid at therapeutic concentrations.[173] Because in vitro cross-reactivity is not predictive of adverse outcome,[173] danaparoid should be given without preceding in vitro testing for cross-reactivity.[148] The success rate is high (approximately 85–90%), as defined by platelet count recovery without new thrombosis.[148,173,174] The anticoagulant effect of danaparoid is monitored with a chromogenic anti-Factor Xa assay, which must be performed using a standard curve prepared with danaparoid. The target range is generally 0.5–0.8 anti–Factor Xa U/mL, although levels of 1.0 U/mL or higher are used by some in the treatment of patients with severe thrombosis. Recommended therapeutic dosing includes an initial intravenous bolus followed by continuous infusion (usually 200 U/hour with monitoring of anti–Factor Xa levels, if available). Danaparoid does not interfere with INR measurements. This is an advantage in the care of patients with venous thromboembolism in whom overlapping warfarin anticoagulation usually is performed after resolution of thrombocytopenia. Danaparoid is approved therapy for HIT in the European Union, Canada, and elsewhere, but it is neither approved for HIT management nor currently available in the United States.

Fondaparinux (Arixtra, GlaxoSmithKline) is a synthetic pentasaccharide anticoagulant modeled after the antithrombin-binding region of heparin; it has exclusive anti–Factor Xa activity. Although fondaparinux is associated with formation of anti-PF4/H antibodies at a frequency similar to that seen with LMW heparin, it is uncommon for fondaparinux to increase platelet activation by HIT antibodies (i.e., it has a low frequency of in vivo "cross-reactivity").[175] Although not approved to treat HIT, fondaparinux is frequently used "off-label" for treatment of HIT with or without thrombosis.[176] Indeed, observational studies of patients with well-characterized HIT suggest a high success rate (at least 90%) with fondaparinux.[156,177,178] Anticoagulant monitoring is not required, and thus the aforementioned problem of "aPTT confounding" seen with DTIs such as argatroban is not seen with fondaparinux.[166]

There are several important contraindications to therapy for acute HIT, including warfarin monotherapy and LMW heparin.[148,163] Warfarin therapy can lead to acute depletion of protein C, which can cause microvascular thrombosis in HIT and lead to venous limb gangrene.[158] However, once thrombocytopenia has resolved, it is reasonable to overlap warfarin cautiously with one of the agents that can reduce thrombin generation in HIT (danaparoid, fondaparinux, and argatroban). Use of LMW heparin is contraindicated because of a high chance of treatment failure (approximately 50% of patients have further thrombocytopenia or thrombosis).[148] Prophylactic platelet transfusion is relatively contraindicated because even patients with severe thrombocytopenia do not usually have evidence of hemostatic dysfunction, such as petechiae, and platelet transfusions theoretically may contribute to increase risk of thrombosis.[148] However, recent observational studies have questioned whether platelet transfusion in HIT is associated with thrombotic events.[179,180]

Management of isolated heparin-induced thrombocytopenia

Isolated HIT is defined as HIT that is recognized because of thrombocytopenia without evidence of HIT-associated thrombosis.[150] Unfortunately, simply stopping administration of heparin or substituting warfarin for heparin is inadequate treatment for these patients. In a large retrospective cohort study,[150] the risk of thrombosis among these patients was approximately 10% at 2 days, 40% at 7 days, and 53% at 30-day follow-up evaluations. Other investigators[181] with a similar approach subsequently found a 38% rate of thrombotic events despite stopping administration of heparin. The frequency of thrombosis surprisingly was not any lower in the subgroup of patients for whom heparin was stopped fairly promptly (<48 hours) after the onset of thrombocytopenia than it was among patients with later cessation of heparin (45 vs. 34%; $p = 0.26$).

For patients strongly suspected (or confirmed) to have isolated HIT, the authors discontinue heparin, start administration of an alternative rapidly acting anticoagulant, and screen for subclinical DVT by means of compression ultrasonography (approximately

50% of patients are shown to have DVT with this approach).[148] Whether or not thrombosis is found, a therapeutic dose of anti-coagulant is given to these patients. This is because prophylactic-dose anticoagulation appears to have a higher failure rate than does therapeutic-dose anticoagulation.[174] After platelet count recovery, the absence of venous thrombosis is confirmed before discharge. For patients found at initial or follow-up imaging to have venous thrombosis, overlapping warfarin anticoagulation is usually begun for longer term antithrombotic control, although recent reports have indicated subsequent outpatient treatment with one of the new oral anticoagulants (e.g., rivaroxaban or dabigatran).[182,183]

Reexposure to heparin in a patient with a history of heparin-induced thrombocytopenia

Patients who have circulating HIT antibodies can have an abrupt decrease in platelet count if heparin is administered. However, the risk of such abrupt-onset HIT on reexposure to heparin is restricted to the first few months after use of heparin. This is because HIT antibodies begin to decline after heparin is discontinued, and usually they are no longer detectable by the 3-month follow-up evaluation.[184] Under exceptional circumstances (e.g., need to per-form heart or vascular surgery), it is recommended to readminister heparin to a patient with previous HIT, provided that HIT anti-bodies are no longer detectable with a sensitive and reliable assay (e.g., SRA or PF4-dependent EIA).[148,184,185] Such patients often do not form HIT antibodies after the brief reexposure to heparin, and if they do, these antibodies are not formed before Day 5. Nevertheless, it seems prudent to limit the heparin reexposure to the operation itself and to use an alternative anticoagulant for perioperative anticoagulation.

Alloimmune thrombocytopenia

Alloantigens are genetically determined molecular variations of proteins or carbohydrates that can be recognized immunologically by some healthy persons. Exposure to alloantigens occurs during pregnancy, transfusion, or transplantation. If alloantibodies form against platelet alloantigens, alloimmune thrombocytopenia can result from platelet clearance mediated by the reticuloendothelial system. Five alloimmune thrombocytopenic disorders have been described (Table 21.3),[186] the most common being NAIT.

Alloantigens

More than 20 platelet alloantigens have been identified.[186–191] Table 21.4 classifies the platelet alloantigens by glycoprotein local-ization and gene frequency, the latter divided into public and private (or low frequency, arbitrarily less than 0.02). A database of geneti-cally confirmed alloantigens is maintained by the European Bio-informatics Institute with 28 antigens in the current list (http://www.ebi.ac.uk). More than one-half of the alloantigens that have

Table 21.3 Five alloimmune thrombocytopenic syndromes

Classical Alloimmune Thrombocytopenic Syndromes
• Neonatal alloimmune thrombocytopenia
• Posttransfusion purpura
Other Alloimmune Thrombocytopenic Syndromes
• Passive alloimmune thrombocytopenia
• Transplantation-associated alloimmune thrombocytopenia
• Platelet transfusion refractoriness

Source: Warkentin and Smith (1997).[186] Reproduced with permission of Elsevier.

been identified are located on one of the two glycoproteins that constitute the GPIIb/IIIa complex (platelet fibrinogen receptor). One of these alloantigens, HPA-1a (previously, Pl^{A1}), is located on GPIIIa. It is responsible for most alloimmune thrombocytopenia in populations of European ancestry, including almost all patients with severe alloimmune thrombocytopenia. The other major platelet glycoprotein complex (GPIb/IX, von Willebrand factor–binding complex) is rarely implicated in alloimmune thrombocytopenia. However, the GPIa/IIa complex (platelet collagen receptor), which bears the HPA-5a/5b (Br$^{a/b}$; Zav$^{a/b}$) alloantigen system, is a rela-tively common cause of moderately severe alloimmune thrombo-cytopenia.[192] The HPA-15a/15b (Gov$^{a/b}$) alloantigen system is expressed on CD109. It has been shown to be a relatively common cause of alloimmune thrombocytopenia that, like HPA-5a/5b, tends not to be severe.[193]

Immunogenetics and frequency of alloimmune thrombocytopenia

The HPA-1a alloantigen is far more immunogenic than its corre-sponding allele, HPA-1b. For example, consider the frequency of NAIT caused by either anti-HPA-1a or anti-HPA-1b alloantibodies in relation to the genotype frequency of HPA-1a (0.85) and HPA-1b (0.15). Thus, a homozygous HPA-1bb (Pl^{A1}-negative) female, representing approximately 2% (0.15 × 0.15) of the population, would have an 85% probability of being exposed to the HPA-1a alloantigen during pregnancy. In contrast, a homozygous HPA-1aa female, representing approximately 72% (0.85 × 0.85) of the popu-lation, would have a 15% probability of being exposed to the HPA-1b alloantigen during pregnancy. Thus, if both alloantigens were equally immunogenic, one would expect anti-HPA-1b to occur approximately six times more often than anti-HPA-1a: (0.72 × 0.15)/(0.02 × 0.85) = 6.4. However, the opposite is actually observed: anti-HPA-1a is far more common than anti-HPA-1b (Table 21.5).[192,194] In a study of 348 cases of suspected NAIT,[192] only one case caused by anti-HPA-1b was found, compared with 144 cases of proven or suspected NAIT secondary to anti-HPA-1a. Thus, the observed ratio of NAIT caused by anti-HPA-1a/anti-HPA-1b (1:144, or 0.007) is almost 1000 times less than predicted by the theoretical ratio (6.4).

Immunogenetics is a major factor determining alloimmunization against HPA-1a. There is a strong association between formation of anti-HPA-1a and *HLA-DRB3*0101* and *HLA-DQB1*0201* (odds ratio, 25 and 40, respectively).[195] In contrast, no HLA association exists for immunization against HPA-1b.[196] Thus, it appears that persons with certain HLA genotypes are much more likely to generate an alloimmune response when GPIIIa bears the leucine[33] substitution that determines the HPA-1a phenotype.

Overall, on the basis of the observed allelic frequencies, the expected theoretical ratio of NAIT for anti-HPA-5b, compared with anti-HPA-5a, should be approximately 8 (Table 21.5). A similar ratio (47:3, or 15.7) has been observed. However, although the expected and observed ratios are similar (contrasting the HPA-1a/1b system), a role for immunogenetics and alloimmunization exists also for the HPA-5a/5b system.[197]

Severity of alloimmune thrombocytopenia

In general, the severity of thrombocytopenia is greater for alloim-mune thrombocytopenia that involves the GPIIb/IIIa complex, compared with the GPIa/IIa complex (Table 21.6).[186,192,194,198] Because there are approximately 20 times more GPIIb/IIIa mole-cules compared with GPIa/IIa complexes (40,000 vs. 2000), this

Table 21.4 Platelet antigens classified according to glycoprotein location and gene frequency

Platelet-Specific Alloantigen (Alternative Nomenclature)	GP	Gene Frequency in Whites	NAIT	PTP	PAT	TAT	PTR
GPIIb/IIIa: Public (Gene Frequency > 0.02)							
HPA-1a (Pl^{A1}, Zw^a)	IIIa	0.85	++	++	+	+	(+)
HPA-1b (Pl^{A2}, Zw^b)	IIIa	0.15	+	+	—	—	(+)
HPA-3a (Bak^a, Lek^a)	IIb	0.61	+	+	—	—	(+)
HPA-3b (Bak^b)	IIb	0.39	?	+	—	—	(+)
HPA-4a (Pen^a, Yuk^b)	IIIa	>0.99	+	+	—	—	(+)
GPIIb/IIIa: Private/Low-Frequency (Gene Frequency < 0.02)							
HPA-4b (Pen^b, Yuk^a)	IIIa	<0.01	+	—	—	—	—
HPA-6b (Tu^a, Ca^a)	IIIa	0.003	+	—	—	—	—
HPA-7b (Mo^a)	IIIa	<0.01	++	—	—	—	—
HPA-7c (Hit^a)	IIIa	<0.01		-	-	-	-
HPA-8b (Sr^a)	IIIa	<0.003	+	—	—	—	—
HPA-9b (Max^a)	IIb	0.002	+	—	—	—	—
HPA-10b (La^a)	IIIa	<0.01	+	—	—	—	—
HPA-11b (Gro^a)	IIIa	<0.001	+	—	—	—	—
HPA-14b (Oe^a)	IIIa	<0.005	+	—	—	—	—
HPA-16b (Duv^a)	IIIa	<0.01	+	—	—	—	—
Va^a	IIb/IIIa	<0.002	+	—	—	—	—
GP Ia/IIa: Public							
HPA-5a (Br^b, Zav^b)	Ia	0.89	+	?	—		(+)
HPA-5b (Br^a, Zav^a, Hc^a)	Ia	0.11	++	+	+	+	(+)
GP Ia/IIa: Private							
HPA-13b (Sit^a)	Ia	0.0025	+	—	—	—	—
Swi^a	Ia	<0.002	+	—	—	—	—
GP Ib/IX: Public							
HPA-2a (Ko^b)	Ibα	0.89	—	—	—	—	?
HPA 2b (Ko^a, Sib^a)	Ibα	0.11	+	?	—	—	(+)
GP Ib/IX: private							
HPA-12b (Iy$_a$)	Ibβ	<0.01	+	—	—	—	—
CD109: public							
HPA-15a (Gov^b)	CD109	0.53	+	?	—	—	—
HPA-15b (Gov^a)	CD109	0.47	+	—	—	—	(+)
GP38							
Dy^a	38 kD	<0.01	+	—	—	—	—
Platelet Nonspecific Alloantigens							
ABO			—	—	—	—	++
HLA			—	—	—	—	++

GP, glycoprotein; NAIT, neonatal alloimmune thrombocytopenia; PTP, posttransfusion purpura; PAT, passive alloimmune thrombocytopenia; TAT, transplantation-associated alloimmune thrombocytopenia; PTR, platelet transfusion refractoriness.

++, relatively common; +, established but rare; —, not reported; (+), probable association, but definitive link inconclusive; ?, possible association but not established. Also see the current list of polymorphisms on the European Bioinformatics Institute website (http://www.ebi.ac.uk/ipd/hpa/table1.html).

Source: Warkentin and Smith (1997).[186] Reproduced with permission of Elsevier.

Table 21.5 Observed frequencies of neonatal alloimmune thrombocytopenia and posttransfusion purpura in relation to expected (theoretic) frequency of the HPA-1ab (Pl$^{A1/A2}$), HPA-5ab (Br$^{a/b}$), and HPA-3ab (Bak$^{a/b}$) alloantigen systems

Target Alloantigen	Percentage of Pregnancies at Theoretic Risk of NAIT[†] (Descending Order)	Observed Cases of NAIT[‡]	Observed Cases of PTP[§]
HPA-3b	14.5	0	0
HPA-1b	10.8	0	29
HPA-3a	9.3	1	9
HPA-5b	8.7	6	11
HPA-1a	1.9	44	105
HPA-5a	1.1	0	7

[†] Percentage of pregnancies at theoretic risk of NAIT for a given target alloantigen is determined as follows: $x(1 - x)^2 \times 100$, where x is the gene frequency of the target alloantigen. Note the lack of correlation between the theoretical and observed risk for NAIT.

[‡] Data are from Mueller-Eckhardt et al.[192] and represent serologic investigations using a defined protocol over an 18-month period ending June 30, 1988.

[§] For comparison, the serologic findings for cases of PTP are shown for which only one platelet alloantigen specificity was identified (from January 1990 to August 2006 at the Blood Center of Wisconsin).[194]

NAIT, neonatal alloimmune thrombocytopenia; PTP, post transfusion purpura.

Source: Warkentin and Smith (1997).[186] Reproduced with permission of Elsevier.

suggests that greater numbers of alloantibodies binding to the more numerous GPIIb/IIIa receptors result in greater platelet destruction. Similarily, thrombocytopenia is less severe when alloimmunization is to HPA-15 on CD109 (2000 receptors).[199]

Neonatal alloimmune thrombocytopenia

NAIT is a transient but potentially life-threatening thrombocytopenic disorder limited to fetal and neonatal life. It is caused by maternal IgG alloantibodies that cross the placenta and cause premature destruction of platelets bearing paternally derived platelet alloantigens (analogous to hemolytic disease of the fetus and newborn). NAIT occurs in approximately 1 to 1.5 per 1000 live births.[200]

Approximately 75% of cases in a population of European ancestry are caused by fetomaternal incompatibility for the platelet-specific alloantigen HPA-1a, and 20% by HPA-5b.[192] Other alloantigens implicated in NAIT, including private alloantigens identified in only one or a few families (e.g., HPA6b [Tu^a/Ca] and HPA-7b [Mo^a]), are shown in Table 21.4. In East Asian populations, anti-HPA-4b (Pen^b) is more common than anti-HPA-1a. Although HLA or ABO alloantibodies have been claimed to cause NAIT, in most

Table 21.6 Severity of thrombocytopenia by platelet count nadirs (×1000/µl) in relation to target glycoprotein for various alloimmune thrombocytopenic syndromes

Glycoprotein	NAIT	PTP	PAT	TAT
GPIIb/IIIa				
HPA-1a (IIIa)	17 (n = 81)	6 (n = 43)	8 (n = 9)	8 (n = 4)
HPA-1b (IIIa)	9 (n = 2)	5 (n = 4)	—	—
HPA-3ab (IIb)	10 (n = 5)	3 (n = 4)	—	—
HPA-4ab (IIIa)	13 (n = 7)	6 (n = 1)	—	—
Mean	16	6	8	8
GPIa/IIa				
HPA-5b	44 (n = 48)	26 (n = 1)	35 (n = 1)	43 (n = 1)
HPA-5a	35 (n = 5)	—	—	—
Mean	43	26	35	43

*Data from Warkentin and Smith[197] and Brunner-Bolliger et al.[198]
The data show that alloimmune thrombocytopenic syndromes that involve GPIIb/IIIa are more likely to cause severe thrombocytopenia than are those involving GPIa/IIa. The data are combined for alloimmune thrombocytopenic syndromes involving either allele of the HPA-3ab and HPA-4ab alloantigen systems, whereas the data are shown separately for the alleles of the HPA-1ab and HPA-5ab systems.
NAIT, neonatal alloimmune thrombocytopenia; PTP, posttransfusion purpura; PAT, passive alloimmune thrombocytopenia; TAT, transplantation-associated alloimmune thrombocytopenia.

cases, undetected platelet-specific alloantibodies or another diagnosis caused the thrombocytopenia.[201]

The typical clinical presentation of NAIT is isolated severe thrombocytopenia in an otherwise healthy neonate, especially if fetomaternal incompatibility involves an alloantigen on the GPIIb/IIIa complex (Table 21.6). Petechiae are found in 90%; gastrointestinal tract hemorrhage in 30%; and hemoptysis, hematuria, and retinal bleeding in fewer than 10% of patients. Isolated intraocular hemorrhage is rare.[202] Approximately 15% have intracranial hemorrhage.[192] The thrombocytopenia usually resolves within 1–3 weeks. Serious sequelae of fetal and neonatal intracranial bleeding include hydrocephalus, porencephalic cysts, and epilepsy. First-born offspring constitute approximately one-half of patients. This suggests that, unlike the situation for hemolytic disease of the fetus and newborn, sensitization can occur early during the first pregnancy.[192] Subsequently affected siblings usually have thrombocytopenia to a similar or greater extent, an observation used to emphasize preventive treatment in subsequent pregnancies. In the case of heterozygous fathers of affected children, an antigen risk assessment should be performed using fetal cells in future pregnancies.

Laboratory investigation of suspected NAIT involves three steps. Firstly, there must be a high index of suspicion: Isolated thrombocytopenia in an otherwise well infant should be assumed to indicate NAIT until proved otherwise. The second step is to type maternal and paternal platelets to determine whether they are incompatible for a major platelet alloantigen. Commonly, the mother lacks certain platelet alloantigens that often are associated with alloimmune thrombocytopenia; for example, maternal homozygous HPA-1bb (PlA1-negative) status confers risk of NAIT caused by anti-HPA-1a. The third step is to determine whether the mother has platelet alloantibodies in her serum. Sometimes, no alloantibodies can be detected in maternal serum despite severe neonatal thrombocytopenia. Indeed, for approximately one-fourth of HPA-1bb mothers with infants believed to have had NAIT, anti-HPA-1a cannot be detected.[192] The potential for low-incidence platelet-specific alloantigens to explain fetomaternal incompatibility means that maternal serum should be tested against paternal platelets whenever possible. Although maternal immunization to low-frequency antigens can explain some cases of NAIT,[203] evidence from large studies indicates that low-frequency antigens account for only a minority of NAIT cases unresolved following investigations for the common HPA antigens.[204]

Debate continues as to whether the titer of alloantibodies predicts severity of fetal thrombocytopenia. The maternal alloantibody is sometimes detectable for years following the birth of the child with NAIT. Patients with a history of NAIT must not donate blood because their plasma can trigger passive alloimmune thrombocytopenia. It is possible that these patients may also be at risk for transfusion reactions and PTP should they receive incompatible blood products in future.

Neonatal treatment

The optimal treatment of a neonate in whom NAIT is suspected because of severe thrombocytopenia is to increase the platelet count urgently to safe levels, even before serologic confirmation of the diagnosis. In some centers (e.g., National Blood Service in the United Kingdom), HPA-1bb and HPA-5bb platelets can be obtained upon request. These should be effective for more than 95% of patients.[205] When matched platelets are not available, washed and irradiated maternal platelets should be given to the neonate. These platelets are obtained by apheresis, and are washed to remove the maternal alloantibodies. Irradiation is performed to prevent graft-versus-host disease caused by maternal lymphocytes. In an emergency, immediate administration of whole blood–derived platelets obtained from random donors may be of benefit to a bleeding infant.[206,207]

Giving high-dose IVIG to the neonate increases the platelet count of approximately 65% of patients.[208] This treatment should be combined with maternally derived platelets. Corticosteroids are not recommended.

Prenatal management

About one-half of the time, NAIT is suspected during the prenatal period, usually because the mother previously bore an affected infant, although the diagnosis sometimes is suggested in utero when fetal ultrasonography shows cerebral hemorrhage, hydrocephalus, or hydrops fetalis. One tenet of management is that thrombocytopenia in a subsequently affected offspring is generally as severe as, or more severe than, a previously affected sibling. Neonatal alloimmune thrombocytopenia caused by anti-HPA-1a is more likely to cause fetal morbidity and mortality than that caused by anti-HPA-5b and usually requires more aggressive treatment. When the father is known to be heterozygous for the implicated alloantigen (a situation that occurs approximately 25% and 20% of the time for

NAIT involving the HPA-1a/1b and HPA-5a/5b systems, respectively), prenatal fetal typing is important, because it identifies the infant who is homozygous for the maternal antigen and is not at risk, obviating further treatment. For pregnancies at risk, general advice to the mother includes avoiding aspirin and nonsteroidal anti-inflammatory medications.

The general approaches that have been taken to manage pregnancies at high risk of severe NAIT[205,209] are regular administration of high-dose IVIG, repeated in-utero platelet transfusions, or both. The initial step is to obtain a fetal platelet count by means of percutaneous umbilical blood sampling, generally starting at 20–24 weeks of gestation. Because of the risk of fetal exsanguination, maternal platelets should be on hand for transfusion if the fetal platelet count is shown to be less than 50,000/μL.[209] IVIG is given at a dosage of 1 g/kg/week starting within one week of documentation of fetal thrombocytopenia. Fetal blood sampling is repeated 4–6 weeks later; if no response is seen, glucocorticoid salvage treatment (prednisone, 60 mg/day) is started.[209] However, not all fetuses respond to this approach.

Another approach, which has been used in certain European centers, involves regular intrauterine platelet transfusions by means of percutaneous umbilical blood sampling, including a short time before delivery. This approach has led to good outcomes in situations in which previous siblings were severely affected.[210] However, each fetal platelet transfusion carries risk of hemorrhage and death[211] that likely depends on the experience of the fetomaternal unit. There is no consensus on which approach is preferred.

Regardless of the antenatal management, there is consensus that delivery should be by means of elective cesarean section, performed as soon as fetal maturity is documented. The major reason for this mode of delivery is that it allows an organized, multidisciplinary approach to the peripartum care of the newborn. This approach includes urgent determination of the cord platelet count; provision of washed, irradiated maternal platelets (or antigen-negative platelets); and, usually, the use of high-dose IVIG (1 g/kg/day for two consecutive days) to treat severe neonatal thrombocytopenia.

Posttransfusion purpura

Posttransfusion purpura is a very rare disorder that typically manifests as severe thrombocytopenia and bleeding that begin 5–10 days after blood transfusion—usually red blood cells (RBCs)—in a patient previously sensitized by pregnancy or transfusion.[194] In 85–95% of cases, women are affected; the median age is 52 years. The observation that previous blood transfusions can be sensitizing explains why, on occasion, males develop PTP. Sometimes the presumably sensitizing transfusion occurs only a few weeks earlier; consequently, PTP can present after just a few weeks of intermittent transfusions.[194]

Although thrombocytopenia usually lasts 1–4 weeks, the duration can be as short as three days[212] to as long as four months or more. The platelet count usually is less than 10,000/μL (Table 21.6). Mucocutaneous bleeding (wet purpura, petechiae, epistaxis, gastrointestinal, and urinary tract) is common, and approximately 5–10% of patients die, usually because of intracranial hemorrhage. Because effective treatments are available (discussed further in this chapter), it is important to diagnose PTP promptly to minimize morbidity and mortality. Diagnostic confusion with HIT can result because both syndromes can present 5–10 days following surgery, and sometimes PF4/heparin antibodies are present because of concomitant exposure to heparin.[213–215]

Pathogenesis

Almost invariably, high-titer, platelet-specific alloantibodies are found in the patient's serum or plasma. Anti-HPA-1a is detected in 60% of cases, although several other platelet alloantigens have been implicated (HPA-1b, -2b, -3a, -3b, -4b, -5a, -5b, and -15b, and the isoantigen CD-36 [Nak[a]]).[194] More than one specificity is observed in approximately 15% of cases. As in NAIT, the HLA-DRB3∗0101 antigen is found in most HPA-1a-negative patients with PTP. As reported for NAIT, antibodies to HPA-3a may be difficult to detect in some patients with PTP.[216]

Although platelet-specific alloantibodies are causative, the pathogenesis of PTP remains obscure, and the quandary is that autologous platelets are destroyed. The currently favored hypothesis is that PTP represents a situation in which alloantibodies resulting from reexposure to an incompatible platelet alloantigen have autospecificity ("pseudospecificity"). Although the platelet-specific alloantibodies are detectable for years following an episode of PTP, the autoreactive (or panreactive) antibodies are detectable only during the acute (thrombocytopenic) phase of PTP. In keeping with this view, Taaning and Tønnesen[217] reported that panreactive GPIIb/IIIa antibodies are readily detected during, but not after, an episode of PTP. Kiefel et al.[218] reported that antibody with allospecificity for HPA-1a, but not for HPA-1b, could be eluted from both autologous and donor HPA-1bb platelets that had been sensitized with acute-phase serum from a PTP patient, suggesting that use of adsorption and elution methods may help distinguish a reactivity profile of PTP sera from that seen with NAIT. One report[219] suggests that such alloantibodies with autoreactivity could arise spontaneously, because a woman with HPA-1bb platelets and no history of blood transfusion developed "ITP" with antibodies showing specificity for HPA-1a. Cure of the thrombocytopenia by splenectomy was accompanied by disappearance of the HPA-1a-like antibodies. Studies by another group of investigators[220] indicate that two distinct types of antibodies—some with alloreactivity and others with autoreactivity—develop during the acute phase of PTP.

Treatment

High-dose IVIG is the treatment of choice for PTP. More than 90% of patients respond, attaining a platelet count greater than 100,000/μL in an average of four days.[221] Plasmapheresis may also be used. Although some physicians also give corticosteroids, this agent probably does not influence the course of disease and should be considered adjunctive rather than primary therapy. In rare instances, splenectomy may be considered for a patient refractory to IVIG, corticosteroids, and compatible platelet transfusion.[222]

Whole blood–derived (unselected) platelets—which are likely to bear the HPA-1a antigen—are usually destroyed quickly, and can cause febrile or even anaphylactoid reactions. Antigen-negative platelets are the preferred component; however, the efficacy of HPA-1a-negative platelet transfusions (for patients with PTP caused by anti-HPA-1a) is also uncertain. Some reports indicate lack of benefit.[223] RBC units should be washed[224] or filtered[223] before administration to remove platelet antigens. Only four patients are known to have developed recurrent PTP with subsequent transfusions.[194] Accordingly, for a patient who has recovered from PTP, future precautions usually include avoidance of incompatible blood components (only autologous, washed, or platelet alloantigen-compatible RBCs are given, or platelet alloantigen-compatible plasma or platelet products are given). However, PTP recurrence is uncommon even if incompatible blood is given, possibly because residual high-titer platelet alloantibodies immediately clear the alloantigens. Patients with a history of PTP must not donate blood because their plasma can trigger passive alloimmune thrombocytopenia (PAT).

Passive alloimmune thrombocytopenia

PAT is characterized by an abrupt onset of thrombocytopenia within a few hours after transfusion of a blood component, most often RBCs or plasma.[186] PAT is caused by the passive transfer of platelet-reactive alloantibodies in the component that rapidly clear the incompatible recipient platelets. In one study, glycoprotein-specific platelet-antibody studies confirmed that the alloantibodies were bound to the recipient's platelets in vivo.[225] Furthermore, although the alloantibody can be detected in the blood donor's plasma, it may not be detectable in the recipient's plasma. This finding suggests that almost 100% of the transfused alloantibody binds to target platelets soon after transfusion.[198,225] Although anti-HPA-1a is most commonly implicated, antibodies to HPA-3a and -5b have also been reported in this syndrome.[186,198,225] In general, the severity of bleeding parallels the degree of thrombocytopenia; thus, spontaneous mucocutaneous bleeding usually occurs only in patients with severe thrombocytopenia caused by anti-HPA-1a. The duration of thrombocytopenia is generally less than one week. It is important to investigate suspected passive alloimmune thrombocytopenia, because the risk that numerous recipients can develop this syndrome means that the implicated blood donor must not donate blood in the future.

Transplantation-associated alloimmune thrombocytopenia

In rare instances, alloimmune mechanisms explain thrombocytopenia that occurs in the setting of HSCT or transplantation of solid organs.

Hematopoietic transplantation

Panzer et al.[226] reported a 32-year-old man with chronic myeloid leukemia who had severe thrombocytopenia (platelet count, 17,000/μL) beginning 18 months after allogeneic marrow transplantation from his HLA-matched sister. High-dose IVIG produced transient increases in platelet count, and persisting remission followed splenectomy. Antibodies with HPA-1a specificity were eluted from the patient's platelets. This led to further investigations, which showed that a small number of residual, non-neoplastic lymphoid cells of host origin produced anti-HPA-1a against the HPA-1a-positive platelets formed by donor-derived megakaryocytes. Thus, host-versus-donor alloimmune thrombocytopenia resulted from mixed chimerism, in which residual host lymphoid cells derived from the HPA-1a-negative individual developed an alloimmune response against platelets derived from the engrafted HPA-1a-positive marrow.

A similar situation attributable to anti-HPA-5b after allogeneic marrow transplantation for chronic myeloid leukemia has been reported.[227] However, in this patient, HPA-5b alloantibodies were detectable both before and after transplantation, and the early posttransplantation thrombocytopenia gradually improved as elutable anti-HPA-5b became more difficult to detect.

Alloimmune thrombocytopenia may have played a role in two cases with transfusion-refractory thrombocytopenia associated with a rise in titer of anti-HPA-1a (compared with the pretransplantation

state) that developed following autologous HSCT performed for metastatic carcinoma of the breast. However, these reports are not conclusive, because it is difficult to distinguish a PTP-like illness (which implies destruction of engrafted autologous donor marrow–derived platelets) from typical posttransplantation platelet transfusion refractoriness.[228]

Solid-organ transplantation

In rare instances, immunocompetent lymphoid cells within a transplanted solid organ cause alloimmune thrombocytopenia in the recipient of the organ. A dramatic scenario was reported by West et al.[229] All three-organ recipients (two of a kidney and one of a liver) had severe thrombocytopenia and bleeding within 5–8 days after transplantation from a multiparous female organ donor with normal platelet counts. The two recipients of renal transplants had thrombocytopenia refractory to high-dose IVIG and platelet transfusions. One of these patients died, but the other recovered after splenectomy performed 50 days after transplantation. The liver transplant recipient had organ rejection, which was accompanied by correction of the platelet count when he received a new liver allograft. HPA-1a alloantibodies were detected in the organ donor and posttransplant (but not pretransplant) recipient serum. These cases illustrate that passenger immunocompetent lymphoid cells occasionally induce severe alloimmune thrombocytopenia when introduced into an alloincompatible recipient.

Platelet transfusion refractoriness

Platelet transfusion refractoriness, which is failure to achieve the expected platelet increment after two consecutive platelet transfusion episodes, has several explanations (Table 21.7). Refractoriness is primarily due to anti-MHC class I antibodies produced by the recipient following multiple transfusions. However, nonimmune, patient-dependent factors are probably the most important, which means that poor platelet count recoveries can persist even when HLA alloimmunization is prevented with leukocyte-reduced blood components[230] and when HLA- or ABO-compatible platelets are given. High-titer anti-HLA antibodies can cause transfusion refractoriness in a surgical setting, and their effect is not removed by hemodilution or absorption with multiple platelet transfusions.[231]

There is anecdotal evidence that platelet-specific alloantibodies sometimes cause refractoriness. However, prospective studies have shown that this is a relatively infrequent occurrence. For example, Novotny et al.[232] found that even when HLA alloantibody formation was largely prevented with blood components filtered before storage, platelet-specific alloantibodies at most explained 4 of 79 (5%) cases of refractoriness. There are occasions, however, on which

Table 21.7 General causes of platelet transfusion refractoriness, listed in probable descending order of frequency

- Nonimmune mechanisms
- Septicemia, fever, disseminated intravascular coagulation, amphotericin B therapy, hypersplenism, and fixed platelet count requirements in severe thrombocytopenia
- Platelet-nonspecific alloantibodies
  HLA alloantibodies
  ABO alloantibodies
- Platelet-specific alloantibodies
- Drug-dependent antibodies (e.g., vancomycin)
- Platelet-reactive antibodies

Source: Warkentin and Smith (1997).[186] Reproduced with permission of Elsevier.

the transfusion service needs to provide HLA- and platelet-specific antigen-compatible platelet products to manage some of these patients.[233] In one study, antibodies to HPA-15 were found in 2.3% of multiply transfused patients, and were implicated in failure to obtain an adequate platelet count in one patient.[234]

Summary

A variety of platelet–antibody assays have improved the ability of the clinician to make an accurate diagnosis of immune thrombocytopenia in many diverse clinical settings that can involve pathogenic autoantibodies, alloantibodies, and drug-dependent antibodies. The treatment decisions that arise depend upon several relevant factors, including the nature of the specific diagnosis, the expected prognosis, and the presence of clinically evident bleeding or thrombosis.

Acknowledgment

We thank Natalie Ramsay for her help organizing the reference list for this chapter.

Key references

A full reference list for this chapter is available at: http://www.wiley.com/go/simon/transfusion

2 Warkentin TE, Levine MN, Hirsh J, *et al.* Heparin-induced thrombocytopenia in patients treated with low-molecular weight heparin or unfractionated heparin. *N Engl J Med.* 1995 May 18;**332**(20):1330–5.

9 Kelton JG, Murphy WG, Lucarelli A, *et al.* A prospective comparison of four techniques for measuring platelet-associated IgG. *Br J Haematol* 1989;**71**(1): 97–105.

31 Harrington WJ, Minnich V, Hollingsworth JW, Moore CV. Demonstration of a thrombocytopenic factor in the blood of patients with thrombocytopenic purpura. 1951. *J Lab Clin Med* 1990;**115**(5): 636–45.

33 Olsson B, Andersson P-O, Jernås M, *et al.* T-cell-mediated cytotoxicity toward platelets in chronic idiopathic thrombocytopenic purpura. *Nat Med* 2003;**9**(9): 1123–4.

37 Rodeghiero F, Stasi R, Gernsheimer T, *et al.* Standardization of terminology, definitions and outcome criteria in immune thrombocytopenic purpura of adults and children: report from an international working group. *Blood* 2009;**113**(11): 2386–93.

39 Neunert C, Noroozi N, Norman G, *et al.* Severe bleeding events in adults and children with primary immune thrombocytopenia: a systematic review. *J Thromb Haemost* 2015 Mar;**13**(3):457–64.

128 Arnold DM, Kukaswadia S, Nazi I, *et al.* A systematic evaluation of laboratory testing for drug-induced immune thrombocytopenia. *J Thromb Haemost* 2013; **11**(1):169–76.

184 Warkentin TE, Kelton JG. Temporal aspects of heparin-induced thrombocytopenia. *N Engl J Med* 2001;**344**(17): 1286–92.

230 The Trial to Reduce Alloimmunization to Platelets Study Group. Leukocyte reduction and ultraviolet B irradiation of platelets to prevent alloimmunization and refractoriness to platelet transfusions. *N Engl J Med* 1997;**337**(26): 1861–9.

CHAPTER 22

Neutrophil production and kinetics: neutropenia and neutrophilia

Lawrence Rice[1] & Miho Teruya[2]

[1]Department of Hematology, Houston Methodist Hospital and Weill Cornell Medical College, Houston, TX, USA
[2]Department of Hematology/Oncology, Baylor College of Medicine, Houston, TX, USA

Introduction

Neutrophils are the body's primary defense against bacterial pathogens. Changes in neutrophil count are frequently encountered in clinical medicine in that increased or decreased neutrophil counts are common with infections and other disorders. Thus, neutrophil changes most often represent a response to an underlying disorder, and they may be the first clue to its presence. At other times, high or low neutrophil counts can be a crucial indicator of a primary hematologic disorder. Increased neutrophils are characteristic of chronic myeloid leukemia and other myeloproliferative disorders, and decreased neutrophils can signal aplastic anemia, myelodysplastic syndrome, acute leukemia, or other disorders perturbing bone marrow function. This chapter will not focus on primary hematologic disorders, but rather will deal with normal neutrophil kinetics and more common aberrations, and will briefly consider esoteric disorders that primarily affect myeloid cells.[1]

Normal neutrophil kinetics

Production in marrow

Neutrophils are produced in the bone marrow, one of the most highly proliferative organs of the body, and they are among the most numerous cells being produced. About 10^{11} are generated daily under baseline circumstances with a capacity to increase several-fold when stressed.[2] Production and differentiation of neutrophils and other granulocytes are termed *granulopoiesis* or *myelopoiesis* and occur in the extravascular space of the bone marrow. Mature cells are stored there until mobilized and released.

Granulopoiesis is regulated by hemopoietins, cytokines that have the ability to stimulate colony formation from progenitor cells in the bone marrow. These hematopoietins include stem cell factor, interleukin-3 (IL3), granulocyte macrophage colony-stimulating factor (GM-CSF), and granulocyte colony-stimulating factor (G-CSF). In addition to stimulating progenitor cells, GM-CSF and G-CSF directly enhance neutrophil function. The IL3 receptor expression is lost once neutrophils mature. G-CSF is the principle cytokine regulating granulopoiesis, because it stimulates granulopoiesis at

several stages of granulocytic differentiation.[3] G-CSF induces commitment of multipotential progenitor cells down the myeloid lineage and stimulates the proliferation of granulocytic precursors. It also reduces the average transit time through the granulocytic compartment, and stimulates release of neutrophil from the bone marrow. G-CSF markedly expands the marrow neutrophil mitotic pool and shortened the transit time of the postmitotic pool. Mean marrow neutrophil transit time of a postmitotic pool in healthy volunteer was 6.4 days, whereas with G-CSF it was 2.9 days.[4]

Once committed to the granulocyte line, precursor cells differentiate along morphologicially recognizable myeloblast, promyelocyte, myelocyte, metamyelocyte, band neutrophil, and then segmented neutrophil stages. The mitotic compartment includes the myeloblast, promyelocyte, and myelocyte stages, and the maturation compartment includes the metamyelocyte to segmented neutrophil stages, defining the postmitotic stage. Total transit time from myeloblast to mature neutrophil is about 10–12 days in vitro.[5] Differentiation of granulocytes is regulated mainly by myeloid transcription factors PU.1, members of the CCAT enhancer binding protein family, and GFI-1. In the promyelocyte stage, primary granules appear containing myeloperoxidase and serine proteases. In myelocytes, secondary and tertiary granules appear. Secondary granules in neutrophils contain lactoferrin and collagenase; tertiary granules contain gelatinase. Secretory vesicles appear near maturity. Other changes during the maturation process include increases in adherence capabilities, deformability, responsiveness to chemoattractants, and the development of the characteristic segmented nucleus.

Mobilization of neutrophils

Mature neutrophils remain in the bone marrow for 4–6 days as a storage pool, poised to respond to microbial invaders. Such cells are estimated to number 4.4×10^9/L under basal conditions, with 0.87×10^9 cells/kg released daily into the circulation. The half-life of neutrophils in the circulation is 6–8 hours, and they then survive longer in tissues, up to 1 or 2 days.[6] The number of neutrophils produced and released from the bone marrow greatly increases in response to stimuli such as corticosteroids, exercise, cytokines such as G-CSF, chemokines, or bacterial products.[4] Only

Rossi's Principles of Transfusion Medicine, Fifth Edition. Edited by Toby L. Simon, Jeffrey McCullough, Edward L. Snyder, Bjarte G. Solheim, and Ronald G. Strauss.

about 2% of neutrophils circulate in the bloodstream at any given time, with about 90% retained in the bone marrow. The retention, mobilization, and homing of neutrophils to and from the bone marrow are regulated by molecular mechanisms involving CXCR4 (C-X-C motif receptor 4), CXCR2 (C-X-C motif receptor 2), and CXCL12 (C-X-C motif ligand 12). CXCR4 is a cytokine receptor essential for the homing of stem cells and more mature neutrophils to the bone marrow. When deleted, it causes a shift in the pool of mature neutrophils from bone marrow to the circulation with no change in the lifespan of circulating neutrophils.[7] A mutation in CXCR4 underlies the WHIM syndrome (warts, hypogammaglobulinemia, infections, and myelokathexis) in which there is deficiency of neutrophils in the circulation with accumulation of mature neutrophils in the bone marrow. The CXCR4 antagonist plerixafor can treat leukopenia in patients with WHIM syndrome, and it is FDA-approved to mobilize stem cells to the peripheral blood for collection and transplantation. CXCR2 is a chemokine receptor expressed on myeloid cells that, when deleted, causes retention of mature neutrophils in the bone marrow. Thus, CXCR4 seems to be necessary to maintain neutrophils in the bone marrow, whereas CXCR2 is necessary for their release. CXCL12, also known as stromal cell–derived factor 1α, is a ligand of CXCR4. Bone marrow stromal cells, including vascular endothelial cells and osteoblasts, express CXCL12.[8] CXCL12 expression is high in the bone marrow during normal steady state, acting to retain neutrophils in the bone marrow by binding the CXCR4 on the neutrophils.

Inflammation causes an increase in cytokine levels, including G-CSF, in the bloodstream. This decreases CXCL12 expression in the bone marrow, allowing egress of neutrophils toward circulation where there is a higher level of cytokine. G-CSF treatment decreases CXCL12 mRNA in the bone marrow, decreasing the CXCL12 protein expression. G-CSF also decreases the surface expression of CXCR4 on neutrophils over 5–18 hours. With less CXCR4 receptors on neutrophils and less CXCL12 expression in the bone marrow, more neutrophils are mobilized into circulation. A study published in 1961 showed administration of prednisone increased the size of both the circulating and marginating pools, whereas exercise and administration of adrenaline caused a shift of cells from the marginating pool to the circulating pool.[9]

After release from the bone marrow, neutrophils become distributed between the circulating and marginal pools, freely exchangeable pools of approximately equal size.[10] Cells in the circulating pool are readily sampled by drawing blood. Cells in the marginal pool are loosely adherent to the endothelium of blood vessels, often slowly rolling along endothelial surfaces.[11,12] They are prepared for rapid egress into the tissues at times of need. Some studies suggest that the marginal pool is not diffusely distributed throughout the vasculature, but is largely localized to the liver, spleen, and lungs.[6]

Migration into tissues

Neutrophils must cross the vascular wall to get to sites of inflammation. P-selectin and E-selectin on endothelial cells capture neutrophils and mediate rolling by binding platelet sialoglycoprotein ligand-1 (PSGL1), L-selectin, and CD44. This activates neutrophil integrins that interact with intracellular adhesion molecules (ICAMs) on endothelial cells. Migration through the endothelium is mostly paracellular, but 20% is thought to be transcellular.[7] In paracellular migration, neutrophils loosen the tight junctions by presenting alternative binding partners, platelet-endothelial cell adhesion molecule-1 (PCAM1), JAM-A, and β_2 integrins (LFA1 and Mac1), facilitating the ability to squeeze through the tight

junctions. Integrin $\alpha3\beta1$ is upregulated and appears crucial to neutrophil diapedisis.[13] In transcellular migration, transmigratory cups expressing high ICAM-1 and VCAM-1 capture the crawling neutrophils, which allows neutrophils to go through the endothelial cells. Leukocyte adhesion deficiency, the lack of ligand on the neutrophil surface, causes an inability to deliver neutrophils to sites of infection. Patients with this disorder have neutrophilia and recurrent bacterial infections.

Once in the tissue, neutrophils initiate the generation of cytokines, including IL8 and Groα, allowing recruitment of more inflammatory cells. Neutrophils then can phagocytose microorganisms and undergo apoptosis. Neutrophils in tissues are more actively phagocytic than neutrophils in the circulation.

Neutrophil clearance

To prevent neutrophil-mediated tissue damage, a negative feedback mechanism controls the influx of neutrophils. Apoptotic neutrophils are phagocytosed by macrophages, which reduces proinflammatory chemokine production and stimulates the release of anti-inflammatory mediators such as prostaglandin E_2 and transforming growth factor-β_1.

Spleen, liver, and the bone marrow clear circulating neutrophils that have not migrated into the tissues. As mentioned in this chapter, neutrophils have a half-life of about 6–8 hours in circulation. The CXCR4–CXCL12 chemokine pathway mediates the homing of neutrophils to the bone marrow. Circulating neutrophils upregulate expression of CXCR4 and become "senescent" within a few hours of their release in blood. A chemotactic gradient of CXCL12 created by bone marrow stromal cells allows the neutrophils with upregulated CXCR4 to home back to the bone marrow. In the bone marrow, senescent neutrophils become apoptotic and are phagocytosed by macrophages.[8]

NETosis

Neutrophils may extend their antimicrobial activity beyond their lifespan by forming neutrophil extracellular traps (NETs). During this process called NETosis, the nuclear and granule membranes dissolve, decondense chromatin and extrude into the extracellular space along with proteins that were contained in the cytosol and granules.[14] One difference between NETosis and apoptosis is that neutrophils undergoing NETosis do not get cleared by anti-inflammatory cells. It is also a slow process, usually taking over 2–4 hours. NETs can trap pathogens within the sticky meshwork of chromatin and expose pathogens to highly concentrated antimicrobial enzymes trapped within the chromatin. It is unclear what stimuli drive NETosis versus apoptosis, but NETosis occurs with a variety of inflammatory mediator stimuli, including TNF, IL8, immune complexes, and pathogens. Although NETs may help clear infections, excessive formation of NETs has been linked to various neutrophil-mediated pathologies, including vasculitis and significant thrombosis and vascular injury.

Neutrophilia

Neutrophilia, defined as a neutrophil count greater than 7.5×10^9/μL, may be acute or chronic. In infants <1 month old, a normal neutrophil count can be much higher (up to 26×10^9/μL). Table 22.1 summarizes causes and mechanisms of acute and chronic neutrophilia. The great majority of neutrophilias are reactive phenomena, with only a small minority representing a primary hematologic disorder.[15]

Table 22.1 Causes and mechanisms of neutrophilia

	Cause	Mechanism
Acute	Stress Epinephrine	Decreased margination
	Exercise	Decreased margination Mobilization from marrow
	Infection Inflammation Stress	Mobilization from marrow
	Corticosteroids Granulocyte colony-stimulating factor	Mobilization from marrow Prolonged survival
	Rebound from neutropenia	Increased marrow proliferation
Chronic	Corticosteroids Leukocyte adhesion deficiency	Prolonged survival
	Myeloproliferative disorders	Prolonged survival Increased marrow proliferation
	Infection Inflammation	Increased marrow proliferation

Neutrophilic leukocytosis is commonly equated by primary care and emergency room physicians with the presence of infection and may even decide whether hospital admission is required. Although neutrophilic leukocytosis is the rule with most bacterial infections, it should be recognized that this is a very nonspecific finding that can occur with any cause of stress or inflammation. Mild chronic neutrophilia can even be due to smoking or obesity, where it has been associated with elevated leptin levels.

The evaluation of neutrophilic leukocytosis begins with a history focused on potential causative factors, particularly infections. This would include systemic symptoms such as fevers, night sweats, and weight loss. History is further directed to possible foci of infection such as cough, shortness of breath, dysuria, and abdominal symptoms. Medication history particularly assesses glucocorticoid use. Special attention on physical examination should be devoted to oropharyngeal and lung exam, lymph nodes, and spleen. As with any abnormality of blood cell counts, review of the peripheral blood smear may be crucial to expeditiously pinpoint the diagnosis. For one thing, eosinophils should be decreased with bacterial infection, and an increase in eosinophils and basophils points to a primary hematologic disorder (or possibly a parasitic, allergic, or vasculitic disorder).

Pseudoneutrophilia may occur during exercise or time of stress due to the effect of epinephrine, where marginal pool cells are shifted to the circulating pool. It occurs rapidly but is short-lived, and should no more than double or triple the neutrophil count. Neutrophil counts quickly return to normal, and immature neutrophils should not be seen.

Neutrophil left shift refers to circulation of relatively immature cells such as band neutrophils. When there is a marked left shift, myelocytes and metamyelocytes circulate. Left shift may occur with infection or with any cause of neutrophilia, so it is nonspecific.

Glucocorticoids cause neutrophilia by decreasing the uptake of neutrophils from the intravascular space. This is similar to the mechanism of neutrophilia in patients with leukocyte adhesion deficiency (CD11/CD18 deficiency). Drugs such as catecholamines and lithium are known to cause neutrophilia: The former affects neutrophil demargination, and lithium may cause G-CSF release.

Leukemoid reaction is a nonclonal neutrophilic leukocytosis with white blood cells (WBCs) >50,000/mm^3. It is generally seen with an uncontrolled inflammatory state, cancer, asplenia, infection, recovery from neutropenia with or without the administration of colony stimulation factor, or some combination of these causes. In chronic infection and/or inflammation, the neutrophil production rate can increase threefold. G-CSF or GM-CSF administration can further increase neutrophil production, with a maximum response requiring 7 to 10 days. There is commonly overshoot when patients recover from neutropenia, as with myelosuppressive chemotherapy.

Leukoerythroblastosis is defined as the presence of immature myeloid cells (myelocytes) and nucleated RBCs in the peripheral blood, often with giant platelets as well. Leukocytosis is usually present. Two-thirds of patients with this finding have an underlying infiltrative disorder of the bone marrow, such as fibrosis, granuloma, necrosis, or metastatic tumor. Leukoerythroblastosis may commonly accompany brisk hemolytic anemia. In about one-tenth of cases, it may result from hypoperfusion of the bone marrow (shock from sepsis, hemorrhage, anaphylaxis, and cardiac failure) causing disruption of the microenvironment. If an underlying cause of leukoerythroblastosis is not readily apparent, a bone marrow biopsy is warranted. In the past, a major differential diagnosis was with chronic myelogenous leukemia (CML), and helpful to differentiate these were the clinical situation, splenomegaly, eosinophilia, and basophilia. Leukocyte alkaline phosphatase, which is high with reactive neutrophilia but low with CML, was sometimes a final arbiter, but this test has become obsolete with the availability of molecular tests for the Philadelphia chromosome t(9,22) (and for Jak2 mutations).

Chronic neutrophilic leukemia is a very rare myeloproliferative disorder characterized by sustained neutrophilia and splenomegaly. It occurs mainly in the elderly and carries a poor prognosis. Bone marrow biopsy shows neutrophilic hyperplasia without excess of myeloblasts.[16]

Neutropenia

An absolute neutrophil count (ANC; the percentage of neutrophils multiplied by the WBC count) of less than 1500/m^2 is considered to be neutropenia. ANC of 1000–1500/m^2 is considered mild neutropenia, 500–1000/m^2 moderate, and below 500/m^2 severe neutropenia. The risk of infection is greatly increased with severe neutropenia, more so below 100/m^2. Agranulocytosis is a condition of acute severe neutropenia with markedly diminished or absent white cell precursors in the bone marrow.

Neutropenia is commonly encountered in clinical practice. Like neutrophilic leukocytosis, the clinical significance of neutropenia varies greatly, starting with conditions that have no impact on overall health and longevity and that may require no evaluation beyond history, physical exam, and review of the blood smear. On the opposite end of the spectrum are neutropenic disorders that can severely challenge health and survival. Acute neutropenia with fever can be a life-threatening medical emergency. Other than the ANC, critical factors in determining the importance of neutropenia and the evaluation warranted include whether it is an affected child or adult, if it can be determined to be congenital or acquired, if it is encountered in an inpatient or in the clinic, whether there have been infectious sequelae, what are the concordant symptoms and signs (e.g., arthritis, skin rash, and/or splenomegaly), and whether the patient is acutely ill. On physical exam, careful attention to lymph nodes, oropharynx, and spleen is warranted.

Review of the peripheral blood smear is invaluable in the initial approach to neutropenia. Helpful findings may include neutrophil inclusions such as Döhle bodies, and hypogranularity (pale cells due to a paucity of secondary granules). Normal neutrophils have 3.2 ± 0.15 lobes in their nucleus; 5% with five or more lobes indicates hypersegmentation. This is constantly found in megaloblastic processes, and may also occur with antimetabolite drugs and with uremia. Changes in other cell lines may bear on the cause of neutropenia, such as large granular lymphocytes (LGLs) or other atypical lymphoid cells. Reactive lymphs can be a clue to viral infection. Blast cells may indicate leukemia.

Beyond the blood smear, tests commonly helpful in the evaluation of neutropenia include rheumatoid factor and antinuclear antibodies when there is reason to suspect an autoimmune problem. A direct Coombs test may help confirm an autoimmune diathesis. Flow cytometry may clarify the etiology of neutropenia in a number of disorders, particularly when there are reasons (such as blood smear findings or splenomegaly) to suspect LGL syndrome/T-NK leukemia or other clonal proliferations. Bone marrow exam is often performed and may be valuable, particularly in more severe neutropenic disorders, although it should be realized that morphologic findings may be nonspecific and compatible with differing pathogenic mechanisms. As an example, a hypercellular marrow with "maturation arrest" could be compatible with a stem cell maturation defect, antibodies to late precursors, early release in times of stress, or recovery from a toxic insult.

Conditions commonly resulting in neutropenia are listed in Table 22.2, and they are briefly discussed below.

Congenital neutropenias

The molecular mechanisms underlying severe congenital neutropenias (SCNs) have been greatly clarified in recent years, and the prognosis for these patients has improved due to advances in supportive care, the use of granulocyte growth factors, and allogeneic bone marrow transplantation.[17] These patients have suffered from recurrent severe infections starting in infancy, and oral ulcerations and painful gingivitis by two years of age. As enumerated in Table 22.2, there are many defined conditions causing such neutropenia. Notable congenital neutropenias include:

- SCN1 is an autosomal dominant disorder caused by mutation in the neutrophil elastase gene on the ELANE gene on chromosome 19p13.3.
- The same ELANE gene is mutated in cyclic neutropenia.[18]
- Kostmann syndrome is an autosomal recessive disorder linked to mutations in HAX1. It is associated with mental retardation.
- Myelokathexis is caused by a mutation in the CXCR4 chemokine receptor, part of the WHIM syndrome mentioned in this chapter. It consists of severe neutropenia in the setting of hypercellular marrow containing hypersegmented neutrophils.
- Shwachman–Bodin–Diamond syndrome (SBDS) is an autosomal recessive disorder usually with mutations in the SBDS gene, consisting of exocrine pancreatic insufficiency, bone marrow dysfunction, skeletal abnormalities, and short stature. There is a variable degree of neutropenia.
- Chediak–Higashi syndrome patients have cutaneous and ocular hypopigmentation, and mild neutropenia with large abnormal granules in the neutrophils. Neutrophil dysfunction leads to frequent pyogenic infections.
- Cyclic neutropenia is characterized by recurrent fevers, mouth ulcers, with infections due to regularly recurring severe neutropenia. G-CSF can be used to treat cyclic neutropenia.
- MonoMAC syndrome is an autosomal dominant disorder due to mutations in the GATA2 transcription factor. It may be associated with mild chronic neutropenia and persistent severe monocytopenia, leading to opportunistic infections and a high risk of eventual leukemic progression.

Table 22.2 Some conditions causing neutropenia

Hereditary Neutropenia
Severe congenital neutropenia (SCN)
- SCN1: ELANE gene mutation
- SCN2: GFI1 gene mutation
- SCN3 (Kostmann disease): HAX1 mutation
- SCN 4: G6PC3 gene mutation
- SCN 5: VPS45 gene mutation
- X-linked SCN: WASP gene mutation
Shwachman–Bodin–Diamond syndrome
Cyclic neutropenia
Benign ethnic neutropenia
Myelokathexis (WHIM syndrome)
Chediak–Higashi syndrome
P14 deficiency syndrome
Glycogen storage disease type 1 (von Gierke)
Barth syndrome
Cohen syndrome
Charcot–Marie–Tooth disease
Hermanski–Pudlak syndrome
Gricelli syndrome
GATA2 deficiency (MonoMAC syndrome)

Infection
Overwhelming bacterial sepsis (typhoid, ehrlichiosis, brucellosis, rickettsia)
Measles, rubella, varicella
HIV, EBV, CMV, hepatitis A, hepatitis B
Other viruses (granulomatous marrow infection [e.g., histoplamosis and TB])

Drugs
(See Table 22.3.)

Autoimmune Conditions
Systemic lupus erythematosus
Evan's syndrome (ITP and AIHA)
Felty syndrome

Malignancies
Acute leukemias
LGL leukemia
Hairy cell leukemia
Myelodysplastic syndromes

Dietary
Global caloric malnutrition
Copper deficiency
Alcoholism
Vitamin B_{12} and folate deficiency

Other Conditions
Hypersplenism
Hyperthyroidism

- The p14 deficiency syndrome, lacking an adaptor protein involved in mitogen-activated protein kinase signaling, is characterized by severe neutropenia, partial albinism, short stature, and recurrent infections.

Neutropenias in adults

In the hospital, the most common causes of neutropenia are medication reactions or sepsis, and these two are especially suspect if the neutropenia has its initial onset during hospitalization. Although almost any drug can rarely cause neutropenia, this side effect is highly associated with certain medications and classes. It is important to consider whether there is agranulocytosis (sudden- and severe-onset neutropenia) versus a gradual decline in ANC, as the former is characteristic of few drugs. Table 22.3 reviews more common drug associations.[19]

Sepsis characteristically leads to increased neutrophil count, but neutropenia may also be seen, particularly in those with compromised marrow reserve such as those who have underlying

Table 22.3 Drugs commonly causing neutropenia and/or agranulocytosis

Antimicrobials	Vancomycin TMP-SMX Dapsone	Cephalosporins Semisynthetic penicillins Ganciclovir	Chloramphenicol Flucytosine
Cardiovascular	Ticlopidine	Captopril	Procainamide
Anti-epileptics	Carbamazepine Valproate	Phenytoin	Ethosuximide
Psychotropic agents	Clozapine	Phenothiazines	
Antithyroid drugs	Methimazole	Propylthiouracil	
Anti-inflammatory agents	Sulfasalazine Phenylbutazone	Diclofenac	Indomethacin
Others	Levamisole	Deferiprone	Rituximab

hematologic disorders, chemotherapy, or malnutrition. Neutropenia in this context augurs a high mortality rate. Other infections that may be characterized by neutropenia include bacteria such as typhoid fever and brucellosis, and nonbacterial infections such as anaplasmosis, ehrlichiosis, and rickettsia. Neutropenia or pancytopenia is seen with granulomatous marrow involvement by histoplasmosis or mycobacteria. Transient neutropenia is very common with viral infection, so intensive evaluation of a low neutrophil count should ordinarily be delayed in those where an acute viral etiology seems likely. Viruses with a particular predilection to cause this include HIV, hepatitis A, hepatitis B, Epstein–Barr virus (EBV), cytomegalovirus (CMV), measles, rubella, and varicella.

Neutropenia is an expected and dose-limiting side effect of many cytotoxic and/or immunosuppressive drugs, such as those used for cancer chemotherapy or to prevent transplanted organ rejection. Prophylaxis with growth factors and/or antibiotics is recommended if the risk of developing febrile neutropenia is greater than 20%, where the risk is calculated from age, extent of primary cancer, comorbidities, and the known myelotoxicity of the chemotherapy regimen (according to the National Comprehensive Cancer Network [NCCN], Multinational Association of Supportive Care of Cancer [MASCC] score, and Infectious Diseases Society of America [IDSA] risk assessment). G-CSF should begin 24–72 hours after the completion of myelotoxic chemotherapy.

Other medications may cause neutropenia with variable frequency, severity, and mechanisms.[20] Neutropenia is sometimes sudden and severe. Dose- and duration-related myelosuppression may be seen with chlorpromazine, ticlopidine, and valganciclovir. Chloramphenicol can cause neutropenia by both dose-related and idiosyncratic mechanisms. Clozapine has been shown to induce apoptosis of myeloid precursors. Immune mechanisms have been implicated in neutropenia from antithyroid drugs and aminopyrine. An epidemic of severe neutropenia was appreciated in 2007 in intravenous cocaine abusers and was linked to levamisole adulteration. Also increasingly recognized in recent years is neutropenia related to rituximab. This is unusual for its late onset, typically three months after the last dose, and may be related to imbalanced recovery of B-lymphocyte subsets with resultant deficiency of stromal-derived factor 1.

Immune mechanisms may be implicated relatively commonly in neutropenia, sometimes in the context of autoimmune disorders such as systemic lupus erythematosus (SLE) or rheumatoid arthritis (RA). Immune neutropenia can vary from mild to severe. Antineutrophil antibodies are classically imputed, but autoreactive cytotoxic lymphocytes can also play a role. Bone marrow examination most often shows normal cellularity to hypercellularity with maturation arrest, but this picture is nonspecific (see above). Available antineutrophil antibody tests are not clinically reliable, creating substantial challenges to validate the diagnosis. Sometimes,

empiric immunosuppressive therapy (e.g., methotrexate) may enlighten in retrospect as to whether immune factors were at play. Felty syndrome is a complication of RA with splenomegaly and neutropenia that may be severe, and it is traditionally blamed on antineutrophil antibodies. This occurs in 1% of patients with RA and may be complicated by severe infections. There may be a continuum of mechanisms underlying Felty syndrome, including large granular lymphocyte proliferation (see below). The mainstay of treatment for Felty syndrome is methotrexate, cyclosporine, or cyclophosphamide. G-CSF engenders a risk of exacerbating underlying inflammatory problems, and it should be used cautiously and at the lowest effective dose.

Splenomegaly can be a cause of leukopenia, anemia, thrombocytopenia, or any combination of these. The degree of cytopenia is generally proportional to the degree of splenic enlargement. Additional factors such as drugs or autoimmune diseases should be considered if neutropenia is out of proportion to the splenomegaly and reduction in other cell lines.

T-cell LGL leukemia and other natural killer (NK) cell proliferations should be considered in adults with neutropenia. NK cell proliferations can vary from nonclonal reactive processes, to indolent clonal proliferations, to very aggressive neoplasms. Reactive LGLs can be idiopathic, or they can be seen in autoimmune disorders and postorgan transplant or during therapy with dasatinib, a tyrosine kinase inhibitor.[21] Similarly, clonal T-NK-cell/LGL leukemia can be associated with rheumatoid arthritis or can be idiopathic. Felty syndrome can be associated with increases in T-NK cells. Peripheral blood smear shows large lymphocytes with mature chromatin, excess cytoplasm, and usually prominent cytoplasmic granules; and flow cytometry shows CD3 and CD57 positive cells with T-cell receptor gene rearrangement in the common form of LGL leukemia. This frequently responds to methotrexate, cyclosporine, or cyclophosphamide therapy. Pure NK cell proliferations are generally CD3 negative and CD56 positive.

Benign ethnic neutropenia is mild to moderate. African Americans have lower average ANC than Caucasians, with 5% falling in the neutropenic range, but they do not experience recurrent infections. Other populations in which ethnic neutropenia may be seen include some in the Middle East and Asia.

Chronic idiopathic neutropenia is the default diagnosis in adults who have acquired the problem but do not meet diagnostic criteria for established etiologies.[18] Most often, this runs a benign course. Some patients require growth factor support at times of illness.

Beyond specifically addressing the cause of neutropenia (e.g., methotrexate for RA or withdrawing suspicious medications), G-CSF has facilitated successful therapy for many neutropenic disorders, hastening recovery in acute situations and improving health and longevity in patients with chronic afflictions. This does not come without a price. After 10 years of G-CSF therapy, the risk of death from MDS and AML was reported as 21% in patients with SCN.[22] This is unfortunately much higher than the previously reported data of 13% after eight years of G-CSF therapy from the Severe Chronic Neutropenia International Registry in 2003.[23] The discrepancy may be due to the difference in sizes of the cohorts of patients, but the study by Rosenberg *et al.* did observe a statistically significant association between the dose of G-CSF and the risk of MDS and AML in SCN. Prompt empiric initiation of appropriate antibiotics can also be life-saving in the situation of fever with severe neutropenia. As stressed in this chapter, changes in neutrophil counts are most often reactive phenomena, but occasionally they are manifestations of a primary hematologic process. Accelerated progress continues in our ability to understand and address these disorders.

Key references

A full reference list for this chapter is available at: http://www.wiley.com/go/simon/transfusion

1 Price TH. Neutrophil production and kinetics: neutropenia and neutrophilia. In: Simon TL, Snyder EL, Stowell CP, *et al.*, Eds., *Rossi's principles of transfusion medicine*. 4th ed. Wiley-Blackwell, 2009: 211–18.

2 Day RB, Link DC. Regulation of neutrophil trafficking from the bone marrow. *Cell Mol Life Sci* 2012; **69**: 1415–23.

4 Price TH, Chatta GS, Dale DC. Effect of recombinant granulocyte colony-stimulating factor on neutrophil kinetics in normal young and elderly humans. *Blood* 1996; **88** (1): 335–40.

7 Borregaard N., Neutrophils, from marrow to microbes. *Immunity* 2010; **33**: 657–70.

8 Strydom N, Rankin SM. Regulation of circulating neutrophil numbers under homeostasis and in disease. *J Innate Immun* 2013; **5**: 304–14.

15 Rice L, Jung M. Neutrophilic leukocytosis, neutropenia, monocytosis, and monocytopenia. In: Hoffman R, Benz EJ, Silberstein LE, *et al.*, Eds., *Hematology: basic principles and practice*. 6th ed. Philadelphia: Churchill Livingstone, 2013: 640–6.

18 Germeshausen M, Deerberg S, Peter Y, *et al.* The spectrum of ELANE mutations and their implications in severe congenital and cyclic neutropenia. *Hum Mutat* 2013; **34**; 905–14.

19 Gibson C, Berliner N. How we evaluate and treat neutropenia in adults. *Blood* 2014; **124** (8): 1251–8.

22 Rosenberg PS, Alter BP, Bolyard AA, *et al.* The incidence of leukemia and mortality from sepsis in patients with severe congenital neutropenia receiving long-term G-CSF therapy. *Blood* 2006; **107** (12): 4628–35.

23 Dale DC, Cottle TE, Fier CJ, *et al.* Severe chronic neutropenia: treatment and follow-up of patients in the Severe Chronic Neutropenia International Registry. *Am J Hematol* 2003; **72**: 82–93.

CHAPTER 23

Neutrophil collection and transfusion

Ronald G. Strauss

LifeSource/Institute for Transfusion Medicine, Chicago, IL, USA

Life-threatening infections with bacteria, yeast, and fungus continue to be a consequence of severe neutropenia (fewer than 500/µL blood neutrophils) and disorders of neutrophil (PMN) dysfunction. The most frequent situation is neutropenic fever and infection with yeast or fungus during either hematopoietic progenitor cell (HPC) transplantation or intense chemotherapy for hematologic malignant disease. Neutropenic infections cause considerable morbidity, occasionally are fatal, and add considerable cost to the treatment of these patients.

Previous attempts to prevent infection in severely neutropenic patients by transfusing PMN concentrates – commonly called prophylactic granulocyte transfusions (GTXs)—achieved only questionable success. Although rates of certain infections were significantly reduced with prophylactic GTX compared to antibiotics only, many adverse effects including pulmonary infiltrates and cytomegalovirus infection were reported, and GTXs were expensive. Similarly, use of therapeutic GTX to resolve existing infections has not gained broad acceptance, despite many reports documenting benefit.[1,2] This lack of enthusiasm for GTX can be explained by the continuing development of effective antimicrobial drugs to prevent and manage infection, by the availability of recombinant hematopoietic growth factors to quicken PMN recovery, by preference for peripheral blood HPC over marrow-derived HPC transplantation to hasten patient recovery from myelotoxic therapy and to shorten the period of severe neutropenia, and by lack of familiarity/experience by most physicians with the markedly improved PMN concentrates—containing higher numbers of neutrophils/granulocytes due to granulocyte colony-stimulating factor (G-CSF) + dexamethasone donor stimulation—now available for transfusion.

Historically, PMN concentrates, collected for transfusion from unstimulated donors or those stimulated only with corticosteroids, contained woefully inadequate numbers of PMNs. Currently, much larger numbers of PMNs can be collected from healthy donors by means of G-CSF plus corticosteroid marrow stimulation followed by large-volume leukapheresis.[2] This chapter discusses the current technology of PMN collection and provides a critical assessment of the potential for use of therapeutic and prophylactic GTX.

Collection of neutrophils for transfusion

Donor marrow stimulation

A limitation of GTX has been the inability to transfuse satisfactory numbers of adequately functioning neutrophils. To ensure adequate numbers and quality of PMNs for transfusion, PMNs must be collected from optimally stimulated donors by automated leukapheresis using an erythrocyte-sedimenting agent, such as hydroxyethyl starch (HES).[2] Under the stress of a severe bacterial infection, the marrow of an otherwise healthy adult will produce between 10^{11} and 10^{12} PMNs in 24 hours. Granulocyte (PMN) concentrates collected from healthy donors who are not stimulated with corticosteroids or G-CSF will contain between 0.2 and 0.8×10^{10} PMNs—about 1% of a healthy marrow's output. Hence, donor stimulation to increase the blood PMN count is mandatory to achieve even a hope of a reasonable PMN dose per GTX.

Donor stimulation with properly timed corticosteroids ($\geq$4 hours before leukapheresis) will increase the yield to about 2×10^{10} PMNs.[3] Stimulation with G-CSF, alone or in combination with corticosteroids, will produce higher but variable PMN yields that vary with G-CSF dose and schedule of administration. Currently, PMN donors are optimally stimulated using 300–480 µg G-CSF given subcutaneously, plus 8 mg dexamethasone taken orally, approximately 12 hours before beginning leukapheresis.[4] Yields of 4 to 8×10^{10} PMNs are achieved regularly, and post-transfusion blood PMN counts in the patient frequently increase to 1000–3000/µL, with PMNs detected in the bloodstream for several hours after GTX (often >24 hours).

Adverse effects following G-CSF and dexamethasone are frequent. Most donors experience minor pain in muscle, bone, or head that is readily relieved with acetaminophen or ibuprofen.[5] Donors given G-CSF for PMN collection have no long-term adverse effects, and it is unusual that they refuse to donate again.[6] A recent report suggested that adrenal corticosteroids might cause posterior subcapsular cataracts in PMN donors.[7] Although this report appeared not to be confirmed by statistically significant findings in a study of larger numbers of PMN donors,[8] many trends—all suggesting possible adverse effects of corticosteroids—were worrisome in

Rossi's Principles of Transfusion Medicine, Fifth Edition. Edited by Toby L. Simon, Jeffrey McCullough, Edward L. Snyder, Bjarte G. Solheim, and Ronald G. Strauss.
© 2016 John Wiley & Sons, Ltd. Published 2016 by John Wiley & Sons, Ltd.

the results.[9] Thus, questions of potential donor risk still remain, and it seems logical to include this cautionary information in donor consent forms or to stimulate PMN donors using G-CSF without corticosteroids—not the author's choice because PMN yields will be decreased by about 25%—until the issue is resolved.

Although they are known to alter PMN function, G-CSF and corticosteroids such as dexamethasone have relatively minor effects at the doses administered to donors for PMN collection.[5] The functional properties of PMNs collected from donors stimulated with G-CSF do not deviate greatly from those of normal PMNs and cause no unusual reactions in recipients when transfused. After transfusion, PMNs from G-CSF-stimulated donors have long intravascular survival times explained by multiple factors, including shift of young PMNs from the storage compartment of donor marrow into the bloodstream for collection, an alteration in expression of several membrane proteins on donor PMNs associated with neutrophil adherence to vascular endothelium and egress from the circulation into the tissues, and possibly by specific anti-apoptotic effects of G-CSF on PMNs.[5] Although it has been suggested that G-CSF-mobilized PMNs might exhibit decreased migration into tissue sites because of their prolonged intravascular circulation, studies with transfused PMNs indicate that they migrate satisfactorily into areas of inflammation and infection.[6,10]

The ability to collect and store PMNs differs when donors are stimulated only once during a course of GTX therapy compared with when they serve as a dedicated donor for the recipient and are stimulated repeatedly on a daily or every-other-day schedule for GTX. PMNs collected after several days of G-CSF stimulation are qualitatively different from PMNs collected after a single dose of G-CSF.[5] They are younger, exhibit increased metabolic activity and different surface markers, may possess enhanced antifungal properties, and do not have the same separation characteristics during centrifugation leukapheresis. Because the functional properties and possibly the efficacy and toxicity of PMNs may differ when collected under conditions of single versus repeated G-CSF and corticosteroid stimulation, additional studies are needed to define optimal donor stimulation and GTX therapy.

Hydroxyethyl starch

Use of an erythrocyte-sedimenting agent, such as HES, during centrifugation leukapheresis is mandatory. The optimal formulation of HES to be used for PMN collection is controversial. In an uncontrolled multicenter trial, pentastarch appeared to be an efficacious and safe erythrocyte-sedimenting agent for use during centrifugation leukapheresis because PMN concentrates, prepared by centrifugation leukapheresis techniques with pentastarch in four cytapheresis centers, were found to contain quantities of PMNs comparable with concentrates prepared previously with hetastarch at participating centers.[3] Later, the efficacy of pentastarch for PMN collection was challenged by a study[11] in which steroid-stimulated donors underwent paired PMN collections, separated by two weeks to seven months, during which they received 500 mL of either 10% pentastarch or 6% hetastarch during centrifugation leukapheresis (7 L donor blood processed at a 1:13 starch–donor blood ratio). In 92% of the donors, hetastarch procedures were more efficient. The PMN yield per collection was $2.3 \pm 0.7 \times 10^{10}$ with hetastarch versus $1.4 \pm 0.076 \times 10^{10}$ with pentastarch.

It is unclear why pentastarch performed so poorly in the later study[11] compared with its performance in the initial multicenter trial.[3] Despite the desirable safety profile of pentastarch (i.e., more rapidly eliminated from the bloodstream than is hetastarch to avoid

the problem, with repeated leukapheresis, in which hetastarch blood levels accumulate and increase in a stairstep manner,[12] and exerting lesser effects on coagulation than does hetastarch[13]), pentastarch should be replaced by hetastarch.

Neutrophil transfusion in clinical medicine

Historical overview of therapeutic granulocyte transfusion

To obtain a historical perspective regarding the efficacy of therapeutic GTX (i.e., collected without donor G-CSF), seven controlled studies are analyzed briefly.[14-20] In these seven studies, the response of infected neutropenic patients to treatment with GTX plus antibiotics (study group) was compared with that of comparable patients given antibiotics alone (control group) evaluated concurrently. The design, size, and results of these seven studies are presented in Tables 23.1 and 23.2. Three of the seven studies reported a significant overall benefit for GTX.[17-19] In two additional studies,[14,16] overall success was not demonstrated for GTX, but certain subgroups of patients were found to benefit significantly. Thus, some measure of success for GTX was evident in five of the seven controlled studies (Table 23.1). However, this success was counterbalanced by four studies that reported negative results in some respect—two with negative overall results[15,20] and two with negative results for some types of patients.[14,16]

An explanation for these inconsistent results is evident on critical analysis of the adequacy of GTX support (Table 23.2). Patients in the three successful trials received relatively high doses of PMNs (generally $\geq 1.7 \times 10^{10}$/day), and donors were selected to be both erythrocyte and leukocyte compatible.[17,19] By contrast, the four controlled studies reporting overall or partial negative results can legitimately be criticized. Two of the four studies with negative findings used PMNs collected by filtration leukapheresis for some patients.[14,16] It is now established that such PMNs are defective, and they are no longer transfused. In the negative studies using PMNs collected by centrifugation leukapheresis,[14,16,20] the dose was extremely low (0.41 to 0.56×10^{10} per GTX). As another factor, investigators in two of the four negative studies[14,20] made no provision for the possibility of leukocyte alloimmunization, as donors were selected solely on the basis of erythrocyte compatibility. Finally, control subjects responded particularly well to antibiotics alone in three of the four negative studies,[14,15,20] suggesting that these patients fared relatively well with conventional treatment alone, and it was not possible to document additional benefit by adding GTX.

Table 23.1 Historical controlled trials of therapeutic granulocyte transfusions

| Investigators | Success | Survival | | | |
| | | Study Group | | Control Group | |
		N	(%)	N	(%)
Higby et al.[18]	Yes	17	76	19	26
Volger and Winton[19]	Yes	17	59	13	15
Herzig et al.[17]	Yes	13	75	14	36
Alavi et al.[14]	Partial	12	82	19	62
Graw et al.[16]	Partial	39	46	37	30
Winston et al.[20]	No	48	63	47	72
Fortuny et al.[15]	No	17	78	22	80

Table 23.2 Design of historical therapeutic granulocyte transfusion controlled trials

| Investigators | Randomized | Characteristics of Neutrophil Concentrates | | | |
		Collection Method	Dose (× 10¹⁰)	Schedule	HLA/WBC*
Higby et al.[18]	Yes	Filtration	2.2	Daily	Yes
Vogler and Winton[19]	Yes	Centrifugation	2.7	Daily	Yes
Herzig et al.[17]	Yes	Filtration	1.7	Daily	Yes
		Centrifugation	0.4	Daily	
Alavi et al.[14]	Yes	Filtration	5.9	Daily	No
Graw et al.[16]	No	Filtration	2	Daily	Yes
		Centrifugation	0.6	Daily	
Winston et al.[20]	Yes	Centrifugation	0.5	Daily	No
Fortuny et al.[15]	No	Centrifugation	0.4	Daily	Yes

*Donors selected to be compatible with recipient by HLA typing (A and B loci matched, at least in part) and/or by leukocyte crossmatching. WBC, white cell.

The results of the seven controlled GTX trials have been analyzed by formal meta-analysis,[21] and conclusions were that the low doses of PMNs transfused and the relatively high survival rate of the nontransfused control subjects were primarily responsible for the differing success rates of these studies. In clinical settings in which the survival rate of nontransfused control subjects was low,[16–19] study subjects benefited from receiving adequate doses of GTX—prompting the authors to suggest that severely neutropenic patients with life-threatening infections should be considered for GTX given in high doses.[21]

Historical overview of prophylactic granulocyte transfusion

Based on historical reports, prophylactic GTXs were of marginal value. Some measure of success was found in seven of 12 studies.[22–28] Five studies failed to show a benefit for prophylactic GTXs.[29–33] In none of these five negative studies were large numbers of PMNs obtained from matched donors and transfused daily. In a situation analogous to that for the negative therapeutic GTX trials, the failure of prophylactic GTX might be explained, as least in part, by inadequate transfusions.

In 1997, data from eight of the 12 controlled trials of prophylactic GTX were analyzed quantitatively by means of formal meta-analysis.[34] The findings of the meta-analysis confirmed that variability in the dose of PMNs transfused, inconsistent attempts to provide leukocyte-compatible GTX, and the varying durations of severe neutropenia in different patient groups were primarily responsible for the differing success rates in the reported controlled trials. It was recommended that high doses of compatible PMNs be transfused, if future trials are conducted.[34]

Assessment of modern granulocyte transfusion
Therapeutic granulocyte transfusions

A modern therapeutic GTX is defined as a transfusion in which PMNs are obtained from donors stimulated with G-CSF with or without corticosteroids and collected by means of centrifugation leukapheresis with an erythrocyte-sedimenting agent during the processing of relatively large volumes of donor blood. Specifically, the requirements of an ideal PMN collection should include (1) at least 300 µg G-CSF given subcutaneously (popular dose is to give the entire 480 µg vial) plus 8 mg dexamethasone given orally to the donor approximately 12 hours before leukapheresis is begun; (2)

pentastarch or, preferably, hetastarch infused throughout the leukapheresis procedure at a ratio of 1 part starch to 12–14 parts donor blood; and (3) processing of 8–10 L of donor blood. The goal should be to transfuse 6 to 8×10^{10} neutrophils per GTX, with a lower limit of 4×10^{10}.

At this time, no satisfactorily designed and conducted randomized clinical trials of modern therapeutic GTX collected after G-CSF and dexamethasone donor stimulation have been reported to establish either the efficacy or the potential toxicity of modern GTX. Two randomized clinical trials have been reported or presented, but, as discussed later, both have shortcomings and flaws that preclude firm conclusions or guidelines for clinical practice. Accordingly, practices must be based on an assessment of the overall literature.

To begin, many case reports, which must be viewed with caution, suggest success for modern GTX. As examples, Clark et al.[35] and Catalano et al.[36] each reported single patients with aplastic anemia, undergoing progenitor cell transplantation, with fungus infections that responded favorably. Ozsahin et al.[37] and Bielorai et al.[38] each reported single patients with chronic granulomatous disease and fungal infections that responded favorably to GTX during the transplantation period. Bielorai et al.[39] reported a single patient with acute leukemia and sepsis with vancomycin-resistant *Enterococcus* that cleared slowly with GTX. Similarly, Lin et al.[40] reported a single patient with multidrug-resistant *Pseudomonas* sepsis who underwent a successful HPC-A transplantation supported by GTX. It is impossible, in these single reports of very complicated patients, to firmly ascribe the good outcome to the GTX.

Studies of larger numbers of infected, neutropenic patients given GTX from G-CSF-stimulated donors are listed in Table 23.3. Even with investigation of larger numbers of patients, the benefits of GTX are unclear because of the lack of concurrent control patients treated with antibiotics alone. Hester et al.[41] transfused 15 patients with hematologic malignancies and infections. PMNs were collected from donors stimulated only with G-CSF and selected without regard for leukocyte compatibility. Although GTXs were successful in most patients, it was not possible to distinguish responses of fungus versus yeast infections. Grigg et al.[42] transfused 11 patients. Eight patients had hematologic malignancies and progressive infections—five of the eight underwent HPC transplantation, and three received chemotherapy. Three additional patients who were undergoing HPC transplantation had stable fungus infections. PMNs were collected from donors stimulated only with G-CSF and selected without regard for leukocyte compatibility. Success was excellent for bacterial and stable fungus infections, but was quite poor for progressive fungus infections with organ dysfunction—a troubling pattern reported later by others.[6,43] Peters et al.[44] transfused 30 patients with hematologic disorders—18 undergoing HPC transplantation. PMNs were collected from donors stimulated with G-CSF or prednisolone and selected without regard for leukocyte compatibility. The exact PMN dose transfused is uncertain, but values from 0.9×10^{10} to 14.4×10^{10} were estimated from data reported. It was impossible to distinguish the success of GTX from G-CSF-stimulated versus prednisolone-stimulated donors. However, the outcome of bacterial infections overall appeared to be superior to that of fungus infections.

Price et al.[6] transfused 19 patients (Table 23.3) with hematologic malignancies, 16 of whom had received HPC transplants and three who were scheduled for transplantation. PMNs were collected from donors stimulated with G-CSF and dexamethasone. Although

Table 23.3 Neutropenic patients treated with GTX collected from G-CSF-stimulated donors

Investigators	PMNs ×10^{10} per Each GTX	Stimulation	Leukapheresis	Outcomes
Hester et al.[41]	4.1	G-CSF 5 µg/kg	Pentastarch 7 L processed	60% (9 of 15) Success with fungus (11 patients) and yeast (4 patients)
Grigg et al.[42]	5.9*	G-CSF 10 µg/kg	Dextran 10 L processed	100% (3 of 3) Success with bacterial infection
Peters et al.[44]	3.5*	G-CSF 5 µg/kg or prednisolone	Hetastarch 6.4 L processed	0% (0 of 5) Success with progressive fungus 67% (2 of 3) Success with stable fungus 82% (14 of 17) Success with bacterial infection
Price et al.[6]	8.2	G-CSF 600 µg/kg plus dexamethasone 8 mg	Hetastarch 10 L processed	54% (7 of 13) Success with fungal infection 100% (4 of 4) Success with bacterial infection
Hubel et al.[43]	4.6–8.1	G-CSF 600 µg/kg with or without dexamethasone 8 mg	Hetastarch or pentastarch 10 L processed	0% (0 of 8) Success with invasive fungus 57% (4 of 7) Success with yeast infection 55% (unrelated donor) Success with bacterial infection 75% (family donor) Success with bacterial infection 70% (unrelated donor) Success with yeast infection 40% (family donor) Success with yeast infection 15% (unrelated donor) Success with fungal infection 25% (family donor) Success with fungal infection
Lee et al.[45]	5.1–10.6	G-CSF 5 µg/kg and/or dexamethasone 3 mg/m²	Pentastarch 6–10 L processed	40% (10 of 25) Success with multiple-organism infections

* Assumptions made as PMN dose expressed ×10^{10} unclear in these reports. PMN dose calculated using values for the total number and differential count of leukocytes collected, and the volume of units collected (Grigg et al.[42]). Dose calculated that would be given to a 70-kg recipient for Peters et al.[44] GTX, granulocyte transfusion; G-CSF, granulocyte colony-stimulating factor; PMNs, granulocytes.

Rates of documented infections were not reported.

donors were selected without regard for leukocyte compatibility, recipients were documented not to exhibit evidence of leukocyte alloimmunization at study entry. Bacterial infections responded well, and yeast infections responded modestly. Despite very high PMN doses, success for invasive fungus infections was dismal. Hübel et al.[43] expanded the study of Price et al.[6] to a total of 74 patients receiving HPC transplants. Comparisons were made to historical control patients ($n = 74$) who did not receive GTX. PMNs were collected either from unrelated donors given G-CSF alone or in combination with dexamethasone, or from family members given G-CSF only. Hetastarch was used for single leukapheresis procedures, and pentastarch was used when donors experienced repeated leukapheresis procedures. Comparative success in nontransfused historical control patients was approximately 90% for bacterial, 40% for yeast, and 30% for fungal/mold infections—values similar to those achieved by GTX recipients. Nontransfused controls actually had better success than PMN recipients for bacterial infections ($p = 0.04$). As a potential adverse effect, allogeneic transplant recipients given GTX from unrelated donors experienced significantly more ($p = 0.04$) Grade IV graft-versus-host disease (GVHD) than controls who were not given GTX. However, relatively few patients were assessed for this endpoint, and firm conclusions are not warranted.

Lee et al.[45] transfused 25 patients with hematologic malignancies, many of whom were infected with multiple organisms. Thus, the outcome of infections with specific types of individual organisms could not be determined. PMNs were collected from donors stimulated with G-CSF alone (66% of donors), G-CSF plus dexamethasone (25% of donors), or dexamethasone alone (8% of donors). Of patients with sepsis, 50% (two of four) responded favorably, and 38% (8 of 21) of patients with progressive localized infections responded favorably.

Two studies reported results in ways that did not lend themselves to tabulation, and they will be briefly described. Illerhaus et al.[46] transfused 42 neutropenic patients with GTX collected from donors stimulated with 5 µg/kg G-CSF. Eighteen of the patients had severe

infections with a variety of organisms, and each received a median of three GTX each containing a median of 2.6×10^{10} leukocytes. Of these 18 patients, eight (44%) improved, four (22%) stabilized, and six (33%) deteriorated—with four of these last six dying of pulmonary aspergillosis. Rutella et al.[47] transfused 20 patients with hematologic malignancies and neutropenic infections. Donors were HLA-identical siblings, and each received 5 µg/kg G-CSF. Favorable responses were seen in 54% of patients with bacterial and 57% of fungal infections. Underlying cancer status (i.e., complete or partial remission achieved) and recovery of blood PMN counts to 500/µL or more were significantly correlated with a favorable response to GTX.

No firm conclusions can be drawn from these larger, but still somewhat anecdotal reports of modern therapeutic GTX for several reasons: (1) No concurrent control subjects were included (i.e., randomly assigned to receive antimicrobial drugs, but no GTX); (2) the number of patients reported, generally, was quite small; and (3) PMN collection methods were variable with a broad range of PMN doses transfused. Based on these preliminary findings, bacterial infections appeared to respond quite well to modern GTX, and relatively mild fungus and yeast infections responded modestly well. However, serious fungus infections with tissue invasion often resisted even the large doses of PMNs transfused with modern GTX.[6,42–46]

Three more recent studies are of special interest and, although they do not provide definitive information to establish clinical practices, they will be discussed in more detail. The first randomized clinical trial of "modern" GTX contained many shortcomings and, accordingly, provided no definitive guidelines for transfusion practices.[48] Problems with the trial included: (1) it was never completed due to poor enrollment; (2) donors were stimulated only with G-CSF without combination with dexamethasone, resulting in relatively low PMN doses; and (3) GTXs were given only every other day, rather than daily, again resulting in low PMN doses. Thus, the trial failed to adequately test the efficacy of modern "high-dose" GTX.[48]

The second, and most recent, randomized clinical trial has been published only as an abstract,[49] and like the earlier trial, it was stopped before completion and, accordingly, failed to provide definitive guidelines for clinical practice. However, it will be discussed as it provides the latest information from randomized clinical trials. RING is a multicenter randomized clinical trial in which 114 infected neutropenic (<500 neutrophils/μL blood) patients were randomly allocated to treatment either with daily GTX collected from donors stimulated with G-CSF + dexamethasone plus antibiotics ($N = 56$) or with antibiotics alone ($N = 58$). The primary endpoint was a composite of survival at 42 days after randomization plus microbial response determined by a blinded adjudication panel. Results by intention-to-treat analysis were nearly identical ($p > 0.99$), with 42% in the GTX arm versus 43% of controls having a favorable response. Similarly, by per protocol analysis (i.e., patients actually treated as intended), results were not different ($p = 0.64$): 49% favorable in the GTX arm versus 41% of controls. No differences in success rates were noted when analyzed per specific types of infection. Although results appeared to be "negative" (i.e., no advantage for GTX), 32% of patients in the GTX arm did not receive the intended dose of PMNs/granulocytes, and when patients given high-dose GTX were compared with those given low-dose GTX, the high-dose GTX patients had significantly higher success rates ($p = 0.01$). The reason(s) for the poor PMNs/granulocyte doses were not determined, but it is clear that the potential benefits of high-dose GTX still remain a possibility—provided high-dose GTXs (at least 4×10^{10} per transfusion) are actually given.[49] Importantly, blood suppliers must document that the high-dose PMNs/granulocyte concentrates they prepare from donors stimulated with G-CSF + dexamethasone do, in fact, contain at least 4×10^{10} PMNs/granulocytes per unit.

The RING clinical trial has been published on-line (Price T, McCullough J, Ness P, Strauss R, Harrison R, Hamza T, Assman S. A randomized controlled trial on the efficacy of high-dose granulocyte transfusion therapy in neutropenic patients with infection (RING). Blood First Edition paper, September 2, 2015; DO110.1182/blood-2015-05-645986.) and reported that the subset of 26 patients given at least three granulocyte transfusions with an average dose per transfusion of at least 5×10^{10} granulocytes had a success rate of 58% contrasted with 11% success in the nine patients given lower granulocyte doses.

As a case in point, in a retrospective review of patients with invasive Fusarium infections, 11 patients with severe neutropenia due to marrow disease and failure to respond to antifungal drugs received a median of seven GTXs containing a mean of 6.84×10^{10} granulocytes per GTX.[50] Ten of the 11 patients (91%) had a favorable response, compared to an expected response of <50% when antifungal drugs are given without GTX. Eight of the 11 patients (73%) survived 90 days after GTX, but survival fell to 45% at discharge, with survival strongly correlated with hematopoietic recovery. The authors concluded that high-dose GTX may effectively control life-threatening infections to "bridge" periods of severe neutropenia until marrow function is restored.[50]

Despite the reports of two attempts[48,49] to perform a properly designed and conducted randomized clinical trial to test the efficacy of high-dose GTX collected from donors stimulated with G-CSF + dexamethasone, the definitive/proven role of GTX in the management of infected, neutropenic, oncology/transplant patients awaits definition by a successfully completed randomized clinical trial—something that seems elusive to date.

Prophylactic granulocyte transfusions

The role of modern prophylactic GTX (i.e., from G-CSF-stimulated donors) has not been established by definitive clinical trials. However, two factors suggest possible success: (1) Rapid recovery from myeloablation, hastened by HPC-A transfusions and treatment of patients with recombinant growth factors, has shortened the period of severe neutropenia to as brief as one week; and (2) this relatively brief period of severe neutropenia might literally be eliminated by transfusing large doses of PMNs collected from donors stimulated with G-CSF plus corticosteroids. A few studies have begun to explore this possibility (Table 23.4).

Bensinger et al.[51] transfused seven allogeneic marrow recipients with PMNs collected from their HLA-identical or syngeneic marrow donors after G-CSF stimulation. Because donors experienced leukapheresis on consecutive days, collection techniques were quite variable in terms of quantities of HES-infused and liters of donor blood processed, and the number of PMNs per GTX varied from 0.3 to 14.4×10^{10}. Recipients received an average of 7.6 GTXs while awaiting marrow recovery, and recipients were given 5 μg/kg G-CSF daily to maintain a mean blood PMN count of 950/μL, measured 24 hours after transfusion. The goals of this study were to evaluate the feasibility and safety of collecting and transfusing PMNs from G-CSF-stimulated donors; patient outcomes were not reported.

Adkins et al.[52] transfused 10 allogeneic marrow recipients with PMNs collected from their HLA-matched sibling marrow donors. Leukapheresis was performed on Days 1, 3, and 5 after transplantation, and GTXs were administered on these days. Recipients

Table 23.4 Prophylactic GTX using PMNs from G-CSF-stimulated donors in hematopoietic progenitor cell recipients

Investigator	PMNs×10^{10} per Each GTX	Stimulation	Leukapheresis	Outcomes
Bensinger et al.[48]	4.2	G-CSF 3.5-6 μg/kg	Variable	Not reported
Adkins et al.[49]	4.1 (Day 1) 5.1 (Day 3) 6.1 (Day 5)	G-CSF 5 μg/kg×5 days after transplantation	Hetastarch 7 L processed Days 1, 3, and 5	60% (6 of 10) Afebrile 40% (4 of 10) Febrile Three culture positive
Adkins et al.[50]	5.6 (Day 2) 7.0 (Day 4) 8.5 (Day 6) 9.9 (Day 8)	G-CSF 10 μg/kg	Hetastarch 7 L processed Days 2, 4, 6, and 8	Reduction of fever and antibiotics if no leukocyte antibodies
Oza et al.[51]	5.9 (Days 3 and 5) 5.2 (Days 6 and 7)	GCSF 10 μg/kg	Hetastarch 7 L processed Days 3 and 6 or Days 5 and 7	Less fever and antibiotics when GTX given; no effect on hospital stay or survival

GTX, granulocyte transfusion; PMNs, granulocytes; F-CSF, granulocyte colony-stimulating factor.

were given 7.5 µg/kg G-CSF every 12 hours until blood PMNs were greater than or equal to 1500/µL. Recipient blood PMNs were maintained at greater than 500/µL throughout the five days of posttransplant GTX. By comparison, a historical group of control recipients treated with G-CSF, but no GTX, exhibited mean blood PMN counts less than 500/µL following transplantation. Prophylactic GTX seemed promising in this setting and, perhaps, would have been even more effective (i.e., higher recipient blood PMN counts and fewer infections) if given daily. In another study, Adkins et al.[53] transfused 23 autologous HPC-A recipients with PMNs collected from first-degree relative donors. Leukapheresis was performed on posttransplant Days 2, 4, 6, and 8, and GTXs were given on those days. Recipients were given 5 µg/kg G-CSF daily until the blood PMN count was greater than or equal to 1500/µL. Recipients were studied for the effects of lymphocytotoxic antibodies (i.e., leukocyte alloimmunization) on GTX effectiveness. The 15 recipients who did not exhibit lymphocytotoxic antibodies during the 10-day study period experienced a mean of 4.1 febrile days and required 7.3 days of antibiotics. Values for the eight recipients with lymphocytotoxic antibodies were less desirable—6.3 febrile days and 10.5 days of antibiotics.

In a later report from the same group,[54] 151 donor–recipient pairs, consisting of HLA-matched sibling donors of peripheral blood progenitor cells and the recipients of their progenitor cells, were initially allocated to either a GTX group or a non-GTX group based on ABO matching of red cells. For several reasons, the final allocation was 53 ABO-matched donor–recipient pairs assigned to GTX and 98 pairs assigned to the non-GTX group. PMNs were collected for GTX on either Days 3 and 6 or Days 5 and 7 after transplantation (different days due to enrollment in two different studies). Thus, recipients received two GTXs on an every-other-day schedule. Recipients also received G-CSF (10 µg/kg/day) beginning one day after transplantation and continuing until a blood PMN count was equal to or greater than 1500/µL for three days. The percentage of recipients with posttransplant fever was 64% with GTX versus 83% without GTX ($p = 0.03$). The median number of days that intravenous antibiotics were given was 9 with GTX versus 11 without GTX ($p = 0.03$). No significant differences were found for length of hospital stay, 100-day survival, or rates of acute GVHD (Table 23.4).

No firm conclusions can be drawn from these reports of modern prophylactic GTX because few nontransfused control subjects were included (none randomly assigned before the studies); relatively few patients were studied; and most patients were given GTXs every other day, rather than daily—possibly providing a less than optimal dose of PMNs. Modern prophylactic GTXs appear promising, but their efficacy, potential adverse effects, and economic analysis await definition by randomized clinical trials of sufficient numbers of patients.

Pediatric granulocyte transfusion

Therapeutic GTXs are prescribed for children with marrow failure and severe neutropenic infections using the same criteria as for adults. In a study by Sachs et al.,[55] 27 children with hematologic/oncologic disorders and neutropenic infections received GTXs every other day. PMNs were collected from crossmatch-compatible donors stimulated with G-CSF only. The average dose of PMNs per each GTX was 8×10^8 PMN/kg recipient body weight. This corresponds to 5.6×10^{10} PMNs for a 70-kg adult. GTXs were very successful, with 93% of patients able to clear infections—including all with invasive pulmonary aspergillosis infections—and with 82% survival one month later.

Most patients with congenital disorders of PMN dysfunction have adequate numbers of blood PMNs, but they are susceptible to serious infections because their PMNs fail to kill pathogenic microorganisms. Patients with severe forms of PMN dysfunction are relatively rare, and no randomized clinical trials have been reported to establish the efficacy of therapeutic GTX in their management. Firm recommendations about the use of GTX to treat patients cannot be made. However, several patients with chronic granulomatous disease, complicated by progressive life-threatening fungal infections, have been reported to benefit.[56–64] Because of the possibility of alloimmunization to leukocyte and red cell antigens, particularly to the Kell blood group, plus the risk of transfusion-transmitted infections, therapeutic GTXs are recommended only for progressive infections that cannot be controlled with antimicrobial drugs. Because of lifetime problems with infections, prophylactic GTXs are impractical.

Neonates (infants within the first month of life) are another group of patients who may suffer life-threatening bacterial infections caused, at least in part, by PMN dysfunction and neutropenia. Neutropenia must be viewed differently in neonates than in older patients, because in the latter, GTXs are considered usually when the blood PMN count falls to less than 500/µL. By contrast, because normal neonates exhibit a physiologic neutrophilia, absolute blood PMN counts as high as 3000/µL (i.e., relative neutropenia due to age) might prompt consideration of GTX in neonates. Six controlled trials (reviewed in Strauss[65]) have assessed the role of GTX in treating neonatal infections. Although four of the six found a significant benefit for GTX, the controlled studies, when assessed by meta-analysis, were insufficiently homogeneous to permit clear recommendations regarding the efficacy of GTX.[21] Thus, the role of therapeutic GTX for neonatal infections is unclear at present and, because they are transfused only rarely at this time, they will not be discussed further.

Summary and recommendations for clinical practice

The use of G-CSF + dexamethasone to stimulate PMN donors has brought GTX therapy into a new era. It is now possible to collect relatively large numbers of PMNs/granulocytes ($>4 \times 10^{10}$) by modern leukapheresis techniques. To determine whether a local need exists for therapeutic GTX, physicians should survey the outcome of neutropenic infections at their own institutions. If these infections respond promptly to antibiotics alone and the survival rate approaches 100%, therapeutic GTXs are unnecessary and should not be used, because possible benefits are too small to outweigh the risks and expense. In contrast, if patients with infection and neutropenia (<500 PMN/µL) do not respond quickly and completely to antibiotics alone, the addition of therapeutic GTX should be considered along with other modifications of therapy, such as selection of different antibiotics, closer monitoring of antibiotic blood levels, intravenous γ-globulin therapy, and treatment with recombinant myeloid growth factors.

Once the decision has been made to provide either therapeutic or prophylactic GTX, PMNs must be collected and transfused optimally as follows:

Collect PMNs from allogeneic donors with a goal to transfuse 6 to 8×10^{10} PMNs per GTX with an absolute lower limit of 4×10^{10}. Develop and refine methods to consistently ensure desired yields. The need to select donors who are leukocyte compatible with recipients has not been established for modern (high-dose PMNs) GTX, despite the historical importance of doing so when lower doses of PMNs were transfused.[34] In studies of modern GTX, Price et al.[6] found no apparent adverse effects of several leukocyte antibodies (granulocyte agglutinating, granulocyte immuno-fluorescent, lymphocytotoxic, and lymphocyte immunofluorescent) that became detectable in the recipient's blood during GTX therapy (i.e., not preexisting antibodies). Adkins et al.,[53] however, found the presence of lymphocytotoxic antibodies to be a poor prognostic factor, in general—although actual donor–recipient incompatibility for individual GTX was rare. Until more data are available, it seems prudent to select donors who are leukocyte compatible (e.g., as done to select platelet donors by HLA matching or leukocyte cross-matching) whenever easily feasible, but never to delay or deny GTX therapy if selecting donors is not readily accomplished.

Stimulate donor neutrophilia by giving 300–600 μg G-CSF sub-cutaneously plus dexamethasone orally 12 hours before beginning leukapheresis. A regimen reported to produce high PMN yields with reasonable adverse effects on the donor is one 480 μg vial G-CSF given subcutaneously plus 8 mg dexamethasone given orally 12 hours before leukapheresis.[4]

Process 8 to 10 L of donor blood using a continuous-flow, centrifugation blood separator with citrated HES (hetastarch pre-ferred) solution infused throughout the entire collection at a starch–donor blood ratio of 1:13.

Transfuse PMN/granulocyte unit as soon as possible after col-lection to minimize storage damage. Data suggest deterioration of PMN function begins within a few hours of storage. Until the efficacy of stored neutrophils from G-CSF-stimulated leukapheresis donors is documented, it seems wise to transfuse within six hours or so of collection. This timing may require agreement by the patient's physician to perform infectious disease testing on the donor before actual PMN collection (e.g., at the time G-CSF is administered before leukapheresis) or accept a donor who has been tested recently for a previous donation (e.g., within the preceding 10–30 days), but has not been tested for the PMN collection in question.

Give GTX daily until resolution of infection—as evidenced by clearing of tissue lesions, negative cultures, or resolution of fever—or until marrow function recovers to produce adequate numbers of endogenous PMNs. Determining marrow recovery may be difficult because PMNs collected from G-CSF-stimulated and dexametha-sone-stimulated donors and transfused at doses of $6{-}8 \times 10^{10}$ PMNs may elevate the recipient's blood PMN count to more than 1000/μL for more than 24 hours. Accurate differentiation of transfused PMNs from those produced endogenously is challenging, and marrow recovery must be based on a sustained increase in blood PMN count after GTX is discontinued.

Disclaimer

The author has disclosed no conflicts of interest.

Key references

A full reference list for this chapter is available at:
http://www.wiley.com/go/simon/transfusion

2 Strauss RG. Granulocyte (neutrophil) transfusions. In: McLeod BC, Szczepior-kowski ZM, Weinstein R, Winters JL, Eds. *Apheresis: principles and practice.* 3rd ed. Bethesda, MD: AABB Press, 2010: 215–28.

4 Liles WC, Rodger E, Dale DC. Combined administration of G-CSF and dexameth-asone for the mobilization of granulocytes in normal donors: optimization of dosing. *Transfusion* 2000; **40**: 642–4.

9 Strauss RG, Lipton KS. Glucocorticoid stimulation of neutrophil donors: a medical scientific, and ethical dilemma. *Transfusion* 2005; **45**: 1697–9.

11 Lee JH, Leitman SF, Klein HG. A controlled comparison of the efficacy of hetastarch and pentastarch in granulocyte collections by centrifugal leukapheresis. *Blood* 1995; **86**: 4662–6.

21 Vamvakas EC, Pineda AA. Meta-analysis of clinical studies of the efficacy of granulocyte transfusions in the treatment of bacterial sepsis. *J Clin Apher* 1996; **11**: 1–9.

34 Vamvakas EC, Pineda AA. Determinants of the efficacy of prophylactic granulocyte transfusions: a meta-analysis. *J Clin Apher* 1997; **12**: 74–81.

65 Strauss RG. Current status of granulocyte transfusions to treat neonatal sepsis. *J Clin Apher* 1989; **5**: 25–9.

CHAPTER 24

Leukocyte-reduced blood components: laboratory and clinical aspects

Tor Hervig[1] & Jerard Seghatchian[2]

[1]Department of Immunology and Transfusion Medicine, Haukeland University Hospital, Bergen, Norway
[2]International Consultancy in Blood Components Quality/Safety Improvement, Audit/ Inspection and DDR Strategies, London, UK

From a semantic viewpoint, it is obvious that "red cell concentrates" should contain red cells only, and the same is true for platelet concentrates—they should contain platelets and no other cells (e.g., contaminating leukocytes). Viable donor leukocytes contaminate blood components and are linked to a wide variety of acute and long-term transfusion complications, including febrile transfusion reactions, alloimmunization, transfusion-associated graft-versus-host disease (TA-GVHD), immunomodulation, and transmission of infectious diseases.[1] Consequently, removal of leukocytes from these concentrates should be an obvious consideration to diminish these complications.

By definition, a unit of leukocyte-reduced (LR) blood or blood component must contain no more than 1×10^6 according to European requirements and less than 5×10^6 according to US requirements.[2] In practice, there is no easy method to fulfil these requirements. For cellular blood components, an additional in-production step as filtration is needed to obtain a low level of contaminating leukocytes. For apheresis methods, some techniques provide significant leukocyte depletion of the red cell and platelet units collected, although all subsets of leukocytes are not reduced to the same degree.

The indications for prescribing LR blood components are not universally accepted. The guidelines for patients needing LR cellular blood components include patients who need chronic transfusions, patients with severe febrile transfusion reactions, patients with acute leukemia, patients needing cytomegalovirus (CMV)-negative blood components, and patients undergoing cardiac surgery. Some centers also include patients undergoing surgery in general in the guidelines, and some hospitals provide LR components to all pediatric transfusions. As the list of indications for LR components increases, many centers have implemented universal leukocyte reduction (ULR) to avoid difficulties with having two different inventories. Some countries in Europe opted for prestorage leukoreduction as a precautionary measure against variant Creutzfeldt–Jakob disease (vCJD), thus implementing ULR. In other countries, it was considered that more research was needed to justify the cost related to leukocyte reduction of all cellular components. The cost issue is essential, and some scientists argue that increased cost is the only argument against ULR.[3] In the developing countries, the increased cost makes implementation of filtration procedures impossible.

In summary, even among countries with high healthcare costs, various guidelines are followed concerning indications for LR cellular blood components. Thus, there is a need to highlight different aspects of leukocyte contamination of cellular blood components.

How do leukocytes affect red cell and platelet storage?

It is well known that both red cells and platelets undergo changes that reduce their functional capabilities during storage. As these changes may occur due to both internal conditions as well as cell-to-cell interactions, leukocyte reduction of cellular components should provide an ideal environment for studying red cell–leukocyte and platelet–leukocyte interactions. After a regular whole blood donation, the unit normally contains $2–5 \times 10^9$ leukocytes. The number of leukocytes in a standard red cell concentrate is $5 \times 10^{8,1}$ and after buffy coat removal around 0.8×10^8. With modern filtration techniques, leukocyte contamination far below 1×10^6 may be achieved.

During the red cell storage, severe disturbances in cellular metabolism, rheological properties, oxidation and carboxylation stress, and cellular aging processes occur.[4] Although the clinical importance of these changes is controversial, there are strong indications that the cell detritions as hemolysis, potassium release, and microvesicle formation cause reduced survival and increased adverse reactions in the recipients.[5,6]

Antonelou and her group have published an extensive paper on the effects of prestorage leukocyte reduction on stored red blood cells (RBCs), with the limitation that platelets were present in the nonfiltered group. They found significantly increased hemolysis, irreversible echinocytosis, microvesiculation, removal signaling, reactive oxygen species (ROS) and calcium accumulation, band 3–related senescence modifications, membrane proteome stress biomarkers, as well as the emergence of a senescence phenotype in the lower density RBCs in the non-LR concentrates.[4] These results are in line with several earlier publications focusing on separate areas of red cell lesion. Reduced hemolysis in LR red cell concentrates has been reported in a large international study. Leukodepletion of AS-3 red cell concentrates prior to storage resulted in reduced glycolytic activity—and posttransfusion recovery of red cells stored for 42 days was significantly better in the prestorage leukocyte reduction group (84% vs. 82% in the group

Rossi's Principles of Transfusion Medicine, Fifth Edition. Edited by Toby L. Simon, Jeffrey McCullough, Edward L. Snyder, Bjarte G. Solheim, and Ronald G. Strauss.

receiving nonfiltered components).[7] A Dutch group has published that red cell rheology is well preserved in LR red cell concentrates.[8] However, it should not be forgotten that the impact of storage and leukocyte burden on adhesion molecules, glycophorin A, and annexin V is also influenced by red cell age. Older RBCs showed significantly reduced expression of glycophorin A during storage, and increasing annexin V concentrations were found in the supernatant of old red cells stored in the presence of leukocytes.[9] In an in vitro study on procoagulant activity of fresh frozen plasma, leukocyte reduction resulted in lower hemostatic potential defined by thromboelastography (TEG) values and coagulation factor concentrations.[10]

Techniques for leukocyte removal from cellular blood components

Centrifugation

Standard centrifugation techniques for cellular component production do not provide results comparable with those of true leukocyte reduction. However, just by removing the buffy coat from whole blood after centrifugation, the residual leukocyte content in the corresponding red cell concentrate may be reduced by 70–80%. In combination with more sophisticated methods for leukocyte reduction for special patient groups, this may be a safe and low-cost alternative.[11]

Filtration

Filtration has become the dominating method for leukocyte reduction of cellular blood components. Filters are made by cotton wool, cellulose acetate, polycarbonate, polyester, or polyurethane. The filters may be positively or negatively charged—or neutral. As the platelets and red cells adhere differently to foreign materials, filters for red cell concentrates and platelet concentrates cannot be used randomly. A whole blood platelet-sparing filter that also reduces leukocyte content in line with the requirements is available.[12] Because of the introduction of leukocyte removal filters, the efficiency has improved from 1–2 log removal to 4–5 log removal of leukocytes. The filters may also, to some extent, remove bioactive substances and bacteria.

Mechanisms of filtration

The plastic housing that contains the filtration medium is designed so that blood encounters a large surface area of medium, the volume of blood retained by the filter (holdup volume) is minimal, and the medium fits tightly enough within the housing so that blood entering the device cannot bypass the filtration medium. Depletion of leukocytes results primarily from barrier retention in which the pore size of the filter medium is large enough to allow passage of red cells and platelets but small enough to impede passage of leukocytes. To achieve the small pore sizes required, manufacturers have used three different fabrication strategies. In one method, polyester is melted and extruded through fine nozzles into a turbulent gas stream at high velocity. In the process, akin to the formation of cotton candy, the polyester is stretched and cooled to form fine threads of microfibers. These fibers are matted together (like teased hair) and compressed to a controlled fiber density. An alternative approach produces coral-reef-like structures of porous polyurethane with an open-cell geometric configuration containing interconnecting channels that necessitate a circuitous path of flow.

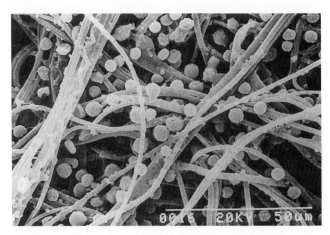

Figure 24.1 Electron micrograph shows fibers from the fine filter (downstream layer) of a leukocyte reduction filter designed for RBCs. The caliber of the fibers relative to that of individual cells is evident. (Source: Nishimura et al., 1989 [Brozovic B, Ed. The role of leucocyte depletion in blood transfusion practice. Oxford, UK: Blackwell, 1989:35—40.])

Polyester fiber filters consist of a series of layers of fiber material. At the upstream end of the filter, the fiber diameter and effective pore size are large. As blood passes through the layers of medium, the fiber diameter becomes smaller, and the pore size decreases to approximately 4 microns (Figure 24.1). Red cells, which are more deformable than leukocyte nuclei, can traverse these small pores. Because synthetic materials are naturally hydrophobic, they do not become "wet" easily in aqueous solutions. As a result, surface tension would prevent blood from flowing through very fine pore spaces under gravity. To overcome this obstacle, manufacturers have modified the surface of the filter medium fibers to increase their "wettability."

Factors affecting filter performance—and clinical implications

Because of the complex physical and biologic forces involved in leukocyte retention by the filter medium, it is not surprising that several factors have been shown to affect the degree of leukocyte reduction obtained (Table 24.1).

The different filters have different optimal operating conditions and different capacities. It is therefore essential to perform filtration in a controlled laboratory or blood center environment according to the manufacturer's instructions. In the first years of blood filtration, most filtration procedures had to be performed at refrigerated temperatures,[13,14] but at present many procedures may be conducted at ambient temperature. The cellular composition of the blood also affects retention of leukocytes. Blood from donors with sickle cell trait often does not become adequately leukocyte reduced when filtered. Results of studies suggest that approximately 50% of

Table 24.1 Factors affecting filter performance

- Capacity of the filter
- Input number of leukocytes
- Temperature (viscoelasticity)
- Flow rate, pressure, priming, and rinsing
- Presence of hemoglobin S
- Number and function of platelets
- Holding time between blood collection and filtration
- Plasma content of cell suspension media

units from donors with hemoglobin AS clog the filter and do not flow.[15] Of the remaining 50%, approximately half of these flow normally but do not undergo adequate leukocyte reduction. The speed of filtration also has been shown to affect leukocyte reduction. If temperature is held constant, faster flow rates may result in decreased performance. This is presumed to result from high shear rates and decreased contact time with the medium. The filtration procedure may also have clinical consequences.

The most obvious effect is the loss of active substances: hemoglobin reduction of LR red cell concentrates and platelet loss from LR platelet concentrates. In a large French quality control database, the average hemoglobin content was 57.6 g in the nonfiltered versus 50.9 g in the LR red cell concentrates.[16] The clinical significance of this difference may, however, be overshadowed by other factors that influence hemoglobin content and patient hemoglobin increment.[17] In a clinical study, Sweeney et al. found a significant lower platelet dose in the LR platelet concentrates (3.3×10^{11}) versus the nonfiltered concentrates (4.0×10^{11}), but there was no significant effect on the corrected count increment (CCI).[18] This observation is in line with the later outcome of a large platelet dosing study.[19]

Significant clinical side effects are observed as a result of leukocyte reduction by filtration. Severe hypotensive reactions are the most prominent. The reactions are induced by generation of vasodilators as bradykinin, probably by donor plasma activation during filter transfer.[20] For several years, this side effect was related to bedside leukocyte reduction procedures, but hypotensive reactions have also been reported after prestorage leukocyte reduction.[21] In the beginning of the filtration era, the *red eye syndrome*, which also included eye pain, photophobia, and sometimes more generalized symptoms, occurred.[22] This syndrome was linked to a cellulose acetate membrane that was used in some filters. When these filters were withdrawn, the syndrome disappeared.

Apheresis devices to reduce leukocyte content

Manufacturers of apheresis devices have modified the machines to collect platelets with low levels of residual donor leukocytes that require no further filtration to meet standards as LR platelet concentrates. These devices achieve a high degree of separation between the donor platelets and the donor leukocytes as a result of several design principles. Flow path geometry, counterflow centrifugation, elutriation, and fluid particle bed separation all are used to separate platelets from leukocytes on the basis of differences in cell mass. Despite advanced design, apheresis systems can fail to collect platelet concentrates that meet standards for being considered LR

Prestorage, poststorage, or bedside leukocyte reduction

Leukocyte filtration may be performed in the blood bank prestorage or after storage of cellular blood components. Prestorage leukocyte reduction during or soon after component preparation has become the preferred method of leukocyte reduction and is ideally suited to process control. The leukocyte filtration is incorporated in the production process, whether this is performed on the donation day or after overnight holding of whole blood. For platelet concentrates, numerous investigators have documented that inflammatory cytokines, including interleukin-1 (IL1), tumor necrosis factor (TNF), and IL6, can accumulate during storage in some units. The extent of cytokine accumulation correlates with the leukocyte content of the unit and the duration of room temperature storage.

For some transfusion recipients, the passively transferred cytokines result in febrile nonhemolytic transfusion reactions. Prestorage leukocyte reduction of platelet concentrates prevents accumulation of these cytokines. There is speculation that prestorage leukocyte reduction would have additional advantages by preventing transfusion of leukocyte fragments that would otherwise develop during storage. Results of laboratory studies and preclinical animal studies have suggested that leukocyte breakdown may contribute to HLA alloimmunization,[23] release of intracellular viruses,[24] and immunosuppression.[25] However, none of these effects has been documented in clinical trials. Results of a large, randomized controlled study conducted in Europe with patients undergoing cardiac surgery showed no advantage of prestorage LR RBCs over poststorage LR RBCs for the prevention of postoperative infection, multiple organ failure, or death.[26]

Poststorage leukocyte reduction is filtration of components shortly before issue from the blood bank. Poststorage filtration is easy to standardize, can be incorporated into the laboratory procedure in a manner similar to that for other manipulations of blood components, and is easily adapted into a program of process control. For whole blood–derived platelet concentrates, poststorage leukocyte reduction has the key disadvantage that cytokines that accumulate during storage are not removed by filtration. For RBCs, there is no known disadvantage to poststorage leukocyte reduction.

In the beginning of the filtration era, bedside filtration procedures were common. However, quality control of the procedure was in practice impossible, and this came in conflict with the Good Manufacturing Practice requirements. Even more important was the publication of a large randomized study that showed that bedside filtration did not prevent HLA immunization.[27] Moreover, for some recipients taking angiotensin-converting enzyme (ACE) inhibitors, bedside filtration has been associated with hypotensive transfusion reactions. For these reasons, bedside leukocyte reduction is no longer recommended.

Process control of leukocyte-reduced components

The concentration of white blood cells (WBCs) in a 300-mL LR blood component with 10^6 WBCs per unit is only 3.3 WBCs/μL. Because traditional automated cell counters are not accurate at leukocyte concentrations less than 100 WBCs/μL, special techniques are required to accurately count residual WBCs in LR components. Several methods have been evaluated for their abilities to count such low numbers of leukocytes accurately. In a large comparison study, the Nageotte hemocytometer and four platforms based on fluorescent staining of nuclei were tested.[28] Although there were significant variances in performance between the automated methods, the flow cytometry–based testing platforms performed best, and the Nageotte method performed poorly in terms of accuracy and precision. However, the use of larger volumes, the concentration of leukocytes, and accurate methodology may improve the performance of the Nageotte method.[29] Recently, a new microscopic method for counting of residual leukocytes in filtered blood components has been evaluated.[30]

As the testing for leukocyte contamination is laborious and costly—and it is important to ensure the stability of the process—strict validation and process control are necessary. A practical guideline for these purposes has been developed by the Biomedical Excellence for Safer Transfusion (BEST) society.[31]

Clinical indications for leukocyte reduction

In the first years, leukocyte reduction was selectively used for special patient groups: to avoid HLA immunization in patients receiving multiple platelet transfusions during cytotoxic therapy, to avoid transmission of CMV, and to prevent febrile transfusion reactions. Later, several other clinical indications were introduced, leading to increased use of leukocyte reduction filters. When it was speculated that leukocyte reduction could reduce risk for vCJD, ULR was implemented in many countries. Thus, it may be argued that ULR sometimes was introduced because it was logistically difficult to administer two parallel inventories—and that the scientific rationale was weak.[3]

HLA immunization

The threshold level of leukocytes needed to provoke primary HLA alloimmunization is not well defined. During the 1990s, the standard for LR blood components was set to 5×10^6 WBCs per transfusion, and this threshold value is still used in the United States. However, in Europe, maximum leukocyte contamination was set at 1×10^6 WBCs per transfusion.

Mechanism

Decades of research provide unequivocal evidence that passenger leukocytes, which express donor HLA antigens, are a prime cause of recipient sensitization to HLA alloantigens. Experiments by Claas et al.[32] with a rodent transfusion model showed that residual donor leukocytes provoked major histocompatibility complex (MHC) alloimmunization and that leukocyte reduction could decrease the incidence of primary sensitization to MHC antigens. These investigators further documented that even very low numbers of donor leukocytes in previously sensitized animals induced secondary immunization, suggesting that leukocyte reduction would be less effective in the previously sensitized patient. The importance of donor leukocytes was confirmed in experiments by Kao[33] and Blajchman et al.,[23] who also provided evidence for the possible role of antigens on microparticles in plasma.[34]

Alloimmunization can occur by means of both direct and indirect immune recognition.[35] Direct allorecognition is the process by which recipient immune cells respond directly to donor HLA antigens without the processing of donor antigens by recipient antigen-presenting cells (APCs). The mixed lymphocyte reaction is an in vitro example of direct T-cell recognition. Direct allosensitization requires at least three fundamental elements—binding of the antigen to the antigen receptor, binding of costimulatory molecules mediating cell–cell contact, and local elaboration of cytokines and appropriate cytokine receptors. Recipients may recognize intact Class I structures on the surface of donor leukocytes (Figure 24.2). Alternatively, Class II–positive donor APCs may carry, within the peptide-binding groove, oligopeptides that represent the cell's own HLA Class I antigen (Figure 24.3). In either case, depletion of Class II–positive donor APCs would reduce the chance of direct HLA immunization to Class I antigens. The failure of the recipient to recognize donor Class I antigens on platelets may reflect the fact that platelets lack critical costimulatory molecules required for direct allostimulation.

Indirect allorecognition is the process by which recipient APCs first engulf donor cells and then process donor antigen for redisplay to the recipient immune system. Donor cells, cell fragments, or soluble donor antigens are engulfed and degraded within lysozymes of the recipient APCs. Small peptide fragments corresponding to the alloantigenic region of donor HLA are then deposited in the peptide-binding groove of Class II structures on recipient APCs (Figure 24.4).[36] Recipient T and B cells then interact with recipient APCs in an MHC-restricted manner and respond to the donor peptide antigens displayed by the APCs. Recipient helper T-cell receptor-mediated recognition of this complex results in elaboration of cytokines by the donor APC (IL1 and IL12), which in turn results in APC surface expression of CD80 and CD86. These molecules bind to CD28, the central costimulatory molecule on helper T cells. T cells are further activated and elaborate cytokines such as CD40 ligand, IL4, IL5, and IL10, which provide the critical help to B lymphocytes for their proliferation and antibody production.[35] Ultraviolet-B (UVB) irradiation of APCs disrupts costimulatory signals[33] and thus may account for the effectiveness of this method for reducing the rate of HLA alloimmunization observed in

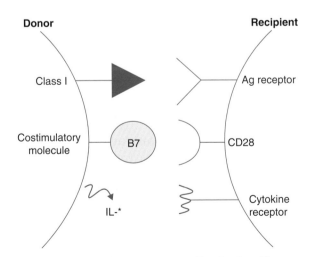

Figure 24.2 Direct HLA alloimmunization to Class I antigen. The recipient cell directly recognizes the foreign Class I provided that a second costimulatory molecule also is expressed and provided that the appropriate cytokine is locally present. Ag, antigen; IL, interleukin.

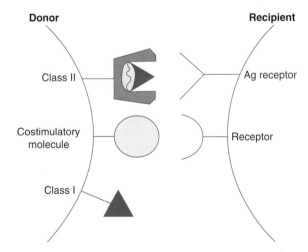

Figure 24.3 Direct HLA alloimmunization to Class I antigen. The donor cell carries a fragment of its Class I molecule within the peptide-binding groove of its own Class II molecule. This model, suggested by Dzik, provides one hypothesis to explain the frequency with which transfusion of unmodified cellular components results in antibodies to HLA Class I. Ag, antigen.

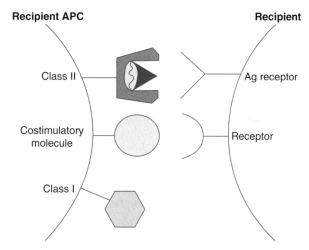

Recipient APC

Class II

Costimulatory
molecule

Class I

Recipient

Ag receptor

Receptor

Figure 24.4 Indirect HLA alloimmunization to Class I antigen. Recipient antigen-presenting cells (APCs) have digested donor cells or cell fragments and deposited a fragment of donor Class I antigen in the peptide-binding groove of the recipient Class II molecule.

a large clinical trial.[37] Indirect immune recognition is unlikely to account for the initial response in an in vitro mixed leukocyte reaction. However, the indirect pathway may be particularly relevant for alloimmune responses observed in vivo after transfusion.[35] In addition, the indirect pathway may account for experimental evidence in favor of alloimmunization by donor cell microparticles.

There are many clinical studies that have investigated primary and secondary HLA immunization in patients receiving leukocyte-depleted cellular blood components or not. Although the studies vary substantially in study design, including different levels of leukocyte depletion, meta-analysis has identified a reduction in alloimmunization with leukocyte reduction for patients with hematologic malignant disease.[38,39] The Trial to Reduce Alloimmunization to Platelet (TRAP) study group published a large randomized clinical study in 1997.[37] The 530 patients undergoing initial therapy for acute leukemia were randomly assigned to one of four arms—whole blood–derived platelets (control), LR whole blood–derived platelets, LR apheresis platelets, and UVB-irradiated pooled platelets. All red cell components were LR. Patients were evaluated for eight weeks. The main finding was a significant reduction in cytotoxic HLA antibodies in patients receiving platelet concentrates with leukocyte reduction by filtration or apheresis technology and platelet concentrates that were UVB irradiated compared with the standard product. However, this study highlights two important issues: In many patients, the cytotoxic antibodies did not cause platelet refractoriness—and there was no benefit of leukocyte reduction concerning clinical outcomes. In a large randomized study (the Viral Activation Transfusion Study), 531 patients were randomized to receive LR red cell concentrates or standard concentrates. The endpoint in this study was not HLA-antibody formation, but although a significant proportion of the patients also received platelet transfusions, there was no benefit from leukocyte reduction.[40] Thus, the conclusions in a Dutch review paper on clinical effects of leukocyte reduction of blood transfusion seem well founded: Leukocyte reduction of platelet concentrates leads to significant reduction in HLA antibodies, but a similar effect is not found for leukocyte reduction of red cell concentrates—and the alloimmunization rate against red cell antigens is not influenced.[11]

Will leukocyte reduction prevent secondary alloimmunization?

Because a secondary or anamnestic immune response requires a far smaller antigenic challenge than does a primary response, the secondary antibody recall to MHC antigens is difficult to prevent with LR blood components. The issue of secondary alloimmunization was directly addressed in the study by Sintnicolaas et al.[41] Female patients ($n = 75$) with hematologic malignant disease and a history of previous pregnancy were randomly assigned to receive platelet concentrate support with either unmodified or LR apheresis platelet concentrates. Among the evaluable patients, HLA alloimmunization developed in 43% (9 of 21) of the standard platelet concentrate group and in 44% (11 of 25) of the filtration group. Refractoriness occurred in 41% (14 of 34) of women in the standard platelet concentrate group and in 29% (8 of 28) of the filtration group ($p = 0.52$). The time to development of refractoriness was similar in the two groups. The authors concluded that leukocyte reduction to less than 5×10^6 WBCs per transfusion did not prevent alloimmunization and refractoriness among previously sensitized recipients.

In the TRAP study, however, analysis of patients who had been pregnant showed some benefit, albeit decreased, from the use of LR blood. In that study, 62% of patients with a history of pregnancy had HLA alloantibodies after transfusion of routine components; 33% did so after transfusion of LR components. Seftel et al.[42] analyzed 106 women with hematologic malignancy and a history of pregnancy treated before and after the introduction of ULR in Canada. They found that leukocyte reduction did not significantly change the rate of alloimmunization (15% vs. 10%) or platelet refractoriness (11% vs. 9%), although the surprisingly low rate of alloimmunization in control patients may have accounted for the lack of observed benefit of leukocyte reduction. However, when previous transfusion was studied as an immunizing event, leukocyte reduction was highly effective in reducing the rate of alloimmunization (29% vs. 2%). Thus, it appears that patients with hematologic malignant disease and a history of exposure to foreign HLA antigens from a previous pregnancy derive diminished benefit from the use of LR components.

Whether leukocyte reduction reduces alloimmuzation to platelet-specific antigens or red cell antigens is unclear. In the Canadian study that concluded that ULR reduces alloimmunization and refractoriness, platelet-specific antibodies were not included.[42] Concerning red cell alloimmunization, a retrospective cohort study by Blumberg et al. reported a significant decrease in alloimmunization in acute myeloid leukemia patients.[43] In a Dutch study, these results could not be reproduced,[44] but this study was related to universal leukocyte reduction, and the "nonfiltered" units were buffy coat-depleted.

Nonhemolytic febrile transfusion reactions

The nonhemolytic febrile transfusion reaction is the most common transfusion reaction as reported from many hemovigilance systems. The febrile transfusion reaction involves patient antibodies reacting with donor lymphocytes, causing release of cytokines from the donor cells, inflammatory cytokines released from recipient cells in response to antigen–antibody complex formation, and passive transfer of cytokines accumulated in the blood component. Among the cytokines involved are IL1β, IL6, IL8, TNFα, and CD40 L.[11]

Given these mechanisms, it seems obvious that the febrile transfusion reactions should be reduced by leukocyte reduction, especially if the filtration is performed prestorage.

Several clinical trials have confirmed that prestorage leukocyte reduction is effective in reducing the rate of FNHTRs to red cells by approximately 50%, with residual rates well below 1%.

A major disadvantage is the small number of randomized clinical trials evaluating effects of leukocyte reduction. Another difficulty is that the components investigated in the studies differ (e.g., it is probable that the leukocyte reduction obtained by buffy coat removal by itself reduces febrile reactions compared with standard cellular concentrates). In their review article, Bilgin et al.[11] accordingly refer to large "before and after universal leukocyte reduction" observational studies from the United States (35,000 RBC transfusions) and Canada (140,000 RBC transfusions and 57,000 platelet transfusions) to conclude that the number of febrile transfusion reactions is reduced by over 50%—provided prestorage leukocyte reduction is performed. Studies based on bedside filtration do not show the same effects, and these studies also contributed to the discontinuation of this procedure.[45,46]

Immunomodulation

For many years, it has been known that exposure of large amounts of allogeneic cells may lead to hyporesponsiveness as easy as antibody formation.[47] Studies on effects of allogeneic transfusions have led to the term *transfusion-related immunomodulation* (TRIM). Originally, the effects were described as beneficial—such as increased renal transplant survival. Later, deleterious effects have been attributed to TRIM—like increased recurrence rate of malignancies, increased rate of postoperative bacterial infections, and increased short-term mortality.[48] The mechanisms behind TRIM are complex, and the effects may be mediated by allogeneic mononuclear cells, leukocyte-derived soluble mediators, and soluble HLA peptides.[48]

Clinical studies on immunomodulation
Posttransfusion infection
Several randomized controlled trials (RCTs) have been performed to examine postoperative infection rates among recipients of LR or non-LR blood. These studies have provided conflicting results; some show benefits of leukocyte reduction, and others do not. An "intention to treat" meta-analysis of eight studies (excluding the report of Van Hilten et al.[50]) indicated that there was no significant TRIM effect.[49] However, when the three cardiac surgery studies were analyzed separately, a statistically significant TRIM effect was observed with a summary odds ratio (OR) of 1.39 (95% CI, 1.08–1.80), indicating that cardiac surgery patients transfused with non-LR components had a 39% higher risk of postoperative infection. A subsequent meta-analysis of these eight studies and the additional RCT by van Hilten[50] included only those patients who were *actually transfused* and found a statistically significant ($p = 0.005$) OR of 0.52 across all studies, indicating a nearly 50% reduction in the risk of postoperative infection associated with the use of LR components.[51] Subset analysis indicated that the three studies in patients undergoing cardiac surgery were the primary contributors to the overall statistical significance. One limitation of these meta-analyses is that the studies differed in the type of component assigned to the non-LR control with some using standard red cells and others using buffy-coat-depleted red cells. Overall, however, these data increasingly suggest a beneficial role of LR blood in reducing the risk of postoperative infections, particularly in patients undergoing cardiac surgery.

Pretransplantation blood transfusion
Several lines of evidence have suggested that recipient exposure to donor WBCs can result in improved survival of subsequent renal transplants. For example, the original studies of Opelz and Terasaki[52] showed that the use of frozen-deglycerolized (and thus LR) blood did not protect against rejection of renal transplants as well as did other RBC preparations. In 1993, a prospective, double-blind, randomized trial showed that patients given postoperative transfusions of non-LR fresh RBCs had better renal allograft survival than did patients given frozen deglycerolized RBCs.[53] Because cyclosporine and tacrolimus have become widely adopted as immunosuppressive agents for organ transplantation, the contribution of transfusion to graft survival has declined. Because the risk of HLA alloimmunization associated with using leukocyte-rich blood components outweighs any benefit from potential immune tolerance, LR components are indicated for organ transplant candidates.

Morbidity and mortality after surgery
LR blood components have been reported to be associated with improved patient outcomes, specifically reduced mortality and/or hospital length of stay unrelated to postoperative infection. This effect has been primarily studied in cardiac surgery patients. A prospective study of three serial periods of transfusion strategies in cardiac surgery patients using non-LR components, LR components, and then non-LR components showed that hospital length of stay declined from 10.1 to 9.5 days with the use of LR components and then returned to 10.8 days with the reintroduction of non-LR components. There was no change in length of stay in control patients who did not require transfusions.[54] A meta-analysis of three RCTs studying LR components in cardiac surgery showed that leukocyte reduction was associated with reduced mortality as well as a reduced risk of postoperative infection.[55] Later, numerous publications indicated a significant benefit of LR components for patients undergoing cardiac surgery, with a short-term mortality reduction of up to 50%.[26] Although the explanations for the beneficial effects may be complex, these data provide convincing evidence in support of the use of LR components in patients undergoing cardiac surgery.

Transfusion-associated graft-versus-host disease
TA-GVHD results from clonal expansion of allogeneic donor leukocytes (see Chapter 54). Patients who experience TA-GVHD either do not eliminate donor leukocytes because of severe immunosuppression or do not recognize donor cells as foreign because of HLA similarity between the donor and recipient. The threshold number of donor leukocytes required to provoke human TA-GVHD cannot be determined and likely varies among different donor–recipient pairs. Because TA-GVHD depends on recipient exposure to viable allogeneic donor leukocytes, it might be anticipated that sufficient leukocyte reduction would reduce the risk of TA-GVHD. However, there are no conclusive clinical data to support this notion,[56] and TA-GVHD has been reported among isolated patients who received transfusion of LR blood components.[57] Therefore, γ-irradiation is a necessary means to prevent TA-GVHD. The pathogen reduction technologies available for platelet concentrates disable leukocyte DNA replication, and these technologies therefore also protect efficiently against TA-GVHD.[58]

Transmission of CMV infection
When it became known that deadly CMV infection in premature children and immunosuppressed patients could be related to transmission from blood donors, this became a major driving force for

leukocyte reduction of cellular blood components.[59] After CMV infection, the virus is lifelong present in mononuclear lymphocytes.

Studies were performed to document the effectiveness of leukocyte depletion to prevent CMV transmission to at-risk neonates. Gilbert et al.[60] conducted a prospective, randomized, blinded trial in which 515 newborns were randomly assigned to receive transfusion support with either unmodified RBCs or RBCs filtered through an IG500 (Terumo Corporation) filter capable of 1–1.5 log leukocyte removal. In the control arm, 29 infants weighed less than 1500 g, and CMV infection developed in nine (33%). In the filtration arm, among 24 neonates weighing less than 1500 g who were CMV seronegative and received CMV-seropositive filtered blood, none acquired CMV infection. In another study, Eisenfield et al.[61] used less advanced filtration technology and documented prevention of CMV transmission to at-risk neonates. In contrast, Ohto et al.[62] performed a prospective randomized study of LR blood components in 52 newborn infants, of whom 43 weighed <1500 g. There was no effect of leukocyte reduction on the rate of CMV infection; however, the geographic region in Japan where this study was conducted had a high rate of CMV among the mothers (89%) and the blood donors (89%), and, importantly, CMV infection likely was due to breastfeeding by mothers secreting the virus into their milk—an observation made by others.[63]

As patients undergoing cytotherapy for hematological malignancies and bone marrow transplantation are severely immunosuppressed, it is important to clarify if leukocyte reduction of cellular blood components transfused to these patients is sufficient to protect against CMV infection. Bowden et al.[64] conducted a large, randomized, prospective trial with CMV-negative patients who received transplants of CMV-negative marrow. The investigators compared support with CMV-seronegative blood with support with filtered blood from untested donors. They randomly assigned 502 CMV-seronegative patients undergoing autologous or allogeneic marrow transplantation to two treatment groups. Among 252 patients receiving CMV-seronegative blood components, two had CMV infection; none had CMV disease. Among 250 patients receiving filtered CMV-untested components, three CMV infections (three with CMV disease) were observed. Two additional CMV infections in the seronegative group and three in the filtration group occurred within 21 days of entrance to the study and were considered the result of transfusions before enrollment. The survival rate was equal in the two study arms.

Because current filters are considerably more effective at leukocyte reduction than were those used in the published studies, most centers use leukocyte reduction as the only preventive measure against CMV infection, and this policy is supported by several recent studies.[65–67] As there is a relatively high "seroconversion rate" in the donor population, the collection of blood from donors with negative test results for antibodies to CMV is not completely safe. Sensitive polymerase chain reaction (PCR) techniques are needed to demonstrate the CMV genome in the blood of seropositive healthy donors. Studies on blood from infected donors showed that the CMV PCR signal is lost or greatly reduced when blood was leukocyte reduced by means of filtration or apheresis processing. However, as the use of CMV-seronegative donors or leukocyte reduction does not completely eliminate the risk of CMV infection, the term *reduction of risk* should be used—as in *leukocyte reduction* and *pathogen reduction technologies*.[68]

Another concern is that transfusion of donor leukocytes could reactivate endogenous viral infection. The clinical relevance of these observations was specifically addressed in a large, multicenter RCT—the Viral Activation by Transfusion Study (VATS). The study was conducted to evaluate the ability of LR blood to prevent either HIV or CMV activation among a cohort of patients with HIV infection undergoing therapy for the infection. The study showed no beneficial effect of leukocyte reduction for prevention of early death, virus activation, or time to first infection-related complication.[40]

Vamvakas has published a systematic review of studies related to bone marrow recipients, and the conclusion was that both CMV screening of the donors and leukocyte reduction of the components reduced the transfusion-associated infection rate by 92–93%.[69] Based on the clinical data available, leukocyte reduction alone seems to be the most practical and economical method for prevention of CMV infection.[70] CMV-antibody testing is of uncertain value, sensitive PCR techniques are expensive, and the testing may delay the transfusions.

Transfusion-related acute lung injury (TRALI)

TRALI is an acute, immune-mediated transfusion reaction characterized by dyspnea, hypoxia, pulmonary edema, low pulmonary capillary wedge pressure, and alveolar infiltrates on chest radiographs (see Chapter 59). Two different mechanisms may contribute to the development of TRALI. First, results of serologic investigations suggest that TRALI occurs when donor plasma contains antibodies reactive against the recipient's HLA type or against recipient non-HLA leukocyte antigens. Some have postulated that TRALI may result when recipient leukocyte antibodies react with residual donor leukocytes, although solid evidence is lacking. However, an FNHTR reaction is more common in this setting. A second mechanism proposes a two-hit model involving lipid agents in donor blood that prime recipient neutrophils in the presence of specific cytokine activation. Thus, leukocyte reduction is not expected to play an important role in the prevention of TRALI. However, in a large "before-and-after" study of acute transfusion reactions, Blumberg et al. found an 83% reduction in TRALI after ULR (2.8 cases per 100,000 components vs. 0.48 after ULR).[71]

Bacterial overgrowth

It is unlikely that prestorage removal of leukocytes would have any measurable effect on the incidence of bacterial overgrowth in blood components. The mechanisms by which leukocyte reduction filters may deplete blood components of low levels of contaminating bacteria have been reviewed. In a European multicenter study, Seghatchian et al. found that leukocyte reduction was not effective to protect against bacterial contamination of cellular components, even if the filtration process were postponed for eight hours to allow for phagocytosis.[72] Because bacterial overgrowth is infrequent, a clinical study would require an enormous number of observations. The hemovigilance network in France reported an analysis of reported cases of bacterial sepsis before and after introduction of ULR. The study found that bacterial sepsis decreased from 3.8% to 1.7% ($p < 0.001$) of all reported adverse events.[73]

Cost-effectiveness of leukocyte reduction

Since the 1990s, there has been a substantial debate about whether leukocyte reduction should be implemented as a universal measure (ULR) or if leukocyte reduction of cellular blood components should be reserved for special clinical indications. In many Western countries, the ULR approach has been implemented.[2] In economically poorer countries, the cost of the procedures has made ULR completely irrelevant.

The main disadvantage of the leukocyte reduction procedure is, accordingly, the cost. The filter and processing costs will differ, but reasonable ranges are US$20–40 and EUR 20–35 per unit. The literature on cost-effectiveness is very heterogeneous. In a review paper on estimating the cost of blood, Shander et al. have found that the cost per quality-adjusted life years (QALYs) ranges from US $2470 if the risk is high (1.85 relative risk) to US$3.4 million if there is no infection risk.[74] In 1995, Blumberg et al. conducted a cost study on transfusion of LR red cell concentrates in a patient population with malignant diseases, and reported a "significant cost reduction" due to leukocyte filtration.[75] A study on the cost-effectiveness of leukoreduction for prevention of febrile nonhemolytic transfusion reactions (REFs) concluded that the cost per prevented FNHTR was EUR 6916.[76] In a review of blood transfusion practices in Spain 1997–2007, Garcia-Erce et al.[77] concluded against ULR, "which has led to an incremental cost for unknown, but probably slight, benefits for patients."

Despite the uncertainties concerning the cost-effectiveness issue, the trend is in favor of ULR in economically wealthy countries. In Europe, the blood directive is focusing on maximal patient safety, and this leukocyte reduction is regarded by many as a step to achieve this goal. In the United States, the trend is that the larger hospitals support ULR. Canada has implemented ULR; a publication based on retrospective data reported significantly reduced in-hospital mortality and suggested that one life was saved for every 120 patients who received LR blood compared with standard blood components.[78]

In the less economic-rich countries, ULR is not implemented. A paper from India[79] concludes that despite the advantages of leukocyte reduction, it is not practically feasible to implement this policy in developing countries and other underresourced nations.

Summary

The majority of cellular blood components transfused in the Western world are leukocyte reduced. High-performance blood filters and low-leukocyte apheresis devices have made LR components available to all transfusion facilities. The technology represents an important advance in the preparation of blood components. Several European nations and Canada have adopted ULR of the blood supply. However, leukocyte reduction represents a large increase of cost in blood component production. Although experimental data point to many possible advantages for the patients, the clinically proven beneficial indications for LR are relatively few. Because ULR already is so widespread, it is possible that the desired, large randomized control studies to evaluate the full clinical picture of leukocyte reduction of cellular blood components will never be conducted. For blood component production in developing countries and other underresourced nations, buffy coat removal or similar leukocyte reduction steps could provide a good and cheap alternative to reduce donor-leukocyte-associated transfusion complications.

Acknowledgments

We highly appreciate the work of Darrel J. Triulzi and Walter H. Dzik, the earlier authors of this chapter. Their extensive literature research is still valid, and our main goals have been to adjust the chapter to a smaller format and to add references that provide additional information.

Key references

A full reference list for this chapter is available at: http://www.wiley.com/go/simon/transfusion

2 Bassuni WY, Blajchman MA, Al-Moshary MA. Why implement universal leukoreduction? *Hematol Oncol Stem Cell Ther* 2008; **1** (2): 106–23.

11 Bilgin YM, van de Watering LM, Brand A. Clinical effects of leucoreduction of blood transfusions. *Neth J Med* 2011; **69** (10): 441–50.

26 van de Watering LM, et al. Beneficial effects of leukocyte depletion of transfused blood on postoperative complications in patients undergoing cardiac surgery: a randomized clinical trial. *Circulation* 1998; **97** (6): 562–8.

27 Williamson LM, et al. Bedside filtration of blood products in the prevention of HLA alloimmunization—a prospective randomized study. Alloimmunisation Study Group. *Blood* 1994; **83** (10): 3028–35.

31 Dumont LJ, et al. Practical guidelines for process validation and process control of white cell-reduced blood components: report of the Biomedical Excellence for Safer Transfusion (BEST) Working Party of the International Society of Blood Transfusion (ISBT). *Transfusion* 1996; **36** (1): 11–20.

37 Leukocyte reduction and ultraviolet B irradiation of platelets to prevent alloimmunization and refractoriness to platelet transfusions. The Trial to Reduce Alloimmunization to Platelets Study Group. *N Engl J Med* 1997; **337** (26): 1861–9.

72 Seghatchian J. Universal leucodepletion: an overview of some unresolved issues and the highlights of lessons learned. *Transfus Apher Sci* 2003; **29** (2): 105–17.

CHAPTER 25

Composition of plasma

Peter Hellstern

Institute of Hemostaseology and Transfusion Medicine, Academic City Hospital, Ludwigshafen, Germany

The first part of this chapter describes the composition of plasma, focusing on those protein components that are important for treatment with plasma or its derivatives. The second part addresses individual factors influencing plasma levels of therapeutic plasma proteins. The regulation of blood coagulation and fibrinolysis and clinically useful blood coagulation and fibrinolysis screening tests are then discussed.

Plasma composition

Plasma is the cell-free part of blood composed of water, proteins, electrolytes, lipids, and carbohydrates. It is the transportation medium through which nutrients, hormones, waste products, and drugs are transported through the body. In vivo, the fluidity of plasma is maintained through complex interactions between its procoagulant and anticoagulant proteins and between these proteins, circulating blood cells, and the endothelium. Coagulation activation in plasma is prevented and its fluidity maintained in vitro by the addition of anticoagulants. Citrate is presently the only anticoagulant used for collecting therapeutic plasma and plasma for fractionation, the starting material for the manufacture of plasma protein concentrates. Although proteomics based on two-dimensional gel electrophoresis and mass spectrometry has revealed about 10,000 different human plasma proteins,[1,2] the number of constituents important for transfusion medicine is small, comprising albumin, immunoglobulins G (IgG) and M (IgM), alpha-$_1$-antitrypsin, C1 inhibitor, von Willebrand factor (vWF), vWF-cleaving protease, blood coagulation factors, and the blood coagulation inhibitors antithrombin (AT) and protein C. The plasma levels and biological half-lives of these plasma proteins are subject to large interindividual variation. Plasma is either prepared from citrate–phosphate–dextrose-anticoagulated whole blood units or collected by automated plasmapheresis. As a consequence of lower final citrate concentrations and lower dilution due to lower anticoagulant-to-blood ratios, apheresis plasma contains higher concentrations of clotting factors V, VIII, IX, and XI than plasma from whole blood.[3,4] A dilution of 1:7 to 1:9 for plasma from whole blood and of 1:16 for apheresis plasma has to be considered when plasma protein concentrations are given that are related to circulating undiluted plasma. IgG levels in plasma from whole blood are significantly greater than in apheresis plasma because of a decrease in IgG when individuals donate apheresis plasma repeatedly at short intervals.[4,5]

Albumin

Albumin is a 66.4-kD protein synthesized in the liver. Considering a total plasma volume of 3 L, about 120–140 g or 40% of the total body content of albumin circulates in the plasma at concentrations between 35 and 50 g/L (Table 25.1), which is more than 50% of the total plasma protein concentration, ranging from 64 to 88 g/L. The albumin concentration in the interstitial space of 10–12 L is about 14 g/L. The intravascular albumin compartment is responsible for 80% of plasma oncotic pressure, thus mainly contributing to maintaining blood volume. An intact liver synthesizes 12 g of albumin per day. In a steady state, the same amount of albumin is eliminated per day. The biological half-life of albumin in plasma is 17–20 days. Compensatory reduction of albumin metabolism occurs when plasma levels decrease because of reduced synthesis in the liver or capillary leakage.[6] A marked acquired hypoalbuminemia is a nonspecific marker of severe illness and strongly indicates poor prognosis.[7,8]

The functions of albumin are as follows:

- Maintenance of the intravascular oncotic pressure;
- Binding and transportation of drugs, vitamins, minerals, bilirubin, uric acid, hormones, amino acids, and fatty acids; and
- Binding of toxic metabolites, among them free fatty acids, and radical scavenging.

Despite all of these important functions of albumin, it is remarkable that congenital analbuminemia causes only mild clinical symptoms (e.g., hypotension or discrete pretibial edema at all ages) or no symptoms at all.[9]

Commercially available albumin preparations are obtained from plasma fractionation, according to Cohn and Oncley[10] or Kistler and Nitschmann,[11] as fraction V and are subsequently pasteurized for virus inactivation.[12] These solutions contain either 3.5–5% or 20–25% (w/v) albumin at a purity of 95–98%. Albumin is also added to many drugs and plasma protein concentrates to stabilize the respective active ingredients.

Rossi's Principles of Transfusion Medicine, Fifth Edition. Edited by Toby L. Simon, Jeffrey McCullough, Edward L. Snyder, Bjarte G. Solheim, and Ronald G. Strauss.
© 2016 John Wiley & Sons, Ltd. Published 2016 by John Wiley & Sons, Ltd.

Table 25.1 Therapeutic plasma proteins: albumin, immunoglobulins, Alpha-$_1$-Antitrypsin, and C1 inhibitor

Plasma Protein	Plasma Concentration	Biological Half-Life	Main Functions
Albumin	35–50 g/L	17–20 days	Maintenance of intravascular oncotic pressure; transportation protein; radical scavenger
Immunoglobulin G	6–17 g/L	23 days	Humoral immunity
Immunoglobulin M	0.5–2.5 g/L	5 days	Humoral immunity
Alpha-$_1$-antitrypsin	1.5–3.0 g/L	4–7 days	Inhibits neutrophil elastase
C1 inhibitor	0.2–0.3 g/L	30–60 hours	Inhibits complement C1 activation

Plasma concentrations represent the 5th and 95th percentiles; biological half-lives represent the means or the 5th and 95th percentiles of elimination half-lives.

Immunoglobulins G and M

IgG and IgM are glycoproteins synthesized in plasma cells and circulating in plasma at concentrations between 6 and 17 g/L and between 0.5 and 2.5 g/L, respectively. The molecular weights are 150 kD for IgG and 971 kD for IgM, and the half-lives are about 23 and 5 days, respectively.

Polyvalent intravenous immunoglobulin (IVIG) preparations can also be administered subcutaneously and are prepared from fraction II during plasma fractionation.[12] Current virus inactivation and elimination procedures are low pH incubation, pasteurization, solvent–detergent treatment, caprylic acid treatment, and nanofiltration. Although most IVIG preparations are primarily IgG with only trace amounts of other immunoglobulin isotypes, some IgM-enriched IVIGs contain up to 15% IgM and have been used for treatment of severe sepsis and septic shock.[13]

Hyperimmune immunoglobulin preparations are obtained from the plasma of actively immunized donors using ethanol fractionation or chromatography.[12] They can be administered intravenously or intramuscularly and are used to prevent postexposure infections, intoxication by tetanus toxoid, and immunization to Rh-positive red cells. For more details, see Chapter 29.

Alpha-$_1$-antitrypsin

Alpha-$_1$-antitrypsin synthesized in the liver is the most abundant serine protease inhibitor (serpin) in plasma. It inhibits a variety of serine proteases of which neutrophil elastase is the most important target. The molecular weight is 52 kD, the plasma concentration is 1.5–3 g/L, and the half-life is 4–7 days.[14,15] Hereditary alpha-$_1$-antitrypsin deficiency resulting in plasma levels lower than 0.8 g/L occurs at a prevalence between 1 in 1,600 and 1 in 5,000.[16] It is associated with lung emphysema and liver disease in childhood. Plasma-derived alpha-$_1$-antitrypsin concentrates are indicated for treatment of patients with emphysema secondary to congenital deficiency.

C1 inhibitor

C1 inhibitor is a 105-kD serpin synthesized in the liver. The plasma concentration is 0.24 g/L, and the half-life ranges from 30 to 60 hours.[17,18] C1 inhibitor affects early activation of the classical complement pathway by blocking activated C1 and subsequent C2,4 complex formations.[19] It also inhibits activated factors XI and XII and plasmin, and the formation of factor XIa, kallikrein, and bradykinin.

An inherited or acquired deficiency of C1 inhibitor may cause angioedema, which is characterized by subcutaneous or mucosal swelling in any part of the skin or the respiratory and gastrointestinal tracts.[19] The prevalence of hereditary angioedema is from 1 in 10,000 to 1 in 50,000. C1 inhibitor concentrates purified by chromatography from the cryoprecipitate-reduced plasma produced during plasma fractionation are used successfully for the treatment of acute attacks of angioedema or for prophylaxis before surgery.[17,20]

von Willebrand factor–cleaving protease

The vWF-cleaving protease (a disintegrin and metalloprotease with a thrombospondin type 1 motif, member 13, ADAMTS13) is a 70-kD protein[21] expressed in the liver, platelets, and other tissues,[22,23] and circulates in plasma at concentrations between 0.7 and 1.3 mg/L.[24] The elimination half-life is 2–3 days.[25] The plasma enzyme cleaves the A2-domain of vWF. A defective cleaving protease results in unusually large vWF multimers, which are associated with thrombotic thrombocytopenic purpura (TTP). Therapeutic plasma contains normal vWF-cleaving protease activities and is effective for treatment of TTP through therapeutic plasma exchange.[26,27]

Clotting factors, coagulation factor inhibitors, and von Willebrand factor

The coagulation proteins discussed here are responsible for normal hemostasis (Table 25.2). Except for factor V, virus-inactivated plasma-derived concentrates have been developed for preventing or treating bleeding caused by hereditary or acquired vWF or any clotting factor deficiency states.[12] Antithrombin and protein C concentrates are also available and are used mainly for prophylaxis or treatment of thromboembolic complications in patients with hereditary deficiency of the respective blood coagulation inhibitor.[12] Because not all clotting factor and inhibitor concentrates are available in all developed countries, factor V deficiency, for which a concentrate has not yet been produced, and other clotting factor deficiency states (e.g., factor XI deficiency) are alternatively treated with plasma.[28]

Fibrinogen is the precursor of fibrin. Thrombin converts fibrinogen into fibrin monomers by cleaving fibrinopeptides A and B. Fibrin monomers polymerize to form an unstable fibrin clot, which is stabilized by factor XIIIa–induced cross-linkage. Fibrinogen is also necessary for supporting platelet function. Prothrombin (factor II); clotting factors VII, IX, X, and XI; and protein C are proenzymes of respective serine proteases. After activation by thrombin, factor V accelerates activation of prothrombin, factor VIII, and factor X. Factor XIII is activated by thrombin to form a transglutaminase, which stabilizes fibrin clots by cross-linkage. vWF is essential for platelet–subendothelium adhesion and platelet aggregation, and for transportation of factor VIII in plasma. vWF protects factor VIII from early proteolysis. Antithrombin is a stoichiometric serpin that strongly inhibits thrombin and factors IXa, Xa, and XIa. Once activated by thrombin–thrombomodulin, activated protein C inhibits factors Va and VIIIa.

Most clotting factors, AT, and protein C are synthesized in the liver. Other sites of protein expression are megakaryocytes and endothelial cells for factor V and for the α-chain of factor XIII. vWF is synthesized in megakaryocytes and endothelial cells.

Table 25.2 Clotting factors, von Willebrand factor, antithrombin, and protein C

Plasma Protein	MW (kD)	Plasma Concentration (mg/L)	Plasma Activity (U/dL)	Half-Life (Hours)	Main Functions	Replacement by Plasma-Derived Concentrates[12] or Plasma
Fibrinogen	340	2.5 g/L	1.5–4 g/L[28]	96[28]	Clot formation, precursor of fibrin; supports platelet function	Fibrinogen concentrate, cryoprecipitate, plasma; locally, fibrin sealant[29]
Factor II	72	150[30]	70–130	60[31,32]	Proenzyme of thrombin	Prothrombin complex concentrates (PCCs), plasma[28,31]
Factor V	330	7[33,34]	70–125	12[35]	Cofactor of prothrombin activation by factor Xa	Plasma[28]
Factor VII	50	1[36]	70–150	5[31,27]	Proenzyme of factor VIIa, which activates factor IX and factor X	Factor VII concentrates,[37] factor VII containing PCC
Factor VIII	330	0.15[38]	60–200	14[39]	Cofactor of factor X activation by factor IXa	Factor VIII concentrates, factor VIII/vWF concentrates
vWF	600–2 × 10^4	8[40]	50–180	12[41,42]	Platelet-subendothelium adhesion; platelet aggregation; transports factor VIII and protects it from proteolysis	Factor VIII/vWF concentrates, vWF concentrates
Factor IX	57	5[40]	60–140	30[39]	Proenzyme of factor IXa, which activates factor X	Factor IX concentrates
Factor X	59	10[40]	70–130	30[31]	Proenzyme of factor Xa, which activates prothrombin	PCC, plasma[28]
Factor XI	143	5[43]	65–130	50[44,45]	Proenzyme of factor XI, which activates factor IX	Plasma, factor XI concentrates[28,43]
Factor XIII	320	20[46]	60–220	170[28]	Proenzyme of factor XIIIa, which stabilizes fibrin by cross-linkage	Factor XIII concentrates
Antithrombin	58	150[47]	75–120	72[47]	Stoichiometric serpin, inactivates thrombin, factor IXa, factor Xa, and factor XIa	Antithrombin concentrates[48]
Protein C	62	44[40]	70–170	9[49]	Proenzyme of activated protein C, which inactivates factor Va and factor VIIIa	Protein C concentrates[50]

Plasma concentrations represent the means or medians; plasma activities represent the 5th and 95th percentiles; half-lives represent the mean or median elimination half-lives; PCC, prothrombin complex concentrate; vWF, von Willebrand factor.

The synthesis of functionally active prothrombin complex factors II, VII, IX, and X and protein C in the liver requires vitamin K–mediated gamma-glutamyl carboxylation. Impairment of carboxylation occurs in vitamin K deficiency, in the presence of vitamin K antagonists, and in some cases of liver dysfunction. This results in synthesis of functionally impaired or inactive prothrombin complex factors, called *proteins induced in vitamin K absence or antagonism* (PIVKA).

Factors influencing individual plasma composition

Age and gender
The physiologic aging process is accompanied by an increase in plasma levels of fibrinogen; factors V, VII, VIII, IX, XI, and XIII; protein C; and protein S in both genders.[51] A significant decrease of prothrombin activity levels with increasing age has been found in men but not in women.[52] Young women have significantly lower AT plasma levels than males of similar age. Because of a marked increase after menopause, AT levels in older women exceed levels in male contemporaries.[53] Gradually declining AT plasma levels have been observed in males older than 45 years.[53] Pregnancy is associated with marked increases in levels of fibrinogen, prothrombin, factors VII and VIII, vWF, and factor X, whereas factor V, factor IX, AT, and protein C levels are largely unchanged.[54]

ABO blood group
Individuals with blood groups O, A_2O, and A_2A_2 have on average about 20–25% lower factor VIII and vWF plasma levels when compared with other ABO blood group constellations.[55–57]

Acute phase reaction
An acute phase response caused by any trigger of inflammation results in an increase in plasma levels of alpha-1-antitrypsin, C1 inhibitor, fibrinogen, prothrombin, factor VIII, and vWF and a decrease of albumin levels.[58] Smoking causes a low-grade systemic inflammatory response and concomitant increases in plasma fibrinogen.[59–61]

Physical exercise and mental stress
Both acute severe physical exercise and acute mental stress cause increases in fibrinogen, factor VII, factor VIII, and vWF levels.[62–66] In contrast, prolonged severe physical exercise results in a decrease in factor VII levels, whereas fibrinogen levels continue to be increased during observation.[67]

Hormones
Danazol, a weak androgen, improves the synthesis of C1 inhibitor, factor VIII, AT, and protein C.[68] Combined oral contraceptives induce increases in plasma fibrinogen; prothrombin; factors VII, VIII, IX, X, and XI; alpha-1-antitrypsin; and protein C, whereas AT and protein S levels decrease.[69–71] Progestogen-only preparations lead to a decrease in factor VIII and an increase in protein S.[72]

Desmopressin (DDAVD)
DDAVP has been used successfully to increase factor VIII and vWF levels in plasma donors.[73,74] The yields of these plasma proteins were markedly improved when cryoprecipitate or factor VIII concentrates were produced from plasma collected after pretreatment of donors with DDAVP.

The influence of storage and freezing on plasma composition
Prolonged storage reduces factor VIII levels regardless of hold at 4 °C or at room temperature.[75,76] Storage at room temperature does,

however, affect protein S activity, which is substantially less when compared to hold at 4 °C. Slow freezing at −20 °C reduces factor VIII and protein S activities markedly in comparison to rapid freezing to a core temperature of below −30 °C within 1 hour.[76] Factor VIII levels decline by 24% even when fresh plasma samples are frozen in liquid nitrogen, stored at −70 °C, and thawed at 37 °C for 10 min.[77]

Regulation of blood coagulation and fibrinolysis

Hemostasis encompasses all processes of clot formation, clot lysis, and wound healing with the aim of maintaining vessel wall integrity. The mechanisms of hemostasis incorporate the vascular endothelium and subendothelium, platelets, leukocytes, red cells, pro- and anticoagulant, and pro- and antifibrinolytic proteins. Primary

hemostasis is characterized by the formation of a platelet plug at the site of vessel wall injury. vWF forms a bridge between platelets and vascular subendothelial structures and promotes platelet aggregation. Secondary hemostasis is achieved by formation of a stable fibrin clot, followed by fibrinolysis and tissue repair. Abnormal bleeding can result from impaired thrombin generation, clot formation, and clot stabilization, or hyperfibrinolysis. Conversely, increased coagulation and diminished fibrinolysis may provoke thrombosis.

Previous models have suggested two independent pathways of coagulation activation, via the intrinsic and extrinsic cascades. But it is now recognized that the generation or exposure of tissue factor (TF) at the site of vessel injury is the first physiologic step in initiating blood coagulation.[78] There are three closely linked phases of coagulation, comprising the initiation, amplification, and propagation processes (Figure 25.1). Clotting is mainly controlled by

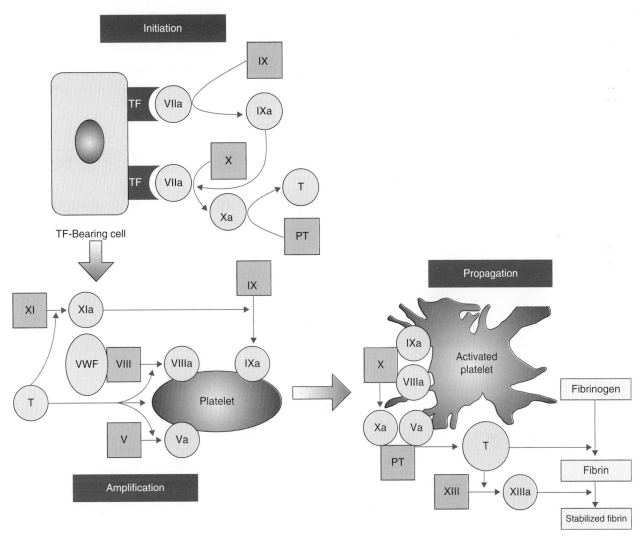

Figure 25.1 Cell-based model of coagulation activation. Inactive clotting factors are in squares, and active factors in circles. The coagulation cascade is initiated by tissue factor (TF) release at the sites of cell injury. During the initiation phase, TF complexes with factor VIIa (FVIIa) at the site of cell injury. TF–factor VIIa activates factor IX and factor X. Factor Xa generates small amounts of thrombin, which activates platelets, factor XI, and cofactors V and VIII, allowing multiple positive feedback loops during the amplification phase. The tenase complex (factor VIIIa–factor IXa) generates large amounts of factor Xa on the surface of activated platelets. The prothrombinase complex (factor Va–factor Xa) converts prothrombin to thrombin, which forms fibrin from fibrinogen and activates factor XIII. PT, prothrombin; T, thrombin; TF, tissue factor.

several circulating inhibitors. Activation of fibrinolysis results in fibrin cleavage by plasmin and subsequent restoration of vessel patency. The central role of thrombin in hemostasis by exerting both procoagulant and anticoagulant effects is illustrated in Figure 25.2.[79]

Initiation and amplification of coagulation

Clotting is initiated by TF–factor VIIa complexes after TF is exposed to the circulating blood by smooth muscle cells, fibroblasts, disrupted or activated endothelial cells, or activated monocytes (Figure 25.1). Circulating factor VIIa represents approximately 1% of total factor VII and can be generated from the inactive zymogen by an autocatalytic mechanism. Factor VIIa does not express its full procoagulant activity until it is bound to TF.[80] TF–factor VIIa activates factors IX and X, and factor Xa generates thrombin by activating prothrombin (*initiation phase*). These small amounts of thrombin ensure that coagulation activation and further thrombin formation are maintained (*amplification phase*). Thrombin activates factors V, VIII, and XI, and platelets that provide the surface on which the *propagation phase* of coagulation occurs.

Propagation of thrombin generation, fibrin clot formation, and fibrin stabilization

The *tenase complex* consisting of platelet membrane–bound factor IXa, factor VIIIa, and ionized calcium cleaves factor X much more effectively than TF–factor VIIa or factor IXa alone. Factor Xa binds to platelet surfaces and complexes with factor Va and calcium to form the *prothrombinase complex*, which rapidly generates large amounts of thrombin. Fibrin monomers resulting from thrombin-induced splitting of fibrinopeptides A and B from fibrinogen polymerize spontaneously to an unstable fibrin clot. Thrombin also activates factor XIII to the transglutaminase factor XIIIa, which stabilizes fibrin polymers by cross-linkage.[81]

Inhibition of blood coagulation and termination of clotting

Several circulating inhibitors terminate the coagulation process (Table 25.3). The stoichiometric heparin-binding serpin AT mainly inhibits thrombin and factor Xa and, less strongly, factors IXa and XIa.[47] Thrombin binds to endothelial thrombomodulin, and this complex activates protein C to the serine protease, activated protein C (APC).[82] Endothelial cell protein C receptor augments protein C activation by the thrombin–thrombomodulin complex. Together with its vitamin K–dependent cofactor protein S, APC inactivates factors Va and VIIIa. Tissue factor pathway inhibitor (TFPI) downregulates blood coagulation by forming a quaternary complex with TF–factor VIIa/factor Xa. Heparin cofactor II is a specific inhibitor of thrombin in the presence of dermatan sulfate or heparin.[47] The protein Z–dependent protease inhibitor is a serpin inhibiting factor Xa in the presence of the vitamin K–dependent protein Z, phospholipids, and calcium.[47] Protein C inhibitor, a heparin-binding serpin, predominantly inhibits APC and thrombin.[47]

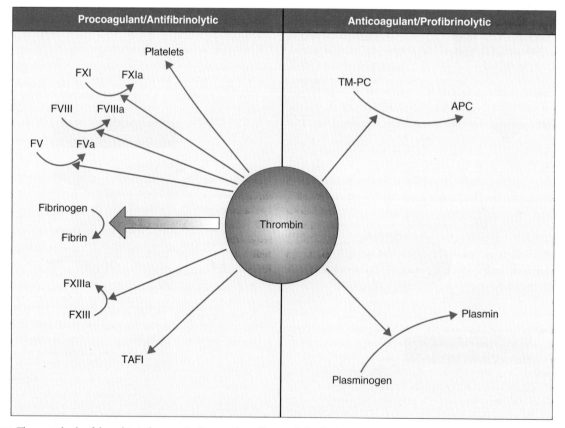

Figure 25.2 The central role of thrombin in hemostasis. Procoagulant effects include platelet activation; the activation of clotting factors V, VIII, XI, and XIII; and subsequent formation of a stable fibrin clot. Thrombin acts as an anticoagulant by activating protein C after complexing with thrombomodulin. It promotes fibrinolysis by activating plasminogen and inhibits fibrinolysis by activating TAFI. APC, activated protein C; F, factor; PC, protein C; TAFI, thrombin activatable fibrinolysis inhibitor; TM, thrombomodulin.

Table 25.3 Inhibitors of blood coagulation and their main functions

Plasma Protein	Main Functions
Antithrombin	Heparin-binding serpin; inhibits thrombin, factor Xa, factor IXa, and factor XIa
Protein C	Serine protease; inhibits factor Va and factor VIIIa
Protein S	Vitamin K–dependent glycoprotein; cofactor of activated protein C
Thrombomodulin	Endothelial cell-surface glycoprotein; complexes with thrombin and activates protein C
Endothelial cell protein C receptor	Endothelial cell-specific transmembrane protein; augments protein C activation
Tissue factor pathway inhibitor (TFPI)	Trivalent protease inhibitor; inhibits TF–factor VIIa by forming a quarternary complex of TFPI, TF, factor VIIa, and factor Xa
Heparin cofactor II	Dermatan sulfate-binding serpin; inhibits thrombin
Protein Z–dependent protease inhibitor	Serpin; inhibits factor Xa in the presence of protein Z

Fibrinolysis and its inhibition

The role of the fibrinolytic system is to restore vessel patency once wound healing has maintained vessel wall integrity (Figure 25.3). The serine protease plasmin cleaves fibrin (and fibrinogen) at multiple sites, resulting in fibrin and fibrinogen degradation products. Once tissue plasminogen activator (tPA) is released by endothelial cells, it is activated by plasmin, transforming from its single-chain form (sc-tPA) to its two-chain form (tc-tPA), both of which are able to activate plasminogen to plasmin. Two-chain urokinase plasminogen activator (tc-uPA; urokinase), which results from the activation of single-chain urokinase plasminogen activator (sc-uPA) synthesized in endothelial and kidney cells, also activates plasminogen to plasmin.[83] Along with plasmin and kallikrein, factor VII activating protease is another potent activator of sc-uPA.[84] Plasmin cleaves not only fibrin but also fibrinogen and other plasma proteins. Fibrin specificity of plasmin is achieved by binding of plasminogen and tPA to the lysine binding sites of fibrin. Both plasminogen activators are mainly inhibited by plasminogen

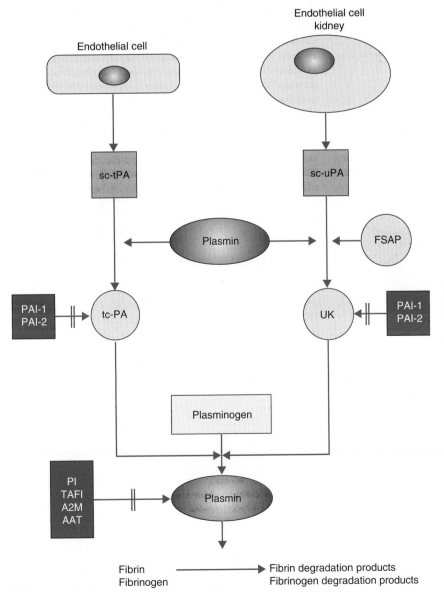

Figure 25.3 Activation of fibrinolysis. Endothelial cells release sc-tPA or sc-uPA, which are activated by plasmin to tc-tPA and tc-uPA (urokinase), respectively. sc-uPA can also be activated to urokinase by FSAP. Both activators are able to generate plasmin from plasminogen. Plasmin cleaves fibrin and fibrinogen to degradation products. tPA and urokinase are inhibited by PAI-1 and PAI-2 and plasmin by PI, A2M, and AAT. TAFI inhibits plasmin-induced cleavage of fibrin by removing lysine residues from fibrin. AAT, alpha-1-antitrypsin; A2M, alpha-2-macroglobulin; FSAP, factor VII activating protease; PAI-1, plasminogen activator inhibitor 1; PAI-2, plasminogen activator inhibitor 2; PI, plasmin inhibitor; ProUK, pro-urokinase; sc-tPA, single-chain tissue plasminogen activator; sc-uPA, single-chain urokinase plasminogen activator; TAFI, thrombin activatable fibrinolysis inhibitor; tc-tPA, two-chain tissue plasminogen activator; tc-uPA, two-chain urokinase plasminogen activator; UK, urokinase.

activator inhibitor type 1 (PAI-1) released from endothelial cells and platelets. Large amounts of plasminogen activator inhibitor type 2 (PAI-2) are synthesized in the placenta. Plasmin is predominantly inhibited by the very fast-acting plasmin inhibitor (alpha-2-antiplasmin) and to a lesser extent by alpha-2-macroglobulin. Plasmin inhibitor cross-linked to fibrin by factor XIIIa inhibits plasmin binding to fibrin. The thrombin-activatable fibrinolysis inhibitor (TAFI) is activated by thrombin–thrombomodulin complexes and protects clots from plasmin-induced degradation by removing lysine residues from fibrin.[85,86]

Clinically useful coagulation and fibrinolysis screening tests

Coagulation and fibrinolysis screening tests are used for detecting disorders of secondary hemostasis caused by coagulation factor deficiencies, dysfunctional coagulation factors, inhibitors against coagulation factors, anticoagulants, or hyperfibrinolysis. In addition to a detailed clinical history and examination and laboratory investigation of disorders of primary hemostasis, coagulation and fibrinolysis screening tests are included in approaches to bleeding patients and to exclusion of bleeding disorders before operations or other invasive procedures.[87] Further applications of these tests are as follows:

- Monitoring of anticoagulant therapy;
- Monitoring of treatment with fresh frozen plasma or clotting factor concentrates;
- Detection of lupus anticoagulants; and
- Detection of hypercoagulable states.

The historical division of coagulation activation and subsequent fibrin formation into an *intrinsic pathway* comprising surface-contact factors and an *extrinsic pathway* (TF–factor VIIa) can be used for a better understanding of blood coagulation screening tests (Figure 25.4). The intrinsic pathway begins with the activation of factor XII and prekallikrein at negatively charged artificial surfaces,

as found on activated platelets and endothelial cells and at subendothelial collagen. Factor XIIa activates factor XIa and further prekallikrein to kallikrein. Factor XIa and kallikrein accelerate factor XII activation through a positive feedback mechanism. Factor XII and factor XI activation is amplified by high-molecular-weight (HMW) kininogen. Factor XIa activates factor IX, and factor IXa activates factor X. The extrinsic pathway starts with the formation of the TF–factor VIIa complex, also resulting in production of factor Xa.

The common pathway begins with factor X activation, where the intrinsic and extrinsic pathways converge. Factor Xa converts prothrombin (factor II) to thrombin (factor IIa) in the presence of factor Va. Thrombin cleaves fibrin to form fibrin monomers, which polymerize spontaneously to an unstable fibrin clot.

Coagulation screening tests use fibrin polymerization as a measuring signal and have limited sensitivity to detect mild coagulation factor deficiencies or weak inhibitors against coagulation factors. Their specificity is also limited by the fact that several causes of abnormal clotting times are not associated with bleeding or thrombosis. Therefore, coagulation screening tests must be combined with the clinical history and symptoms when assessing the individual risk of bleeding or thrombosis.[87–90] Laboratories performing coagulation screening tests must consider the different sensitivities of reagents to clotting factor deficiencies, therapeutic anticoagulants, or lupus anticoagulants. Each laboratory should establish its own reference ranges, which depend not only on the reagents but also on the instruments used for analyses. It is also important to define a gray area of borderline assay results that should prompt specific coagulation assays despite a lack of clearly abnormal screening test results.

The *activated partial thromboplastin time* (aPTT) measures the intrinsic and common pathways of coagulation activation. The recalcification clotting time of citrated plasma is determined after addition of kaolin, celite, micronized silica, or ellagic acid, providing a large artificial surface area, and phospholipids functioning as a

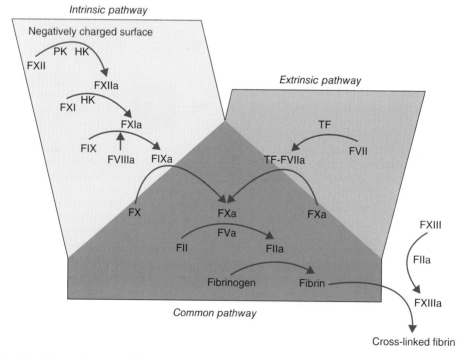

Figure 25.4 Classical model of the coagulation cascade, with intrinsic, extrinsic, and common pathways. F, factor; HK, high-molecular-weight kininogen; PK, prekallikrein; TF, tissue factor.

platelet substitute. The *prothrombin time* (PT) is performed by adding brain tissue or recombinant thromboplastin and calcium to citrated plasma and recording the clotting time. This screening test assesses coagulation activation via the extrinsic and common pathways. The *thrombin time* (TT) measures the time for clot formation to occur in citrated plasma after addition of thrombin. It reflects the amount and quality of fibrinogen and the rate of fibrin formation. The reasons for abnormal aPTT, PT, and TT values and their clinical relevance are shown in Table 25.4.

The main use of aPTT is for screening coagulation defects and inhibitors. The test is relatively sensitive to factor VIII, IX, XI, and XII deficiencies and to prekallikrein and HMW kininogen deficiencies. It may also be prolonged by more severe defects of fibrinogen, factors V and X, and fibrin polymerization. Factors affecting the clotting response of the aPTT test include the composition and concentration of phospholipids, the type of contact activator and buffer, and the length of incubation with the plasma. An aPTT should be sufficiently sensitive to record single clotting factor deficiencies of 30% of normal or less.[91] Some aPTT reagents fail to detect individual coagulation factor deficiencies as low as 20%. When used as a screening test for lupus anticoagulant, the detection sensitivity is predominantly determined by the type and concentration of the phospholipid reagent. The aPTT is still the most widely used method for monitoring treatment with unfractionated heparin. Therapeutic thrombin and Factor Xa inhibitors also prolong the aPTT. Conditions associated with a prolonged aPTT but not with any increased risk of bleeding include factor XII, prekallikrein, and HMW kininogen deficiencies; lupus anticoagulants; transient phospholipid antibodies; increased hematocrit resulting in citrate anticoagulant excess; and heparin contamination of samples. Recent findings suggest that moderate factor XII deficiency might be associated with vascular mortality.[92] Transient phospholipid antibodies and concomitant prolonged aPTT without any clinical symptoms are frequently observed in children suffering from repeated infections.[93] Increased plasma levels of fibrinogen, factor VIII, and factor IX sometimes cause an abnormally short aPTT, which has been associated with overall poor prognosis and venous thromboembolism.[94,95]

The PT reflects changes in the three vitamin K–dependent clotting factors (prothrombin and factors VII and X) and the non-vitamin-K-dependent factor V. Its sensitivity to clotting factor deficiencies or to vitamin K deficiency or antagonism by oral anticoagulants strongly depends on the source and type of TF thromboplastin reagent. PT prolongations not associated with clotting factor deficiencies may be caused by lupus anticoagulants, increased hematocrit, or impaired fibrin polymerization. Because the heparin sensitivity of PT reagents is reduced by adding heparin-neutralizing substances, only very high unfractionated heparin concentrations may cause prolonged PT. The PT is still the most widely used test for monitoring treatment with warfarin or other oral anticoagulants. For this purpose, the PT is calibrated against the international reference thromboplastin and given as an international normalized ratio (INR).[96] Therapeutic thrombin and factor Xa inhibitors also prolong the PT.

The TT detects an impaired fibrin polymerization resulting from fibrin(ogen) degradation products, monoclonal gammopathies, or

Table 25.4 Reasons for an abnormal activated partial thromboplastin time, prothrombin time, and thrombin time

Abnormal aPTT	Prolonged PT	Prolonged TT
Associated with Hemorrhage, Prolonged • Fibrinogen, prothrombin, factor V, X, VIII, IX, or XI deficiency • Vitamin K deficiency or antagonism by oral anticoagulants or beta-lactam antibiotics • Specific clotting factor inhibitors • Unfractionated heparin and low-molecular-weight heparins • Factor Xa inhibitors (e.g., apixaban, edoxaban, fondaparinux, rivaroxaban) • Thrombin inhibitors (e.g., hirudins, argatroban, dabigatran)	Associated with Hemorrhage • Fibrinogen, prothrombin, factor V, X, or VII deficiency • Specific clotting factor inhibitors • Vitamin K deficiency or antagonism by oral anticoagulants or beta-lactam antibiotics • Factor Xa inhibitors (e.g., apixaban, edoxaban, fondaparinux, rivaroxaban) • Thrombin inhibitors (e.g., hirudins, argatroban, dabigatran) • High doses of unfractionated heparin • Inhibition of fibrin polymerization: fibrin(ogen) degradation products, monoclonal gammopathies, dysfibrinogenemia	Associated with Hemorrhage • Unfractionated heparin and low-molecular-weight heparins • Thrombin inhibitors (e.g., hirudins, argatroban, dabigatran) • Inhibition of fibrin polymerization: fibrin(ogen) degradation products, monoclonal gammopathies, 30% of hereditary dysfibrinogenemias • Hypofibrinogenemia No Association with Hemorrhage or Associated with Thrombosis • Inhibition of fibrin polymerization: 50% of hereditary dysfibrinogenemias
No Association with Hemorrhage or Thrombosis, Prolonged • Prekallikrein or high-molecular-weight kininogen deficiency, severe factor XII deficiency • Transient phospholipid antibodies, predominantly in children with infections • Increased hematocrit • Heparin contamination • Partially activated sample Associated with Thrombosis *Prolonged:* • Lupus anticoagulant • Moderate factor XII deficiency? *Shortened:* • Increased plasma levels of fibrinogen, prothrombin, factors V, VIII, IX, and X; coagulation activation	No Association with Hemorrhage • Increased hematocrit • Inhibition of fibrin polymerization: dysfibrinogenemia Associated with Thrombosis • Lupus anticoagulant • Inhibition of fibrin polymerization: dysfibrinogenemia	Associated with Thrombosis • Inhibition of fibrin polymerization: 20% of hereditary dysfibrinogenemias

Hereditary dysfibrinogenemia may be associated with bleeding or thrombosis or both, or not associated with any symptoms. aPTT, activated partial thromboplastin time; PT, prothrombin time; TT, thrombin time.

dysfibrinogenemias more sensitively than the aPTT and PT. Hereditary dysfibrinogenemia is heterogeneous and may be associated with bleeding and/or thrombosis, or it may be asymptomatic.[28] Unfractionated heparin and therapeutic thrombin inhibitors such as hirudins, argatroban, and dabigatran cause a marked prolongation of the TT. The *reptilase time* performed by adding the snake venom reptilase to citrated plasma is unaffected by heparin and even more sensitive to impaired fibrin polymerization than is the TT. Because none of the coagulation screening tests are usually prolonged until the fibrinogen level falls below 0.5 g/L, a specific assay for *clottable fibrinogen* should be included in the basic screening tests for detecting coagulation factor deficiencies. Functional fibrinogen is either measured by the Clauss method on the basis of thrombin-induced clotting or calculated from the change of turbidity during measurement of the PT (PT-derived fibrinogen).

Coagulation screening tests do not detect factor XIII deficiency, which must be confirmed by appropriate assays.

There is presently no simple and adequately sensitive screening test for detecting mild *hyperfibrinolysis*. D-dimer latex agglutination, and turbidimetric and enzyme-linked immunosorbent assays quantify the plasmin-degraded products of cross-linked fibrin in plasma using monoclonal antibodies. However, elevated D-dimer levels are found in numerous clinical conditions that are not inevitably associated with hyperfibrinolysis-induced bleeding. Severe hyperfibrinolysis can be diagnosed easily by markedly elevated D-dimers, prolonged TT and reptilase time, thrombelastography/thrombelastometry, and low fibrinogen, plasminogen, and plasmin inhibitor levels. However, the detection of mild hyperfibrinolytic states associated with bleeding continues to be a diagnostic challenge.

The need for "global screening tests" allowing on-site assessment of the overall hemostatic potential has resulted in further developments of old viscoelastic tests using new technologies. Thromboelastography originally described by Hartert[97] and rotational thrombelastometry (ROTEM™) are able to detect thrombocytopenia, platelet dysfunction, coagulopathies, impaired fibrin stabilization, and hyperfibrinolysis when performed in whole blood.[98] Although these tests have been used successfully in guiding blood component administration in hepatic and cardiac surgery and in trauma,[99–101] validation studies are lacking on their sensitivity and specificity to detect mild disorders of hemostasis in all clinical settings. Studies demonstrated a low sensitivity of thromboelastography to detect platelet dysfunction and vitamin K–dependent coagulation factor deficiency.[102,103] The endogenous thrombin potential as measured by a thrombin generation curve invented by Hemker[104] may be a useful tool for estimating the risks of both bleeding and thrombosis. However, data justifying its use in clinical routine are still lacking.

Summary

Plasma is used therapeutically or as starting material for manufacturing albumin, immunoglobulins, protease inhibitor, clotting factor, and coagulation inhibitor concentrates. Plasma protein levels are subject to wide intra-individual and interindividual variation. Age, gender, ABO blood group, acute phase reactions, physical exercise, mental stress, and hormones substantially influence the plasma levels of therapeutically used plasma proteins. Hemostasis is now understood to involve complex interactions between vessel walls, platelets, blood cells, proteins circulating in blood or being fixed to cells, and other humoral factors such as ionized calcium. Clinically useful coagulation screening tests include activated partial thromboplastin time, prothrombin time, and thrombin time. The detection of mild hyperfibrinolysis and of mild coagulation disorders requires additional specific assays, a clinical history, and an examination.

Disclaimer

The author has disclosed no conflicts of interest.

Key references

A full reference list for this chapter is available at: http://www.wiley.com/go/simon/transfusion

1 Hu S, Loo JA, Wong DT. Human body fluid proteome analysis. *Proteomics* 2006; **6**: 6326–53.

12 Burnouf T. Modern plasma fractionation. *Transfus Med Rev* 2007; **21**: 101–17.

66 Austin AW, Wissmann T, von Kanel R. Stress and hemostasis: an update. *Semin Thromb Hemost* 2013; **39**: 902–12.

78 Hoffman M, Monroe DM. Rethinking the coagulation cascade. *Curr Hematol Rep* 2005; **4**: 391–6.

CHAPTER 26

Plasma and cryoprecipitate for transfusion

Simon J. Stanworth[1] & Alan T. Tinmouth[2,3,4]

[1]NHS Blood & Transplant and Oxford University Hospitals, John Radcliffe Hospital, Headington, Oxford, UK
[2]Departments of Medicine, and Laboratory Medicine & Pathology, University of Ottawa, Ottawa, ON, Canada
[3]General Hematology and Transfusion Medicine, Division of Hematology, The Ottawa Hospital, Ottawa, ON, Canada
[4]University of Ottawa Centre for Transfusion Research, Ottawa Hospital Research Institute, Ottawa, ON, Canada

Plasma for transfusion

Plasma for transfusion can be collected through centrifugation of whole blood or by plasma apheresis. It can then be stored frozen as whole plasma or used to produce more purified constituents, including concentrates of coagulation factors and fibrin sealant, immunoglobulins (normal or specific, e.g., Rh immune globulin), anticoagulants (e.g., antithrombin and protein C), complement-related proteins (C1-esterase inhibitor), and albumin. Fresh frozen plasma (FFP) is human donor plasma frozen within a short specified time period after collection (often eight hours) and then stored at a defined temperature, typically −30 °C. Plasma frozen at slightly later intervals (typically up to 24 hours) after collection is referred to as *frozen plasma* (or FP24). Both components are usually considered clinically equivalent, and for the purposes of this chapter will be covered (interchangeably) by the common term *frozen plasma* (FP), unless otherwise stated.

After thawing for transfusion, FP contains near normal levels of most plasma proteins, including procoagulant and inhibitory components of the coagulation system, although all levels will be further diluted by citrate anticoagulant solution. Factor VIII is typically the main (or only) plasma protein whose level is quality controlled for the specification of the product, for example by UK[1] guidelines,[2] and this threshold needs to be met for a proportion of units (typically 75%). Coagulation factor content is well maintained in thawed FP up to five days but with evidence of a fall in factors V and VIII.

A typical unit of plasma derived from a collection of whole blood has a volume of just under 300 ml, and local and national guidelines for usage generally specify a dose of around 10–20 ml/kg. The composition of FP can be influenced by many factors. These would include gender, age, genetic, dietary, and other environmental factors, all potentially modifying levels of individual proteins. The composition of collected plasma would also be affected by the processing procedure, including how quickly the plasma is collected and then stored. Although clinicians tend to assume approximate equivalence in clinical effectiveness between individual units of FP, it is likely that there is heterogeneity, reflecting not only this biological variation in constituents between donors (e.g., vWF and FVIII levels being lower in Group O donors), but also differences in processing, storage, and preparation for administration. Such variation might be expected to be less marked for pooled plasma components such as solvent–detergent FP.

To illustrate this variation, Figure 26.1 shows data for procoagulant factor content from 66 units of (white cell–depleted) FP.[3,4]

Which patients are transfused FP?

Clinical use of FP has grown steadily over the last two decades in many countries. There is evidence of variation in usage both within and between countries. In a comparison of FP use in five countries, the ratio of FP units to red blood cell units transfused varied from 1:3.6 in the United States to 1:8.5 in France.[5] Two studies have reported a wide variation in the use of FP among centers within the same country for patients undergoing cardiac surgery[6,7] and critical care patients.[7] Interestingly, in the latter study, lower use of FP in critical care patients did not correlate with lower use in cardiac surgery patients, which suggests that important variation in the use of FP within hospitals also exists.[7]

FP is given primarily for two indications: to prevent bleeding (prophylaxis) or stop bleeding (therapeutic). Prophylactic transfusions, which may account for over 50% of all FP transfusions, are often given prior to surgery or an invasive procedure.[8] In a subset of Finnish hospitals, over 6000 FP units were tracked to 1159 transfused patients, revealing that FP was transfused most often to surgery patients, especially cardiac.[9] This is consistent with other reports of FP transfusions in other countries[10–16] Local audits in many countries additionally identify other recipients of FP as including patients requiring reversal of warfarin over-anticoagulation, or patients with disseminated intravascular coagulation (DIC), massive transfusion, or thrombotic thrombocytopenic purpura (TTP).

Further information on FP use is summarized in Tables 26.1 and 26.2. Table 26.1 describes studies that reported on the indications for FP transfusions. Table 26.2 provides information on the use of FP by medical and surgical specialties and by study.

The side effects of FP

Crucial to recommendations in guidelines for FP transfusion practice is the need for a clear understanding of the risk of harm. FP is not without risk, and indeed may be among the most "high risk" of all blood components.[17,18] More immediate and serious complications of FP are transfusion-related acute lung injury (TRALI) and transfusion-related circulatory overload (TACO), although there are ongoing issues of reporting and

Rossi's Principles of Transfusion Medicine, Fifth Edition. Edited by Toby L. Simon, Jeffrey McCullough, Edward L. Snyder, Bjarte G. Solheim, and Ronald G. Strauss.
© 2016 John Wiley & Sons, Ltd. Published 2016 by John Wiley & Sons, Ltd.

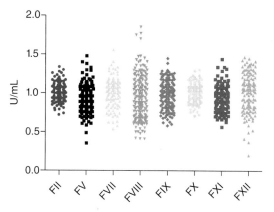

U/mL axis with values 0.0, 0.5, 1.0, 1.5, 2.0; x-axis labels FII, FV, FVII, FVIII, FIX, FX, FXI, FXII

Figure 26.1 Coagulation factor concentration in individual units of fresh frozen plasma tested in the Component Development Laboratory of NHS Blood and Transplant. Source: Rebecca Cardigan, NHSBT. Reproduced with permission.

Fluid overload may be a greater issue if larger doses of FP are transfused to attempt (full) reversal of abnormal coagulation tests (discussed later in this chapter). The risks related to circulatory overload are poorly understood, but could be important for critically ill patients, for example in Intensive Care units (ICUs). Other risks are transfusion-transmitted infections, including an unquantifiable risk of prion disease. Allergic reactions to FP are relatively common, with a frequency of around 1–3% of all transfusions, and they can be extremely troublesome or, rarely, life-threatening for some multi-transfused patients.

Understanding risks of FP transfusion is important when considering use of FP as prophylaxis, which as stated is a common indication for FP in clinical practice. A prophylactic policy should only be justified if the risk of bleeding is greater than the risk of harmful effects. Without evidence of benefit, such a policy aimed at preventing (uncommon) bleeding complications could involve transfusing (harmful) FP to a large number of patients, many of whom might not bleed even if prophylactic FP were not given.

diagnosis of these conditions that make accurate estimation of prevalence difficult.[19,20] In the United Kingdom, an association between cases of TRALI and female donors has been identified through the Serious Hazards of Transfusion hemovigilance scheme, and the use of predominantly male donors for the production of FP has been associated with a reduction in the incidence of TRALI.[21]

Main recommendations for the use of FP

Recommendations for the transfusion of FP have remained relatively consistent over the years, including: (1) active bleeding, or prior to surgery or an invasive procedure in patients (adults and neonates) with acquired deficiencies of one or more coagulation factors as demonstrated by an increased international normalized

Table 26.1 Studies reporting reasons for frozen plasma transfusions (Percentage of Transfusion Episodes)

Indication for Frozen Plasma	Tinmouth[16]	Stanworth[15]	Iorio[14]	Hui[13]	Dzik[8 ***]	Tobin[11]	Metz[10]	Tuckfield[14]	Shanberge[12]
Therapeutic	—	—	—	—	35	—	—	—	89
Prophylactic	11.9[+]	31	—	—	48	—	—	—	11
Bleeding	8.4	54	41.2	—	—	27[*]	27[*]	31[*]	—
Perioperative	34.6	—	—	—	—	22[*]	41[*]	47[*]	—
Coagulopathy	14.3	—	25.8	13	8	—	4	10	—
Liver Disease	—	19	—	13.5[#]	—	8.5[**]	—	—	14.4
Warfarin	20.2	14	2.4	32.5[##]	21	36.5	11.5	4	24.0
Cardiac Sx	—	13	—	6.5[#]	—	—	—	—	16.5
AAA	—	—	—	—	—	—	—	—	7.0
Massive Transfusion	7.3	13[#]	—	24[#]	—	—	16[#]	7.5[#]	2.1
ICU Coagulopathy	—	—	—	—	—	—	—	—	3.9
DIC	—	3	8.1	8.5[#]	—	—	—	—	—
Other	6.5	—	22.5	—	8	—	—	—	23.6
Trauma	—	3	—	—	—	—	—	—	—

[+] Only prior to invasive procedures.
[*] Correct coagulopathy.
[**] Prophylactic associated with warfarin or liver disease.
[***] Does not include operating room requests.
[#] With bleeding.
[##] Immediate reversal required.

Table 26.2 Studies reporting frozen plasma transfusions utilization by Medical/Surgical Specialty (Percentage of Transfusion Episodes)

Medical Specialty	Tinmouth[16]	Stanworth[15]	Iorio[14]	Hui[13]	Shanberge[12]	Tobin[11]	Metz[10]
Medical	29	22	22.9	13	48.8	27.5	35
Oncology	—	2[#]	—	—	—	3	8
Surgical	25.1[*]	36	51.4	36	46	24.5[*]	31[*]
Cardiac Surgery	73	—	—	6	—	8.5	23
Orthopedics	—	—	—	—	—	3.0	2
Obstetrics/Gynecology	2	—	—	—	1.8	—	1
Critical Care	11	32	25.7	39	—	39.5	—
Emergency	12.6	6	—	14	—	5	—
Pediatrics	3	—	—	—	3.1	—	—

[*] Not including cardiac and/or orthopedic surgery.
[#] Hematology and oncology.

ratio (INR), prothrombin time (PT), or activated partial thrombo-plastin time (aPTT), when no alternative therapies are available or appropriate; (2) immediate correction of vitamin K deficiency or reversal of warfarin effect in patient with active bleeding, or prior to surgery or an invasive procedure (in conjunction with use of prothrombin complex concentrates [PCCs]); (3) DIC or consump-tive coagulopathy with active bleeding; (4) TTP; and (5) active bleeding, or prior to surgery or an invasive procedure in patients with a congenital factor deficiency when no alternative therapies are available or appropriate. Variations of these indications will be found in most national guidelines.[22–26] Previous common uses of FP that are now considered inappropriate include: volume replace-ment, correction of hypoalbuminemia or nutritional support, and immunoglobulin replacement.

Evidence for indications

This section will explore in more detail what levels of evidence exist to support these indications—in other words, whether the *presumed* benefits really outweigh the *real* risks. The clearest evidence for a direct beneficial effect of FP would be expected to come from randomized controlled trials (RCTs) of FP compared with no FP/plasma. Studies of interventions comparing FP with a nonblood product (e.g., solutions of colloids and/or crystalloids) may also assess effectiveness, but these studies would need to be separately evaluated given that these solutions have variable effects on in vivo or in vitro coagulation.[27]

A update of an earlier systematic review was recently pub-lished.[28,29] Since the earlier 2004 systematic review of RCTs on FP use, 21 new RCTs have been published in the literature, with an additional eight ongoing and four recently completed RCTs expected to be published in the next few years. This makes a total of 80 completed and published RCTs in this area in the past 50 years, which one might expect to represent a sufficient body of evidence to inform the safe and effective use of plasma for transfu-sion. Most of the research activity identified in this updated review has covered the same groups of patients as reported in the original systematic review, with most new trials continuing to recruit patients with liver and cardiac disease. Of the new identified trials, eight evaluated prophylactic use of plasma and 13 therapeutic plasma use in patients with bleeding and active disease. Many of the identified studies in the update suffered from the same limita-tions and risks of bias that were highlighted in the first systematic review. For example, 15 of the 21 additional included trials had fewer than 30 participants in each arm. Small sample sizes com-promise the ability of randomization to achieve equivalence of baseline characteristics. When considered as a whole, there was no evidence of any consistent benefit from using FP infusion in either the prophylactic or therapeutic setting.

In two large, well-conducted trials, evidence for a lack of benefit for prophylactic use of FP was reported. Both were designed to evaluate carefully the effectiveness of FP in a large group of patients, and provided information about the sample sizes required to allow adequate power to detect clinically important differences between the groups of patients. In the first trial, the Northern Neonatal Nursing Initiative (NNNI) Trial Group randomized 776 neonates to FP or to volume expanders (gelofusin or dextrose–saline) and did not show any differences in the prevention of intraventricular hemorrhage.[30] Allocation concealment and blinding of outcome assessors (to monitor clinically relevant long-term developmental outcomes) were reported. Of note, the study did not include measurement of coagulation tests. In the other trial, the

effectiveness of FP was evaluated in patients with acute pancreati-tis,[31] and, in total, 275 patients were randomized to receive either FP or a colloid solution. No evidence for benefit was reported.

The next sections provide additional information about the use of plasma in selected clinical settings.

1. Cardiac surgery

Epidemiological evidence indicates that FP given before or during cardiac surgery accounts for approximately 5–10% of all use (Tables 26.1 and 26.2). Variation in practice remains a hallmark of plasma transfusion practice. A recent UK audit aimed to describe transfusion practice for all adult patients undergoing cardiac sur-gery during a three-month period in 2010.[32] Data on each patient were obtained from the Central Cardiac Audit Database (CCAD) and blood transfusion laboratories. Clinical data were received from 25/38 (66%) of cardiac centers in the United Kingdom, and data on 6140 cardiac procedures were collected. Of these 6140 procedures, 3374 (55%) were coronary artery bypass graft (CABG), 1231 (20%) were cardiac valve, and 784 were CABG plus valve (13%). The range of usage of red blood cells and blood components was very wide across the different centers; for example, for patients undergoing CABG, the mean use of red cells was 2.98 units (range 0–32) and FP 1.98 units (range 0–22). Figure 26.2 graphically illustrates this variation in FP practice between hospital centers for one type of surgery. Although there may be some variation in the clinical profiles of patients between different cardiac surgical centers whom participated in this audit, it seems unlikely to provide a full explanation for the differences between centers in transfusion rates, which also were seen for other cardiac procedures.

When considering RCTs comparing prophylactic-use FP to either no FP or nonplasma product after cardiopulmonary bypass (CPB), the findings have not shown evidence of a consistent significant beneficial effect on blood loss or transfusion requirement; meta-analysis indicated no statistically significant difference for FP use for the outcome of postoperative blood loss.[29] The hemostatic changes related to cardiac bypass are multifactorial, and not solely related to coagulation factor deficiency, and perhaps it is not surprising that FP use prophylactically fails to provide benefit.

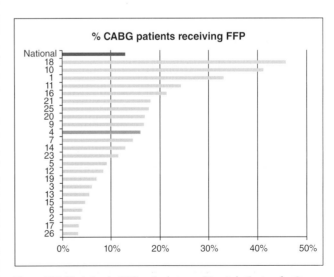

Figure 26.2 Variation in FP Practice between Hospitals Centers for One Type of Surgery

2. Massive transfusion: trauma

Few trials have evaluated the effects of therapeutic FP in patients with bleeding who have multiple or global deficiencies of coagulation factors, for example DIC or massive transfusion, presumably in part reflecting the difficulties of trial design in this setting. One study identified in the systematic review was aimed at addressing the effectiveness of FP in DIC in a group of neonates, using defined criteria for a diagnosis of DIC.[33] In this small three-way controlled trial, neonates were randomly allocated to receive either exchange transfusion (using whole blood), FP (and platelet) infusions, or no plasma in a control group. Although there were no differences in rates of improvement for coagulation tests or in survival in either treatment group, the size of the trial was small (a total of 33 patients across three arms).

Injury remains a leading cause of death worldwide for younger patients, and uncontrolled hemorrhage is a primary cause of death in 40% of cases. Transfusion therapy is an integral part of supportive treatment for major blood loss.[34,35] Current approaches to *hemostatic resuscitation* now typically specify early empiric delivery of plasma (FP) alongside red cells (packed red blood cells [PRBCs]). The rationale for early use of plasma is that around one-quarter of all trauma patients who present to hospital have a coagulopathy (acute traumatic coagulopathy), which leads to increased risks of major hemorrhage, massive transfusion, and a 3–4-fold increased risk of death. Waiting for laboratory tests including standard coagulation tests can often delay the administration of FP in the setting of acute bleeds, which may be an additional reason why formulaic transfusion policies have been promoted in settings such as trauma.[36] However, the exact benefit of these different transfusion strategies has not been evaluated in high-quality randomized trials. The role of higher doses of plasma (and platelets) has been addressed in the PROPPR randomized trial (NCT01545232) in North America. The main results have just been reported for a composite main outcome of 24-hour and 30-day all-cause mortality, which revealed no significant differences between patients receiving plasma, platelets, and red cells in different blood component ratios (1:1:1 vs. 1:1:2). Strategies describing more "aggressive" use of FP and platelets have also been recently reported in surgical practice.[37]

3. Intensive care

In the ICU setting, there are some data on the frequency with which FP is given as prophylaxis, for example prior to central venous cannulation or other invasive procedures. A large observational study of coagulopathy in intensive care (ISOC-1) illustrates the clinical uncertainties surrounding the use of FP. In this study of just under 2000 ICU admissions, one-third of patients had a prolonged PT and around a third of these patients received FP. Overall, 50% of patients received FP in the absence of evidence of clinical bleeding, and many had only mild or moderate prolongation of PT. The dose of FP administered was also highly variable. The use of FP prior to central venous calculation is debatable; the evidence would suggest that the rate of important hemorrhagic complications associated with central venous cannulation is very low, even in patients with normal or abnormal coagulation test results.[38–41]

Dara *et al.* reported a single-center retrospective cohort study of FP use in medical ICU patients.[42] They identified patients in whom an INR ≥1.5 was found during ICU stay and evaluated FP use in the subgroup who were not actively bleeding. In addition to variability in FP transfusion practice, the authors observed that patients who received FP had a similar rate of hemorrhage to matched cases, but had a higher incidence of "acute lung injury" during the 48 hours

after transfusion (18% vs. 4%; $p = 0.02$). This association raises the possibility that critically ill patients, many with concurrent inflammatory problems, may be more susceptible to TRALI after receiving plasma-rich blood products, although distinguishing TRALI from other clinical problems such as volume overload remains problematic. These findings do not prove cause and effect, but again emphasize a need for concern about inappropriate use of FP, in view of the real risk of harm.[43]

The Transfusion of Fresh Frozen Plasma in Nonbleeding ICU Patients (TOPIC) trial was a recent multicenter RCT to investigate whether it is safe to withhold FP transfusion to coagulopathic critically ill patients undergoing an invasive procedure.[44] This study described a noninferiority, prospective, multicenter, randomized, open-label, blinded end point evaluation trial. In the intervention group, a prophylactic transfusion of FP prior to an invasive procedure was omitted compared to transfusion of a fixed dose of 12 ml/kg in the control group. The primary outcome measure was relevant bleeding; other outcomes included minor bleeding, correction of INR, onset of acute lung injury, length of ventilation days, and duration of ICU stay. Due to slow inclusion, the trial was unfortunately stopped before the predefined target enrollment was reached. At the time of study analysis, 81 patients had been randomly assigned, 42 to FP and 41 to no FP transfusion prior to procedures. The results indicated that the incidence of bleeding did not differ between the groups with a total of one major and 13 minor bleedings ($p = 0.08$ for noninferiority for all bleeding). FP transfusions resulted in a small reduction of INR to less than 1.5 in 54% of the transfused patients. Of note, there were no differences in lung injury scores between the two groups, but there was an increased duration of mechanical ventilation in patients receiving FP. In summary, although a small study, the findings did not support a difference in bleeding complications irrespective of whether FP was prophylactically transfused before procedures or not. The study was consistent with the wider literature, indicating a lack of effectiveness of plasma prophylactically to reduce bleeding risk prior to procedures.[28,29]

4. Liver disease

The coagulopathy of liver disease is complex, with abnormalities of platelets, fibrinolysis, and inhibitors of coagulation as well as coagulation factor deficiency. Where possible, deficiency of vitamin K should always be corrected first before considering the role of plasma transfusion. There is evidence that FP continues to be administered in patients with cirrhosis. 85 out of 110 (77%) hospitals who registered to participate in a recent national UK audit undertaken to describe use of blood components in patients with cirrhosis submitted data on a total of 1333 consecutive cases.[45] Overall, 391/1313 (30%) of patients were transfused at least one blood component during their admission. 34/45 (76%) patients who received FP for prophylaxis received it prior to a procedure, with variable pretransfusion results for PT/INR. 60% (49/81) of patients who were bleeding and transfused FP had a pretransfusion INR of >1.5.

Recent evidence has changed our understanding about hemostasis in cirrhosis, suggesting there is not hypocoagulability in stable cirrhosis, but a "resetting" of the pro- and anticoagulation factors such that clot formation remains normal.[46] Transfusion of plasma blood components based upon perceived coagulopathy indicated by conventional coagulation indices may be not only inappropriate but also harmful, by potentially increasing the risk of thrombotic complications and exacerbating already elevated portal pressures resulting in an increased risk of bleeding from varices.[46] This is of particular consequence when assessing the need for transfusion of prophylactic FP for which there is no agreed threshold for transfusion.

No recent RCT data are available in the setting of adult cirrhosis. One early randomized trial[47] attempted to assess the effects of regular prophylactic transfusions of FP in patients with paracetamol overdose. Twenty patients were evaluated, and no effects on bleeding, morbidity, and mortality were observed. However, the small size of the study and the crossover design were not optimal for detecting differences between the two groups.

Other studies to investigate FP transfusion practice in patients with liver disease have been uncontrolled and observational. Youssef *et al.*[48] reported the effects of FP transfusion in 100 patients with liver disease, and found that it was difficult to correct abnormalities of coagulation screening tests unless large volumes of FP were transfused, and that the effects of transfusion were short-lived. Lack of evidence for an association between bleeding and laboratory tests of coagulation in liver disease has also been reported in a number of studies, for example the retrospective study of McVay and Toy.[49] Although these studies contain no control group data, there is again a consistent theme of lack of evidence for benefit for FP when transfused to patients with liver disease. Of note, the lack of bleeding in cirrhotic patients despite diminished procoagulant synthesis (and abnormal PT/aPTT) may be explained by a parallel reduction in the production of anticoagulant proteins, such as proteins C and S, leading to equivalent thrombin generation potential on activation of both pro- and anticoagulant pathways.[43]

In summary, guidelines for plasma transfusion typically include the multiple coagulation factor deficiency state of liver disease associated with bleeding or prior to invasive procedures. However, the number of relevant studies published to support these statements is very limited, and it is far from clear just how effective this transfusion policy is. In particular, observational studies evaluating common invasive procedures such as liver biopsy, paracentesis, or central venous cannulation indicate that moderate disturbances of coagulation tests are in fact not predictive for bleeding risk.[49–51]

5. Reversal of warfarin effect

In addition to vitamin K, guidelines recommend FP or PCCs for reversal of over-anticoagulation but only in patients with major bleeding.[52] However, there is continuing controversy over which component is preferable, and this, in part, reflects a lack of clinical trials directly comparing the two components. PCCs are produced by fractionation of pooled plasma and contain coagulation factors II, IX, and X at a significantly higher concentration than FP. But not all PCCs are the same, and factor VII levels do vary between products. In a prospective RCT comparing the safety and effectiveness of a four-factor PCC and FFP ($n = 202$), Sarode reported a rapider reduction in the INR in patients receiving PCC.[53] However, there were no differences in hemostatic efficacy or safety in patients receiving PCC or FFP. Further evaluation is required to ascertain whether the rapider improvements in coagulation screening tests translate into clinical benefit in specific populations (e.g., intracranial hemorrhage) and if there are any increased risks of thromboembolic complications. In the absence of major bleeding associated with over-anticoagulation due to vitamin K antagonists, primary treatment should be initiated with oral/IV vitamin K.

6. Therapeutic apheresis: thrombotic thrombocytopenic purpura

FP is frequently used as a replacement fluid in patients undergoing therapeutic apheresis procedures.[54] Based on the findings of one RCT,[55] plasma exchange with FP is the first-line treatment of choice for TTP,[56] the FP providing a source of ADAMTS13 (A Disintegrin And Metalloprotease with ThromboSpondin type 1 motif 13). However, definitive randomized studies to define the optimal dose and schedule of FP or type of plasma (e.g., cryo-supernatant, or solvent–detergent treated) for therapeutic apheresis in patients with TTP have not been undertaken. Of interest, early studies investigating plasma exchange for conditions other than TTP have reported that despite repeated procedures with coagulation factor–free replacement fluids, no bleeding complications occurred, even though marked reductions of coagulation factor levels were seen.[57]

Is there an optimal dose of FP?

As described in the section on patients with liver disease, there are important questions about what is the optimal dose of FP, and not infrequently only large volumes achieve correction of coagulation test results. However, questions about appropriate or optimal dose for FP transfusion generally presuppose that evidence of dose-dependent effectiveness exists in the first place. Much of the evidence for informing appropriate dose comes from a derived synthesis of physiological assessments of coagulation factor content and effects of plasma infusion.[58]

There is evidence that FP may be ineffective in correcting mild-moderate abnormalities of coagulation screen tests. Abdel-Wahab *et al.* prospectively evaluated the effects of plasma transfusions on PT/INR in hospital patients with prolonged INRs.[59] They followed patients with a pretransfusion PT between 13.1 seconds and 17 seconds (INR equivalent 1.1–1.85). 324 plasma units were evaluated in 121 patients. Fewer than 1% of patients had normalization of PT/INR post transfusion, and only 15% demonstrated a correction of halfway to normal. Of interest, there was also no meaningful correlation with clinical bleeding, as recorded retrospectively by patient chart review. Finally, when all cases of transfusion were reviewed for correction, there was little evidence for dose–response effect.

In another study, 22 critically ill adult patients were allocated in consecutive groups to receive lower dose FP (median volume 12.2 ml/kg) or higher dose FP (median volume 33.5 ml/kg), with the aim to increase hemostatic coagulation factor levels to >30 IU/dl (based on experience of treating patients with hemophilia).[60] The lower dose only increased the coagulation factor levels above the desired threshold in one of five patients as compared to all seven patients achieving the target levels with the higher dose. Many patients who received the lower (standard) dose, but not larger dose, of FP failed to achieve the target level of coagulation factor replacement. Another study[61] reported on 103 adult patients with minimally prolonged INRs, and found that adding FP to their treatment failed to change the decrease in INR that occurred over time. When other studies or trials do report apparent "correction," the overall absolute or mean changes again appear very small. For example, in one RCT of patients with liver disease, the median reduction in INR attained after FP was 0.2 (range 0–0.7).[62]

It should be appreciated that the outcomes for many studies of plasma, including dose, are laboratory-based and particularly centered on the PT/aPTT. But correlations between these coagulation screen tests and coagulation factor levels are poor and nonlinear, with limitations in expectations of achieving correction, particularly as factor levels approach normal.[63] The laboratory tests of aPTT and PT were developed to investigate coagulation factor deficiencies in patients with a bleeding history by providing an end assessment of thrombin generation by fibrin formation, and therefore the important issue of their applied clinical validity continues to be raised. The PT and aPTT results may be abnormal for a number of reasons not associated with bleeding risk, not least normal variation for some individuals. Some laboratories report the INR, and physicians then base decisions to transfuse plasma on results above a certain threshold, typically 1.5 times the control. But again, the INR is based on PT and was developed to monitor warfarin therapy, by standardizing results to account for different sensitivities of thromboplastins. The extrapolation of PT to INR may really only be valid for monitoring anticoagulation in those patients stably anti-coagulated with vitamin K antagonists.[65]

An important study by Deitcher[65] showed that over the INR range of 1.3–1.9 inclusive, mean factor levels ranged from 31% to 65% (factor II), from 40% to 70% (factor V), and from 22% to 60% (factor VII). All of these levels are consistent with adequate con-centrations of factors to support hemostasis. These results would be consistent with the findings from observational studies mentioned earlier, pointing to a lack of predictive effect for bleeding risk in patients with mild or moderate abnormalities of coagulation tests.[45]

Clinical effectiveness of cryoprecipitate

Fibrinogen (Fg) is the key final component of the clotting pathway and forms fibrin—an insoluble protein that is the foundation of a stable clot. Fg is one of the earliest coagulation proteins to fall in major bleeding,[66,67] and when levels fall, patients have a reduced ability to form clots and may bleed for longer periods. Cryoprecipitate has been used since 1965 in the United Kingdom as a standard source and treatment for low fibrinogen concentrations, and is used in other countries such as the United States and Canada. Cryoprecipitate is prepared by controlled thawing of frozen plasma to precipitate higher molecular weight proteins, including factor VIII, von Willebrand factor, and fibrinogen. Risks from cryoprecipitate transfusion are small but include those common to all blood components (i.e., infection, transfusion-associated acute lung injury, and transfusion-associated circulatory overload).[21]

An adult dose of around 10 single donor units of cryoprecipitate typically raises the plasma fibrinogen level by up to 1 g/l. Cryoprecipitate should not therefore be considered for transfusion solely as a more concentrated form of FP (e.g., when there are concerns about fluid overload), as it predominantly contains only factor VIII,

von Willebrand factor, fibronectin, factor XIII, and fibrinogen. The remaining product, following the removal of cryoprecipitate, is termed *cryosupernatant* (cryopoor plasma) and has been used in the treatment of TTP, because of the theoretical benefit of its reduced content of von Willebrand factor high-molecular-weight multimers, although the added benefit of cryosupernatant has not been proven.[65]

A specific solvent–detergent purified fibrinogen concentrate is now available, and it may represent a safer concentrate for direct fibrinogen replacement in isolated deficiencies, for example inher-ited hypofibrinogenemia. This product is not licensed for broader clinical use in many countries; however, its use has been reported in other clinical situations, including trauma, cardiac surgery, and obstetrical hemorrhage (see below). The clinical effectiveness of cryoprecipitate as compared to the fibrinogen concentrate has not been evaluated.

Trauma hemorrhage remains the clinical setting where much of the research on fibrinogen replacement has been conducted. Low levels of Fg and increased breakdown of Fg are key components of the early coagulopathy in trauma, and low Fg levels on admission to hospital are independent predictors of early mortality in trauma patients.[67] Fibrin strands that form in a low-Fg environment are more susceptible to clot breakdown (fibrinolysis), and this process is both overactivated and ubiquitous in major trauma.[68]

Early clinical data suggest that Fg supplementation using concen-trates may improve outcomes for trauma hemorrhage, by improving clot strength[69] and reducing blood loss;[70] but to date no definitive trauma trials have been completed to confirm these findings. In an uncontrolled observational study of 131 hemorrhagic patients, mor-tality rates fell by 14% after fibrinogen treatment.[71] Two observational cohort trauma studies[72,73] have also reported reduction of mortality in patients receiving higher fibrinogen content during massive trans-fusion therapy. Despite very high doses of Fg (up to 12 g), plasma levels did not increase beyond the normal range in health, and there were no reported adverse events.[71]

Use of guidelines for plasma transfusion

Although practice guidelines produced by national and professional organizations for FP transfusion are readily available in many countries, there continues to be evidence for variation in practice.

Table 26.3 Studies evaluating appropriateness of frozen plasma transfusions

Study (Country)	Period of Study	Number of Patients	Number of Frozen Plasma Transfusion	Number of Units	Percentage of Inappropriate Transfusions (Source of Guidelines)
Pahuja et al.[75] (India)	2010	560	877	NR	78% (Local)
Tinmouth et al.[16] (Canada)	2008	NR	573	2012	29% (Adjudicated)
ANZICS[76] (Australia/New Zealand)	2008	340	NR	NR	29% (National)
Moylan et al.[77] (Australia)	2006	1158	375	950	11% (National)
Iorio et al.[14] (Italy)	2006	109	221	615	32% (Local)
Makroo et al.[78] (India)	2005	821	821	2915	30% (National)
Liumbruno et al.[79] (Italy)	2003–2005	NR	NR	24918	25% (Local)
Hui et al.[13] (Australia)	2002–2003	NR	NR	793	10% (National)
Pentti et al.[83] (Finland)	2001	NR	181	NR	34% (Local)
Scholfield et al.[80] (Australia)	2000	NR	NR	669	37% (National)
Tobin et al.[111] (Australia)	1999	NR	100	411	57% (National)
Luk et al.[74] (Canada)	1999	358	671	2372	53% (National)
Prathiba et al.[84] (India)	1998	NR	931	2665	69% (National)
Jones et al.[81] (UK)	1996	41	NR	216	34% (National)
Metz et al.[10] (Australia)	1993–1994	NR	200	944	31% (National)
Cheng et al.[82] (Hong Kong)	1994	NR	1152	5635	43% (Local)

NR, Not reported.

The result is that FP appears to have the highest rate of inappropriate utilizations (up to 50%[74]) among standard blood components with evidence of inappropriate practice based on local audits. Table 26.3 summarizes results from a number of studies or audits that have been published that evaluate the appropriateness of transfusion of FP, according to local or national guidelines.

The reasons for poor compliance with guidelines are not entirely clear. In part, it may reflect misunderstandings about the limitations of coagulation tests; it may also reflect on difficulties defining appropriate use in the face of a limited evidence base, and that much transfusion medicine for physicians is based on practice passed down from mentors, who used blood components in a more liberal way. Perhaps now a more systematic approach is required to understand the determinants of this prescribing pattern and barriers to practice change.[85–87] This would include identifying better strategies for delivery and uptake of evidence-based healthcare all of which are clearly demonstrated as unpredictable for FP. A systematic review of the RCT evidence for the effectiveness of different educational strategies operating in transfusion medicine has pointed out the very weakness of the evidence itself for the success of these approaches to deliver sustained and effective behavioral change.[88,89]

Key references

A full reference list for this chapter is available at: http://www.wiley.com/go/simon/transfusion

7 Dzik W, Rao A. Why do physicians request fresh frozen plasma? *Transfusion* 2004; **44**: 1393–4.

15 Stanworth SJ, Walsh TS, Prescott RJ, Lee RJ, Watson DM, Wyncoll D, Intensive Care Study of Coagulopathy (ISOC) investigators. A national study of plasma use in critical care: clinical indications, dose and effect on prothrombin time. *Crit Care* 2011; **15** (2): R108.

28 Stanworth SJ, Brunskill S, Hyde CJ, McClelland DBL, Murphy MF. What is the evidence base for the clinical use of FFP: a systematic review of randomised controlled trials. *Brit J Haematol* 2004; **126**: 139–52.

29 Yang L, Stanworth S, Hopewell S, Doree C, Murphy M. Is fresh-frozen plasma clinically effective? An update of a systematic review of randomized controlled trials. *Transfusion* 2012 Jan 18. doi: 10.1111/j.1537-2995.2011.03515.x

44 Muller MC, Arbous MS, Spoelstra-de Man AM, *et al.* Transfusion of fresh-frozen plasma in critically ill patients with a coagulopathy before invasive procedures: a randomised clinical trial. *Transfusion* 2015; **55**: 26–35.

51 Segal JB, Dzik WH. Paucity of studies to support that abnormal coagulation test results predict bleeding in the setting of invasive procedures: an evidence-based review. *Transfusion* 2005; **45**: 1413–25.

70 Nienaber U, Innerhofer P, Westermann I, *et al.* The impact of fresh frozen plasma vs. coagulation factor concentrates on morbidity and mortality in trauma-associated haemorrhage and massive transfusion. *Injury* 2011; **42**: 697–701.

CHAPTER 27

The purification of plasma proteins for therapeutic use

Joseph Bertolini

CSL Behring, Broadmeadows, Victoria, Australia

Introduction

It has been noted that blood plasma is the largest human proteome.[1] As it is part of the circulation system, plasma contains other tissue proteomes as subsets through its contact with all organs of the body and their diverse cellular components. In addition it contains specific plasma cells involved in the immune response and homeostasis. In one study 289 proteins were detected in plasma, while in another 3700 protein spots were identified by two-dimensional electrophoresis, and 325 distinct proteins identified.[1,2] Proteins found in plasma can constitute proteins secreted by solid tissues that act in plasma; immunoglobulin (Ig); "long-distance" receptor ligands, such as hormones; "local" receptor ligands, such as cytokines and growth factors; and tissue leakage products. If there is an existing disease state, there may be aberrant secretions and foreign proteins as a result of cell damage, or the presence of a tumor or infectious organism.[1]

The true plasma proteins are considered to be those that carry out their functions in circulation.[3] These constitute a number of proteins predominantly produced by the liver and, the immunoglobulins from the bone marrow.[4,5] The hepatic derived plasma proteins encompass key proteins that constitute:

- The coagulation pathway and its regulation; these include the clotting factors (fibrinogen [factor I] and factors V, VII, VIII, IX, X, XI, XII, and XIII) and the regulatory factors or protease inhibitors (antithrombin III, heparin cofactor H, and proteins C, S, and Z);
- Components of the immune response and reaction to foreign bodies via the classic and nonclassic pathway, consisting of the complement factors and mannose binding lectin;
- Acute phase reactants such as, α_1-acid glycoprotein, C-reactive protein, serum amyloid protein, serum amyloid A, and α_2-HS glycoprotein, constitute part of the body's response to injury and infections; increased production of several hundredfold can occur;
- Plasma proteinase inhibitors, which regulate the action of key proteolysis enzymes such as plasmin cathepsin G, elastase, and kallikrein and include α_1-antichymotrypsin, α_2-macroglobulin, inter-α-trypsin inhibitor, C1 inhibitor, and α_1-antitrypsin;
- Carrier proteins, which are involved in the transport of iron, copper, hemoglobin, heme, bilirubin, and fatty acids; these include albumin transferrin, ceruloplasmin, transthryretin, retinal binding protein, haptoglobin, hemopexin, and vitamin binding protein.

- Biochemical regulators involved in immune cell regulation such as interleukins, interferons, and growth factors; for example tumor necrosis factor and transforming growth factor β.

The immunoglobulins, produced in the bone marrow exist as a number of subtypes—IgG, IgM, IgA, IgE, and IgD. IgG and IgM are in the highest concentration, and have the prime role in immune surveillance, the sequestration of foreign bodies and the initiation of subsequent immune cellular and humoral responses.[6]

With increased understanding of the biochemical basis of disease, researchers see plasma proteins as possible therapeutic agents in a number of conditions either as a means of supplementation in cases of deficiency, or to regulate biochemical pathways to achieve desired therapeutic outcomes. The biochemistry, clinical use, and production of these proteins have been reviewed recently.[7,8] Of the many identified plasma proteins, 20 therapeutic products have been developed and are in clinical use, with approximately another five in various stages of development.[9–30] These are tabulated in Table 27.1.

The production of plasma proteins for therapeutic use has led to the development of a large global industry involving the complex activities of collecting blood and plasma donations and applying bioprocessing procedures to produce products with validated efficacy and pathogen safety.[31]

It is generally agreed that the start of plasma fractionation can be traced to the work of Cohn in his Harvard Laboratory in the 1940s, where he developed an ethanol-based precipitation process for the purification of albumin to be used as a resuscitative fluid in theatres of war.[32]

This chapter will describe the manufacture of plasma proteins for therapeutic use and make extensive use of divergent examples to illustrate the range of approaches that can be taken. In addition, it will detail the expected specifications of the final product. This information will be of use to the reader involved in the assessment, purchase, or use of plasma products, who is often confronted with literature on products containing unfamiliar concepts and terminology relating to plasma fractionation, viral removal procedures, and product specifications. An increased understanding of the production of plasma protein therapeutics will facilitate communication with plasma products manufacturers and aid in the assessment of existing products and the exploration of possibilities for future development.

Rossi's Principles of Transfusion Medicine, Fifth Edition. Edited by Toby L. Simon, Jeffrey McCullough, Edward L. Snyder, Bjarte G. Solheim, and Ronald G. Strauss.
© 2016 John Wiley & Sons, Ltd. Published 2016 by John Wiley & Sons, Ltd.

Table 27.1 Plasma proteins with established clinical use or under active investigation

Protein or Therapeutic Product	Clinical Use
Established Clinical Use	
Albumin	Fluid replacement in trauma, burns, sepsis, and cirrhosis
Immunoglobulins:	
- Intravenous	Replacement therapy in primary and secondary immunodeficiency, immunomodulation in certain autoimmune diseases including immune thrombocytopenia purpura, Kawasaki disease, Guillain–Barré syndrome, autoimmune polyneuropathy, and myasthenia gravis
- Hyperimmune to viral and bacterial antigens	Treatment of hepatitis A, hepatitis B, cytomegalovirus, varicella–zoster, and tetanus infections
- Anti RH(D) immunoglobulin	Prevention of Rh(D) isoimmunization due to fetus–maternal rhesus D incompatibility, treatment of immune thrombocytopenia purpura
Factor VIII	Replacement in hemophilia A–factor VIII deficiency; induction of immune tolerance for anti–factor VIII antibodies
Von Willebrand factor (vWF)	Treatment of vWF deficiency
Factor IX	Replacement in hemophilia B–factor IX deficiency
Activated prothrombin complex concentrate (aPCC)	Treatment of patients with inhibitory antibodies to factor VIII or factor IX
Composed predominantly of prothrombin and factors VIII, VII, VIIa, IX, X, Xa; and protein C. Brand name: Factor VIII Inhibitor Bypassing Activity (FEIBA®)	
Prothrombin complex concentrate (PCC); factors II, VII, IX, and X; and regulatory proteins: protein C, S, and Z	Treatment of the rare conditions of factor VII and factor X deficiencies, reversal of the anticoagulant activity of warfarin and prevention of massive bleeding, often in combination with fibrinogen
Fibrinogen	Replacement in congenital fibrinogen deficiency and in acquired deficiency following massive bleeding
Factor XI	Treatment of Factor XI deficiency; incidence: $1:10^6$
Factor XIII	Treatment of Factor VIII deficiency; incidence: $1:2 \times 10^6$
Factor X	Treatment of Factor X deficiency; incidence: $1:1 \times 10^6$
Fibrin glue (fibrinogen and thrombin components)	Used in surgery as a sealant to achieve hemostasis, as a surgical glue and to promote wound healing
Alpha$_1$-proteinase inhibitor	Treatment of alpha$_1$-proteinase inhibitor deficiency
Antithrombin III	Treatment of acquired and hereditary deficiency of Antithrombin III
C1-esterase inhibitor	Treatment of hereditary angioedema
Under Investigation	
Plasmin	Dissolution of clots by direct application in peripheral arterial occlusion, stroke, deep vein thrombosis, myocardial infarction, and clotted intravascular devices
Reconstituted plasma-derived high-density lipoprotein (derived from Apolipoprotein A)	Atherosclerotic plaque stabilization in acute coronary syndrome through reduction in lipid content and other anti-inflammatory and antithrombotic mechanisms
Transferrin	Treatment of hypotransferrinemia, enhancing erythropoiesis, and reducing anemia in β-thalassemia. Used in hematological stem cell transplantation to sequester free iron-binding of iron reduces free-iron-mediated ischemia/reperfusion injury in transplanted organs
Plasminogen	Treatment of ligneous conjunctivitis related to plasminogen deficiency
Haptoglobin	Removal of free hemoglobin arising from hemolysis in burns, trauma, and surgical intervention
Ceruloplasmin	Use in Ukraine and Russia has been as an adjunct therapy in cancer therapy, emergency medicine indications, and infection; outcomes thought to be enhanced by the antioxidant and ferroxidase activity of ceruloplasmin

Key components of the manufacture of plasma protein therapeutics

Plasma for fractionation

The manufacture of plasma protein therapeutics commences with the collection of plasma. This is a logistically and technically complex activity due to the need to ensure product quality and safety.[33] The viral safety of plasma collected for fractionation is ensured by what has been referred to as a "Five Layer Safety."[34] These layers are donor screening, blood testing, donor referral, quarantine, and investigation. Details of these activities are provided in Chapters 44, 55 and 56.

Plasma used in the United States for manufacture is either recovered plasma—plasma derived from whole blood collection, or source plasma collected by plasmapheresis. No specific monograph exists in the United States that details the handling conditions to be applied to collected plasma. However, the pharmacopeia of the European Union (European Pharmacopeia) specifically details the freezing conditions applicable for labile and nonlabile proteins.[35] Thus, it recommends that plasma to be used in the manufacture of labile proteins needs to be frozen within 24 hours of collection, and that the rate of freezing be such that −25 °C is attained in 12 hours of

being placed in the freezing apparatus. For the recovery of nonlabile proteins the plasma must be frozen to −20 °C or below within 24 hours of collection. During storage and transportation, the temperature of the plasma can exceed −20 °C for not more than a total of 72 hours, it must not transiently exceed −15 °C on more than one occasion and at no time must the temperature exceed −5 °C.

The Cohn process

The procedure that continues to have a pivotal role in plasma fractionation was developed by Cohn in the 1940s. It is based on the differential precipitation of plasma proteins by manipulation of ethanol concentration and pH of a low-ionic-strength solution maintained at a subzero temperature.[32] The original process, known as the *Cohn method*,[6] is presented in Figure 27.1 and shows the conditions for the generation of specific fractions. Also shown is the recovery of cryoprecipitate from freeze-thawed plasma by centrifugation, typically incorporated in the processing of plasma. In addition the source of current therapeutic proteins or those under development, listed in Table 27.1, are detailed. An example will be considered to specifically illustrate the principle of the Cohn process: If one takes Supernatant I, adding ethanol to a final concentration of 25% (v/v) and adjusting the solution to pH 6.9,

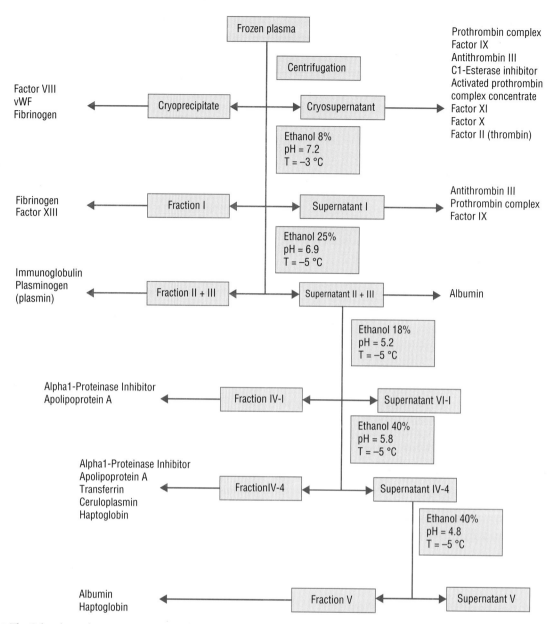

Figure 27.1 The Cohn plasma fractionation process with the fractions indicated that are the source of various therapeutic proteins.

while ensuring the ionic strength and temperature remain at approximately I = 0.09 and −5 °C respectively, results in the generation of the immunoglobulin-enriched Fraction II + III and Supernatant II+III containing albumin.

It is important to have an understanding of the Cohn process as the terminology associated with the process is often used in literature associated with various plasma-derived products. Each Cohn fraction is an enriched, albeit crude, source of various plasma proteins that can be further purified to generate a therapeutic product. How this is achieved will be covered in the subsequent sections. Prior to this however, a description of viral removal procedures commonly used in manufacturing processes will be undertaken. These need to be incorporated in any manufacturing process to ensure the viral safety of the product.

Viral removal procedures

To ensure the viral safety of plasma protein therapeutics, as has been discussed in this chapter, a safe plasma supply is required, achieved

through careful donor selection and screening and testing of donations. A third important determinant is the presence of inactivation or removal procedures in the manufacturing process. This is covered extensively in Chapter 56.

The purification of plasma proteins typically results, at various process steps, in the partitioning of virus away from the protein of interest. Thus, for example in the Cohn process, virus removal is achieved with the precipitation of Fractions III, I/III, II/III, and Fraction IV-I/IV-4 in the manufacture of immunoglobulin and albumin, respectively.[36] Regulatory requirements, however, require the inclusion of at least two dedicated orthogonal viral removal procedures that are effective against both enveloped and non-enveloped viruses.[37–41]

There is an ongoing interest in identifying effective yet convenient means of achieving viral removal. Viral filtration is a preferred option as it can, in many cases, be added to an existing process and is usually benign with respect to its effect on product integrity.[42–44] The preferred pore size for viral filters is 15 or 20 nm, thereby ensuring the removal of small non-enveloped viruses such as parvovirus B19 and hepatitis A.[45] This can limit the size of the protein that can be filtered. Immunoglobulins with a molecular weight of 150,000 d, can readily be filtered.[46,47] For larger proteins, viral filters with 35 nm pore size need to be used, although this would only be effective in removing large enveloped viruses such as hepatitis B and C and HIV. Examples of this include von Willebrand factor (vWF) which has a molecular weight of 500,000 d but exists as a series of multimers to a molecular weight of 20,000 kd.[48] Factor VIII–vWF has been filtered through a 20 nm filter by using specific conditions to dissociate the complex prior to filtration and subsequent inducing reassembly.[49] Viral filtration of fibrinogen, with a molecular weight of 340,000 d, through a 20 nm filter has also been achieved.[50]

Chromatographic procedures

The Cohn fractionation process can generate highly purified albumin and immunoglobulin products.[32,51] Today, albumin is still predominately purified by the Cohn procedure, and this was the case until the late 1990s for the production of immunoglobulin products. The purification of other therapeutic proteins from enriched Cohn fractions has only been able to be achieved by the application of chromatographic techniques.[52]

Details of the purification of the major plasma-derived therapeutic proteins will be provided in this chapter. However, an appreciation and understanding of these processes requires knowledge of the principles of chromatography and the orthogonal approaches that need to be applied to obtain highly purified preparations.

Chromatographic techniques allow the purification of proteins because of their differences in molecular weight, charge, hydrophobicity, and specific affinity for ligands. This involves the use of size exclusion, ion exchange, hydrophobic interaction (HIC), and affinity chromatography, respectively.[53–56] Chromatography is typically performed with columns packed with resin beads of about 80 μm in diameter and derivatized with particular functional groups to allow the particular chromatographic separation to be performed.

Size exclusion separation occurs as proteins percolate through the beads. Smaller proteins enter the pores of the beads, and hence their passage through the column is retarded, leading to the separation of proteins on the basis of molecular weight, with higher molecular weight proteins eluting first followed by the smaller species.

Ion exchange chromatographic resins exist in either the anion (positively charged) or cation (negatively charged) forms. Typical ion exchange ligands include dietlylaminoethyl (DEAE), quaternary amino ethyl (QAE), quaternary ammonium (Q), carboxymethyl (CM), sulfopropyl (SP), and methyl sulfonate (S) for anion and cation exchange chromatography, respectively. As proteins are zwitterion molecules, the net charge of the molecule can be modulated by changing the pH of the protein environment. Proteins have different pI values-the pH at which the net charge of the protein is zero.[56] Therefore, the net charge of a protein depends on pH, and this determines the degree of interaction with an ion exchange resin. Interaction can be further modulated by changes in ionic strength. Thus, by utilizing conditions that promote differential binding to ion exchange resins, coupled with defined elution conditions—again involving specific conditions of pH and conductivity—fractionation of a mixture of proteins can be achieved.

Proteins exhibit differences in their hydrophobic profile, reflecting differences in the composition of amino acids with hydrophobic (nonpolar) or hydrophilic (polar) properties.[56] This difference is exploited in hydrophobic interaction chromatography (HIC).

Solution conditions can be manipulated so that the more hydrophobic proteins are retained on a column while less hydrophobic proteins flow through.

Proteins exhibit unique surface epitopes and functional domains.[56] Immobilized antibodies and specific ligands on chromatographic resins, which can specifically interact with these parts of proteins, can be the basis of affinity chromatography for the purification of proteins from complex mixtures. Immobilized monoclonal antibodies, heparin, and metal affinity ligands are used in the purification of several plasma proteins.[52]

Manufacturing processes for plasma protein therapeutics

In this section, specific processes used in the recovery of all the major plasma proteins for therapeutic use will be described. The focus will be on illustrating the range of techniques that can be used in the manufacture of these products, and exposing the reader to a wide range of concepts underpinning the fractionation of plasma proteins. In addition, the expected pharmacopeial specifications of the final product, that ensure desired product safety and efficacy, will be detailed.

Albumin

The Cohn process remains the dominant process for the manufacture of albumin (Figure 27.1).[32] Details on the production of albumin by the Cohn process in a modern facility and the required quality attributes expected of the product have been reviewed elsewhere.[19]

As previously described, the Cohn process involves manipulation of ethanol concentration and pH of solutions at low ionic strength, while maintaining subzero temperatures, to achieve differential precipitation of proteins. The recovery of albumin involves the generation of Supernatant I, II+III, IV-1, IV-4, and finally the precipitation of pure albumin as Fraction V at 40% (v/v) ethanol, pH 5.8, with temperature maintained at −5 °C. A variation to the Cohn process was reported by Kistler and Nitschmann in 1962.[57] The aim was to maximize albumin yield and decrease the use of ethanol. Fraction I is generated as by the Cohn process. Precipitate A, the equivalent of Fraction II+III in the Cohn process, is produced with 19% (v/v) ethanol, pH 5.85, and allows the recovery of the albumin containing Supernatant A. This then progresses through the generation of Supernatant IV (40% v/v ethanol, pH 5.85, −8 °C) and Precipitate C (40% v/v ethanol, pH 4.8, −8 °C). Resuspension of Precipitate C and recovery of Supernatant D (10% v/v ethanol, pH 4.6, −3 °C) provide the final purified albumin. This process was initially used by the Swiss manufacturer ZLB, and continues to be used following its incorporation into CSL Behring.[31] The albumin recovered by ethanol fractionation is highly purified, although trace amounts of residual plasma proteins—typically, haptoglobin, ceruloplasmin, $α_2$-macroglobulin, acid$_2$-glycoprotein, hemopexin, and transferrin—can be detected[58,59] (CSL data on file).

An alternative chromatographic process, based on the method of Curling et al., was developed by CSL Behring (Australia) in the 1990s.[58,60,61] The process was initially developed for the purification of albumin from Supernatant II + III but was later adapted for the processing of Supernatant I.[62] The process is shown in Figure 27.2. The process incorporates three chromatographic steps—anion and cation exchange chromatography with DEAE and CM Sepharose®, respectively, and size exclusion chromatography using Sephacryl® S200 resin. This last step markedly contributes to the purity of the recovered albumin, removing residual proteins and aggregates.

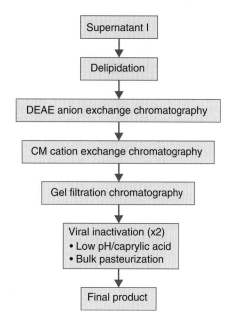

Figure 27.2 Chromatographic process for the purification of albumin—Albumex® (CSL Behring, Australia).

Chromatographically purified albumin is purer than that derived by ethanol fractionation and also exhibits a lower aggregate content.[58] This increased purity has been associated with a decreased rate of adverse reactions with chromatographically purified albumin.[62]

The Cohn process for the manufacture of albumin contributes to the viral safety of the product through partitioning virus away from the product stream.[63–66] With the alternative chromatographic process, similar partitioning is achieved at the chromatographic steps.[67,68] In addition, a specific viral inactivation step is included in the manufacturing process—pasteurization at 60 °C for 10 hours.[63–66] This has been part of the production of albumin from the very beginning and undoubtedly accounts for the fact that there has never been a viral transmission from an albumin product.[69] The pasteurization of albumin was possible due to the finding that N-acetyl tryptophanate and sodium octanoate (caprylate), or sodium octanoate alone, stabilized the molecule during heating.[70,71]

The European Pharmacopoeia (EP) and US regulations (CFR21) stipulate that pasteurization be performed in the final container following dispensing in order to completely remove the risk of recontamination.[72,73] Reflecting advances in bioprocessing execution and control, CSL Behring (Australia), in addition to developing a novel chromatographic manufacturing process, obtained approval from the Australian regulatory authority to implement bulk pasteurization of its albumin product prior to dispensing.[58] This product (Albumex®) is registered and used in Australia, New Zealand, Hong Kong, Singapore, Taiwan, Malaysia, and Indonesia (CSL data on file). Albumex® has an additional viral inactivation step consisting of incubation at low pH in the presence of caprylic acid at 30 °C for 10 hours.[74] This step was introduced to add further viral safety to the product and reflected the regulatory expectations that plasma protein products have at least two dedicated viral inactivation or removal steps.[37]

The specifications of the product are governed by EP and US Pharmacopeia and National Formulary (USP) or CFR pharmacopeial requirements, which provide limits for physical properties, biological safety, purity, excipients, and contaminants.[72,73,75] Purified albumin solutions are supplied by various manufacturers as 4,

4.5, 5, 20, and 25% (w/v) solutions and typically exhibit a shelf-life of up to five years at room temperature (25–30 °C).[19] It is a requirement that solution must be clear and can be almost colorless, yellow, amber, or green (EP). The variation in color reflects differences in the presence of residual heme as well as colored protein impurities such as haptoglobin, ceruloplasmin, transferrin, and hemopexin.[59,76] Chromatographically purified albumin is typically a greenish color, reflecting its higher purity. It contains only a small amount or absence of colored proteins and heme, but increased levels of albumin bound bilirubin and the green oxidized derivative—biliverdin.[76] The product should not change in appearance with heating at 57 °C for 50 hours (CFR21).

The product should have a pH (at 20 °C) of 6.7–7.3 (EP) or 6.4–7.4 (USP). Osmolality should be equivalent to that of plasma (USP). With respect to excipients, sodium should not exceed 160 mmol/L (EP) or 130–160 mmol/L (USP). Sodium caprylate (sodium octanoate) should be 0.16 mmol/g albumin if it is the single stabilizer (CFR21). In preparation where dual stabilizers, sodium caprylate and N-acetyl tryptophanate, are used, the concentration of each should be 0.08 mmol/g albumin (CFR21).

Albumin purity should be at least 95% (EP) or 96% (USP), with aggregate content not more than 10% as determined by the area of the chromatogram determined by adsorption at 280 nm. Heme levels as determined by adsorption at 403 nm should not exceed 0.15 AU (EP). Chromatographically purified albumin contains no detectable heme-related absorbance.[76]

Prekallikrein activator (PKA) activity should not be more than 35 IU/mL (EP). This is an important specification as PKA (also known as factor XIIa or Hageman factor fragment), if present, can lead to a clinical hypotensive reaction.[77]

Contaminant levels, of which potassium and aluminum are specified, should be 0.05 mmol/g albumin (EP) or 2 meq/L (USP) and 200 µg/L (EP), respectively. The limit for aluminum was introduced into the British Pharmacopoeia in 1993 to ensure albumin safety for use in renal dialysis and with premature babies.[78] Another concern was the accumulation of aluminum with the treatment of burn patients.[79] The source of aluminum is from the glass containers used for the product. Leaching of aluminum is abetted by even very low concentrations of citrate (<0.1 mmol/L), which originates from the anticoagulant used during plasma collection.[80] Through optimization of diafiltration processes used in manufacturing, to minimize citrate content, current albumin products meet the required aluminum pharmacopeial limit.[19,81]

The solution should be sterile, nonpyrogenic, and with endotoxin levels not more than 0.5 EU/mL (EP/USP). The pharmacopeias also specify that the final product be incubated for a period prior to final inspection to provide additional assurance of product sterility. CFR21 requires incubation for at least 14 days at 20–35 °C, and the EP states not less than 14 days at 30–32 °C, or not less than four weeks at 20–25 °C.

Immunoglobulins

The Cohn process also served as the starting point for the purification of immunoglobulins.[32] Oncley developed a process for the recovery of purified immunoglobulins from Cohn Fraction II + III.[51] In the process, the fraction is resuspended and reprecipitated with 20% v/v ethanol, at pH 7.6 (modifications exist with pH 6.7), and temperature at −5 °C. The recovered precipitate is then resuspended, and the solution adjusted to 17% v/v ethanol, at pH 5.2, with temperature maintained at −6 °C. This results in precipitation of IgM and other impurities (Fraction III), whereas IgG remains in the supernatant (Supernatant III). IgG is then recovered as Fraction II by precipitation with 25% v/v ethanol, pH 7.4, with the temperature at −5 °C.

A modification of the Oncley process was developed by Kistler and Nitschmann in 1962.[57] The aim was to increase the yield of IgG and reduce ethanol use. In this process, Precipitate A (corresponding to Cohn Fraction I + II + III) is obtained at 19% v/v ethanol, pH 8.5, temperature −5 °C. Following resuspension of the precipitate in water, the solution is adjusted to pH 5.1 and ethanol is added to 12% v/v while maintaining the temperature at 5 °C. This results in the precipitation of impurities, including IgM (Precipitate B), with IgG remaining in the supernatant (Supernatant b) (equivalent of Cohn Supernatant III). The IgG is recovered by precipitation at 25% v/v ethanol, pH 7.0, at −7 °C. This precipitate G corresponds to Cohn Fraction II. These processes, with various modifications, for many years, have accounted for the bulk of commercially produced immunoglobulins.[82,83] The Kistler–Nitschmann process was particularly identified with the ZLB (later CSL Behring) facility in Bern, where the process was used for the production of Sandoglobulin®.[84]

The development of new immunoglobulin manufacturing processes from the mid-1990s has reflected the desire of manufacturers to improve product characteristics and safety. This has led to the increase in final formulation protein concentration in order to increase the convenience of use, the introduction of viral inactivation steps to improve safety; and the introduction of procedures to improve yield and manufacturing efficiency.[82,83,85] A number of companies have developed hybrid processes where the crude IgG precipitate generated by ethanol precipitation (Fraction II + III or Precipitate A) is subjected to further chromatographic processing to recover the purified immunoglobulin.[20,82,83,85,86] CSL Behring (Australia) developed a unique completely chromatographic procedure, and in 2000, its use commenced for the production of immunoglobulin for the Australian market and other toll customers, which included New Zealand, Hong Kong, Singapore, and Taiwan.[87–89] A key feature of this process was the increased yield in IgG that was achieved when compared to the Cohn-based process.[90]

In the following, a brief description is presented of the manufacturing processes of all the major immunoglobulin products currently produced and the expected pharmacopeial specifications of immunoglobulin products. This area has also been reviewed extensively elsewhere.[20]

A number of products are purified essentially by the complete application of the Oncley ethanol fractionation process. In the manufacture of Octagam® (Octopharma), purified IgG is recovered as Fraction II (Figure 27.3). In addition to the viral partitioning that occurs during the fractionation process, there is solvent–detergent (S/D) treatment and low-pH incubation, as described above, for viral inactivation. The oil/solid phase extraction step is a means of removing the S/D used during the viral inactivation procedure.[20,91,92]

In the BIVIGAM® (Biotest, AG) process, pure IgG as Supernatant III is produced by the Oncley process.[93] This is then subjected to the first viral inactivation procedure involving S/D treatment. It is then further purified by Q anion exchange chromatography before undergoing viral filtration through a 35 nm pore filter (Figure 27.4). The specific viral inactivation procedures in this process target inactivation and removal of enveloped viruses (HIV, hepatitis B, and hepatitis C). Removal of non-enveloped viruses (parvovirus B19 and hepatitis A) relies on partitioning into the discarded Fraction III during the recovery of Supernatant III.[93]

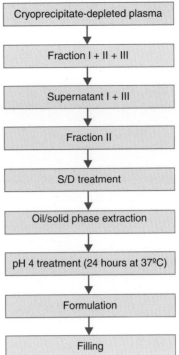

Octagam®

Figure 27.3 Process steps for Octagam® (Octapharma).

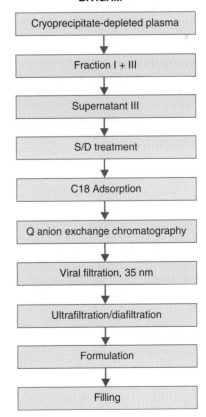

BIVIGAM®

Figure 27.4 Process steps for BIVIGAM® (Biotest).

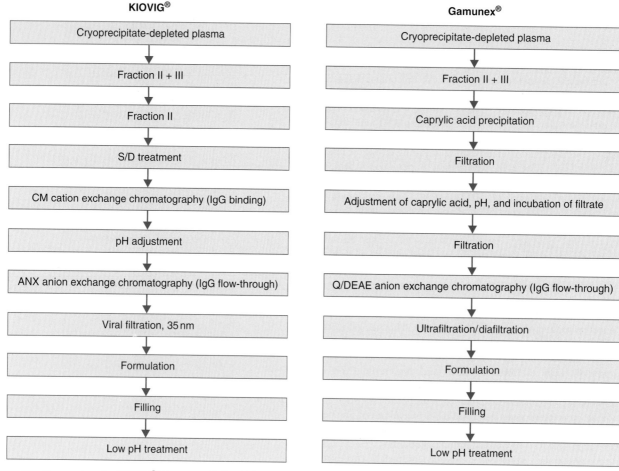

Figure 27.5 Process steps for KIOVIG®/Gammagard® (Baxalta).

Figure 27.6 Process steps for Gamunex® (Grifols).

KIOVIG® or Gammagard® produced by Baxalta (European and US trade names, respectively) is also produced by the Oncley process resulting in the generation of purified IgG as Fraction II[94] (Figure 27.5). The purified immunoglobulin is then subjected to three viral inactivation or removal procedures—S/D treatment, viral filtration with a 35 nm filter, and low-pH formulation and incubation of the dispensed product. The cation exchange chromatography step is used to bind the immunoglobulin and thereby allow the removal of the S/D used in the viral inactivation procedure. Passage through the anion exchange column retains impurities and results in further purification of the immunoglobulins.

The manufacture of Gamunex® (Grifols) is one of a number of hybrid manufacturing processes that involves the generation of a crude IgG fraction by ethanol precipitation followed by further purification by chromatography[108,109] (Figure 27.6). Cohn Fraction II + III is suspended and caprylic acid added to precipitate impurities. The caprylic acid concentration is adjusted in the recovered filtrate and incubated at 25 °C for one hour. This constitutes the first viral inactivation procedure in the manufacturing process. The generation of pure IgG is achieved by sequential passage through a strong (Q) and a weak (DEAE) anion exchange chromatographic columns. Following buffer exchange, concentration, and formulation, where pH is adjusted approximately 4.25, the product is dispensed and then incubated at 28 °C for 21 days. This constitutes the second viral inactivation step. The viral inactivation procedures of Gamunex® are effective for enveloped viruses

(HIV, hepatitis B, and hepatitis C) but are not recognized for use against non-enveloped viruses (hepatitis A and parvovirus B19). The virus clearance for non-enveloped virus in the Gamunex® process is accounted for by caprylic acid precipitation, depth filtration following the caprylate incubation, and partitioning during anion exchange chromatography.[85]

In the manufacture of Flebogamma DIF®, Cohn Fraction II+III is resuspended, partially purified by precipitation of impurities by the addition of polyethylene glycol (PEG), and then further purified by anion exchange chromatography under conditions whereby impurities are retained. The purified immunoglobulin recovery is subjected to three validated viral removal or inactivation procedures: pasteurization, S/D treatment, and viral filtration through 20 nm filters. The PEG precipitation of the resuspended Cohn Fraction II + III is also associated with significant viral clearance. There is a second PEG precipitation after the low-pH treatment, pasteurization, and S/D treatment, which serves to remove immunoglobulin aggregates and facilities passage of the solution in the subsequent viral filtration step[60,95] (Figure 27.7).

The purification of Clair Y g® (LFB) involves the use of Cohn Fraction I + II + III. Following resolubilization, impurities are removed by caprylic acid precipitation. The filtrate is ultrafiltered to remove caprylic acid and the retenate is subjected to S/D treatment. The immunoglobulin is then captured on an anion exchange column allowing the solvent and detergent of the viral inactivation procedure to be removed. The eluted immunoglobulin

Flebogamma DIF®

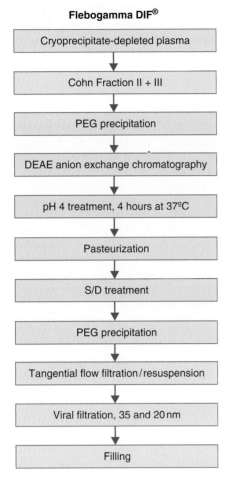

Figure 27.7 Process steps for Flebogamma DIF® (Grifols).

ClairYg®

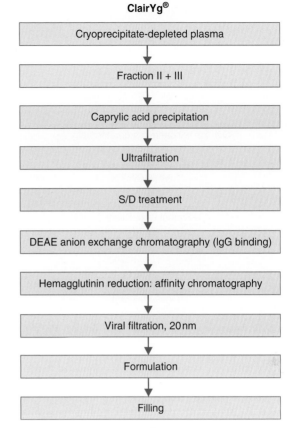

Figure 27.8 Process steps for ClairYg® (LFB).

Privigen®

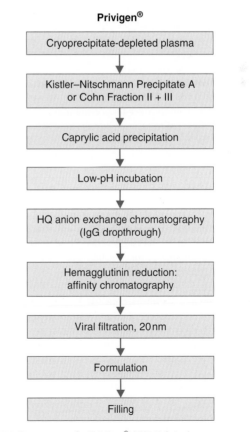

Figure 27.9 Process steps for Privigen® (CSL Behring).

is then passed through an affinity resin to reduce the anti-A and anti-B isoagglutinin titer. The immunoglobulin then undergoes viral filtration, the second viral removal step, prior to formulation and filling[96] (Figure 27.8).

The manufacture of Privigen® (CSL Behring) is also a hybrid manufacturing process that involves the generation of a crude IgG fraction by ethanol precipitation followed by further purification by chromatography.[97] Kistler–Nitschmann precipitate A or Cohn Fraction II + III is resuspended, and caprylic acid addition is used to precipitate impurities. The recovered partially purified immunoglobulin solution is subjected to low-pH incubation in the presence of a low concentration of detergent as part of the first viral inactivation procedure incorporated in the process. Final purification of the immunoglobulins is achieved by passage through a Q anion exchange chromatographic column under conditions where impurities (predominantly IgM and IgA) are bound and IgG flows through. This in turn is passed over an affinity column to decrease the anti-A and anti-B hemagglutinin titers.[98] The recovered immunoglobulin solution is then subjected to viral filtration the second viral removal procedure in the process, prior to formulation and dispensing (Figure 27.9).

The final manufacturing process to be described is a completely chromatographic process used by CSL Behring (Australia) to manufacture Intragam P®[87,88] (Figure 27.10). As has been mentioned in this chapter, a key feature of this process is the achieved increased recovery of immunoglobulins. Supernatant I, which is

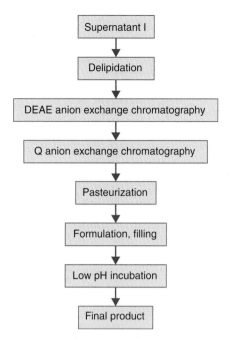

Figure 27.10 Process steps for Intragam P® (CSL Behring, Australia).

essentially fibrinogen-depleted plasma, is delipidated to minimize chromatographic resin fouling, prior to being passed through a DEAE anion exchange column. Albumin, a protein of interest, adheres to the resin while immunoglobulins drop through. As has been discussed in the albumin section, albumin is eluted and undergoes further processing. The recovered immunoglobulin fraction undergoes further purification by passage through a Q anion exchange chromatographic column at a pH that promotes the binding of the major protein impurities, IgA, IgM, and transferrin, but results in the flow-through of the IgG immunoglobulins. The process includes pasteurization as the first viral inactivation procedure. Following formulation at a low pH (pH 4.25) and filling, the dispensed product is incubated at 27 °C for 14 days as the second viral inactivation procedure of the process.

Gamimune N® (Miles Cutter/Bayer) in 1992 was the first immunoglobulin for intravenous use to be available as a 10% (w/v) formulation.[99] There has been a consistent trend over the last 20 years of moving from a final protein concentration of 5 or 6% (w/v) to 10% (w/v). The increased protein concentration reduces the volume that needs to be infused and hence, is more convenient for the patient.[100] Today, all the major immunoglobulin products on the market that have been described here are available at the 10% w/v formulation.[101] CSL Behring has developed a 20% w/v formulation immunoglobulin product called Hizentra® intended for subcutaneous administration.[102]

A key challenge in the development of an immunoglobulin preparation suitable for intravenous use was identifying a means of preventing the development of anti-complementary activity in the product arising from the formation of aggregates. These led to spontaneous activation of the complement system and caused severe adverse reactions.[103] Early success in inactivating anti-complementary aggregates was achieved in 1962 by Barandum and Isliker through mild proteolysis with pepsin at pH 4.0.[103] Improvements in processing, such as the use of ultrafiltration and diafiltration at pH 4.0 for the removal of ethanol from Supernatant III and for the concentration of IgG, instead of precipitation and lyophilization, minimized aggregate formation and generated a clinically

tolerated product.[104] It was then shown that formulation of the immunoglobulin at approximately pH 4.25 generated a liquid stable product with low anti-complementary.[105,106] The stability of immunoglobulin at low pH is due to the fact that this is below their isoelectric point, and results in non-interacting positively charged molecules. Consequently, many immunoglobulin products are now formulated at less than pH 5.0.[101,105,107] This is the case for many of the products described above—Privigen®, Hizentra®, KOIVIG® (Gammagard®), BIVIGAM®, Intragam P®, and Gammunex®. Formulation pH of Flebogamma DIF® and Octogam® is still much lower than neutral at pH 5–6.0 and pH 5.1–6.0, respectively.

Excipients are used in the formulation of immunoglobulins. These serve to stabilize the immunoglobulin molecules in solution by minimizing protein–protein interactions to ensure the clinically acceptable tonicity of the product.[108,109] Most immunoglobulin products in fact can be stored at room temperature for up to 36 months.[101,110] Currently used excipients comprising of amino acids, sugars and sugar alcohols have a long history of use and are known to be well tolerated.[108] Glycine is most commonly used, but as illustrated by the products described above, proline, maltose, sorbitol, and mannitol are also used. Low concentrations of sodium chloride and polysorbate detergent may also be added to adjust tonicity and enhance stability.[111–115]

As immunoglobulins for intravenous use are manufactured by varying processes, the properties of the different products produced have been examined.[96,116] In addition, consideration has been given to whether formulation differences could affect clinical tolerability.[111–115] Although differences have been noted, there is no evidence that they significantly correlate with differences in product efficacy and tolerability. As registered products, these immunoglobulin products meet the standards as prescribed by relevant regulatory authorities.

The European Pharmacopoeia has a comprehensive monograph on immunoglobulins for intravenous use.[117] The product is expected to be sterile and free of pyrogens and endotoxins. A liquid formulation is expected to be clear or slightly opalescent, colorless, or pale yellow. The allowable pH is 4.0–7.4. Osmolality must be greater than 240 mOsmol/kg. The minimum allowable protein concentration of a formulation should not be less than 30 g/L (3% w/v). As modern immunoglobulin products are typically formulated at 10% (w/v), this limit is not usually relevant. Purity is expected to be greater than 95%—with the currently used manufacturing processes, this is readily achieved. Aggregate content must not exceed 3% of total protein. This is an important quality attribute as aggregates typically result in complement activation-mediated adverse reactions. Any propensity for this is monitored through the measurement of anti-complementary activity, with the specification set at <1 CH_{50}/mg IgG. Specifically, this means that an aliquot of immunoglobulin solution will not sequester more than 50% of a given amount of complement.

The allowable maximum limit of prekallikrein activator (PKA) (factor XIIa), which can mediate the formation of the vasoactive peptide bradykinin from kinnogen and lead to hypotensive reactions, is set at 35 IU/mL.[118]

Hemagglutinins, anti-A and anti-B antibodies to red cell antigens, can result in hemolytic reactions with the infusion of immunoglobulins. Therefore, the EP stipulates a maximum allowable titer of 1:64. Given that high-volume administration of immunoglobulins is required in some indications, specifically those associated with achieving immune modulation, manufacturers are introducing specified hemagglutinin removal steps in manufacturing their process to lower the titer in their products.[96,116] Therefore, the titer of some products will be considerably lower than this limit.

The EP does not define a maximum level of IgA allowed in immunoglobulin products but the product must comply with the level stated on the label. The range for the products described here is 5–200 μg/mL.[101] Knowledge of the IgA content of an immunoglobulin product is important for a clinician when confronted with an IgA deficient patient who could exhibit an anaphylactic reaction if infused with a higher IgA concentration immunoglobulin product.[119]

Although not prescribed in the EP, immunoglobulin products are expected to exhibit a subclass distribution comparable to that normally found in plasma.[119] Partial depletion of IgG$_3$ and IgG$_4$ is, however, encountered in a number of manufacturing processes.[20] There is no evidence that this affects the efficacy of the product. The EP requires that a developed immunoglobulin purification process maintain the integrity of the Fc portion of the immunoglobulin molecule—key to its immunomodulatory role through interaction with the Fc receptor and its effector role in complement activation.[119] Monitoring of Fc function is not a product release requirement but is part of process validation. An immunoglobulin product should exhibit an Fc function of >60% of that of an EP standard. However, current products typically have values of 100%.[20]

The EP also stipulates that antibody titer to hepatitis B be at least 0.5 IU/g IgG. There is no limit for antibodies to hepatitis A, but regulatory authorities expect levels to be above 10 IU/ml. This may be increasingly difficult to maintain due to the consistent decline in population titers from at least 2003 due to increased hygiene and the availability of an effective hepatitis A vaccine.[20,120] Product specifications for the United States also include minimum antibody levels for measles, diphtheria, and polio.[121] With respect to measles, there are interesting trends suggesting that as disease prevalence is decreasing as a result of increased vaccination, antibody titer in plasma and hence immunoglobulin products is decreasing.[122]

In 2010, increased incidences of thromboembolic events were reported in patients using Octogam®.[123] Analysis showed this was due to increased levels of factor XIa caused by a process change. The regulatory agencies requested that manufacturers confirm that their processes have the capability of removing thrombogenic activity and generate a product low in procoagulant activity.[117,124,125] Procoagulants have been shown to be partitioned away from the product during purification and inactivated by pasteurization and exposure to low pH.[123–125] The most commonly used methods are non-activated partial thromboplastin time (NaPTT) and the thrombin generation assay (TGA). The latter is typically calibrated relative to factor XIa concentration. NaPTT values with clotting time >150 seconds are considered acceptable. With respect to TGA-derived results, existing products typically have very low to nondetectable levels of factor XIa.[126,127]

Factor XIII

The development of manufacturing processes for factor XIII has been extensively reviewed.[15] The focus here will be on describing the production of a major commercial factor XIII product, Fibrogammin P® (in Europe) and Corifact® (in the United States), as undertaken by CSL Behring. The process utilizes Cohn Fraction I precipitate derived from cryoprecipitate-depleted plasma. Following resolubilization and removal of fibrinogen by treatment with aluminum hydroxide and Vitacel® (a cellulose fiber), the clarified solution is subjected to DEAE anion exchange chromatography.

The purified factor XIII is then subjected to two viral inactivation and removal procedures—pasteurization (60 °C for 10 hours) and viral filtration with 20 nm filters. These dedicated viral removal procedures, together with viral partitioning achieved during the chromatography procedure, result in excellent viral clearance through the manufacturing process. Following formulation to the target potency and with the addition of albumin, glucose, and sodium chloride, the solution is sterile filtered, dispensed, and lyophilized.[128,129] There is no monograph for factor XIII product, but these products have been extensively characterized with respect to purity, function, and factor XIII integrity. This includes factor XIII activity, specific activity, factor XIII subunit A content, fibrinogen clotting time, PKA, and activated factor XIII.[15]

Factor X

The manufacture of a therapeutic factor X produced by BPL (UK) is shown in Figure 27.11. The key steps in the process are adsorption of factor X from cryoprecipitate-depleted plasma by DEAE anion exchange chromatography. Further purification is achieved by

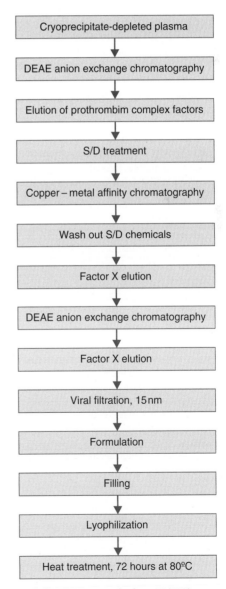

Figure 27.11 Manufacturing process for factor X (BPL).

metal affinity chromatography with a copper chelate resin. Viral removal of enveloped and non-enveloped viruses is achieved by S/D treatment and viral filtration with 15 nm filters. In addition, the lyophilized product is subject to heat treatment at 80 °C for 72 hours.[15] The product has been shown to comply with required toxicity, thrombogenicity, and immunogenicity requirements. In addition, in vitro tests confirm the product is potent, highly purified, and free of potentially hazardous residues. The testing includes determination of factor X potency, specific activity, the presence of factor II, factor IX, proteins C and S, and NaPTT.[15]

Activated prothrombin complex concentrate (aPCC)

aPCC, known as factor VIII inhibitor bypassing activity (FEIBA®), is manufactured by Baxalta. Details on the development, production, mechanism of action, and clinical use of the product have recently been reviewed.[11] The manufacturing process is shown in Figure 27.12. It involves purification of prothrombin complex factors (II, VII, IX, and X) from cryoprecipitate-depleted plasma by DEAE anion exchange chromatography. The recovered material undergoes viral filtration with a 35 nm filter. The factors are then contact activated, generating activated Factor VII and some activated factor X. These activated factors, together with prothrombin, are thought to be important for the clinical efficacy of the product.[11,130] The product undergoes a second viral inactivation treatment involving vapor heat treatment at 60 °C and 80 °C for at least 8.5 hours and 1 hour, respectively, on the lyophilized product. This step is effective against both enveloped and non-enveloped viruses. The product is then formulated with sodium citrate and sodium chloride, and dispensed in 500, 1000, and 2500 arbitrary FEIBA units. One unit of activity is defined as that amount of product that shortens the activated partial thromboplastin time (aPTT) of a high-titer factor VIII inhibitor reference plasma to 50% of the blank value. The final product is a lyophilized preparation.[131]

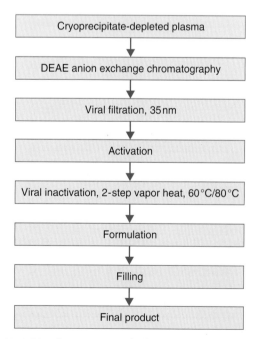

Figure 27.12 Manufacturing process for factor VIII bypassing activity (FEIBA®) (Baxalta).

Alpha₁-proteinase inhibitor

The manufacturing processes for the four major alpha₁-proteinase inhibitor (API) products on the market, Aralast NP® (Baxalta), Zemaira® (CSL Behring), Prolastin C® (Grifols), and Glassia® (Kamada), are presented in Figure 27.13.[132–136] A comprehensive examination of these manufacturing processes is available elsewhere.[23]

Cohn Fraction IV-I is the source material. The Aralast NP® process utilizes a unique step involving, an extended thaw of the paste and dissolution in pH 6.0 buffer that allows the recovery of an API-enriched precipitate. The generated initial crude API solutions undergo an initial "activation hold" step at approximately pH 9 and at an elevated temperature of approximately 45 °C. This results in increased recovery of functional protein, which could be related to refolding of denatured protein. The commencement of the purification process typically involves polyethylene glycol (PEG) precipitation of impurities, destabilization of unwanted proteins by reduction with dithiothrietol (DTT), and adsorption with fumed silica (Aerosil®). This treatment takes advantage of the fact that there are no disulfide bonds in the API molecule.[137] All processes utilize anion exchange chromatography for further purification. Further polishing is achieved by adsorption with bentonite (aluminum phyllosilicate clay), hydrophobic interaction chromatography, or cation exchange chromatography. The Aralot NP®, Glassia®, and Prolastin-C® processes all incorporate S/D treatment as the first viral inactivation procedure. Pasteurization is used in the Zemaira® process. All processes include viral filtration as the second viral removal step, and this is effective for both enveloped and non-enveloped viruses. Aralast NP®, Zemaira®, and Prolastin C® are presented as lyophilized final products, whereas Glassia® is a liquid product.[23]

The EP prescribes certain product qualities for API preparations.[138] The specific activity should not be less than 0.35 mg of active API per mg of total protein. The ratio of API activity to antigen should not be less than 0.7. With respect to appearance, the liquid preparation should be clear or slightly opalescent, colorless, or pale yellow, pale green, or pale brown; the freeze-dried preparation should be a powder or solid friable mass, hygroscopic, and white, pale yellow, or pale brown.

It is required that the pH be in the range of 6.5–7.8, that the preparation be completely soluble, and that osmolality be greater than 240 mOsmol/kg. In addition, the water content of the freeze-dried preparation must be within the limits approved for the product by the competent authority. The product must be sterile and free of pyrogens and bacterial endotoxins.

Factor XI

The manufacture of factor XI is undertaken by LFB Biotechnologies (France).[14] Cryoprecipitate-depleted plasma (cryosupernatant) is passed through a negatively charged filter to capture the factor XI. It is then eluted with 1 M NaCl containing antithrombin III (ATIII), which inhibits any proteolytic activity that could degrade the product. Following buffer exchange by ultrafiltration, the solution is subjected to viral inactivation treatment with S/D. The solution is passed through a sulfate(S) cation exchange chromatographic resin to capture the protein and allow the washing away of the virus-inactivating chemicals. The factor XI is recovered with eluate buffer containing lysine and arginine by increasing the salt content and pH to 170 mM and 7.5, respectively. Heparin and ATIII were added to the eluate, and then it was sterile

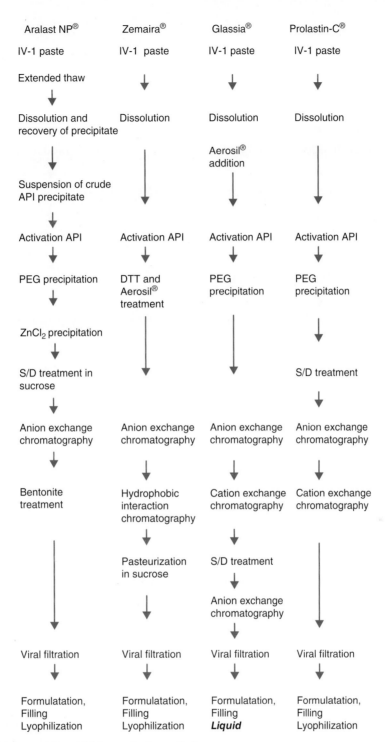

Figure 27.13 Comparison of alpha$_1$-proteinase inhibitor production methods.

filtered, dispensed, and lyophilized. The product is highly purified, containing only trace amounts of fibrinogen, albumin, C1-esterase inhibitor, fibronectin, alpha$_2$-macroglobulin, and IgG. The levels of other coagulation factors, kinin system components, and proteases are also low or nondetectable.[139]

The EP required that the freeze-dried final product be white or almost white powder or friable solid. The water content must be within the limits approved by the competent authority. It should completely dissolve within 10 minutes. The potency must be within 80–120% of that stated on the label. The reconstituted product should be of pH 6.8–7.4 and have a minimum osmolality of 240 mOsmol/kg. Heparin and ATIII added as stabilizers must comply with the level stated on the label. Ensuring the absence of activated coagulation factors, the NaPTT coagulation time should not be less than 150 seconds. There should not be any significant presence of anti-A and anti-B hemagglutinins, with no agglutination occurring at a 1:64 dilution of the product. The product must be sterile and free of bacterial endotoxins.[140]

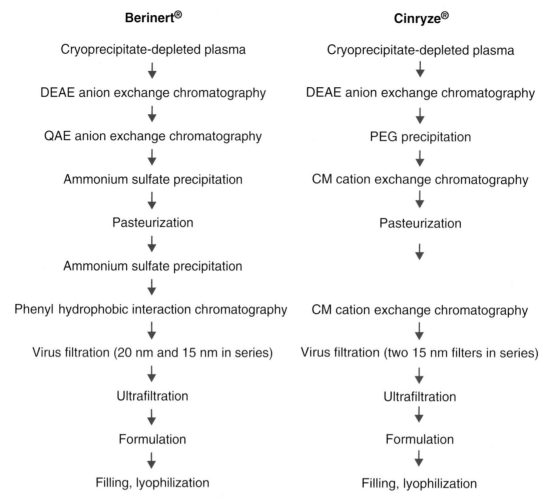

Figure 27.14 Processes for the manufacture of C1-esterase inhibitor.

C1-esterase inhibitor

A recent review comprehensively deals with the biology, purification, and clinical use of C1-esterase inhibitor.[24] This section will focus on describing the manufacturing processes of two of the major C1-esterase inhibitor products on the market: Berinert® (CSL Behring), and Cinryze® (US) or Ceton® (Europe) (Sanguine).[24,141,142] As can be seen in Figure 27.14, the processes are quite distinct in the use of chromatographic processes. In the production of Berinert®, cryo-precipitate-depleted plasma is initialed; passed through a DEAE anion exchange column, under conditions in which the C1-esterase inhibitor flows through; and subsequently captured on a QAE anion exchange resin. Further purification is achieved by ammonium sulfate precipitation steps and hydrophobic interaction chromatography (HIC). In the Cinryze® process, the C1-esterase inhibitor is captured from the starting material by anion exchange chromatography, and further purification is achieved by PEG precipitation and two procedures involving cation exchange chromatography. In both processes, viral removal involves pasteurization and virus filtration requiring two filters in series.[141,143] The recovered virally filtered product is formulated, dispensed, and lyophilized. In the case of Berinert®, excipients used in its formulation are glycine, sodium chloride, and sodium citrate.[144]

There are no pharmacopoeial requirements for C1-esterase inhibitor concentrates. However, as with other lyophilized therapeutic protein products, it must have an acceptable appearance in the lyophilized state and comply with registered residual moisture content. The product must readily dissolve and present as a colorless and clear solution with clinically acceptable osmolality and insoluble particle count. It must be sterile and free of bacterial endotoxins. Manufacturers determine and report the potency of the product.[144] The integrity of the product is determined by monomer content, which is a quality control release specification. Thus, for example, Berinert® must have a monomer content of >89% to meet release specifications (CSL data on file). Recently, a biochemical and purity comparison of four commercially available C1-esterase inhibitor products (Berinert®, Cinryze®, Cetor®, and Ruconest® [transgenic product]) was published consisting of characterization of molecular weight, determination of specific activity, and quantitation and identification of residual proteins. It was the hope of the authors that the work would contribute to the establishment of regulatory requirements for determining purity and setting allowable threshold levels.[145]

Antithrombin III

As examples of manufacturing processes for Antithrombin III (ATIII), the processes for Kybernin P® (CSL Behring), Thrombotrol® (CSL Behring [Australia]), and Thrombate III® (Grifols) are

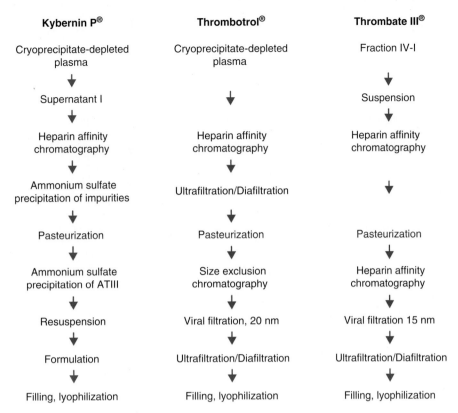

Figure 27.15 Comparison of Antithrombin III manufacturing processes.

described and shown in Figure 27.15.[146,147] Further information on the biology, purification, and clinical indications for ATIII is available in a recent review.[18]

From either Supernatant I, cryoprecipitate-depleted plasma, or a Fraction IV-I suspension, ATIII is captured by heparin affinity chromatography. The Kybernin P® process then uses sequential ammonium sulfate steps to remove impurities and to concentrate the ATIII by precipitation. All processes incorporate pasteurization as a viral inactivation step. In the Kybernin P® process, a subsequent ammonium precipitation of ATIII allows the removal of pasteurization stabilizers and the production of a concentrated solution, which is formulated, dispensed, and lyophilized. In the Thrombotrol® and Thrombate III® processes, further purification is achieved by size exclusion and heparin affinity chromatography, respectively. Both processes incorporate viral filtration. The recovered filtrate is then concentrated and diafiltered prior to formulation, dispensing, and lyophilization. Thrombotrol® and Thrombate III® processes incorporate two dedicated viral inactivation and removal steps that are effective for both enveloped and non-enveloped viruses. The Kybernin P® process has only one dedicated viral inactivation step—pasteurization, which is effective against both enveloped and non-enveloped viruses. In addition, viral clearance is achieved by precipitation at the first ammonium sulfate precipitation step.[146]

The EP prescribes a number of product specifications.[148] At least a 60% fraction of the product must bind heparin. The specific activity of the product should not be less than 3 IU ATIII per mg of protein (excluding albumin excipient). The lyophilized product should be a white or almost white, hygroscopic, friable solid or powder. The water content must be within limits approved by the competent authority. The product should completely dissolve within 10 minutes with gentle swirling, giving a clear or slightly turbid, colorless or almost colorless solution. The limits for pH and osmolality are 6.0–7.5 and >240 mOsmol/kg, respectively. The maximum allowed heparin content is 0.1 IU per IU ATIII. The product must be sterile and free of bacterial endotoxins.

Fibrinogen

Riastap® (US) or Haemocomplettan® (Europe) produced by CSL Behring is the leading fibrinogen concentrate available on the market. The product is derived from cryoprecipitate residue after extraction of factor VIII. The manufacturing process is based on a series of glycine-based precipitations—a procedure initially described by Bromback and Bromich in 1956.[149,150] The cryoprecipitate extract is initially adsorbed with aluminum hydroxide, and then the fibrinogen is precipitated with high-concentration glycine. The reconstituted fibrinogen is then pasteurized. Following the addition of glycine to promote precipitation of residual proteins, a purified fibrinogen is recovered by precipitation by increasing the concentration of glycine. The pure fibrinogen precipitate is redissolved, concentrated and diafiltered, formulated, dispensed, and lyophilized. The pasteurization step is effective against enveloped and non-enveloped virus. Further viral clearance is obtained at the cryoprecipitation and glycine precipitation steps.[151,152]

The EP requires that the lyophilized product be white or pale yellow, in a hygroscopic powder or friable solid; that the water content is within approval limits; and that it dissolves within 30 minutes at room temperature, forming an almost colorless, slightly opalescent solution. The solution should contain not less than 10 g/l fibrinogen with pH of 6.5 to 7.5 and a minimum osmolality of 240 mOsmol/kg. The product should be sterile and free of bacterial endotoxins.[153]

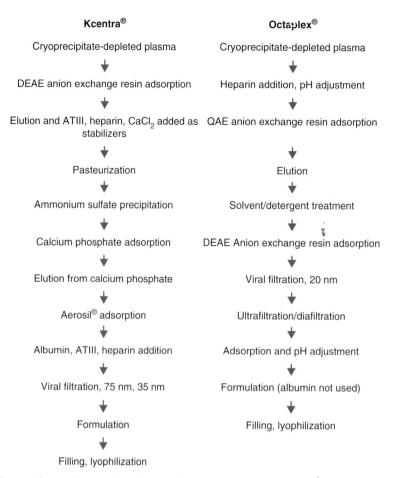

Figure 27.16 Comparison of the manufacture of two prothrombin complex concentrate products.

The development of another fibrinogen product by Octapharma, called Octofibrin®, which is highly purified and incorporates two dedicated viral removal procedures (S/D treatment and viral filtration), has been reported. It is currently undergoing clinical trial.[154]

Prothrombin complex concentrate

The manufacture of commercially available prothrombin complex concentrates (PCC) is predominantly achieved by the use of anion exchange chromatography. Incorporated viral removal procedures include S/D treatment, heat pasteurization, vapor heat or dry heat, and viral filtration. The final formulation may involve the addition of heparin and antithrombin (ATIII) as specific clotting factor stabilizers (for the prevention of activation), and albumin as an excipient.[12,155]

A manufacturing process for PCC should ensure the generation of a product with a balanced content of vitamin K–dependent factors (II, VII, IX, and X) and the presence of physiologically relevant amounts of the regulatory inhibitory proteins, proteins C, S, and Z.[12] The properties of various PCCs have been compared. All had similar levels of coagulation factors, but there were differences in purity and content of the inhibitory proteins.[156]

To specifically illustrate the principles of the manufacture of PCC, the process used for the production of Kcentra® (CSL Behring) (Beriplex® in Europe) and Octaplex® (Octapharma)—two commercial products in wide use—will be examined (Figure 27.16). The manufacture of Kcentra® is initiated by the adsorption of the PCC

factors from cryoprecipitate-depleted plasma with DEAE anion exchange resin. The factors are eluted and stabilized by the addition of ATIII, heparin, and $CaCl_2$. The eluate is pasteurized to ensure viral safety. Further purification involves ammonium precipitation of impurities, binding to calcium phosphate, followed by elution and Aerosil® (fumed silica) adsorption of the eluate. The recovered solution is formulated by the addition of albumin, ATIII, and heparin to stabilize the active components, and then subjected to viral filtration through two 20 nm filters. Following dilution to a targeted factor IX concentration and the adjustment of the final albumin concentration, the product is dispensed and lyophilized[157] (CSL information on file). In the Octaplex® process, PCC factors are adsorbed from cryoprecipitate-depleted plasma with a Q anion exchange chromatographic resin following pH addition and heparin addition to prevent factor activation. The recovered eluate undergoes S/D treatment for viral inactivation. Subsequent binding to a DEAE anion exchange resin allows the washing away of the viral inactivation chemicals, and provides further purification. The product is then subjected to viral filtration with a 20 nm filter. Following ultrafiltration, the product is formulated with the addition of heparin (but no albumin), then dispensed and lyophilized.[12,158]

Both processes generate highly a purified PCC with balanced factor content and regulatory proteins.[181–183] The dedicated viral removal steps and partitioning of virus, which occur at specific process steps, ensure the viral safety of these products.[159,160]

There is an EP monograph for PCC products.[161] It stipulates that a product must contain factor IX together with variable

Table 27.2 Examples of manufacturing processes for Factor IX

Brand Name (Manufacturer)	Purification Process	Specific Viral Removal Steps
Alphanine® (Grifols)	DEAE anion exchange chromatography Barium citrate adsorption Dextran sulfate affinity chromatography (x2)	Solvent/detergent treatment Viral filtration (15 nm)
Betafact® (LFB)	DEAE anion exchange chromatography(x2) Heparin affinity chromatography	Solvent/detergent Viral filtration (15 nm)
Berinin P® (CSL Behring)	DEAE anion exchange chromatography Ammonium sulphate precipitation of residues Ca_2PO_4 adsorption/elution Heparin affinity chromatography	Pasteurisation (60 °C, 10 h)
Mononine® (CSL Behring)	DEAE anion exchange chromatography Monoclonal affinity chromatography, Amino-hexanoic affinity chromatography	Viral filtration (15 nm)

amounts of factor II, VII, and X. The preparation may contain stabilizers (e.g., albumin, heparin, and ATIII). The lyophilized product should be a white or slightly colored, very hygroscopic powder or friable solid. Water content should be within approved limits. The preparation must dissolve completely within 10 minutes with gentle swirling. The potency of the reconstituted preparation should be not less than 20 IU of factor IX per milliliter. The pH of the solution should be between 6.5 and 7.5, and osmolality not less than 240 mOsmol/kg. If the content of any of the other factors is stated, it should not be less than 80% or more than 120% of the stated range. The specific activity of factor IX should not be less than 0.6 IU/mg of total protein (before addition of any stabilizer). The presence of any activated coagulation factors should not result in the coagulation time in a NaPTT assay to be less than 150 seconds. If heparin has been used in the formulation, the amount should comply with that on the label and not be more than 0.5 IU per IU of factor IX. The preparation must be sterile and free of bacterial endotoxins.

Factor IX

The approaches taken for the purification of high-purity factor IX has recently been extensively documented, and the key process stages have been collated for all the registered factor IX products.[13,155] Predominantly, the process commences with the initial capture of prothrombin complex factors (factors II, VII, IX, and X). The isolation of factor IX can then involve the use of ion exchange, affinity, hydrophobic, or metal-chelating chromatography, or adsorption with insoluble metal salts. The manufacturing processes incorporate specific viral removal procedures, usually S/D treatment and viral filtration.[13,155]

Details of the manufacture of four products—Alphanine® (Grifols), Betafact® (LFB), Berinin P® (CSL Behring), and Mononine® (CSL Behring)—are shown in Table 27.2. It can be seen that all products involve initial adsorption of factor IX (and the other PCC factors II, IX, and VIII) from cryoprecipitate-depleted plasma by DEAE anion exchange chromatography. In the manufacture of Alphanine®, final purification involves adsorption to a barium citrate precipitate, followed by two sequential dextran sulfate affinity chromatography steps. Viral removal is achieved by S/D treatment and viral filtration.[13,162] The recovery of purified factor IX in the Betafact® process involves further purification by DEAE anion exchange chromatography and heparin affinity chromatography. Viral removal is achieved by S/D treatment and viral filtration.[13,163]

In the Berinin P® process, the crude preparation initially obtained by DEAE anion exchange chromatography, undergoes a viral inactivation procedure—pasteurization—and then is partially purified by ammonium sulfate precipitation, prior to recovery of factor IX by calcium phosphate adsorption and final purification by heparin affinity chromatography (CSL data on file). The purification of Mononine® involves passage of a DEAE anion exchange chromatography eluate, which contains PCC factors adsorbed from cryosupernatant, through a specific anti–factor IX monoclonal antibody affinity resin. The pure factor IX is eluated with sodium thiocyanate and is then diafiltered. The material is then passed through a viral removal filter. Subsequent passage through an amino-hexanoic affinity column removes any leached monoclonal antibody ligand from the previous column.[164–167] The products are then formulated dispensed and lyophilized.

The required properties of a purified factor IX product are detailed by an EP monograph.[168] The lyophilized product should be a white or pale yellow hygroscopic powder or friable solid. The water content should be within limits approved by the competent authority. The preparation should dissolve completely with gentle swishing within 10 minutes. The reconstituted product should have a pH between 6.5 and 7.5, and a minimum osmolality of 240 mOsmol/kg. Potency should be not less than 20 IU/mL, and specific activity not less than 50 IU/mg of total protein. Any presence of activated factors should not cause the coagulation time in the NaPTT test to exceed 150 seconds. If heparin has been used in the formulation, it should be stated on the label but in all cases should not exceed 0.5 IU of heparin per IU of factor IX. The product should be sterile and free of bacterial endotoxins.

von Willebrand factor

Haemate P®/Humate P® (CSL Behring) was one of the first developed intermediate-purity factor VIII-vWF products. Since its licensing in Germany in 1981 for the treatment of hemophilia A, it has also been used to this day for the treatment of von Willebrand disease.[169] The manufacture of the product is from cryoprecipitate and involves initial adsorption of impurities from the reconstituted solution with aluminum hydroxide and then purification of the factor VIII–vWF complex by a series of glycine- and sodium chloride–mediated precipitation steps. Pasteurization is incorporated as a viral inactivation step[155] (CSL data on file).

In the late 1980s, new purification processes were developed incorporating chromatographic procedures to improve the efficiency of manufacture, improve product purity, and facilitate the introduction of viral inactivation procedures. A detailed examination of the chromatographic approaches that can be used to purify vWF, and an overview of the manufacturing processes and the viral removal procedures utilized for registered vWF products has been published elsewhere.[10,155] They show that a

Table 27.3 Examples of manufacturing processes for von Willebrand factor

Brand Name (Manufacturer)	Purification Process	Specific Viral Removal Steps
Haemate P®/Humate P® (CSL Behring)	Aluminum hydroxide treatment Glycine precipitation Sodium chloride precipitation NaCl/glycine precipitation	Pasteurization (60 °C for 10 hours)
Alphanate® (Grifols)	Polyethylene glycol precipitation Heparin affinity chromatography	Solvent/detergent treatment. Dry heat (80 °C for 72 hours)
Wilate® (Octapharma)	DEAE anion exchange chromatography Size exclusion chromatography	Solvent/detergent treatment. Dry heat (10 °C for 2 hours)
Wilfactin® (LFB)	Alumina gel treatment DEAE anion exchange chromatography (X2) Gelatin affinity chromatography	Solvent/detergent treatment Viral filtration, 35 nm. Dry heat (80 °C for 72 hours)

range of chromatographic procedures are used consisting of anion exchange, size exclusion, and affinity chromatography. Viral removal procedures include S/D treatment, pasteurization, dry heat treatment, and viral filtration.

The purification processes and viral removal procedures for some specific vWF products are shown in Table 27.3. The starting material in all cases is cryoprecipitate. The manufacture of Alphanate® involves an initial purification involving PEG precipitation to remove impurities, followed by heparin affinity chromatography to recover the purified vWF.[10,170] The manufacture of Wilate® and Wilfactin® involves the use of size exclusion chromatography and gelatin affinity chromatography respectively, to further purify the DEAE anion exchange chromatographic fraction obtained through the processing of a cryoprecipitate solution.[10,171,172] The manufacturing processes incorporate S/D treatment and dry heat as viral inactivation steps. In the Wilfactin® process, viral filtration is included.

The manufacturing process for a vWF product must deliver a consistent product with respect vWF multimer composition. The EP requires that during process development, quantitative analysis of the product must be undertaken using electrophoretic and densitometric techniques to confirm that the product closely approximates the multimer distribution of a plasma reference preparation.[173–175] The dispensed product must contain not less than 20 IU/ml of vWF, and the measured value must be within 20% of that stated on the label. Factor VIII must be tested if there is greater than 10 IU of factor VIII per 100 IU of vWF. The measured value must be within 40% of the stated value. vWF potency must only be measured by the ristocetin cofactor assay. vWF products are characterized on the basis of specific activity and a vWF activity–FVIII ratio. For the former, it must be greater than 1 U vWF/mg of total protein excluding any protein stabilizer. A value greater than 80 U vWF/mg protein is usual, although products with lower specific activity exist.[155] The vWF activity–FVIII ratio is not prescribed but must comply with the approved limit for the product with the competent authority. Values for the various products are from 0.75 to 2.4. The exception is Wilfactin, where the ratio is approximately 60.[155] This reflects the design of the manufacturing process which reduces the co-purification of factor VIII, thereby producing a predominantly vWF product.[171]

With respect to other product characteristics, the EP requires that the lyophilized final product be a white or pale yellow, hygroscopic powder or friable solid with a water content that is within the approved limits of the competent authority and that dissolves completely with gentle swirling within 10 minutes, giving a clear or slightly opalescent, colorless yellow solution.

Some products allow for filtration to remove flakes or particles present after reconstitution. If this is the case, it must be shown in validation studies that there is no impact on product potency. The reconstituted product must have a pH between 6.5 and 7.5, an osmolality greater than 240 mmol/kg, and no anti-A- or anti-B-mediated agglutination at a 1:64 dilution at a defined dilution of the reconstituted preparation. The product must be sterile and endotoxin free.[175]

Factor VIII

The production of cryoprecipitate for clinical use by Judith Pool in 1965 was a pivotal event in the treatment of hemophilia as it provided a high-potency product and an alternative to what hitherto had been used-fresh frozen plasma.[176] In the following years, purification processes were developed that further improved the purity and viral safety of factor VIII products. Haemate P®/Humate P®, in Germany in 1981, was the first registered intermediate-purity product containing a dedicated viral inactivation procedure. The product contained both factor VIII and vWF, and it became a recognized therapeutic for both hemophilia A and von Willebrand disease.[169] The purification process increased the specific activity of vWF from 1 IU/mg of protein for cryoprecipitate to approximately 38 IU/mg of protein in Haemate P®/Humate P®.[155]

In subsequent years, the application of chromatographic steps further increased the purity of factor VIII products.[9] Commonly referred to as *high-purity products*, the specific activity was typically greater than 100 IU/mg and for some products as high as 180 IU/mg.[9,155] The different manufacturing processes resulted in a variation in the vWF content, which in some cases limited their use to the treatment of hemophilia A and the exclusion of von Willebrand disease. With the development of these new processes, the opportunity was also taken to introduce two specific viral removal procedures. Typically, these were S/D treatment and dry-heat treatment of the lyophilized final product. Vapor heat and viral filtration have also been applied.[9,155] The use of monoclonal affinity chromatography allowed the generation of factor VIII concentrates with higher specific activity: >3000 IU/mg. These products, of course, do not have vWF.[9,155]

Table 27.4 presents the manufacturing process of a number of commercially available factor VIII products. The aim is to specifically present details to illustrate the range of processes that have been used to purify Factor VIII and ensure viral safety. In the manufacture of the high-purity products BeriateP® (CSL Behring), Factane® (LFB), and Immunate® (Baxalta), there is typically an initial Al(OH)$_3$ adsorption step. This serves to remove vitamin K–dependent prothrombin complex factors. Further purification then

Table 27.4 Representative manufacturing processes for factor VIII

Brand Name (Manufacturer)	Purification Process	Specific Viral Removal Steps	Specific Activity (IU/mg)
Intermediate-Purity Product			
Haemate P®/Humate P® (CSL Behring)	Aluminum hydroxide treatment Glycine precipitation Sodium chloride precipitation NaCl/glycine precipitation	Pasteurization (60 °C for 10 hours)	38
High-Purity Products			
Beriate P® (CSL Behring)	Al(OH)$_3$ adsorption Al(OH)$_3$/QAE anion exchange resin adsorption DEAE anion exchange chromatography	Pasteurization Viral filtration, 20 nm	170
Factane® (LFB)	Al(OH)$_3$ adsorption DEAE anion exchange chromatography FVIII/vWF dissociation-0.3 M CaCl$_2$ FVIII/vWF reassociation	Viral filtration, 35 nm, 15 nm	>100
Immunate® (Baxalta)	Al(OH)$_3$ adsorption DEAE anion exchange chromatography	Solvent/detergent treatment Vapor heat (60 °C for 10 hours, 7–8% moisture, 190 bar)	75
Alphanate® (Grifols)	PEG precipitation Heparin affinity chromatography	Solvent/detergent treatment Dry heat (80 °C for 72 hours)	>100
Very-High-Purity Products			
Hemofil M® (Baxalta)	Recovery of cryoprecipitate Anti–factor VIII affinity chromatography QAE anion exchange chromatography	Solvent/detergent treatment Viral filtration, 20 nm	>3000
Monoclate® (CSL Behring)	Al(OH)3 adsorption Anti-vWF affinity chromatography Amino hexanoic affinity chromatography	Pasteurization	~2000

occurs by anion exchange chromatography.[177–179] Factane® has a unique viral filtration step involving passing the product through a 15 nm filter. It had been thought that the factor VIII–vWF complex was too large to be able to be successfully filtered. However, this was achieved by dissociating the complex prior to filtration by exposure to calcium chloride and then reassociating the complex by its removal from the filtrate. The manufacturing process for Alphanate® differs in that there is an initial PEG precipitation step that is effective in removing fibrinogen and fibronectin. Final purification utilizes heparin affinity chromatography.[180–182]

The examples of the manufacture of very-high-purity factor VIII products offer some interesting and distinct differences. In the case of Hemofil M®, following a cold precipitation clarification step of the cryoprecipitate suspension, the solution undergoes S/D treatment to effect viral inactivation. Factor VIII purification is achieved by anti–factor VIII immunoaffinity chromatography. This step is very effective in achieving the removal of fibrinogen, fibronectin, and vWF. There is then a viral filtration step. A subsequent Q anion exchange chromatographic step binds factor VIII eluted from the affinity column and allows any leached monoclonal antibody affinity ligand to flow through.[183,184] In the Monoclate® process, the cryoprecipitate suspension is treated with aluminum hydroxide for clarification and removal of vitamin K–dependent clotting factors. The recovered solution is then pasteurized to provide a viral inactivation step. The factor VIII–vWFr complex is captured by an immobilized anti-vWF antibody. Factor VIII is dissociated with the used elution conditions, recovered, and passed over an amino hexanoic affinity column to remove any possible leached monoclonal antibody affinity ligand[185,186] (CSL data on file).

All factor VIII products are lyophilized. Various excipients are used and can include amino acids, sugar alcohols, sugars, and salts. In some cases, albumin is also included.[155]

The required properties of factor VIII are detailed in the EP.[187] The specific activity should not be less than 1 IU of factor VIII per milligram of total protein before the addition of any protein stabilizer. But, as has been noted, with modern purified products this is readily achieved. The potency of the preparation as stated on the label should result in not less than 20 IU factor VIII per milliliter. With respect to the appearance of the lyophilized preparation, water content, solubility, pH, osmolality of the reconstituted material, anti-A and anti-B hemagglutinin titer, sterility and endotoxin content, the requirements previously described for the vWF product apply.

Conclusion

The production of plasma protein-based therapeutic products is a complex process commencing with the collection of plasma by a system incorporating donor selection, viral testing and quality assurance measures that ensure the viral safety of the plasma for fractionation.[33] Starting with the work of Cohn, and through the subsequent application of knowledge of protein chemistry, bioprocessing technology, and virology, processes have been developed for the production of therapeutic products for a range of clinical indications, which meet the high standards of safety and efficacy prescribed by the regulatory authorities.[7]

Today, the production of plasma protein therapeutic products is a large global industry.[31,188] Despite the development of many recombinant alternatives, the production of products by fractionation of plasma remains cost-effective and continues to grow.[189] There is particular growth in the provision of albumin and immunoglobulins.[190] Albumin is required in large amounts, and immunoglobulins have unique biological properties. These factors make it commercially unattractive or scientifically unjustifiable to produce these products by recombinant means, and therefore they will most likely continue to be produced from plasma for the foreseeable future.[19,189,191]

Plasma fractionators are continuing to explore the clinical utility of additional plasma proteins and improve existing products. Proteins with therapeutic potential that are being investigated are shown in Table 27.1. Plasmin and reconstituted HDL are the most advanced in the clinical development pathway.[19,25]

With respect to existing products, the focus is on improving formulations and addressing issues that can lead to adverse reactions. The development of high-concentration immunoglobulins for subcutaneous use, ensuring that procoagulant activity is removed during the manufacture of immunoglobulins, the introduction of a procedure to remove anti-A and anti-B hemagglutinins from immunoglobulin products and the development of a liquid formulation for alpha$_1$-protease inhibitor are examples of these activities.

Plasma manufacturers are confronted with a limited and expensive starting raw material—plasma.[192] An efficient means of producing plasma-derived products that is high yielding and cost-effective would be of commercial benefit to the manufacturer and welcomed by the healthcare community, which is seeking an affordable and adequate supply of products. Recent trends in the use of disposable technologies and the developing concept of continuous processing may help to decrease the costs of establishing and operating a manufacturing facility.[193–195]

The developed countries are well served for fractionation capacity. Many developing countries such as China and Brazil are extending and improving their capabilities.[31] However, there are many developing countries that do not have adequate access to plasma protein products and cannot afford to purchase the requirements for their population.[196] Arguments for and against the establishment of a localized fractionation facility have been discussed.[192,197] The adoption of improvements in bioprocessing approaches could make the design and establishment of a fractionation facility less complex, cheaper and hence feasibile for construction and operation in a developing country.

The challenge for the future is aptly captured by the following reflection: "Nearly 2 billion people—or a third of the world's population—lack access to essential medicines. We need to ask ourselves: what use is our scientific endeavour and innovation when they do not come to the aid of people who need it the most? Should a drug be described a 'blockbuster' by a billion-dollar label or a billion-patients label?"[198]

The plasma fractionation industry will continue to deliver unique therapeutics essential for human health. It is likely that the future will be as eventful as the period from Cohn to the present day.

Key references

A full reference list for this chapter is available at: http://www.wiley.com/go/simon/transfusion

7 Bertolini J, Goss N, Curling J, Eds. *Production of plasma proteins for therapeutic use*. Hoboken, NJ: John Wiley and Sons Inc., 2013.

8 Lundblad RL. *Biotechnology of plasma proteins*. Boca Raton, FL: CRC Press, 2012.

117 European Directorate for the Quality of Medicines and Healthcare (EDQM). Normal immunoglobulin for intravenous use. In: *European Pharmacopoeia*. 8th ed. Strasbourg, France: EDQM, 2013.

155 Brooker M. *Registry of clotting factor concentrates*. 9th ed. Montreal: World Federation of Hemophilia, 2012.

188 Burnouf T. Plasma fractionation in the world: current status. *Transfus Clin Biol* 2007;**14**:41–50.

190 Robert P. *The worldwide plasma proteins market 2012*. Orange, CT: Marketing Research Bureau Inc., 2013.

CHAPTER 28

Recombinant products for the treatment of hemophilia: recent advances

Michael Wilson,[1] Andrew Nash,[1] Iris Jacobs,[2] & Arna Andrews[1]

[1]CSL Behring, Broadmeadows, Victoria, Australia
[2]CSL Behring, King of Prussia, PA USA

There are a number of heritable bleeding disorders that result from mutations in the genes encoding key components of the blood coagulation cascade. The most common is von Willebrand disease, whereas hemophilia A and B, which are attributable to mutations in the genes encoding coagulation factors VIII (FVIII) and IX (FIX) respectively, are perhaps the most well characterized. This chapter focuses on recombinant products that have been approved or are currently in human clinical trials to treat hemophilia A and B.

The genes encoding FVIII and FIX are located on the X chromosome, and hemophilia A and B are recognized as X-linked recessive disorders occurring almost exclusively in hemizygous males, with incidence rates of 1/5000 (hemophilia A) and 1/30,000 (hemophilia B). The disorders manifest most often as uncontrolled internal bleeding into joints and muscles, with prolonged and frequent joint bleeds leading to hemophilic arthropathy and significant morbidity. Intracranial hemorrhage occurs at a substantially lower frequency but can have the most severe consequences, including a mortality rate of up to 30% and long-term neurological sequelae in more than 50% of survivors.[1] The mainstay of treatment for these patients over the past 50 years has been on-demand replacement therapy with intravenous administration of FVIII or FIX concentrates. Treatment at the first onset of symptoms can limit both bleeding and the extent of local inflammation and tissue damage, and this has resulted in a marked improvement in both life expectancy and quality of life. For patients with severe disease, prophylaxis from an early age has been demonstrated to be the most effective approach to preventing arthropathy;[2] however, the requirement for frequent intravenous dosing (up to four times/week) has made this therapeutic strategy problematic.[3]

Factor VIII and FIX concentrates derived from pooled human plasma were first used to treat hemophilia patients in the late 1960s,[4] and although very effective at controlling bleeds, their use was subsequently associated with the widespread transmission of viral infections throughout the hemophilia community, most notably hepatitis C and HIV.[5] Although improved donor screening and the use of effective virus reduction steps in the manufacturing process have resolved this issue and these products continue to be used very effectively, recombinant coagulation factors produced through genetic engineering and in vitro mammalian cell culture techniques have emerged as an important and widely used alternative. The gene encoding FVIII was first cloned in 1984,[6,7] and the first recombinant FVIII product became available in 1992. Similarly, the gene encoding FIX was cloned in 1982,[8] and a recombinant form of this molecule was available for the treatment of hemophilia B patients by 1997. In addition to recombinant FVIII and FIX, a recombinant factor VIIa (FVIIa) has also been developed, primarily for the treatment of hemophilia A patients who develop inhibitor antibodies directed against therapeutic recombinant FVIII.[9]

Subsequent to the first introduction of recombinant coagulation factors, there have been a number of incremental innovations, including the development of formulations free of human albumin (stabilizer) and the use of fermentation culture media free of extraneous animal proteins. Although these innovations have provided a notional benefit in terms of patient safety, more recent efforts have focused on the development of products that require less frequent dosing and are less immunogenic. Less frequent dosing through improved pharmacokinetics has been of particular interest as this would enable more effective and sustained prophylaxis and improved quality of life. For both FVIII and FIX, the principal technologies that have been applied in order to generate products with these characteristics include:

1 *Pegylation:* The addition of polyethylene glycol (PEG) is a well-characterized strategy to improve the half-life of proteins by either increasing their molecular weight to prevent renal clearance or masking epitopes that are involved in binding to clearance receptors.[10]

2 *Fc and albumin fusion proteins:* In-line immunoglobulin Fc or albumin fusion proteins are able to harness the neonatal Fc receptor (FcRn) recycling pathway to bypass lysosomal degradation (see Figure 28.1A). This salvage system is used by IgG and albumin, which have the longest half-lives of all serum proteins.[11]

Recombinant FVIII

Coagulation FVIII is a member of the ferroxidase family of proteins and is made up of A1–A3 ferroxidase domains, with a B domain between A2 and A3, and carboxy terminal discoidin domains (C1 and C2) that facilitate binding to thrombocytes. FVIII is expressed primarily by the liver and/or the reticuloendothelial system, and intra- and extracellular processing, including cleavage at the amino terminus of the B domain and the addition of N- and O-linked glycan structures, generates the mature form that incorporates a

Rossi's Principles of Transfusion Medicine, Fifth Edition. Edited by Toby L. Simon, Jeffrey McCullough, Edward L. Snyder, Bjarte G. Solheim, and Ronald G. Strauss.

light-chain (LC) (A3–C1–C2) and heavy-chain (HC) (A1–A2–B) linked by a divalent metal ion (Me^{2+}). Once secreted into the plasma, FVIII binds noncovalently to von Willebrand factor (vWF) via the acidic a3 domain located at the carboxy terminus of the B domain, stabilizing and protecting FVIII from degradation and thereby prolonging its serum half-life.[12]

FVIII is activated to FVIIIa following thrombin cleavage resulting in the release of the B and a3 domains and dissociation from vWF. Once activated, FVIIIa acts as a coagulation cofactor that drives the rate of conversion of FX → FXa by facilitating the interaction of FIXa and FX on a phospholipid surface. FVIIIa interaction results in a conformational change in the active site of FIXa that favors cleavage of FX → FXa.[12]

Hemophilia A is the consequence of mutations in the F8 gene that result in insufficient levels of active FVIII protein. For the most part, these mutations lead to decreased FVIII production; however, mutations leading to otherwise normal levels of a dysfunctional protein are also observed. The first-generation rFVIII products were based on the full-length FVIII sequence, and products such as Recombinate (Baxter), Advate (Baxter), Kogenate FS (Bayer), and Helixate FS (CSL Behring) are functionally similar to plasma-derived FVIII.[13] Since they were first introduced, these rFVIII products have undergone subtle process improvements; for example, Baxter developed Advate by modifying the manufacturing process used for Recombinate to exclude the use of all animal and human-derived material[14,15] (Table 28.1).

Table 28.1 Summary of recombinant therapeutic molecules on the market or in clinical development for the treatment of hemophilia A or B

Trade/Project Name Scientific Name	Features	Phase Completed	Manufacturer	References
Recombinate Octocog alpha	Wild-type FVIII	Market	Baxter	17
Advate Octocog alpha Plasma-free-method	Wild-type FVIII	Market	Baxter	15
Kogenate FS/Helixate FS Sucrose-formulated Octocog alpha	Wild-type FVIII	Market	Bayer/CSL Behring	14
BAY81-8973	Wild-type FVIII	Ph III	Bayer/CSL Behring	
Refacto Monoctocog alfa	BDD FVIII	Market	Pfizer	17
Novoeight Turoctocog alfa	BDD FVIII	Market	Novo Nordisk	18
Eloctate Efraloctocog alfa	rFVIIIFc In-line Fc fusion	Market	Biogen Idec	28–30
Greengene F Berocotog alfa	BDD FVIII	Ph II/III	Green Cross	20
Nuwiq Simoctocog alfa	BDD FVIII	Market	Octopharma	21
N8-GP Turoctocog alfa pegol	BDD FVIII O-linked pegylation	Ph II/III	Novo Nordisk	23
BAX 855	Full length FVIII Lysine linked pegylation	Ph II/III	Baxter	24
BAY 94-9027 Damoctocog alfa pegol	BDD FVIII site specific pegylation	Ph I	Bayer	22, 25, 26
CSL627 rVIII-SingleChain	Single chain FVIII	Ph III	CSL Behring	31, 32
Benefix nonacog alfa	Wild-type FIX	Market	Pfizer	36
Rixubis nonacog gamma	Wild-type FIX	Market	Baxter	37
IXinity trenonacog alfa	Wild-type FIX	Ph III	Emergent BioSolutions	—
Alprolix Eftrenonacog alfa	FIX fused to Fc	Market	Biogen Idec	42, 43
CSL654IX-FP	FIX fused to recombinant albumin with cleavable linker	Ph III	CSL Behring	46, 47
GlycoPEGylated rFIX Nonacog beta pegol	FIX N-linked pegylation	Ph III	Novo Nordisk	44
Novoseven Eptacog alfa	Wild-type FVIIa	Market	NovoNordisk	49
BAX817	Wild-type FVIIa	Ph III	Baxter	—
LR769	Wild-type FVIIa Manufactured from milk of transgenic rabbits	Ph III	rEVO Biologics/LFB	—
CSL689 rVIIa-FP	FVIIa fused to recombinant albumin	Ph I	CSL Behring	54
CB-813d/PF-05280602	FVIIa analog with enhanced activity	Ph I	Catalyst Biosciences/Pfizer	—

The observation that deletion of the heavily glycosylated B domain significantly improved the yield of rFVIII in cell lines whilst having no deleterious effect on the function or half-life of the protein has given rise to modified versions of rFVIII.[16] The first of the B domain–deleted (BDD) rFVIII products on the market was ReFacto (Pfizer), which has all but 12 of the wild type B domain amino acid residues deleted and is manufactured in a Chinese hamster ovary (CHO) cell line.[17] More recently, Octapharma, Novo Nordisk, and Green Cross have reported on the development of BDD rFVIII molecules[18–20] with some specific nuances. For example, Octapharma have developed a BDD rFVIII (simoctocog alfa or Nuwiq) using a human embryonic kidney cell line rather than the industry standard CHO cell system. They speculate that production from a cell of human origin may reduce the risk of immunogenicity via two potential mechanisms: (1) increased sulfation of key tyrosine residues, which are known to be important for high-affinity interaction with vWF; and (2) more "human-like" glycosylation patterns.[21] Although the initial clinical trial data are promising, data from the key patient group of previously untreated patients (PUPs) have not yet been published, so it is difficult to gauge the success of this approach. Simoctocog alfa has been approved for use in Europe. Novo Nordisk's turoctocog alfa (Novoeight) has recently been approved for use in Europe, Japan, and the United States,[18] and berocotog alfa (Greengene F), being developed by Green Cross, is in Phase II/III trials (ClinicalTrials.gov identifier NCT02027779) (Table 28.1).

More recently, there has been increasing interest in the engineering of rFVIII proteins that improve patient convenience through an extended half-life and, as a consequence, less frequent dosing. There is also interest in trying to develop molecules with lower immunogenicity as well as lower cost of goods through the use of higher yielding expression systems. Technologies that have been successfully employed to improve the half-life of FVIII include pegylation, in-line recombinant FVIII–Fc fusions, and single-chain FVIII proteins, and these are discussed in more detail in this section.

Engineered recombinant FVIII proteins

The addition of PEG is a well-characterized strategy to improve the half-life of proteins by either increasing their molecular weight to prevent renal clearance or masking epitopes that are involved in binding to clearance receptors.[10] For FVIII, given the larger molecular weight, it is most likely the latter mechanism that is responsible for the increase in half-life observed with a number of pegylated rFVIII proteins. Bayer have generated a BDD rFVIII (BAY-9027) with site-specific pegylation through the introduction of an unpaired cysteine residue on the light chain.[22] Similarly, N8-GP (Novo Nordisk) is pegylated via a unique O-glycan located in the partially truncated B domain of the parental molecule Novoeight (turoctocog alfa). In this instance, a 40 kDa PEG molecule was added.[23] Baxter has developed a pegylated version of the recombinant FVIII product Advate (BAX 855), which has 20 kDa PEG molecules added via linkage to lysine residues with ~60% of the PEG molecules linked to the B domain following a manufacturing process that resulted in a ratio of 2 moles of PEG per FVIII.[24] In all three instances, biochemical assessment of the pegylated FVIII molecules, including FIXa cofactor activity, thrombin generation, thrombin-mediated activation, and binding to vWF, indicated that the modified rFVIII proteins retained activity similar to that of their respective unpegylated versions. In addition, binding to the clearance receptor, low-density lipoprotein receptor-related protein (LRP), was significantly lower with the pegylated proteins compared with their respective parental rFVIII molecules, suggesting that this

may be the mechanism that accounts for the improved pharmacokinetics[18,24–26] (summarized in Table 28.1).

Clinical trial data have confirmed that pegylation will extend the half-life of rFVIII by ~1.5-fold in humans. For example, Novo Nordisk reported a first-in-human single-dose escalation study (25, 50, and 75 U kg^{-1}) with N8-GP. Twenty-six patients with severe hemophilia A received their previous FVIII product, then, following a washout period, were treated with the same dose of N8-GP. The therapeutic was well tolerated with no new inhibitor development observed.[27] Similarly, Bayer reported data from a Phase I clinical trial in 14 patients with severe hemophilia A demonstrating that BAY 94-9027 was well tolerated with no evidence of immunogenicity and a half-life of ~19 hours versus 13 hours for rFVIII.[22] Finally, a Phase II/III study has recently been completed assessing BAX 855 in severe hemophilia A patients, but no data have been published to date.

Biogen Idec has developed a BDD rFVIII–Fc fusion protein (rFVIIIFc) using HEK293H cells co-expressing an rFVIII-Fc in-line fusion with an Fc fragment to create an Fc FVIII-Fc heterodimer. Fc fusion proteins are able to harness the neonatal Fc (FcRn) recycling pathway to bypass lysosomal degradation.[11] Extensive in vitro characterization of rFVIIIFc exemplified by the one-stage clotting assay, activation of the FXase complex, clotting activation by ROTEM, inactivation by APC, and binding affinity to vWF demonstrated equivalency to BDD rFVIII.[28] Preclinical in vivo data showed a half-life improvement of ~twofold in FVIII −/− mice and nonhuman primates and ~1.4-fold in rabbits. Cessation of bleeding in the mouse tail clip model was found to be comparable to BDD rFVIII.[29]

Data from a Phase III pivotal clinical trial were recently reported evaluating the safety, efficacy, and pharmacokinetics of rFVIIIFc in 165 previously treated males patients aged ≥12 years with severe hemophilia A. The study had three arms: arm 1, individualized prophylaxis (25–65 IU/Kg) every 3–5 days; arm 2, weekly prophylaxis (65 IU/Kg); and arm 3, episodic treatment (10–50 IU/Kg). The median annualized bleeding rates (ABRs) observed in arms 1, 2, and 3 were 1.6, 3.6, and 33.6, respectively. Consistent with the pegylated rFVIII products and the preclinical animal model data, the half-life was extended ~1.5-fold for rFVIII-Fc versus rFVIII. No patients developed inhibitors. This study demonstrated that rFVIIIFc was well tolerated and efficacious in the prevention and treatment of bleeding events, including within the setting of major surgery, in adolescents and adults with severe hemophilia A.[30]

CSL Behring has developed a recombinant single-chain rFVIII (rVIII-SingleChain), which is composed of a BDD rFVIII with the HC and LC covalently bonded. This molecule is significantly more stable than endogenous FVIII, which circulates with the LC and HC held together by a labile metal ion bridge. Once activated, the rFVIIIa is structurally comparable to that formed from the two-chain endogenous FVIII. The single-chain FVIII has been shown to have comparable haemostatic activity to both a full-length and a BDD rFVIII in the tail clip bleeding model in FVIII −/− mice.[31] Detailed analysis using thromboelastography, thrombin generation, aPTT, and FVIII activity assays in FVIII −/− mice dosed with 20 IU/kg of either Advate or rVIII-SingleChain showed equivalent activity for the two products.[31] Interestingly, in preclinical PK studies in a number of species including mice, rats, rabbits, and cynomolgus monkeys, an improvement in half-life for rVIII-SingleChain compared with Advate was observed. The extent of this improvement was similar to what has been observed with the pegylated rFVIII and rFVIII-Fc molecules, and this was attributed to the higher affinity of rVIII-SingleChain binding to vWF.[32] A

Phase I trial has been completed, but no data have been reported to date.

vWF as a rate-limiting factor for FVIII half-life extension

The half-life of FVIII appears to be driven by that of its cognate binding partner, vWF, which has a half-life of 16 hours. Consequently, and as described in both preclinical animal models of hemophilia A and in patients treated with either pegylated FVIII, Fc-BDD-FVIII fusion protein, or a single-chain BDD-FVIII molecule, there is an upper limit of a ~1.5-fold half-life improvement that can be achieved through direct modification of rFVIII. The modest half-life improvement of these modified rFVIII therapies translates into a requirement for twice-weekly dosing in order to achieve effective prophylaxis. This contrasts with what has been achieved with rFIXFc or rFIX-albumin in-line fusion proteins with three- to fivefold improvements in half-life translating to once-weekly or even once-fortnightly dosing for effective prophylaxis (see below for more detail). As hypothesized by Yee et al., co-administration of a rFVIII with a modified recombinant vWF to enable decoupling from endogenous vWF in hemophilia A patients may be required to overcome the limitations on rFVIII half-life observed to date.[33] Recent data reported at the 2014 WFH Congress with a novel BDD rFVIII-vWF D′D3 fragment-Fc fusion protein support this hypothesis.[34] These types of approaches coupled with the ability to engineer improvements in affinity between rFVIII and vWF, as exemplified with the rVIII-SingleChain described in this chapter, may provide further options for addressing the current limitation on half-life extension.

Recombinant FIX

Factor IX is a 55 kDa vitamin K–dependent serine protease that circulates as a zymogen. Upon cleavage by FXIa (intrinsic pathway) or the FVIIa/tissue factor (TF) complex (extrinsic pathway), the disulfide bridged activated form, Factor IXa (FIXa), in conjunction with FVIIIa in the presence of phospholipid and calcium is able to convert FX to FXa, leading to prothrombin activation.[35] Loss-of-function mutations in the FIX gene located on the X chromosome result in hemophilia B, which accounts for about 20% of all cases of hemophilia and has a clinical manifestation almost identical to that of the more prevalent hemophilia A.

As with hemophilia A, treatment options for hemophilia B were severely limited before the introduction of freeze-dried powdered concentrates in the 1970s; however, the impact of HIV and hepatitis C infection on the bleeding disorders community in the 1980s and early 1990s tempered this advance. The subsequent implementation of stricter screening protocols and advances in viral inactivation methods has resulted in safer plasma-derived products, but the introduction of recombinant versions of FIX heralded a new era in treatment for hemophilia B patients. The first commercial recombinant FIX (rFIX) product, Nonacog alfa (Benefix®, Pfizer Inc.), received approval in 1997 and is indicated for the control and prevention of bleeding episodes in adult and pediatric patients, including perioperative management.[36] Surprisingly, it was not until 2013 that a second product, nonacog gamma (Rixubis, Baxter Healthcare Corp.), was approved by the US Food and Drug Administration (FDA), and this product is the first rFIX specifically indicated for the routine prevention of bleeding in hemophilia B patients (both children and adults).[37,38] In addition to routine prophylaxis (prevention or reduction in frequency of bleeding

episodes), Rixubis is also indicated for the control of bleeding episodes and perioperative management in these patients. A number of other companies are developing biosimilar recombinant FIX products, and the most advanced, trenonacog alpha (IXinity, Emergent BioSolutions), is currently in Phase III clinical trials.

In developed countries, the availability of rFIX has increased safety and supply, enabling a prophylaxis regime for patients with severe hemophilia. Prophylaxis is now standard of care for children and an increasing number of adults, resulting in an improved quality of life and reducing complications with hemophilic arthropathy.[39,40] In reality, however, the half-life of recombinant FIX products (18–24 hours) necessitates rigorous regimens to maintain desired factor levels, with frequent injections (up to 2–3 times weekly) required.[41]

Engineered recombinant FIX proteins

Over the last decade, a number of promising new approaches designed to prolong the half-life of FIX have been pursued, and the first of these, a long-acting recombinant Fc fusion FIX (rFIXFc) named eftrenonacog (Alprolix, Biogen Idec), was approved by the FDA in March 2014. This product comprises a single molecule of FIX covalently fused to the dimeric Fc domain of IgG1 to generate a Fc FIX–Fc heterodimer.[42] As noted in this chapter, Fc fusions to recombinant protein therapeutics prolong half-life by harnessing the FcRn recycling pathway. Following successful early-stage safety and PK studies, a Phase III, nonrandomized, open-label study in 123 previously treated male patients aged 12 to 71 years with severe hemophilia B (FIX ≤2 IU/dL) was able to demonstrate the safety, improved PK, and efficacy of rFIXFc. This study encompassed four treatment groups: (1) weekly dose-adjusted prophylaxis (50 IU/kg starting dose), (2) interval-adjusted prophylaxis (100 IU/kg every 10 days to start), (3) on-demand treatment (20 to 100 IU/kg) dosing regimens, and (4) a perioperative treatment group. The primary efficacy endpoints, the median ABRs, were 3.0, 1.4, and 17.7, and mean ABRs were 3.12, 2.4, and 18.67, respectively, in groups 1, 2, and 3. In the interval-adjusted prophylaxis group of 26 patients who received 100 IU/kg of rFIXFc, 14 (54%) had dosing intervals of 14 days or more during the last three months of the study with an averaged median interval of 12.5 days during the efficacy period. No inhibitors were detected following treatment with rFIXFc, and adverse events were consistent with those expected from this patient population.[43]

A sequential pharmacokinetic assessment demonstrated that rFIXFc exhibited a threefold increase in half-life compared with rFIX (82.1 h, rFIXFc: 33.8 h, rFIX) with the time to reach a 1% FIX level following a 50 IU/kg dose improving from 5.1 days (rFIX) to 11.2 days (rFIXFc).[43] A further study to assess the safety and efficacy of rFIXFc in previously untreated patients with hemophilia B is currently in progress (NCT0223431).

Two further FIX molecules, each using alternative strategies to extend product half-life, are in late-stage clinical development. The first is a recombinant glycoPEGylated form of FIX (nonacog beta pegol [N9-GP]) from Novo Nordisk. This molecule has a 40 kDa PEG moiety attached to the FIX activation peptide by site-directed glycoPEGylation. During the activation process, this peptide and the associated PEG are removed to leave native activated FIX.[44] Clinical data from a Phase III study in 74 previously treated male patients aged 13 to 70 years with severe hemophilia B (FIX ≤2 IU/ dL) have shown that weekly prophylaxis at doses of 40 IU/kg resulted in median and mean annualized bleeding rates of 1.04 and 2.51, respectively; weekly prophylaxis at doses of 10 IU/kg resulted in median and mean annualized bleeding rates of 2.93 and

4.56, respectively. During the 52-week trial period, 10 of 15 (66.7%) patients with target joints at trial entry had no treatment-requiring bleeding episodes in their target joints during prophylaxis with 40 IU/kg, compared with 1 of 13 (7.7%) in the 10 IU/kg arm. The higher dose regimen resulted in significantly higher FIX trough levels, which may be the reason for the observed differences in lower bleeding rates, improved responses to treatment of bleeds, and increased likelihood of target joint resolution in the higher dose arm patients. Throughout the trial, the mean FIX trough activities were significantly above the FIX activity level for mild hemophilia B; 8.5

IU/kg with 10 IU/kg weekly and 27.3 IU/dL with 40 IU/kg weekly. Nevertheless, spontaneous bleeding episodes were higher than the expected bleeding phenotype of mild hemophilia B, and the reason for this requires further investigation. PK analyses suggested the steady-state mean half-life of nonacog beta pegol was between 107 and 111 hours.[45]

A further half-life extended molecule in clinical development is a FIX -albumin fusion (rIX-FP) from CSL Behring, which utilizes the same FcRn-mediated recycling pathway as rFIXFc to prolong half-life. This molecule is a genetic fusion of recombinant human FIX to

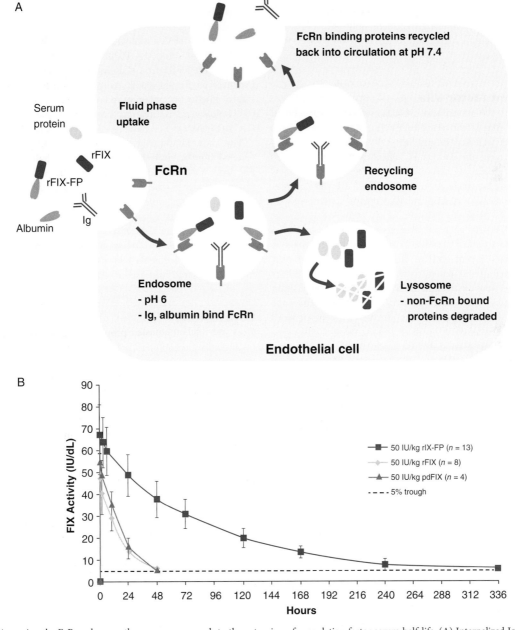

Figure 28.1 Accessing the FcRn salvage pathway as an approach to the extension of coagulation factor serum half-life. (A) Internalized Ig, albumin, and rIX-FP bind to FcRn in an acidic endosomal compartment and are subsequently recycled back into the circulation after release from FcRn at neutral pH. Serum proteins that do not interact with a recycling receptor are degraded in the lysosomal compartment. (B) FIX activity levels in hemophilia B patients following infusion of 50 IU/kg rFIX-FP, 50 IU/kg rFIX, and 50 IU/kg plasma-derived FIX (pdFIX). Activity is reported in international units per decaliter. The horizontal dotted line represents the 5 IU/dL FIX activity level. Mean $t_{1/2}$ for rIX-FP was 5.8 or 5.3 times longer compared with pdFIX or rFIX, respectively. Source: Santagostino *et al.* (2012).[47] Reproduced with permission of American Society of Hematology.

human albumin with a connecting linker sequence derived from the FIX activation peptide.[46] Upon activation by either FXIa or FVIIa/TF, the albumin moiety is removed in parallel to the activation of FIX itself. A Phase I PK study of rIX-FP demonstrated a 5.3-fold longer half-life (93 hours) compared to rFIX, an approximately 45% higher incremental recovery, and a sevenfold slower clearance. As shown in Figure 28.1B, administration of rIX-FP at 50 IU/kg resulted in FIX trough levels above 5% for more than 240 hours.[47] This observation strongly supports the possibility that rIX-FP will enable dosing intervals of more than two weeks in some patients. The outcome of recently completed Phase III trials will confirm the PK and efficacy of this promising new therapy.

Taken together, the available clinical data for these half-life extended FIX products provide legitimate hope for a hemophilia B prophylaxis regimen requiring treatment only once every two weeks and of maintaining higher FIX trough levels for patients with more active lifestyles.

Recombinant factor VIIa

Factor VII is a 406-amino-acid, 50 kDa, vitamin K–dependent serine protease that is converted to FVIIa upon cleavage of the peptide bond between Arg152 and Ile153. FVIIa consists of a two-chain molecule with the 20 kDa LC disulfide bonded (Cys135–Cys262) to the 30 kDa HC. Upon vessel damage, FVIIa interacts with TF, initiating the coagulation cascade. The FVIIa–TF complex catalyzes the conversion of FIX and FX into the active proteases FIXa and FXa.[48]

Congenital FVII deficiency is a relatively rare recessive condition that is estimated to affect between 1 in 300,000 to 1 in 500,000 people. The major use of FVII in factor replacement therapies, however, is in hemophilia patients who have developed inhibitors through their treatment with either FVIII or FIX. Due to its position within the coagulation cascade, treatment with FVIIa bypasses the need for FVIII or FIX and provides an alternative on-demand therapy for these patients.

At present, the only plasma-derived product widely used for the treatment of inhibitor patients is FEIBA-NF, a FVIII inhibitor bypass activity (FEIBA) complex that contains a mix of Factors II, IX, and X (mainly nonactivated) and Factor VII (mainly in the activated form) plus traces of FVIII. Plasma-derived FVII is also available as part of four-factor prothrombin complex concentrates (PCCs), which contain prothrombin and factors VII, IX, and X. PCCs are commonly used for anticoagulation reversal but not generally in the treatment of hemophilia.

The only recombinant FVIIa product currently available is NovoSeven (eptacog alpha, Novo Nordisk),[49] which was initially approved in the European Union in 1996 and in the United States in 1999 and is now licensed for hemophilia patients with inhibitors, patients with acquired hemophilia (a disease caused by the spontaneous development of inhibitors to FVIII), patients with congenital FVII deficiency, and patients with Glanzmann's thrombasthenia. Although safe and effective, the short half-life of recombinant FVIIa (2.6 hours)[50] results in the need for short-term repeat dosing and limits the potential for a prophylaxis treatment option.

A number of further recombinant FVIIa products, both plasma equivalent and modified molecules, have progressed into human clinical trials. The investigational products still in clinical development are listed in Table 28.1, whereas the development of three further, initially promising products have subsequently been halted. A Phase II trial with N7-GP, a glycoPEGylated FVIIa from Novo Nordisk, failed to establish a dose–response relationship despite an observed reduction in the annualized bleeding rate;[51] a recombinant FVIIa analog from Bayer (BAY 86-6150), engineered with a number of amino acid changes for increased activity and longer half-life, was halted in a Phase II/III trial due to the induction of antidrug antibodies;[52] and development of a third product, Vatreptacog alpha, another recombinant FVIIa analog (NN-1731, Novo Nordisk) with three amino acid substitutions that increased activity, was also halted as a result of antidrug antibodies.[53]

Two short-acting recombinant FVIIa products, rFVIIa (BAX817) from Baxter and rhFVIIa (LR769, made from the milk of transgenic rabbits) from rEVO Biologics, are currently in Phase III trials (NCT01757405 and NCT02020368, respectively). A modified recombinant FVIIa from Catalyst Biosciences (CB-813d, licensed to Pfizer as PF-05280602), with preclinical data demonstrating improvements in potency and duration of effect as compared to NovoSeven, is nearing completion of a Phase I study (NCT01439971).

The only long-acting recombinant FVIIa molecule to have reached human clinical trials is a FVIIa albumin fusion (rVIIa-FP) from CSL Behring. The results from a Phase I safety and pharmacokinetics study in healthy volunteers showed that the drug was safe and well tolerated with dose-responsive FVIIa plasma activity. The median half-life was between 6.1 to 9.7 hours with rVIIa-FP showing a reduced clearance compared to the commercially available rFVIIa. When compared to reported pharmacokinetics for the licensed rVIIa, rVIIa-FP is estimated to provide a three- to fourfold increase in half-life.[54]

Conclusions

Over the past 25 years, therapeutic options available for the treatment of hemophilia have expanded to include plasma-derived coagulation factors, recombinant wild-type coagulation factors, and, most recently, recombinant coagulation factors engineered in order to extend serum half-life and improve patient convenience. This latter approach has been most successful in respect to engineered rFIX for the treatment of hemophilia B. With respect to hemophilia A, improvements in PK characteristics of rFVIII have been far more modest, and there remains significant scope for further innovation. As an example, researchers have recently reported on clinical data from a bispecific antibody that can act as a FVIII mimetic for the treatment of hemophilia A patients with some promising early data from a small number of subjects ($n = 6$) in a Phase II study.[55] Novo Nordisk have developed an anti-TFPI (tissue factor pathway inhibitor) mAb, and Alnylam have a small interfering RNA (siRNA) approach to targeting ATIII in an effort to decouple the coagulation cascade from the natural endogenous inhibitors.[56] Both these approaches have shown potential in preclinical models, but the risk of thrombosis suggests a cautious approach to development. Finally, gene therapy has made some steps forward, particularly in the hemophilia B space.[57] The likely outcome in the longer term will be greater benefit to patients with a suite of products available depending on the nature of the disease.

Key references

A full reference list for this chapter is available at: http://www.wiley.com/go/simon/transfusion

5 Mannucci PM. Back to the future: a recent history of haemophilia treatment. *Haemophilia* 2008 Jul; **14** (Suppl. 3): 10–8. PubMed PMID: 18510516.

6 Toole JJ, Knopf JL, Wozney JM, *et al.* Molecular cloning of a cDNA encoding human antihaemophilic factor. *Nature* 1984 Nov 22–28; **312** (5992): 342–7. PubMed PMID: 6438528.

7 Gitschier J, Wood WI, Goralka TM, *et al.* Characterization of the human factor VIII gene. *Nature* 1984 Nov 22–28; **312** (5992): 326–30. PubMed PMID: 6438525.

8 Choo KH, Gould KG, Rees DJ, Brownlee GG. Molecular cloning of the gene for human anti-haemophilic factor IX. *Nature* 1982 Sep 9; **299** (5879): 178–80. PubMed PMID: 6287289.

9 Scharrer I. Recombinant factor VIIa for patients with inhibitors to factor VIII or IX or factor VII deficiency. *Haemophilia* 1999 Jul; **5** (4): 253–9. PubMed PMID: 10469179.

49 Persson E, Bolt G, Steenstrup TD, Ezban M. Recombinant coagulation factor VIIa—from molecular to clinical aspects of a versatile haemostatic agent. *Thrombosis Res* 2010; **125** (6): 483–9.

56 Oldenburg J, Albert T. Novel products for haemostasis—current status. *Haemophilia* 2014 May; **20** Suppl 4: 23–8. PubMed PMID: 24762271.

CHAPTER 29

Coagulation factor concentrates for inherited bleeding disorders

Gary M. Woods[1] & Amy L. Dunn[2,3]

[1]Division of Pediatric Hematology/Oncology, Children's Hospital of the King's Daughters, Norfolk VA, USA
[2]Department of Pediatrics, The Ohio State University, Columbus, OH, USA
[3]Hemophilia and Bleeding Disorder Program, Hemophilia Treatment Center, Division of Hematology/Oncology/BMT, Nationwide Children's Hospital, Columbus, OH, USA

Introduction

Congenital bleeding disorders can be categorized broadly into primary hemostatic defects (platelet disorders and von Willebrand disease) and secondary hemostatic defects (coagulation factor defects). Mucocutaneous bleeding, including easy bruising, epistaxis, and menorrhagia, is associated with a primary hemostatic defect, whereas secondary hemostatic defects are associated with deep, delayed bleeding, especially into the joints and muscles.[1] Congenital bleeding disorders have historically led to significant disability in children, but advancements in the last 20 years have improved both the morbidity and mortality associated with these conditions. Continuing research is underway, and promising advancements in management modalities continually provide hope for ongoing improvements in the care of patients with congenital bleeding disorders.

Hemophilia

Hemophilia A and hemophilia B are the most common X-linked bleeding disorders and result due to a deficiency in plasma clotting factors VIII (FVIII) and IX (FIX), respectively.[2] The gene for FVIII is located on the Xq28 band of the long arm of the X chromosome, and the FIX gene is on the Xq27 band. Hemophilia A accounts for about 80% of all cases of hemophilia. Hemophilia is present throughout the world and affects all races and ethnic groups. The incidence of hemophilia A is 1:5000 and hemophilia B is 1:20,000–30,000 live male births.[3] Approximately one-third of all new cases occur in families with no history of hemophilia and are due to spontaneous mutations.[2,4]

FVIII and FIX activity levels generally correlate well with clinical bleeding severity and can help predict bleeding risk. Generally, all affected members of a family will exhibit similar bleeding phenotypes and factor activity levels.[2] Severe disease is classified as FVIII or FIX activity of <1%, moderate is 1–5%, and mild is 6–40%.[2,4] Approximately 20,000 individuals in the United States are affected by hemophilia, 43% of which are considered severe, 26% moderate, and 31% mild.[3] However, mild cases may be underrepresented.

Hemophilia A and B are clinically indistinguishable and are characterized by prolonged bleeding, hemarthroses, and soft tissue/muscle hematomas. Although clinically they appear similar, FIX deficiency tends to be a milder disease with less significant handicaps.[2,5,6] Laboratory screening results are similar in both disorders. Patients with hemophilia A and B will have normal prothrombin time (PT), platelet count, and platelet function analyzer 100 (PFA-100), whereas their activated partial thromboplastin time (aPTT) will be prolonged and will correct with a mixing study. Mild cases may be missed due to aPTT sensitivity issues. Performance of FVIII and FIX activity assays will distinguish between the two diseases.

Genetics in hemophilia

As previously noted, the genes for FVIII and FIX are located on the long arm of the X chromosome. The FVIII gene is 186 kb long and consists of 28 exons.[1] Over 2000 unique mutations have been described, with intron 22 inversion being the most common, affecting almost 45% of individuals with severe disease.[7–9] FVIII is a complex glycoprotein containing 2351 amino acids separated into six domains: three A domains (A-1, A-2, and A-3), a connecting B domain, and two C terminal domains (C-1 and C-2).[2,10,11] The B-domain function is not well understood, but it is not necessary for hemostatic activity.[2] Intracellular proteolytic cleavage by thrombin at the Arg1689 site results in the formation of a heterodimer with an N-terminal heavy chain (A-1, A-2, and partially proteolyzed B domain) bound to a C-terminal light chain (A-3, C-1, and C-2).[1,2] This heterodimeric FVIII circulates in the blood bound via the C2 domain with von Willebrand factor (vWF). VWF protects it from proteolytic degradation and concentrates FVIII at sites of injury.[2] Thrombin activates FVIII by cleaving sites in both the heavy and light chains to release FVIII from vWF.[11] The half-life ($t_{1/2}$) of VWF-bound FVIII in the plasma is about 12 hours.

FIX is shorter in length, only 34 kb long, and consists of eight exons.[12,13] Mature FIX is a serine protease that contains 415 amino acids, is synthesized in the liver, and requires a posttranslational vitamin K–dependent γ-carboxylation to become active. It has a $t_{1/2}$ of about 24 hours.[12,14] Depending on the genetic defect, FIX deficiency may reflect a quantitative or qualitative abnormality in the FIX molecule. About 70% of FIX mutations are of the missense type.[13] Hemophilia B Lyden, a rare variant, occurs due to point mutations in the promoter region of FIX. These patients have severe deficiency in childhood; however, postpubertal andro-

Rossi's Principles of Transfusion Medicine, Fifth Edition. Edited by Toby L. Simon, Jeffrey McCullough, Edward L. Snyder, Bjarte G. Solheim, and Ronald G. Strauss.

gen production results in increased FIX promoter activity and thus increased FIX production, effectively correcting their disease.[15]

Hemophilia A and B are X-linked recessive conditions that can also occur due to spontaneous mutations. Seventy percent of mild and moderate hemophilia cases have been shown to be familial on pedigree analysis, whereas only 57% of severe hemophilia B and 45% of severe hemophilia A are clearly familial. Half of the patients with familial mild to moderate hemophilia or severe hemophilia B had an affected direct male ancestor, and only 28% of those with familial severe hemophilia A had an affected direct male ancestor. In sporadic cases, 88% of mothers of affected individuals were found to carry the mutation, whereas only 19% of maternal grandmothers carried the mutation.[16] Many sporadic cases of the characteristic FVIII inversion originate from a *de novo* mutation found in the maternal grandfather's male germ cells.[8]

Hemophilia A can be diagnosed early in life by measuring FVIII levels on cord blood in individuals at risk for inheriting the disease. Prenatal diagnosis is now usually accomplished through molecular biological techniques analyzing various polymorphic markers from DNA obtained by chorionic villous sampling. These modern techniques, like restriction fragment length polymorphism analysis, denaturing gradient gel electrophoresis, single-strand conformation polymorphism, and DNA sequencing, are accurate and can be obtained early in pregnancy.[17] The intron 22 inversion responsible for about half of the FVIII mutations can be detected by polymerase chain reaction on a potential carrier or using chorionic villous cells. This technique will diagnose almost all of the intron 22 inversions seen in severe hemophilia, but has been shown to miss up to 4% of moderate and 12% of mild hemophilia A.[18] FIX levels are physiologically low at birth, and thus a low FIX level in the cord blood must be repeated at 6–12 months of age to confirm the severity of the hemophilia B diagnosis.[1]

Clinical features

The clinical hallmark of hemophilia is bleeding, especially into the joints, muscles, and soft tissue, but the site of bleeding and pattern of bleeding are widely varied based on disease severity and age.[2,10] Although clinical manifestations are almost exclusively seen in males, women may be affected if they inherit mutated genes from both parents, have a new mutation, have chromosomal abnormalities like Turner syndrome, or are symptomatic carriers. Factor activity of <50% has been associated with increased bleeding in female carriers.[19]

Individuals with mild hemophilia (activity 6–40%) usually have clinically mild disease and may only bleed after a hemostatic challenge such as surgery or trauma.[4] Those with moderate hemophilia have prolonged bleeding with surgery and trauma, but spontaneous bleeding is uncommon. Severe hemophilia is associated with recurrent mucocutaneous bleeding, hemarthroses/deep soft tissue bleeds with minimal or no identified trauma, and severe postsurgical bleeding. Some patients with severe disease have a milder clinical disease, whereas some with mild and moderate disease have a more severe phenotype. It has been postulated that this considerable phenotypic heterogeneity might be related to the co-presence of factor V Leiden mutation and other pro-thrombotic conditions that counteract the bleeding tendency, differences in physical activity levels, and structural integrity of joints.[10,20–23] Additionally, some patients have a markedly different FVIII level if performed via one-stage versus chromogenic assay.[24]

The first hemostatic challenge experienced by hemophilia patients is birth. Up to 53% of patients experience a bleed by one month of age, with postcircumcision bleeding the most common (47.9%), followed by head bleeds (19.4%) and bleeding from heel sticks (10.4%).[25] The rate of intracranial hemorrhage (ICH) experienced in neonates with hemophilia is reported at 1–4%, much higher than the rate experienced in neonates without bleeding disorders, and these hemorrhages have been associated with seizures, psychomotor retardation, and cerebral palsy.[25–27] Generally, prolonged labor and instrumentation during delivery, including forceps, vacuum assistance, and scalp electrodes, should be avoided in infants born to known hemophilia carriers to decrease the risk of ICH.[26]

Children become symptomatic more often after the newborn period and before two years of age.[28] The first symptomatic bleeding leading to the diagnosis of severe hemophilia has been shown to occur at a median of about 10 months of age (19 months with the presence of a prothrombotic risk factor), and as late as 22 months in moderate hemophilia; mild hemophilia may go undetected for many years until a significant hemostatic challenge is encountered.[20–22,29–31] ICH is a serious complication in hemophilia at all ages, with 2% of patients older than 2 years facing this problem with an associated 20% mortality rate. Severe hemophilia and high-titer inhibitors are independent risk factors for ICH development.[32]

Hemarthrosis is characteristic of severe hemophilia. The age range for the first joint bleed in severe hemophilia varies significantly and has been reported as 0.2 years to 5.8 years.[33] The factors that initiate the hemorrhage are often unknown, and the onset can be random, occurring spontaneously or after minimal injury. Joint bleeds become more prevalent after individuals begin to weight bear. All synovial joints are at risk, but ankles are most commonly affected in children, and the knees, elbows, and ankles are more affected in adolescents and adults. Usually one joint is affected at a time, but a joint that experiences repeated bleeds is referred to as a *target joint*. Repeated hemorrhages into a joint leads to hemophilic arthropathy, which is associated with synovial hyperplasia, articular cartilage degradation, cystic changes in the subchondral bone, loss of joint space, and atrophy of the surrounding muscles, eventually leaving a deformed joint with contractures, pain, and decreased range of motion.[10,34,35]

Muscle hematomas are the second most common type of bleeding experienced in hemophilia, accounting for 10–25% of all bleeds.[36] Quadriceps, iliopsoas, and forearm muscles are commonly affected and, if the bleeds are large enough, can result in compartment syndrome. Iliopsoas bleeding is a primary concern in hemophilia because significant blood loss can occur into this large muscle and nerve compression might follow.[37] Other bleeding encountered in hemophilia includes epistaxis, oral mucosal, gastrointestinal tract, and hematuria.

Management of hemophilia

Hemophilia management is complex. It requires multidisciplinary comprehensive care focused on preventative care, factor replacement management, and treatment of disease complications.[38] Preventative care includes standard dental care to reduce gingival disease; education on wearing MedicAlert bracelets and avoidance of aspirin, nonsteroidal anti-inflammatory drugs, and other platelet-modifying medications; avoidance of contact sports; and vaccinations against blood-borne pathogens.[1] Before factor replacement therapy, most patients with severe disease developed arthropathy before the age of 20 and the mortality rate due to ICH was significant. In the 1920s and 1930s, life expectancy in developing countries, like Finland and Sweden, was only 8–11 years, and as

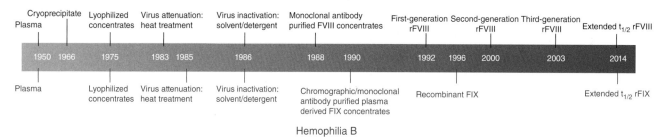

Figure 29.1 Evolution timeline of hemophilia A and hemophilia B treatment modalities.

recently as the 1960s life expectancy was still <30 years.[39–41] Many advancements in the medical management of hemophilia have been made since the 1960s (Figure 29.1). As advancements were made in hemophilia management, setbacks were encountered. Transmission of hepatitis C virus (HCV) and human immunodeficiency virus (HIV) complicated blood component therapy.[42,43] With factor replacement therapy came inhibitor development and rising cost of treatment, which is especially an issue in developing countries.[44] Even with these setbacks, advancements in the last 30 years, including the emergence of comprehensive hemophilia treatment centers, recombinant factor concentrates, and a more widespread adoption of prophylactic home replacement therapy, have led to improved outcomes in individuals with hemophilia.[45]

Blood component therapy

Fresh frozen plasma (FFP) and whole blood were the only preparations that could treat FVIII or FIX deficiency until 1964, when a method for concentrating FVIII into a cold-insoluble precipitate, or cryoprecipitate, was discovered.[46] Cryoprecipitate prepared from single plasma units contains about 50% of the FVIII, vWF, fibrinogen, and factor XIII (FXIII) of the original plasma unit, or about 100 IU of FVIII and 0.2 g of fibrinogen in 8–10 mL. Cryoprecipitate made elective surgery and outpatient treatment of bleeding episodes possible for patients with hemophilia A. Cryoprecipitate is still used in many developing countries, but it has disadvantages over the newer commercially prepared concentrates, including increased risk of blood-borne pathogen transmission, marked variations in FVIII and vWF content, larger volume, and required storage temperatures of <20–30 °C.

In the 1970s, fractionation methods were developed that produced plasma-derived lyophilized concentrates of both intermediate-purity (containing vWF in addition to FVIII) FVIII as well as prothrombin complex concentrates (PCCs), which contain the vitamin K–dependent clotting factors II, VII, IX, and X and protein C and S. These new products led to the adoption of home self-infusion replacement therapies for both hemophilia A and B and led to reduced morbidity compared to untreated patients. This even led to the pioneering of primary prophylaxis in Sweden, which achieved the goal of preventing bleeding episodes.[47] Hemophilia centers were able to develop comprehensive care programs because they were no longer overwhelmed with providing emergency treatments.[48] The discovery of the effect of desmopressin on FVIII and vWF in 1977 provided a relatively inexpensive and safe treatment option for many patients with mild hemophilia A. This synthetic drug increases FVIII and vWF plasma levels by releasing them from Weibel Palade bodies and endothelial cells and reduced the use of plasma-derived products in this population.[4,49]

The late 1970s and early 1980s were devastating in the care of hemophilia. Approximately half of the population with hemophilia in the United States, or 9300 individuals, became infected with HIV, and 80% with hepatitis C.[50] As many as 90% of patients with hemophilia became seropositive for hepatitis B surface antigen. The first reported case of acquired immunodeficiency syndrome in individuals with hemophilia was reported in the early 1980s, and it became apparent that it was being transmitted via blood and blood components, including factor concentrates.[51] Approximately 90% of persons who received FVIII concentrates and 55% of those who received PCCs prepared in the United States between 1979 and 1984 became seropositive for HIV.[52] Fortunately, HIV proved to be heat labile; thus, by late 1984, almost all hemophilia patients were receiving heat-treated concentrates. By 1984, solvent/detergent processes for treating blood products were developed that drastically reduced the transmission of both hepatitis B and C.[53] By 1985, HIV seropositivity screening for blood and plasma donors was also in place. In addition to better virus attenuate products, FVIII concentrates purified using murine monoclonal antibodies and immunoaffinity chromatography became commercially available in 1987. The purification process eliminated several logs of virus, and these products were then further virus attenuated by pasteurization or solvent/detergent treatments.[54] These measures greatly improved the safety of plasma-derived FVIII and FIX products, and since 1987 there has not been a new HIV or hepatitis case from blood-borne transmission from factor concentrates reported in the North American population.[52]

Even with these advancements, transmission of blood-borne viruses or novel infectious agents remained a concern. One of the most important innovations in hemophilia care came with the cloning of the FVIII gene in 1982 and the FIX gene in 1984, which allowed for the development and production of recombinant factor products, which were first shown to be clinically effective in 1989.[55]

Recombinant factor VIII

Recombinant FVIII (rFVIII) was developed quickly after the molecular cloning of complementary DNA encoding human FVIII and the expression of human FVIII from recombinant DNA clones.[56,57] Three generations of standard half-life rFVIII products are commercially available with differences in their preparation. First-generation products utilized animal-derived proteins in cell culture, and stabilization of FVIII in the final formulation was accomplished with human serum albumin. Second-generation products eliminated animal products during fermentation, and nearly all of the human albumin is eliminated in the final formulation. No human-derived protein is used in the culture medium or final formulation of third-generation products.[58] The commercially available rFVIII products are summarized in Table 29.1.

Table 29.1 Summary of the commercially available recombinant factor VIII products.

	Recombinant Factor VIII Product Features					
	Recombinate	Kogenate FS	Helixate FS	Advate	Xyntha	Eloctate
Host Cell	CHO	BHK	BHK	CHO	CHO	HEK
Purification and Virucidal Techniques	ION Exchange Chromatography Mouse Monoclonal Antibody (Mab) Immunoaffinity Chromatography	ION Exchange Chromatography Mouse Monoclonal Antibody (Mab) Immunoaffinity Chromatography Solvent Detergent	ION Exchange Chromatography Mouse Monoclonal Antibody (Mab) Immunoaffinity Chromatography Solvent Detergent	ION Exchange Chromatography Mouse Monoclonal Antibody (Mab) Immunoaffinity Chromatography Solvent Detergent	Synthetic Peptide Affinity Chromatography Immunoaffinity Chromatography Solvent Detergent Nanofiltration	Synthetic Peptide Affinity Chromatography Solvent Detergent Nanofiltration
Stabilizer	Albumin	Sucrose	Sucrose	Mannitol Trehalose	Sucrose	Sucrose
Available vial Sizes (IU)	250 500 1000 1500 2000	250 500 1000 2000 3000	250 500 1000 2000 3000	250 375 500 750 1000 1500 1700 2000 2500 3000 4000	250 500 1000 2000 3000	250 500 750 1000 1500 2000 3000 4000
Diluent volume	10 ml	2.5 ml up to 100 units 5 ml for 200 units +	2.5 ml up to 100 units 5 ml for 200 units +	2 ml up to 1700 units 5 ml for 2000 units+	4 ml	3 ml
Dosage calculation	1 IU/kg raises level by 2%	1 IU/kg raises level by 2%	1 IU/kg raises level by 2%	1 IU/kg raises level by 2%	1 IU/kg raises level by 2%	1 IU/kg raises level by 2%
T1/2	9.7–19.5 hours	7.8–15.3 hours	7.8–15.3 hours	8–14 hours	3.5–10.6 hours	12–16.4 hours
Storage	Room temperature, until expiration Not to exceed 86 °F Can refrigerate at 36 °F–46 °F	Room temperature, 12 months Not to exceed 77 °F Should refrigerate at 36 °F–46 °F	Room temperature, 12 months Not to exceed 77 °F Should refrigerate at 36 °F–46 °F	Room temperature, 6 months Not to exceed 86 °F Should refrigerate at 36 °F–46 °F	Room Temperature, 3 months Not to exceed 77 °F Can refrigerate at 36 °F–46 °F	Room temperature, 6 months Not to exceed 86 °F Should refrigerate at 36 °F–46 °F

BHK, baby hamster kidney; CHO, Chinese hamster Ovary; °F, degree Farenheit; HEK, human embryonic kidney; IU, international unit; kg, kilogram; ml, milliliter.

The only first-generation rFVIII product that remains on the market in the United States is Recombinate (Baxter, USA), and it has demonstrated the same pharmacokinetics and clinical effectiveness as plasma-derived FVIII products.[59,60] Most, if not all, patients in the United States and many other developed countries were switched to rFVIII despite its cost, but concern did arise for the potential for blood-borne pathogen transmission with first-generation products due to its stabilization with human serum albumin.

Second-generation rFVIII products include Kogenate FS (Bayer, USA) and Helixate FS (CSL Behring, USA). Third-generation products include full-length (Advte, Baxter) and truncated (Xyntha, Pfizer, USA) preparations. The truncated preparations are B-domain-deleted (BDD), as the heavily glycosylated B domain seems to be dispensable for the hemostatic activity of FVIII.[61] BDD products have been shown to be safe, effective in the treatment of bleeding episodes, and well tolerated.[62] The important advancement with these products is that no human proteins are utilized in the initial preparation stages or in the final formulation. Most recently, the US Food and Drug Administration (FDA) approved the use of the first extended $t_{1/2}$ rFVIII product (Eloctate, Biogen USA). BDD rFVIII is fused to the Fc portion of immunoglobulin G subclass 1 (IgG$_1$).[63,64] This product has been proven to have prolonged circulation in the body compared to other rFVIII products.[65,66] Other technologies, including PEGylation and single-chain technology, are currently being investigated to prolong the $t_{1/2}$ of rFVIII products.

Dosage and administration of factor VIII

FVIII concentrates are routinely used to treat acute bleeding episodes in individuals with moderate or severe hemophilia and for those with mild hemophilia with poor response to desmopressin. Factor replacement can be given "on demand" (after a bleeding episode) to treat a hemorrhage, or as "prophylaxis" (scheduled infusions to prevent or decrease the frequency or intensity of hemorrhages). Acute hemarthrosis, intramuscular bleeding, and surgical prophylaxis are common indications for factor replacement, and prompt treatment can prevent or reduce complications like chronic joint disease, and can reduce the need for additional factor infusions (Table 29.2 and Table 29.3).[67] Usually, 1 U/kg of FVIII will increase the plasma FVIII concentration by 2% (0.02 IU/dL).[10] The $t_{1/2}$ of FVIII is about 12 hours, but varies greatly among patients with ranges of 6–25 hours described.[68] The $t_{1/2}$ may be shorter in patients that are younger, are febrile, have ongoing extensive bleeding, or have an inhibitor.

Factor replacement can be achieved using bolus dosing or may require continuous infusions. Continuous infusions are often utilized in operative and postoperative situations, as well as for managing central nervous system (CNS) hemorrhage.[2] A bolus

Table 29.2 Suggested plasma factor peak level and duration of administration (when there is no significant source restraint).

Type of Hemorrhage	Hemophilia A		Hemophilia B	
	Desired Level (IU/DL)	Duration (Days)	Desired Level (IU/DL)	Duration (Days)
Joint	40–60	1–2, may be longer if response is inadequate	40–60	1–2, may be longer if response is inadequate
Superficial muscle/no NV compromise (except iliopsoas)	40–60	2–3, sometimes longer if response is inadequate	40–60	2–3, sometimes longer if response is inadequate
Iliopsoas and deep muscle with NV injury, or substantial blood loss				
▪ INITIAL	80–100	1–2	60–80	1–2
▪ MAINTENANCE	30–60	3–5, sometimes longer as secondary prophylaxis during physiotherapy	30–60	3–5, sometimes longer as secondary prophylaxis during physiotherapy
CNS/head				
▪ INITIAL	80–100	1–7	60–80	1–7
▪ MAINTENANCE	50	8–21	30	8–21
Throat and neck				
▪ INITIAL	80–100	1–7	60–80	1–7
▪ MAINTENANCE	50	8–14	30	8–14
Gastrointestinal				
▪ INITIAL	80–100	7–14	60–80	7–14
▪ MAINTENANCE	50		30	
Renal	50	3–5	40	3–5
Deep laceration	50	5–7	40	5–7
Surgery (major)				
▪ Preop	80–100		60–80	
▪ Postop	60–80	1–3	40–60	1–3
	40–60	4–6	30–50	4–6
	30–50	7–14	20–40	7–14
Surgery (minor)				
▪ Preop	50–80		50–80	
▪ Postop	30–80	1-5, depending on type of procedure	30–80	1-5, depending on type of procedure

Note: This table was used with permission of the WFH. NV, neurovascular. Source: Oldenburg and Albert (2014).[66] Reproduced with permission of Wiley.

Table 29.3 Suggested plasma factor peak level and duration of administration (When there is significant resource restraint).

Type of Hemorrhage	Desired Level (IU/DU)	Hemophilia A Duration (Days)	Desired Level (IU/DL)	Hemophilia B Duration (Days)
Joint	10–20	1–2 may be longer if response is inadequate	10–20	1–2, may be longer if response is inadequate
Superficial muscle/no NV compromise (except iliopsoas)	10–20	2–3, sometimes longer if response is inadequate	10–20	2–3, sometimes longer if response is inadequate
Iliopsoas and deep muscle with NV injury, or substantial blood loss				
▪ INITIAL	20–40		15–30	
▪ MAINTENANCE	10–20	3–5, sometimes longer as secondary prophylaxis during physiotherapy	10–20	3–5, sometimes longer as secondary prophylaxis during physiotherapy
CNS/head				
▪ INITIAL	50–30	1–3	50–80	1–3
▪ MAINTENANCE	30–50	4–7	30–50	4–7
	20–40	8–14	20–40	8–14
Throat and neck				
▪ INITIAL	30–50	1–3	30–50	1–3
▪ MAINTENANCE	10–20	4–7	10–20	4–7
Gastrointestinal				
▪ INITIAL	30–50	1–3	30–50	1–3
▪ MAINTENANCE	10–20	4–7	10–20	4–7
Renal	20–40	3–5	15–30	3–5
Deep laceration	20–40	5–7	15–30	5–7
Surgery (major)				
▪ Preop	60–80		50–70	
▪ Postop	30–40	1–3	30–40	1–3
	20–30	4–6	20–30	4–6
	10–20	7–14	10–20	7–14
Surgery (minor)				
▪ Preop	40–80		40–80	
▪ Postop	20–50	1-5, depending on type of procedure	20–50	1-5, depending on type of procedure

Note: This table was used with permission of the WFH. NV, neurovascular. Source: Oldenburg and Albert (2014).[66] Reproduced with permission of Wiley.

dose of 50 U/kg of FVIII should be administered followed by a continuous infusion of 2–5 IU/kg/hour as initial dosing, but intermittent FVIII monitoring should be obtained and infusion rates should be adjusted accordingly to ensure FVIII activity is in the desired hemostatic range.[2,69,70]

Prophylaxis

Primary prophylaxis refers to beginning factor replacement before a pattern of recurrent bleeding begins. *Secondary prophylaxis* refers to beginning the therapy after recurrent joint bleeds or muscle bleeding has occurred.[67] The idea for prophylactic treatment started in Malmö, Sweden, after the observation that patients with moderate hemophilia had a significantly lower incidence of chronic arthropathy.[71] Patients with severe hemophilia A were monitored for 2–25 years on prophylactic factor infusions and were shown to have fewer bleeding events and less joint disease than those receiving on-demand treatment.[72,73] Randomized trials have proven that prophylaxis administration improves outcomes and reduces joint disease in children with severe hemophilia when compared to episodic on-demand treatment.[74] Thus, prophylactic administration of factor to prevent bleeding episodes has become the standard of care for patients with severe hemophilia.

Full-dose prophylaxis in hemophilia A usually involves administration of FVIII every other day or three days a week at 25–40 U/kg.[75,76] Because prophylaxis is now recommended to start at a young age, the frequent infusions may result in the need for a central venous access device (CVAD). Although factor administration may be easier, placement requires careful consideration due to the risk of infections and thrombosis.[76] It is common to use an escalating dose–frequency schedule in young children that entails starting with once-weekly infusion, and escalating to twice weekly and eventually thrice weekly. Some increase to full-dose prophylaxis regardless of bleeding phenotype, whereas others only increase dosing in those patients with a high incidence of bleeding.[77] It remains to be seen how the introduction of longer acting concentrates will affect prophylactic therapy.

Recombinant factor IX

Until the late 1990s, intermediate-purity PCCs were the mainstay of treatment for hemophilia B. These products contained some inactivated as well as some activated coagulation factors and were associated with thromboembolic complications. Due to this thrombogenic potential, high-purity plasma-derived FIX concentrates (Mononine, CSL Behring; and Alphanine, Grifols, USA) were created, and although more expensive, they were also less thrombogenic.[78] These products were plasma derived, though, and were associated with the same risks seen with other plasma-derived products; thus, recombinant FIX (rFIX) products were created (Table 29.4).

Recombinant FIX products are made using no albumin, human plasma, or animal-derived protein, but are made in a mammalian cell line. There are now three available rFIX products, summarized in Table 29.3. There are two standard-acting products that have similar efficacy (Rixubis, Baxter; and Benefix, Pfizer). Most recently, the FDA approved an extended $t_{1/2}$ rFIX product (Alprolix, Biogen Idec, USA). Similar to Eloctate, rFIX is fused to the Fc portion of IgG_1, which significantly prolongs the circulating plasma $t_{1/2}$ of the FIX.[79] Other technologies are currently being explored to prolong the $t_{1/2}$ of FIX, including glycopegylation and albumin fusion.

Dosage and administration of factor IX

FIX requires a higher dose to achieve the same plasma concentrations when compared with FVIII replacement. The recommended dosage for hemorrhage treatments varies based on the type and severity of bleed (Table 29.2 and Table 29.3).[67] The $t_{1/2}$ of FIX is about 24 hours.[68] Plasma-derived FIX products will raise the FIX activity by 1% (0.01 IU/dL) when 1 U/kg is administered. Generally, 1 U/kg of rFIX will raise the plasma FIX activity by 0.8–1% (0.008 IU/dL).[10] Thus, to obtain 100% replacement in a severe hemophilia B patient, they must receive 100–120 IU/kg. Factor IX concentrates may be given in bolus or continuous infusions, with continuous infusions usually utilized perioperatively and with CNS bleeding. A bolus dose of 100–200 U/kg should be infused followed by 4–8 U/kg/hour with periodic FIX activity measurements to maintain appropriate hemostatic levels.[2,69,70,80]

Ancillary therapeutic options
Desmopressin

Desmopressin is the treatment of choice for individuals with mild hemophilia A whenever an appropriate two- to fourfold increase in FVIII activity is seen 30–60 minutes after administration, and these levels are adequate for the type of bleeding episode.[49,67,81] Not all

Table 29.4 Summary of the commercially available recombinant factor IX.

	Recombinant Factor IX Products		
Host Cell	BeneFIX	Rixubis	Alprolix
	CHO	CHO	HEK
Purification and Virucidal Techniques	Immunoaffinity Chromatography Nanofiltration	Ion Exchange Chromatography Nanofiltration Solvent Detergent	Column Chromatography Nanofiltration
Stabilizer	Sucrose	Sucrose	Sucrose
Available vial sizes (IU)	250	250	
	500	500	500
	1000	1000	1000
	2000	2000	2000
	3000	3000	3000
Diluent volume	5 ml	5 ml	5 ml
Dosing calculation	1.2–1.4 IU/kg raises plasma level by 1%	1.1 IU/kg raises plasma level by 1%	1 IU/kg raises plasma level by 1%
1/2 Life	14–28 hours	16–27 hours	~87 hours
Storage	Room temperature not to exceed 86 °F for 6 months	Room temperature not to exceed 86 °F for 6 months	Room temperature not to exceed 86 °F for 6 months
	Should refrigerate at 36 °–46 °F	Should refrigerate at 36 °–46 °F	Should refrigerate at 36 °–46 °F

Products CHO, Chinese hamster Ovary; °F, degree Farenheit; HEK, human embryonic kidney; IU, international unit; kg, kilogram; ml, milliliter.

patients with mild hemophilia will respond to desmopressin, so a trial dose using 0.3 μg/kg IV/subcutaneous (SC) dosing or a fixed dose of 150 μg (one spray) or 300 μg (one spray in each nostril) by intranasal spray for <50 kg or >50 kg, respectively, must be administered and FVIII activity levels are monitored. Desmopressin may be dosed every 12–24 hours, but 3–4 repeated doses over a short period can result in decreased responsiveness, or tachyphylaxis. Desmopressin side effects are generally mild and include tachycardia, headache, and flushing. Significant fluid retention resulting in hyponatremia and seizures can occur, and patients must be fluid restricted for at least 24 hours following administration.[82]

Antifibrinolytic agents

Antifibrinolytic agents, like lysine analogs ε-aminocaproic acid and tranexamic acid, inhibit plasminogen activation and are usually used as an adjuvant therapy to maintain hemostasis. These agents can be useful in preventing lysis of a formed clot, especially when bleeding occurs in areas of high fibrinolytic activity like the oral mucosa.[67,83] The recommended dose of ε-aminocaproic acid is 50–100 mg/kg IV or orally every 6–8 hours, whereas the dose of tranexamic acid is 10 mg/kg IV q6–8 hours or 15–25 mg/kg orally every 6–8 hours. For invasive dental procedures, therapy should be started the evening prior to the procedure and continued for 7–10 days.[83] The use of tranexamic acid mouthwash has been shown to be effective at decreasing postoperative bleeding and transfusion requirements in hemophilia patients following oral surgery when used in conjunction with systemic antifibrinolytic therapy.[84] The recommended dosing is 10 mL of 4.8% tranexamic acid solution for two minutes four times a day.

Vaccinations

Despite the current low risk of posttransfusion hepatitis, all persons with hemophilia should receive both hepatitis A and B immunizations. All blood products are screened for hepatitis, but testing may not be 100% effective. The risk of transmission is greatly increased with plasma-derived products, in which 2500–20,000 plasma donors are used to produce one lot of concentrate. The Centers for Disease Control and Prevention did investigate seroconversion to hepatitis A or B of people with bleeding disorders and found none could be attributed to factor products.[85] These vaccines should be given subcutaneously due to the risk of intramuscular (IM) bleeding associated with IM vaccines.[67]

Avoidance of drugs that cause platelet dysfunction

Certain drugs can induce platelet dysfunction, which can exacerbate bleeding in patients with congenital bleeding disorders. Aspirin irreversibly inhibits platelet cyclooxygenase, resulting in the inhibition of prostaglandin synthesis, and thus should be avoided. Other medications known to induce platelet dysfunction include antihistamines, phenothiazines, and nonsteroidal anti-inflammatory agents (indomethacin and ibuprofen). Acetaminophen can be used to relieve mild pain in conjunction with rest, cooling, and elevation. Cyclooxygenase 2 (COX-2) inhibitors have also been shown to be effective in managing hemophilic arthropathy pain without interfering with platelet function, and are thus considered a safe alternative for pain management in this population.[86]

Inhibitors in hemophilia

One of the most serious complications associated with hemophilia is the development of a neutralizing IgG allo-antibody, or inhibitors, to their deficient factor.[87] Approximately 20–30% of patients with severe hemophilia A, 5–10% of mild and moderate hemophilia A, and 2–5% of patients with hemophilia B will develop an inhibitor.[88–90] The significant difference in inhibitor rates is potentially explained by cross-reactive material (CRM). Many patients with hemophilia B will have evidence of FIX antigen despite low activity because many FIX mutations are missense. The presence of this FIX antigen could potentially explain the lower risk of inhibitor development in that population.[91] Inhibitors usually develop in early childhood, within the first 50 exogenous factor exposure days, and the risk declines after 150 treatment days.[92] Inhibitor formation in hemophilia is a complex multifactorial process, and associated risk factors include family history of inhibitors, hemophilia genotype, race, and immune regulatory polymorphisms (tumor necrosis factor-α, interleukin-10, and cytotoxic T-lymphocyte antigen-4). Inhibitor development rate is also dependent on the type of genetic mutation. In hemophilia A, 88% of patients with a large deletion will develop an inhibitor, 25–41% with moderate deletions, 16–21% with minor deletions, 20% with intron 22 inversions, and 5% with missense mutations.[7,93] In hemophilia B, large deletions or minor deletions associated with a stop codon are associated with an inhibitor rate of 50–100%.[94,95] Immunogenicity differences between plasma-derived and recombinant factor products have been debated, but no conclusive evidence has shown a significant difference in inhibitor development between these products.[96–99]

These antibodies are measured in Bethesda units. A Bethesda unit is the amount of antibody present that will reduce the expected factor level by 50%. Presence of <5 BU/mL represents a low titer or low-responding inhibitor, and >5 BU/mL represents a higher titer or high-responding inhibitor. High-responding inhibitors tend to be more persistent, and even though they can become undetectable after long periods of no treatment, they usually have a recurrent anamnestic response 3–5 days after a challenge with factor products.[67] Inhibitors complicate hemophilia treatment because of diminished responsiveness to exogenous factor concentrates. Progressive joint disease and significant mobility impairment are more prevalent in patients with inhibitors than those without.[100] Also, life-threatening anaphylaxis has been reported in up to 50% of hemophilia B patients with FIX inhibitors upon exposure to exogenous factor concentrates.[101]

Management of inhibitors in hemophilia

Management of patients with inhibitors is twofold: management or prevention of acute bleeding, and attempting to eliminate the inhibitor. Bleeding in patients with low-titer inhibitors can often be managed with FVIII concentrates in typical or high doses if hemostatic levels of FVIII can be achieved. However, patients with high-titer (>5 BU) inhibitors require alternative therapies. Bypassing agents, like activated prothrombin complex concentrate (aPCC), factor VIII inhibitory bypass activity (FEIBA), and activated recombinant factor VII (rFVIIa), have been used and are equally efficacious.[102]

aPCCs, a combination of the vitamin K–dependent factors II, VII, IX, and X and protein C and S at varying concentrations, have been used in the management of both FVIII and FIX inhibitor patients for many years. The recommended dose of FEIBA is 50–75 IU/Kg every 12–24 hours, but repeated doses of more than 3–5 days should be monitored carefully due to thromboembolic risks.[103] FEIBA has been shown to be effective at treating acute bleeding, at controlling perioperative bleeding, and for prophylaxis in hemophilia patients with inhibitors.[103–105]

The development of rFVIIa (Novo Seven, Novo Nordisk, Denmark) was an important landmark in the management of hemophilia patients with inhibitors. It has been demonstrated that rFVIIa at concentrations much higher than normal circulating concentrations mediate a tissue-factor-independent conversion of factor X to its activated form on a phospholipid surface.[106] In the absence of FVIII and FIX, rFVIIa induces hemostasis likely by enhancing thrombin generation on activated platelet surfaces. This leads to thrombin activation, which recruits more platelets and enhances platelet adhesion. This thrombin also recruits factor XIII, leading to a tighter fibrin clot structure.[107]

The first successful use of rFVIIa in patients with hemophilia was during and following an open synovectomy.[108,109] Although the $t_{1/2}$ is short (2–3 hours), rFVIIa has been used with clinical success in patients with inhibitors presenting with life- or limb-threatening bleeds, as prophylaxis for joint bleeding, and as prophylaxis for elective surgical procedures.[101,110–113] Dosing is typically 90 µg/kg with repeated dosing every 2–3 hours until hemostasis is achieved followed by increasing intervals thereafter. Clearance rates may be higher in younger children. Despite its short $t_{1/2}$, daily prophylactic doses of 90 or 270 µg/kg have been shown to be effective in decreasing the frequency of joint bleeding.[113,114] For the majority of patients with hemophilia B who have had severe allergic reactions to FIX products, rFVIIa is regarded as their treatment of choice.[115]

Another option for the management of hemophilia patients with inhibitors could be the use of nonhuman (porcine) FVIII protein. Porcine FVIII has limited cross-reactivity with the antihuman FVIII antibodies. A recombinant porcine FVIII concentrate (Obizur, Baxter) was recently approved by the FDA to treat bleeding episodes in adults with acquired hemophilia A, but further studies are needed to evaluate its safety and efficacy in the treatment of patients with congenital hemophilia A and inhibitors.[116,117]

Staphylococcal protein A immunoabsorption columns are available outside of the United States to rapidly to reduce a very high-titer inhibitor to FVIII and FIX. Due to the availability of bypassing agents, these columns are rarely used, but they may have some benefit especially in reducing the incidence of nephrotic syndrome in hemophilia B patients if used prior to immune tolerance therapy.[118]

Immune tolerance therapy

The ultimate goal in the management of inhibitors is complete eradication, and this is achieved between 60% and 80% of the time with immune tolerance induction (ITI).[118] ITI is costly and requires good venous access as well as patient compliance to be successful. Deferring ITI until the inhibitor titer is <10 BU is preferable, but if the titer does not decline after a 1–2-year period and/or the inhibitor is associated with a severe or life-threatening bleed, ITI should be considered earlier.[119] Inhibitors are divided into good-risk and poor-risk features. *Good-risk features* include an inhibitor titer of <10 BU, a maximum inhibitor titer of <199 BU, and ITI started less than 5 years since inhibitor diagnosis. *Poor-risk inhibitors* do not meet all three criteria.

Currently, there are no strong recommendations for the optimal dose and frequency for ITI, and protocols vary by institution.[119] The International Immune Tolerance Study showed that high dose (200 IU/kg/day) and low dose (50 IU/kg/3 times/week) were equally efficacious in achieving tolerance in "good-risk" patients with high-titer inhibitors, but the high-dose group achieved a negative titer faster and had less bleeding.[120]

The success rate for ITI in hemophilia B patients with inhibitors is much less than that for hemophilia A.[121] The success rate seemed to be mired by the development of nephrotic syndrome of unclear etiology about 8–9 months after the start of ITI. The nephrotic syndrome generally resolves after FIX product avoidance, thus complicating any further ITI.[122]

Gene therapy

Gene therapy replaces the missing factor or protein with a nucleic acid rather than the protein, with the goal of transfecting certain targeted tissue with the nucleic acid to replace the mutated area of the genome. Hemophilia is a monogenic hereditary disorder with well-understood genetics, making it a potential target for gene therapy.[123] Gene therapy has been in clinical trials in hemophilia B for many years with limited success using adeno-associated viral vector serotype 2 (AAV2), but the response was not able to be sustained.[124]

Recent gene therapy clinical trials for severe hemophilia B used adeno-associated viral serotype 8 vector (AAV8), which encoded for a codon-optimized FIX. The AAV8 serotype was chosen because it transduces hepatocytes well, without the efficient interactions with antigen-presenting cells and cross-reactivity with preexisting anti-AAV2 antibodies. Six subjects received low-, intermediate-, or high-dose vector doses, and all subjects expressed between 2% and 11% FIX activities many months after therapy. Some were able to stop prophylaxis therapy altogether, whereas the others required less frequent FIX infusions.[124,125] Although sustained improvement in FIX levels was obtained, the levels achieved were not sufficient to prevent bleeding in the setting of a severe trauma or surgery. Ongoing efforts are underway to optimize gene therapy in hemophilia B.

Utilizing the AAV for the larger FVIII transgene is more challenging due to its large size. However, a codon-optimized FVIII has been created using a BDD FVIII, and injection into hemophilia A mice using a spleen focus forming virus promoter within a self-inactivating HIV-based lentiviral vector showed a sustained 29–44-fold increase in expression of FVIII levels.[126] The gene size used would be small enough to fit into an AAV vector, suggesting a potential gene delivery system.

von Willebrand disease (vWD)

vWD is the most common autosomally inherited bleeding disorder. The estimated prevalence of vWD is about 1%, but clinically significant vWD prevalence is about 1 in 1000.[127,128] vWD usually presents with mucocutaneous bleeding and postoperative hemorrhage, but bleeding to a less severe degree than in hemophilia. No geographical or ethnic predilection exists, and females outnumber males almost 2:1 in most populations, despite autosomal inheritance.[129] This likely represents a diagnosis bias due to the hemostatic challenge of menses. vWD occurs secondary to a quantitative deficiency or qualitative deficiency in vWF.

vWF is a large multimeric glycoprotein that has many roles in both primary and secondary hemostasis. vWF mediates platelet adhesion to exposed endothelium by binding to GPIB/IX/V platelet surface glycoprotein, assists in platelet aggregation by binding to the GPIIb/IIIA platelet surface glycoprotein, and binds to circulating FVIII to prevent protein C–mediated proteolytic degradation.[1]

The gene for vWF is located on the short arm of chromosome 12, spanning 178 kb with 52 exons that code for a 2813-amino-acid-containing protein.[1,130,131] Megakaryocytes and vascular endothelial cells are responsible for synthesizing pro-vWF subunits that dimerize in the endoplasmic reticulum.[132] The pro-vWF dimers form multimers within the Golgi bodies, and the final product protein can be released directly into the plasma or stored either in the Weibel–Palade bodies or within platelet α-granules. vWF in circulation ranges from 500 kDa up to 20 million (high-molecular-weight) Da, with the higher molecular weight vWF more physiologically active.[1,132] Under high shear stress, the larger multimers bound to platelets may stretch and expose a Tyr[1605]-Met[1606] bond in the A2 domain of vWF, where ADAMTS13 (a disintegrin and metalloprotease with thrombospondin 1 motif, member 13) cleaves vWF into its characteristic cleavage products.[1,130,132] vWF, irrespective of multimer size, has a circulating $t_{1/2}$ of about 20 hours.[132]

vWF levels are influenced by many factors. VWF is an acute-phase reactant, rising with stress, infection, and exercise. Chronic elevations in vWF are seen in hyperthyroidism as well as diseases with chronic endothelial damage, like diabetes. Increased estrogen levels, as seen with hormonal contraception, hormone replacement, and pregnancy, have been reported to increase vWF levels as high as 300–400%. Age is another significant factor, as vWF levels naturally increase 1–2% per year.[133] Race also affects vWF levels, with African Americans having higher average levels than Caucasian populations.[134,135] Hypothyroidism has been shown to decrease circulating levels of vWF, and ABO blood groups influence vWF levels, with the lowest levels found in blood type O and the highest in blood type A; and certain variants, like the exon 28 D1472H polymorphism, have artificially low VWF:RCo without affecting GpIbα binding.[133,136–138]

Clinical manifestation

Bleeding symptoms are generally mild in type 1 disease and increase in severity with types 2 and 3. Mucocutaneous bleeding, including easy bruising, epistaxis, and menorrhagia, is the most common manifestation. Postoperative bleeding, especially following oral procedures, is frequently seen. Hemarthroses are uncommon in type 1, but can be seen in types 3 and 2N due to the associated reductions in FVIII activity.[131]

Classification and diagnosis

vWD has been classified into three main categories: type 1 (quantitative deficiency), type 2 (qualitative defects, including subtypes A, B, M, and N), and type 3 (complete vWF deficiency).[132] Laboratory evaluation for suspected vWD should initially include nonspecific hemostasis tests, including a complete blood count (CBC), PT, aPTT, thrombin time (TT), and fibrinogen to evaluate for other potential bleeding diathesis.[1] Platelet dysfunction has similar presentations and should also be considered. Specific vWF quantification and function testing includes circulating levels of VWF:Ag, measurement of vWF function through either ristocetin-based platelet aggregation (VWF:RCo) or von Willebrand collagen binding assays, ratio analysis of VWF:RCo/VWF:Ag, vWF multimer analysis, and FVIII levels (Figure 29.2).[131,139]

Type 1 vWD

Type 1 vWD accounts for 75–80% of all vWD cases.[1,130,133] It is inherited in an autosomal dominant fashion with incomplete penetrance.[131] It is characterized by equivalent mild to moderate reductions in both VWF:Ag and VWF:RCo, with a VWF:RCo/VWF:Ag ratio >0.6, normal or prolonged PFA-100 closure, normal vWF multimeric analysis, and normal PT and CBC.[1,131,132] Currently, there is no consensus on the plasma level of vWF that qualifies as vWD, with upper limit cutoffs ranging from 0.15 to 0.5 IU/dL reported in the literature, with widely varied bleeding

	Normal	Type 1	Type 2A	Type 2B	Type 2M	Type 2N	Type 3	PLT-VWD
vWF:Ag	N	L, ↓ or ↓↓	↓ or L	↓ or L	↓ or L	N or L	Absent	↓ or L
vWF:RCo	N	L, ↓ or ↓↓	↓↓ or ↓↓↓	↓↓	↓↓	N or L	Absent	↓↓
FVIII	N	N or ↓	N or ↓	N or ↓	N or ↓	↓↓	1-9 IU/dL	N or L
RIPA	N	Often N	↓	Often N	↓	N	Absent	Often N
LD-RIPA	Absent	Absent	Absent	↑↑↑	Absent	Absent	Absent	↑↑↑
PFA-100 CT	N	N or ↑	↑	↑	↑	N	↑↑↑	↑
BT	N	N or ↑	↑	↑	↑	N	↑↑↑	↑
Platelet count	N	N	N	↓ or N	N	N	N	↓
vWF Multimer pattern	N	N	Abnormal	Abnormal	N	N	Absent	Abnormal

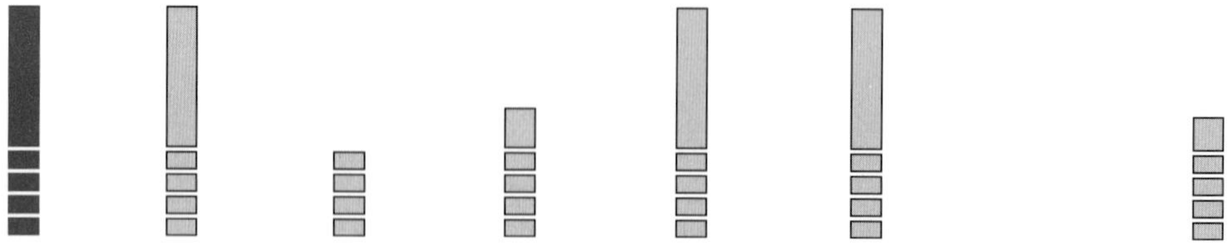

Figure 29.2 Expected laboratory values in von Willebrand disease based on subtype. L, 30–50 IU/dL; ↓, ↓↓, ↓↓↓, relative decrease; ↑, ↑↑, ↑↑↑, relative increase; BT, bleeding time; FVIII, factor VIII activity; LD-RIPA, low-dose ristocetin-induced platelet aggregation (concentration of ristocetin ≤0.6 mg/mL); N, normal; PFA-100® CT, platelet function analyzer closure time; RIPA, ristocetin-induced platelet aggregation; VWF, von Willebrand factor; VWF:Ag, VWF antigen; VWF:RCo, VWF ristocetin cofactor activity. Source: Sukhu et al. (2003).[135] Reproduced with permission of Wiley.

symptoms described at these levels. aPTT may be prolonged due to decreased FVIII activity when VWF:Ag is <0.35 IU/dL, but a normal aPTT does not rule out vWD.[1]

Vicenza type vWD is a type 1 vWD subtype (commonly referred to as *type 1C*) and is inherited in an autosomal dominant manner. It is characterized by low plasma vWF levels, normal platelet vWF content, and supranormal multimers.[140] Although not usually present in the plasma, the larger multimers are observed after DDAVP administration. Despite larger than normal multimers, the functional vWF activity and hemostatic function are decreased. It is unclear if the abnormal function is due to a quantitative or qualitative defect.[140]

Type 2 vWD

Type 2 vWD accounts for 20–25% of all vWD cases and is associated with a qualitative defect in vWF. It is clinically similar to type 1vWD, and all subtypes are characterized by a VWF:RCo/VWF:Ag ratio <0.6.[1,130]

Type 2A vWD

Type 2A vWD is inherited mainly in an autosomal dominant pattern and is associated with loss of the HMW and intermediate-weight von Willebrand multimers.[130–132] The loss of multimers is either due to a defect in their synthesis or due to increased sensitivity to cleavage by ADAMTS13.[1,132,133] Bleeding diathesis described is usually mild to moderate, but can have significant gastrointestinal bleeding secondary to arteriovenous malformations, and generally these patients have a poor response to desmopressin.[132,141–143]

Type 2B vWD

Type 2B vWD is characterized by mutations in the A1 domain that result in enhanced affinity of vWF for platelet receptor GpIb.[132,144] Many individuals will have mild to moderate thrombocytopenia due to the increased platelet aggregation that can be exacerbated by stress and desmopressin, and these individuals will have significantly increased ristocetin-induced platelet aggregation at low concentrations of ristocetin.[145,146] Although vWF is synthesized normally, type 2B vWD shows decreased large-molecular-weight multimers because large multimers bind platelets spontaneously upon secretion and are subsequently cleaved by ADAMTS13.[146,147] The cleaved multimers are small and do not mediate platelet adhesion or connective tissue binding well.[147]

Type 2M vWD

Type 2M vWD is characterized by decreased vWF affinity for platelets without the loss of HMW molecules.[132] These patients usually have a mutation within the A1 domain that impairs vWF binding to the GpIb platelet receptor.[148,149] Recent evidence suggests that individuals with 2M subtypes experience a milder bleeding phenotype than other subtypes.[142]

Type 2N vWD

Type 2N or Normandy variant vWD is associated with mutations in the region of the vWF gene (exons 18–21 or 24–27) that is involved in binding vWF to FVIII.[150,151] These mutations result in decreased or absent vWF binding to FVIII, which in turn results in premature degradation of FVIII.[150] VWF:Ag and VWF:RCo can be normal or borderline low, but the FVIII activity is disproportionally decreased (5–40%). Bleeding symptoms mimic those of hemophilia A, and the decreased FVIII levels make the diagnosis difficult to make.

Diagnosis is made either by genetic analysis of vWF gene or by enzyme-linked immunosorbent assay-based VWF:FVIII binding assay.[1]

Type 3 vWD

Type 3 vWD has almost a complete deficiency of vWF. It is inherited in an autosomal recessive manner, and heterozygous relatives have mild or no bleeding symptoms.[152–154] This type is characterized by vWF:Ag of <5%, VWF:RCo of <5%, and FVIII levels of <10%.[132] These individuals can have a more severe bleeding tendency than the other subtypes, including mucocutaneous hemorrhage as well as hemarthroses and hematomas, similar to that of moderate hemophilia.[131] Due to the lack of vWF, these patients do not respond to desmopressin.

Platelet-type vWD

Platelet-type vWD is similar to type 2B in both clinical presentation and laboratory features. It is also characterized by platelet hyper-responsiveness, but it is associated with a gain-of-function mutation in the platelet GPIBA gene, which codes for the vWF receptor GPIbα.[155]

Treatment

Treatment for vWD is dependent on the subtype. FVIII and vWF levels of >50% are generally considered to be sufficient for maintaining hemostasis except in the setting of severe trauma or invasive procedures.[82]

Desmopressin can be used to increase vWF and FVIII plasma concentrations because it promotes their release from endothelial stores.[82] Typically, a 2–4-fold increase above basal levels is seen in 30–60 minutes, and hemostatic levels of vWF and FVIII are present for 6–8 hours after administration.[131] Over 80% of patients with type 1 vWD will respond to desmopressin with the likelihood of response dependent on their initial VWF:Ag level. Baseline VWF:Ag of <10 U/dL often does not have substantial responses.[81,141,156,157] Patients with Vicenza variant show a promising initial response to DDAVP, but the response is not sustained, with VWF:Ag levels near pre-baseline levels at about 240 minutes following administration.[140] Except for some patients with 2A disease, type 2 vWD usually does not respond to desmopressin, and in fact can exacerbate thrombocytopenia in type 2B. Individuals with type 3 disease are considered unresponsive.[81,157] Desmopressin is administered using 0.3 µg/kg IV/SC dosing or a fixed dose of 150 µg or 300 µg by intranasal spray for weights of <50 kg or >50 kg, respectively. A desmopressin trial is needed to confirm adequate response in all patients. Repeated doses over a short period can result in decreased responsiveness, or tachyphylaxis, and fluid restriction is required for 24 hours following doses to avoid hyponatremia.[82]

Plasma-derived VWF:FVIII concentrates should be used for major bleeding events and as prophylaxis for major surgeries, in patients for whom desmopressin is not beneficial (type 3 and nonresponsive type 1 and 2 patients) and desmopressin is contraindicated (type 2B patients, patients with seizure disorders, and infants).[1] There are three commercially available licensed plasma-derived products for vWF replacement in the United States that are FDA approved: Humate-P (CSL Behring), Alphanate SD/HT (Grifols), and Wilate (Octapharma, USA). These products are not interchangeable as they have differing ratios of vWF to FVIII.

Humate-P contains 50–100 IU/mL of VWF:RCo and 20–40 IU/mL of FVIII activity, and the median $t_{1/2}$ of the VWF:RCo activity is about 11 hours.[158] Alphanate SD/HT contains a higher FVIII activity of 40–180 IU/mL and >16 IU/mL of VWF:RCo activity. Its median WF:RCo $t_{1/2}$ is about seven hours. Wilate contains 90 IU/mL of VWF:RCo activity as well as 90 IU/mL of FVIII activity, with a median $t_{1/2}$ of VWF:RCo of 13–16 hours.[159] Dosing is usually based on the VWF:RCo units. Major surgeries can require as many as 7–14 days of hemostasis, where minor procedures may only need 1–5 days. Minor procedures and spontaneous bleeds may only require a single dose of 20–40 u/kg of VWF:RCo to adequately control bleeding. Major spontaneous bleeding or surgical procedures require more aggressive management. Major spontaneous bleeding may require doses of 50–60 IU/kg of VWF:RCo. The goal of major surgical prophylaxis is generally to obtain peak VWF:RCo levels of 80–100 IU/dL for up to three days and a nadir of 50 IU/dL for at least 5–7 days.[131,139] A loading dose of 50 IU/kg of VWF:RCo can be given 30–60 minutes before surgery with doses of 20–60 IU/kg of VWF:RCo every 8–24 hours to follow to maintain hemostasis depending on the severity of the procedure. Monitoring VWF:RCo and FVIII trough and peal levels will aid in determining the subsequent dosing schedule.[131] Continuous infusions after initial boluses have been shown to successfully achieve surgical hemostasis and may be required in certain situations.[160]

Adverse reactions associated with these concentrates are rare, but include allergic/anaphylactic symptoms like rash, edema, chest tightness, and pruritus.[161] Venous thromboembolism has been reported with the use of these concentrates, so caution should be used with their use in patients with known risk factors for thrombosis. In patients requiring ongoing replacement therapy, monitoring FVIII levels has been recommended to ensure FVIII levels remain in a safe range.[162–164] vWD patients who may require replacement therapy should be vaccinated against hepatitis A and B due to the risk of acquiring blood-borne pathogens, although there has not been a documented case of viral transmission with these products in many years.[165]

There is no consensus on the use of prophylactic infusions in severe vWD, but currently there are ongoing investigations into weekly prophylaxis for severe vWD. One particular study is the vWD International Prophylaxis (VIP) study. This is a nonrandomized study with dose escalation based on bleeding symptoms, and any of the vWF concentrates may be used. An interim retrospective review evaluating one year prior to initiating prophylaxis to at least six months after has shown a significant decrease in the number of annual bleeding events (12 to 3) in the 55 evaluated patients.[166]

Recombinant vWF (rVWF) products are currently under development. A recent phase 1 prospective trial for an rVWF product was completed and showed promising data. Endogenous FVIII was stabilized following the infusion of a rVWF:rFVIII, and in vivo cleavage of HMW rVWF multimers by ADAMTS13 was demonstrated. The product was well tolerated and had no serious adverse events, including no thrombotic events or inhibitor formation.[167]

Historically, cryoprecipitate has been used in the management of vWD. This product is rarely used today due to the risk of blood-borne pathogens, fluid overload, and increased thrombotic risk. Cryoprecipitate use is discouraged by the National Hemophilia Foundation except for life- or limb-threatening situations in which no vWF concentrates are available.[67]

Antifibrinolytics may be used solely to treat mild mucocutaneous bleeding. Using these medications in conjunction with desmopressin or vWF concentrates may be useful in controlling bleeding, especially in the oral cavity, gastrointestinal tract, and genitourinary tract. Menorrhagia is a common complaint among women with vWD and can be severe enough to cause symptomatic anemia. Treatment may require a combination of hormonal contraception, desmopressin when indicated, as well as antifibrinolytic therapy.[139]

Other rare congenital clotting protein disorders

Prothrombin deficiency

Prothrombin (FII), a vitamin K–dependent glycoprotein synthesized in the liver, is the inactive zymogen of thrombin, an enzyme that cleaves fibrinogen into fibrin and activates factor XIII (FXIII) to covalently crosslink fibrin into a stable sheath.[168,169] Congenital prothrombin deficiency is one of the rarest congenital bleeding disorders, with an estimated incidence of 1 in 2,000,000 births, with higher incidences in consanguineous marriages.[169] The inheritance pattern is autosomal recessive with more than 40 mutations described within the 20.3 kb prothrombin gene on chromosome 11p11–q1212, which is only clinically relevant in those who inherit abnormal alleles from both parents.[169,170] Defects are classified as quantitative, or hypoprothrombinemia (homozygotes and compound heterozygotes); qualitative, or dysprothrombinemia (homozygotes or heterozygotes); or combined.[169]

Clinical manifestations

Bleeding severity seems to correlate with prothrombin levels in hypoprothrombinemia, but a discrepancy in bleeding severity and genotype exists in dysprothrombinemia. Prothrombin deficiency may be classified as severe if levels are <5, moderate if 5–10, and mild if >10%, respectively.[171] Patients with prothrombin activity levels of 20–40% are usually asymptomatic, and the $t_{1/2}$ of prothrombin is about three days.[172,173] Patients with homozygous and compound heterozygous prothrombin gene defects can have moderate to severe bleeding. Bleeding manifestations include easy bruising, mucosal bleeding (epistaxis, gingival bleeding, and menorrhagia), hemarthroses, subcutaneous/muscle hematomas, and postoperative bleeding. Gastrointestinal bleeding is less common.[169,172] In the neonatal period, intracranial hemorrhage, severe umbilical cord bleeding, hematomas, and increased bleeding after circumcision have all been reported.[172,174] Heterozygotes are usually asymptomatic, but mucocutaneous bleeding and bleeding following tonsillectomy and tooth extraction have been described.[169,172]

Diagnosis

Typically, prothrombin deficiency will result in the prolongation of both the PT and aPTT, but results are reagent dependent and abnormalities could be minimal. Prothrombin antigenic and activity assays are required for diagnosis after vitamin K deficiency and liver disease have been excluded.[169,174]

Management

Fresh frozen plasma (FFP) and PCCs are the treatments of choice, as no pure prothrombin concentrates are available.[169] These modalities can be used individually or simultaneously. FFP at 15–20 ml/kg, which should raise prothrombin levels by 25%, can be used to treat acute bleeds. For more severe bleeding episodes and surgical prophylaxis, consider a loading dose of 10–20 ml/kg of FFP, followed by 3 ml/kg every 12–24 hours to maintain adequate hemostasis.[169,172] Dosing for PCCS is based on the amount of each factor in the specific product, and it is important to note that the amount of factors varies not only between products but also between manufacturer-produced lots. Typical dosing for PCCs is 20–50 units/kg.[169] Antifibrinolytic agents (aminocaproic acid and tranexamic acid) have been used for mild bleeding. Due to the long $t_{1/2}$ of prothrombin, prolonged courses of treatment should be dosed based on prothrombin activity assays to maintain an activity >25%.[172]

Factor V deficiency

Factor V (FV) is a large glycoprotein synthesized in the liver that is activated by thrombin to serve as a cofactor for activated factor X (FXa) in the prothrombinase complex (FVa/FXa) to covert prothrombin to thrombin.[175,176] Congenital FV deficiency is a rare autosomal recessive bleeding disorder, with a reported incidence of about 1 in 1,000,000.[174] The FV gene is located on the long arm of chromosome 1p23, and the inherited defect can be either homozygous, which is more prevalent in consanguineous families; compound heterozygote; or heterozygote.[175,176] Mutations can result in either quantitative (type 1) or qualitative (type 2) defects.[175]

Clinical manifestations

Bleeding severity correlates poorly with FV activity levels, but severely affected patients (<5–10% activity) tend to be more predisposed to severe bleeding episodes.[171,175,176] This is likely due to the fact that 20–25% of circulating FV is stored within platelet α-granules, which is released upon platelet activation, and seemingly binds immediately to surface receptors forming the prothrombinase complex.[171] The bleeding phenotype in FV deficiency is clinically heterogeneous.[171,175,176] Severe deficiency can present at birth or in early childhood with easy bruising and mucosal membrane bleeding, like epistaxis and oral cavity bleeding, but ICH and umbilical stump bleeding have also been reported. Other bleeding manifestations may include muscle hematomas, hemarthroses, menorrhagia, and postsurgical bleeding. Heterozygote individuals and those with activity levels >10–15% are generally asymptomatic, but may have mild bleeding phenotypes.[171,174–176]

Diagnosis

FV deficiency is associated with both a prolonged PT and aPTT. Measurement of FV activity and/or antigen is required to confirm the diagnosis after liver disease has been ruled out.[175]

Management

There is no commercially available purified FV concentrate. Antifibrinolytic agents alone may be sufficient to control minor bleeding episodes.[175] Severe bleeding episodes or perioperative management should be managed with FFP, dosed at 15–20 ml/kg, to maintain FV activities >20%. The $t_{1/2}$ of FV is 13–36 hours, so daily FFP dosing is generally sufficient.[175,176]

Combined factor V and factor VIII deficiency

Combined FV and FVIII (FV/FVIII) deficiency is a rare autosomal recessive disorder with a reported incidence of less than 1 in 1,000,000 in the general population, with the highest prevalence in those of Middle Eastern Jewish and non-Jewish Iranian decent (1:100,000). There is a higher prevalence in consanguineous marriages.[177,178] The molecular basis for this disorder is a mutation in either the LMAN1 (lectin mannose binding 1) gene on chromosome 18q21 in 70% of the cases or MCFD2 (multiple coagulation factor deficiency gene 2) gene on chromosome 2p21 in 30% of the cases. These genes encode proteins essential for the intracellular transport of both FV and FVIII.[179–181]

Clinical manifestations

No strong association between activity levels and clinical bleeding has been established, but individuals with <20% activity are more likely to have spontaneous bleeding and those >40% are generally asymptomatic.[171] The combined deficiency of FV and FVIII does not lead to more significant bleeding than a similar isolated deficiency of FV or FVIII alone.[182] FV/FVIII deficiency is usually associated with a mild bleeding phenotype, and common bleeding symptoms include epistaxis, easy bruising, oral cavity bleeding, menorrhagia, and postsurgical bleeding. Bleeding after circumcision has also been frequently reported. Less frequently, ICH, umbilical cord bleeding, hemarthroses, and gastrointestinal bleeding have been reported.[182,183]

Diagnosis

Both PT and aPTT will be prolonged in FV/FVIII deficiency and correct with mixing studies. A decrease in the plasma activity of both FV and FVIII to between 5% and 30% is usually seen. Liver disease and systemic consumptive processes (i.e., DIC) need to be excluded.[182] Diagnosis is confirmed by genetic testing for LMAN1 or MCFD2 mutations.

Management

Bleeding episode treatment requires a source of both FV and FVIII. FV replacement is achieved with FFP; FVIII replacement is achieved with FFP, desmopressin, and plasma-derived or recombinant FVIII. FFP should not be utilized solely for FVIII replacement due to its shorter $t_{1/2}$ as compared to FV.[182,183] Recombinant FVIIa has been successfully used to control severe bleeds, but the safety of this off-label use has not been established.[184] Monitoring of replacement treatment can be done with FV and FVIII assays.

Factor VII deficiency

Factor VII (FVII) is a vitamin K–dependent serine protease that, when activated, binds to exposed tissue factor (TF) to form the tissue factor complex, which activates FIX and FX and initiates the formation of a stable fibrin clot.[185] Congenital FVII deficiency is an autosomal recessive condition and is considered the most common rare congenital bleeding disorder, with an incidence of 1 in 500,000.[173,186] To date, over 130 mutations have been described in the FVII gene, located on chromosome 13q34.[185,186]

Clinical manifestations

Bleeding symptoms do not correlate well with FVII activity levels, and there is a poor association between laboratory phenotype and clinical severity.[171,173,186] Heterozygotes are typically asymptomatic, whereas compound heterozygotes and homozygotes have bleeding symptoms ranging from asymptomatic to severe hemorrhagic diathesis.[185,186] Individuals with FVII activities >25% usually remain asymptomatic, whereas FVII activity of <5–10% may be associated with more severe spontaneous bleeding.[171,186] Commonly reported bleeding symptoms include epistaxis, easy bruising, oral cavity bleeding, and postoperative bleeding.[185] Menorrhagia is also a frequent complication and can be quite severe.[186] Muscle hematomas and hemarthrosis have less frequently been reported, and CNS and GI bleeding, although rarely encountered, can be severe.[185]

Diagnosis

An isolated prolongation of the PT that corrects with mixing study is characteristic of FVII deficiency. A FVII activity assay is required to confirm the diagnosis after vitamin K deficiency and liver disease have been excluded.[185]

Management

Many interventions are available to manage FVII deficiency, and therapies should be individualized based on clinical situations due to the short in vivo $t_{1/2}$ (6–8 hours) of FVII. Recombinant FVIIa is the treatment of choice, but its short in vivo $t_{1/2}$ and increased clearance in children influence the frequent dosing schedule of 15–30 μg/kg every 4–6 hours in certain clinical situations. It is notable that much lower dosing and decreased frequency of infusions is needed for FVII deficiency as compared to patients with hemophilia and inhibitors.[185–187] Single intermediate rFVIIa doses (60 μg/kg) have been shown to be effective in many mild to moderate bleeding episodes.[188] Although rFVIIa therapy has been associated with an increased thrombosis risk, recent studies have shown that the use of a minimally effective dose of rFVIIa is both safe and efficacious at obtaining and maintaining hemostasis in bleeding episodes and as surgical prophylaxis.[187,188]

Plasma-derived FVII concentrates are similar to PCCs except for the higher content of FVII. Although effective in obtaining FVII activity sufficient for adequate hemostasis, the concentrations of the other vitamin K–dependent factors are higher than that of FVII, inferring an increased thrombosis risk.[185] FFP, 10–15 ml/kg, is an inexpensive and readily available treatment modality, and often is the only treatment available in many developing countries. Limitations to FFP, including increased risk of blood-borne pathogens, limited effectiveness, fluid overload, and the need for repeated administrations every 6–8 hours, have limited its use in clinical practice. aPCCs and PCCs can also be used, but their use is limited in practice due to concerns similar to the use of FPP.[185,186]

Prophylaxis in FVII deficiency is generally limited to certain clinical situations. Menorrhagia and associated iron deficiency are common complications in FVII-deficient women. If menorrhagia is not well controlled with antifibrinolytics and hormonal contraception, rFVIIa prophylaxis could be considered.[185] Prophylaxis should also be considered in patients with a severe bleeding phenotype and recurrent bleeding episodes.[186]

Monitoring replacement therapy is accomplished by following FVII activity levels. FVII activity of 50% is associated with a normal PT.[185]

Factor X deficiency

Factor X (FX) is a liver-synthesized vitamin K–dependent plasma glycoprotein that is essential for thrombin formation, as it binds with FVa to form the prothrombinase complex.[189,190] Congenital FX deficiency is a rare autosomal recessive disorder with a reported incidence of 1 in 1,000,000, with 1 in 500 being carriers. There is a higher prevalence in consanguineous marriages.[177,190] The FX gene is located on chromosome 13q34, and 105 distinct mutations have been described in individuals with FX deficiency, resulting in either a quantitative (type 1) or qualitative (type 2) defect.[189]

Clinical manifestations

FX deficiency has been classified into three groups: severe (<1% activity), moderate (1–5% activity), and mild (6–10% activity).[190] Activity levels of <10% have been associated with spontaneous bleeding and bleeding symptoms seem to correlate with activity levels as severe patients tend to have more significant bleeding histories. Individuals with activities of 10–40% only have minor spontaneous or triggered bleeding if they have any symptoms, and those >40% are generally asymptomatic.[171] Compared to other rare congenital bleeding disorders, severe FX deficiency tends to be associated with more severe bleeding symptoms. Easy bruising, epistaxis, oral cavity bleeding, menorrhagia, GI bleeding, hematomas, and hemarthroses are commonly reported. Intracranial hemorrhage, bleeding after circumcision, and umbilical cord bleeding have been reported in the neonatal period.[189,190]

Diagnosis

The PT and aPTT are typically both prolonged in FX deficiency because it serves as the first enzyme in the common pathway. They both correct on mixing studies, and vitamin K deficiency and liver disease need to be excluded. Both immunologic and functional assays are required to classify FX deficiency. Reductions in both FX activity and antigen suggest a type 1, or quantitative, defect, whereas a reduction in activity with normal antigen concentrations suggests a type 2, or qualitative, defect.[189]

Management

An FX activity of 10–40% is generally accepted as hemostatic and should be the goal for replacement therapy, keeping in mind the relatively long FX $t_{1/2}$ of 20–40 hours.[190] Currently, there is no FX purified concentrate available in the United States, but a phase 3 clinical trial for a plasma-derived FX concentrate is currently ongoing. FX replacement therapy can therefore be accomplished with FFP or aPCCs/PCCs. Single doses of FFP (15–20 ml/kg) or aPCCs/PCCs are usually sufficient to control most bleeding symptoms, but daily doses may be required if prolonged hemostasis is required. Due to thrombosis concerns with these factor replacement therapies, individuals should be monitored clinically for symptoms of thrombosis, and monitoring with FIX levels and D-dimers should be considered in those receiving prolonged treatments.[189] Minor bleeding symptoms may be controlled with just topical therapies and/or antifibrinolytics.[190]

Prophylaxis is generally limited to certain situations. Menorrhagia that is uncontrolled with hormonal therapy and antifibrinolytics may benefit from prophylaxis with FFP or aPCCs/PCCs. Prophylaxis should be considered in patients with severe deficiency and repeated bleeding episodes, especially CNS bleeds, hemarthrosis, and hematomas. Prophylaxis for a child born to a family already with one severely affected child may prevent complications like ICH.[189]

Factor XI deficiency

Factor XI (FXI) is a plasma glycoprotein synthesized in the liver that circulates as the zymogen of a serine protease (FXIa) bound in a complex with high-molecular-weight kininogen (HMWK). Once activated by FXIIa, FXIa activates FIX, which maintains thrombin production at vascular injury sites.[191] Congenital FXI deficiency is generally inherited as an autosomal recessive trait, but the structure of circulating FIX could result in a dominant negative effect, leading to a dominant inheritance pattern. More than 220 mutations have been described in the FXI gene, located on the long arm of chromosome 4 (4q35.2).[192] The estimated prevalence is about 1 in 1,000,000 in most populations, but is substantially higher at 1 in 450 among the Ashkenazi Jewish population.[192]

Clinical manifestations

FXI activity levels do not correlate well with bleeding tendencies.[171,192] Severe FXI deficiency is defined as activity levels <20%, whereas activities between 20% and the lower limit of the normal activity (65–80%) are considered mildly deficient.[192] Overall, FXI deficiency is associated with a mild bleeding diathesis, but bleeding may occur at the time of the injury or hours later. Spontaneous bleeding is rare in even severely deficient FXI patients.[171,192,193] Epistaxis and menorrhagia may occur. Postoperative and posttrauma bleeding is common, especially in areas with high fibrinolytic activity like the oral cavity, nose, and genitourinary tract.[192,193] Bleeding is less common at other trauma sites, including circumcisions, cutaneous lacerations, orthopedic surgery, and appendectomy.[194] Mild deficiency is generally associated with an asymptomatic state, but a low risk of postoperative bleeding still exists.[171]

Inhibitor development has been described in congenital FXI deficiency following exposure to FFP or FXI concentrates. Although these individuals still rarely have spontaneous bleeds, they may suffer prolonged bleeding during surgery even with appropriate therapy. FXI inhibitors should be suspected in individuals receiving appropriate therapy that continue to bleed and continue to have prolonged aPTTs.[192] Also, FXI deficiency likely conveys a decreased ischemic stroke risk as well, as recent evidence showed FXI activity >95% was a potential risk factor for ischemic strokes, but it does not protect against myocardial infarctions, as postulated in hemophilia A and B.[192,193]

Diagnosis

Factor XI deficiency is characterized by an isolated prolonged aPTT. The aPTT will be greater than two standard deviations above normal values in homozygotes, and may be normal or only slightly prolonged in heterozygotes; however, this depends upon the sensitivity of the PTT reagent utilized. After liver disease is excluded, confirmation of FXI deficiency is achieved by demonstration of reduced FXI activity. Because FXI deficiency can remain asymptomatic until an injury occurs, patients of Ashkenazi Jewish descent undergoing surgery or invasive procedures should consider screening with an aPTT, and FXI activity should be measured if it is abnormal.[194]

Management

Perioperative replacement therapy should be utilized for higher risk surgical procedures in areas of high fibrinolytic activity. FXI replacement is achieved with the use of FFP or FXI concentrates. FFP is typically dosed at 15–20 ml/kg, but again caution must be used as the potentials for fluid overload, transmission of infectious agents, and allergic reactions are all present.[192,194] Plasma-derived FXI concentrates have been available since the 1980s.[194,195] Each FXI concentrate also contains antithrombin, so caution must be applied with use in the elderly, those with cardiovascular disease, and those with other thrombotic risk factors due to the 10% risk of arterial and venous thrombosis after FXI concentrate administration.[192,194,195] The goal of FXI replacement therapy for severe FXI deficiency is to attain approximately 40–45% activity for seven days with major surgery and approximately 30% for day days for minor procedures.[192,194] Because the $t_{1/2}$ of FXI is about 45 hours, prolonged courses of therapy can be managed with bolus dosing on alternating days.[195]

In individuals with FXI inhibitors, rFVIIa has been used off label in small single and repeated doses (15–30 μg/kg) with concurrent antifibrinolytic use successfully to manage major surgeries, including open heart for dissecting aortic repair. Caution must be again applied as both of these agents do have an associated thrombotic risk. Fibrin sealants may be an appropriate alternative to antifibrinolytic therapy in some situations.[192]

Minor procedures (i.e., tooth extraction, colonoscopy with biopsy, and skin biopsy) do not usually require factor replacement therapy. These situations can typically be managed with antifibrinolytic therapy. Fibrin sealants may also be used in some situations.[192,194,195]

Factor XIII deficiency

Factor XIII (FXIII) is a transglutaminase heterotetramer consisting of two catalytic subunits (A) and two carrier subunits (B). Thrombin, along with cofactors fibrinogen and calcium, cleave the activation peptide from the A subunit of FXIII to initiate its activation. The major function of FXIIIa is the cross-linking of fibrin chains, resulting in a mechanically stronger thrombus. Congenital FXIII deficiency is a rare autosomal recessive bleeding disorder with a reported incidence of about 1 in 2,000,000, with severe disease present in individuals who are homozygotes or compound heterozygotes. Congenital FXIII deficiency is more commonly seen in consanguineous marriages. FXIII-A deficiency is much more common than FXIII-B deficiency, for which there are only a few reported cases in the literature.[196–198] The gene coding for FXIII-A is on chromosome 6p24–25, and over 100 mutations have been described so far.[197] FXIII deficiency type I results from decreased synthesis of the protein, and the type describes a qualitative defect of a normal concentration of defective FXIII-A.[199]

Clinical manifestations

Factor XIII activity levels correlate well with bleeding symptoms experienced in FXIII deficiency.[171] The deficiency is considered severe when activity levels are <5%, moderate if 5–10%, and mild when >10%.[196] The first and most clinically characteristic bleeding symptom experienced is bleeding from the umbilical cord days after birth.[196–198] Easy bruising and subcutaneous hematomas, intramuscular bleeds, hemarthroses, delayed bleeding after surgery or trauma, and ICH (the most common cause of disability or death) have all been reported. FXIII deficiency also has associated nonbleeding symptoms, including recurrent spontaneous abortions and impaired wound healing and scar formation.[196,197] Individuals with mild and moderate deficiency may only have mucocutaneous bleeding or might be completely asymptomatic.[171]

Diagnosis

Standard coagulation screening labs of PT, aPTT, TT, and fibrinogen are all normal in FXIII deficiency. The following algorithm has been recommended for the diagnosis of FXIII deficiency:[199]

1 First-line screening to detect all forms of FXIII deficiency should be obtained with a quantitative function FXIII activity assay, either by the measurement of ammonia released during the transglutaminase reaction or by the measurement of labeled amine incorporated into a protein substrate.

2

   A. If the FXIII quantitative screen is abnormal, then:
   • Measure FXIII-A_2B_2 antigen; if decreased, measure FXIII-A and FXIII-B antigens.
   • Measure FXIII activity and FXIII-A antigen in the platelet lysate.
   B. If the FXIII quantitative screen is normal, then:
   • Perform a mixing study to evaluate for neutralizing antibodies.
   • If there is high suspicion of FXIII deficiency, consider a type II defect.

3 Perform molecular genetic studies, and use sodium dodecyl sulfate–polyacrylamide gel electrophoresis (SDS-PAGE) to evaluate fibrin crosslinking.

The urea clot solubility test has been traditionally used to screen for FXIII deficiency, but it can only detect individuals with severe deficiency, so this screening test is no longer routinely recommended.[199]

Management

Due to the clinical severity of the bleeding in FXIII deficiency, once factor activity of <1% is confirmed, prophylactic factor replacement therapy is the standard of care.[199] Prophylactic therapy should also be considered in individuals with factor activity <4–5% with severe bleeding phenotypes.[200] Treatment decisions should take into account that activity levels of 3–5% are usually sufficient to prevent spontaneous bleeding and the $t_{1/2}$ of plasma FXIII is 11–14 days, meaning a monthly dosing schedule should be sufficient.[196]

FFP and cryoprecipitate are easily available sources of FXIII, providing 1 and 3 units/mL of FXIII, respectively, that can be used in the management of FXIII deficiency. FFP is dosed at 15–20 ml/kg every 20–30 days, and cryoprecipitate is 1 unit per 10 kg of body weight. Plasma-derived pasteurized FXIII (pdFXIII) concentrate (Corifact, CSL Behring) is preferred over FFP and cryoprecipitate because of the higher concentration of FXIII and lower risk of blood-borne virus transmission.[196] Prophylactic dosing of pdFXIII is recommended at 10–35 units/kg every 4–6 weeks.[196,197,199] For major surgery, FXIII activity levels should be maintained >5% until wound healing is complete. Prophylactic FXIII therapy ideally should be started before 5–6 weeks of gestation in pregnancy to prevent spontaneous abortions and miscarriages.[196]

A recombinant FXIII (rFXIII) product (Tretten, Novo Nordisk) has recently been FDA approved for prophylactic therapy in the United States. It has been shown to be both safe and effective in preventing bleeding episodes in children and adults with congenital FXIII-A deficiency. Although about 10% of patients developed non-neutralizing antibodies to FXIII, none of these patients had bleeds that required treatment, and these antibodies eventually became undetectable despite further rFXIII exposure.[201] It is important to note that this product is not effective for the rare case of FXIII subunit B deficiency.

Fibrinogen disorders

Fibrinogen is the soluble glycoprotein precursor to insoluble fibrin. It is synthesized in the liver and consists of two sets of three polypeptide chains.[202] The three chains (Aα, Bβ, and γ) coding for fibrinogen are coded by different genes located in a 50-kb region on chromosome 4.[203,204] Normal circulating plasma fibrinogen concentration is about 150–350 mg/dl, and it is constitutively secreted into circulation where it has a $t_{1/2}$ of about four days. Fibrinogen levels of about 100 mg/dl are associated with adequate hemostasis.[186,202] Fibrinogen is converted into fibrin in three phases: (1) Thrombin cleaves fibrinogen to produce fibrin monomers, (2) an organized polymeric structure forms from self-assembly of fibrin units, and (3) FXIIIa covalently crosslinks fibrin.[202] Along with fibrin clot formation, fibrinogen also has a role in nonsubstrate thrombin binding, platelet aggregation, and fibrinolysis.[203,204]

Congenital fibrinogen deficiency is a rare bleeding disorder that affects the quantity of fibrinogen (afibrinogenemia or hypofibrinogenemia), its quality and activity (dysfibrinogenemia), or both (hypodysfibrinogenemia).[186,202,204] Clinical manifestations vary according to the type of deficiency, and a strong association exists between clinical bleeding severity and fibrinogen levels.[171,204]

Afibrinogenemia

Afibrinogenemia is a rare autosomal recessive disorder with a reported prevalence of 1 in 1,000,000, with a higher incidence in consanguineous marriages.[202] Over 80 distinct mutations, with a majority in the Aα chain, have been identified in afibrinogenemia, and individuals are homozygotes or compound heterozygotes.[171] It is characterized by an undetectable plasma fibrinogen level.

Many individuals are diagnosed in the neonatal period, as up to 85% of cases of afibrinogenemia present with umbilical stump bleeding. Some present later in life following a significant bleeding challenge. Mucocutaneous bleeding, muscle hematomas, oral cavity bleeding, prolonged bleeding after venous puncture, GI bleeding, and hemarthroses have all been reported in afibrinogenemia. ICH is a major cause of death in this population.[202] Afibrinogenemic women have gynecologic complications, including menorrhagia, spontaneous recurrent abortions, as well as antepartum and postpartum hemorrhage.[186,202] Issues with wound healing and wound dehiscence have also been reported.[203] Importantly, both arterial and venous thromboembolic events have been reported in afibrinogenemia both before and after replacement therapy, so close monitoring and high clinical suspicion are warranted.[186,202,203]

Hypofibrinogenemia

Hypofibrinogenemia is inherited in an autosomal fashion and is associated with heterozygous fibrinogen gene mutations; thus, it is more prevalent than afibrinogenemia.[202,204] Hypofibrinogenemia is characterized by a fibrinogen level <100 mg/dl. Patients are often asymptomatic, but may have a mild bleeding phenotype. Many are only diagnosed after a major hemostatic challenge. Bleeding after trauma, hematomas, menorrhagia, and GI bleeding are the most frequently reported bleeding symptoms, and wound healing can also be an issue.[171,202,203]

Dysfibrinogenemia and hypodysfibrinogenemia

Dysfibrinogenemia and hypodysfibrinogenemia are rare autosomal dominant disorders caused by heterozygous missense mutations in one of the three fibrinogen genes, making them more prevalent than type 1 disorders.[202] Patients are frequently asymptomatic, but can present with a bleeding diathesis (usually bleeding after trauma/surgery or postpartum) or thrombosis.[186,202,203] Women can suffer from spontaneous abortions, stillbirths, and postpartum thrombosis.[202,203]

Diagnosis

Any test that depends on fibrin as the endpoint (PT, aPTT, and TT) will be prolonged in hypofibrinogenemia or afibrinogenemia.[202,203] Erythrocyte sedimentation rates are determined mainly by fibrinogen and thus will be low. The absence of immunoreactive fibrinogen must be demonstrated to diagnose afibrinogenemia, whereas a proportional decrease in functional and immunoreactive fibrinogen is required to diagnose hypofibrinogenemia.[202]

For dysfibrinogenemia, screening should include a TT, reptilase time, as well as an immunologic and functional fibrinogen assay. Classically, TT will be prolonged, but the immunologic fibrinogen assay will be normal and the functional fibrinogen assay will be low.[202,203] With normal functional fibrinogen present, a prolonged reptilase time is consistent with dysfibrinogenemia. Hypodysfibrinogenemia will show both a qualitative defect as well as a quantitative defect with fibrinogen levels of 50–120 mg/dl.[203] Mutation analysis should be obtained if possible as it can provide useful information for carrier testing and prenatal diagnosis.

Management

Fibrinogen levels of 100–150 mg/dl are generally considered to be sufficient for hemostasis, so <100 mg/dl is typically used as the trigger for fibrinogen replacement.[205] FFP, cryoprecipitate, and fibrinogen concentrates are all available for fibrinogen replacement. Because the $t_{1/2}$ of fibrinogen is so long, every-other-day replacement is usually sufficient for prolonged courses of treatment.

A plasma-derived fibrinogen concentrate (RiaSTAP, CSL Behring) has a standardized concentration, relatively small volume, and a minimal risk of blood-borne viral transmission. The risk of thrombosis is low and has been shown to have a better clinical efficacy profile than FFP.[205] Initial pediatric dosing should be 70 mg/kg with a goal fibrinogen level of 100 mg/dl.[205,206] Life-threatening bleeds may require higher initial doses, as well as maintaining higher fibrinogen levels.[206] FFP dosed at ~15 ml/kg can be used for fibrinogen replacement, noting an average fibrinogen concentration of 2.5 g/L although with significant variations.[205] Cryoprecipitate contains about 15 g/L of fibrinogen, and one unit of cryoprecipitate per 5–10 kg of body weight should increase the fibrinogen concentration by 50–100 mg/dl. Again, these products do share similar limitations due to fluid overload, exposure to blood-borne viruses, and increased thrombotic risk.

Weekly prophylactic fibrinogen replacement may be appropriate in certain situations. Primary prophylaxis to prevent bleeding episodes should be considered in patients with afibrinogenemia. Secondary prophylaxis could be considered in individuals with recurrent severe bleeding, like hemarthroses and hematomas, or after a life-threatening bleed (ICH). Prophylaxis plans should be individualized due to the associated potential thrombotic risk.[204]

Antifibrinolytic therapy may also be helpful in certain situations. Particularly, it may be useful following dental procedures or to treat mucosal bleeding. Fibrin glue is another option to aid in the treatment of superficial wounds.[202]

Women with congenital afibrinogenemia can conceive, but pregnancies usually end in spontaneous abortion by 5–8 weeks.[202] It is recommended that fibrinogen levels should be maintained >50 mg/dl during the first two trimesters, >100 mg/dl during the third trimester, and >150 mg/dl during labor.[207]

Key references

A full reference list for this chapter is available at: http://www.wiley.com/go/simon/transfusion

4   Mannucci PM, Tuddenham EG. The hemophilias—from royal genes to gene therapy. *N Engl J Med* 2001; **344** (23): 1773–9.

67   Srivastava A, Brewer AK, Mauser-Bunschoten EP, *et al.* Guidelines for the management of hemophilia. *Haemophilia* 2013; **19** (1): e1–47.

72   Nilsson IM, Hedner U, Ahlberg A. Haemophilia prophylaxis in Sweden. *Acta Paediatr Scand* 1976; **65** (2): 129–35.

74   Manco-Johnson MJ, Abshire TC, Shapiro AD, *et al.* Prophylaxis versus episodic treatment to prevent joint disease in boys with severe hemophilia. *N Engl J Med* 2007; **357** (6): 535–44.

88   Astermark J, Altisent C, Batorova A, *et al.* Non-genetic risk factors and the development of inhibitors in haemophilia: a comprehensive review and consensus report. *Haemophilia* 2010; **16** (5): 747–66.

139   Nichols WL, Hultin MB, James AH, *et al.* von Willebrand disease (VWD): evidence-based diagnosis and management guidelines, the National Heart, Lung, and Blood Institute (NHLBI) Expert Panel report (USA). *Haemophilia* 2008; **14** (2): 171–232.

171   Peyvandi F, Di Michele D, Bolton-Maggs PH, *et al.* Classification of rare bleeding disorders (RBDs) based on the association between coagulant factor activity and clinical bleeding severity. *J Thromb Haemost* 2012; **10** (9): 1938–43.

CHAPTER 30

Coagulation factor concentrates and pharmacologic therapies for acquired bleeding disorders

Neil Shah[1] & Lawrence Tim Goodnough[1,2]

[1]Department of Pathology, Stanford University, Stanford, CA, USA
[2]Division of Hematology, Stanford University, Stanford, CA, USA

Introduction

Acquired disorders of hemostasis may occur in association with specific clinical conditions or may arise spontaneously in otherwise healthy patients. Unlike inherited coagulation disorders, acquired coagulation disorders are often diagnosed in adult patients, although they may present at any age. Bleeding symptoms can vary from mild bruising and mucosal bleeding to prolonged postoperative bleeding and severe hemorrhage. If the patient does not have a history of significant hemostatic challenge such as surgery or trauma, it may be difficult to distinguish an acquired coagulation defect from an undiagnosed congenital disorder such as mild hemophilia or von Willebrand disease. Management of bleeding in patients with acquired coagulation disorders requires prompt recognition of the underlying disorder to guide therapy.

The acquired coagulation defects discussed in this chapter, and their characteristic effects on laboratory tests of hemostasis, are summarized in Table 30.1. Congenital disorders of coagulation are considered in Chapter 30, and hemostatic support for patients with blood loss in the perioperative setting and trauma is also reviewed in Chapters 48 and 49, respectively.

Reducing and/or avoiding blood loss is a key component of patient blood management.[1] Under physiologic conditions, hemostasis is achieved through constriction of damaged vessels, formation of a platelet plug, and activation of coagulation factors, resulting in formation of a stabilized fibrin clot at the site of bleeding. Parallel to this, the fibrinolytic system is activated to control clot formation and propagation and dissolve the unnecessary (and potentially dangerous) clots.[2] Hemostatic and prothrombotic agents exploit these physiologic pathways to tip the balance toward forming and maintaining clots, thereby reducing bleeding.[3] There have been significant advances in the efficacy of clotting factor concentrates and pharmacologic therapies as alternatives to plasma and cryoprecipitate therapy in the management of patients with hemorrhage due to acquired coagulopathies, and these will be reviewed in this chapter.

We acknowledge the contributions of the three previous authors, Thomas J. Raife, Jeffrey S. Rose, and Steven R. Lentz, for contribution in the previous edition of this chapter.

Prothrombin complex concentrates (PCCs)

Currently approved PCCs are summarized in Table 30.2.[4] PCCs contain variable levels of factors II, VII, IX, and X, and they are either activated (i.e., to allow for bypassing inhibitors to factor VIII or factor IX in the treatment of patients with hemophilia A or B) or non-activated. The non-activated PCCs are further categorized based on the presence (four-factor) or absence (three-factor) of sufficient levels of factor VII.[5] Commercial preparations of PCCs that contain all four (including factor VII) of the vitamin K–dependent clotting factors are approved in the United States, the European Union, and various other countries such as Canada and Australia.[6,7]

PCCs are historically standardized according to their levels of factor IX for treatment of hemophilia B but are now also approved for acute reversal of warfarin toxicity, and they show some evidence of benefit for reversal of oral Xa inhibitor (but not thrombin inhibitor) therapy.[8] The relative roles of PCC therapy relative to plasma therapy in treating acquired coagulopathies are in part related to the variability in the contents and levels of clotting factors in these preparations; their regulatory approval status in different countries; their availability among hospital formularies, particularly in smaller community hospitals; and their potential risks of thrombogenicity.[5,9]

Safety concerns have focused on thrombotic events. A prospective study found that 4.6% of patients had a thrombotic event, but it attributed these adverse events to cessation of anticoagulant therapy for underlying and ongoing risks of thrombosis.[10] Thrombogenicity has been a recognized problem for patients, in part related to the presence of activated clotting factors (for which heparin and antithrombin III have been added to some preparations)[11] and also due to presence of other, preexisting thromboembolic risk factors that resulted in anticoagulation for these patients (e.g., venous thrombosis and atrial fibrillation). Reported incidence of thromboembolic events published between 1998 and 2008 ranged from 0% to 7% (overall weighted mean of 2.3%), with higher and repeated dosing potentially associated with higher risk.[12] A recent review[13] of eight clinical studies identified a thromboembolic event rate of 0.9% associated with PCC therapy. Studies of optimal dosing strategies for PCCs, including fixed versus variable (weight-based) dosage, provide a basis for future research.[14,15,16]

Product information for activated PCCs such as factor VIII inhibitor bypass activity (FEIBA) (VH Immuno, Vienna, Austria)

Rossi's Principles of Transfusion Medicine, Fifth Edition. Edited by Toby L. Simon, Jeffrey McCullough, Edward L. Snyder, Bjarte G. Solheim, and Ronald G. Strauss.
© 2016 John Wiley & Sons, Ltd. Published 2016 by John Wiley & Sons, Ltd.

Table 30.1 Laboratory tests of hemostasis in patients with acquired coagulation defects

Disorder or Therapy	PT	aPTT	TT	Fibrinogen	Platelet Count
Liver disease	↑	(↑)	↑	(↓)	(↓)
Vitamin K deficiency or warfarin therapy	↑	↑	N	N	N
Disseminated intravascular coagulation	↑	↑	↑	↓	↓
Inhibitor to factor VIII (acquired hemophilia)	N	↑	N	N	N
Acquired von Willebrand syndrome	N	(↑)	N	N	N
Inhibitor to factor V	↑	↑	N	N	N
Acquired factor X deficiency	↑	↑	N	N	N
Lupus anticoagulant	(↑)	(↑)	N	N	N
Warfarin therapy	↑	(↑)	N	N	N
Heparin therapy	N	↑	↑	N	N
Direct thrombin inhibitor therapy	↑	↑	N	N	N
Fibrinolytic therapy	↑	↑	↑	↓	N

PT, prothrombin time; aPTT, activated partial thromboplastin time; TT, thrombin time. Test results are indicated as normal (N), increased (↑), or decreased (↓). Parentheses indicate a mild or variable effect.

and Autoplex-T (Baxter, Roundtree, IL) state they "must be used only for patients with circulating inhibitors to one or more coagulation factors and should not be used for the treatment of bleeding episodes resulting from coagulation factor deficiencies in the absence of inhibitors to Factors VIII or IX."[17] Additionally, the presence of DIC is a stated contraindication to their use.[18] In one study, 7% of FEIBA-treated patients suffered potentially related adverse events.[19]

Recombinant activated factor VII (rVIIa)

Recombinant FVIIa acts via two mechanisms to increase coagulation activation at the site of tissue damage.[20] Firstly, rFVIIa complexes directly with tissue factor (TF) released from the subendothelium at sites of vascular disruption. The TF–rFVIIa complex then activates the remainder of the common coagulation cascade via activated factor X. rFVIIa can also bind to activated platelets, which concentrates factor X activation to sites of tissue injury. The factor Xa generated by these two mechanisms drives the thrombin burst, initiating the formation of the fibrin meshwork critical to secondary coagulation and clot stabilization. The potential role for rFVIIa in tissue factor–independent clotting has raised concern for its site specificity and the risk for off-target thrombosis. Accordingly, a black box warning was added to the package insert in 2005 warning of the risk of thromboembolic complications, along with continued uncertainty regarding its level of efficacy for use in off-label settings.

Approved indications of rFVIIa in the US and EU include treatment in patients with congenital hemophilia A or B who have inhibitors to factors VIII or IX, and in patients with congenital factor VII deficiency. Additionally, it is approved in the European Union and is of value in patients with inherited qualitative platelet defects (Glanzmann's thrombasthenia).[21] However, these approved indications accounted for only 4.2% of cases using rFVIIa in the United States from 2000 to 2008.[22]

Off-label use of rFVIIa in a variety of other clinical settings has risen rapidly (Figure 30.1). Use of rFVIIa in patients who had

Table 30.2 Prothrombin complex concentrates

Products	Factor Levels (IU/ml)			
	II	VII	IX	X
Available in the USA				
Four Factor				
Kcentra (CSL Behring)	17–40	10–25	20–31	25–51
Three-factor (II, IX, and X)				
Profilnine SD (Grifols)	≤150	≤35	≤100	≤100
Bebulin VH (Baxter)	24–38	<5	24–38	24–38
Available outside the USA				
Four-factor (II, VII, IX, and X)				
Beriplex (CSL Behring)[a]	20–48	10–25	20–31	22–60
Octaplex (Octapharma)[b]	14–38	9–24	25	18–30
Cofact (Sanquin)[c]	14–35	7–20	25	14–35
Prothromplex T (Baxter)[d]	30	25	30	30
PPPSB-Th[e]	20	20	20	20
Three-factor (II,IX,X)				
Prothromplex HT (Baxter)[f]	30	—	30	130

The values given are the number of units per 100 factor IX units (IU/ml) in each 20 ml vial.
[a] UK and EU.
[b] UK, Canada, and EU.
[c] EU.
[d] Austria.
[e] Japan.
[f] Australia.
Source: Goodnough and Shander (2011).[4] Adapted with permission from American Society of Hematology.

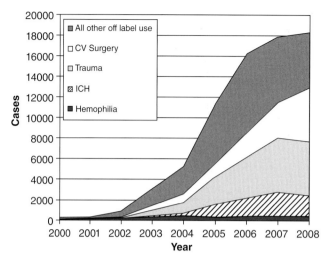

Figure 30.1 Estimated annual in-hospital cases of recombinant factor VIIa use for hemophilia and off-label indications. Cases signify the number of hospitalizations during which recombinant factor VIIa was used. All cases for each year are depicted. The width of each segment represents the number of cases for each category, as indicated by differential shading. Hemophilia includes hemophilia A and B, and trauma includes body and brain trauma. ICH, intracranial hemorrhage. Source: Logan et al. (2011).[22] Reproduced with permission of American College of Physicians.

spontaneous intracranial hemorrhage (ICH) increased eightfold, accounting for 11% of all off-label rFVIIa usage. A large dose-seeking clinical trial in patients with spontaneous ICH initially showed promise[23] in reducing the volume of hemorrhage and improved patient outcomes (reduced mortality and long-term disability); however, the subsequent trial,[24] although confirming reduced hematoma growth, did not demonstrate improved patient outcomes. Other off-label use includes cardiovascular surgery and trauma.[25] Gill et al. reported significant reductions in bleeding, transfusion requirements, and reexploration when used post-operatively in high-risk bleeding cardiac surgical patients.[26] A subsequent literature review found only limited available evidence for efficacy in five off-label clinical settings (Figure 30.1).[27]

The potential role of rFVIIa therapy remains undefined in patients on oral antithrombin or Xa inhibitors who have hemorrhagic complications. A case report suggested that the combination of rFVIIa and hemodialysis was effective in management of dabigatran-associated bleeding in a patient after cardiac surgery.[28]

The uncertainty over whether the demonstrable effects of rFVIIa on international normalized ratio (INR) correction are accompanied by adequate restoration of in vivo hemostasis compared with PCCs,[29] or improvement in bleeding times in reversal of warfarin in normal subjects,[30] has led to two guidelines[31,32] and one evidence-based review[29] to recommend against the routine use of rFVIIa for acute warfarin reversal.[31]

The safety profile of rFVIIa in controlled trials suggests that an increased risk of thrombotic arterial events may be underreported by treating physicians.[33] Thromboembolic events associated with rFVIIa were reported to the US Food and Drug Administration in approximately 2% of treated patients in clinical trials.[34] A review of 285 trauma patients revealed that 27 (9.4%) had thromboembolic complications after administration of rFVIIa.[35] Levi et al. [36] analyzed 35 randomized trials of rFVIIa with 4,468 subjects and found that 11.1% had thromboembolic events. Rates of venous thromboembolic events were similar for subjects who received rFVIIa compared with placebo (5.3% and 5.7%, respectively); however, arterial events were significantly higher (5.5% vs. 3.2%, $p < 0.003$) in subjects receiving rFVIIa, when analyzed for older (age >75) patients.

Antifibrinolytic agents

Antifibrinolytics agents act by inhibiting the physiologic fibrinolytic pathway, limiting and dissolving clots. Aprotinin is a serine protease inhibitor that directly inhibits plasmin (and many other serine proteases), whereas lysine analogs—ε-aminocaproic acid (EACA) and tranexamic acid (TXA)—act through interfering with activation of plasminogen to plasmin and through the binding to fibrin clots.[37] Additionally, aprotinin inhibits the contact activation pathway and may attenuate the inflammatory response in cardiopulmonary bypass.[38] Aprotinin was removed from marketing in 2007, but a reexamination of the Blood Conservation Using Antifibrinolytics in a Randomized Trial (BART)[39] led to a reversal of this decision and reintroduction of aprotinin in Canada and the European Union for cardiac surgery.

Renewed interest in TXA arose from the CRASH-2 (Clinical Randomization of an Antifibrinolytic in Significant Haemorrhage) trial in which over 20,000 trauma patients were randomized to receive adjuvant TXA versus placebo. Treatment with TXA compared to placebo was associated with a risk of death of 14.5 vs. 16%, respectively.[40] Another prospective study evaluating 900 combat cases found TXA was independently associated with survival, with a lower unadjusted mortality rate (17.4%) compared to the no-TXA group ($p = 0.03$).[41] Many European and Canadian massive transfusion protocols (MTPs) include TXA as part of their management.

In other perisurgical settings, patients undergoing radical retropubic were randomized to TXA versus placebo, and a perioperative transfusion rate of 34% versus 55%, respectively, was observed with no increased risk of thromboembolic events.[42] A study of patients undergoing surgery for hip fracture and reported significantly lower red blood cell transfusion rates in patients randomized to TXA versus placebos; however, the rate of occurrence of postoperative vascular events was 16% in the TXA arm versus 6% in the placebo arm (not statistically significant).[43] Investigation of TXA therapy in a large randomized trial of postpartum hemorrhage, is in progress.[44] A systemic review of trials in off-pump coronary artery bypass graft (CABG) surgery concluded that TXA administration (1–2 g loading dose and 200–400 mg/h) was associated with significantly fewer transfusions, with no increased risk of complications.[45] A meta-analysis focusing primarily on the safety of TXA confirmed lower mortality in patients treated with TXA, compared to no treatment.[46]

Fibrinogen concentrates

Commercial fibrinogen concentrates are available as pasteurized, lyophilized products from pooled donors that undergo purification, viral inactivation, and removal processes, and they have been recently reviewed.[47] In a systematic review of 91 eligible studies (70 plasma and 21 fibrinogen concentrates), the evidence did not support the clinical effectiveness of plasma for surgical and/or trauma patients; perioperatively, fibrinogen concentrate was associated with improved clinical outcomes.[48]

Fibrinogen can be dosed based upon the severity of bleeding and initial fibrinogen concentration.[49] One to two grams should be administered initially if hemorrhage occurs with low fibrinogen levels.[50] Subsequent dosing depends upon clinical response and laboratory or point-of-care test results. The use of point-of-care testing with ROTEM®/TEG® technology facilitates targeted coagulation factor repletion[51,52] based on using fibrinogen levels to calculate dosing. A model has been developed that evaluates management of fibrinogen levels with plasma, cryoprecipitate, or fibrinogen concentrate therapy.[53] High-quality prospective studies are required before definitive conclusions can be drawn.

There are concerns that excessive fibrinogen therapy may increase microthrombogenicity. A randomized clinical trial of fibrinogen concentrate found that fibrinogen therapy was not associated with significant alterations of hemostatic parameters.[54] In a porcine model of fibrinogen administration (600 mg/kg), no hypercoagulability or thromboembolism followed fibrinogen therapy.[55]

Emerging factor concentrates

Various concentrated or recombinant coagulation factors are routinely used in treatment of congenital deficiencies; some of these have also been considered as potential hemostatic agents in acquired coagulopathies. Fibrinogen concentrates are currently approved in the European Union and in United States for treatment of bleeding in patients with congenital fibrinogen deficiency. In a pilot study, thromboelastometry-guided administration of fibrinogen concentrate to patients undergoing aortic valve operation and ascending aorta replacement, to achieve a high-normal plasma level, resulted in lower blood loss and fewer transfusions.[56] Another study reported that administration of fibrinogen concentrate in patients with decreased platelet function with bleeding after CABG surgery was associated with less transfusion of allogeneic blood components.[57] Encouraging reports have been published on use of fibrinogen concentrate as a hemostatic agent in trauma patients, but the evidence remains inconclusive.[48,58,59] Fibrinogen concentrates have also been reported to be an effective addition to conventional treatments for obstetrical hemorrhage associated with hypofibrinogenemia.[60,61]

Factor XIII is primarily used for prophylactic treatment of patients with congenital deficiency of factor XIII. However, its cross-linking of fibrin and improvement in clot firmness may promote hemostasis in procedures associated with extensive blood loss. In a preliminary study in patients undergoing cardiopulmonary bypass, administration of factor XIII was effective in reducing postoperative blood loss and transfusions in patients with lower-than-normal factor XIII.[62] A randomized trial in patients undergoing elective gastrointestinal (GI) cancer surgery indicated that early administration of factor XIII during surgery may promote

fibrin clot firmness and reduce fibrinogen consumption and blood loss.[63] Guidelines from the Society of Thoracic Surgeons and the Society of Cardiovascular Anesthesiologists recommended factor XIII as a hemostatic agent to stabilize the clots in bleeding patients undergoing cardiac surgery when other treatments are ineffective.[64] However, a randomized trial on safety and efficacy of recombinant factor XIII in reducing transfusions in patients undergoing heart surgery with cardiopulmonary bypass did not indicate any benefit.[65]

Clinical settings

Liver disease
Pathophysiology

Liver disease and liver transplantation are associated with multiple hemostatic defects. The liver produces the soluble coagulation factors and many of the regulatory proteins, including α_2-macroglobulin, antiplasmins, antithrombin, tissue factor pathway inhibitor, ADAMTS13 metalloprotease, protein C, and protein S. Plasma levels of antihemophiliac factor, or factor VIII, are determined by its release along with von Willebrand factor (vWF) from endothelium; therefore, levels may be elevated, rather than decreased, in patients with liver disease. The liver also plays a key role in clearance of activated coagulation factors and fibrinolytic fragments that interfere with hemostatic mechanisms. Significant liver dysfunction can, therefore, lead to both bleeding and thrombosis from impaired biosynthesis of multiple hemostatic factors, failed clearance of inhibitory factors, and fibrinolysis.

In both acute and chronic liver disease, the extent of hepatocellular damage generally correlates with the magnitude of the hemostatic defect, as assessed by laboratory tests and clinical bleeding. Deficiency of factor VII usually precedes that of other factors because of its short (6-hour) biological half-life. Levels of factor IX tend to be less depressed than other vitamin K–dependent factors. Levels of factor V are variably decreased in acute hepatitis and are often decreased in chronic liver disease. Levels of fibrinogen are usually elevated in acute hepatitis as part of the acute phase response. In cirrhosis, levels of fibrinogen are typically normal or mildly decreased, with levels less than 100 mg/dL indicative of end-stage liver disease and poor prognosis.

Impaired vitamin K utilization results in the production of nonfunctional vitamin K–dependent factors. Production of abnormal fibrinogens (dysfibrinogenemia) and accumulation of fibrin degradation products (FDPs) also impair coagulation. Dysfibrinogenemia caused by abnormal posttranslational processing of fibrinogen is common in chronic active hepatitis and cirrhosis. The abnormal fibrinogens have been shown to have antithrombin activity and to impair fibrin polymerization, which may result in the formation of fibrin clots with impaired stability. Impaired hepatic clearance of FDPs is seen in patients with disseminated intravascular coagulation (DIC).

Management of bleeding

Bleeding associated with severe liver disease can be a clinical challenge. Because the hemostatic defect invariably includes deficiency of coagulation factors, transfusion of plasma has been the mainstay of therapy.[66] However, a reassessment of hemostasis in patients with chronic liver disease has challenged dogma that the major coagulopathy in these patients consistently leads to bleeding.[67] The main culprits for bleeding tendencies in this setting are portal hypertension, infection, and renal failure.[68]

The INR is a very poor predictor of bleeding in conjunction with surgical procedures.[69] The prophylactic transfusion of plasma to correct modest elevations (1.1–1.85) of the INR has not been demonstrated to have a significant impact on either the INR[70] or clinical outcomes, and should be discouraged.[71,72] Plasma may be transfused to treat active bleeding when the INR is greater than 1.7–1.8.[73] In bleeding patients, the recommended initial dose of plasma is 15 mL/kg, with doses up to 30 mL/kg in patients with severe coagulopathy.[4,74] The hemostatic benefit of plasma transfusion is often quite transient, necessitating frequent dosing and volume overload.[75] Due to the short half-life of factor VII, the poor recovery of factor IX from transfused plasma, and the loss of transfused clotting factors into third-space fluid, repeated administration may be required.

Fibrinogen levels are seldom decreased enough from liver dysfunction to cause major bleeding. However, severe hypofibrinogenemia (fibrinogen level <100 mg/mL) in a patient with active bleeding should be treated with cryoprecipitate.[76] Each unit of cryoprecipitate contains 150–250 mg of fibrinogen. A typical initial dose of 10–15 units should increase the plasma concentration of fibrinogen by 50–75 mg/dL. Fibrinogen concentrate therapy can also be considered.

Vitamin K (5–10 mg for adults, 1–2 mg for children) should be administered to most patients with coagulopathy and liver disease, but its effectiveness is often poor; even if the prothrombin time (PT) is shortened, clinical bleeding may persist. Desmopressin acetate (DDAVP), which stimulates release of vWF (and possibly factor VIII) from endothelial cells, is sometimes used. However, factor VIII and vWF are often elevated in liver disease, so the value of DDAVP is uncertain and has not been rigorously tested.[77] PCCs, which contain vitamin K–dependent coagulation factors, are gaining renewed interest for treating the coagulopathy of liver disease.[11]

An evolving approach to the rapid treatment of the coagulopathy of liver disease in life-threatening bleeding is the use of recombinant activated factor VII (rFVIIa).[6] Doses of rFVIIa ranging from 5 to 120 μg/kg have been tried before liver biopsy, with prompt normalization of the PT occurring in most patients. However, normalization of the PT associated with the use of rFVIIa has not been demonstrated to prevent bleeding or improve clinical outcomes in any number of controlled clinical trials, including patients with liver disease and GI bleeding or in liver transplant patients.[33] Thus, the utility of rFVIIa in treating the coagulopathy of liver disease remains unproven.

Vitamin K deficiency
Pathophysiology
Vitamin K comprises a group of fat-soluble vitamins that are available from many dietary sources and from GI flora. Because there are two independent sources of vitamin K, deficiency solely from inadequate dietary absorption or inadequate production by GI flora is rare. Deficiency usually arises from disruption of both sources.

Vitamin K is a coenzyme in the hepatocellular pathway that synthesizes coagulation factors II, VII, IX, and X, as well as the regulatory factors protein C, protein S, and protein Z. Vitamin K is required for the γ-carboxylation of several amino terminal glutamyl residues that serve as the Ca(2+)-binding site for these Ca(2+)-dependent coagulation proteins. In conditions of vitamin K deficiency, plasma levels of vitamin K–dependent coagulation factors are quantitatively decreased, and production of dysfunctional non-carboxylated factors further contributes to impaired hemostasis.

Hemorrhagic disease of the newborn
Hemorrhagic disease of the newborn is a bleeding disorder caused by inadequate production of vitamin K–dependent coagulation factors. A transient physiologic decrease in coagulation factors normally occurs during the newborn period because of synthetic limitations of the immature liver. With maternal or newborn vitamin K deficiency, plasma concentrations of vitamin K–dependent factors can decline to levels that are inadequate to maintain hemostasis. Bleeding in hemorrhagic disease of the newborn can be severe and can include melena, intracranial hemorrhage, bleeding from circumcision, generalized ecchymosis, and intramuscular hemorrhage. Factors that predispose to hemorrhagic disease of the newborn include prematurity, delayed bacterial colonization of the gut, liver disease, inadequate maternal or infant vitamin K intake, and prenatal exposure to warfarin or anticonvulsant drugs. Because breast milk is a poor source of vitamin K, postnatal deficiency of vitamin K tends to be more severe in breastfed infants who do not receive vitamin K supplementation.

Prophylactic administration of vitamin K_1 to newborns (1 mg parenterally or 2 mg orally) diminishes the transient decrease in vitamin K–dependent factors and prevents hemorrhagic disease of the newborn. This practice is mandated by law in many countries, which accounts for the rarity of the disorder in the developed world.

Other causes of vitamin K deficiency
Malabsorption syndromes, including celiac disease, sprue, inflammatory bowel disease, and parasitic infestations, can impair absorption of dietary vitamin K. Absorption of vitamin K also can be impaired in severe biliary stasis or after ingestion of bile acid sequestering resins. Ingestion of high-dose aspirin, high-dose vitamin E, warfarin, or other anticoagulants is a common cause of vitamin K deficiency, either from decreased absorption or from vitamin K antagonism. Antibiotic therapy contributes to vitamin K deficiency by inhibiting the synthetic capacity of vitamin K–producing bacteria. Certain antibiotics, such as cephalosporins that contain an N-methyl thiotetrazol ring, interfere directly with vitamin K activity. The combination of inadequate dietary intake of vitamin K and use of broad-spectrum antibiotics is an insidious cause of vitamin K deficiency in hospitalized patients.

Treatment
A single oral dose of 5–10 mg of vitamin K_1 usually restores adequate levels of vitamin K–dependent coagulation factors within 24 hours. Larger doses may be required in patients with severe deficiency, particularly those associated with warfarin or other anticoagulants. In cases of ingestion of warfarin-like rodent poisons, doses of vitamin K_1 up to 100 mg daily (orally or intravenously) may be required because of the potency and extremely long biological half-lives of these poisons. Guidelines for the reversal of warfarin anticoagulation, in addition to vitamin K administration, are summarized in this chapter.

Disseminated intravascular coagulation
Pathophysiology
DIC is a syndrome of diverse etiology that is characterized by pathologic activation of procoagulant and fibrinolytic pathways. Systemic activation of these pathways creates two seemingly paradoxical clinical problems: tissue injury caused by disseminated microvascular thrombosis, and hemorrhage caused by consumption of coagulation factors and accelerated fibrinolysis. Some patients, such as those with DIC caused by meningococcemia,

experience severe thrombosis of the skin and other organs but have little clinical evidence of bleeding. Other patients with DIC present with bleeding from surgical sites, severe ecchymosis, and diffuse oozing from phlebotomy sites and mucosal surfaces. Still other patients have clinical manifestations of both thrombosis and hemorrhage.

DIC is usually a secondary phenomenon, and the clinical entities that underlie its development are impressively diverse. They include obstetric accidents, intravascular hemolysis, sepsis, viral illnesses, crush injuries, burns, head injuries, autoimmune and inflammatory disorders, malignancies, toxins, and medications. The most common causes of DIC in the developed world are obstetric accidents and infection. Worldwide, venomous snake bite is estimated to be among the most common causes of DIC.

DIC often occurs in patients who have features of the systemic inflammatory response syndrome (SIRS). In SIRS, pathologic processes evoke the production of inflammatory mediators that stimulate expression of tissue factor and release of plasminogen activators from endothelial cells.[78] Tissue factor initiates coagulation pathways, leading to the production of thrombin, which in turn stimulates platelet aggregation, activation of coagulation factors V and VIII, and cleavage of fibrinogen to form fibrin matrices. Generalized production of thrombin can lead to diffuse microvascular deposition of fibrin and subsequent organ failure. Thrombin is normally regulated by the thrombomodulin–protein C anticoagulant system, but this regulatory system is impaired in DIC because of downregulation of thrombomodulin and consumption of protein C. Plasminogen activators activate plasmin, which proteolytically cleaves both fibrin clots (fibrinolysis) and soluble fibrinogen (fibrinogenolysis). Generation of plasmin in the systemic circulation causes proteolytic consumption of fibrinogen and accumulation of FDPs, both of which contribute to bleeding in DIC.

Platelet activation and aggregation lead to thrombocytopenia and bleeding in DIC. Consumption of platelets in DIC can be extremely rapid, overwhelming the capacity of the marrow to replenish the circulating pool of platelets. In addition, partial activation of platelets and accumulation of FDPs may produce a functional defect in the platelets that remain in the circulation. Severe deficiency of the vWF-cleaving metalloprotease ADAMTS13 has been reported in DIC and may contribute to platelet microvascular thrombosis.[79]

Clinical features

DIC is a spectrum of disorders with acute and chronic manifestations. In fulminant acute DIC, thrombosis and hemorrhage often produce multi-organ failure manifested by renal, pulmonary, hepatic, cutaneous, and central nervous system dysfunction. Metabolic instability, hypotension, fever, proteinuria, and hypoxia are common. Hematologic signs include generalized ecchymosis, petechiae, or skin necrosis, and bleeding from mucosal surfaces, venipuncture sites, and surgical sites. In DIC associated with meningococcemia, the appearance of rapidly progressing retiform skin lesions is a poor prognostic sign. The skin lesions in these patients are caused by widespread thrombosis of dermal and subdermal vessels. The thrombotic diathesis of DIC also can include significant large-vessel thrombosis.

Chronic DIC reflects low-grade systemic activation of hemostatic pathways and is associated with underlying vascular disease, autoimmune disorders, chronic inflammatory disorders, malignancies, and chronic liver disease. Because hemostatic compensatory mechanisms usually keep pace with consumption, bleeding may be less prominent than thrombotic complications, except with severe thrombocytopenia. Clinical manifestations are variable and may include deep venous thrombosis or migratory thrombophlebitis as well as epistaxis and ecchymosis.

Treatment

Treatment of DIC requires control of the triggering pathologic process. Management of bleeding and thrombosis is an important adjunctive measure, and can provide time for definitive therapies, such as antimicrobial therapy, surgery, or cancer treatment, to become effective. Prevention of ischemic organ injury is of paramount concern. Other supportive measures may include volume expansion and correction of hypotension to improve microcirculation and optimize tissue oxygenation.

The use of heparin in DIC highlights the dilemma of a disorder that simultaneously produces bleeding and thrombosis. Although it may be counterintuitive to consider using an anticoagulant in the face of pathologic bleeding, the devastating consequences of systemic thrombosis make heparin a rational treatment for DIC. Moreover, by slowing consumption of coagulation factors, heparin may paradoxically improve the bleeding diathesis. Heparin inhibits thrombin activity and slows the consumptive process while reducing microvascular fibrin deposition. Heparin has been found to prevent complications of DIC in certain syndromes such as DIC associated with acute promyelocytic leukemia or solid tumors, but its value in treating DIC in other clinical settings is less certain. The initial dose of heparin in DIC is usually relatively low (e.g., 8 U/kg/hour by continuous intravenous infusion). Declining levels of FDPs and D-dimer, rising levels of fibrinogen, and shortening of the activated prothrombin complex concentrate (aPTT) demonstrate the efficacy of heparin in slowing consumption of coagulation factors and decreasing fibrin formation.

In patients with active bleeding or impending biopsy and laboratory evidence of severe consumption of fibrinogen (fibrinogen level less than 100 mg/dL) or other coagulation factors (PT greater than 1.5 × control value), transfusion of cryoprecipitate (0.2 unit/kg) or plasma (15 mL/kg) is indicated. It is important to remember that many patients who have definitive laboratory evidence of DIC may not have clinically significant thrombosis or hemorrhage. Such patients typically do not require any specific therapy other than treatment of the underlying process.

When bleeding associated with DIC is refractory to heparin and transfusion therapy, antifibrinolytic agents such as EACA are occasionally used. In addition to stabilizing clots, antifibrinolytic agents also reduce FDP production. However, inhibition of fibrinolysis has the potential to exacerbate fibrin deposition, resulting in severe thrombotic complications. Therefore, antifibrinolytic agents should be reserved for life-threatening hemorrhage, and should be considered for use only in conjunction with heparin in the setting of DIC.

Potential therapeutic agents for DIC include antithrombin and activated protein C, as well as small molecules that directly inhibit thrombin or factor Xa.[80] Antithrombin is a serine protease inhibitor that inactivates thrombin, factor Xa, and other coagulation factors. Heparin is a cofactor for antithrombin, and if antithrombin becomes depleted in DIC, the effectiveness of heparin anticoagulation may be limited. Antithrombin has been reported to be beneficial as an adjunctive to heparin therapy in DIC when its levels are depleted to less than 70% of normal.[80,81] Protein C is an anticoagulant agent that inhibits thrombin production by inactivating factors Va and VIIIa. Protein C and activated protein C have shown efficacy in clinical trials of DIC associated with bacterial sepsis.[82,83] These agents and others in development offer the promise of improved treatment of DIC in the future.[80]

Coagulation factor inhibitors

Normal blood plasma contains several proteins that inhibit activated coagulation factors. These natural coagulation factor inhibitors include antithrombin, heparin cofactor II, α_1-protease inhibitor, α_2-macroglobulin, C1 inhibitor, plasminogen activator inhibitors, and tissue factor pathway inhibitor. They function to limit the extent of hemostatic and fibrinolytic reactions and thereby localize thrombi to sites of vascular injury.

In contrast to natural coagulation factor inhibitors, pathologic inhibitors (also known as *circulating anticoagulants*) may occur as an immunologic response to coagulation factor therapy in patients with hereditary hemophilia, or may arise spontaneously as autoantibodies in patients without a history of abnormal hemostasis. Patients who spontaneously develop inhibitors of coagulation factor VIII often present with a severe bleeding diathesis, and are said to have *acquired hemophilia*. Spontaneous inhibitors of other coagulation factors are encountered less frequently, but also can cause abnormal bleeding. When a coagulation factor inhibitor is suspected, it is essential to distinguish between an inhibitor of a specific coagulation factor, which often causes bleeding, and a nonspecific inhibitor such as a lupus anticoagulant, which may predispose to thrombosis rather than bleeding.

Factor VIII inhibitors (acquired hemophilia)

Acquired hemophilia is a rare disorder that is caused by the spontaneous development of an autoantibody inhibitor of coagulation factor VIII. The annual incidence has been estimated to be about one case per million.[84] Autoantibodies to factor VIII occur mainly in adults; they may arise in the postpartum period or in association with immunologic disorders such as systemic lupus erythematosus, rheumatoid arthritis, inflammatory bowel disease, or lymphoproliferative disorders. Approximately 50% of cases occur in elderly patients without any underlying medical condition.

The characteristic clinical presentation of acquired hemophilia is the appearance of pathologic hemorrhage in a patient with no history of abnormal bleeding. Patients may present with rapidly enlarging ecchymosis, soft tissue hematoma, gross hematuria, hemarthrosis, or GI bleeding. Bleeding is sometimes severe and life threatening. With no known history of a bleeding disorder, the presence of an inhibitor is often not recognized before surgical procedures, and some patients are diagnosed only after experiencing excessive postoperative bleeding.[84]

The presence of a circulating inhibitor to factor VIII can be readily detected in the hemostasis laboratory. Typically, the aPTT is prolonged, and it does not correct to the normal reference range when repeated on a 1:1 mixture of the patient's plasma with normal plasma. Occasionally, the 1:1 mixture must be incubated for up to two hours to allow the inhibitor to completely inactivate factor VIII before the aPTT is performed. The PT is usually normal. The factor VIII activity level is low (often less than 10% of normal), but levels of other coagulation factors (e.g., factors IX, XI, and XII) are normal. If multiple coagulation factors are affected, a nonspecific inhibitor (lupus anticoagulant) should be suspected. The diagnosis of a specific factor VIII inhibitor is confirmed by a quantitative assay of the inhibitor level (often expressed in *Bethesda units* [BU]). One BU is defined as the amount of inhibitor that neutralizes half the factor VIII activity in a 1:1 mixture with normal plasma.

The natural history of acquired hemophilia is variable. In some cases, such as those that present in the postpartum period, the inhibitor disappears spontaneously within weeks to months.[85] In other cases, the inhibitor persists for many years. In patients with active bleeding, the immediate goal of treatment is to control acute hemorrhage (Table 30.3). Invasive procedures, intramuscular injections, and the use of antiplatelet agents should be avoided if possible. If the bleeding is mucosal, an antifibrinolytic agent such as EACA should be given.

If the inhibitor level is low (less than 10 BU), large doses of recombinant (most commonly used in developed countries) or plasma-derived human factor VIII (starting dose of 100–150 U/kg, followed by a continuous infusion of 10 U/kg/hour) can overwhelm the inhibitor.[84] Factor VIII levels should be measured frequently to assess the response to treatment; the usual goal of factor VIII replacement in a patient with active bleeding is to maintain a factor VIII activity level that is greater than 50% of normal.

Patients with very low inhibitor levels (less than 3 BU) may respond to DDAVP, which acts by stimulating release of endogenous vWF and factor VIII from endothelial storage sites. DDAVP is administered either intravenously or nasally, and can be repeated every 24 hours for up to three days. Side effects of DDAVP include fluid retention and hyponatremia; therefore, this drug should not be used in elderly patients with a history of cardiovascular disease. Repeated use of DDAVP for more than three doses may result in loss of its hemostatic effectiveness because of depletion of vWF from storage sites.[77]

If the inhibitor level is high (greater than 10 BU), the likelihood of achieving a therapeutic response to human factor VIII is low, and alternative treatments such as rFVIIa therapy should be considered. Plasmapheresis or immunoadsorption columns have been used to acutely decrease the plasma level of a circulating inhibitor to allow successful treatment with human factor VIII.[86] Some patients respond well to porcine factor VIII concentrate (starting dose of 50–100 U/kg), because most acquired inhibitors have low cross-reactivity with porcine factor VIII. However, continuous or repeated use of porcine factor VIII often results in the development of inhibitors of porcine factor VIII, which limits therapeutic options for management of future episodes of bleeding. It is recommended, therefore, that use of this product be restricted to life- and limb-threatening emergencies. Other therapeutic options for the

Table 30.3 Management of acute bleeding episodes in patients with acquired factor VIII inhibitors

Low inhibitor level (<10 BU)
- Desmopressin acetate (DDAVP)
- Human factor VIII concentrate
- Recombinant human factor VIII

High inhibitor level (>10 BU)
- Recombinant human factor VIIa
- Porcine factor VIII concentrate
- Prothrombin complex concentrate
- Activated prothrombin complex concentrate
- Plasmapheresis or immunoadsorption, followed by human factor VIII concentrate or recombinant human factor VIII

Adjunctive measures
- Immobilization
- Compression
- Avoid aspirin and other antiplatelet agents
- ε-aminocaproic acid (if bleeding is mucosal)

management of acute bleeding in patients with acquired hemophilia include rFVIIa or FEIBA (activated PCCs).

The long-term management of patients with acquired factor VIII inhibitors should be directed toward eradication of the inhibitor. Although some inhibitors disappear spontaneously, even after many years, a trial of immunosuppressive therapy should be considered in most patients. Some patients respond to corticosteroids alone.[84] Other immunosuppressive treatments include cyclophosphamide, azathioprine, cyclosporin A, intravenous immunoglobulin, and rituximab.[85]

Lupus anticoagulants

Lupus anticoagulants are autoantibodies that nonspecifically inhibit phospholipid-dependent coagulation reactions in vitro. Although first recognized in patients with systemic lupus erythematosus, nonspecific inhibitors are actually encountered more frequently in patients without lupus. Lupus anticoagulants are induced by certain medications, including procainamide, hydralazine, quinidine, and chlorpromazine, or may occur in association with human immunodeficiency virus infection. Lupus anticoagulants also arise spontaneously in patients who are otherwise healthy.

Lupus anticoagulants represent a subset of a larger group of "antiphospholipid" autoantibodies that recognize phospholipid–protein complexes. Antiphospholipid antibodies are usually either IgG or IgM; other immunoglobulin classes are rare. Lupus anticoagulants often prolong the aPTT but rarely prolong the PT. The aPTT usually does not correct completely to normal when the patient's plasma is mixed 1:1 with normal plasma, but correction in mixing studies can be observed with lupus anticoagulants of low titer or low avidity. Some lupus anticoagulants do not prolong either the aPTT or PT. Several alternative clotting assays, including the dilute Russell viper venom time and kaolin clotting time, have been developed as high-sensitivity screening tests for lupus anticoagulants. Regardless of whether the aPTT or one of the alternative assays is used to detect the lupus anticoagulant, a confirmatory test should be performed to establish that the inhibitor is phospholipid dependent.[87]

Paradoxically, although lupus anticoagulants prolong clotting times in vitro, they are often associated clinically with thrombosis rather than with bleeding. Thrombotic events in patients with lupus anticoagulants can be either venous (e.g., deep venous thrombosis and pulmonary embolism) or arterial (e.g., myocardial infarction, stroke, and peripheral arterial occlusion). A syndrome of severe microvascular thrombosis resulting in acute multi-organ failure (the *catastrophic antiphospholipid antibody syndrome*) has been described in some patients.[88] In addition to thrombosis, patients with lupus anticoagulants may experience pregnancy loss, thrombocytopenia, neurologic symptoms, and livedo reticularis. The mechanisms by which lupus anticoagulants predispose to these clinical conditions are incompletely understood, but may involve autoantibody-mediated activation of procoagulant cell surface receptors[89] or disruption of the anticoagulant properties of annexin A5.[90]

Individual patients with antiphospholipid antibodies usually have positive laboratory test results for lupus anticoagulants, anticardiolipin antibodies, anti-β_2-glycoprotein I antibodies, or a combination. However, none of the currently available laboratory tests for antiphospholipid antibodies predict with certainty which patients have an increased risk for clinical complications, and it is likely that only a subset of individuals with abnormal test results are actually predisposed to thrombosis. Patients with lupus anticoagulants, either with or without anticardiolipin antibodies, have a higher risk for thrombotic complications than those with isolated anticardiolipin antibodies.[91] Women with persistence of antiphospholipid antibodies also have an increased risk for miscarriage and other complications of pregnancy.

Identification of a lupus anticoagulant in a bleeding patient is important for several reasons. Firstly, because most lupus anticoagulants do not cause a bleeding diathesis (with the rare exception of those associated with severe thrombocytopenia or hypoprothrombinemia; discussed further in this chapter), a search for another abnormality of hemostasis should be undertaken. Secondly, recognition that prolongation of the aPTT is caused by a lupus anticoagulant may prevent inappropriate transfusion of plasma and other blood components. Thirdly, all patients with lupus anticoagulants should be considered to be at high risk for thrombosis, particularly in the settings of surgery, trauma, or pregnancy.

Patients with lupus anticoagulants may have coexistent autoimmune thrombocytopenia. The thrombocytopenia is often mild, but it can be associated with abnormal bleeding if the platelet count decreases to less than $50,000/\mu L$. Another circumstance in which lupus anticoagulants are directly associated with increased risk of bleeding, rather than thrombosis, is the hypoprothrombinemia–lupus anticoagulant syndrome. Patients with this syndrome appear to have an autoantibody inhibitor that causes accelerated clearance of prothrombin from plasma.[92] The PT is typically prolonged out of proportion to the aPTT. The diagnosis can be confirmed by performing a specific assay for prothrombin (factor II) activity or antigen. A prothrombin level below 20% of normal can produce severe hemorrhage. Treatment of bleeding in such patients is challenging. Transfusion of plasma may be ineffective. Treatment options for acute bleeding include intravenous IgG and rFVIIa.[93,94] Immunosuppressive therapy with corticosteroids, danazol, or rituximab may be effective for long-term management.[95,96]

In patients with venous or arterial thrombosis, anticoagulant therapy with heparin followed by long-term anticoagulation with warfarin is usually indicated. The presence of a lupus anticoagulant may interfere with monitoring of heparin using the aPTT, and alternative monitoring methods such as factor Xa inhibition assays may be needed to measure the heparin level. Alternatively, fixed-dose low-molecular-weight (LMW) heparin can often be used without laboratory monitoring. Lupus anticoagulants also can influence the INR in patients who are treated with warfarin. In such patients, it may be necessary to monitor warfarin therapy by measuring the level of a specific vitamin K–dependent factor (e.g., factor II or X).[97]

Acquired von Willebrand syndrome

Acquired deficiency of vWF arises spontaneously in previously healthy individuals or occurs in association with neoplastic, rheumatologic, or hematologic disorders. Up to 50% of patients have monoclonal gammopathies or lymphoproliferative disorders.[98] The clinical presentation of acquired von Willebrand syndrome is similar to that of congenital von Willebrand disease, except that it occurs in individuals with no personal or family history of abnormal bleeding. Symptoms vary from mild cutaneous and mucosal bleeding (ecchymosis, epistaxis, gingival hemorrhage, or menorrhagia) to severe, life-threatening hemorrhage. The diagnosis should be suspected in patients who have a prolonged bleeding time or a prolonged platelet function analyzer (PFA-100) closure time. The aPTT is either prolonged or normal. Levels of vWF activity (ristocetin cofactor activity), vWF antigen, and factor VIII are often depressed. Most cases are caused by autoantibody inhibitors of vWF. The inhibitors cause rapid clearance of vWF from the circulation, and inhibitory activity often cannot be demonstrated in the patient's plasma by mixing studies. Variant forms of acquired von Willebrand syndrome occur in some patients with solid tumors, particularly Wilms' tumor. In these patients, the deficiency of vWF is not mediated by autoantibodies, but is caused instead by absorption of vWF to malignant cells or cell products.[99] Selective loss of high-molecular-weight multimers of vWF can be seen in patients with aortic valve stenosis.[100]

Management of bleeding in patients with vWF inhibitors can be difficult. As in patients with other bleeding disorders, invasive procedures, intramuscular injections, and the use of antiplatelet agents should be avoided if possible. In patients with an underlying hematoproliferative disorder, treatment with chemotherapeutic or cytoreductive agents may lead to resolution of the long-term bleeding diathesis.[32] In patients with acute bleeding, therapeutic options include DDAVP, infusion of factor VIII concentrates that contain large quantities of vWF (e.g., Humate P or Haemata P [CSL Behring, King of Prussia, PA; and CSL Behring GMBH, Marburg, Germany], Alphanate (Grifols, Los Angeles, CA), and Wilate [Octaparma, Lachen, Switzerland]), or purified vWF concentrates. Highly purified factor VIII concentrates or recombinant human factor VIII cannot be used, because these products generally contain little or no vWF. Cryoprecipitate can also be given as a source of vWF. Replacement therapy may be only transiently effective because of the short half-life of vWF caused by excessive clearance from the circulation. Antifibrinolytic agents such as EACA may be beneficial, particularly in patients with mucosal bleeding. Treatment with rFVIIa may be efficacious in some patients with vWF inhibitors.[101] Administration of high-dose intravenous IgG (2 g/kg over 2–5 days) may result in a rapid increase in vWF levels. Repeated administration of intravenous IgG every three weeks may be effective in controlling chronic bleeding.[102]

Inhibitors of factor V

Autoantibody inhibitors of factor V can arise in patients following surgery, transfusions, or antibiotic therapy. The majority of cases have been reported in patients who were exposed to topical hemostatic agents, such as bovine thrombin or fibrin sealant, that contain trace amounts of bovine factor V. The inhibitor presumably arises as an alloantibody to bovine factor V that cross-reacts with human factor V.[37] Inhibitors to factor V may occur after a single exposure to fibrin sealant, but re-exposure appears to increase the likelihood of inhibitor development.[103] Typically, both the PT and aPTT are prolonged, and do not correct to normal when performed on a 1:1 mixture of the patient's plasma with normal plasma. The thrombin time also is prolonged because of the presence of a coexisting inhibitor to bovine thrombin. The diagnosis can be confirmed by performing a quantitative assay of the factor V inhibitor level. The clinical presentation is quite variable, ranging from apparently normal hemostasis to severe hemorrhage, possibly because of differential effects of the inhibitor on plasma and platelet pools of factor V. Treatment options for acute bleeding are limited; some patients respond to transfusion of platelets, immunoadsorption, or plasmapheresis.[104] In a majority of patients, the inhibitor disappears within weeks to months, and immunosuppressive therapy does not appear to influence the time course of the disease.

Acquired factor X deficiency

Acquired deficiency of factor X can occur in patients with primary amyloidosis. The deficiency arises from accelerated clearance of factor X from the circulation resulting from adsorption of factor X to amyloid fibrils.[105] Both the PT and the aPTT are prolonged, but unlike the situation in patients with circulating inhibitors, the PT and aPTT usually correct to normal when performed on a 1:1 mixture of the patient's plasma with normal plasma. The hemostatic defect in these patients is multifactorial; in addition to factor X deficiency, patients with amyloidosis may have excessive fibrinolysis and amyloid infiltration of blood vessels. Management of bleeding in such patients is problematic. Replacement therapy in the form of plasma or prothrombin complex concentrate is often ineffective, and antifibrinolytic agents such as EACA are of limited benefit.

Other coagulation factor inhibitors

Autoantibody inhibitors of other coagulation factors are rarely encountered. As with inhibitors of factor V, inhibitors of prothrombin prolong both the PT and the aPTT. Inhibitors of factors IX or XI prolong only the aPTT. Specific factor and inhibitor assays can be performed to distinguish the type of inhibitor present. Depending on the inhibitor, treatment options for bleeding episodes include plasma, PCCs, factor IX concentrates, or rFVIIa. Adjunctive treatment with antifibrinolytic agents such as EACA also may be beneficial.

Inhibitors of factor XIII do not affect either the PT or aPTT; specific assays of fibrin stabilization (e.g., the urea clot lysis assay) are necessary to identify these inhibitors.[41] In patients with acute bleeding, large doses of cryoprecipitate or factor XIII concentrate can be given to try to overwhelm the inhibitor, but this approach may have limited effectiveness.

Acquired platelet function disorders

Acquired disorders of platelet function occur much more frequently than congenital platelet abnormalities. Acquired platelet dysfunction is caused by drugs such as aspirin, medical conditions such as chronic renal insufficiency, or procedures such as cardiopulmonary bypass. The risk of bleeding in patients with acquired platelet dysfunction is variable and unpredictable, and abnormal bleeding generally occurs only in the presence of additional hemostatic defects. Signs of platelet dysfunction manifest typically as mucocutaneous bleeding with excessive bruising, gingival bleeding, or epistaxis. Diagnostic tests of platelet function include the bleeding time and the PFA-100. Although useful as screening tests, these tests lack diagnostic specificity, and they cannot be used to predict bleeding risk. The bleeding time may be prolonged because of abnormalities of cutaneous connective tissue, and both the bleeding time and the PFA-100 test results may be abnormal in the presence of anemia (hematocrit <30%) or thrombocytopenia (platelet count <100,000/μL). Many medications can alter platelet function and lead to a delayed PFA-100 closure time or prolonged bleeding time, so a thorough medication history must be obtained before these tests are performed. Formal platelet aggregation testing may be useful in the evaluation of selected patients.

Drug-induced platelet dysfunction

A large number of drugs and medications have been reported to impair platelet function (Table 30.4). Among the most frequently encountered are aspirin, nonsteroidal anti-inflammatory drugs, and antiplatelet agents such as ticlopidine, clopidogrel, and abciximab. The antiplatelet effects of aspirin are irreversible, so recovery of normal hemostasis relies on the release of new platelets into the circulation rather than the disappearance of the drug from the plasma. The ability of platelets to aggregate is partially restored

Table 30.4 Some drugs that cause impairment of platelet function

Aspirin	Nitroglycerin
Nonsteroidal anti-inflammatory drugs	Isosorbide dinitrate
Ticlopidine	Nitroprusside
Clopidogrel	Nitroglycerin
Abciximab	Isosorbide dinitrate
Eptifibatide	Nitroprusside
Tirofiban	Nitroglycerin
β-Lactam antibiotics	Isosorbide dinitrate
Prostacyclin	Nitroprusside
Dipyridamole	Nitroglycerin
Dextrans	

within 4–5 days after aspirin ingestion is stopped, but platelet dysfunction may persist for up to 7 days after aspirin is discontinued.[106] If possible, aspirin should be discontinued 7–10 days before a surgical or endoscopic procedure, unless it has been prescribed for the secondary prevention of stroke or myocardial infarction.[107] Most other nonsteroidal anti-inflammatory drugs inhibit platelet reactivity in a reversible manner, and platelet function usually returns to normal within 24 hours after the drug is discontinued. Nonsteroidal anti-inflammatory drugs that selectively inhibit cyclooxygenase-2, such as celecoxib, appear to have very little effect on platelets and can be used to treat pain in patients with preexisting bleeding disorders such as hemophilia. The risk of clinical bleeding caused by aspirin or other nonsteroidal anti-inflammatory agents is generally low, and platelet transfusions should not be given prophylactically. However, ingestion of these drugs can increase the risk for serious bleeding in patients who also have additional hemorrhagic risk factors. If severe hemorrhage caused by defective platelet function is suspected, transfusion of platelets can rapidly restore normal hemostasis.

The thienopyridines, ticlopidine and clopidogrel, are platelet adenosine diphosphate (ADP)-receptor antagonists that inhibit platelet function by disrupting interactions with ADP and fibrinogen. Similar to aspirin, these drugs produce a persistent antiplatelet effect that lasts for up to a week after the drug is discontinued.[106] Therefore, these drugs usually should be discontinued 5–7 days before invasive procedures.

Abciximab is the prototype of a class of antiplatelet drugs that directly block the binding of fibrinogen to its platelet receptor, glycoprotein (GP) IIb/IIIa (integrin αIIbβ3). Other drugs in this class include eptifibatide and tirofiban. These agents are indicated for use in acute coronary syndromes and to prevent thrombosis of intravascular stents. They are often given in conjunction with other antithrombotic agents such as heparin.[108] Abciximab has an extended biological half-life because of its high affinity for GPIIb/IIIa; its antiplatelet effects can therefore persist for several days. In contrast, the antiplatelet effects of eptifibatide and tirofiban are transient, and usually resolve within a few hours of discontinuation in patients with normal renal function.[109] Management of bleeding in patients receiving GPIIb/IIIa antagonists may be complicated by the development of acute thrombocytopenia (platelet count less than 50,000/μL), which occurs in up to 5% of patients.[110] In cases of severe bleeding, platelet transfusions are an effective approach to control hemorrhage, in either the presence or absence of thrombocytopenia.

Many other drugs can impair platelet function (Table 30.4). The antiplatelet effects of β-lactam antibiotics are generally apparent only in patients receiving large parenteral doses of penicillins or cephalosporins. The frequency of clinically important bleeding in patients

taking β-lactam antibiotics appears to be low, and is not predicted by the bleeding time or other laboratory tests of platelet function. Prostacyclin and dipyridamole inhibit platelet aggregation by elevating the intracellular concentration of cyclic adenosine monophosphate. Infusion of dextran inhibits platelet aggregation and enhances fibrinolysis through multiple mechanisms. Nitrovasodilators (nitroglycerin, isosorbide dinitrate, and nitroprusside) inhibit platelet function through nitric-oxide-dependent mechanisms. Both tricyclic antidepressants and selective serotonin reuptake inhibitors can alter platelet function, but the risk of serious clinical bleeding appears to be low.[111] Phenothiazines such as chlorpromazine, promethazine, or trifluoroperazine also have been reported to have mild antiplatelet effects. Consumption of ethanol can produce platelet dysfunction as well as thrombocytopenia, and may contribute to clinical bleeding in patients with alcoholic liver disease.

Uremia

Chronic renal insufficiency is associated with both hemorrhagic and thrombotic manifestations. Bleeding often manifests as ecchymoses, epistaxis, or GI or genitourinary bleeding. The primary hemostatic abnormality in uremia is thought to be a defect in platelet function, but the pathophysiology of the platelet function defect remains poorly understood. Both dialyzable and nondialyzable substances contribute to the defect. As in many other acquired disorders of platelet function, the clinical importance of platelet dysfunction in uremia is uncertain. The bleeding time and PFA-100 closure time are prolonged, and platelet aggregation studies reveal defects in aggregation with ADP and epinephrine. In general, abnormalities of the bleeding time or platelet aggregation responses do not correlate with the severity of renal insufficiency or the degree of bleeding.

Management of bleeding in uremia is directed by the clinical circumstances rather than the results of laboratory tests of platelet function. Many patients with chronic renal failure do not have significant problems with bleeding despite a prolonged bleeding time and abnormal platelet aggregation responses. If bleeding is encountered in a patient with uremia, assessment of hemoglobin and hematocrit, platelet count, PT, and aPTT is necessary to evaluate for other potential causes of defective hemostasis. Coexisting anemia contributes to a bleeding propensity, and patients with bleeding may benefit from transfusion of red cells, or treatment with erythropoietin or darbopoietin, to maintain the hematocrit above 30%. Treatment with DDAVP or estrogens improves the bleeding time and prevents clinical bleeding in some patients with uremia.[112] Transfusion of cryoprecipitate may partially correct the hemorrhagic diathesis of uremia. Transfusion of platelets is usually not recommended in the absence of thrombocytopenia (platelet count less than 50,000/μL), because uremic plasma can induce dysfunction in transfused platelets. Patients with uremia may be unusually sensitive to anticoagulants or antiplatelet medications such as aspirin, which should be discontinued if possible. The benefit of intensive dialysis in correcting abnormal platelet function and diminishing bleeding is uncertain.[112]

Cardiopulmonary bypass

Abnormal platelet function, often in conjunction with thrombocytopenia, is a frequent cause of bleeding in patients undergoing cardiopulmonary bypass. The risk of perioperative bleeding varies depending on the type of surgical procedure, the age of the patient, preoperative renal function, and the duration of bypass. Prior exposure to antiplatelet agents and other antithrombotic medications increases the risk of bleeding.

The platelet defect caused by cardiopulmonary bypass is thought to result from activation of platelets within the extracorporeal circulation. Platelet activation is stimulated by multiple mediators, including thrombin generated from activation of the intrinsic and extrinsic coagulation pathways, mechanical stress, complement activation, hypothermia, and exposure of platelets to the blood–air interface.[113] Partial activation and degranulation lead to desensitization and decreased adhesiveness of residual circulating platelets. The severity of platelet dysfunction correlates with the duration of bypass. Platelet function abnormalities usually resolve within five hours, but can persist for 24 hours or longer following complicated surgery.[114] Bleeding from platelet dysfunction is often exacerbated by thrombocytopenia caused by hemodilution and consumption of platelets. Consumption of coagulation factors, increased fibrinolytic activity, and inadequate neutralization of heparin with protamine sulfate also contribute to bleeding.

Management of bleeding associated with cardiopulmonary bypass is generally based on clinical considerations rather than laboratory testing. Bleeding times and PFA-100 closure times are frequently prolonged but are not predictive of perioperative blood loss.[114] Routine prophylactic administration of plasma or platelets is discouraged.[115] In the setting of excessive perioperative or early (within 24 hours) postoperative bleeding, however, platelet transfusions may be indicated even in the absence of severe thrombocytopenia. Several drugs have been used to decrease the risk of perioperative bleeding during cardiopulmonary bypass. These include DDAVP and antifibrinolytic agents such as EACA or TXA. The use of point-of-care testing such as thromboelastography (TEG) to guide targeted therapy is being studied.[115,116]

Antithrombotic therapy

Use of antithrombotic drugs has increased in recent years because of growing recognition of the efficacy of these medications for the prevention and treatment of venous thromboembolism, embolic stroke, and other thrombotic disorders. Although warfarin, heparin, and aspirin continue to be the most commonly prescribed antithrombotic medications, several new antithrombotic drugs are making their way into routine clinical use. These new drugs include LMW heparins, direct thrombin inhibitors, fibrinolytic agents, pentasaccharides, clopidogrel, and platelet GPIIb/IIIa antagonists.[117] The major complication of all these medications is bleeding. In this section, the management of bleeding associated with warfarin, heparin, LMW heparins, pentasaccharides, direct thrombin inhibitors, and fibrinolytic therapy is considered. Management of bleeding associated with antiplatelet medications was discussed in the "Drug-induced platelet dysfunction" section.

Warfarin

Warfarin and other vitamin K antagonists produce their antithrombotic effects by inhibiting the hepatic synthesis of vitamin K–dependent coagulation factors. Warfarin inhibits the cyclic regeneration of active vitamin K by blocking the action of vitamin K epoxide reductase and vitamin K reductase.[118]

Warfarin has a narrow therapeutic range with wide interindividual dosing requirements. Its metabolism is influenced by diet, patient compliance, genetic factors, liver dysfunction, and interactions with other medications. Numerous drugs influence the pharmacokinetics of warfarin by altering its absorption or metabolic clearance, or by altering the production of vitamin K by intestinal flora. As a general rule, any change in medication

regimen, including nonprescription medications and dietary supplements that contain vitamin K, should be presumed to have a potential effect on the anticoagulant response to warfarin. The risk of bleeding is highest during the initial phase of anticoagulation, within the first few weeks after initiation of therapy. Dosing algorithms that consider multiple parameters, such as gender, age, weight, height, race, and use of other medications, offer promise for decreasing the risk of early bleeding. Newer dosing algorithms incorporate pharmacogenomic information derived from genotyping two polymorphic genes (*CYP2C9* and *VKORC1*) that are involved in warfarin metabolism.[119] The clinical utility of these pharmacogenomic approaches is being tested in several clinical trials.[120]

The most common laboratory method for monitoring the anticoagulant effect of warfarin is the INR. The INR compares the ratio of the patient's PT to the mean PT of a group of normal individuals. Because the response of the PT to depletion of vitamin K–dependent coagulation factors is highly variable when measured in different laboratories, the INR has been widely adopted as a method to standardize monitoring of oral anticoagulant therapy. The ratio is adjusted for the sensitivity of the PT reagent used in each laboratory. The target therapeutic INR for most indications is 2.0–3.0, although different therapeutic ranges are recommended for some indications.[118]

The risk of major bleeding in patients on chronic warfarin therapy has been estimated to be 1–5% per year.[121] Intensity of anticoagulation is probably the most important risk factor for hemorrhage, particularly when the INR is greater than 5.0. Clinical conditions that increase risk of hemorrhage include advanced age, hypertension, cerebrovascular disease, heart disease, renal insufficiency, a history of GI bleeding, and concomitant use of antiplatelet agents. The risk of hemorrhagic complications resulting from warfarin therapy is decreased when patients are enrolled in coordinated programs for management of anticoagulation.[122]

Reversal of the anticoagulant effects of warfarin can be achieved through discontinuation of warfarin, administration of vitamin K₁, transfusion of plasma, or PCCs. Management should be guided by the degree of elevation of the INR and the presence or absence of clinical bleeding (Table 30.5). Minor or moderate elevation of the INR (above the therapeutic target but less than 9.0) in the absence of bleeding can often be managed safely by decreasing or omitting several doses of warfarin until the INR approaches the therapeutic range. Major elevation of the INR (greater than 9.0), even in the absence of clinically evident bleeding, should be treated by temporary discontinuation of warfarin and administration of vitamin K₁ (5–10 mg orally). Vitamin K₁ also can be administered by slow intravenous infusion. A meta-analysis found that oral and intravenous vitamin K₁ were equally effective in achieving a therapeutic INR at 24 hours in patients with excessive oral anticoagulation.[123] Subcutaneous administration of vitamin K₁ is associated with an unpredictable response and is therefore not recommended.[123] In patients with active major bleeding, four-factor PCC therapy is indicated.[7] Published guidelines from medical societies on acute reversal of warfarin are listed in Table 30.6.[31,32,124–127] The clinical effectiveness of rFVIIa in the setting of warfarin-associated hemorrhage has not been subjected to randomized controlled trials, and rVIIa has been associated with an elevated risk of arterial thromboembolic complications in patients >75 years of age.[36]

Approaches that can be used to manage warfarin anticoagulation in patients who require elective surgery have been reviewed.[128] For

Table 30.5 Guidelines for reversal of warfarin anticoagulation

INR	Bleeding	Recommendation
<5.0	None	Decrease or omit warfarin dose
	Minor	Discontinue warfarin
		Consider vitamin K_1 (2.5 mg orally)
	Major	Discontinue warfarin
		Vitamin K_1 (10 mg by slow intravenous infusion*)
		Fresh frozen plasma (15 mL/kg) or prothrombin complex concentrate
5.0–9.0	None	Omit one or two doses of warfarin; resume at lower dose
	Minor	Discontinue warfarin
		Vitamin K_1 (2.5–5.0 mg orally)
>9.0	None	Hold warfarin
		Vitamin K_1 (5–10 mg orally)
	Minor	Discontinue warfarin
		Vitamin K_1 (5–10 mg orally)
		Consider fresh frozen plasma (15 mL/kg)
	Major	Discontinue warfarin
		Vitamin K_1 (10 mg by slow intravenous infusion*)
		Fresh frozen plasma (15 mL/kg) or prothrombin complex concentrate

* Intravenous administration of vitamin K_1 may produce (but rarely) an anaphylactic reaction.
INR, International normalized ratio.

many patients, a reasonable approach is to discontinue warfarin 4–5 days before surgery and begin heparin or a LMW heparin along with warfarin in the postoperative period. Heparin or LMW heparin can then be discontinued when the INR returns to the target therapeutic range. Patients who require major surgery urgently (within 24 hours) should receive plasma (15 mL/kg) and vitamin K_1 (2.5–5 mg orally or parenterally).

Heparin

The antithrombotic effect of heparin is mediated by its ability to potentiate the inhibition of activated coagulation factors by antithrombin. In the presence of heparin, antithrombin irreversibly inactivates thrombin and factor Xa. Heparin is often administered intravenously, although it also may be given subcutaneously.

Weight-based dosing of heparin appears to improve clinical outcomes in patients with venous thromboembolism.[129] A common dosing schedule utilizes an intravenous bolus dose of 80 U/kg followed by 18 U/kg/hour by continuous infusion. The dosage is then adjusted to maintain a therapeutic aPTT. The therapeutic range may vary between different laboratories that utilize different reagents for measuring the aPTT. In many laboratories, prolongation of the aPTT to a value that is 1.5- to 3.0-fold higher than the control value corresponds to a therapeutic heparin level. For certain indications, such as cardiopulmonary bypass surgery, higher doses

of heparin are required and monitoring is performed using the activated clotting time rather than the aPTT.

The major side effect of heparin therapy is hemorrhage. In clinical studies of heparin administered for short-term treatment of venous thromboembolism, rates of major bleeding have ranged from 0% to 7%.[57] In some patients, bleeding is exacerbated by thrombocytopenia or platelet dysfunction. Because heparin has a short biological half-life of about one hour, the primary approach to management of bleeding is to discontinue the drug. In patients with therapeutic levels of heparin, recovery from its anticoagulant effects can be expected within two hours after discontinuation of heparin infusion. In cases of major hemorrhage, or when very large doses of heparin have been given (e.g., for cardiopulmonary bypass or through a medication error), protamine sulfate should be administered.

Protamine sulfate is a strongly basic protein that neutralizes the anticoagulant effects of heparin within minutes. It is given by slow intravenous injection. The recommended dose of protamine sulfate is 1.0 mg for every 100 units of heparin remaining in the patient, which can be calculated based on the 60-minute half-life of heparin. For example, a patient receiving 1000 units of heparin per hour by continuous intravenous infusion should be given enough protamine to neutralize all of the heparin administered within the last hour (1000 units), plus half of the heparin administered in the preceding hour (500 units), plus a quarter of the heparin administered in the hour prior to that (250 units). Therefore, the total dose of protamine sulfate would be 17.5 mg. Protamine sulfate itself has a weak anticoagulant effect, and overdosage may exacerbate bleeding.

Low-molecular-weight heparins

LMW heparins are derived from heparin by chemical or enzymatic fragmentation.[129] Several LMW heparins, including dalteparin, enoxaparin, and tinzaparin, are available for prevention or treatment of venous thromboembolism, unstable angina, and other indications. Danaparoid sodium is not derived from heparin, but it is a mixture of LMW heparin-like glycosaminoglycans. Although danaparoid sodium is considered to be a "heparinoid," its effects are very similar to those of the LMW heparins.

Compared with heparin, LMW heparins have less inhibitory activity against thrombin and greater relative inhibitory activity against factor Xa. The LMW heparins produce a more predictable anticoagulant response than heparin, reflecting their better bioavailability, longer half-life, and dose-independent clearance. These properties allow LMW heparins to be given subcutaneously once or twice daily, usually without laboratory monitoring. Because LMW heparins are cleared through a renal route, dosages need to be adjusted in patients with renal insufficiency.

Table 30.6 Published guidelines for acute reversal of warfarin coagulopathy in patients with intracerebral hemorrhage

Society (Year)	Vitamin K	Plasma (ml/kg)		PCC (U/kg)
Australian (2004)	IV (5–10 mg)	Yes (NS)	AND	Yes (NS)*
EU Stroke (2006)	IV (5–10 mg)	Yes (10–40)	OR	Yes (10–50)
AHA (2010)	IV (NS)	Yes (10–15)	OR	Yes (NS)
French (2010)	Oral or IV (10 mg)	Yes (NS)†	OR	Preferred (25–50)
British Standards (2011)	IV (5 mg)	No		Yes (NS)
ACCP (2012)	IV (5–10 mg)	Yes		Preferred

* If a three-factor PCC is administered, FFP is also recommended as a source of factor VII.
† Use of plasma only when PCCs not available.
PCC, prothrombin complex concentrate; rFVIIa; NS, not specified; IV, intravenous.

Source: Goodnough and Shander (2013).[6] Reproduced with permission of Lippincott, Williams & Wilkins.

A large number of randomized clinical trials have demonstrated that LMW heparins are at least as safe and effective as heparin for most indications.[129] The incidence of heparin-induced thrombocytopenia is lower with LMW heparins than with heparin.

Despite the favorable safety profile of LMW heparins, bleeding remains a major side effect. In clinical trials evaluating LMW heparins for treatment of venous thromboembolism, the rates of major bleeding have ranged from 0% to 3%.[121] Epidural bleeding and spinal hematoma have been reported in patients receiving LMW heparins concurrently with spinal or epidural anesthesia.[130] Management of bleeding is complicated by the long half-life of these medications. Unlike heparin, the anticoagulant effects of LMW heparins cannot be reversed completely by administration of protamine sulfate. Protamine sulfate can be administered in an attempt to control active bleeding in patients who have received LMW heparin within eight hours, but large doses (20 to 50 mg) may be required.[129]

Pentasaccharides

The pentasaccharides, fondaparinux and idraparinux, are synthetic analogs of the antithrombin-binding region of heparin.[131] These drugs selectively inhibit factor Xa without having any appreciable inhibitory effect on thrombin. Fondaparinux has a half-life of 18–22 hours and is usually administered subcutaneously once daily. It is used for the prevention and treatment of venous thromboembolism and in acute coronary syndromes. Idraparinux is an investigational pentasaccharide that has a substantially longer half-life of 130 hours and can be administered in a fixed dose once weekly.[131] The pentasaccharides have no specific antidotes, and their anticoagulant effects are not reversed by administration of plasma, PCCs, or protamine sulfate.

Direct thrombin inhibitors

The direct thrombin inhibitors include desirudin, lepirudin, bivalirudin, and argatroban. Because the direct thrombin inhibitors are structurally unrelated to heparin, one major indication for their use is in the treatment of heparin-induced thrombocytopenia. They also are being evaluated for use in prophylaxis of deep venous thrombosis, cardiopulmonary bypass surgery, and acute coronary syndromes.[131]

Most of the direct thrombin inhibitors are administered parenterally, and are monitored using the aPTT. They have short half-lives (less than two hours) when given by intravenous infusion. Because lepirudin, desirudin, and bivalirudin are cleared renally, their half-lives may be prolonged dramatically in renal failure. Clearance of argatroban is not influenced by renal impairment, but may be decreased in the presence of hepatic dysfunction. The risk of bleeding in patients receiving direct thrombin inhibitors appears to be dose dependent.[132] Management of bleeding relies on prompt discontinuation of the drug.

Fibrinolytic agents

Pharmacologic lysis of fibrin thrombi is a commonly used strategy for treatment of acute myocardial infarction and stroke, and also is used in selected cases of peripheral arterial occlusion and venous thromboembolism. Most fibrinolytic agents in clinical use are plasminogen activators, which include streptokinase, urokinase, and recombinant forms of tissue plasminogen activator such as alteplase and reteplase. Plasminogen activators produce thrombolysis by converting plasminogen to plasmin, which then degrades fibrin into soluble FDPs. Fibrinolytic agents can be administered systemically by intravenous infusion, or delivered in proximity to sites of thrombi via catheter-directed approaches. Contraindications to the use of fibrinolytic therapy include recent hemorrhagic stroke or major surgery, prolonged cardiopulmonary resuscitation, uncontrolled hypertension, and active GI bleeding.[133]

In addition to producing therapeutic lysis of pathologic thrombi, fibrinolytic agents generate plasmin in the systemic circulation, resulting in bleeding from lysis of hemostatic plugs at surgical sites and other locations.[133] Bleeding, therefore, is a major complication of fibrinolytic therapy. Because circulating plasmin degrades fibrinogen, hypofibrinogenemia can contribute to bleeding. The extent of systemic fibrinogenolysis varies with different fibrinolytic agents and different routes of administration.[134]

The risk of major hemorrhage associated with fibrinolytic therapy is influenced by the age of the patient and concomitant use of additional antithrombotic agents such as heparin, direct thrombin inhibitors, or antiplatelet agents. In the absence of invasive procedures or simultaneous heparin therapy, treatment of acute myocardial infarction with fibrinolytic agents generally is associated with a low incidence of major bleeding (less than 5%). Intracranial hemorrhage is a rare, but potentially devastating, complication of fibrinolytic therapy. In large clinical trials of streptokinase, or alteplase for treatment of acute coronary ischemia, the incidence of intracranial hemorrhage has ranged from 0.2% to 0.8%.[133]

Bleeding that occurs in association with fibrinolytic therapy can often be managed by discontinuing infusion of the plasminogen activator and replacing fibrinogen by transfusion of cryoprecipitate (0.2 unit/kg) or (in Europe) by infusion of fibrinogen concentrates. The goal of transfusion therapy with cryoprecipitate is to maintain a plasma fibrinogen level of >100 mg/dL. Adjunctive treatment with antifibrinolytic agents such as EACA or aprotinin may be beneficial when rapid reversal of bleeding is desired.

Target-specific oral anticoagulants (TSOACs)

Although vitamin K antagonists (VKAs) have formed a cornerstone in the therapy of venous thromboembolism (VTE) and atrial fibrillation (AF), concerns around dietary and drug interactions, therapy monitoring, and risk of major bleeding have led to the ushering in of a wave of direct oral anticoagulants (TSOACs).[135] These include targeted therapies against thrombin (dabigatran) and factor Xa (rivaroxaban, apixaban, edoxaban, betrixaban, and darexaban)[136] that have showed superior or non-inferior outcomes while having lower rates of major bleeding. The RE-LY trail showed that, compared to warfarin, the rates of stroke and systemic embolism were lower in the higher dose dabigatran group (150 mg) and non-inferior in the lower dose group (110 mg).[137] Side effects such as major hemorrhage compared to warfarin were lower in the low-dose dabigatran group (110 mg) and equivalent in the higher dose 150 mg group. The ARISTOTLE trial showed that apixaban was superior to warfarin in preventing both stroke and systemic embolism, and had lower rates of major bleeding.[138] The ROCKET-AF trial showed that rivoraxaban compared to warfarin was non-inferior for prevention of stroke or systemic embolism while having lower rates of intracranial and fatal bleeding.[139] Since these initial trials, subsequent meta-analyses have confirmed that TSOACs have lower rates of major bleeding, particularly intracranial and fatal bleeding episodes.[136,140]

Although TSOACs are associated with lower rates of major bleeding, treatment of life-threatening bleeding such as intracranial hemorrhage remains a challenge, as there is no standard antidote and an absence of high-quality trials.[141] The current framework for reversal strategies relies on studies from animal models, case reports, small case series, and crossover trials in healthy volunteers.[142] The decision to pursue reversal should take into account a number of variables that include patient presentation, time since last dose, short half-life of TSOACs, and patient renal and hepatic functions. Standard coagulation assays do not conclusively help aid therapy decisions as they may not be informative, provide only a qualitative rather than quantitative assessment, and require complex interpretation based on time of last dose.[143] There should be a focus on elimination of the drug from systemic circulation[144] through discontinuation, activated charcoal if last dose was ingested within two hours since presentation,[145,146] and dialysis for dabigatran; rivaroxaban and apixaban are not amenable to dialysis as they are highly plasma–protein bound.[142] Reversal with factor concentrates should be pursued in those with life-threatening bleeding, whereas supportive and adjunct therapy may be sufficient in many other cases.[147] Four-factor PCC was shown to correct thrombin potential in patients receiving rivaroxaban but not in those receiving dabigatran.[8] Activated PCCs such as FEIBA (factor VIII inhibitor bypassing activity) have been shown to be correct abnormalities for dabigatran, apixaban, and rivaroxaban in in vitro studies, animal studies, and a handful of case reports.[147] As activated factor VII has shown variable performance in controlling bleeding or correcting coagulation assays in animal and in vitro studies, it is generally not recommended for the reversal of TSOACs. Among limited data, for correction of life-threatening bleeding, four-factor PCC is preferred for reversal of rivaroxaban and apixaban, whereas activated PCC is preferred for reversal of dabigatran; although there are no data of use for adjuncts such as desmopressin and antifibrnolytic agents, they may be considered due to low thrombotic potential.[147] Specific antidotes against TSOACs are in development with varying mechanisms such as competing inactive molecular mimics or monoclonal antibody fragments.[148–150]

Disclaimer

The authors have disclosed no conflicts of interest. Lawrence Tim Goodnough has been a consultant for CSL Behring.

Key references

A full reference list for this chapter is available at: http://www.wiley.com/go/simon/transfusion

1 Goodnough LT, Shander A. Patient blood management. *Anesthesiology* 2012;**116**: 1367–76.

4 Goodnough LT, Shander A. How I treat warfarin-associated coagulopathy in patients with intracerebral hemorrhage. *Blood* 2011;**117**: 6091–9.

6 Goodnough LT, Shander A. Current status of pharmacologic therapies in patient blood management. *Anesth Analg* 2013;**116**: 15–34.

49 Levy JH & Goodnough LT. How I use fibrinogen replacement therapy in acquired bleeding. *Blood* 2015;**125**: 1387–1393.

149 Lu G, DeGuzman FR, Hollenbach SJ, *et al.* A specific antidote for reversal of anticoagulation by direct and indirect inhibitors of coagulation factor Xa. *Nat Med* 2013;**19**: 446–51.

CHAPTER 31

Immunoglobulin products

Melvin Berger

Medical Research Strategy, CSL Behring, King of Prussia, PA, USA

Plasma-derived immunoglobulin (Ig) is used for an astonishingly wide range of autoimmune and inflammatory diseases, in addition to its traditional uses for prevention of infection and as antibody replacement and augmentation therapy in immune deficiency diseases[1,2] (Figure 31.1). Increased recognition and treatment of immune deficiencies in the developing world have added to the global demand for IgG. However, the major reason for the continued strong growth in demand for IgG products is the increased use of "high-dose" therapy, particularly in autoimmune neurologic diseases.[1,2] Long-term treatment of adults with doses in the range of 1–2 gr/kg or even more per month is the major contributor to the continuously growing global utilization of Ig products, which exceeded 143 metric tons in 2014 (Figure 31.2).[3] Indeed, the demand for Ig is the major driver of the increased demand for plasma and growth in fractionation capacity.

Structure and origin of Ig molecules

In order to understand the many uses for serum immunoglobulin preparations, it is necessary to understand the major difference between immunoglobulins and most other plasma proteins: diversity.[4–7] The prototypic immunoglobulin molecule is a tetramer composed of two identical heavy chains, each with a molecular mass of approximately 55 kD and two identical light chains of 22 kD, giving an overall molecular mass of 155 kD.[4,6] There are four major classes, or *isotypes*, of immunoglobulins in plasma: IgA, IgE, IgG, and IgM, with IgG accounting for 75% of all of the immunoglobulin in plasma. These classes are defined by the heavy chains α, ε, γ, and μ, respectively. Gamma heavy chains are actually a family of four types, γ1–γ4, which are grossly related but contain differences that result in different effector functions (Table 31.1). Depending on which chain a particular IgG molecule contains, it is assigned to "subclass" 1–4. Besides IgA, IgE, IgG, and IgM, there is a fifth class, IgD, composed of molecules with δ heavy chains. These play an important role in B-cell differentiation, but are only a minor component of the total plasma Ig pool. There are two types of light chains, κ and λ, and only one type is used in any individual Ig molecule. In addition, there are loci in the γ and κ chain genes at which different individuals may have different alleles or markers called Gm1-17 and Km1-3. These are useful as markers termed *allotypes* in genetic studies, but their clinical significance is not known.

The four chains are arranged into a pair of dimers linked together with varying numbers of interchain disulfide bonds and sugar chains at characteristic positions in each class or subclass. Immunoglobulin molecules are generally depicted as having a Y-like structure (Figure 31.3).[4,6] Each light chain contains a single variable region and a single constant region, whereas each heavy chain also has a single variable region, but three to four constant regions. The junction between the first and second constant regions of the heavy chain is considered a "hinge" that gives some flexibility to the arms. The variable regions of the light and heavy chains are aligned together to form the antigen-binding sites, whereas the heavy chain constant domains align to form a "handle," which binds receptors and other proteins that facilitate the effector functions and determine the metabolic fate of each class of molecules. IgA and IgM may contain an extra *joining* (J) *chain*, which binds to the heavy chains and holds together two of the four-chain units in the former, and five in the latter.

Ig molecules are cleaved into characteristic fragments by proteolytic enzymes such as papain or pepsin (Figure 31.3): The dimer containing the second and third constant domains of each of the heavy chains from all members of a class is crystallizable, and it has therefore been termed *Fc*. In contrast, because of the diversity of the variable regions, the fragments containing the antigen-binding sites are not crystallizable. With papain, the cleavage occurs toward the amino terminus side of the "hinge," and two separate but identical antigen-binding fragments (Fab) are released. With pepsin, cleavage occurs toward the carboxyl side of the hinge, and a single fragment with two identical antigen-binding sites (F[ab′]₂) is produced. The antigen-binding specificity of each immunoglobulin molecule is determined by the sequences of several short stretches of amino acids in the N-terminal domain of each heavy and light chain, which are called *hypervariable* or *complementarity-determining* regions.

Each person's immune system can make approximately 10^{12} different antibody specificities. This remarkable diversity initially arises by *rearranging* or splicing together multiple DNA segments for different variable and constant region domains at slightly different junctions, to make a single antibody gene unique to that particular immature B cell.[4–7] Upon exposure to an antigen, a naïve B-lymphocyte with a complementary binding site is selected and stimulated to proliferate, forming a germinal center in a lymph node or the spleen. Among the progeny of that B cell, in the appropriate milieu of antigen, helper T cells, and cytokines, some cells undergo further cutting and splicing of their heavy chain genes, resulting in isotype switching. Somatic hypermutation can also occur in their variable region genes,[4,5] resulting in *affinity maturation*. At any point, some cells may stop differentiating and become

Rossi's Principles of Transfusion Medicine, Fifth Edition. Edited by Toby L. Simon, Jeffrey McCullough, Edward L. Snyder, Bjarte G. Solheim, and Ronald G. Strauss.
© 2016 John Wiley & Sons, Ltd. Published 2016 by John Wiley & Sons, Ltd.

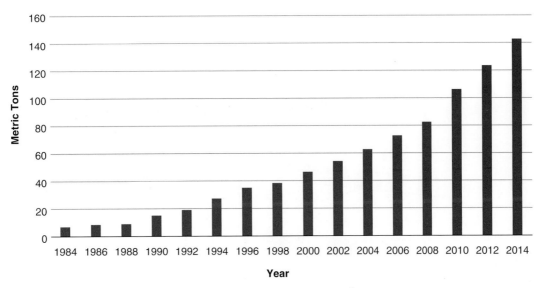

Figure 31.1 Global demand for IgG products (IVIG and SCIG). Source: Data from Bult (2014).[3]

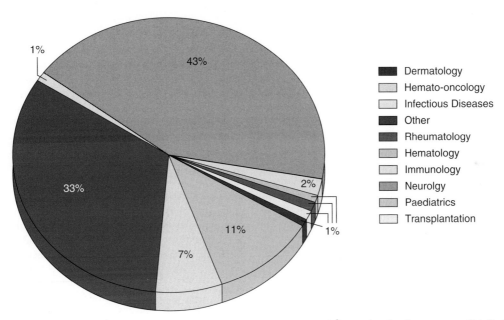

Figure 31.2 Use of IgG for diseases in different specialities. Source: O'Shaughnessy *et al.* (2012).[2] Reproduced with permission of Medical Data Services and Solutions (www.mdsas.com).

Table 31.1 Mechanisms of action of IgG

Dependent on Antigen-Binding (Fab') Region
- Precipitation, agglutination, and neutralization of toxins and antigens
- Sensitizing targets for phagocytosis, complement, and cell-mediated cytolysis
- Neutralize viral adhesion
- Neutralizing superantigens
- Elimination of complement-activating circulating immune complexes
- Neutralizing autoantibodies (anti-id)

Dependent on Fc Interactions with Effectors/Receptors
- Binding to cellular receptors and activating phagocytosis and cell-mediated cytolysis
- Binding C1q and activating complement
- Increasing catabolism of autoantibodies by saturating FcRn
- Inhibiting C3 deposition or further activation
- Downregulation of B– and T-cell function
- Cytokine regulation
- Fc receptor blockage, altering phagocyte function

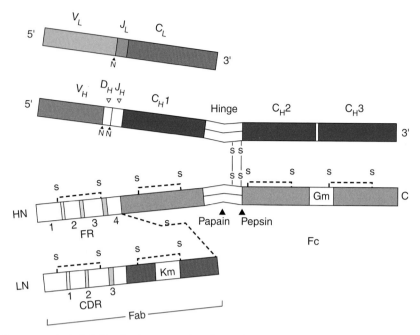

Figure 31.3 Diagram of IgG structure: A single IgG molecule consists of two heavy chains and two light chains. The upper pair show regions of the proteins encoded by different DNA segments: 5′ = 5′ end of the DNA segment coding for that part of the protein, and 3′ = 3′ end of the DNA segment. VL, light chain variable region; JL, light chain joining region; CL, light chain constant region; VH, heavy chain variable region; DH, heavy chain variable region; JH, heavy chain joining region; CH1, first heavy chain constant region; CH2, second heavy chain constant region; CH3, third heavy chain constant region. The lower pair show structural features of the protein chains: HN and LN, amino terminus of heavy and light chains, respectively; C, carboxy terminus; S–S, disulfide bonds. The hinge region is shown in white. Sites of cleavage by papain and pepsin are shown by arrows above labels inside red boxes. Papain cleavage results in formation of two monovalent F(ab) fragments and a disulfide-linked Fc fragment. Pepsin cleavage yields a bivalent disulfide-linked F(ab′)2 fragment. CDRs, complementarity determining regions (1–3, also known as *hypervariable regions*). FRs, framework regions (1–4), which are conserved. Note that FRs and CDRs are found in both heavy and light chains, as illustrated by white versus colored regions, but the labels are attached to only one chain each for readability. Gm is an allotypic region on the heavy chain; Km is an allotypic region on the κ-light chain. Source: Schroeder *et al.* (2010).[4] Reproduced with permission of Elsevier.

plasma cells, which are totally devoted to producing antibodies of a single isotype and specificity. Other cells may become quiescent "memory" cells, which can be rapidly stimulated on re-exposure to antigen. Upon initial exposure to an antigen or vaccine, the "primary" antibody response usually consists of IgM and relatively low-affinity IgG. Upon re-exposure, however, or during progression of an infection, class switching and affinity maturation will result in an increase of the ratio of IgG to IgM and an increase in the *avidity*: a product of the affinity, specificity, and quantity or "titer" of the overall antibody response. High-avidity IgG production is characteristic of "secondary" responses to vaccines and convalescent sera following infections.

The unique combination of light and heavy chain hypervariable regions that form the antigen-binding sites of any given antibody molecule may, in turn, seem "new" to the body and can serve as an antigen itself. Each unique antigen-binding site is called an "idiotype" because it belongs only to that specificity. An antibody that recognizes or blocks the antigen-binding site of another antibody is therefore called an "anti-idiotype" (anti-id).[4,7] Thus, the circulating pool of IgG contains thousands or even millions of different antibody and anti-id specificities (Figure 31.4). Anti-ids are believed to be important in regulating B- and T-cell responses, forming a major component of the "network" hypothesis for which Jerne received a Nobel Prize in 1984.[7] Anti-idiotypic neutralization of autoantibodies may be a major mechanism by which therapeutic IgG ameliorates autoimmune diseases (discussed further in this chapter).

A short history of commercial IgG production

Although sera from vaccinated animals had been used for passive immunity since the late 1800s, and convalescent human sera and placental extracts were used in the 1920s and 1930s, large-scale purification of immunoglobulins from plasma did not begin until the 1940s. With a grant from the US Navy, Edwin Cohn, a physical biochemist at Harvard University, developed a process for fractionating plasma using sequential precipitations with increasing concentrations of cold ethanol to produce large amounts of purified, stable albumin (fraction V) for treatment of shock on the battlefield during World War II.[8] The globulins containing most of the antibody activity were found in fractions II and III, which also contained clotting factors and lipoproteins. Oncley modified the procedure by manipulating the pH, ionic strength, and ethanol concentration, and succeeded in recovering most of the 7 s gamma globulins (now recognized as IgG) in fraction II, with the clotting factors and faster sedimenting globulins in fraction III. During the 1940s, intramuscular injections of fraction II *immune serum globulin* (ISG) were studied for prevention of hepatitis and measles. Janeway *et al.* in Boston and Barandun in Switzerland attempted to give ISG intravenously, but their efforts were abandoned because of severe immediate reactions, including hypotension, chills, and fever. IM injections of 16% plasma-derived ISG were routinely used for antibody replacement in immune deficiency patients and for prophylaxis against infectious disease until the 1980s, but the doses that

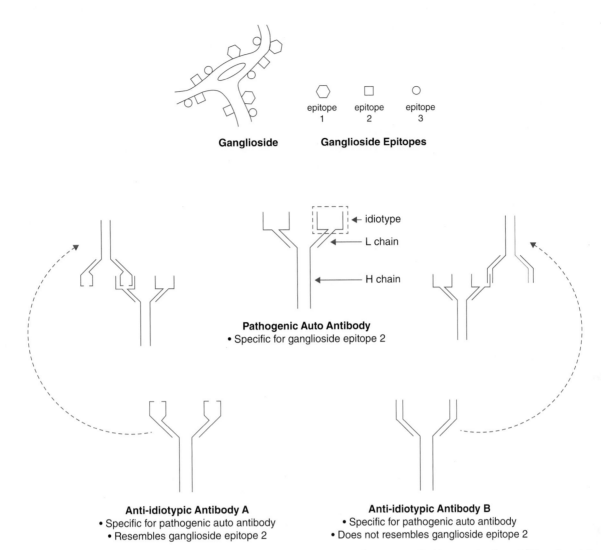

Figure 31.4 Idiotypic antibodies produced against different determinants on antigen—in this case, ganglioside sugars in a bacterial lipo-oligosaccharide, and different anti-idiotypes produced in response to a single idiotypic antibody. Source: Berger *et al.* (2013).[63] Reproduced with permission of Wiley.

could be tolerated by this route were limited, and efficacy in immune deficiencies was far from ideal.

Studies through the 1960s and 1970s suggested that the majority of vasomotor reactions and other immediate adverse effects that accompanied the early trials of intravenous (IV) administration of ISG were attributable to complement activation by aggregates of the 7 s globulins. Barandun *et al.* showed that these could be removed by ultracentrifugation or dissociated by treatment with low concentrations of pepsin, incubation at pH 4, and/or reduction and alkylation of disulfide bonds.[9] Other protein modifications such as S-sulfonylation and treatment with β-propiolactone were also studied. The first commercial IVIGs were pepsin- or plasmin-treated preparations that contained fragmented IgG molecules that sedimented slower than intact IgG (i.e., at 5–6.5 s) and had shortened half-lives and decreased effector function compared to the IgG in the IM preparations.

By the late 1970s, combined treatments including mild reduction and alkylation, reconstitution in 0.3 M glycine, and/or treatment at pH 4 with low concentrations of pepsin were introduced to prevent aggregate formation while leaving the IgG molecules intact. These processes eventually led to the first preparations that could safely be

given by the IV route, Gamimune® and Sandoglobulin®, respectively. The most important contribution to the tolerability of these preparations, however, was arguably the use of high concentrations of sugars as stabilizers: maltose in Gamimune and sucrose in Sandoglobulin.

Despite minimization of complement-binding aggregates, early IVIG preparations still frequently caused hypotension and/or other signs associated with vasodilatation and increased capillary permeability, which were shown to be associated with the presence of contaminating amounts of proteins such as pre-kallikrein activator and kallikrein itself.[10] Contamination with factor XIa was also found to be responsible for procoagulant activity in many ISG and early IVIG preparations.[10] In addition, other studies showed that isolated Fc fragments, IgG aggregates, and antigen–antibody complexes induced secretion of prostaglandin E_2 from monocytes, suggesting that this mediator might also be contributing to pain and other adverse effects of early IVIG preparations.[11]

In 1981, the World Health Organization published a set of "Desirable Characteristics of IVIG Preparations":[12]
- IVIG should be extracted from a pool of at least 1000 individual donors.
- IVIG should contain as little IgA as possible.

- The IgG should be modified biochemically as little as possible and possess opsonizing and complement-fixing activities.
- IVIG should be free from preservatives or stabilizers that might accumulate in vivo.

These characteristics were not fully achieved until the most recent generation of IVIG products were developed in the new millennium. Because there is no suitable alternative to polyclonal human IgG for antibody replacement therapy in immunodeficient patients, and because of the critical role of IVIG in treating a number of other diseases, the WHO includes IgG in its "Model List of Essential Medicines."[13]

Current IgG products

Additional methods to increase the yield of IgG per liter of plasma, improve the convenience of administration, and minimize AEs resulted in liquid IVIG preparations that are >95% pure IgG are readily available in most countries. Many manufacturers now utilize modified purification procedures which employ only a single ethanol precipitation step and substitute precipitation with fatty acids such as caprylate, or medium-chain alcohols, together with depth filtration for the serial Cohn–Oncley ethanol steps.[14] Anion exchange column chromatography is used to improve the purity by decreasing the concentrations of IgA and potentially vasoactive and/or thrombogenic protein contaminants, and some manufacturers also add cation exchange chromatography to further purify the IgG.

To improve the convenience of preparing and administering IVIG, most manufacturers have developed IVIG preparations that are available as 10% liquids and can be kept at room temperature for at least part of their shelf life.[15] Currently, three products—Gammagard® (Baxter), Gamunex® (Grifols), and Privigen® (CSL Behring)—dominate the US market. Gammagard and Gamunex are stabilized with glycine, and Privigen is stabilized with L-proline. All are available as 10% liquids, none contain any sugars, and none contain more than 50 mcg/ml IgA. IM ISG is rarely used in the United States, but Gammagard, Gammunex, and Gammaked® are labeled for subcutaneous administration, and CSL Behring markets a 20% proline-stabilized product, Hizentra®, specifically for subcutaneous use.

Prevention of pathogen transmission

Although clotting factor concentrates prepared by Cohn fractionation were known to have transmitted what is now known as hepatitis B, fraction II ISG had been given to hundreds of children for measles prophylaxis with only one case of apparent transmission of that virus. The subsequent widespread use of fraction II ISG provided confidence that this product carried little risk of transmission of blood-borne infectious agents. Unfortunately, that turned out to be false confidence. Even after the recognition of AIDS, complacency persisted because HIV (then termed HTLV III) was inactivated and/or partitioned out by the ethanol precipitation procedure.[16] In the late 1980s, reports of "non-A, non-B" hepatitis, (now termed *hepatitis C*, caused by hepatitis C virus [HCV])[17] began to appear among recipients of IVIG and other plasma products, and further, dedicated steps were added to assure safety of these products (see Chapter 56). To date, there have been no reports of virus or prion transmission by current IgG products, but we must continue to be vigilant because of the threat of emerging pathogens.

Pharmacokinetics and metabolism of IgG

Conventional-dose IVIG therapy (for immune deficiencies)

As recognition of primary immune deficiencies increased in the 1950s, a study by the British Medical Research Council resulted in the recommendation that most patients with hypogammaglobulinemia could be successfully treated with 25 mg/kg/week of IM ISG.[18] Within a few years after IVIG became available in the early 1980s, this was increased to 400–500 mg/kg at intervals of 3–4 weeks, which kept the serum IgG levels in most recipients at or above the lower limit of normal, approximately 500 mg/dl, at the "trough" just before the next dose was given.[19,20] An intravenous bolus of 400 mg/kg of IgG given intravenously immediately raises the serum IgG level by about 1000–1200 mg/dl. The levels then drop by 40–50% over 48–72 hours, because IgG is distributed into the total extracellular fluid volume, of which only about 50% is intravascular.[19,21] After this equilibration phase, the IgG is catabolized with first-order kinetics and a half-life of 21–30 days, which differs in different individuals, so it is usually repeated every 3–4 weeks.[21] A major reason for this relatively long half-life of IgG, compared to IgA, IgM, and other plasma proteins, is due to a specific, saturable receptor on the surface of endothelial cells termed FcRn because it is also found in the placenta and is responsible for facilitated transport of IgG into the fetus.[22,23] IgG, which binds to FcRn, is internalized into recycling endosomes in which it is protected from lysosomal degradation, returned to the apical surface, and exocytosed back into the circulation. Because IgG is not sequestered into other compartments such as intracellular or lipid-bound pools, *two compartment models* are traditionally used to describe its kinetics, although *single-compartment models* are sometimes used as an alternative. Early studies with radioactively labeled IgG showed that after equilibration, 45–50% of the IgG remained intravascular.[Rev. in 21] Because the ratio of total extracellular fluid volume to body mass index shows excellent linearity ($r = 0.97$, $p < 0.001$) across a range of BMIs from 15 to 40,[24] there seems little justification for limiting the dose of IVIG according to the "ideal body weight" in obese individuals, as some pharmacies and committees have recommended.[25]

Subcutaneous IgG therapy

Although first introduced in the late 1970s as an alternative to IM injections of ISG,[26] the use of small portable pumps to deliver concentrated IgG solutions subcutaneously has increased in popularity in the past decade and is now employed by more than half of the PID patients in several countries. There are two fundamental differences between the subcutaneous route of administration of IgG (SCIG) and the intravenous route (IVIG), which lead to most of the practical differences between the two routes. The first of these is the lack of a requirement for venous access with SCIG; the second is the relatively slow adsorption of SCIG into the intravascular compartment, which was described in detail more than a hundred years ago.[27] In contrast, a trained professional is usually required to administer IVIG, and rapid infusion may contribute to systemic adverse events (AEs).[27] The doses of IgG that are practical to give by the subcutaneous (SC) route are smaller than those by the IV route, so SCIG is usually given weekly or even more frequently. These differences result in a number of other effects that may lead to a preference for one route versus the other in a variety of different individual situations. With SCIG, the initial direction of the movement of IgG is opposite that of IVIG: The IgG must first diffuse from a subcutaneous depot into lymphatics, from which it reaches the bloodstream indirectly via the thoracic duct.[27] Equilibration of the IgG from the subcutaneous sites into the total intravascular and extracellular fluid space requires about the same amount of time as equilibration of IVIG out of the intravascular compartment.[21,26–28] Thus, with SCIG, the intravascular IgG concentration increases more gradually, peaking at 36–72 hours after the end of an infusion. Most other features of SCIG are consequences of this difference in kinetics. For example, many of the systemic AEs of IVIG are related to the rate of the infusion and resolve when the infusion is slowed. The $Cmax$ achieved with SCIG is, on average, only 61% of the peak achieved with IV infusions.[21,28] In recent studies comparing IVIG and SCIG in PID patients, the mean peak serum C_{max} immediately after IV infusions was 2303 mg/dl.[29–31] In contrast, the mean peak with SCIG was 1410 mg/dl, and the interval (t_{max}) between beginning an SCIG infusion and the peak IgG concentration was 62.6 h (2.61 days).[29–31] The slower rate of rise toward the peak and the truncation of its height are believed to be responsible for the much lower incidence of systemic AEs with SCIG.[26,27,32,33] This is consistent with observations that many AEs of IVIG infusions are rate related,[32,33] and it has been repeatedly confirmed. No differences have been reported in the half-life ($t_{1/2}$) of IgG given by the subcutaneous versus IV routes, which is about 30–35 days.[21] With weekly SCIG, there are only about four days between the t_{max} of one dose and the administration of the next dose, suggesting that only about 10–20% of the administered IgG is metabolized before the serum level starts to rise again. In contrast, with IVIG dosing intervals of 3–4 weeks, approximately 36–48% of the IgG may be metabolized by the time the next dose is due. These differences in the dosing intervals used in most SCIG-versus-IVIG regimens result in increased trough (C_{min}) serum IgG levels with SCIG. Pooled data from seven studies in which equivalent monthly IgG doses were given as weekly SCIG infusions versus IVIG infusions every 21–28 days showed that trough serum IgG levels were 10–20% (mean, 12.7%) higher with weekly SCIG.[28,35] After 6–12 weekly infusions, SCIG results in near-steady-state IgG levels, with differences between C_{min} and C_{max} ≤5–10% of the overall mean. (This steady state can also be achieved by "loading" the patient with five or six consecutive daily infusions of what will then be the weekly SCIG dose.)[34] In contrast, with IVIG, the trough-to-peak difference is often ≥100% of the overall mean.[21,26]

Another approach to subcutaneous IgG therapy involves the use of recombinant human hyaluronidase to temporarily depolymerize the hyaluronan chains that cross-link the subcutaneous tissue.[36] This increases the dispersion and absorption of medications delivered into the subcutaneous space and allows full monthly doses of 10% IVIG (in the range of 200–500 ml) to be given as a single SC infusion into a subcutaneous site.[36,37] The C_{max} is between that of standard SCIG and an IV bolus, but the C_{min} (trough) is not changed from that experienced with conventional 3–4 weekly IVIG dosing. The combination product, containing one vial of recombinant hyaluronidase and one of 10% Gammagard, is marketed as HyQvia by Baxter. In clinical studies in immune-deficient patients, HyQvia was well-tolerated and efficacious,[36,37] but because experience with this form of therapy is limited, its label includes cautions and restrictions about use in children and during pregnancy.[36]

The area under the curve (AUC) of serum concentration versus time of a drug after a single intravenous infusion is defined as 100% bioavailability.[38] The bioavailability of the drug when given by any other route is generally lower, so this is not unexpected with subcutaneous versus IV administration of IgG, and it is also found with therapeutic fusion proteins containing its Fc domains.[39] In licensing studies of SCIG, the US Food and Drug Administration (FDA) mandated determination of the bioavailability of SCIG as compared to IVIG and calculation of the dose adjustment which would be necessary to achieve an AUC with SCIG equal to that previously measured with IVIG in the same patients. Multiple studies and different lines of evidence demonstrated that the bioavailability of SCIG is about two-thirds of that of IVIG, regardless of the preparations being compared.[38] Interestingly, and in close agreement with the results of the SCIG licensing trials, the results of pooled analyses including 500 subjects and 20 different IgG preparations show that the slopes of regression lines for IgG level versus monthly dose indicate an increment of 87 mg/dl for every 100 mg/kg increase in monthly SCIG dose compared to an increment of 121 mg/dl in the trough level of IgG for every 100 mg/kg increment in monthly IVIG dose, suggesting a bioavailability of 71.9%.[40,41] The decreased bioavailability may involve degradation in the tissues and/or local binding in the intercellular matrix, but seems to be a general property of IgG. The European Medicines Agency does not require dose adjustment for SCIG as compared to IVIG, and analyses of large payor databases in the United States suggest that equivalent or even slightly lower total monthly doses of SCIG versus IVIG are given to PIDD patients.[42]

High-dose IVIG therapy for autoimmune and inflammatory diseases

The initial dose of IVIG used for most autoimmune/inflammatory diseases is 2 g/kg given over 2–5 days, followed by maintenance doses of 1–2 g/kg every 3–4 weeks. This regimen is based on the serendipitous 1981 observation that five consecutive daily repetitions of the monthly dose of IVIG for immune deficiencies at that time (400 mg/kg) normalized the platelet counts in immune-deficient patients who also had immune thrombocytopenia.[43,44] Infusion of 2 g/kg of IVIG increases the serum IgG level greater than fourfold, from pretreatment means of 700–1060 mg/dL to peaks well over 3000 mg/dL,[44] and IgG levels as high as 5000–7000 mg/dl have been reported.[45,46] These extremely high levels may contribute to vaso-occlusive AEs due to hyperviscosity in some patients.[45,46] The distribution phase of the IVIG is not expected to be altered by the IgG level, but if serum levels are sufficient to saturate FcRn, the catabolic rate may be increased.

Drug interactions

Standard polyclonal IVIG is not known to bind or influence the distribution or metabolism of small molecules; neither does conventional drug therapy alter the levels or metabolism of IgG. Although not formally studied, high-dose IVIG might be expected to increase the catabolism of IgG monoclonal antibodies and fusion proteins containing the Fc of IgG, due to saturation of FcRn,[23,39] as explained further in this chapter. IgG therapy, whether given by the IV or SC route, may decrease the antigenicity of live virus vaccines such as measles, mumps, and rubella (MMR); varicella; and Zostavax, so it is recommended that a period of six months be allowed to elapse between the last IgG therapy and administration of any of these vaccines.[47] If a patient has not been immunized and has received IgG therapy more than one month before potential exposure to MMR or varicella, passive immunization with IgG would be recommended.

Adverse reactions to IVIG and SCIG

Immediate reactions

Mild reactions to IVIG infusions are common, occurring in 15–20% of infusions and in 50% of patients at one time or another.[32,33] These AEs are mostly uncomfortable and/or unpleasant but rarely serious. Symptoms may include headache, nausea, musculoskeletal pain, and flushing and tachycardia. When severe, IVIG infusion reactions may resemble anaphylaxis, but they usually do not involve IgE and should be termed *anaphylactoid*.[33] A key difference between these anaphylactoid reactions that accompany IVIG infusions and true IgE-mediated anaphylaxis is that the former are usually associated with hypertension, rather than hypotension. Furthermore, anaphylactoid IVIG reactions often are less severe with subsequent infusions rather than more severe as would be expected with true allergy. In most cases, symptoms during IVIG infusions can be easily managed by slowing or temporarily stopping the infusion until the symptoms subside and/or by treatment with acetaminophen, nonsteroidal anti-inflammatory drugs (NSAIDs), and/or antihistamines.[32,33] Some patients may require corticosteroids; and many patients are given NSAIDs or steroids prophylactically. Most AEs are related to the rate of infusion and can be avoided by beginning the infusion slowly (0.01 ml/kg/min) and gradually increasing the rate stepwise as tolerated.

Patients who are naïve to IVIG replacement, have had interruptions in their therapy, and/or who are actively or chronically infected have an increased risk of infusion-related AEs.[48] This may be related, in part, to formation of antigen–antibody complexes as the IgG is being given, and/or the rapid release of lipopolysaccharide or other components of pathogens already present in the recipient. The risk of these reactions can be reduced by making sure patients are afebrile and that those with active infections are on antibiotics before giving an IVIG dose. The incidence of reactions may increase when patients already on therapy are given a different brand of IVIG,[32,33] so whenever this occurs, it is prudent to begin the infusion slowly and/or to premedicate the patient.[48]

True anaphylaxis may occur in patients receiving IVIG (discussed further in this chapter), particularly in those who are deficient in IgA but still have the capacity to produce IgE. This occurs very rarely, but may be life threatening, and can be avoided by slow administration of low-IgA products[32,33] and/or by administering the IgG subcutaneously.[49]

Systemic reactions to SCIG infusions are rare. Gardulf *et al.* reported only 30 systemic reactions in 25 immunodeficient patients given 3232 infusions (0.93%).[23,50] A subsequent review, which included additional studies totaling over 40,000 infusions, showed that only one study reported a rate of systemic AEs >1%.[26] Although nearly 75% of patients may have some local discomfort associated with the swelling and redness at the site of the infusions, the swelling and local symptoms usually subside within 24–48 hours, and do not usually deter patients from continuing with their SCIG regimen. Because of the infrequency of systemic side effects with SCIG, premedication is rarely necessary, nor is close monitoring required during the infusion. SCIG has thus emerged as an ideal route for home use in many patients.[35,50]

The increasing use of IVIG, particularly with large doses for inflammatory and autoimmune diseases, has resulted in other serious adverse events, including transmission of hepatitis C, aseptic meningitis, renal failure, thromboembolism, and hemolytic anemia.[32,33,52–54] This has led to the requirement (in the United States) that all IVIG products contain a "Black Box" warning about acute renal dysfunction/failure, and "Warnings and Precautions" about the risk of thromboembolic events, hemolytic anemia, aseptic meningitis syndrome, and transfusion-associated acute lung injury (TRALI).[53] Most reports of acute renal failure or dysfunction were due to osmotic nephrosis related to the use of sucrose as a stabilizer in certain products.[54] The risk of aseptic meningitis seems to be highest in patients receiving high-dose IVIG for neurologic diseases, and TRALI seems very rare.[52]

Thromboembolic events (TEEs)

Determining the true rates of TEEs and hemolytic incidents are difficult because the FDA and manufacturers' pharmacovigilance efforts rely on voluntary efforts of patients/providers and because there are little data with which to calculate a denominator such as the numbers of doses given or patients treated. Hyperviscosity due to high-dose IVIG and slow blood flow in critical vascular beds may contribute to TEEs in some patients; and endothelial cell and/or platelet activation also likely play a role. There are multiple reports of myocardial infarction, transient cerebral ischemic attacks, and strokes related to high-dose IVIG therapy.[53] Best estimates suggest a baseline incidence of 0.16–0.6 TEEs for every one million grams of IVIG sold.[56–58] Considering 50 grams as a median adult dose, these rates represent roughly 0.8–3 cases per 100,000 doses. In a recent well-investigated episode, TEEs were reported in nine patients involving seven different lots of a single product.[55]

Subtle changes in the procedure used to fractionate the plasma and produce that product, including the use of resins to isolate certain clotting system proteins, apparently increased contact activation of factor XI, which had co-purified with the IgG during the initial ethanol precipitation.[55] Because the total factor XI plus XIa was still within acceptable limits by the assays in use at that time, the affected product was within specifications. Only recently developed thrombin-generation assays have sufficient sensitivity to detect activated FXIa. Factor XI and kallikrien are difficult to separate from IgG because their isoelectric points are similar to IgG's, and they co-precipitate during ethanol precipitation.[10] On one hand, the results suggest that contamination of one or two individual lots was not responsible for the increase in factor XIa, because many lots were affected. On the other hand, even with the affected lots, TEEs were extremely rare, suggesting that multiple risk factors in the individual affected patients also contributed.

Better chromatographic purification methods, and the use of specific immunoadsorbents to remove FXI/FXIa from products that are made by multiple precipitations without ion exchange chromatography, should decrease the risk of factor XIa–related AEs. Furthermore, the use of the new thrombin generation assays should insure the absence of procoagulant activity in current and future IgG products.

Hemolytic reactions

An analogous problem is the presence of antibodies to erythrocytes (isoagglutinins), resulting in positive Coombs' tests, occasional cases of clinically significant hemolytic anemia, and extremely rare episodes of acute severe intravascular hemolysis.[56,57] In the original Cohn–Oncley fractionation scheme, isoagglutinins, which have higher isoelectric points than other IgGs, were greatly reduced by removing fraction III and continuing with fraction II alone.[58] Several recent production schemes combine the fraction II and III precipitates as the starting material for IgG purification, and many manufacturers have substituted caprylic acid or fatty alcohols for the ethanol steps that removed more of the isoagglutinins, resulting in 2–4-fold increases in isoagglutinin titers in the final products.

As with thromboembolic events, true rates of Coombs' positivity, hemolytic anemia, and acute severe hemolysis in relation to IVIG therapy are difficult to estimate. However, risk factors that have been identified include non-O blood group, underlying associated inflammatory state, and high cumulative doses of IVIG over several days. Some studies of high-dose IVIG therapy report that as many as 20% of patients may convert to Coombs' positivity shortly after infusions, but the incidence of clinically significant anemia or acute severe hemolysis is significantly lower than that.[33,52,53] Analysis of recent US and Canadian series reported clinically significant hemolysis after IVIG in a combined total of 37 patients, including 23 patients with blood type A, nine with type B, four with type AB, and only one with type O.[56,57]

Prescreening of donors to avoid using plasma units with high isoagglutinin titers in the pools from which the IVIG is prepared,[59] and the use of specific immunoadsorbents[60] to lower the titers of Anti-A and Anti-B, are steps now being introduced to decrease this problem.

Mechanisms of action of IVIG

IgG has both Fc-dependent and Fc-independent mechanisms that contribute to defense against infection[61-63] (Table 31.1). Fc-independent functions include neutralization of toxins, which are important virulence factors in several types of bacterial infection, agglutination, and precipitation of infectious particles, and neutralization of adhesion and attachment molecules. Fc-dependent functions include activating complement, facilitating phagocytosis (both locally at sites of tissue invasion and in bloodstream clearance by macrophages in the reticuloendothelial organs), and enhancing direct cell-mediated cytotoxicity. In general, all of these mechanisms involve stoichiometric interactions between the IgG and antigens and/or effector molecules such as C1q and Fcγ receptors. Therefore, it is not surprising that most studies comparing the efficacy of different doses of IgG replacement therapy in immune-deficient patients show fewer infections in groups that received higher doses. Pooled analyses of recent licensing studies of IVIG and SCIG clearly show that the incidence of pneumonia and other infections decreases as serum IgG levels increase.[40,41]

A broad array of mechanisms of action of IVIG of potential relevance to the use of high-dose therapy have been demonstrated in vitro and in animal models.[61-63] However, it is rarely clear which effects are most important in any given disease *in vivo*, because the pathogeneses of most autoimmune or inflammatory diseases are incompletely understood. Therefore, it is difficult to know whether any given effect demonstrated in vitro or in a model is really relevant in the diseased patient in vivo. One useful way to categorize mechanisms of action in these diseases is by considering whether they are likely to involve direct competition between normal molecules in therapeutic IgG and pathogenic autoantibodies.[63] Clues suggesting situations in which competitive effects are likely include strong dependency on the dose of therapeutic IgG or the amount of therapeutic IgG in the circulation at any point in time, "wearing off" of the IVIG effect as its concentration wanes, and efficacy of plasmapheresis or immunoadsorption to remove pathologic antibodies. Several mechanisms of this type are detailed below. In contrast, true "immunomodulatory effects" on the underlying disease process may be indirect, with more complex pharmaco-dynamics and dose–responses characteristics. This difference is illustrated by a recent study in myasthenia gravis patients that showed that high-dose IVIG temporarily ameliorated the effects of anti-acetyl choline receptor antibodies but did not decrease their production and did not exert a "disease modifying effect" on the underlying immunopathogenesis of the autoimmune process.[64]

Anti-idiotypic binding

Because each individual's immune repertoire arises randomly, it is readily understandable that some individuals respond to a given pathogen with antibodies that cross-react with self-antigens (e.g., *Campylobacter jejuni* and myelin gangliosides in Guillain–Barré syndrome [GBS]), whereas other individuals recognize different epitopes. Furthermore, it is easy to speculate that individuals who mount rigorous anti-id responses will rapidly bring a self-reactive response under control, whereas those whose anti-id response is weak or ineffective may continue to produce clinically significant amounts of autoantibodies.[65] Because IVIG contains the antibodies from tens of thousands of healthy donors, it follows that it likely contains many different anti-ids.

Shortly after its introduction, IVIG was found to neutralize "inhibitors" of the clotting protein factor VIII in hemophilia patients receiving replacement therapy.[66] These "inhibitors" are in fact antibodies against factor VIII (FVIII). Furthermore, F(ab′) fragments of the IVIG neutralized the inhibitors, suggesting anti-id binding. Subsequent studies have shown that IVIG contains a wide variety of anti-ids,[Rev. in 63] consistent with Jerne's network theory of anti-id suppression of potential autoimmunity,[7] and suggesting that this is actually quite common in normal physiology. The most important support for an anti-id mechanism of IVIG in vivo would be the observations that F(ab′) or F(ab′)$_2$ fragments from IVIG neutralize the autoantibody in vitro and/or can remove it by affinity chromatography, that removal of the autoantibodies by plasma-pheresis has a similar effect, and that autoantibodies recovered from patients reproduce the disease physiology in vitro or in animals.

FcRn saturation increases catabolism of endogenous antibodies

As noted above, FcRn on endothelial cells maintains the relatively high normal concentration and long half-life of IgG in the circulation.[22,23,67] In FcRn knockout mice and in patients with FcRn mutations, the half-life of IgG is very short, and its plasma concentration is quite low.[68,69] Furthermore, it is difficult to passively transfer IgG-mediated pathology in FcRn knockout mice, because the half-life of the pathologic IgG is so short.[69] By analogy, if FcRn is saturated by high doses of *exogenous* IVIG, the catabolism of *endogenous* pathologic IgG is greatly increased. In wild-type mice, high-dose IgG dramatically increases the catabolism of path-ogenic IgG; whereas, in FcRn knockout mice, high-dose IgG does not further enhance the already rapid catabolism of the exogenous pathologic IgG.[23,69] Thus, by saturating FcRn with normal anti-bodies, IVIG increases degradation of pathogenic IgG. This thera-peutic effect of IVIG therefore requires that the total IgG concentration exceeds the binding capacity of FcRn and depends on the ratio of the serum concentration of normal IgG to the concentration of pathogenic autoantibodies.

Complement scavenging

Complement components C4 and C3 contain a unique internal thioester bond that can transfer to the target during complement activation, forming a covalent bond.[70] Covalent binding of C4b and/or C3b provides increases the stability of convertases and the likelihood that the initial activation will be amplified. The CH1 domain in IgG has particularly good acceptors for this reaction, and high concentrations of soluble IgG can compete with surface-bound IgG for newly activated C3b. Inhibition of complement deposition by IVIG at concentrations readily achieved during high-dose therapy has been demonstrated in vitro and in animal models, and in humans being treated for dermatomyositis.[71] Clinical improvement following IVIG treatment in that condition is accompanied by decreased activation of C3 and decreased deposition of C3b and C5-9 on endomysial capillaries.[71] Basta *et al.* (2003) also showed that IgG could bind C3a and C5a noncovalently, thereby diminishing pro-inflammatory effects of complement activation.[72]

Indirect actions of IVIG that do not involve competition *per se*

Most recent reviews of "the" mechanism of action of IVIG focus on putative immunomodulatory effects involving networks of T cells, B cells, and cytokines.[61,62] Modulation of activities of macrophages or self-reactive T cells are more likely to be important when these cells, rather than autoantibodies, are directly responsible for the end-organ pathology. Furthermore, many of these immunomodulatory effects of IVIG have prolonged time courses, and are therefore not likely to be responsible for therapeutic effects that "wear off" before a dose of IVIG has reached its half-life.[61–63,73] Analysis of the pharmacodynamics of IgG therapy in any given disease may thus shed light on the mechanism by which the therapeutic IgG is acting, and also on the immunopathogenesis of the disease.[63]

IVIG can interfere with maturation of dendritic cells in vitro, and can inhibit expression of HLA–antigen complexes and the co-stimulatory molecules CD80 and CD86.[61,74,75] It certainly seems possible that decreasing or altering dendritic cell activity would decrease antigen presentation and alter the pattern of cytokine production, modulating the role of the dendritic cells in stimulating different types of T cells. IVIG can decrease the production of pro-inflammatory cytokines like interleukin-1 (IL1), IL12, and interferon-γ and increase production of regulatory molecules like IL10 and IL1 RA.[61,76] In this way, IVIG could alter the balance between regulatory (CD25+) and effector (CD4+ or CD8+) T cells,[76] and could also decrease the inflammatory activity of macrophages. However, when the pathology involves direct effects of antibodies and/or complement on target tissues, it is not clear how modulating T cells or macrophages could produce dramatic beneficial effects. One report showed that IVIG decreased a B-cell activating cytokine that was elevated in sera from chronic idiopathic demyelinating polyneuropathy (CIDP) patients; but the clinical correlation was poor, the time course of changes in cytokine levels was not reported, and the role of that cytokine (and autoantibodies, for that matter) in CIDP is not clear.[77] A recent report that IVIG decreases the number of circulating "natural killer" (NK) cells; their expression of the low affinity Fc receptor, CD16; and their cytotoxic activity more likely represent in vitro blockade of CD16 than a genuine physiologic downregulation,[78] and the role(s) played by NK or other cells that can mediate antibody-dependent cellular cytotoxicity has not been established in the diverse autoimmune diseases for which IVIG is used.

Putative effects of IVIG in ameliorating autoimmune disease by modulating programmed cell death have been proposed, but this remains a very controversial area. Some studies suggest that anti-Fas antibodies in IVIG can induce apoptosis in B cells.[79] However, other results suggesting that IVIG has limited or only transient effects on autoantibody production (or alloantibody, in the case of transplant rejection) would not be consistent with induction of apoptosis as a major mechanism by which IVIG acts in autoimmune disease. Because the level of Fas expression and the sensitivity of cells to pro-apoptotic signals vary with the degree of activation and physiologic state of the cells in question, however, it is not difficult to see how

different results could be obtained in different experimental systems. Further compounding the issues are observations suggesting not only that IVIG preparations may contain antibodies against Fas and another important family of proteins that regulate cell death called *Siglecs*, but also that dimers in IVIG preparations may contain anti-idiotypic antibodies that can complex with and neutralize these autoantibodies.[80] Thus, a number of factors such as low-pH treatment during preparation and storage (which tends to dissociate dimers), stabilizers, and the percentage of dimers in any IgG preparation may also influence the results of laboratory studies, and perhaps the results with different preparations in vivo.

In the past decade, there has been intense focus on increased expression of the inhibitory receptor FcRIIB, as a mechanism of action of a small subset of molecules in IVIG that have fully sialylated carbohydrate side chains.[81,82] These heavily sialylated IgG molecules are proposed to bind to a distinct receptor termed DC-SIGN, inducing the cytokine IL32, which increases FcRIIB expression and inhibits activity of inflammatory macrophages.[81] This putative mechanism would explain why high doses of IVIG are necessary for anti-inflammatory effects, because only a small percentage of the IgG molecules are sialylated. Although a mouse model showed that merely 33 mg/kg of a highly sialylated Fc analog could replicate the effects of 1 g/kg of standard IVIG,[82] these effects appear to depend on the mouse strain and model used.[83,84] Thus, their relevance to specific human diseases is not clear.

Dosing and scheduling IgG treatment regimens

Immune deficiencies

Antibody replacement therapy in immune deficiencies is typically initiated at doses of 400–600 mg/kg of IVIG every 3–4 weeks, or 100–200 mg/kg/week subcutaneously. Doses in this range usually yield trough (in the case of IVIG) or steady-state (in the case of SCIG) serum IgG levels toward the low end of the normal range, and are quite effective in preventing sepsis or other serious bacterial infections.[40,41] However, based on results of clinical observations and a few controlled studies,[85,86] patients with chronic lung and/or sinus disease, and those suffering frequent breakthough infections, are usually given higher doses. Several lines of evidence suggest that the resistance to acute infections is directly related to the serum (and tissue) IgG level at any point in time.[40,41] Analyses of large pooled datasets suggest that patients receiving IVIG every four weeks are more likely to experience infections and hospitalizations in the last week of their dosing cycle,[87,88] before their next dose is due. In a survey performed by the US immune deficiency foundation before the use of SCIG was common, two-thirds of respondents on IVIG answered positively to a question about whether they could feel their IVIG "wearing off" before the next dose was due.[89] A small case series illustrated that different patients require different "biologic IgG trough levels" to remain infection free,[90] and results from a cohort of 90 patients with X-linked agammaglobulinemia or common variable immunodeficiency followed at a single center for over 20 years showed that the range of IgG doses needed to keep the patients free from breakthough infections varied widely: from 0.2 to 1.2 gr/kg/mo, resulting in trough serum IgG levels varying from 500 to 1700 mg/dl (5–17 g/l).[91] Thus, although guidelines can be used to recommend starting doses in previously untreated patients, dose, dosing interval, and route of administration should be individualized based on the clinical results for each patient.[90,91]

Acute autoimmune or inflammatory diseases

In contrast to immune deficiencies, in which the frequency of infection can be used to monitor and individualize IgG treatment, there are few such metrics available for guiding therapy in most acute inflammatory or autoimmune diseases treated with IVIG, so the regimen of 2 grams of IVIG per kg is usually used.

Kawasaki syndrome is an acute, severe inflammatory vasculitis syndrome of uncertain etiology that is most common in young children.[92] IVIG is the major treatment used, and a meta-analysis of studies in which different doses of IVIG were co-administered with aspirin showed a correlation between the dose of IVIG and its efficacy in terms of preventing coronary artery aneurysms, which were present at the convalescent phase in only 3.8% of patients who received the highest dose studied: 2 g/kg.[93] Furthermore, a randomized trial in 549 subjects[94] and the meta-analysis cited above both reported that administering the IVIG as a single infusion over 8–12 hours led to more rapid resolution of symptoms and was more effective than giving it as five consecutive daily doses of 400 mg each. Thus, the commonly used first-line treatment for Kawasaki syndrome is 2 gr/kg of IVIG given as a single large bolus over 8–12 hours. The observation that more rapid administration of the large infusion increases its efficacy suggests that the peak IgG level achieved—rather than the total dose, AUC, or trough level—is the most important determinant of efficacy in this particular situation. This conclusion, in turn, may be most consistent with the hypothesis that the target of IVIG in Kawasaki syndrome is intravascular, perhaps involving endothelial cells per se and/or circulating leukocytes.

Guillain-Barré syndrome is acute autoimmune polyneuropathy causing flaccid paralysis that frequently follows resolution of an infectious disease, most notably gastroenteritis due to *C. jejuni*.[95] The leading hypothesis for the pathogenesis of GBS is that the antibodies produced by the host's immune system in response to the lipo-oligosaccharide of the infectious agent cross-react with ganglioside antigens on myelin, activating complement and causing dysfunction and demyelination of peripheral nerves.[95,96] As such, GBS is frequently cited as a leading example of the *molecular mimicry* theory of autoimmune disease. Although GBS is generally considered an acute, monophasic disease, as many as 5% of patients succumb during the acute episode, and up to 20% may have slow recovery and/or prolonged disability.[95,97,98] First-line treatments for GBS include high-dose IVIG and/or plasma exchange. Laboratory evidence supports hypotheses that IVIG acts predominantly by blocking the binding of autoantibodies to the nerves, presumably due to the presence of anti-idiotypes and/or by blocking complement deposition.[63,99,100] It is likely that plasmapheresis also acts primarily by removing autoantibodies. However, different antibodies targeting different epitopes may be involved in different patients and different clinical variants, and neither measurements of autoantibodies nor in vitro determinations of the ability of IVIG to neutralize them are used to select or adjust the dose or schedule of IVIG treatment. Practice parameters of the American Academy of Neurology consider plasma exchange and IVIg as equally effective first-line treatments.[101] A recent *Cochrane Review* reached the same conclusion but noted that the full course of IVIG treatments was more likely to be completed than the series of plasma exchanges, and that there was little additional benefit of combining the two modalities.[102] The most common dose of IVIG is 2 g/kg, usually given over 2–5 days. One study of 39 subjects suggested that six days of 0.4 g/kg (total dose = 2.4 g/kg) was preferable to three days of 0.4 g/kg (total dose = 1.2 g/kg) in terms of the number of days until

subjects could walk with assistance, but the difference did not reach significance except in a smaller subgroup.[103] A more recent study showed that the serum IgG levels achieved by patients receiving 0.4 gr/kg/day for five days were quite variable, and that patients with the highest increments in IgG level from baseline to day 14 showed the best response in terms of the percentage able to walk unaided six months after the acute episode, and vice versa.[104]

These results suggest that caution should be used in institutions in which the maximum dose of IVIG is restricted to a preset total number of grams, or in which dosing is based on lean or ideal body mass rather than actual body mass, because such rules may result in underdosing GBS patients, and their efficacy in this situation has not been established. Some investigators have suggested that high-risk patients may benefit from a "second dose" (or course) of IVIG, but this has not yet been formally studied. The International GBS Outcomes Study (IGOS) is being carried out to determine how to identify patients at high risk of death or long-term disability and who might benefit from more rigorous treatment.

Immune thrombocytopenic purpura (ITP), as noted in this chapter, was the first condition in which beneficial effects of IVIG in an autoimmune disease were reported (in ITP, autoantibodies mediate destruction of the patient's own platelets). ITP patients may suffer or be at risk for clinically important bleeding episodes, including acute severe blood loss and intracerebral hemorrhage. Corticosteroid therapy is frequently sufficient to increase the platelet count enough to control symptoms such as nosebleeds and menorrhagia. However, when more severe and/or acute bleeding requires a faster increase in the platelet count, IVIG is often used at a dose of 1–2 g/kg given over several consecutive days.[105,106] In general, this will increase the platelet count to >50,000 within seven days of beginning a course of therapy in >80% of patients. IVIG may also be used preoperatively to raise the platelet count and decrease the risk of bleeding in ITP patients. In patients with Rh+ red cells, anti-Rh(D) immune globulin (Rhophylac®, WinRho®, and RhoGAM®) may be used as an alternative to IVIG, obviating many of the potential adverse effects of high-dose IVIG.[107] The Rh(D) immune globulin is believed to act by creating immune complexes with the recipient's red cells that then saturate phagocytic receptors in the reticuloendothelial organs, sparing the platelets. This, in turn, is associated with some destruction of the antibody-coated red cells, but the resulting hemolysis is rarely clinically significant. IVIG is repeated at monthly intervals in some patients, but many individuals with chronic ITP are managed with corticosteroids, splenectomy, rituximab, and/or thrombopoietin receptor agonists.

IVIG may be expected to have effects in autoimmune neutropenia, autoimmune hemolytic anemia, and alloimmune thrombocytopenia (sensitization of baby's platelets with maternal IgG transferred across the placenta) similar to those in ITP, but these disorders are less common than ITP. Furthermore, if IVIg is used, it would frequently be given together with corticosteroids, with which it should have synergistic effects. High-dose IVIG is used as a treatment for pure red cell aplasia secondary to parvovirus B19 infection.[108] In that situation, the IVIG likely helps the host control the infection.

Chronic autoimmune or inflammatory diseases

*Chronic idiopathic demyelinating polyneuropathy:*In many ways, CIDP resembles a chronic form of GBS.[109,110] CIDP differs in that few patients recall preceding infections or other triggering events. CIDP is considered by many to be an autoantibody-mediated disease, and plasma exchange is very effective.

However, unlike the putative role of antiganglioside antibodies in GBS, no single major target antigen(s) has been identified in CIDP.[63] Based upon results of a randomized, placebo-controlled trial of IVIG in 117 CIDP patients (the ICE study), the FDA approved IVIG for CIDP using a loading dose of 2 g/kg followed by maintenance dosing of 1 g/kg every three weeks.[111] In many patients, the effects of IVIG in CIDP are transient, suggesting a mechanism of action involving competition with autoantibodies rather than inhibition of their production, and "wear-off" effects are common.[63] Guidelines call for individualization of therapy, and prescribing regimens other than those used in the ICE trial are prevalent.[112–114] A recent prospective study found that 60% of CIDP patients required IVIG more often than once every two weeks to stably maintain optimal strength.[114] Anecdotal reports and small series suggest that continuously maintaining high serum IgG levels by the use of SCIG may result in more stable maintenance of strength, and a large, randomized, controlled multicenter study of SCIG therapy is now underway.[115]

Multifocal motor neuropathy (MMN): MMN is characterized by multiple motor nerve conduction blocks with sparing of sensory nerves.[116,117] The electrophysiology is consistent with segmental demyelination, but recent studies suggest immunologic target(s) on axons rather than, or in addition to, Schwann cells or myelin. Unlike GBS and CIDP, corticosteroids and PLEx are usually not effective in MMN,[118–120] raising questions about its immunopathogenesis. About half of MMN patients have IgM antibodies against the ganglioside GM1, and these seropositive patients tend to have more severe weakness, disability, and eventual axon loss than seronegative patients. Efficacy of IVIG was demonstrated in multiple anecdotal and case series reports in the mid-1990s. Small controlled studies soon followed, and the results of a 44-subject, randomized, double-blinded, placebo-controlled crossover trial were reported by Hahn *et al.* in 2013.[121] Mean maximal grip strength declined 31% during placebo treatment and increased 3.75% during IVIG treatment ($p = 0.005$).[121] IVIG was recommended as first-line treatment by a European Federation of Neurological Sciences/Peripheral Nerve Society task force in 2006[122] and 2010,[123] and it is usually given in doses of 1–2 g/kg every 3–4 weeks. Interestingly, even early reports noted that improvement in strength and conduction began within a few days after the IVIG, but lasted only 1–2 months, at best.[124–126] As with CIDP, many patients complain that their strength deteriorates in the third or fourth week after an IVIG dose. Small case series suggest that SCIG may help to ameliorate these "wear-off effects" and promote more constant activity, but long-term follow-up studies of SCIG are needed to determine if this will prevent the slow deterioration that now characterizes most MMN patients.

Autoimmune mucocutaneous bullous (blistering) diseases: Autoimmune mucocutaneous bullous (blistering) diseases are a family of conditions including multiple subtypes of pemphigus and pemphigoid in which separation of intraepidermal or subepidermal layers of skin occurs because of antibodies against intercellular adhesion molecules such as desmoglein.[127] Most of these disorders have relapsing-remitting courses, and subtypes are characterized by differences in the locations and depth of the blisters, which in turn are probably related to differences in the specific targets of the autoantibodies. In general, corticosteroids are first-line therapies, and most patients are also given cytotoxic drugs such as cyclophosphamide or azathioprine. "High-dose" IVIG is often added as an alternative or addition to steroids in patients who develop complications of steroid treatment, and is regarded as a "steroid-sparing" therapy.[128] IVIG may also be preferentially used in patients with poor tolerance of cytotoxic agents. A major effect of IVIG seems to be reduction of autoantibody titer, although this has been reported to take several months,[128] so it is not clear whether the mechanism is competitive or mediated by other pathways. In cases of severe mucosal and/or ocular involvement, high-dose IVIG may be used to achieve a more rapid remission of acute attacks or exacerbations.

IgG in transplantation

IgG therapy has three main uses in solid organ transplantation. High-dose IVIG is employed along with plasmapheresis and rituximab in regimens designed to "desensitize" or remove preformed anti-HLA antibodies ("panel reactive antibodies" [PRA]) before transplantation in patients who have developed these antibodies in response to exposure to alloantigens in their fetuses, in the case of multiparous women, or in a previous transplant.[130] In this situation, the IVIG is likely acting by anti-idiotype blocking, exchanging with endogenous IgG in the extravascular spaces, so the latter can be removed by plasmapheresis, and saturating FcRn to increase the catabolism of the endogenous anti-HLA antibodies. Particularly with kidney transplant patients, caution must be used in selecting the IVIG product and scheduling the infusions to avoid adverse effects due to isoagglutinins or sucrose. The newer IVIG preparations with reduced isoagglutinin content and nonsugar stabilizers should ameliorate these concerns. The second major use also involves high-dose IVIG, which is used to treat acute antibody mediated rejection.[131] In this situation, part of the effect of the IVIG is undoubtedly to neutralize and/or accelerate the catabolism of the antibodies against the graft that are causing the rejection. However, immunomodulatory and inflammatory activities, including inhibiting complement, blocking Fc receptors, and altering the cytokine milieu, are also likely important. Many recipients of solid organ transplants become at least transiently hypogammaglobulinemic as a result of their immunosuppressive regimen, because of GI losses in visceral transplants[132,133] and/or because of preexisting hypogammaglobulinemia or specific antibody deficiency that may have been undiagnosed before the transplant (particularly in lung transplant recipients). Such patients may benefit from antibody replacement, which may be given by the IV or subcutaneous routes, using regimens like those used for patients with primary antibody deficiency. Formerly, cytomegalovirus (CMV) hyperimmune globulin was used prophylactically after transplants, especially in antibody-negative recipients of organs from CMV+ donors (so-called D+/R− transplants). This has become much less common in the current era in which antiviral chemotherapy with Gancyclovir and Valgancyclovir is available, but it may still be used in patients who do not tolerate those agents and/or who develop active CMV disease.

In recipients of hematopoietic stem cell transplantations (HSCTs) for severe combined immune deficiency (SCID), particularly the X-linked form due to mutations in the cytokine receptor common γ chain, B-cell reconstitution frequently occurs much slower than hematopoietic and T-cell reconstitution.[134] Most SCID patients are given IgG replacement for at least a year after transplantation, and some require it for life.

Based on the results of a large, randomized, double-blind, placebo controlled study in France;[135] an independent meta-analysis in Canada;[136] and a *Cochrane Database Review*[137] IVIG is not recommended for routine prophylaxis of infection after allogeneic

HSCT. However, in some lymphoproliferative diseases, especially when rituximab is used in combination with conventional chemotherapy (e.g., CHOP [cyclophosphamide, hydroxydaunorubicin, oncovin, and prednisone or prednisolone], and in some cases in which rituximab is used (with or without cytotoxic agents) for nonmalignant antibody-mediated disorders, prolonged depletion of circulating B cells and significant hypogammaglobulinemia may occur, resulting in severe and/or recurrent infections. Such patients should be evaluated for IgG and/or specific antibody deficiency, and IgG replacement therapy using regimens similar to those used for primary immune deficiency should be considered.[138,139]

Hyperimmune globulins

Hyperimmune immune globulins are made from plasma obtained from normal subjects with high titers of antibodies to the desired microbe or antigen detected by screening, or because they have been immunized or are convalescing.[140,141] Plasma is processed as for regular (IM) ISG or IVIG, and the final product is tested to assure an adequate antibody titer to the microbe or other antigen. In general, hyperimmunes contain about fivefold higher titers of specific antibodies to the microbe or antigen for which they are labeled than standard IVIG preparations (on the basis of a unit of specific antibody per gram of IgG).[140,141] Thus, to get the same amount of specific antibody, fivefold higher doses of standard IVIG would have to be given, constituting an extremely high dose of the latter. For example, to get the recommended amount of specific IgG for protection against respiratory syncytial virus required 750 mg/kg of the hyperimmune RespiGam® but would require 3750 mg/kg of "standard" IVIG. To put this in a current perspective, the same amount of specific IgG is contained in 15 mg/kg of the monoclonal anti-RSV antibody palivizumab (Synagis®), which can be given as a simple IM injection.[141] Other hyperimmunes target the Rh(D) red cell antigen (RhoGAM, PhoPhylac, etc.) to prevent sensitization of Rh(D)-negative women to Rh(D)+ fetal erythrocytes, and also for ITP in Rh(D)+ individuals, CMV (CytoGam® and Cytotect®), botulism toxins (BIG-IV® and Baby-BIG®), hepatitis B virus (HepaGamB, HyperHepB S/D), rabies virus (BayRab, Imogam-Rabies HT), tetanus (HyperTet), and varicella–zoster virus (VariZIG®). The same adverse effects may occur with the hyperimmunes as with standard IgG preparations. However, the doses of IV hyperimmunes are generally lower than the high doses of IVIG used for immunomodulatory effects, and so are less likely to produce serious adverse effects unless they are administered too rapidly.

Antivenoms used for spider and snake bites[142] and anti-thymocyte globulin used for immunosuppression (i.e., in transplant recipients) are usually animal antisera and may be associated with anaphylaxis and/or serum sickness.

Summary

Given the diversity of the immune repertoire and the multiple interactions of its Fc domains with receptors and other effector systems, it is not really surprising that polyclonal IgG, pooled from tens of thousands of individuals, has a broad multiplicity of uses. Modern preparations are highly purified and contain stabilizers designed to prevent aggregate formation, and thus can be given intravenously or subcutaneously with relative freedom from severe systemic adverse reactions. Caution and monitoring are still necessary as occasional serious and/or life-threatening AEs still occur, especially individuals with identifiable risk factors. Doses in the range of 600–1000 mg/kg/month are generally used for replacement therapy for immune-deficient patients. This may be given in IV boluses every 3–4 weeks, or fractionated into smaller increments given by the subcutaneous route weekly or even more often. Although the former require venous access and are frequently monitored by trained medical personnel, the latter are frequently self-administered in the home, greatly facilitating the convenience of long-term IgG therapy and the quality of life for patients and their families. High-dose IVIG therapy (1–2 g/kg, usually every 2–4 weeks) is used for a growing number of autoimmune/inflammatory diseases, generally in clinical settings, and accounts for a continuously increasing global demand for IgG products.

Key references

2 O'Shaughnessy D, Hollingsworth R, Kane P, Foster M. UK NHS Third National Immunoglobulin Database Report. 2012. http://www.ivig.nhs.uk/documents/Third_National_Immunoglobulin_Database_Report_2011_2012.pdf.

21 Bonilla FA. Pharmacokinetics of immunoglobulin administered via intravenous or subcutaneous routes. *Immunol Allergy Clin North Am* 2008;**28**:803–19.

26 Berger M. Subcutaneous immunoglobulin replacement in primary immunodeficiencies. *Clin Immunol* 2004;**112**:1–7.

33 Berger M. Adverse effects of IgG therapy. *J Allergy Clin Immunol Pract* 2013;**1**:558–66.

52 Pierce LR, Jain N. Risks associated with the use of intravenous immunoglobulin. *Transfus Med Rev* 2003;**17**(4):241–51.

61 Ballow M. The IgG molecule as a biological immune response modifier: mechanisms of action of intravenous immune serum globulin in autoimmune and inflammatory disorders. *J Allergy Clin Immunol* 2011;**127**:315–23.

Apheresis, transplantation, and new therapies

CHAPTER 32

Apheresis: principles and technology of hemapheresis

Edwin A. Burgstaler & Jeffrey L. Winters

Therapeutic Apheresis Treatment Unit, Mayo Clinic, Rochester, MN, USA

Terminology and definitions

Apheresis is derived from a Greek word that means *separate* or *remove*, and it was first used in 1914 by Able, Rowntree, and Turner to describe a procedure where blood was withdrawn from dogs and separated into cells and plasma, with the plasma being discarded and the cells returned with a replacement fluid.[1] Apheresis procedures can be divided into two categories, *cytapheresis*, where the cellular elements are removed, and *plasmapheresis*, where plasma is removed. Table 32.1 defines various apheresis procedures.

Basic concepts common to all apheresis procedures

Blood component separation

Separation of blood components is performed by centrifugation, filtration, or a combination.[3] Centrifugation uses centrifugal force and blood component–specific gravity to separate the elements in the blood. The elements are then removed by siphoning off the desired component or spilling the lighter components over a barrier that retains the heavier components. In some systems, elutriation is also used. Two opposing forces—centrifugal force that pushes heavier elements away from the centrifuge center, and pump withdrawal force that pulls the elements to the centrifuge center—separate based on size rather than specific gravity. Effective separation by centrifugation is dependent on the centrifuge g-force, determined by the rotations per minute and rotor radius, and the time that blood is exposed to the centrifugal force.[3]

Filtration separates elements based upon size.[3] The filter can be a bundle of hollow fibers with pores in their walls or a membrane surface with pores.[3] The pore size determines what passes through the filter and what is retained. Cascade or double-membrane filtration systems can remove substances from the plasma by using two filters, a primary membrane plasma separator to separate the plasma from the cells and a plasma fractionator with smaller pores to remove proteins, such as immunoglobulins.[4]

The Autopheresis C (Fenwal Inc., a Fresenius-Kabi Company, Lake Zurich, IL, USA) combines centrifugation and filtration to increase plasma collection efficiency. A grooved cylinder covered with a filter membrane is encased within a larger cylinder. Whole blood enters the larger cylinder and surrounds the rotating grooved cylinder. The rotation moves the cells away from the filter toward the inner wall of the larger cylinder while the plasma moves toward the rotating filter. Pressure causes the plasma to flow through the filter to a collection bag while cells exit the bottom of the larger cylinder and are returned. The rotation improves efficiency by keeping platelets and cells from plugging the membrane pores.[3]

Anticoagulation

Contact between the plastic disposables and the blood activates the coagulation cascade and clots the circuit in the absence of anticoagulation. To prevent this, blood is anticoagulated prior to extensive contact with the tubing. In the United States, citrate or heparin are the primary anticoagulants with additional medications available in other countries.[5,6]

Citrate anticoagulants contain citric acid, which binds calcium so that it cannot participate in the coagulation cascade.[6] It is necessary to lower the ionized calcium concentration to 0.2 to 0.3 mmol/L to inhibit coagulation. This would be incompatible with life, yet citrate anticoagulation is safely used due to compensatory mechanisms that increase calcium through release from albumin, mobilization from bone stores, and resorption by the kidneys.[6] Citrate is also rapidly metabolized by the liver, kidneys, and skeletal muscle releasing the chelated calcium.[6] Citrate anticoagulation produces regional anticoagulation, anticoagulation of the blood within the apheresis device but not in the patient-donor.

Heparin anticoagulates blood by increasing antithrombin activity.[6] It is not used as widely as citrate due to systemic anticoagulation and the risk of heparin-induced thrombocytopenia.[6] Heparin is used in procedures where citrate interferes with the mechanism of action of the apheresis device, and it is frequently used in therapeutic plasma exchange (TPE, another term for plasmapheresis) performed with filtration-based devices. The use in filtration TPE is related to plasma removal efficiency. In a centrifugal device, the plasma extraction ratio is higher (80%), resulting in the removal of most of the administered anticoagulant. The lower plasma extraction ratio (30%) of filtration devices means a large percentage of the anticoagulant is returned to the patient, causing a greater risk of toxicity.[5]

Heparin and citrate may be used in combination to minimize the side effects of both by reducing the amount of citrate needed and its electrolyte disturbances and reducing heparin dose to minimize the length of systemic anticoagulation. This dual anticoagulation is used in procedures on low-weight patients, such as children, where the total volume of anticoagulant administered during the procedure may be large relative to the individual's blood volume.

Rossi's Principles of Transfusion Medicine, Fifth Edition. Edited by Toby L. Simon, Jeffrey McCullough, Edward L. Snyder, Bjarte G. Solheim, and Ronald G. Strauss.
© 2016 John Wiley & Sons, Ltd. Published 2016 by John Wiley & Sons, Ltd.

Table 32.1 Definitions of apheresis procedures

Procedure	Definition	Donor	Therapeutic
Cytapheresis			
Leukocytapheresis	Blood from a patient or donor is separated, and the white blood cells are collected (e.g., granulocytes in donors, leukemic blasts in patients, or hematopoietic progenitor cells in either), returning the remainder of the blood to the patient or donor.	Yes	Yes
Adsorptive cytapheresis	Blood is passed through a column or filter that selectively adsorbs activated monocytes or granulocytes, with the remainder of the blood returned to the patient.	No	Yes
Extracorporeal photopheresis	Blood is separated, with a "buffy coat" containing white blood cells and platelets being collected. This is mixed with a photoactivating agent, exposed to ultraviolet A light, and returned to the patient.	No	Yes
Plateletpheresis	Blood is separated, with the platelets collected for transfusion.	Yes	No
Thrombocytapheresis	Blood is separated, with the platelets removed and discarded while the remaining components are returned to the patient.	No	Yes
Erythrocytapheresis	Blood is separated, with the red blood cells being collected for transfusion (red cell donation) or discarded in the case of some patients with an elevated red cell mass. The volume of red cells removed is limited such that it does not require replacement of the red blood cells.	Yes	Yes
Red cell exchange	Blood is separated, with the red blood cells being removed and discarded. The volume of red blood cells collected requires replacement with donor red blood cells.	No	Yes
Plasmapheresis			
Plasmapheresis	Blood is separated, and the plasma is collected. The volume collected is such that a replacement fluid is not needed.	Yes	No
Therapeutic plasma exchange	Blood is separated, and the plasma is collected and discarded. The volume of plasma collected is large enough that a replacement fluid consisting of colloid or colloid and crystalloid is required.	No	Yes
Double filtration plasmapheresis	Blood is separated into the cellular components and plasma. The plasma is then further processed, utilizing a filter with a pore size selected to remove a substance of interest in the plasma, such as LDL cholesterol or immunoglobulins. The treated plasma is then returned to the patient.	No	Yes
Rheopheresis	This is a type of double-filtration plasmapheresis where the pore size of the filter removes high-molecular-weight substances such as IgM, fibrinogen, or LDL cholesterol with the goal of enhancing blood flow and improving oxygen delivery to tissues.	No	Yes
Immunoadsorption	Blood is separated into the cellular components and plasma with the plasma passed through a column which removes immunoglobulins.	No	Yes
Lipid apheresis	The selective removal of LDL cholesterol, lipoprotein(a), and other potentially pathologic lipids. A variety of devices are available that can remove these substances based upon size, electrical charge, chemical precipitation, or using antibodies that recognize apolipoproteins.	No	Yes

Source: Schwartz et al. (2013).[2] Reproduced with permission of Wiley.

Vascular access

In donor apheresis, vascular access is obtained through peripheral venipuncture. A large-bore steel needle (17 gauge or greater) is inserted into an antecubital vein as the draw while an intravenous catheter (18 gauge or larger) is inserted into a peripheral vein of the opposite arm to serve as the return.[8] In blood donors, this is effective and safe.

Underlying disease, previous medical treatment, previous IV insertion, hypovolemia, and multiple apheresis procedures may make peripheral access difficult in patients, and it may be necessary to insert a central venous catheter. Central venous catheters capable of supporting apheresis must have a large diameter and short length to minimize resistance to flow and have rigid walls to prevent collapse under negative pressure in order to allow adequate flow rates.[8] Catheters used for dialysis are acceptable for apheresis.

Central venous catheter placement represents the greatest risk for apheresis complications,[9] with complications including pneumothorax, bleeding, thrombosis, and infection.[5] Deaths due to these complications have been reported.[10] Studies have found adequate access can be obtained in patients using peripheral veins. One TPE study involving multiple sclerosis patients found inadequate peripheral access in only 4.5% of patients.[11] To minimize risks, each patient should have their peripheral access evaluated and used, if possible.

Blood donor apheresis

The 2011 National Blood Collection and Utilization Survey demonstrated a continued shift from whole blood to apheresis donation.[12] Compared to 2008, there was a decrease in red blood cell (RBC) units produced from whole blood donation by 9.7% with an increase in apheresis production of 2.7%. Similarly, there was a decline in whole blood–derived platelets by 10.3% with a corresponding increase in apheresis platelet collections by 18.1%.[12] In 2011, 91.1% of platelet doses were collected by apheresis.[12] This shift is a result of the ability to optimize the products collected based upon the donor's characteristics and inventory needs. For example, although AB plasma is in high demand as the universal plasma product, AB red blood cells are only compatible with 4% of the population and are therefore of limited use. Collecting only plasma from an AB donor allows that donor to donate plasma more frequently and does not generate a low-demand product likely to outdate. Multicomponent collections (e.g. a platelet collection with a concurrent collection of plasma) can also be performed, allowing even greater optimization. Table 32.2 lists the various blood

Table 32.2 Blood components collected by apheresis

Granulocytes
Hematopoietic progenitor cells
Plasma: Multiple doses may be collected depending upon donor characteristics
Platelet: Single, double, or triple
Double platelet and single plasma
Platelet and single or double plasma
Red blood cell: Single or double
Red blood cell and plasma
Red blood cell and platelet
Red blood cell, platelet, and plasma

Table 32.3 Advantages of apheresis collected blood components

- Reduced donor exposure: full transfusion dose collected from one donor
- Frequent repeat donors: "pedigreed" donors with repeated screening and testing
- Higher quality products: more quality control per component collected
- Consistent and standardized product volumes and yields
- Ability to matching donors to patients: HLA matching for platelet transfusions
- Reduced donor reactions
- Double, triple, or multiple full-dose blood component collections
- Safety enhancement for the patient with reduced frequency of certain transfusion reactions

components and their combinations that can be collected. Table 32.3 lists advantages of collecting blood components by apheresis.

Donor apheresis instrumentation

Devices cleared by the US Food and Drug Administration (FDA) and currently available in the United States will be briefly described. Table 32.4 lists the different products that each of these devices can collect.

Alyx (Fenwal Inc., a Fresenius-Kabi Company, Lake Zurich, IL, USA)

The Alyx is a single-needle instrument designed for double red cell and multicomponent collection (Table 32.4). Blood is drawn by the donor pump into an "in-process" bag. Blood is drawn by the in-process pump into the centrifuge. Because the in-process pump is slower than the donor pump, unprocessed blood accumulates in the in-process bag. Plasma is drawn from the centrifuge by the plasma pump and delivered to the plasma bag to be returned to the donor or saved for plasma collection. The packed RBCs are pumped into the RBC bag for collection (or returned during a plasma collection). In RBC collection, when a predetermined amount of blood has been processed, the plasma and saline are returned to the donor by the donor pump. Simultaneously, the in-process pump delivers unprocessed blood from the in-process bag so the centrifuge is continuously processing blood. During RBC collection, when the appropriate amount of RBCs are collected, the extra blood components are returned to the donor. A preservative solution is added to the RBCs, which are pumped through a leukoreduction filter into final storage bags. The extracorporeal volume (ECV) is 110 ml plus the volume of the products. The Alyx is a compact device that can be utilized on mobile blood drives.[3]

Amicus (Fenwal Inc., a Fresenius-Kabi Company, Lake Zurich, IL, USA)

The Amicus can perform single– and multicomponent collections (Table 32.4). Blood is pumped into a double chamber belt wrapped around a spool. Prior to entering the centrifuge, plasma is added to the whole blood to adjust the hematocrit (HCT). When blood enters the centrifuge, the lighter platelets quickly migrate toward the center of the centrifuge and are withdrawn by the platelet-rich pump (PRP) from the inlet side of the separation chamber. As blood flows through the separation chamber, the HCT increases, and mononuclear cells flow to the center of the centrifuge and are drawn by the PRP pump toward the platelet outlet. However, when they encounter the lower HCT of the entering diluted blood, they fall to the outside of the chamber. They continue to circulate in the center of the separation chamber until they are returned to the donor during reinfusion. The packed RBC and granulocytes flow to the far end of the separation chamber and are returned to the donor. The PRP is pumped into the second chamber (collection chamber), where the platelets concentrate and the platelet-poor plasma is directed into a collection bag or returned to the donor.[3]

The interface between the blood components in the separation chamber is monitored by an interface detector and maintained by a microprocessor. The Amicus can perform double– or single-needle procedures, with the later used for multicomponent collections (Table 32.4). RBC leukoreduction is done off-line by manually filtering the product. The ECV without products is 205 ml for double– and up to 329 ml for single-needle procedures.[3]

Autopheresis-C and Aurora (Fenwal Inc., a Fresenius-Kabi Company, Lake Zurich, IL, USA)

The Autopheresis-C and Aurora perform plasma collection (Table 32.4). The centrifugal filtration system described under blood component separation is used by both. The devices are single-needle systems using citrate anticoagulation. Both have ECVs of 200 ml, not including the volume of the products being collected.[3]

COBE Spectra and Spectra Optia (Terumo BCT, Lakewood, CO, USA)

The COBE Spectra and Spectra Optia can be used for granulocyte collection. Both use a circular separation channel with ports positioned at different distances from the outside wall. With the COBE Spectra, the collect line content is monitored visually by the operator and the plasma pump rate is adjusted to alter the collect line appearance and therefore the product content. The Spectra Optia is automated with an interface detector that monitors the collect line content and the product content. The COBE Spectra is capable of multiple procedures but will be retired and replaced by

Table 32.4 Products collected by donor apheresis devices available in the United States

Device	Platelet	cRBC	Double RBC	Plasma	cPlasma	Granulocytes	HPC
Alyx		X	X		X		
Amicus	X	X			X		X
Autopheresis-C/Aurora				X			
COBE Spectra	X				X	X	X
MCS+ LN8150			X		X		
MCS+ LN9000	X				X		
PCS-2				X			
Spectra Optia						X	X
Trima Accel	X	X	X	X	X		

RBC, red blood cell; cRBC, concurrent RBC; cPlasma, concurrent plasma; HPC, hematopoietic progenitor cell.

the Spectra Optia. The Spectra Optia typical ECV during granulocyte collection is 253 ml while the maximum is 297 mL, not including the product volume.[3]

Haemonetics MCS+ LN9000 and LN8150 (Haemonetics Corporation, Braintree, MA, USA)

MCS stands for *mobile collection system*. The LN9000 is used for platelet collection and concurrent plasma, and the LN8150 for double RBC collection and RBC with concurrent plasma (Table 32.4). The LN9000 uses a conical shaped Latham bowl, and the LN8150 uses a bowl with vertical walls.[3]

With the LN9000, blood fills the spinning conical bowl from the bottom, with the RBCs migrating to the outside wall and plasma staying on the inside wall with the buffy coat (white blood cells [WBC] and platelets) lying between. Plasma exits the bowl by first passing through a laser-based sensor. When the plasma–buffy coat interface is detected, plasma is rapidly pumped into the bowl from the bottom, flushing the lighter platelets from the bowl. When they are detected by the line sensor, a valve opens to the collect bag, which then closes when WBCs are detected. At that point, the bowl contains only RBCs, which are returned to the donor along with the plasma. The cycle is then repeated. WBC removal occurs through an on-line leukoreduction filter. When concurrent plasma is collected, the desired volume of plasma is retained during the last reinfusion.[3]

In the LN8150, the vertical-wall centrifuge bowl (blow-molded bowl) also fills from the bottom. Instead of a laser-based sensor at the top of the bowl, the line sensor detects the presence of RBCs in the bowl effluent line and stops the cycle. A small amount of saline is pumped to the donor, and then a predetermined amount of RBCs are transferred to the RBC reservoir bag. The remaining RBCs, plasma, and additional saline are returned to the donor. The cycle is repeated until the programmed RBC volume is collected. The donor is disconnected when all remaining plasma and RBCs have been returned. Additive solution is pumped to the reservoir bag, and the set is disconnected. Leukoreduction is performed by gravity through pre-attached filters as blood drains into two RBC product bags.[3]

The LN9000 and LN8150 ECV is dependent on the size of bowl used, donor HCT, and phase of the cycle. The range is 542 ml (38% HCT) to 391 ml (54% HCT). The instruments are designed to be portable and can be used for mobile blood drives.[3]

Haemonetics PCS-2 (Haemonetics Corporation, Braintree, MA, USA)

The Haemonetics PCS-2 is used for plasma collection (Table 32.4). The LN8150 vertical wall bowl is used with plasma diverted to a collection bag until the bowl fills with RBCs. The bowl contents are then returned to the donor. Cycles are repeated until the target plasma volume is collected. The ECV depends upon the donor hematocrit ranging from 480 ml (38% HCT) to 359 ml (52% HCT). The device is portable.[3]

Trima Accel (Terumo BCT, Lakewood, CO, USA)

The Trima Accel is capable of single and multicomponent collections (Table 32.4). Blood is pumped into a rotating single-stage circular channel. The collect line from the centrifuge is attached to a conical leukocyte reduction chamber. The "collect pump" pumps the product into collection bags. The plasma is collected in the plasma collection bags or is returned to the donor, depending upon the procedure being performed. The packed cells go to the return reservoir or RBC collection bag, again depending upon the procedure being performed. A microprocessor directs component flow from the centrifuge

through a valve system to the proper collection bags. The plasma–cell interface is maintained by algorithms that utilize donor data entered at the procedure beginning. Because of this, there is no interface detector, but there is an RBC detector that will monitor RBC spillover during the collection. The Trima Accel is a single-needle system. Double RBC units can be collected, filtered, and additive solution added, all on-line. The ECV, without products, is 196 ml for the platelet kit and 182 ml for the RBC–plasma kit.

Product and procedure requirements

Granulocytes

Chapter 23, "Neutrophil collection and transfusion," discusses granulocyte collection and clinical use, and the reader is referred to this chapter for procedure and product requirements.

Hematopoietic progenitor cells

Chapter 36, "Hematopoietic stem cells and cord blood," discusses the collection and processing of hematopoietic progenitor cells, including procedure and product requirements. The reader is referred to this chapter.

Plasma

In 2011, 81,000 plasmapheresis procedures were performed in the United States, collecting 205,000 plasma units. An additional 246,000 units were collected as concurrent plasma.[12] These apheresis units, however, represent only 7.6% of the plasma collected for transfusion with the majority collected from whole blood donation.[12] Plasma is also collected as *source plasma*, plasma to be fractionated and manufactured into products such as albumin, intravenous immune globulin, and coagulation factor concentrates (see Chapter 27).

The regulatory and accreditation requirements for plasma collection depend upon donation frequency. Donors may donate more frequently than every four weeks (*frequent*) or less frequently than every four weeks (*infrequent*). In general, frequent donors donate "source plasma" and infrequent donors donate plasma for transfusion. Infrequent plasma donors must fulfill whole blood donor requirements.[13] AABB Standards for Blood Banks and Transfusion Services also require that donors taking warfarin be deferred for one week following their last dose to allow for vitamin K–dependent coagulation factor regeneration.[14] Frequent plasma donors must fulfill criteria outlined in the US Code of Federal Regulations (CFR).[14,15] These require that total serum protein is greater than 6.0 g/dL prior to each donation, a serum protein electropheresis or quantitative immunodiffusion be performed every 4 months, and a physical examination performed by a physician be performed annually.[15] This ensures that "frequent" plasma donation does not deplete plasma proteins that could harm the donor and affect the potency and efficacy of the products.

Both frequent and infrequent plasma donors are limited to the total plasma volume that can be donated in 12 months. Donors weighing 110 to 175 lbs. can donate up to 12 L, and those weighing >175 lbs. can donate up to 14.4 L.[13] Frequent plasma donors are limited to two donations within a seven-day period, with at least two days between the donations.[15]

Platelets

Donor requirements for apheresis platelet donation are the same as whole blood donation.[14,16] Both the AABB and FDA have requirements that address a donor's exposure to antiplatelet medications.

The FDA requires deferral of donors who have ingested aspirin or piroxicam within two days prior to collection.[16] Donors who have taken clopidogrel or ticlopidine, drugs whose metabolites inhibit platelet function and have a longer antiplatelet effect, are deferred for 14 days.[16] AABB Standards require that donors taking "medications known to irreversibly inhibit platelet function" be evaluated prior to donation.[14]

Platelet donors must have a minimum 150,000/μL platelet count. A pre-donation count must be used to program the apheresis instrument and can be a postcollection count from the donor's previous donation or a count on a sample drawn immediately prior to the current donation. If the count is not available prior to the start of collection, the procedure can begin but the count must be entered when available. If a pre-procedure count cannot be obtained, an average of the donor's previous platelet counts, a default count recommended by the instrument manufacturer, or a default count determined by the collection center may be used.[16] When a pre-procedure platelet count cannot be determined on a first-time donor, a triple-platelet product cannot be collected.[14] If capable, the instrument must be programmed to ensure that the donor's platelet count does not fall below 100,000/μL.[16]

Platelet donors have restrictions on donation frequency and the total number of donations that can occur within a 12-month period.[14,16] Donors can donate twice per week but must have two days between donations if they are donating a single dose of platelets. If donating a double or triple product, they are deferred for one week. Donors cannot donate more than 24 times in a rolling 12-month period.[16] This limit arose from the observation that donors collected on early apheresis devices experienced declines in total lymphocyte numbers, T-lymphocyte numbers, and immunoglobulin G (IgG) levels for up to eight months.[17] These findings have not been seen with newer devices.[17] This requirement has persisted, and restrictions on donation intervals were added as studies suggested that long-term platelet donation resulted in baseline platelet count decline and a delay in platelet recovery.[18] These findings have not been seen in other studies.[19]

The FDA has also placed limits on the total amount of plasma removed during a platelet donation and the total amount of RBCs lost within eight weeks.[16] Donors weighing <175 lbs. can have no more than 500 mL of plasma removed, whereas those weighing ≥175 lbs. can have 600 mL removed.[16] RBC loss, from whole blood donation or loss during the apheresis donation, can result in prolonged donor deferral.[14,16] These deferrals are listed in Table 32.5.

The FDA requires that 75% of the apheresis platelet products contain at least 3.0×10^{11} platelets,[15] whereas AABB requires that 90% contain 3.0×10^{11} platelets.[14] The products must also have a

pH >6.2 at issue or the end of storage.[14] If products are leukocyte reduced, then 95% of the units sampled must have $\leq 5 \times 10^6$ residual leukocytes.[14]

Red blood cells

RBCs can be collected as a single or a double unit. Single units are usually collected as part of a multicomponent collection due to the costs associated with the collection. Advantages of apheresis RBC collections include fewer donor reactions, better inventory management, standardized RBC doses, and decreased donor exposure if both units of a double RBC are given to the same patient.[20] Disadvantages include stricter donor criteria that are dependent upon the apheresis device used, longer donation time, and potential apheresis-related complications.[20]

Apheresis RBC donors must meet whole blood donation criteria[14,21] and must also meet criteria defined by the device manufacturer. These criteria define height, weight, and hematocrit requirements based upon the donor's sex.[21] The FDA requires that the hemoglobin/hematocrit method used to qualify the donor be a quantitative method.[21]

The maximum allowed RBC volume removed during the collection is defined in the device operator's manual with no specific requirements from the FDA.[21] AABB standards require that the amount of RBC removed not reduce the donor's hemoglobin below 10 gm/dL or the hematocrit below 30%.[14]

Donation frequency is determined by the type of RBC product donated. Single-unit RBC donors are deferred for eight weeks, whereas those donating two units are deferred for 16 weeks.[21] The deferral length may vary based upon the absolute RBC loss in cases where there is an incomplete procedure or there has been additional RBC loss due to other donations (Table 32.5).[16]

The FDA requires that 95% of the products collected meet the "expected or target RBC volume" and "any other target parameters" defined in the device operator's manual. The FDA defines how the testing to validate and monitor the apheresis RBC collections is performed.[21] For validation, the FDA requires testing 100 consecutively collected units. For monitoring, at least 50 units, consisting of single and double RBCs, must be monitored each month. When a center collects fewer than 50 units, all of the units must be tested.[21] AABB standards require that the method used result in a mean hemoglobin of ≥60 g or 180 mL RBCs. At least 95% of the units must have >50 g of hemoglobin or 150 mL RBCs. If the RBC unit is leukocyte reduced, the method must have a mean hemoglobin ≥51 g or a 153 mL RBC volume and a residual leukocyte count $\leq 5 \times 10^6$. Ninety-five percent of units must have >42.5 g of hemoglobin or 128 mL RBCs.[14]

Multicomponent collections

Multiple different components can be collected by apheresis from a single donor (Table 32.2). With multicomponent collections, the donor and product requirements that apply to the individual products apply to the procedure. Donation frequency requirements seen with plasma donation apply when plasma is collected concurrently with a platelet or RBC product. Red cell loss deferrals given in Table 32.5 and the plasma volume limits described with plasma and platelet donation also apply.

Therapeutic apheresis

The first therapeutic apheresis procedures occurred in the 1950s, when TPE was used to treat hyperviscosity in Waldenström's

Table 32.5 Impact of red cell loss on donor eligibility[16]

First Red Cell Loss	Total of First and Subsequent Red Cell Loss in Preceding 8 Weeks	Eligibility
<200 mL	<200 mL	No deferral
<200 mL	>200 mL but ≤300 mL	Defer for 8 weeks from second loss
>200 mL but ≤300 mL	NA	Defer for 8 weeks from first loss
<200 mL	>300 mL	Defer for 16 weeks from second loss
≥300 mL	NA	Defer for 16 weeks from loss

NA, Not applicable.

macroglobulinemia.[22,23] Since these original reports, apheresis has been used in a variety of diseases, sometimes with limited evidence and unclear rationale supporting its use due to a lack of knowledge of disease pathogenesis and enthusiasm to apply a new therapy to otherwise untreatable conditions.

Therapeutic apheresis instrumentation and selected procedures

Chapters 32 and 33 discuss TPE and specialized apheresis procedures. The specific indications and the treatment protocols will not be described in this chapter. Devices available in the United States capable of performing these procedures will be briefly described. Greater detail is available in apheresis-specific textbooks.[3]

Therapeutic plasma exchange

Amicus (Fenwal Inc., a Fresenius-Kabi Company, Lake Zurich, IL, USA)

The Amicus can perform TPE using a specially designed spool, spool holder, and TPE kit. In the kit, only the separation chamber is used, with the collection chamber used for other procedures (see Amicus in the "Blood Donor Apheresis" section) filled with saline to balance the centrifuge. Blood enters the far end and flows toward two outlet ports on the near side of the separation chamber. A "bump" molded into the spool deflects cells (RBC, WBC, and platelets) so that they flow out the packed cell line to the patient. Plasma is drawn into a 1 L waste container by the plasma pump. The cell–plasma interface is monitored and controlled by a microprocessor-controlled interface detector. Plasma is automatically transferred to larger waste bags as needed. The ECV is 160 ml. The instrument can determine volumes of plasma to remove, replacement volumes, and fluid balance.[3]

Haemonetics LN9000 (Haemonetics Corporation, Braintree, MA, USA)

The Haemonetics LN9000 uses the Latham conical bowl (225 ml or 125 ml) described in the "Blood Donor Apheresis" section. The device is intermittent flow, with the bowl filling with whole blood that is then processed with plasma removal followed by return of the cellular components. During this return phase, bowl contents are mixed with replacement fluid pumped by the plasma pump. An interface detector and line sensor determine when to switch to return mode, detecting when cells begin to exit the centrifuge.[3]

Spectra Optia (Terumo BCT, Lakewood, CO, USA)

The Spectra Optia is a multiple-purpose therapeutic instrument. It uses a circular flexible channel that fits inside a rigid insert. Blood enters the channel with the RBC, WBC, and platelets pushed to the outer wall while the plasma remains on the inner wall. A connector with tubing ports at different distances from the outer wall is used to selectively remove plasma or cells. The plasma port, near the center, is connected to the plasma pump, which delivers plasma to the waste bag. The packed cell port is near the channel outer wall, and cells leave the centrifuge and are combined with replacement fluid in the return reservoir. A return pump delivers the return reservoir contents to the patient. The Spectra Optia has a camera system (Automated Interface Management [AIM]) to monitor the buffy coat. When the buffy coat builds up, it is returned to the patient while plasma removal continues. The Spectra Optia ECV is 185 ml. The instrument can determine volume of plasma to remove, replacement volumes, and fluid balance.[3]

Selective removal of plasma components

Kaneka MA-03 Liposorber (Kaneka Pharma America, LLC, New York, NY, USA)

This system selectively removes low-density lipoprotein (LDL) cholesterol, very-low-density lipoprotein (VLDL) cholesterol, and lipoprotein(a) (Lp^a) with minimal high-density lipoprotein (HDL) cholesterol removal. Heparin anticoagulated blood is pumped into a hollow fiber filter. Cells exit the hollow fibers while plasma passes through the walls and is delivered to one of two affinity columns. The affinity columns contain negatively charged dextran sulfate bound to cellulose beads, which electrostatically bind the positively charged apolipoprotein B containing LDL, VLDL, and Lp^a. Treated plasma then passes through a conductivity meter, to detect the presence of 4.1% sodium chloride and a particle filter. It is mixed with the cells, warmed to 37 °C, and returned to the patient. After the affinity column has been perfused with 500–600 ml of plasma, flow is diverted to the second column and the first column is flushed with Lactated Ringer's solution to remove residual plasma. The column is regenerated with 4.1% sodium chloride, which removes the lipoproteins. The column is perfused with Lactated Ringer's solution to rinse residual 4.1% sodium chloride to the waste bag. Plasma flow is switched to the first column, and the second is regenerated. These cycles continue until 1.5 plasma volumes have been treated. The MA-03 is a double-needle system, and the ECV is 400 ml (230 ml plasma and 170 ml blood).[3]

B Braun Plasmat Futura Heparin-Induced Extracorporeal LDL Precipitation (HELP) System (B. Braun Medical, Inc., Bethlehem, PA, USA)

This system selectively removes LDL, VLDL, and Lp^a with minimal HDL removal. Heparin anticoagulated blood is separated into plasma and cells using a hollow fiber plasma separator. The plasma is diluted with pH 4.84 heparin–sodium acetate solution to lower the pH to 5.1. The negatively charged heparin at the low pH precipitates positively charged LDL, VLDL, and Lp^a as well as some fibrinogen. A filter removes this precipitate with a heparin adsorber, then removes excess heparin, and a dialysis module removes excess volume and adjusts the plasma to a physiologic pH. The plasma is then mixed with the cells and returned to the patient. The system has an ECV of 450 ml (300 ml plasma and 150 ml blood).[3]

Therapeutic cytoreductions

Only one instrument has been cleared by the FDA for therapeutic leukocytapheresis and therapeutic thrombocytapheresis, the COBE Spectra (Terumo BCT, Lakewood, CO, USA). The procedures are modifications of donor WBC and platelet collections performed on this device. For acute leukemia with increased circulating blasts, the mononuclear cell (MNC) program is used. For removal of mature granulocytes, the polymorphonuclear (PMN) program is used. Both allow collection of a larger product volume and processing of a larger blood volume than the corresponding donor procedures. Procedure duration depends upon blood volume treated or processing time. Therapeutic thrombocytapheresis on the COBE Spectra uses a non-leukocyte-reduced platepheresis kit.[3]

The Spectra Optia is approved for therapeutic thrombocytapheresis and leukocytapheresis in Europe and, once FDA clearance has been obtained, will replace the COBE Spectra in the United States.

Extracorporeal photopheresis

UVAR-XTS (Therakos, West Chester, PA, USA)

This device performs extracorporeal photopheresis (ECP) and will be replaced by the CELLEX (see the "CELLEX" subsection). The UVAR-XTS can use two sizes of Latham conical bowls depending upon the patient's blood volume, 225 ml and 125 ml. Heparin anticoagulated blood enters the Latham bowl (see the description of the LN9000 in the "Blood Donor Apheresis" section). Exiting plasma is diverted to the plasma-return bag until the buffy coat (WBC and platelets) reaches the shoulder of the bowl, when an optical sensor triggers an elutriation process. Rapidly flowing plasma enters the bowl, collecting the buffy coat into the recirculation bag. A line sensor measures the hematocrit leaving the bowl, and when a defined hematocrit is reached, the flushing stops and the bowl stops rotating. The plasma in the plasma-return bag is then pumped through the bowl to empty the RBCs. If the large bowl is used, two cycles are processed. If the small bowl is used, then five cycles are processed. During the last cycle, the contents of the recirculation bag are pumped into the empty bowl, and blood from the patient is used to bring the buffy coat to the top of the bowl, where it is harvested into the recirculation bag. The remaining bowl contents are returned. The medication, 8-methoxypsoralen, is added to the recirculation bag, and the contents are pumped into a flat, clear plastic chamber located between ultraviolet-A (UVA) lights that photoactivate the buffy coat. Photoactivation time is dependent on the buffy coat volume, hematocrit, and UVA light intensity. The treated cells are returned after photo activation. The device is unique in that it uses pneumatic pumps, rather than roller pumps. It is capable of only single-needle access. The ECV is variable depending on bowl size, hematocrit, and stage of the procedure, ranging from 220 to 620 ml.[3]

CELLEX (Therakos, West Chester, PA, USA)

This system utilizes a modified Latham bowl that fills from the center rather than the bottom. Plasma is continually pushed out the top of the bowl, and RBCs are drawn from the bottom. This allows continuous flow through the bowl, which is more efficient than the cycles utilized by the UVAR-XTS, reducing procedure time and ECV while allowing double-needle access. Heparinized blood enters the rotating bowl with the red cells migrating to the bottom while plasma rises to the top, where it is pushed into the return bag. The buffy coat is positioned on the shoulder of the bowl by the red cell pump and monitored by a laser optical system. When 1460 ml has been processed, plasma is pumped into the bowl to loosen the buffy coat, which is transferred to the treatment bag. A hematocrit line sensor determines when to stop the harvest by monitoring for red cells entering the line. The buffy coat is then pumped through the line sensor and photoactivation chamber to determine the product hematocrit and volume, which is used to adjust the photoactivation length. The same medication used with the UVAR-XTS is added to the bag and photoactivation is performed, after which the buffy coat is returned. Either double- or single-needle procedures can be performed with the ECV (being 216 ml or 266 ml, respectively).[3]

Evidence supporting therapeutic apheresis use

Between 1976 and 2012, 8433 English language therapeutic apheresis articles were published with 138, less than 2%, representing randomized controlled trials.[24,25] The mean number of enrolled subjects in the randomized controlled trials was only 56 patients, indicating that most were inadequately powered.[24,25] The total

Table 32.6 American Society for Apheresis categories

ASFA Category	Definition
I	First-line therapy, either stand-alone or in conjunction with other therapies.
II	Second-line therapy, either stand-alone or in conjunction with other therapies.
III	Optimum role of apheresis is not established; therefore, decision making should be individualized based upon the patient's clinical situation.
IV	Evidence demonstrates or suggests that apheresis is ineffective or harmful.

ASFA, American Society for Apheresis.

Source: Schwartz *et al.* (2013).[2] Reproduced with permission of Wiley.

number of articles and randomized controlled trials published per year increased between the periods of 1976–1999 and 2000–2012, but the number of subjects enrolled in the randomized trials did not.[25]

Given the limited quality of the apheresis medical literature, what resources are available to determine appropriate evidence-based practice? Three therapeutic apheresis practice guidelines have been published.[2,26,27] In 2011, the American Academy of Neurology published TPE guidelines for neurologic diseases.[26] These examined randomized controlled trials and assessed their quality. They did not provide treatment guidance concerning patient care issues (e.g., frequency, treatment duration, replacement fluid, etc.).[26] In 2014, the European Academy of Dermatology and Venereology published guidelines on ECP use.[27] These include recommendations concerning patient selection, treatment schedule, and response assessment for 10 ECP indications.[27] In 2013, the American Society for Apheresis (ASFA) published their sixth edition of guidelines covering the therapeutic procedures listed in Table 32.1.[2]

ASFA guidelines are published every three years and review the English language therapeutic apheresis literature. They consider all of the available literature, not just randomized controlled trials. The 2013 document provided guidance on 78 conditions, those for which sufficient published evidence existed.[2] For each, the ASFA guidelines provide an ASFA Category (Table 32.6) that describes the role of apheresis in disease treatment and a recommendation grade.[2] Based upon the GRADE system,[28] the recommendation is either a strong (Grade 1) or weak recommendation (Grade 2) to perform or, in the case of Category IV indications (see Table 32.6), not perform the procedure. It also includes an assessment of published evidence quality (A, *high*; B, *moderate*; and C, *low to very low*).[28] The 2013 ASFA Categories and recommendations are given in Table 32.7. The ASFA guidelines also provide a standardized, single-page "fact sheet" for each indication that includes the elements listed in Table 32.8.[2]

Therapeutic apheresis clinical decision making

How does one determine if a patient should undergo a procedure? For each patient, a series of questions, as described by Shaz *et al.*[29] and listed in Table 32.9, should first be considered. These questions can be answered by utilizing the ASFA Guidelines or by reviewing the relevant medical literature, and assessing the patient. This determines the likelihood that the procedure will benefit the patient. After considering the published evidence and determining the patient is similar to those described in the literature, the next step is to consider individual patient characteristics that will influence the risk–benefit ratio. Factors to considered are given in

Table 32.7 2013 ASFA category and recommendation grades[2,30]

Disease	Apheresis Treatment	ASFA Category	Recommendation Grade
ABO-incompatible hematopoietic stem cell transplantation			
Bone marrow (major ABO incompatible)	TPE	II	1B
Apheresis (major ABO incompatible)	TPE	II	2B
Apheresis (major ABO incompatible)	Red cell exchange	III	2C
ABO-incompatible liver transplantation			
Living donor	TPE	I	1C
Deceased donor	TPE	III	2C
Humoral rejection	TPE	III	2C
ABO-incompatible renal transplantation			
Living donor	TPE	I	1B
Deceased donor, non-A1	TPE	IV	1B
Humoral rejection	TPE	II	1B
Acute disseminated encephalomyelitis	TPE	II	2C
Acute inflammatory demyelinating polyneuropathy (Gullain-Barré syndrome)			
Prior to IVIG	TPE	I	1A
IVIG failure	TPE	III	2C
Acute liver failure	TPE	III	2B
Age-related macular degeneration	Rheopheresis	I	1B
Amyloidosis, systemic	TPE	IV	2C
Amyotrophic lateral sclerosis	TPE	IV	1C
ANCA-associated rapidly progressive glomerulonephritis (polyangitis, Wegner granulomatosis)			
Dialysis dependent	TPE	I	1A
Diffuse alveolar hemorrhage	TPE	I	1C
Dialysis independent	TPE	III	2C
Antiglomerular basement membrane antibody disease (Goodpasture syndrome)			
Dialysis dependent	TPE	III	2B
Diffuse alveolar hemorrhage	TPE	I	1C
Dialysis independent	TPE	I	1B
Aplastic anemia	TPE	III	2C
Autoimmune hemolytic anemia			
Severe warm autoimmune hemolytic anemia	TPE	III	2C
Severe cold agglutinin disease	TPE	II	2C
Babesiosis			
Severe	Red cell exchange	I	1C
High-risk population	Red cell exchange	II	2C
Burn shock resuscitation	TPE	III	2B
Cardiac transplantation			
Rejection prophylaxis	ECP	II	2A
Cellular rejection	ECP	II	1B
Desensitization due to donor-specific HLA antibodies	TPE	III	2C
Antibody-mediated rejection	TPE	III	2C
Catastrophic antiphospholipid antibody syndrome	TPE	II	2C
Chronic focal encephalitis (Rasmussen encephalitis)	TPE	III	2C
	IA	III	2C
Chronic inflammatory demyelinating polyradiculopathy	TPE	I	1B
Coagulation factor inhibitors			
Alloantibody	TPE	IV	2C
	IA	III	2B
Autoantibody	TPE	III	2C
	IA	III	1C
Cryoglobulinemia, severe/symptomatic	TPE	I	2A
	IA	II	2B
Cutaneous T-cell lymphoma/Sézary syndrome			
Erythrodermic	ECP	I	1B
Non-erythrodermic	ECP	III	2C
Dermatomyositis/polymyositis	TPE	IV	2A
	Leukocytapheresis	IV	2A
Dilated cardiomyopathy, idiopathic: NYHA II–IV	TPE	III	2C
	IA	II	1B
Familial hypercholesterolemia			
Homozygous	Lipid apheresis	I	1A
Heterozygous	Lipid apheresis	II	1A
Homozygous with small blood volume	TPE	II	1C
Focal segmental glomerulosclerosis, recurrent after transplantation	TPE	I	1B
Graft-versus-host disease			
Chronic skin	ECP	II	1B
Acute skin	ECP	II	1C
Acute or chronic nonskin	ECP	III	2B
Hemolytic uremic syndrome, atypical			
Inherited complement pathway regulatory deficiency	TPE	II	2C
Factor H autoantibodies	TPE	I	2C
Inherited MCP deficiency	TPE	IV	1C

Table 32.7 (*Continued*)

Disease	Apheresis Treatment	ASFA Category	Recommendation Grade
Hemolytic uremic syndrome, infection-associated			
Diarrhea-associated	TPE	IV	1C
S. pneumonia-associated	TPE	III	2C
Henoch–Schönlein purpura, severe			
Cresentic glomerulonephritis	TPE	III	2C
Severe extrarenal disease	TPE	III	2C
Heparin induced thrombocytopenia			
Pre-cardiopulmonary bypass	TPE	III	2C
Thrombosis	TPE	III	2C
Hereditary hemochromatosis	Erythrocytapheresis	I	1B
Hyperleukocytosis			
Symptomatic leukostasis	Leukocytapheresis	I	1B
Prophylaxis	Leukocytapheresis	III	2C
Hypertriglyceridemic pancreatitis	TPE	III	2C
Hyperviscosity in monoclonal gammopathies			
Symptomatic	TPE	I	1B
Prophylaxis prior to rituximab therapy	TPE	I	1C
IgA nephropathy			
Crescentic glomerulonephritis	TPE	III	2B
Chronic progressive	TPE	III	2C
Immune thrombocytopenic purpura, refractory	TPE	IV	2C
	IA	III	2C
Immune complex rapidly progressive glomerulonephritis	TPE	III	2B
Inclusion body myositis	TPE	IV	2C
	Leukocytapheresis	IV	2C
Inflammatory bowel disease			
Ulcerative colitis	Adsorptive cytapheresis	II	2B
Crohn disease	Adsorptive cytapheresis	III	1B
	ECP	III	2C
Lambert–Eaton myasthenic syndrome	TPE	II	2C
Lipoprotein(a) hyperlipoproteinemia	LDL apheresis	II	1B
Lung allograft rejection			
Bronchiolitis obliterans syndrome	ECP	II	1C
Antibody-mediated rejection	TPE	III	2C
Malaria, severe	Red cell exchange	II	2B
Multiple sclerosis			
Acute central nervous system demyelination	TPE	II	1B
	IA	III	2C
Chronic progressive	TPE	III	2B
Myasthenia gravis			
Moderate to severe	TPE	I	1B
Pre-thymectomy	TPE	I	1C
Myeloma cast nephropathy	TPE	II	2B
Nephrogenic systemic fibrosis	TPE	III	2C
	ECP	III	2C
Neuromyelitis optica			
Acute demyelination	TPE	II	1B
Maintenance therapy	TPE	III	2C
Overdose, envenomation, poisoning			
Mushroom poisoning	TPE	II	2C
Envenomation	TPE	III	2C
Natalizumab and progressive multifocal leukoencephalopathy	TPE	III	2C
Other compounds	TPE	III	2C
Paraneoplastic neurologic syndromes	TPE	III	2C
	IA	III	2C
Paraproteinemic demyelinating polyneuropathies			
IgG/IgA	TPE	I	1B
	IA	III	2C
IgM	TPE	I	1C
	IA	III	2C
Multiple myeloma	TPE	III	2C
Pediatric autoimmune neuropsychiatric disorders associated with streptococcal infections (PANDAS)	TPE	I	1B
Pemphigus vulgaris	TPE	III	2C
	ECP	III	2C
	IA	III	2C
Peripheral vascular disease	LDL apheresis	III	2C
Phytanic acid storage disease (Refsum disease)	TPE	II	2C
	LDL apheresis	II	2C
Polycythemia vera and erythrocytosis			
Polycythemia vera	Erythrocytapheresis	I	1B

(*continued*)

Table 32.7 (Continued)

Disease	Apheresis Treatment	ASFA Category	Recommendation Grade
Secondary erythrocytosis	Erythrocytapheresis	III	1C
Polyneuropathy, organomegaly, endocrinopathy, M protein, and skin change (POEMS)	TPE	IV	1C
Posttransfusion purpura	TPE	III	2C
Psoriasis			
	TPE	IV	2C
	Adsorptive cytapheresis	III	2C
	Lymphocytapheresis	III	2C
	ECP	III	2B
Pure red cell aplasia	TPE	III	2C
Red cell alloimmunization during pregnancy			
Prior to ability to perform intrauterine transfusion	TPE	III	2C
Renal transplantation			
Desensitization due to donor-specific HLA antibodies, living donor	TPE	I	1B
Desensitization due to donor-specific HLA antibodies, deceased donor	TPE	III	2C
Antibody-mediated rejection	TPE	I	1B
Schizophrenia	TPE	IV	1A
Scleroderma (progressive systemic sclerosis)	TPE	III	2C
	ECP	III	2B
Sepsis with multi-organ failure	TPE	III	2B
Sickle cell disease			
Acute stroke	Red cell exchange	I	1C
Acute chest syndrome, severe	Red cell exchange	II	1C
Hepatic sequestration	Red cell exchange	III	2C
Intrahepatic cholestasis	Red cell exchange	III	2C
Multi-organ failure	Red cell exchange	III	2C
Preoperative management	Red cell exchange	III	2A
Prevention of iron overload	Red cell exchange	II	1C
Priapism	Red cell exchange	III	2C
Prophylaxis for stroke prevention	Red cell exchange	II	1C
Splenic sequestration	Red cell exchange	III	2C
Vaso-occlusive pain crisis	Red cell exchange	III	2C
Stiff-person syndrome	TPE	III	2C
Sudden sensorineural hearing loss	TPE	III	2C
	Rheopheresis	III	2A
	Lipid apheresis	III	2A
Sydenham chorea	TPE	I	1B
Systemic lupus erythematosus			
Nephritis	TPE	IV	1B
Severe extrarenal manifestations	TPE	II	2C
Thrombocytosis			
Symptomatic	Thrombocytapheresis	II	2C
Prophylactic	Thrombocytapheresis	III	2C
Thrombotic microangiopathy, drug-associated			
Ticlopidine	TPE	I	1B
Clopidogrel	TPE	III	2B
Cyclosporine/tacrolimus	TPE	III	2C
Gemcitabine	TPE	IV	2C
Quinine	TPE	IV	2C
Thrombotic microangiopathy, hematopoietic stem cell transplant associated	TPE	III	2C
Thrombotic thrombocytopenic purpura	TPE	I	1A
Thyroid storm	TPE	III	2C
Toxic epidermal necrolysis (Lyell syndrome), refractory	TPE	III	2B
Voltage-gated potassium channel autoantibody disease	TPE	II	1C
Wilson disease, fulminant hemolysis	TPE	I	1C

ASFA, American Society for Apheresis; ECP, extracorporeal photochemotherapy, IA, immunoadsorption; IgA, immunoglobulin A; IgG, immunoglobulin G; IgM, immunoglobulin M; MCP, membrane cofactor protein; NYHA, New York Heart Association; TPE, therapeutic plasma exchange.

Source: Winters and Chun (2014).[30] Reproduced with permission.

Table 32.10.[29] If the benefit outweighs the risk, for ASFA categorized indications, the guidelines can be used to determine the role of apheresis and the frequency, treatment duration, and other parameters.[30]

"Uncategorized" indications

Not all disorders treated with apheresis are included in the ASFA Guidelines due to limited published evidence. How should such an "uncategorized" indication be approached? Figure 32.1 provides a schema for evaluating such indications. The literature should be examined and then considered in the context of McLeod's criteria (Table 32.11).[30,31] If the disorder's pathophysiology is understood or at least hypothesized, and the apheresis procedure could potentially modify this (e.g., the pathologic substance has a molecular weight that allows removal by TPE and is located in the intravascular space) and there is evidence of efficacy in the disorder or a similar disease, then the patient should be evaluated against those factors listed in Table 32.10 to determine the risk–benefit

Table 32.8 Elements included in the ASFA guidelines

Element	Description
Disease incidence	Incidence per 100,000 of the population per year
Apheresis procedure	The procedure used to treat the disorder (e.g., therapeutic plasma exchange), with some diseases having multiple different procedure types utilized
Summary of the literature	A table listing the total number or published reports (including treated patients) broken down by randomized controlled trials, controlled trials, case series, and case reports
Disease description	A description of the disease, including the signs, symptoms, and typical presentation as well as the pathophysiology
Disease management	A description of the non-apheresis therapies used to treat the disorder
Rationale for the use of therapeutic apheresis	A discussion of how the apheresis treatments may modify the pathophysiology of the disorder as well as a discussion of significant published literature, especially randomized controlled trials
Technical notes	A description of the specific disorder treatment, including volume treated, replacement fluid (if applicable), frequency of treatment, and any other relevant information necessary to safely and effective provide apheresis therapy
Duration and discontinuation of apheresis	A description of the usual course of therapy, including indicators, both clinical and laboratory, of therapy response
References	The references reviewed to create the guidance. In addition, the search terms utilized to identify the articles are also provided to allow the interested reader to replicate the search.

Source: Schwartz et al. (2013).[2] Reproduced with permission of Wiley.

Table 32.10 Factors to be considered when prescribing apheresis treatment

Volume status of the patient
Cardiovascular stability of the patient
Vascular access available in the patient
Risk of central venous access if peripheral access is not available
Impact of apheresis on other treatments (i.e., removal of coagulation factors in a patient with a planned surgical procedure)
Removal or interactions with medications (i.e., removal of antibiotics by plasma exchange)
Effect of the apheresis on the accuracy and interpretation of laboratory tests

Source: Winters and Chun (2014).[30] Reproduced with permission of American Society for Apheresis.

Table 32.11 McLeod's criteria for evaluation of apheresis efficacy[30,31]

Mechanism	Current understanding of the disease process supports a rationale use of apheresis as a treatment.
Correction	The abnormality involved in the disease pathogenesis can be corrected with the apheresis treatment.
Clinical effect	There is evidence that apheresis confers a clinical benefit and not just a statistically significant change in a laboratory parameter.

Source: Winters and Chun (2014).[30] Reproduced with permission of American Society for Apheresis.

ratio.[30] If the potential benefit outweighs the risk, then treatment is appropriate.

Apheresis "prescription"

This defines the treatment parameters and includes the blood volume treated, the treatment frequency, the replacement fluid used, and treatment duration and discontinuation. For ASFA categorized indications, this is included in the guidelines (Table 32.8). In determining these for uncategorized indications, evidence-based rational thought should be utilized.

Volume treated

In exchange procedures, the volume removed is not a fixed amount but rather a volume that considers specific patient characteristics. Blood volume varies depending upon sex, height, and weight. Plasma volume is also dependent upon hematocrit. Simply defining a fixed volume fails to consider these variations and may result in over or undertreatment. There are numerous equations,

Table 32.9 Questions to consider prior to performing therapeutic apheresis[29,30]

Is the patient's diagnosis the most likely diagnosis?
Is the patient similar to other patients reported in the medical literature who were treated with apheresis?
Have standard disease treatments failed, or are they contradicted?
Are there alternate treatments to the apheresis procedure that are of equal efficacy but are less invasive, are less expensive, or have more supporting evidence?
What is the risk–benefit ratio in the patient considering the patient's underlying medical problems and current therapy?

Source: Winters and Chun (2014).[30] Reproduced with permission of American Society for Apheresis.

normograms, and rules of thumb available to determine a patient's blood volume, plasma volume, red cell volume, and so on.[6,32,33] However, modern apheresis devices calculate these for the operator. A discussion of these calculations will not be provided, and the interested reader is referred to apheresis textbooks.[6,32,33]

In exchange procedures, the replacement fluid results in the dilution of the substance that is being removed so that 100% of that substance cannot be removed. In TPE, the removal of a substance limited to the intravascular space is defined by the equation $Y = Y_0 e^{-X}$, where Y is the final concentration of the substance, Y_0 is the initial concentration of the substance, and X is the number of plasma volumes exchanged.[34] Because this is an exponential equation, Y never reaches zero. Table 32.12 lists the fraction removed and fraction remaining after the exchange of various plasma volumes. For a substance that distributes in both the intra- and extravascular compartments, such as IgG, the fraction removed will appear to be less than predicted if the plasma concentration is measured after the procedure. This is due to redistribution during the procedure. The fraction of IgG remaining after a 1 to 1.5 plasma volume exchange will be 50% as opposed to

Table 32.12 Plasma volumes exchanged: fraction removed and remaining

Plasma Volume Removed	Fraction Removed (%)	Fraction Remaining (%)
0.5	40	60
1.0	62	38
1.5	78	22
2.0	85	15
2.5	91	9
3.0	94	6

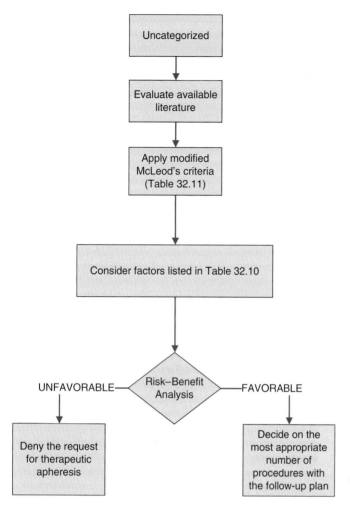

Figure 32.1 Decision making in uncategorized indications. Source: Winters and Chun (2014).[30] Reproduced with permission of American Society for Apheresis.

the 22–38% predicted (Table 32.12). If IgG were measured in the waste plasma, however, more would be present than expected as it is being removed from both the intra- and extravascular space.[34] In TPE, standard practice is to perform a 1.0 to 1.5 plasma volume exchange. The benefit of exchanging additional plasma volumes beyond this does not outweigh the longer procedure risks and exposure to larger replacement fluid amounts.

In red cell exchange procedures, the goal is to reach a defined target, which is referred to as the *fraction of cells remaining* (FCR). The FCR represents the percentage of red cells at the end of the procedure that were not exchanged. In treating sickle cell crises, the target is to reduce the hemoglobin S (HbS) containing red cells to 20–30% of the total circulating red cell mass, which is an FCR of 20–30% if all cells at the procedure start contained HbS. Apheresis devices will calculate the volume of red cells to be exchanged when the patient's sex, height, weight, starting hematocrit, target hematocrit, and target FCR are entered.

For non-exchange procedures, such as hematopoietic progenitor cell collection, ECP, or lipid apheresis, the volume treated is usually determined by a target. In the case of these three procedures, such targets would include the cell dose necessary for a successful transplant, the amount of blood processed to collect a defined buffy coat volume for photoactivation, or a blood volume process defined by the instrument manufacturer.

Replacement fluid

The replacement fluids used in exchange procedures are determined by a number of factors. In a red cell exchange for sickle cell crisis, red cells lacking HbS are utilized, although additional characteristics may be needed such as antigen matching for compatibility or matching to avoid red cell alloimmunization. In TPE, the replacement fluid depends upon the goal of the treatment. In most procedures, the goal is pathologic substance removal (e.g., removal of autoantibodies and immune complexes). The most commonly used replacement is 4–5% human albumin. This colloid has a physiologic solute concentration that avoids fluid shifts seen with crystalloids, avoiding hypovolemia.[32] As 5% albumin is slightly hyperoncotic compared to plasma, saline may be given as a portion of the replacement, usually in a ratio of 70% albumin and 30% normal saline, alternating the two solutions. Albumin has a better side effect profile than plasma as it does not transmit disease, has a lower allergic reaction frequency, and does not produce other reactions associated with plasma (e.g., transfusion-related acute lung injury [TRALI]). Disadvantages are that it is expensive and does not replace all physiologically important substances removed (e.g., coagulation factors).[32]

When the TPE goal is to replace a deficient plasma substance, such as replacing ADAMTS13 in a patient with thrombotic thrombocytopenic purpura or coagulation factors in an individual with acute hepatic failure, plasma is used. In some cases, the final portion of the replacement may consist of plasma to replace the coagulation factors. This is important in bleeding patients, such as pulmonary hemorrhage seen in anti-basement membrane antibody disease, or in patients where a hemostatic challenge will occur, such as surgery or a biopsy.[32] When albumin is used as a replacement fluid, most coagulation factor levels will return to normal within 24 hours except for factors VIII and IX and von Willebrand factor, which reach pre-TPE levels in four hours,[35] and fibrinogen, which reaches 66% of pre-apheresis levels at 72 hours.[36]

In addition to albumin and plasma, there are other replacement fluids that can be used such as starch solutions. However, side effect profiles limit their use.[32] Crystalloid solutions cannot be used as the sole replacement fluid or as more than 40% of the replacement fluid due to a high frequency of hypotensive reactions due to redistribution from the intravascular space.[32]

Frequency

Procedure frequency depends upon a number of factors, including the resynthesis rate, redistribution from the extravascular compartment, and the patient's clinical situation. Procedures are most often performed daily or every other day, with the latter done to allow redistribution of the substance from the extravascular compartment. Every-other-day procedures may also be performed to allow recovery of coagulation factors. In some diseases, where synthesis is slow, greater time between procedures may be possible. In such circumstances, signs and symptoms guide therapy as there is often a lack of correlation between disease severity and laboratory measurement of the pathologic substances involved.

Duration and discontinuation

Treatment duration depends upon the characteristics of the substance being removed. A substance widely distributed in the extravascular compartment will require more procedures than one limited to the intravascular compartment. This can be seen in hyperviscosity due to monoclonal paraproteins. In hyperviscosity in Waldenströms macroglobulinemia, the IgM paraprotein is limited to the intravascular compartment and a single 1 to 1.5 plasma volume exchange will remove approximately 70%. One procedure is usually sufficient to resolve signs and symptoms. In the case of hyperviscosity due to IgG monoclonal paraproteins or IgG autoantibodies, multiple procedures may be required. Simone et al. examined the IgG autoantibody removal in Guillain–Barré syndrome and chronic inflammatory demyelinating polyneuropathy (CIDP). They found that because of the antibody extravascular distribution, in order to deplete the body of 85% of IgG, five 1.25 volume TPEs were necessary.[37] A common treatment schedule for IgG-mediated autoimmune diseases is five 1 to 1.5 plasma volume exchanges over 5–10 days.

For some diseases, specific criteria have been defined for discontinuation. In TTP, the usual criteria are a platelet count ≥150,000/μL, a lactate dehydrogenase level approaching normal, and resolution of neurologic symptoms. Once these are achieved, TPE is continued for two additional days and then either discontinued or weaned, with increasing amounts of time between procedures.[2] There is no published evidence demonstrating the superiority of weaning compared to simply stopping therapy.[2] For other diseases, duration may simply be defined by resolution of symptoms. In CIDP, the goal of treatment is symptom improvement or stabilization, and TPE is continued until this is achieved.[2] For some diseases, published literature has identified fixed procedure numbers. In acute central nervous system demyelinating

disorders such as relapsing and remitting multiple sclerosis, a randomized controlled trial found seven treatments every other day, skipping weekends, to be effective.[38] In Guillain–Barré syndrome, two TPE procedures were found to be superior to none in mild symptoms, four superior to two in moderate symptoms, and six equivalent to four in severely affected patients.[39]

Apheresis complications

Donor reaction overview

Among American Red Cross apheresis donors, the reaction frequencies were 577.5/10,000 for platelet donation and 538.3/10,000 for double red cell donation, compared to 348.9/10,000 for whole blood donation.[40] Severe reactions, requiring outside medical management, occurred in 3.2/10,000 whole blood, 2.9/10,000 platelet, and 2.9/10,000 double red cell donations. The differences were not statistically significant, although the reaction types with severe reactions to whole blood donation were predominantly vasovagal reactions, whereas those due to apheresis donation were phlebotomy related.[40] One study found severe reactions in 0.01% of apheresis platelet donations,[41] a rate 20 times that seen with whole blood donation (0.0005%).[42] Reaction types and frequencies in apheresis and whole blood donors are listed in Table 32.13. Venipuncture-related complications are most frequent with apheresis donation, with first-time donation being the most common risk factor.[40,43]

Therapeutic apheresis reaction overview

Reaction frequencies among patients undergoing therapeutic apheresis vary among studies. McLeod observed reactions in 4.75% of procedures, and Couriel and Weinstein observed reactions in 17%.[10,45] A difference between these studies was that Couriel and Weinstein considered central line complications as an apheresis complication, whereas McLeod did not. In the study by Couriel and Weinstein, all severe reactions, including one patient death, were associated with central line placement.[10] Shemin et al. observed reactions in 36% of TPE procedures.[46] The reactions observed by McLeod were transfusion reactions related to replacement fluids (1.6%), citrate toxicity (1.2%), hypotension (1.0%), vasovagal reactions (1.0%), tachycardia (0.4%), respiratory distress (0.3%), tetany and seizure (0.2%), and chills and rigors (0.2%).[45]

Common apheresis complications
Citrate toxicity

Citrate chelates calcium, making it unavailable for the coagulation cascade. Ionized calcium levels necessary for anticoagulation occur within the apheresis device, not in the patient-donor, due to compensatory mechanisms. Despite this, levels of ionized calcium can reach a point whereby spontaneous neuron depolarization occurs, resulting in the signs and symptoms listed in Table 32.14.[47] The table

Table 32.13 Frequency of reactions among apheresis and whole blood donors

Reaction	Apheresis[43]	Whole Blood[44]
Hematoma	1.15%	9–16%
Citrate toxicity	0.4%	Not applicable
Vasovagal	0.05%	2–5%
Vasovagal with loss of consciousness	0.08%	0.1–0.3%

Table 32.14 Signs and symptoms of hypocalcemia due to citrate toxicity

- Perioral and acral paresthesias
- Shivering
- Lightheadedness
- Twitching
- Tremors
- Nausea and vomiting
- Hypotension
- Carpopedal spasm
- Tetany
- Seizure

Table 32.15 Treatment of hypocalcemia due to citrate

- Perform slow reinfusion to allow metabolism of citrate.
- Increase the blood-to-citrate ratio so that less citrate is given.
- Administer oral calcium carbonate.
- Administer intravenous calcium gluconate or calcium chloride.

Source: Winters (2006).[47] Reproduced with permission of Wiley.

lists these in the order of appearance, so it is possible to avoid more severe reactions by identifying the early, mild symptoms.[47] Hypocalcemia can also suppress myocardial function, induce arrhythmias, and prolong the QT interval.[47] Treatments of hypocalcemia are listed in Table 32.15. Prevention of hypocalcemia includes continuous intravenous calcium administration during the procedure and correction of low levels prior to the start of the procedure.[47]

Although hypocalcemia is commonly thought of as citrate toxicity, citrate anticoagulation results in a variety of electrolyte and acid–base disturbances. The second most common divalent cation in the blood is magnesium, which is also chelated by citric acid. Significant magnesium decline has been seen during apheresis procedures. Signs and symptoms of hypomagnesemia are similar to those of hypocalcemia, including muscle spasms, muscle weakness, decreased vascular tone, and impaired cardiac contractility, and therefore may present as hypocalcemia that fails to respond to calcium supplementation.[47] Treatment consists of procedure discontinuation with magnesium supplementation.

Citrate metabolism generates bicarbonate, producing a metabolic alkalosis.[47] In most circumstances, this is not significant but in the presence of renal impairment and/or increased citrate load when plasma is used as the replacement fluid, severe metabolic alkalosis may occur. Symptoms are nonspecific and present as worsening hypocalcemia, although suppressed respiratory drive can occur as the body tries to compensate. Metabolic alkalosis resolves with time, although in severe cases, dialysis may be necessary.[48]

Metabolic alkalosis can also produce hypokalemia. To buffer the generated bicarbonate, protons leave cells with a resulting net potassium influx to maintain a neutral charge. Significant potassium decline, up to 11% in a large-volume stem cell collection study, can occur.[49] Most patients are asymptomatic, but symptoms can include weakness, hypotonia, and cardiac arrhythmia. Treatment consists of oral or intravenous replacement.[49]

Hypotension

Hypotension is a common reaction during apheresis and can result from numerous mechanisms. As indicated in Table 32.14,

citrate-induced hypocalcemia can cause hypotension. Other causes include hypovolemia, vasovagal reactions, and the presence of angiotensin-converting enzyme inhibitors (ACEIs). In hypovolemia, the amount of blood within the extracorporeal circuit is greater than can be tolerated by the patient-donor. It is characterized by hypotension and tachycardia.[47] Hypovolemia is relatively uncommon among healthy apheresis donors because the total amount of blood withdrawn into the extracorporeal circuit and the collected products is limited to 10.5 mL/Kg.[14] Hypovolemia is common among patients as they may be volume depleted due to underlying disease and poor oral intake. Vasovagal reactions are characterized by low blood pressure with an inappropriately low pulse. Increased parasympathetic output in response to sympathetic drive leads to vasodilation and bradycardia.[50] Both hypovolemia and vasovagal reactions are treated by pausing the procedure, placing the patient-donor in the Trendelenburg position, and infusing fluids.[50]

An uncommon but important cause of hypotension, in patients undergoing TPE with albumin replacement fluid and lipid apheresis with the Kaneka MA-03 Liposorber system, is the use of ACEIs. This reaction is characterized by flushing, hypotension, bradycardia, and dyspnea occurring after a few milliliters of blood is returned to the patient due to bradykinin generation in the apheresis device. Bradykinin may be generated by pre-kallikrein activating factor that is present in some albumin lots.[51] In the Liposorber system, bradykinin is generated when blood comes into contact with the negatively charged dextran sulfate beads within the Liposorber columns.[52] Normally, bradykinin has a short half-life, metabolized by kinase I and kinase II. ACEIs inhibit these, resulting in unopposed bradykinin effects. Treatment options are limited, and when severe reactions occur, procedures must be terminated. Avoiding ACEI administration for 24–48 hours before the procedures can prevent these reactions. ACEIs can be safely administered immediately following the procedures.

Allergic and anaphylactic reactions

In therapeutic apheresis, allergic and anaphylactic reactions are most often triggered by the replacement fluid. Allergic and anaphylactic reactions can occur when either plasma-containing blood products or albumin is used. They can also occur in donor apheresis.[47] In donors, substances present in the disposables or substances used in the procedure trigger histamine release. For example, there have been reports of apheresis platelet donors developing allergic and anaphylactic reactions to residual ethylene oxide present from sterilizing the disposables.[53] In granulocyte collections, hydroxyethyl starch (HES) is used as a sedimenting agent to enhance the product yield. HES can activate the alternate complement pathway generating C3a and C5a, which can trigger mast cell release.[54] Simple allergic reactions can be treated with oral or intravenous antihistamines. In donors, procedures would be discontinued, whereas in patients, they could be resumed after ensuring that the symptoms are not progressing. In severe reactions, procedures should be discontinued but vascular access maintained. Treatment of severe reactions would include administration of epinephrine, fluids, and potentially aminophylline for bronchoconstriction. These patients may also require intubation to maintain their airway. At the end of an apheresis procedure, the contents of the centrifuge are returned to the patient-donor. In the setting of severe allergic or anaphylactic reactions where procedures are stopped early, this should be avoided in order to prevent allergen infusion.

Summary

The term *apheresis* has been used to describe a family of medical procedures for more than 100 years. The use of apheresis to collect blood products for transfusion continues to expand. Apheresis has been used to treat a variety of medical conditions since the 1950s, but its use has been hampered by limited numbers of high-quality randomized controlled trials. Despite this, there continues to be development of new apheresis devices and application of apheresis to new diseases.

Key references

A full reference list for this chapter is available at: http://www.wiley.com/go/simon/transfusion

2 Schwartz J, Winters JL, Padmanabhan A, *et al.* Guidelines on the use of therapeutic apheresis in clinical practice: evidence-based approach from the Apheresis Applications Committee of the American Society for Apheresis. The Sixth Special Issue. *J Clin Apheresis* 2013;**28**:145–284.

3 Burgstaler EA. Current instrumentation for apheresis. In: McLeod BC. Szczepiorkowski ZM. Weinstein R. Winters JL. Eds. *Apheresis: principles and practice*. 3rd ed. Bethesda, MD: AABB Press 2010:95–130.

29 Shaz BH, Winters JL, Bandarenko N, Szczepiorkowski ZM. How we approach an apheresis request for category III, category IV, or non-categorized indication. *Transfusion* 2007;**47**:1963–71.

30 Winters JL, Chun C. Clinical decision making and the American Society for Apheresis guidelines. In: Linz W, Chhibber V, Crookston K, Vrielink H, Eds. *Principles of apheresis technology: technical principles of apheresis medicine*. 5th ed. Vancouver, BC: American Society for Apheresis. 2014:51–75.

32 Introduction to therapeutic apheresis. In: Winters JL, Crookston K, Delaney M, *et al.*, Eds. *Therapeutic apheresis: a physician's handbook*. 4th ed. Bethesda, MD: AABB, **2013**:1–50.

CHAPTER 33

Therapeutic apheresis

Shanna Morgan & Jeffrey McCullough

Department of Laboratory Medicine and Pathology, University of Minnesota Medical School, Minneapolis, MN, USA

Introduction

The pathophysiology or symptoms of some diseases are due to the excessive accumulation of blood cells or plasma constituents. In these situations, blood cell separators ordinarily used to collect blood components by apheresis from normal donors can also be used therapeutically.[1] Therapeutic apheresis includes plasma exchange, red blood cell exchange, therapeutic cytoreduction, photopheresis, and specific selective adsorption. In the United States, in 2006 approximately 112,109 therapeutic apheresis procedures were performed. Subsequent summary data are not available, but therapeutic apheresis is projected to be a $120,000,000 business as of 2015.

Plasma exchange

Techniques of plasma exchange
Instruments

In plasma exchange using blood cell separators, the whole blood enters the instrument, where most of the red cells, leukocytes, and platelets are separated from the cell-poor plasma. This plasma is diverted into a waste bag and is replaced with one or more of several available solutions described in this chapter.

Several instruments can be used, including the Terumo Optia (which is the updated version of the Spectra), Fresenius Kabi Amicus, Fresenius AS104, and Haemonetics MCS. The Terumo and Fresenius instruments are continuous-flow systems that make it easier to control the patient's fluid volume, and the Haemonetics instrument uses repeated cycles of filling and emptying the blood cell separator. In the United States, the Spectra has been the most widely used, and the extent of use of Optia and Amicus instruments is not clear. Details of operating these instruments are not included here. The manufacturer's operating manuals must be used because of the complexity of these procedures. Thorough quality control programs are essential to be sure staff are properly trained, fluids monitored, alarms tested, lines and fluid attachments secured, and medications and replacement solutions used correctly. The plasma removed must be discarded as biohazardous waste.

Vascular access

The majority of therapeutic plasma exchanges (TPEs) will have a withdrawal rate between 60 and 150 ml/minute, allowing most procedures to process one plasma volume in approximately two to three hours. Vascular access for TPE is most commonly via peripheral veins or central venous catheter (CVC), although arteriovenous fistulas or grafts are possible options as well. Factors such as the desired flow rate; the vascular anatomy; patients' mobility and ability to care for a catheter; the urgency, frequency, and anticipated duration of TPE; or whether other treatments that require venous access are needed all help determine the selection of vascular assess.[2] Peripheral venous access is preferable because it can be done immediately and is without the potentially serious risks associated with the use of CVCs. Peripheral venous access is not recommended for children given their small venous caliber.[2] To minimize infusion-related bacteremia, once a vein is selected, a three-inch area of skin should be swabbed with povidone–iodine followed by either isopropyl alcohol or chlorhexidine gluconate.[3,4] In patients who are anxious or particularly sensitive to venipuncture, injected lidocaine 1% or lidocaine/prilocaine anesthetic cream can be of assistance.[5] Forced-air warming blankets, warm compresses, and arm exercises can increase venous blood flow, making venipuncture more successful. The feasibility of using antecubital veins is variable. One study showed only 50% of patients were able to complete a planned course of therapy with only peripheral access.[6] Another study indicated that only 4.4% of patients were considered to have inadequate peripheral venous access.[7] According to the 2007 International Apheresis Registry, peripheral access is more common in Europe and Australia (66–70%) than in Asia and the Americas (2–15%).[8] Unfortunately, CVCs are often required due to small vein caliber, poor vascular tone, or altered mental status or the need for several procedures.[9]

If CVC placement is necessary, the apheresis personnel should be involved to ensure appropriate catheter selection. Poiseuille's equation (in which R is proportional to viscosity × length/radius) states that there are primarily three determinants of resistance to flow in a catheter: radius, length, and viscosity.[10,11] Shorter catheters allow for less resistance to flow with the added benefit of allowing the anticoagulant to reach the blood sooner. A larger diameter offers less resistance and also ensures that a small clot or fibrous sheath will not block the lumen.[10]

Shorter catheters allow for less resistance to flow with the added benefit of allowing the anticoagulant to reach the blood sooner. A larger diameter offers less resistance and also ensures that a small clot or fibrous sheath will not block the lumen.[10] The catheters must have sufficient rigidity so as not to collapse under negative pressure during blood removal.[10,11] A general rule is that if a CVC can

Rossi's Principles of Transfusion Medicine, Fifth Edition. Edited by Toby L. Simon, Jeffrey McCullough, Edward L. Snyder, Bjarte G. Solheim, and Ronald G. Strauss.

support hemodialysis, it will be sufficient for TPE. Double-lumen catheters are most commonly color coded with red for the draw line and blue as the return line. There are potential risks with all catheter tip positions, but it is generally accepted that the tip should be preferentially in the superior vena cava (SVC) or inferior vena cava (IVC), outside the pericardial sac, and should not touch the vein or heart wall at a sharp angle.[12] Radiographic confirmation of the catheter position is necessary prior to use. The majority of evidence-based guidelines on CVC care has been inferred from hemodialysis literature. In order to prevent fibrin sheaths and thrombosis, CVCs must be flushed with saline and locked with an anticoagulant after each use and at regular intervals when not in use. Catheter-locking solutions include heparin, citrate (4%), and tissue plasminogen activator (tPA).[2] Depending on the length of time between catheter flushes, the heparin concentration will range from 100 to 5000 units per mL, with 100 units per mL being used at 24-hour intervals.[2] To reduce the risk of bleeding, the solution should be aspirated if the heparin dose is 1000 units per mL or greater.[2]

Exchange volume

The volume of plasma to be exchanged is usually based on the estimated plasma volume of the patient. Because there is continuous mixing in the patient of replacement solution and patient's plasma, the relationship between the fraction of the unwanted compound remaining and the proportion of the patient's plasma volume exchanged is exponential (Figure 33.1). After exchange equal to the patient's plasma volume, the unwanted component will be reduced to approximately 35% of the initial value. Exchanging two times the patient's plasma volume further reduces the unwanted component only to approximately 15% of the initial value. Because of this diminishing effectiveness, usually one or at most 1.5 times the patient's plasma volume is exchanged. Depending on the size of the patient, this procedure may last between two and four hours.

Because the molecule targeted for removal by TPE is often an immunoglobulin G (IgG) antibody, which is approximately 50% extravascular, and because removal of accessible (i.e., intravascular) IgG becomes progressively less efficient during a TPE procedure, most practitioners limit an exchange to 1–1.5 times the patient's estimated plasma volume. An exchange of this magnitude will remove 60–75% of intravascular material while limiting side effects from depletion of normal plasma components. The intravascular IgG level will rise during the ensuing 1 to 2 days by equilibration with extravascular sources, and further removal by a subsequent exchange can then be undertaken more efficiently. It does not appear that a rebound overshoot in antibody levels occurs after plasma exchange, but rapid re-equilibration of IgG occurs because 50% of IgG is extravascular.[13,14] Because IgG removal is often the goal of TPE, it is worthwhile to consider certain aspects of IgG metabolism. The subclasses IgG1, IgG2, and IgG4 together constitute about 90% of total IgG. Their catabolic rates are proportional to total IgG level, and their half-lives are therefore inversely proportional to concentration. Animal studies concerning levels of specific antibody were interpreted to show that the synthetic rate for IgG exhibits negative feedback, increasing when IgG or specific antibody levels or both are lower.[15] However, Junghans[16] has shown that "knock-out" mice genetically deficient for the FcRn receptor catabolize IgG quite rapidly and maintain very low IgG levels, but they have the same IgG synthetic rate as normal mice. This argues against negative feedback regulation of IgG synthesis and suggests that a reduction in antibody levels induced by TPE would not produce a meaningful "rebound" increase in IgG synthesis.

A reduction of 70% to 85% can be obtained with four to six exchanges in 14 days. The effects of a series of TPEs on extravascular, intravascular, and total IgG are shown schematically in Figure 33.2. Treatment of some patients such as those with TTP or acute Guillain–Barré disease might involve plasma exchange daily for several days.

A model[14] that takes into account the size of the exchange relative to the patient's blood volume, the amount of material available to exchange, the amount of material in both the intravascular and extravascular compartments, the mobility of the material between the pools, and the production and catabolic rate of the material showed good agreement with in vivo observations in patients with hyperbilirubinemia and hypercholesterolemia.

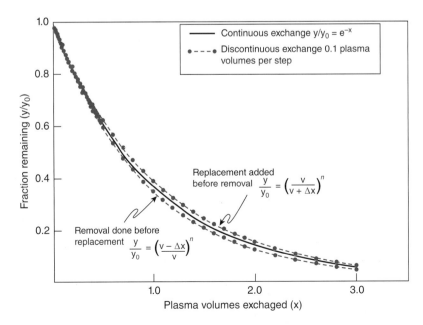

Figure 33.1 Calculated fraction of intravascular substance remaining during a plasma exchange, assuming no equilibration with extravascular material. Source: Chopek and McCullough (1980).[21] Reproduced with permission of American Association of Blood Banks.

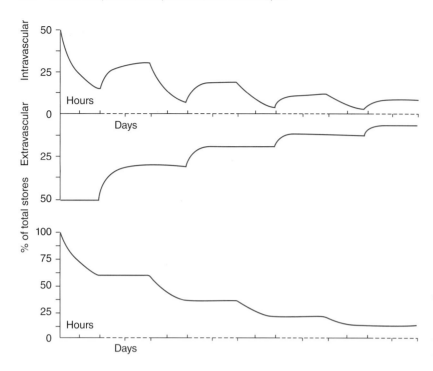

Figure 33.2 Computer-generated curve estimating amounts of intravascular and extravascular immunoglobulin (IgG; upper curves), and total IgG (lower curve) during a course of four one-plasma-volume therapeutic plasma exchanges with an IgG-free replacement medium. Published formulas were used for rates of removal during exchanges and re-equilibration after exchanges. No correction was made for continuing synthesis.

Replacement solutions

Saline replacement alone can suffice when only 500–1000 mL of plasma is removed in a manual plasmapheresis, but in order to maintain intravascular volume, colloid replacement solutions (Table 33.1) are given to the patient that are most commonly equivalent in volume to the amount of plasma removed during the procedure. If a patient is hemodynamically unstable, the management of replacement fluids can be adjusted to compensate. This can be done by infusing the replacement solutions at either (1) less than 100% fluid balance (volume replaced is less than volume removed) if the patient is fluid overloaded, or (2) greater than 100%

fluid balance (volume replaced is greater than volume removed) if the patient is in need of extra fluids.

For the majority of indications, the standard replacement medium is 5% human serum albumin in normal saline;[17] however, substitution of 25–50% of the total with saline has been shown to be well tolerated in certain patient groups.[18] Although it is a pooled product, 5% albumin is preferred over plasma as a source of replacement colloid because (1) it is treated to inactivate blood-borne pathogens, (2) it can be given without regard to blood type, and (3) it does not require thawing or other preparation before use. Transient loss of coagulation factors and other plasma proteins that occurs with albumin solution replacement is mild enough that fresh frozen plasma (FFP) replacement is not typically warranted in patients without known coagulation disorders. An exception to this might be during a series of several daily procedures when it would be prudent to monitor the fibrinogen level and platelet count to assess the need for platelets, FFP, or cryoprecipitate. When there is a need to replace essential plasma constituents, such as with TTP or depleted coagulation factors, FFP should be used. The advantages of plasma include supplementation of immunoglobulins, antithrombin, and fibrinogen, along with other proteins. The disadvantages of plasma include a viral transmission risk, an increased citrate load, ABO incompatibility risk, allergic reactions, and the potential for sensitization. Partial replacement with saline (crystalloid) can be used; however, this should not exceed 25–30% of the replacement volume.[18]

There are a few circumstances in which replacement of patient plasma with donor plasma is used. Patients with ITP customarily receive exchanges with FFP in light of abundant evidence that patients with thrombotic thrombocytopenic purpura (TTP) respond better to plasma than to albumin. Cryoprecipitate-reduced plasma is also effective for this purpose.[19] Some plasma may also be given toward the end of an exchange to patients with preexisting thrombocytopenia or humoral coagulopathy, who are considered to be at increased risk for bleeding complications when the dilutional

Table 33.1 Colloid replacement fluids for TPE

Fluid	Advantages	Disadvantages
5% Albumin	Virus inactivation Ease of use Reactions rare	High cost Most proteins not replaced
Single-donor plasma*	All proteins replaced	High cost Inconvenient† Citrate reactions Urticaria Viral infection risk
Solvent/detergent-treated plasma	All proteins partially replaced‡ Lipid-coated viruses inactivated	Very high cost Inconvenient† Citrate reactions Urticaria Pooled product Unavailable in US
6% Hetastarch	Low cost Viral safety Ease of use Slow catabolism	No proteins replaced Hypotensive reactions Dosage limit

* Fresh frozen plasma or plasma cryoprecipitate reduced.
† Must be thawed before use; must match patient ABO group.
‡ Coagulation factors ≥80% of normal levels.
TPE, therapeutic plasma exchange; US, United States.

coagulopathy of an albumin exchange is superimposed, or to patients with ongoing blood loss regardless of pretreatment coagulation status.

One group reported infusing a solution of hydroxyethyl starch (HES), a less costly volume expander, in the early part of an exchange.[20] They reason that recommended dosage limitations for HES will not actually be exceeded, because much of the infused HES will be removed in exchange for albumin infused later. This group has seen successes, albeit with a higher incidence of side effects. HES is not recommended for patients with renal impairment, underlying coagulopathy, or a history of hypersensitivity to HES.

The apheresis physician should determine whether any combination of replacement fluids is used and, if so, the relative proportions of each fluid. This should be based upon the patient's cardiovascular stability, underlying disease, frequency of procedures, coagulation status, and cost.

Biochemical changes resulting from plasma exchange

Removal of such a large volume of plasma has several biochemical effects (Table 33.2).[21–23] Because some platelets are in the plasma being removed, there is about a 30% decrease in the platelet count, which takes about three days to return to baseline. The changes in the proteins IgG, IgM, IgA, factor V, ferritin, transferrin, lactic dehydrogenase, serum glutamic oxaloacetic transaminase, and alkaline phosphatase follow closely the decrease expected based on the volume of plasma removed.[21,22] When no FFP is used for replacement, coagulation test results are abnormal at the end of the plasma exchange. For instance, the prothrombin time is usually 20 seconds or more, the partial thromboplastin time is more than 180 seconds,

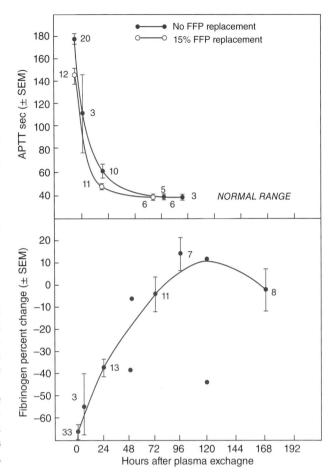

Figure 33.3 Normalization of fibrinogen level and activated partial thromboplastin time after plasma exchange using albumin for replacement.

and the fibrinogen is decreased by about 70%.[21,23] These test values return to baseline in about 24 hours, except fibrinogen, which normalizes in 72 hours[21,22] (Figure 33.3).

Complement components C3, C4, and CH50 can be depleted when albumin is used as the replacement fluid. Because of its rapid rate of synthesis, however, complement is not depleted unless plasma exchange is done daily for several days.[24]

There are no clinically important changes in electrolytes as a result of plasma exchange (Table 33.2). Because citrate is usually used as the anticoagulant, and it exerts its effect by binding calcium, an important consideration is the ionized calcium level. If FFP is used for replacement, this provides additional citrate. Citrate toxicity is the result of the hypocalcemia, not the citrate itself. The hypocalcemia may cause symptoms of paresthesia, muscle cramping, tremors, shivering, lightheadedness, and anxiety; when more severe, it can cause grand mal seizures, tetany, and, most dangerous of all, electrocardiographic abnormalities (Figure 33.4). Very low ionized calcium levels may cause abnormal coagulation tests, but hemorrhage is not a result of hypocalcemia because severe cardiac arrhythmias occur first. Studies of citrate and calcium metabolism during normal-donor plateletpheresis have established that symptoms only begin to occur when the rate of citrate infusion exceeds 60 mg/kg/hour.[25–27] Although there is some reduction in ionized calcium levels even when albumin is used as the

Table 33.2 Comparison of changes induced by plasma exchange of 1.0 to 1.5 plasma volumes with equal volume replacement

	Albumin Replacement	FFP Replacement
Hematology	↓ Platelets (30% to 50%) ↑ Granulocytes (2000 to 3000/mL) ↓ Hemoglobin (10% to 15%)	↓ Platelets (30% to 50%) ↑ Granulocytes (2000 to 3000/mL) No change in hemoglobin
Proteins	↓ Pathological antibodies (60% to 75%) (60% to 75%) ↓ All other proteins (60% to 75%) Long-term effects depend upon TER, FCR, and S (see text)	↓ Pathological antibodies All other proteins change to approximate levels present in FFP
Coagulation	↓ Individual factors (60% to 75%) Transient coagulopathy (24 to 48 hours)	All factors approximate levels in FFP
Electrolytes	Slight ↓ potassium Albumin: Ø Bicarbonate (6 mEq/L) ↑ Chloride (4 mEq/L) PPF: ↑ Bicarbonate ↓ Chloride	↓ Potassium (0.7 mEq/L) ↑ Bicarbonate (3 mEq/L) ↓ Chloride (6 mEq/L)
Citrate and calcium	Slight ↑ citrate (0.2 mM/L) ↓ Total calcium (1.4 mg/dL) ↓ Ionized calcium (0.5 mEq/L)	↑ Citrate (1.1 mM/L) Slight ↓ total calcium (0.3 mg/dL) ↓ Ionized calcium (0.6 mEq/L)

FCR, Fractional catabolic rate; FFP, fresh frozen plasma; PPF, plasma protein fraction; S, synthesis; TER, transcapillary escape rate.

Source: Chopek and McCullough (1980).[21] Reproduced with permission of American Association of Blood Banks.

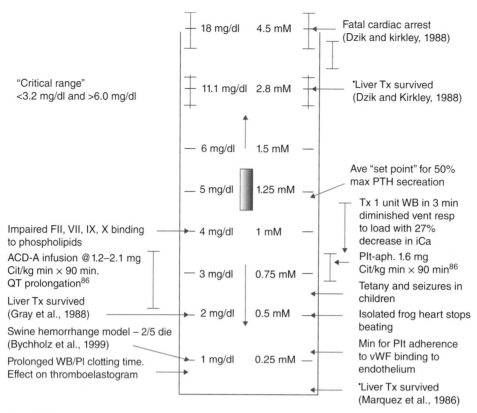

Figure 33.4 Relationship of clinical signs and symptoms to ionized calcium concentration.

replacement solution,[21,28] the citrate infusion rates are below 60 mg/kg/hour and only approach this rate when FFP is used and the flow rates are substantial. Thus, supplementation with calcium during plasma exchange should be based on each patient's situation.

The differences between albumin and FFP as replacement solutions are summarized in Table 33.2.

Complications of plasma exchange

Apheresis of normal donors for the production of blood components is well tolerated with few side effects and only very rare serious complications. However, therapeutic apheresis is carried out in ill patients who should not be expected to react the same as a healthy donor.[29] Deaths have occurred due to therapeutic apheresis, and the mortality rate is estimated to be three per 10,000 procedures.[30,31] Most deaths have resulted from cardiac or respiratory arrest, but deaths due to anaphylaxis, pulmonary embolus, and vascular perforation have also been reported.[30,31] The nature and incidence of complications will depend somewhat on the condition of the patient prior to plasma exchange. In one comprehensive report of complications of plasma exchange, side effects occurred during 12% of procedures and involved 40% of patients.[32] The incidence of severe complications was 0.5% of procedures. A national registry of therapeutic apheresis procedures in the former East Germany reported complications in 22% of 1945 procedures in 419 patients.[33] There were severe complications in 2%, including cardiac arrhythmia, bronchospasm, adult respiratory distress syndrome (ARDS), and thromboembolic problems. Of the 419 patients, 87 died; of these, 64 died of their underlying disease and 19 of related causes not thought to be due to the plasma exchange. Twelve patients died during or immediately after the plasma exchange, and four of these

fatalities were thought to be due to the apheresis procedure.[33] Two of these fatalities resulted from ARDS, one from myocardial infarction, and one from pulmonary embolus. The complication rate was almost twice as great when FFP was used as the replacement solution compared to albumin, although the nature of the complications was not described. The Canadian Apheresis Study Group reported that adverse reactions occurred in about 9% of 58,000 procedures.[34] About two-thirds of these were mild, and only 8% were severe, resulting in a severe reaction rate of 7 per 1,000 procedures.[34]

The complications of plasma exchange are due to vascular access, replacement solutions, or the procedure itself.

Vascular access

Placement of vascular access devices is often required, although peripheral venous access should be used whenever possible. There are numerous complications associated with catheters, some of which can be fatal. Vascular access devices may cause either immediate or delayed adverse effects. Immediate adverse effects include bleeding, arterial puncture, arrhythmia, air embolism, thoracic duct injury, catheter malposition, pneumothorax, and hemothorax.[35–37] Delayed complications include infection, venous thrombosis, venous sclerosis, catheter migration, catheter embolization, myocardial perforation, and nerve injury.[2,35,36,38–40] Complications with CVCs differ with insertion sites and physician experience, with more than 15% of patients experiencing some type of complication.[41–43] In one study of 385 CVC procedures, there was an overall mechanical complications rate of 33%.[36] Another study showed that 11% (3 of 28) of CVCs placed in patients undergoing TPE procedures experienced life-threatening complications associated with catheter use. These complications were pneumothorax, air embolus upon removal, and catheter-related bloodstream infection.[6] Infectious complications range from 5% to 26%; however, the implementation of the Pronovost checklist has been shown to reduce catheter-related bloodstream infections.[41,43,44] The reported rate of vascular access complications associated with TPE procedures is lower when compared to hemodialysis procedures; however, this is likely explained by the longer duration of catheter use along with higher comorbidities in hemodialysis patients.

Replacement solutions

Complications related to replacement solutions include citrate-induced hypocalcemia, coagulation factor depletion, depletion of other functional proteins, electrolyte abnormalities, and transfusion reactions or disease transmission when plasma is used. Adverse reactions to albumin are rare.[45] Exchanges of plasma for albumin produce temporary deficiencies of other plasma proteins, such as coagulation factors; however, these are usually subclinical, and levels are rapidly restored by ongoing synthesis and re-equilibration.[46]

Allergic reactions such as urticaria or mild fevers are rather common even when albumin is the replacement solution. Plasma replacement carries a higher risk of urticarial and hypocalcemic reactions.[47] Progenic reactions can occur to specific lots of albumin.[45,46] An unusual case of hemolysis due to infusion of hypotonic replacement solution has been reported.[48] The 25% albumin was diluted to 5% in sterile water rather than saline, resulting in the hypotonic solution. Depletion of coagulation factors leading to a bleeding diathesis should not occur because this can be prevented by using FFP as the replacement solution. The same is true for other functional proteins and electrolytes. If FFP is used, febrile or allergic reactions are more common because of the proteins in the plasma. Antibodies in the plasma may cause transfusion-related acute lung injury (TRALI),[49] and ABO-incompatible plasma can cause hemolysis.

Adverse effects secondary to any replacement solution include citrate-induced hypocalcemia, citrate-induced metabolic alkalosis, and inadvertent removal of protein-bound medications and therapeutic antibodies. Citrate is used as the anticoagulant in the instrument, and additional exposure will occur if plasma is used as the replacement solution. Citrate-related complications are more likely to occur in patients with liver dysfunction, altered mental status, or pediatric patients, but can occur in any population due to the prolonged exposure throughout the procedure. Mild citrate-induced hypocalcemia may manifest as perioral and distal extremity paresthesias. Patients may also experience gastrointestional issues, such as nausea or vomiting, and muscle cramps. In extreme cases, tetany, prolongation of the QT interval, arrhythmias, or hypotension may occur if the deficiency is not treated (Figure 33.4). It may be prudent to evaluate pre–, intra–, and postprocedural ionized calcium levels and perform electrocardiogram monitoring in patients who are unable to reliably communicate symptoms of hypocalcemia (e.g., pediatric and altered mental status patients). Treatment of citrate-related complications consists of either slowing the rate of the procedure or administration of supplemental calcium. If resolution of symptoms does not occur, evaluation of a magnesium level may be appropriate. The effects of nonplasma replacement solutions have been discussed in this chapter. Hypotonic replacement solutions should not be infused during the procedure as this can cause hemolysis. Donor plasma as the

replacement solution can cause any of the usual reactions to plasma, including hives, anaphylactic reactions, TRALI, and infectious risks. When reactions occur during plasma replacement, it may be difficult to identify the offending unit because of the timing or the reaction in relation to the infusion rate.

Apheresis procedure

Mild reactions are rather common during plasma exchange; they are usually chills (possibly due to infusion of room-temperature replacement solutions) or lightheadedness (possibly due to a vaso-vagal reaction). These can also be symptoms of hypocalcemia due to citrate infusion, and so when the symptoms begin the operator often slows the blood flow rate and the symptoms subside. Another procedure-related complication is hypotension or hypertension due to fluid imbalance. Hypotension can be caused by hypovolemia resulting from the blood required to fill the extracorporeal circuit. Thus, the volume of the circuit in relation to the patient's blood volume must be considered, and for smaller patients it may be desirable to prime the circuit with albumin. If this is done, the dilutional effect of the priming solution must also be considered. Hypertension can occur if the volume of fluid returned exceeds that removed. Thus, it is important that the operator closely monitor the fluid balance during the procedure.

Anaphylactoid reactions consisting of flushing, hypotension, bradycardia, and dyspnea have occurred in patients taking angiotensin-converting enzyme (ACE) inhibitors for hypertension.[50–52] Bradykinin (BK) causes vasodilitation and smooth muscle contraction in some tissues. ACE is the major peptidase that inactivates BK.[52] Patients receiving ACE inhibitor drugs have less ability to inactivate BK. Thus, situations that promote BK release may lead to hypotensive reactions in patients taking ACE inhibitors. This is thought to occur during therapeutic apheresis, possibly due to contact between the patient's blood and the foreign surfaces of plastic bags, tubing, centrifuge systems, and blood filters. Discontinuation of the ACE inhibitor for 24 to 48 hours before therapeutic apheresis prevents these reactions.[52]

Diseases treated by plasma exchange

Three types of plasma molecules may be candidates for therapeutic removal: (1) antibodies that are troublesome because of their binding specificity—these are often autoantibodies; (2) molecules that confer abnormal physical properties, such as hyperviscosity or cold insolubility, on plasma and hence on the blood—these, too, are usually antibodies, although they may be bound in immune complexes; (3) molecules such as low-density lipoproteins (LDLs) that have nonimmune toxicity; and (4) to achieve relatively high levels of a normal plasma constituent that is deficient in the patient's plasma and is not available in a concentrated form for simple infusion. From a theoretic point of view, it is easier to envision a significant therapeutic effect when the molecule to be removed is relatively large and has a relatively long half-life in the circulation, with a correspondingly low rate of synthesis. In practice, the majority of successfully treated disorders are caused by pathogenic IgG, which has these properties.

The American Society for Apheresis (ASFA) has described indication categories for therapeutic apheresis (Table 33.3). The indications are Category I: diseases for which apheresis therapy is a standard first-line therapy, although it may not always be necessary; Category II: diseases in which apheresis is a valuable second-line therapy when first-line measures fail or are poorly tolerated;

Table 33.3 ASFA 2013 indication categories for therapeutic apheresis

Disease Name	TA Modality	Disease Condition	Category	Grade
Acute disseminated encephalomyelitis	TPE		II	2C
Acute inflammatory demyelinating polyneuropathy (Guillain–Barré syndrome)	TPE		I	1A
	TPE	Post IVIG	III	2C
Acute liver failure	TPE		III	2B
Age related macular degeneration, dry	Rheopheresis		I	1B
Amyloidosis, systemic	TPE		IV	2C
Amyotrophic lateral sclerosis	TPE		IV	1C
ANCA (associated rapidly progressive glomerulonephritis) (granulomatosis with polyangiitis; Wegener's granulomatosis)	TPE	Dialysis dependence	I	1A
	TPE	DAH	I	1C
	TPE	Dialysis independence	III	2C
Anti-glomerular basement membrane disease (Goodpasture's syndrome)	TPE	Dialysis dependent and no DAH	III	2B
	TPE	DAH	I	1C
	TPE	Dialysis independence	I	1B
Aplastic anemia; pure red cell aplasia	TPE	Aplastic anemia	III	2C
	TPE	Pure red cell aplasia	III	2C
Autoimmunic hemolytic anemia: WAHA; cold agglutinin disease	TPE	Severe WAHA	III	2C
	TPE	Severe cold agglutinin disease	II	2C
Babesiosis	RBC exchange	Severe	I	1C
	RBC exchange	High-risk population	II	2C
Burn shock resuscitation	TPE		III	2B
Cardiac transplantation	ECP	Rejection prophylaxis	II	2A
	ECP	Cellular or recurrent rejection	II	1B
	TPE	Desensitization, positive crossmatch due to donor specific HLA antibody	III	2C
	TPE	Antibody-mediated rejection	III	2C
Catastrophic antipospholipid syndrome	TPE		II	2C
Chronic focal encephalitis (Rasmussen encephalitis)	TPE		III	2C
	IA		III	2C
Chronic inflammatory demyelinating polyradiculoneuropathy	TPE		I	1B
Coagulation factor inhibitors	TPE	Alloantibody	IV	2C
	IA	Alloantibody	III	2B
	TPE	Autoantibody	III	2C
	IA	Autoantibody	III	1C
Cryoglobulinemia	TPE	Symptomatic/severe	I	2A
	IA	Symptomatic/severe	II	2B
Cutaneous T-cell lymphoma; mycosis fungoides; Sézary syndrome	ECP	Erythrodermic	I	1B
	ECP	Non-erythrodermic	III	2C
Dermatomyositis or polymyositis	TPE		IV	2A
	Leukocytapheresis		IV	2A
Dilated cardiomyopathy, idiopathic	TPE	NYHA II-IV	III	2C
	IA	NYHA II-IV	II	1B
Famalial hypercholesterolemia	LDL apheresis	Homozygotes	I	1A
	LDL apheresis	Heterozygotes	II	1A
	TPE	Homozygotes with small blood volume	II	1C
Focal segmental glomerulosclerosis	TPE	Recurrent in transplanted kidney	I	1B
Graft-versus-host disease	ECP	Skin (chronic)	II	1B
	ECP	Skin (acute)	II	1C
	ECP	Nonskin (acute/chronic)	III	2B
HSCT, ABO incompatible	TPE	Major HPC, marrow	II	1B
	TPE	Major HPC, apheresis	II	2B
	RBC exchange	Minor HPC, apheresis	III	2C
Hemolytic uremic syndrome, atypical	TPE	Complement gene mutations	II	2C
	TPE	Factor H antibodies	I	2C
	TPE	MCP mutations	IV	1C
Hemolytic uremic syndrome, infection-associated	TPE	Shiga toxin associated	IV	1C
	TPE	*S. pneumoniae* associated	III	2C
Henoch–Schönlein purpura	TPE	Crescentic	III	2C
	TPE	Severe extrarenal disease	III	2C
Heparin-induced thrombocytponia	TPE	Pre-cardiopulmonary bypass	III	2C
	TPE	Thrombosis	III	2C
Heritary hemachromatosis	Erythrocytapheresis		I	1B
Hyperleukocytosis	Leukocytapheresis	Leukostasis	I	1B
	Leukocytapheresis	Prophylaxis	III	2C
Hypertriglyceridemic pancreatitis	TPE		III	2C
Hyperviscosity in monoclonal gammopathies	TPE	Symptomatic	I	1B
	TPE	Prophylaxis for rituximab	I	1C
Immune complex rapidly progressive glomerulonephritis	TPE		III	2B
Immune thrombocytopenia	TPE	Refractory	IV	2C
	IA	Refractory	III	2C

Table 33.3 (*Continued*)

Disease Name	TA Modality	Disease Condition	Category	Grade
Immunoglobin A nephropathy	TPE	Crescentic	III	2B
	TPE	Chronic progressive	III	2C
Inclusion body myositis	TPE		IV	2C
	Leukocytapheresis		IV	2C
Inflammatory bowel disease	Adsorptive cytapheresis	Ulcerative colitis	III/II	1B/2B
	Adsorptive cytapheresis	Crohn's disease	III	1B
	ECP	Crohn's disease	III	2C
Lambert–Eaton myasthenic syndrome	TPE		II	2C
Liprotein(a) hyperlipoproteinemia	LDL apheresis		II	1B
Liver transplantation, ABO-incompatible	TPE	Desensitization, live donor	I	1C
	TPE	Desensitization, deceased donor	III	2C
	TPE	Humoral rejection	III	2C
Lung allograft rejection	ECP	Bronchiolitis obliterans syndrome	II	1C
	TPE	Antibody-mediated rejection	III	2C
Malaria	RBC exchange	Severe	II	2B
Multiple sclerosis	TPE	Acute CNS inflammatory demyelinating disease	II	1B
	IA	Acute CNS inflammatory demyelinating disease	III	2C
	TPE	Chronic progressive	III	2B
Myasthenia gravis	TPE	Moderate-severe	I	1B
	TPE	Pre-thymectomy	I	1C
Myeloma cast nephropathy	TPE		II	2B
Nephrogenic systemic fibrosis	ECP		III	2C
	TPE		III	2C
Neuromyelitis optica (Devic's syndrome)	TPE	Acute	II	1B
	TPE	Maintenance	III	2C
Overdose, envenomation, and poisoning	TPE	Mushroom poisoning	II	2C
	TPE	Envenomation	III	2C
	TPE	Natalizumab and PML	III	2C
	RBC exchange	Tacrolimus	III	2C
Paraneoplastic neurological syndromes	TPE		III	2C
	IA		III	2C
Paraproteinemic demyelinating polyneuropahties	TPE	IgG/IgA	I	1B
	TPE	IgM	I	1C
	TPE	Multiple myeloma	III	2C
	IA	IgG/IgA/IgM	III	2C
PANDAS; Sydenham's chorea	TPE	PANDAS exacerbation	I	1B
	TPE	Sydenham's chorea	I	1B
Pemphigus vulgaris	TPE	Severe	III	2C
	ECP	Severe	III	2C
	IA	Severe	III	2C
Peripheral vascular diseases	LDL apheresis		III	2C
Phytanic acid storage disease (Refsum's disease)	TPE		II	2C
	LDL apheresis		II	2C
Polycythemia vera and erythrocytosis	Erythrocytapheresis	Polycythemia vera	I	1B
	Erythrocytapheresis	Secondary erythrocytosis	III	1C
POEMS syndrome	TPE		IV	1C
Posttransfusion purpura	TPE		III	2C
Psoriasis	TPE		IV	2C
	Adsorptive cytapheresis	Disseminated pustular	III	2C
	Lymphocytapheresis		III	2C
	ECP		III	2B
Red cell alloimmunization in pregnancy	TPE	Prior to IUT availability	III	2C
Renal transplantation, ABO compatible	TPE	Antibody-mediated rejection	I	1B
	TPE	Desensitization, living donor, positive crossmatch due to donor-specific HLA antibody	I	1B
	TPE	Desensitization, high PRA deceased donor	III	2C
Renal transplantation, ABO incompatible	TPE	Desensitization, live donor	I	1B
	TPE	Humoral rejection	II	1B
	TPE	Group A2/A2B into B, deceased donor	IV	1B
Schizophrenia	TPE		IV	1A
Scleroderma pProgressive systemic sclerosis)	TPE		III	2C
	ECP		III	2B
Sepsis with multi-organ failure	TPE		III	2B
Sickle cell disease, acute	RBC exchange	Acute stroke	I	1C
	RBC exchange	Acute chest syndrome, severe	II	1C
	RBC exchange	Priapism	III	2C
	RBC exchange	Multi-organ failure	III	2C
	RBC exchange	Splenic sequestration; hepatic sequestration; intrahepatic cholestasis	III	2C
Sickle cell disease, Non-acute	RBC exchange	Stroke prophylaxis/iron overload prevention	II	1C
	RBC exchange	Vaso-occlusive pain crisis	III	2C
	RBC exchange	Preop management	III	2A
Stiff-person syndrome	TPE		III	2C

(*continued*)

Table 33.3 *(Continued)*

Disease Name	TA Modality	Disease Condition	Category	Grade
Sudden sensorineural hearing loss	LDL apheresis		III	2A
	Rheopheresis		III	2A
	TPE		III	2C
Systemic lupus erythematosus	TPE	Severe	II	2C
	TPE	Nephritis	IV	1B
Thrombocytosis	Thrombocytapheresis	Symptomatic	II	2C
	Thrombocytapheresis	Prophylactic or secondary	III	2C
Thrombotic microangiopathy, drug associated	TPE	Ticlopidine	I	1B
	TPE	Clopidogrel	III	2B
	TPE	Cyclosporine/tacrolimus	III	2C
	TPE	Gemcitabine	IV	2C
	TPE	Quinine	IV	2C
Thrombotic microangiopathy, HSCT associated	TPE	Refractory	III	2C
Thrombotic thrombocytopenic purpura	TPE		I	1A
Thyroid storm	TPE		III	2C
Toxic epidermal necrolysis	TPE	Refractory	III	2B
Voltage-gated potassium channel antibodies	TPE		II	1C
Wilson's disease	TPE	Fulminant	I	1C

DAH, diffuse alveolar hemorrhage; HSCT, hematopoietic stem cell transplant; PANDAS, pediatric autoimmune neuropsychiatric disorders associated with streptococcal infections; POEMS, polyneuropathy, organomegaly, endocrinopathy, M protein, and skin changes; PML, progressive multifocal leukoencephalopahty; WAHA, warm-type autoimmune hemolytic anemia.

Source: Guidelines on the Use of Therapeutic Apheresis in Clinical Practice, 2013 [J Clin Apher 28:145–284]. Reproduced with permission of Wiley.

Category III: diseases in which there is uncertainty due to inadequate data or controversy due to conflicting reports; and Category IV: diseases in which there are negative data from controlled trials or anecdotal reports.

The customary intensity (frequency and duration) of TPE therapy can be categorized as follows: aggressive (A), which implies daily TPE until remission or improvement; routine (R), which implies five to seven treatments every other day (or three times per week); prolonged (P), which implies one to three treatments per week for 3–8 weeks; and chronic (C), which implies one treatment every 1–4 weeks, continuing indefinitely. These intensity categories, which need not be mutually exclusive, are summarized in Table 33.4. More than one category may be applicable to a given disease, or even a given patient, depending on extant clinical circumstances.

TPE in neurologic disorders

Immune processes, especially formation of circulating antibody to structures in the nervous system, have been implicated in several neurologic diseases, and TPE has become an important therapy for some of them.[53–55]

Guillain–Barré syndrome

Guillain–Barré syndrome (GBS) affects the peripheral nervous system. A typical clinical course begins with symmetric distal paresthesias, followed by leg and arm weakness. Symptoms spread proximally and reach a peak of severity by 14–30 days after onset. About one-fourth of patients with GBS have mild illness and remain

Table 33.4 Intensity of treatment categories for TPE

Level	Schedule	Duration
Aggressive (A)	Daily	3 treatments to indefinite
Routine (R)	3 times a week	5–7 treatments
Prolonged (P)	1–2 times a week	3–8 weeks
Chronic (C)	Every 1–4 weeks	Indefinite

TPE, therapeutic plasma exchange.

ambulatory throughout. A nerve conduction defect resulting from demyelination is found in most cases, but there are variants in which axonal damage is evident in motor fibers or both motor and sensory fibers. A conduction block indicating demyelination is the usual finding in electrophysiologic studies, although inexcitability may also be seen in the axonal variants.[56]

GBS is often associated with a history of recent infection with *Campylobacter jejuni*, cytomegalovirus, Epstein–Barr virus, *Mycoplasma pneumoniae*, or other organisms. It has been postulated that antibodies are formed in response to a strain-specific lipopolysaccharide that is antigenically similar to one of the myelin gangliosides (e.g., GM1 after *C. jejuni* infection).[56,57] Spontaneous recovery is the usual outcome of GBS and may be associated with the decline in antibody levels expected after recovery from infection. Neither oral nor pulse intravenous steroids are helpful in GBS; however, large randomized controlled trials have documented that TPE can shorten recovery time and reduce disability.

The North American trial enrolled 245 disabled patients, 142 of whom received TPE.[58] At 4 weeks, 59% of treated patients versus 39% of controls had improved by one grade in a clinical grading scale devised for the study. The median time to improve one grade was 19 days in treated patients versus 40 days in controls, whereas median times to walk unassisted were 53 and 85 days, respectively. In the subgroup of ventilated patients, the median times to weaning were 24 and 48 days, respectively. A similar shortening of recovery time in severely affected patients was shown in the French Cooperative Group trial involving 220 patients. In another study of 556 patients, this group showed benefit from TPE in mildly affected patients as well.[60] A typical treatment schedule in these trials consisted of five to six exchanges of 1.0–1.5 plasma volumes over 7–14 days. Patients with GBS are more prone to hemodynamic instability during TPE.

Later studies have shown that intravenous immunoglobulin (IVIG) is also beneficial in GBS. A large multicenter trial compared IVIG, TPE, and TPE followed by IVIG, with 121–130 patients in each treatment group.[61] The trends favored TPE plus IVIG, although none of the differences was statistically significant. Some authorities now favor IVIG for initial treatment, citing its relative simplicity, wider availability, and lower incidence of adverse effects.[56]

Chronic inflammatory demyelinating polyneuropathy (CIDP)

CIDP is an acquired neuropathy that may follow either a continuously progressive or an intermittent, relapsing course. Both weakness and sensory loss are usually present, and both distal and proximal sites may be affected. Nerve conduction studies suggest demyelination, which may be apparent in nerve biopsy tissue if this is obtained. Patchy inflammatory infiltrates may be seen in nerve root biopsies. The cerebrospinal fluid usually has a moderately elevated protein concentration and a cell count less than $10/\mu L$.[62] Although it is usually idiopathic, CIDP may also occur in the context of an associated condition, such as inflammatory bowel disease, chronic active hepatitis, connective tissue disease, Hodgkin's disease, human immunodeficiency virus (HIV) infection, or monoclonal gammopathy.[62]

The precise cause of CIDP remains unknown; however, the disease associations, the clinical similarities to GBS, and the histopathology suggest an immune process. The presence of a monoclonal protein in some cases points to an antibody mediated disorder, as does the finding that an animal model of CIDP (experimental allergic neuritis) can be passively transferred with serum.

Most patients with CIDP will respond to moderately high doses of glucocorticoids.[62] A double-blind, sham-controlled crossover trial[63] showed improvement in five of 15 patients treated with TPE for three weeks; after crossover, a similar proportion responded in the sham group. However, many patients worsened after TPE was stopped. Hahn et al.[64] reported that of 15 patients who completed the trial, 12 improved during the TPE portion. These patients took prednisone for six months after completing TPE, and, following recovery from a brief relapse when TPE was stopped, many maintained good function.[65]

Two studies have compared IVIG to TPE. In a retrospective study by Choudhary and Hughes,[66] 21 of 33 patients (64%) improved after TPE treatment, and a response to IVIG was seen in 14 of 21 patients (67%) treated at the same institution. A prospective observer blinded crossover study of 20 patients at the Mayo Clinic suggested that both therapies were able to produce rapid, statistically significant improvement; the authors concluded that either was appropriate as a primary treatment.[67] Some authorities recommend using IVIG first, based on its relative simplicity, wide availability, and lower incidence of adverse effects.[68] The TPE protocols used in CIDP have tended to specify relatively prolonged treatment. A proposed schedule is three 1-plasma-volume exchanges each week for two weeks, followed by two exchanges each week for another four weeks.[63]

Peripheral neuropathy and monoclonal gammopathy

Myelin antibody activity is expressed by the monoclonal proteins of many patients with neuropathy. Specificity for a carbohydrate epitope on myelin-associated glycoprotein (MAG) can be identified in a majority of IgM-associated neuropathies.

Most clinical features of neuropathies associated with a monoclonal gammopathy are similar to CIDP,[62] and, although progression may be slower overall, it is also more relentless, so that instances of spontaneous improvement are uncommon. The prevalence of neuropathy is higher in patients with IgM paraproteins than in those with IgG or IgA except in osteosclerotic myeloma, where the prevalence of neuropathy with IgG or IgA proteins is quite high, sometimes as a part of the POEMS syndrome (polyneuropathy, organomegaly, endocrinopathy, monoclonal protein, and skin changes). Patients with multiple myeloma or Waldenström's macroglobulinemia should be treated with appropriate chemotherapy and may experience improvement in the neuropathy as a result. However, many patients have neuropathy in addition to a monoclonal gammopathy of undetermined significance (MGUS) and are usually treated with immunosuppressive regimens similar to those used in CIDP.[69]

TPE can be helpful in MGUS-associated neuropathy. In a sham-controlled trial in 39 patients, twice-weekly exchange led to improvement in disability scores, weakness scores, and electrodiagnostic parameters in the blinded portion of the trial. Scores also improved in sham-treated patients who received true TPE in an open follow-up study.[70] In this and other studies, a response was noted more frequently in patients with IgG and IgA paraproteins than in those with IgM.

Myasthenia gravis

About 85% of patients with myasthenia have circulating antibody to a portion of the α-subunit of the acetylcholine (ACh) receptor molecule (AChR) on the motor end plate of muscle cells. A few others have antibody to the muscle cytoplasmic proteins titin or RyR.[71] Because of the relationships between circulating antibody, pathology, and symptoms, TPE has seemed a very reasonable approach to treatment for myasthenia. Although a controlled trial has never been published, numerous open trials have suggested that TPE can lead to rapid symptomatic improvement in concert with lower levels of circulating AChR antibody. TPE has also been effective in patients who test negative for antibody, suggesting that some pathogenic antibodies may not be detected by current assays.[55,71]

As a result of favorable experience, TPE is a widely accepted therapy for myasthenia; however, it is not recommended for all patients. It is instead reserved for those with severe disease and those who are intolerant of, or unresponsive to, other therapies. Patients whose breathing, swallowing, or walking is inadequate are good candidates for the rapid improvement brought about by TPE, even as an initial treatment.[72] An occasional patient will need regular TPE at 2–4-week intervals in addition to maintenance drug therapy for optimal function.

Myasthenia may respond to IVIG. No randomized trials have been conducted to prove efficacy; however, in a controlled study comparing IVIG to TPE in 87 patients, either three or five infusions of 0.4 g/kg IVIG were equivalent to three TPE treatments. The median time to response was shorter for TPE-treated patients (9 days vs. 15 days), but not significantly so ($p = 0.14$).[73] A multicenter retrospective chart review found that ventilatory status at two weeks and functional status at one month were significantly better in patients treated with TPE.[74]

Lambert–Eaton myasthenic syndrome

Lambert–Eaton myasthenic syndrome (LEMS) is also characterized by weakness and fatigue. The syndrome is most often seen in patients with cancer, with almost half of cases being in patients with small cell lung cancer. The pathophysiology of LEMS also involves the neuromuscular junction, but the defect is in the nerve cell ending instead of the muscle cell. Symptoms are caused by circulating antibody against "active zones" in the nerve terminus, which house the voltage-gated calcium channels that mediate electrical events in neuromuscular impulse transmission.

These antibodies reduce the amount of ACh released during depolarization events, causing weakness in affected skeletal muscles as well as dysfunction in autonomic nerves.[75]

Curiously, cholinesterase inhibitors are not as effective in LEMS as they are in myasthenia gravis.[76] More useful are agents that prolong nerve action potentials by blocking voltage-gated potassium channels (VGKCs). Immunosuppressive drugs such as prednisone and azathioprine may also be beneficial in LEMS, and paraneoplastic cases may respond to specific antitumor therapy.[75,76]

TPE has been helpful in LEMS. Responses are usually less dramatic than those seen in myasthenia gravis, perhaps suggesting that a damaged nerve ending needs more time to heal than a motor end plate. IVIG has also been reported to be active in both the short and long term.[75,76]

Neuromyotonia and limbic encephalitis

Neuromyotonia is characterized by muscle cramps, involuntary contractions, fibrillations, and fasciculations. There is evidence to suggest that some cases are caused by the presence of antibodies to VGKC that has a role in terminating action potentials in nerve fibers. TPE has been followed by clinical improvement in individual cases.[77]

Stiff-person syndrome

Stiff-person syndrome (SPS), originally known as stiff-man syndrome, is characterized by progressive rigidity and/or spasms of trunk and proximal limb muscles. About 60% of patients have high titers of circulating antibody to the 65-kD isoform of glutamic acid decarboxylase (GAD-65), which is the rate0limiting enzyme in the synthesis of γ-amino butyric acid (GABA), the neurotransmitter at many inhibitory central nervous system (CNS) synapses. When present, anti-GAD-65 is believed to have a pathogenic role, even though neuronal GAD is a cytoplasmic enzyme. CNS histology is normal in SPS, suggesting that anti-GAD causes functional rather than structural changes. About 5% of cases are associated with cancer, usually breast cancer. Most of these patients have other kinds of antibodies. Symptoms often respond to diazepam or other agents that increase CNS GABA levels. Immunomodulatory therapies such as prednisone, TPE, and IVIG have also seemed beneficial in individual cases, but no controlled trials of TPE have been performed. In paraneoplastic cases, improvement may follow removal of the malignancy.[78,79]

Paraneoplastic neurologic syndromes

In addition to LEMS, several other neurologic syndromes associated with malignant tumors are characterized by circulating antibody to structures in the nervous system. Paraneoplastic encephalomyelitis includes seizures, mental changes, and cerebellar and autonomic dysfunction. It is often associated with anti-Hu (also called ANNA-1), an antibody to a 38- to 40-kD antigen in the nuclei of neurons and of small cell lung cancer cells. Paraneoplastic cerebellar degeneration is characterized by ataxia, dysarthria, and down-beating nystagmus. It may be associated with ovarian, breast, and small cell lung cancers, as well as with Hodgkin's disease. About 40% of these patients have an antibody to 34- and 62-kD antigens in Purkinje cells (anti-Yo). Paraneoplastic opsoclonus–myoclonus syndrome produces both vertical and horizontal dysrhythmic conjugated eye movements. It may occur in children with neuroblastoma and in adults with lung, breast, or other tumors. Cases seen with breast or gynecologic cancers may have circulating anti-Ri (also called ANNA-2), an antibody to 55- and 80-kD antigens in neuronal nuclei. Paraneoplastic SPS is characterized by stiffness and spasm in axial muscles. It is associated with antibody to amphiphysin, a 128-kD synaptic vesicle protein. Cancer-associated retinopathy produces photosensitivity and gradual vision loss. It is associated with anti-CAR, an antibody to antigens shared by retinal neurons and small cell lung cancer cells.[79A]

Treatment of these syndromes is uniformly difficult. They seldom respond well to immunosuppressive drugs or to antitumor measures, even when these are otherwise effective. TPE has been tried in these syndromes, usually with disappointing results.[79A]

Nonneoplastic disorders with central nervous system antibodies

Rasmussen's encephalitis is a rare, acquired disorder that begins in childhood, often following a viral infection. Seizures are a prominent feature; however, unlike patients with idiopathic epilepsy, those with Rasmussen's encephalitis develop progressive, predominantly unilateral neurologic deficits, including hemiparesis and mental retardation. The histopathology includes inflammation and atrophy of brain tissue, usually confined to one hemisphere.[80] Recent studies have revealed circulating IgG antibody to the Glu-R3 receptor for the CNS neurotransmitter glutamate, which may arise in response to a cross-reactive microbial antigen. Treatment with either TPE or IVIG has been followed by temporary improvement.[55] Sydenham chorea is a movement disorder that may follow a group A streptococcal infection in children. Patients with Sydenham chorea may also exhibit obsessive-compulsive symptoms, and children who develop obsessive-compulsive behaviors, tics, and other neurologic symptoms in the absence of chorea may also have evidence of streptococcal infection (pediatric autoimmune neuropsychiatric disorders associated with streptococcal infection [PANDAS]).[81] A cross-reactive antibody response to streptococcal antigens could mediate symptoms in some of these patients, and small controlled trials have indicated that both TPE and IVIG can be beneficial in either Sydenham chorea or PANDAS.[55,82]

Neuromyelitis optica has also been treated effectively by TPE.[83]

Multiple sclerosis

Multiple sclerosis (MS) is a disease characterized by localized neurologic dysfunction that is caused by demyelinated "plaques" in the CNS. Two clinical patterns are observed. About 70% of patients will have acute attacks that resolve fully or partially (relapsing-remitting). The other 30% have slow, continual progression of disease (chronic progressive). The frequency of attacks in relapsing-remitting MS tends to decrease with disease duration, and some patients evolve to a chronic progressive pattern.[84]

Discrete areas or plaques of demyelination in white matter, which are easily visualized with magnetic resonance imaging (MRI), are the hallmarks of MS. Histopathologically, these areas are initially inflammatory but progress to fibrosis.[84] The mechanism of their appearance remains unexplained, but most authorities in the field suspect involvement of the immune system.[55] Most evidence suggests a misdirected cellular immune response in MS, and it has been difficult to assign a primary pathogenic role to circulating antibody. Antibodies to myelin basic protein (MBP) or myelin oligodendrocyte glycoprotein (MOG) can be found both in CNS lesions[85] and in serum[86] in some MS patients. Although they are predictive of progression to MS in patients with a clinically isolated demyelinating event,[88] such antibodies do not produce MS in experimental animals.[89] Also, anti-MOG does not correlate with histopathologic classification or apparent responsiveness to TPE.[90]

The study of treatments for MS is complicated by the natural history of the disease, particularly the tendencies for acute attacks to subside and for attack frequency to decline, but also by other spontaneous fluctuations in disease activity. Immunosuppressive and immunomodulatory agents have been the mainstays of drug therapy in MS. Resolution of acute attacks is thought to be hastened by brief courses of either glucocorticoids or adrenocorticotrophic hormone, both of which may promote faster restoration of normal nerve conduction by decreasing edema and inflammation in and around new plaques. The relentless progression of disability is probably not halted by these measures, although aggressive treatment of optic neuritis with intravenous steroids may delay the onset of frank MS that often follows. Cyclosporine, total lymphoid irradiation, and cytotoxic immunosuppressants such as azathioprine and cyclophosphamide have only modest benefits that may not warrant the risks such drugs entail. Mycophenolate mofetil, low-dose methotrexate mitoxantrone, and interferon-β glatiramer acetate (a mixture of synthetic polypeptides that may modulate immune responses to MBP) have been tried. Some of these agents reduce the frequency of acute attacks and the appearance of new lesions. Immunomodulatory monoclonal antibodies, such as alemtuzumab, daclizumab, natalizumab, and rituximab, are also being investigated.[91–93]

Prophylactic administration of IVIG to patients with MS is reported to reduce the frequency of attacks and may slow clinical deterioration in relapsing-remitting patients. It has not as yet been shown to mediate improvement in chronic visual impairment or motor symptoms.[93]

The rationale for TPE in MS is uncertain, given the paucity of evidence that any circulating factor has a role in the etiology of acute attacks or chronic progression. TPE has nevertheless been used, and encouraging results have been reported from uncontrolled studies. In controlled trials; however, it has been difficult to discern benefit, even with vigorous TPE regimens. The first randomized, double-blind, sham-controlled study in chronic progressive MS was reported to show significant benefit for patients receiving TPE in addition to cyclophosphamide and prednisone.[94] The study was subsequently questioned because of anomalies in statistical analysis, and because dramatic recoveries in several of the TPE patients, not seen in subsequent trials, suggested that some relapsing remitting patients were misclassified and entered into the trial during attacks that would have improved spontaneously.[95] Two later sham-controlled trials have not shown convincing benefit.[96,97] A single trial suggested that TPE could be useful in a subset of patients with MS with prolonged severe demyelination;[98] however, that study combined results of MS patients with those of patients having neuromyelitis optica. As a result, TPE is classified as "of little or no value" in progressive MS and of uncertain value in acute severe demyelination in previously nondisabled individuals (Table 33.3).

TPE in hematologic and oncologic disorders
Monoclonal proteins

In addition to peripheral neuropathy (discussed in this chapter), four other syndromes associated with monoclonal immunoglobulins are regarded as clinical indications for TPE. Hyperviscosity, coagulopathy, and renal failure, which almost always occur in the setting of a malignant B-cell disorder, are discussed here; cryoglobulinemia is covered in a later section of this chapter.

Hyperviscosity was the first condition to be treated successfully with manual plasmapheresis, the precursor to TPE. The full-blown syndrome consists of neurologic symptoms, a bleeding diathesis, a peculiar retinopathy marked by alternating dilated and constricted segments in retinal veins, and hypervolemia caused by expansion of plasma volume. Symptoms are uncommon if the relative serum viscosity is below four and become more likely when it exceeds six. The hyperviscosity syndrome is most often seen in patients with Waldenström's macroglobulinemia, who have IgM paraproteins, but it may also occur in multiple myeloma.[99]

At higher paraprotein levels, a relatively large change in viscosity may follow a relatively small change in concentration. It is this nonlinear relationship that allowed the two-unit manual plasmapheresis technique available in the 1950s to lower viscosity enough to relieve symptoms. Because most IgM paraproteins are roughly 80% intravascular, the same relationship also predicts that a one-plasma-volume automated exchange will provide a wide margin of safety and can therefore be repeated less frequently for hyperviscosity than is necessary for many other conditions. Viscosity measurements should guide therapy, but treatment every 1–2 weeks may be adequate.[99]

Coagulopathy: Paraproteins may interfere in platelet and clotting factor interactions in the absence of hyperviscosity. Such coagulopathies are found in 60% of patients with macroglobulinemia, 40% of patients with IgA myeloma, and 15% of patients with IgG myeloma.[100] In instances that are clinically significant, TPE therapy can help restore adequate hemostasis.

Renal failure: This develops in 3–9% of patients with myeloma and confers a poor prognosis. In many cases, renal biopsy demonstrates accumulation of free light chains in renal tubules. Urinary excretion of light chains will greatly exceed the amount that could be removed by TPE if renal function is normal. The reverse may be true in renal failure; however, light chain levels return to baseline within hours after TPE.[101] Three controlled studies have examined rates of recovery of renal function in myeloma patients who received TPE therapy. In one study, three of seven dialysis-dependent patients who received TPE recovered renal function, whereas none of five control patients did.[102] In another, 13 of 15 patients in the treatment group recovered renal function compared with only two of 14 controls.[103] A more recent controlled study enrolled 104 patients and assessed a composite outcome comprising death, dialysis, or a low glomerular filtration rate. Outcomes were not improved in the patients randomly assigned to receive TPE treatment.[104] Thus, the value of TPE in this circumstance is questionable.

Alloantibodies to blood cells

Alloantibodies to red cells and platelets may be problematic in a number of disease processes. Treatment by antibody removal has been tried in several of these.

Hemolytic disease of the fetus and newborn was one of the first problems to be approached with automated apheresis instruments. In the hope of slowing fetal hemolysis, sensitized D-negative mothers carrying D-positive fetuses underwent TPE to lower anti-D titers. Since the original reports, the number of sensitized mothers has declined as prophylaxis with Rh immune globulin has become more widespread. Furthermore, intrauterine transfusion with D-negative red cells has proven to be a better treatment for affected fetuses. For these reasons, TPE is seldom called for now, but it may still be useful in an occasional pregnancy when there is very early evidence of fetal involvement, because intrauterine transfusion is not feasible before about 18 weeks of gestation.[105,106] Prompt, early institution of TPE was followed by successful delivery after multiple prior abortions in compelling case reports involving mothers with anti-M and anti-P.[107]

TPE has also been used to remove isoagglutinins in the setting of *hematopoietic stem cell transplantation.* Allogeneic transplantation across a major ABO barrier (e.g., group A donor to group O recipient) is feasible if a hemolytic transfusion reaction to red cells in the marrow graft can be avoided. This was first accomplished in marrow transplants by exhaustive pretransplant TPE of the recipient; however, most centers have preferred to simply remove most of the red cells (e.g., <20 mL remaining) from an incompatible marrow graft before transplantation.[108] Peripheral blood stem cell collections include far fewer red cells (usually <10 mL). Such grafts can be infused safely without any manipulation. Red cell engraftment may be delayed in this situation. TPE has been used, both before transplant to avoid delayed engraftment and after transplant to correct it, with uncertain results in both cases.[109]

Transplantation of a solid organ, such as a liver or kidney, across a major ABO barrier can result in hyperacute rejection and is usually avoided for this reason. When organ availability is limited, however, clinical circumstances have sometimes led to transplantation of an ABO-incompatible liver or kidney after extensive TPE of the recipient, often with a satisfactory outcome.[110–114]

Organ transplantation across a minor ABO barrier (eg, group O donor to group A recipient) does not carry an increased risk of rejection. Some patients, however, develop hemolytic anemia caused by isoagglutinins derived from B lymphocytes in the stem cell graft. Red cell destruction mediated by these "passenger lymphocytes" is most often seen in heart, lung, or liver transplantation, in which the volume of lymphoid tissue transplanted is relatively high. Passenger lymphocyte syndrome is usually evident by 1–3 weeks after transplantation.[115] Severe hemolysis may improve after TPE and compatible (e.g., group O) red cell transfusion.[116]

Alloimmunization to HLA or platelet antigens can cause refractoriness to platelet transfusions. To restore responsiveness, antibody removal by means of TPE or a protein A–silica column has been attempted. IVIG has also been tried.[18] However, the results have been inconclusive, and the best option for alloimmunized patients is transfusion of compatible platelets.

Thrombotic thrombocytopenic purpura (TTP) and hemolytic uremic syndrome

Thrombotic thrombocytopenic purpura

TTP is characterized by microangiopathic hemolytic anemia and thrombocytopenia, often severe. Central nervous system changes, fever, and renal abnormalities may be seen in advanced cases, although frank renal failure is unusual. A rare relapsing form begins in childhood, but the majority of cases in adults are sporadic, with women accounting for 70%. TTP is most often idiopathic but may be seen in association with other illnesses, such as systemic lupus erythematosus (SLE) and HIV infection, as well as with certain drugs. Idiopathic TTP was formerly assigned a mortality rate of 90%, but empiric studies in the 1970s and 1980s demonstrated much improved survival in patients receiving daily TPE with plasma replacement. Some patients, including children with the relapsing form of the disease, will respond to simple plasma infusion.[117]

The pathogenesis of TTP has been offered. It involves a plasma enzyme (a metalloproteinase called ADAMTS13 on the basis of structural features) that cleaves ultra-large von Willebrand factor (ULvWF) multimers secreted by endothelial cells, yielding the

smaller vWF polymers found in normal plasma. Children with relapsing TTP have an inherited deficiency of ADAMTS13,[118] whereas in idiopathic adult cases an "acquired deficiency" arises because of the formation of an autoantibody inhibitor to the enzyme.[119,120] In either case, persistence of ultra-high-weight vWF in the circulation promotes inappropriate adherence of platelets to endothelial cells and to each other, leading to consumptive thrombocytopenia and to microvascular obstructions that cause mechanical trauma to red cells and varying degrees of end-organ ischemia. Periodic plasma infusion may abort or prevent attacks in congenitally deficient patients by supplying active enzyme.[118] Idiopathic cases respond better to TPE (78% response rate vs. 63% for plasma infusion),[121] presumably because exchanges remove inhibitory antibody as well as replace the deficient enzyme. Exchanges are usually carried out daily until the platelet count and LDH (as a marker of hemolysis) have normalized.

Various immunosuppressive maneuvers, including glucocorticoid therapy, vincristine, rituximab, and splenectomy, have been advocated as adjunctive treatments. Discovery of a causative autoantibody provides support for their use in idiopathic, but not in congenital, cases.[107]

A syndrome resembling TTP has been identified in some patients taking the antiplatelet drugs ticlopidine[122] and clopidogrel.[123] Antibody to ADAMTS13 has been detected in such case,[124] and TPE has been reported to improve outcome (76% survival vs. 50% for unexchanged patients in a retrospective study of ticlopidine recipients).[122] ADAMTS13 deficiency is generally not found in TTP-like syndromes associated with other drugs such as quinine or cyclosporine.[125]

Hemolytic uremic syndrome

The hemolytic uremic syndrome (HUS) usually involves microangiopathic hemolysis, renal insufficiency, and mild-to-moderate thrombocytopenia. It occurs in children in a self-limited form that follows infection with a verotoxin-producing *Escherichia coli* (diarrhea positive); however, not all pediatric cases have this association (diarrhea negative). Both a familial and a nonfamilial form may be seen in adults. Some nonfamilial cases are associated with prior chemotherapy or stem cell transplantation.

Because of the striking overlap in clinical manifestations, it was long supposed that the pathogenesis of HUS was the same as, or similar to, that of TTP. Largely on this basis, TPE has been recommended for diarrhea-negative childhood HUS and for adult HUS. Responses have generally been less favorable than in TTP, especially in HUS associated with chemotherapy or hematopoietic stem cell transplantation[117,126,127] and TPE is not recommended in these situations.

Studies of ADAMTS13 in adult patients with familial and nonfamilial forms of HUS have revealed neither severe deficiency nor inhibitory activity.[119] Thus, the hypothesis that HUS has the same pathogenic mechanism as TTP has not been substantiated.

Posttransfusion purpura

Posttransfusion purpura (PTP) is a rare syndrome in which the platelet count falls to dangerously low levels about one week after an allogeneic transfusion. Patients who develop the syndrome lack the common allele for one of the platelet-specific glycoprotein antigens, most often the HPA-1a antigen on glycoprotein IIIa. Most patients have had multiple prior transfusions or pregnancies, and have been immunized thereby to the platelet-specific antigen coded by the prevalent allele. The transfusion that precedes the illness appears to stimulate an anamnestic increase in the titer of IgG platelet-specific alloantibody, most often anti-HPA-1a; however, the patient's own antigen negative platelets are also destroyed, causing very low levels of platelets. PTP is self-limited and should resolve without treatment after a few weeks; however, bleeding complications, including fatal CNS hemorrhage, may occur in the interim.[128]

Treatment of PTP is recommended, because many patients will have bleeding complications. High-dose glucocorticoids are usually given empirically and pulse methylprednisolone at 1 g/day has been reported effective. Platelet transfusions, even those from antigen-negative donors, seldom raise the platelet count but are likely to cause severe reactions. Daily TPE usually promotes a rise in platelet count within several days and is thought to be an effective treatment for this reason, even though no controlled trials have been conducted.[129] Exchanges usually include FFP replacement to avoid a superimposed humoral coagulopathy. Intravenous immune globulin produces a similarly rapid increase in platelet count and has become the favored treatment modality for this group of patients.[130]

Idiopathic thrombocytopenic purpura

Idiopathic thrombocytopenic purpura (ITP) is an autoimmune illness affecting platelets. Most patients have an autoantibody of the IgG class directed against a platelet–membrane glycoprotein antigen. ITP is sometimes accompanied by warm-type autoimmune hemolytic anemia (WAIHA; also called Evans syndrome). In pediatric patients, ITP is acute and self-limited; recovery is the rule regardless of treatment. Adults with ITP, most of whom are women, seldom recover without treatment, and their disease often progresses to a chronic form. An ITP syndrome may also be seen in patients with SLE or HIV.[131]

The goal of treatment in ITP is to prevent bleeding. Fortunately, most of the circulating platelets in patients with ITP are relatively young and have above-average hemostatic activity, so a normal platelet count is not needed to avoid hemorrhage. Glucocorticoids, splenectomy, and IVIG are the mainstays of therapy.[131] Large intravenous doses of anti-D will often raise the platelet count in Rh(D)-positive patients because excessive red cell destruction occupies phagocytic cells and inhibits platelet destruction. A few favorable anecdotal reports of TPE in ITP appeared in the 1970s, and one small trial suggested a lower rate of splenectomy in exchanged patients but a later study found no long-term benefit associated with such therapy.[131] Given this experience, enthusiasm for TPE has waned.

Favorable responses to protein A–silica column treatment have been reported in ITP associated with HIV infection,[132] as well as in patients with chronic ITP without HIV.[133] The mechanism of action of protein A in this effect is unknown. A purely subtractive mechanism (i.e., removal of platelet antibody) seems unlikely because responses have been reported when as little as 250 mL plasma per week was treated. Bearing this uncertainty in mind, the protein A–silica column remains an option for chronic ITP refractory to more standard therapies, although this has been used very little because the protein A columns are not approved by the US Food and Drug Administration (FDA) and thus are not available in the United States.

Autoimmune hemolytic anemia (AIHA)

AIHA is caused by autoantibodies to red cells. Such antibodies are classified as either "cold" or "warm" agglutinins, depending on the temperature of maximal activity. Cold agglutinins are usually IgM antibodies directed against the I/i antigens; they bind most strongly at low temperatures and may produce a syndrome of complement-mediated intravascular hemolysis (cold agglutinin disease [CAD]). Warm agglutinins are usually IgG and are often directed against an antigen that does not appear on Rh_{null} cells; they bind better at body temperature and produce a predominantly extravascular hemolytic syndrome, WAIHA. Autoimmune hemolytic anemia can be idiopathic but can also be associated with infections, lymphoproliferative disorders, or other autoimmune diseases.

Most patients need treatment. Standard therapy is aimed at lowering antibody production and inhibiting destruction of sensitized cells. Glucocorticoids, IVIG, and splenectomy are often effective in WAIHA, and other immunosuppressive drugs may be tried if these measures fail. All of these approaches are less successful in CAD.

TPE to deplete circulating antibody has been tried in both WAIHA and CAD when conventional treatments have failed. Because the IgM antibodies in CAD are predominantly intravascular and only loosely bound to cells, their removal by TPE should be relatively efficient. Such therapy, when added to conventional drug treatment, has been reported to lower antibody titers and transfusion requirements, albeit only temporarily. In WAIHA much of the circulating antibody is bound to red cells; TPE has been tried in this disorder also, but it is less likely to be helpful. A nonrandomized study compared responses to red cell transfusions in five AIHA patients who underwent TPE before some transfusions and four other patients who did not. Responses were significantly better in the patients who did *not* receive TPE and were not improved by TPE in the patients who did, suggesting that TPE is not effective for this purpose,[134] although it may be helpful in certain specific situations.[134A]

Pure red cell aplasia and aplastic anemia

Pure red cell aplasia and aplastic anemia are marrow disorders. In the former, there is reticulocytopenic anemia, whereas the latter leads to pancytopenia. At least some cases of both conditions likely have an immunologic basis. Allogeneic marrow transplantation is the preferred treatment for severe aplastic anemia if a suitable donor is available, but immunosuppressive therapies, such as glucocorticoids, cytotoxic drugs, cyclosporine, and antithymocyte globulin, may be effective, especially in milder cases.

In the serum of a minority of patients, it is possible to demonstrate a factor, probably antibody, that inhibits the growth of marrow-derived precursor cells in culture.[135] This provides a rationale for TPE, which has been reported in both disorders in a few cases. Results in aplastic anemia have been mixed; responses appear to be more likely in patients with serum inhibitory activity. All reported instances of TPE treatment for pure red cell aplasia have led to improvement, which is sometimes quite dramatic in patients with serum inhibitory activity. Thus, although TPE is not a primary therapy for either disorder, it can be offered to patients who have failed to improve after receiving conventional treatment, especially those found to have serum inhibitory factors.

Coagulation factor inhibitors

Coagulation factor inhibitors are IgG antibodies to components of the clotting cascade. They interfere with clotting by inactivating the targeted factor. Inhibitors may be autoantibodies that arise in individuals with no prior bleeding. Alternatively, they may be alloantibodies that form in genetically deficient patients after exposure to "foreign protein" in the course of factor replacement therapy. Factor VIII is the clotting protein most often affected by antibodies of either type, and most of the following concerns factor VIII inhibitors.

The two goals of treatment for a patient with an inhibitor are control of individual bleeding episodes and suppression of inhibitor synthesis. Depending on inhibitor titer, the first goal can sometimes be achieved by infusion of high doses of human factor VIII. Porcine factor VIII, which cross-reacts only partially with human factor VIII antibodies, can be effective in the face of somewhat higher inhibitor titers, but its availability in recent years has been uncertain. For patients with the highest titers, factor VIII–bypassing products such as recombinant factor VIIa are needed. TPE or selective immunoadsorption of IgG during a bleeding episode may reduce inhibitor titers enough to allow infused factor VIII to bring about hemostasis. Suppression of inhibitor synthesis is approached with immunosuppressive measures, including high-dose glucocorticoids, cytotoxic agents, cyclosporine, IVIG, and rituximab.[136,137] Tolerance-inducing protocols that include regular infusion of exogenous factor VIII have been devised for patients with alloimmune inhibitors. In the so-called Malmö protocol, extensive TPE or IgG depletion with protein A–sepharose column procedures is used to reduce the inhibitor level at the onset of treatment so that infused "tolerizing" factor can circulate. Frequent, large (two to three plasma volume) exchanges with FFP replacement are recommended for patients with inhibitor. Central venous access is often required; placement of a catheter in a patient with a refractory bleeding diathesis is a challenge for all concerned and often mandates infusion of a factor VIII–bypassing product for wound hemostasis.[138]

TPE has also been reported for treatment of patients with antiphospholipid antibodies, which may interfere with in vitro assays of coagulation, such as the partial thromboplastin time. In contrast to the inhibitory antibodies described above, however, they usually promote inappropriate coagulation in vivo and cause thrombotic events. Patients suffering thrombotic events in three or more organ systems are said to have catastrophic antiphospholipid antibody syndrome.[139,140] Plasma exchange may be helpful in these patients.[140A]

TPE in rheumatic and other immunologic disorders

TPE has been tried in a number of rheumatic diseases and other diseases that are considered to have an immune or autoimmune etiology.

Cryoglobulinemia

Cryoglobulins are abnormal serum proteins that precipitate reversibly at $4\,^{\circ}C$; some will precipitate at higher temperatures. Such precipitates always contain immunoglobulin, and immunoelectrophoretic or immunofixation analysis allows distinction of three types. Type I cryoglobulins consist of a single species of monoclonal immunoglobulin. These are usually found in B-cell lymphoproliferative disorders such as myeloma or Waldenström's macroglobulinemia. Cryoglobulin levels are often quite high (>500 mg/dL) and may cause Raynaud phenomenon or acral necrosis due to microvascular obstruction, as well as other symptoms. Type II cryoglobulins contain both monoclonal and polyclonal immunoglobulins. The former is usually an IgMκ with anti-IgG specificity, and the latter is polyclonal IgG bound to the IgMκ in an immune complex. Most cases occur in the context of chronic hepatitis C infection. They typically manifest a cutaneous vasculitis on the lower extremities and may have visceral manifestations of immune complex disease as well.[141] Type III cryoglobulins are

mixed polyclonal, often with IgM anti-IgG that binds IgG in immune complexes. These may arise in acute infections such as hepatitis B, or in chronic inflammatory states such as severe rheumatoid arthritis. Clinical manifestations resemble serum sickness.

If there is an underlying condition, cryoglobulin levels and related symptoms may decrease with treatment of this primary disorder, for example chemotherapy for myeloma or interferon for hepatitis C virus infection. For idiopathic and secondary cases of mixed cryoglobulinemia, prednisone therapy often relieves symptoms, and alkylating agents may be useful in patients with severe symptoms resistant to prednisone.

TPE will reduce cryoglobulin levels and control symptoms, even in the absence of other treatments,[142,143] but inconvenience and expense mitigate against such use. It should be started promptly for patients who seek treatment for severe acral ischemia or visceral manifestations of vasculitis, in whom it can help achieve control of symptoms until aggressive drug therapy takes hold.[144] Patients with chronic vasculitic skin ulcers may also benefit.[145] In all cases, replacement fluids should be warmed to body temperature before infusion.

Rheumatoid arthritis (RA)

RA is a disease of unknown cause that is more prevalent in women. It is the most common chronic inflammatory joint disease and a leading cause of disability. Most patients have rheumatoid factor, an IgM autoantibody to IgG; however, because this antibody is absent in many clinically typical cases, and because it is also found in patients who do not have arthritis, it is not likely to be directly involved in pathogenesis.

Conservative treatment includes nonsteroidal anti-inflammatory agents, oral glucocorticoids in low doses, and intra-articular steroids. More severely affected patients eventually receive slow-acting *disease-modifying anti-rheumatic drugs* that are probably immunomodulatory, such as antimalarials, gold compounds, and methotrexate. Tumor necrosis factor and interleukin-1 (IL1) inhibitors are also approved for treatment of RA.

TPE was tried for RA in the 1970s and 1980s, but controlled trials did not show benefit. There were subsequent reports of lymphapheresis, with or without accompanying TPE. Some controlled trials investigating this approach showed significant but short-lived benefit, whereas others did not. In practice, the prospect of only a modest chance of modest benefit from a costly, inconvenient therapy has discouraged treatment with therapeutic apheresis.[146]

A sham-controlled trial of 12 weekly protein A–silica column treatments produced improvement in 33% of 48 treated patients versus only 9% of 43 controls. Benefit persisted for about eight months on average, and a subsequent course was again beneficial in seven of nine initial responders.[147] Although its mechanism of action is unclear, this device has gained FDA approval for use in RA, but it is not generally available in the United States and has not gained widespread use.

Systemic lupus erythematosus

SLE has long been regarded as the prototypic autoimmune disease. The most important diagnostic criterion, circulating antibodies to DNA, especially double-stranded DNA (anti-dsDNA), identifies patients who may have a variety of other autoantibodies and a disparate array of clinical syndromes in which skin disease, joint disease, cytopenias, or nephritis may be the sole or dominant problem.

Immunosuppressive measures are the cornerstone of therapy for SLE. Most patients are given prednisone in varying doses, and those with severe disease may also receive azathioprine or cyclophosphamide. The plethora of autoantibodies that seem relevant to clinical signs made SLE an obvious target for TPE. It was one of the first illnesses to be treated with automated TPE in the early 1970s, and early case reports and uncontrolled series suggested a favorable effect.[146]

Lupus nephritis is a particularly devastating manifestation in which glomerular deposition of immune complexes and anti-DNA is believed to have a prominent role in pathogenesis. Thus, it seemed an attractive setting for randomized trials of TPE. A controlled trial with only eight patients suggested benefit.[148] However, in a multi-center randomized controlled trial comparing oral cyclophosphamide plus TPE to oral cyclophosphamide alone, there was no advantage for the patients receiving TPE.[149] A later international trial, which enrolled patients with a variety of severe manifestations, was structured to exploit enhanced sensitivity to a properly timed pulse dose of intravenous cyclophosphamide that was believed to follow pathogenic antibody removal by TPE.[150] This trial also failed to show any advantage for all patients treated with TPE[151] or for a subgroup with nephritis.[152] Thus, large controlled studies have failed to confirm any worthwhile effect of TPE in SLE.

Systemic vasculitis

The term *systemic vasculitis* encompasses a group of disorders that cause inflammation in blood vessel walls and ischemic tissue damage. Vasculitis syndromes are conveniently classified on the basis of the size of vessels typically involved, but most are of unknown etiology. Immune complexes are found in patients with some syndromes, and autoantibodies such as anti-neutrophil cytoplasmic antibodies (ANCA) in Wegener's granulomatosis (c-ANCA) and polyarteritis (p-ANCA) can be demonstrated in others. This has lent credence to the notion that humoral immune factors are somehow involved.[153]

Prednisone is the first-line therapy for most vasculitic syndromes, and cyclophosphamide is often added in more severe cases. Randomized controlled trials in renal vasculitis,[154] as well as in a group of patients with polyarteritis or Churg–Strauss angiitis, have shown little evidence that addition of TPE to drug therapy confers long-term benefit. Nevertheless, it may be requested for patients who are not responding to maximal drug therapy.

Polymyositis and dermatomyositis

Polymyositis and dermatomyositis are inflammatory diseases affecting skeletal muscle. A characteristic dermatitis involving the eyelids, knuckles, neck, and shoulders is also part of the latter condition. The usual clinical picture includes proximal weakness with biochemical evidence of muscle cell enzyme leakage; the diagnosis is confirmed by muscle biopsy. The natural history is progressive fiber loss, eventually leading to profound, irreversible weakness. An autoimmune etiology is suspected, but circulating antibody specific for skeletal muscle has not been implicated. Initial treatment is high-dose prednisone, which can often be tapered to maintenance levels. Resistant disease is treated with azathioprine, methotrexate, an alkylating agent, or a combination. Controlled trials have also shown that IVIG infusion reduces muscle enzyme levels and improves strength temporarily.[55]

Several uncontrolled series were interpreted to show that TPE was beneficial, but they were unfortunately confounded by concurrent escalations in immunosuppressive drug therapy.[55] A randomized controlled trial in which 12 patients received TPE, 12 received lymphapheresis, and 12 received sham apheresis, with no changes in drug therapy, showed no difference in the response rate among the three groups.[155] Thus, despite the successes with IVIG, there appears to be no role for TPE in the treatment of polymyositis.

Goodpasture syndrome (GPS)

GPS is characterized clinically by pulmonary hemorrhage and rapidly progressive glomerulonephritis. Light microscopy of renal biopsies shows crescent formation in many glomeruli, and immunofluorescent and electron microscopy reveal linear subendothelial immune deposits that may also be evident in a lung biopsy. In 95% of cases, there is a circulating antibody that binds to glomerular basement membrane (anti-GBM). Such antibodies are specific for a noncollagenous sequence near the carboxy terminus of the α3 chain of type IV collagen, which is found in appreciable quantities only in renal and pulmonary basement membranes. Untreated GPS progresses quickly and relentlessly, and most patients die of uremia or complications of lung hemorrhage.[156] The preferred treatment for GPS is high-dose prednisone and cyclophosphamide, combined with aggressive TPE, to quickly reduce anti-GBM levels and minimize progression of tissue damage.[111] Exchanges are usually carried out daily and may be continued for up to two weeks. It is prudent to give some FFP replacement in the latter part of each exchange to avoid a dilutional coagulopathy that might cause exacerbation of lung bleeding.

A single controlled trial failed to show an advantage for GPS patients who received TPE; however, this study has been largely discounted because the TPE schedule (every three days) was not sufficiently aggressive and because the extent of renal damage at entry was worse in the TPE group than in controls.[157] Early treatment is recommended because patients who are already dialysis-dependent at the onset of TPE are unlikely to recover renal function.[158] It follows that the subset of patients whose renal biopsies show irreversible lesions are not likely to benefit from TPE unless they also have pulmonary hemorrhage.

Other rapidly progressive glomerulonephritis

In addition to GPS, there are two other categories of rapidly progressive glomerulonephritis (RPGN)—those with an immune complex disease who have granular subendothelial immune deposits, and those with pauci-immune RPGN who have scant immune deposits, if any. Light microscopic findings in both are similar to those found in GPS, with severe glomerular inflammation and crescent formation. Some cases also have associated lung hemorrhage. Patients in either group may have isolated renal disease or may have accompanying features that suggest a diagnosis of systemic vasculitis, mixed cryoglobulinemia, or Henoch–Schönlein purpura for granular-immune complex RPGN, or microscopic polyangiitis or Wegener's granulomatosis for pauci-immune RPGN patients, most of whom test positive for ANCA.

Therapies are similar for these two categories of RPGN, and some trials and series have included patients with both types. Virtually all patients receive prednisone, and most receive either oral or intravenous cyclophosphamide. TPE has been used extensively in patients with both types of disease. Two controlled trials, one published in 1988[159] and the other in 1992,[160] showed no advantage for patients who received TPE in addition to immunosuppressive drugs. However, a subgroup analysis in the second study suggested that patients who have dialysis-dependent renal failure are more likely to recover renal function if they receive TPE. No such trend was noticed in the more recent trial.[154] A prospective, randomized trial[161] compared TPE with immunoadsorption. Among 38 patients with non-GPS RPGN, 87% of whom had ANCA, 70% avoided long-term dialysis. TPE and immunoadsorption were equally effective. In another study of ANCA-positive patients with an elevated creatinine, 54% of dialysis-dependent patients randomly assigned to receive TPE became dialysis independent compared to only 32% of those who received pulse methylprednisolone instead of TPE.[162] Thus, although the role of TPE is not clearly defined in all types of RPGN, current evidence suggests efficacy in ANCA-positive patients who are dialysis dependent.

Hyperthyroidism

TPE may be helpful as adjunctive treatment in patients with severe thyrotoxicosis.[163]

Solid organ transplantation

In organ transplant recipients, TPE has been used both to treat and to prevent rejection, as well as for recurrence of certain diseases in a transplanted organ. The role of photopheresis is described later.

Rejection

Cellular immune mechanisms mediate most organ allograft rejection episodes; however, antibody-mediated rejection may occur rapidly in patients who have preexisting antibodies to ABO or HLA antigens expressed by the graft. Such "hyperacute" rejection is characterized histologically by neutrophil infiltration, fibrin deposition, and endothelial damage in small blood vessels; failure of the graft is mainly caused by ischemic damage. All treatments have been futile in hyperacute rejection, including TPE. So-called vascular changes, which may be seen microscopically in later rejection episodes, were formerly taken to indicate antibody-mediated rejection, even when immunofluorescence microscopy and tests for circulating antibody were negative.[164]

Standard posttransplant management for kidney and heart transplantation consists of prophylactic immunosuppression with glucocorticoids, a calcineurin inhibitor (cyclosporine or tacrolimus), and an antimetabolite such as azathioprine or mycophenolate mofetil. High-risk recipients and those who have rejection episodes in spite of these standard measures are treated with pulse steroids, T-cell antibody preparations, or both.[165,166]

Case reports and uncontrolled series published in the late 1970s and early 1980s suggested TPE was beneficial in renal transplant rejection. Then, five controlled trials[11] were reported in the mid- and late 1980s. Four showed no significant benefit for patients receiving TPE in addition to standard drug therapy, even in the subgroups whose transplant biopsies showed "vascular" histologic changes. In the one study suggesting benefit, the mean treatment time was 10–11 months after transplant, when antibody-mediated rejection is less likely. The last and largest study concluded that TPE therapy for renal transplant rejection could no longer be recommended.[167] Nevertheless, use of TPE for this purpose continued to be reported.[111]

In the more recent past, a new wave of enthusiasm for TPE has focused on patients with clinical and histologic evidence of acute rejection who also have circulating donor-specific antibody and/or deposition of complement component C4d in transplant biopsy tissue, suggesting a humoral mechanism.[168] The antibody can be shown by a positive crossmatch with donor cells or by flow cytometric reactions with donor antigens. C4d deposition is demonstrated by immunofluorescence microscopy.[169]

Observations in the pretransplant period have shown that antibody titers can be reduced by TPE.[138] Furthermore, in open trials, patients with refractory acute rejection who demonstrate donor-specific antibody and/or C4d have relatively good long-term graft survival ($\geq$80%) after treatment regimens that include TPE and IVIG.[170,171] A conference on antibody-mediated rejection recommended that demonstration of circulating antibody be considered an essential criterion for diagnosis of humoral rejection and that the effectiveness of TPE and IVIG in this entity be studied in "rigorous prospective, multicenter" trials.[166,171]

TPE has also been employed in cases of cardiac allograft rejection. Favorable outcomes have been reported in individual patients who were also receiving other therapies, but no controlled trials have been conducted. The criteria for a diagnosis of humoral rejection in this setting continue to evolve. "Vascular" histology is more difficult to detect or exclude in the endomyocardial biopsies performed to monitor cardiac allografts because few blood vessels are found in this part of the heart muscle. Immunofluorescence microscopy for IgG had been considered a reasonable criterion for humoral rejection; however, it has been suggested more recently that this diagnosis be made, and TPE employed, in patients with deteriorating cardiac function whose biopsies lack cellular infiltrates.[172] In some such biopsies, it has been possible to demonstrate capillary endothelial swelling, macrophage influx, and C4d deposition.[173] Controlled data to support the TPE recommendation are lacking, as are any published data correlating this clinical syndrome with circulating donor-specific antibody.

Pretransplant TPE has been tried in organ transplant candidates who are sensitized to HLA antigens. Those whose sera react with lymphocytes from a large fraction of the population are less likely to have a compatible crossmatch with a cadaveric donor and hence have a lower likelihood of receiving a transplant. Prospective immunosuppression, combined with antibody removal by TPE or protein A-sepharose immunoadsorption, has been explored as a means to achieve a compatible crossmatch before transplantation and thereby prevent hyperacute rejection. Several centers have reported groups of patients who received kidney transplants after being prepared in this way and achieved quite respectable graft survival rates.[174] Similar protocols have facilitated successful transplantation of ABO-incompatible kidneys and livers.[111–114] In more recent studies, pretransplant TPE has facilitated elective living donor transplantation of HLA-crossmatch positive as well as ABO-incompatible organs.[110,169]

In summary, evidence from controlled trials has not shown global efficacy for TPE in reversing established rejection episodes in renal allografts. Anecdotal experience focusing on patients with circulating antibody and immunopathologic evidence of humoral rejection seems more promising, but controlled trials in such patients have not been published. Pretransplant antibody removal can make transplantation feasible for otherwise ineligible candidates. It can also facilitate transplantation of kidneys from living donors across ABO and donor-specific crossmatch barriers. Clarification of the role of TPE in cardiac transplantation awaits controlled studies targeting patients with documented humoral rejection and circulating donor-specific antibody.

Role of TPE in recurrence of disease

Focal glomerulosclerosis (FGS) is a disease that causes nephrosis and renal failure, predominantly in children. It recurs in about 30%

of allograft recipients, which suggests that a humoral factor may have a role in its pathogenesis. A 50-kD plasma factor that binds to protein A has been implicated but has not been further characterized.[175] Reduced proteinuria and improved renal function have been reported when recurrence in an allograft is treated with increased immunosuppression and TPE.[176]

GPS may occasionally recur in a transplanted kidney; however, this can usually be avoided by delaying transplantation until the anti-GBM response has subsided spontaneously. If the syndrome recurs in spite of this precaution, it should be treated promptly with TPE and cyclophosphamide.

Allograft vasculopathy, a diffuse coronary artery disease that sometimes develops in transplanted hearts, is the leading cause of morbidity and mortality in heart transplant recipients who survive beyond one year. It may be related either to continuing hyperlipidemia or to chronic rejection. Selective depletion of low-density lipoproteins (LDLs), which is discussed in greater detail in the "Hypercholesterolemia" section, has been reported helpful in a few such patients with persistent lipoprotein abnormalities.[177]

TPE in toxic and metabolic disorders

This section covers conditions in which removal of plasma constituents other than immunoglobulin is potentially beneficial.

Hypercholesterolemia

Familial hypercholesterolemia (FH) is a genetically determined deficiency of cell surface LDL receptors that interferes with cholesterol offloading from LDL into cells and with the normal negative-feedback regulation of LDL synthesis, leading to highly elevated levels of circulating LDL, cholesterol (650–1000 mg/dL), and lipoprotein(a) [Lp(a)]. Skin xanthomas and coronary atheromas develop in the first decade of life in homozygotes, and death from myocardial infarction before age 20 is common. Heterozygotes also have elevated LDL, cholesterol (350–500 mg/dL), and Lp(a) levels; they may develop xanthomas by age 20 and coronary atherosclerosis by age 30.[178,179]

Milder forms of hypercholesterolemia can be influenced by dietary modifications and are amenable to drug treatment. However, FH homozygotes and some FH heterozygotes respond only modestly to these measures and remain at risk for premature death. Drastic surgical measures, such as ileal bypass, portacaval shunt, and liver transplantation, may be recommended for such patients if they have evidence of coronary artery disease.[178,179] Alternatively, removal of LDL and its associated cholesterol from the blood can be accomplished repeatedly by various modalities of therapeutic apheresis.[180,181]

A standard TPE will lower LDL and cholesterol levels by 50% or more, and long-term treatment every 1–2 weeks can lead to shrinkage of cutaneous xanthomas and regression of coronary artery deposits.[182] Although TPE removes both LDL and Lp(a), it also depletes high-density lipoproteins (HDLs), which are believed to have an antiatherogenic action. This disadvantage has stimulated efforts to deplete LDL semiselectively and on-line from patient plasma separated by an apheresis device, and then return the LDL-depleted plasma to the patient.

Refsum's disease

Refsum's disease results from deficiency of the peroxisomal enzyme phytanoyl–CoA hydroxylase, which participates in degradation of phytanic acid by α-oxidation. Accumulation of diet-derived phytanic acid in plasma lipoproteins and in tissue lipid stores leads to

symptoms, which may include peripheral neuropathy, cerebellar ataxia, retinitis pigmentosa, anosmia, deafness, ichthyosis, renal failure, and arrhythmias. Slow progression is the usual course, but rapid deterioration and even sudden death may follow a marked increase in plasma phytanic acid.[183]

Restriction of dietary intake of phytanic acid via dairy products, meats, and ruminant fats is the mainstay of treatment. It leads to gradual clearing of phytanate stores by slow ω- oxidation and gradual symptomatic improvement in most patients. Nutrition must be maintained, however, because mobilization of calories from endogenous fat can increase plasma phytanic acid levels acutely and cause clinical exacerbations. TPE will remove large quantities of phytanic acid incorporated into plasma lipids.[184] Selective lipoprotein depletion is also effective.[185] Apheresis therapy is most appropriate for patients who have very high plasma phytanate levels and an associated exacerbation of symptoms. Skin disease, neuropathic symptoms, and ataxia usually improve as plasma levels drop. Cranial nerve defects usually do not.[184]

Drug overdose and poisoning

Toxic effects may occur after exposure to excessive doses of pharmacologic agents or to harmful agents in the environment. Management techniques for both types of event are similar and may include removal of toxin still in the gastrointestinal tract, enhancement of renal elimination, and direct removal from blood by hemodialysis, hemoperfusion (e.g., over charcoal columns), or TPE.[186] Specific antidotes may also be given if available. Serious events are usually treated with multiple measures.

TPE has been reported to be beneficial, when combined with other therapies, in cases involving substances such as methyl parathion, vincristine, and cisplatin that bind tightly to plasma proteins. It has also been reported for severe hyperthyroidism,[163] either endogenous or exogenous, in which its effectiveness may be limited by extensive binding of L-thyroxine to tissue proteins. TPE has been reported in poisonings due to ingestion of the *Amanita phalloides* mushroom; however, diuresis clears more *Amanita* toxin.[111]

Unfortunately, the literature on this topic is older and entirely anecdotal. Furthermore, TPE has always been used in combination with other therapies that are presumably effective. This complicates the formulation of firm, rational guidelines. Nevertheless, it seems reasonable to offer TPE to a severely affected patient with an overdose or poisoning who has a high blood level of a toxic agent that binds to plasma proteins. It should also be noted that TPE has shown minimal or no beneficial effect in overdosage of drugs known to bind to tissue proteins and lipids, including barbiturates, chlordecone, aluminum, tricyclic antidepressants, benzodiazepines, quinine, phenytoin, digoxin, digitoxin, prednisone, prednisolone, tobramycin, and propranolol.[111]

Acute hepatic failure

Acute hepatic failure may develop after a severe liver insult, such as overwhelming hepatitis B infection or acetaminophen overdosage. Cases may also be caused by drug reactions, Wilson's disease, vascular anomalies, acute fatty liver of pregnancy, and a variety of toxins. Acute hepatic failure results in many metabolic imbalances and synthetic defects. Clinical symptoms include jaundice, coagulopathy, encephalopathy, and renal failure. The treatment of choice is liver transplantation, which leads to 60–80% long-term survival versus >60% mortality for untransplanted patients.

Cerebral edema accounts for fatal outcomes. TPE has been helpful in acute hepatic failure in Wilson's disease.[189]

TPE with plasma replacement has seemed appealing as a means to restore metabolic homeostasis, remove toxic metabolites that may cause cerebral edema, and supply coagulation factors and other deficient plasma proteins in quantity without causing volume overload. Practical evaluations of this approach have produced mixed results.[187] Some investigators have found TPE helpful in stabilizing and maintaining patients until an organ for transplant becomes available. Improvements in blood pressure, cerebral blood flow, and neurologic status were attributed to TPE in one study;[187] however, intracranial pressure, a key prognostic indicator, did not decrease. Hemoperfusion over activated charcoal, which will lower plasma ammonia levels, has also shown no advantage over intensive supportive care alone.

Potential problems with extensive TPE arise from the diminished ability of patients with acute hepatic failure to metabolize the citrate in infused plasma. Accumulation of citrate leads to ionized hypocalcemia and to alterations in arterial ketone body ratios that may interfere with regeneration of hepatocytes.[188] Thus, although TPE can partially reverse coagulopathy and other synthetic deficits in these patients, a favorable net impact on outcome has been difficult to demonstrate.

Therapeutic apheresis in children

TPE or cytapheresis can be performed on even very small children.[190–193] The major consideration is that the instruments are designed for adults, and thus the extracorporeal volume may be too large for small patients. This can be overcome by priming the instrument with red cells, albumin, or other combinations of fluids. The Optia has a small extracorporeal volume and may be more convenient for small patients. The blood flow rates through the instrument are not high for adults but may represent a large portion of a small child's blood volume. Therefore, problems can arise quickly if there are difficulties with the lines or blood flow. Also, the rate of return of blood and solutions can be much greater in relation to the total blood volume of a small child, and thus citrate or other complications can occur more frequently than in adults if adjustments in blood flow are not made to reflect the small patient's blood volume.[194]

Acknowledgment

The authors acknowledge the contribution of this chapter in the prior edition by Bruce McLeod (now retired) in providing a foundation for the current chapter.

Key references

A full reference list for this chapter is available at: http://www.wiley.com/go/simon/transfusion

1   McLeod BC, Price TH, Weinstein R, Eds. *Apheresis: principles and practice.* 3rd ed. Bethesda, MD: AABB Press, 2010.

21   Chopek M, McCullough J. Protein and biochemical changes during plasma exchange. In: *Therapeutic hemapheresis.* Arlington, VA: AABB, 1980:13.

47   McLeod BC, Price TH, Owen H, *et al.* Frequency of immediate adverse effects associated with therapeutic apheresis. *Transfusion* 1999;**39**:282–8.

54   Gwathmey K, Balogun RA, Burns T. Neurologic indications for therapeutic plasma exchange: 2011 update. *J Clin Apher* 2012;**27**:138–45. doi: 10.1002/jca.21219

99   Zarkovic M, Kwaan HC. Correction of hyperviscosity by apheresis. *Semin Thromb Hemost* 2003;**29**:535–42.

114   The critical role of plasmapheresis in ABO-incompatible renal transplantation. *Transfusion* 2008;**48** (11): 2453–60.

146   Koo AP. Therapeutic apheresis in autoimmune and rheumatic disorders. *J Clin Apher* 2000;**15**:18–27.

170   Montgomery RA, Zachary AA. Transplanting patients with a positive donor-specific crossmatch: A single center's perspective. *Pediatr Transplantation* 2004;**8**:535–42.

194   Wong ECC, Balogun RA. Therapeutic apheresis in pediatrics: technique adjustments, indications and nonindications, a plasma exchange focus. *J Clin Apher* 2012;**27**:132–37. doi: 10.1002/jca.21224

CHAPTER 34

Therapeutic phlebotomy and specialized hemapheresis

Jeffrey A. Bailey[1,2,3] **& Robert Weinstein**[1,2]

[1]Departments of Medicine and Pathology, Division of Transfusion Medicine, University of Massachusetts Medical School, Worcester, MA, USA
[2]UMass Memorial Medical Center, Worcester, MA, USA
[3]Program in Bioinformatics and Integrative Biology, University of Massachusetts Medical School, Worcester, MA, USA

The sixth comprehensive, evidence-based analysis of apheresis thera-pies by the American Society for Apheresis (ASFA) recorded 60 disease conditions as Category I (apheresis as first-line therapy) or Category II (apheresis as second-line or adjuvant therapy) indications for therapeutic apheresis.[1] Among these, 37 (62%) were indications for plasma exchange, consistent with prior surveys that found plasma exchange to be the predominant form of apheresis therapy in North America.[2,3] Whereas apheresis procedures have been in wide use for decades,[4] many on the basis of accumulated experience, the approval of new therapeutic indications, devices, and drugs is increasingly dependent on the presentation of carefully acquired supportive evidence in randomized controlled trials.[5,6] This applies to phlebot-omy and apheresis therapies as well[7,8] and ASFA presents its recom-mendations, and the strength of the evidence that underlies them, according to the G.R.A.D.E. system.[1] Accordingly, this chapter, which reviews therapeutic phlebotomy and specialized apheresis procedures that target, for processing, specific fractions of the plasma or cellular compartment of the blood, emphasizes those procedures that are supported by evidence.

Therapeutic red cell apheresis

John J. Abel of the Johns Hopkins University used the term "plas-mapheresis" to describe a method for removing large quantities of plasma from experimental animals.[9] Thus, the removal of red cells for therapeutic purposes can be referred to as *erythrocytapheresis*.[1] This term particularly applies to the removal of red cells using automated blood-processing instruments that are capable of selectively removing erythrocytes while returning the plasma, buffy coat cells, and addi-tional isotonic saline to the patient.[10] The therapeutic replacement of patient red cells for donor red cells is more specifically referred to as *red cell exchange*,[11] although the term erythrocytapheresis is fre-quently used synonomously.[1]

Red cell exchange

Therapeutic red cell exchange can be performed manually or with programmable automated blood-processing (apheresis) instru-ments. Manual exchange is mainly limited to neonates or resource-limited settings. Thus, this discussion focuses on auto-mated red cell exchange.

Basic features of automated blood processors that perform apheresis using centrifugation technology are detailed in Chapter 32. The machine operator enters the patient's gender, height, and weight into the instrument's computer to calculate total blood volume. The operator also inputs the known starting and desired ending hematocrit of the patient, the average hematocrit of red cell replacement units to be used, and the desired fluid balance (a default of 100% may be offered by the instrument). Finally, the operator can choose to enter the desired fraction of the preproce-dure red cells remaining (FCR) within the patient's circulation at the end of the procedure or the volume of replacement fluid (e.g., red cells of average hematocrit as programmed into the instrument's computer) needed for the procedure.

Calculation of the desired FCR is predicated on the targeted therapeutic endpoint over the starting point for the red cell exchange. For manual or automated exchanges where there is no correction for changes in the hematocrit, correction is needed:

$$FCR = 100 \times \left(\frac{\text{starting hematocrit}}{\text{ending hematocrit}}\right) \times \left(\frac{\text{endoint parameter}}{\text{starting parameter}}\right) \quad (1)$$

For example, a sickle cell patient with a hematocrit of 25% and 100% HbS, targeted to an endpoint of HbS 30% and ending hematocrit of 30%, would yield:

$$FCR = 100 \times \left(\frac{25\%}{30\%}\right) \times \left(\frac{30\%}{100\%}\right) = 25\%$$

The replacement volume needed to reach the desired FCR is dependent on the patient's blood volume, the starting hematocrit, the target hematocrit, fluid balance, and the average hematocrit of the replacement RBC units. It is important to remember that modern automated apheresis instruments incorporate the starting and endpoint hematocrit, and thus the machine FCR simply approximates the desired fraction of original parameter of interest.

According to ASFA, red cell exchange is indicated as first- or second-line therapy for treatment of severe manifestations of the protozoal infections (e.g., malaria and babesiosis) and for the management of sickle cell disease (SCD).[1]

Rossi's Principles of Transfusion Medicine, Fifth Edition. Edited by Toby L. Simon, Jeffrey McCullough, Edward L. Snyder, Bjarte G. Solheim, and Ronald G. Strauss.
© 2016 John Wiley & Sons, Ltd. Published 2016 by John Wiley & Sons, Ltd.

Sickle cell disease

Sickled erythrocytes were first described in Western medicine in 1910 by Dr. J.B. Herrick, who noted the abnormally shaped red cells in the peripheral blood film of a dental student from the Caribbean island of Grenada.[12] An underlying mutation results in substitution of valine for glutamic acid as the sixth amino acid residue in the hemoglobin β chain[13] and has arisen multiple times in Africa due to its protective effects from severe falciparum malaria in the heterozygous state.[14] Once at appreciable frequency in a population, the homozygous sickle state leads to SCD. The description of these countervailing forces on survival provided one of the initial examples of balancing selection in evolution.[15]

The fundamental molecular etiology of sickling is due to increased hydrophobic interactions between nearby HbS molecules whereby deoxygenated HbS aggregates into large inflexible polymers and inflexible sickled red cells. This combined with membrane changes increasing sickle cell adhesiveness is the underlying basis for the hemolytic and vaso-occlusive morbidity of SCD.[16,17] The exquisite dependence of polymerization on the proportion of HbS[18] has provided a scientific basis, in concert with the strong clinical basis,[19] for transfusion therapy of normal red cells in sickle cell anemia.

For the most part, clinical studies related to transfusion management of SCD have focused on simple transfusion or manual exchange transfusion.[19–23] The efficacy of manual versus automated red cell exchange in the treatment of SCD has not been directly compared.[24] Although for most SCD complications, simple transfusions may likely be as effective, automated red cell exchange can more rapidly decrease the proportion of HbS red cells during severe acute episodes.[1] In SCD patients who receive chronic transfusion, automated red cell exchange can mitigate iron overload[25,26] while maintaining a low HbS level. Thus, it has entered into routine use in centers where therapeutic apheresis is available. Its indicated roles in the aspects of SCD (Table 34.1)[1,24,27] are discussed here. Exchanges may be performed using isotonic saline, rather than red cells, as the replacement fluid in the early phases of the procedure in order to minimize the number of donor red blood cell (RBC) units required by avoiding the initial removal of the normal replacement red cells.[25,26]

Life- or organ-threatening complications

Red cell exchange is standard therapy (ASFA Category I) for children with acute vaso-occlusive stroke[1] and should be performed shortly following documentation of thrombotic (rather than hemorrhagic) stroke by noncontrast computed tomography.[19,24,27] The treatment goal should be a hemoglobin concentration between 9 and 10 g/dL and less than 30% HbS. Acute intervention, followed by chronic maintenance transfusion therapy, may limit early

morbidity and mortality and prevent recurrence (discussed further in this chapter).[19,27]

In its 2000 report,[22] the National Acute Chest Syndrome Study Group (NACSSG) defined acute chest syndrome, the second most common cause for hospitalization and the leading cause of death in SCD,[27] on the basis of presentation with a new alveolar infiltrate involving one or more complete lung segments (atelectasis excluded) and accompanied by chest pain, a fever >38.5 °C, tachypnea, wheezing, or cough. Although the NACSSG report was not powered to detect a particular advantage of red cell exchange over simple transfusion,[22] the consensus opinion of experts in the field is to recommend red cell exchange for severe ACS (oxygen saturation <90% despite supplemental oxygen).[1,27]

Acute multiorgan failure syndrome is a common cause of death in sickle cell disease,[24,27,28] it may present as an unusually severe pain episode in patients with sickle cell anemia or HbSC disease and is characterized by fever, accelerated hemolysis with a rapid decrease in hemoglobin and platelet count, nonfocal encephalopathy, and rhabdomyolysis.[28] Besides the central nervous system, other organs, including liver and kidney, may be involved.[28] Standard red cell transfusion therapy is likely effective if severe anemia is present. Although evidence is limited to case reports and series, red cell exchange should be considered with higher hemoglobin levels.[24] Red cell exchange can also be considered for hepatic sequestration and intrahepatic cholestasis.[27]

The role of transfusion and exchange transfusion in priapism, which occurs in approximately 30% to 90% of males with SCD,[27,28] has been debated. However, there is increasing consensus that transfusion is not warranted, and the recent NIH expert panel states that transfusion should not be used.[27] Studies have shown no benefit over conventional therapies, the time to resolution is often longer for those transfused, and further interventions such as surgical decompression are often required.[19] In addition, severe neurologic abnormalities have been associated with red cell exchange, as first reported in six boys with sickle cell anemia 1 to 11 days following partial exchange transfusion for priapism unresponsive to conservative therapy.[29] The syndrome was characterized by severe headache at the onset, often associated with increased intracranial pressure, and further neurologic events ranging from seizure activity to obtundation requiring ventilatory support.[29,30] Finally, a comprehensive review of 42 well-documented case reports of transfusion therapy in SCD-associated priapism evaluated the effectiveness of transfusion therapy versus conventional therapies in terms of time to detumescence.[31] The mean time to detumescence with transfusion therapies was 10.8 days (26 cases) versus 8.0 days with conventional therapies (16 cases). Neurologic complications with transfusion therapy were described in nine cases, some with persistent long-term deficits.

Primary and secondary prevention of stroke

Approximately 5% to 10% of untransfused children with SCD will have a clinically evident cerebral infarction by age 20.[32,33] Chronic transfusion therapy, given every 3 to 4 weeks, to maintain the level of HbS below 30% can improve the arteriographic appearance of affected cerebral vessels and reduce the risk of recurrent stroke from 66% to 90% to approximately 10%.[24,27] Chronic automated red cell exchange can be substituted for simple transfusion, with the added potential benefit of preventing or mitigating iron overload.[25,26] Reports of recurrent stroke rates of 50% or greater after discontinuation of transfusion therapy have led most to recommend indefinite prophylactic transfusion regimens.[24,27,34]

Table 34.1 Red cell exchange in sickle cell disease[1,24,27]

Acute or emergent	Acute vaso-occlusive stroke
	Multi-organ failure syndrome
	Hepatic sequestration or intrahepatic cholestasis
	Severe acute chest syndrome
Chronic	Prevention of stroke in high-risk children
	Secondary stroke prevention
	Prevention of iron overload in chronic transfusion recipient

The demonstration that transcranial Doppler ultrasound (TCD) was highly predictive of stroke risk in children with SCD[34] led to the Stroke Prevention Trial in Sickle Cell Anemia (STOP trial),[21] which examined the ability of chronic transfusion therapy to prevent a *first* stroke in high-risk children with SCD. Time-averaged mean blood-flow velocity of at least 200 cm/sec in the internal carotid or middle cerebral artery and a stroke-free history were required for study entry.[21] Over a period of approximately 2 to 3 years, transfusion therapy to maintain HbS below 30% without exceeding a hemoglobin concentration of 12 g/dL reduced the occurrence of stroke in the treatment group by 90% compared to the control group.[21] A follow-up study (STOP2)[35] examined the effect of discontinuation of transfusion therapy after 30 months in children from the first STOP trial whose transcranial Doppler readings had reverted to normal. The study was halted when an interim analysis revealed that, of 41 children randomly assigned to discontinue transfusions, 14 had reverted to elevated TCD findings within nine months after stopping transfusions and two had suffered ischemic strokes. Neither elevated TCDs nor strokes were observed in the controls continuing transfusion. Similarly, the Stroke With Transfusions Changing to Hydroxyurea (SWiTCH) trial comparing transfusions (with chelation) to hydroxyurea was halted when interim analysis revealed reversion to elevated TCD and increased incidence of overt stroke.[36]

As a result of these studies demonstrating no equivalent therapy or safe endpoint for chronic transfusion therapy, the current recommendation is that individuals with a history of elevated transcranial arterial flow or a history of stroke continue transfusion therapy indefinitely.[27] Furthermore, the indication for transfusion in stroke prevention may broaden, given that among children with magnetic resonance imaging (MRI)-demonstrated silent infarcts, but lacking elevated intracranial arterial flow rates, those randomized to receive chronic transfusions had lower rates of both silent infarcts and overt strokes.[37]

Transfusional iron overload

There are no randomized, prospective comparisons of simple transfusion versus automated red cell exchange in the prevention of iron overload in children with SCD who require chronic transfusion therapy. However, four case series of eight to 14 subjects[25,26] have been reported in which children were either converted from a simple transfusion program to monthly red cell exchange or begun on red cell exchange early on. In addition, some in each series were on chelation therapy with desferrioxamine,[27] and some were not. In general, red cell exchange resulted in a 25% to 100% increase in red cell usage and a concomitant increase in donor exposures. However, serum ferritin tended to stabilize in those who were not on chelation therapy and significantly decreased in those who continued on chelation therapy. Some children who were begun on red cell exchange before development of iron overload did not accumulate iron as a result of their red cell exchange treatments.

Protozoan disease

Severe manifestations of malaria and babesiosis are ranked as Category II indications by ASFA, largely on the basis of anecdotal evidence.[1,38,39]

Malaria

Severe malaria is usually caused by *Plasmodium falciparum*.[40] The infection results from injection of sporozoites into the bloodstream by the bite of a female *Anopheles* mosquito. The sporozoites migrate to and infect liver cells, where they asexually reproduce to form numerous merozoites that burst forth and invade RBCs. This initiates the erythrocytic life cycle with repeated rounds of RBC infections and increasing parasitemia, and symptoms such as recurrent fever, which can culminate in life-threatening end-organ dysfunction that defines severe malaria.[41]

The relative severity of *P. falciparum* malaria is due to adherence of falciparum-infected erythrocytes to glycosylated molecules on microvascular endothelium and to platelet CD36 via *P. falciparum* erythrocyte membrane protein-1 (PfEMP-1), an adhesive protein expressed on the surface of infected erythrocytes.[42,43] The sequestration and vasoclusion combined with the elaboration of pro-inflammatory cytokines such as tumor necrosis factor-α (TNFα) and interferon-γ result in the severe manifestations of the disease.[44] Thus, the use of exchange transfusion and automated red cell exchange in the treatment of severe malaria is based on an ability to rapidly reduce the burden of parasitemia and the potential to thereby improve the rheologic properties of the blood and reduce the level of toxic mediators such as cytokines.[1] Case series (16 patients total) and one case report describe lowering of parasitemia by 80% to 90% using automated red cell exchange of 1.0 to 1.5 red cell volumes in approximately two hours, followed by rapid clinical recovery, in cases of severe *P. falciparum* malaria, including cerebral malaria.[1] The exact impact on the number of sequestered infected RBCs remains undetermined. The evidence for improved survival is mixed, with retrospective case control series variably favoring antibiotic therapy alone or adjunct exchange transfusion, but all studies have suffered from poor control for malaria severity.[39]

The US Centers for Disease Control and Prevention (CDC) and American Society for Apheresis (ASFA) have, until recently, both recommended consideration of RBC exchange in cases of severe malaria with parasitemia >10%.[1] However, CDC investigators recently analyzed their malaria reporting data from 1985 to 2010 and compared 101 exchange transfusion cases with 314 propensity-matched non-exchange cases of severe malaria.[45] They found no survival advantage with 17.8% mortality in the exchange-transfused group compared to the 15.9% for the controls. This, along with the lack of high-level evidence in the literature, led the CDC to conclude that exchange transfusion should no longer be recommended.[45] However, their retrospective analysis only had power to assuredly detect a very strong effect (<4.6% mortality in exchange transfused at 90% power, presuming 15.9% in controls) and lacked key data for the vast majority of cases (e.g., <10% of cases reported parasitemia levels, a key trigger for exchange per ASFA guidelines). These study limitations were cited in ASFA's response to this publication saying that the ASFA recommendation for red cell exchange would stand.[46] What is not in dispute is that current artemisinin combination therapies lead to rapid parasite clearance, in line with the rapidity of clearance by apheresis or manual exchange.[47] Given that these drugs also clear sequestered parasites, artemisinin-based therapy (although not first-line therapy in the United States) should limit the need for adjunct red cell exchange to speed parasite clearance.[45,47] However, in the face of the recent emergence and spread of artemisinin resistance in Southeast Asia and the lack of another effective antimalarial,[48] a properly controlled prospective trial to determine the benefit of exchange (e.g., 50% improved survival) probably remains worthwhile.

Babesiosis

Babesiosis in humans is a zoonotic disease and is spread to humans primarily through ticks of the genus *Ixodes*.[49] The first reported case of human babesiosis was in an asplenic individual from Europe.[50] The first case in a patient with an intact spleen was reported in Nantucket.[51] Within the United States, the predominant organism is *Babesia microti*, the reservoir hosts are wild rodents, and the vector is the deer tick *Ixodes scapularis*, which is the same tick that transmits *Borrelia burgdorferi*, the causative agent of Lyme disease.[49] Over the past several decades, the endemic range has expanded, and now encompasses seven states in the Northeast and the Midwest United States, which accounted for >95% of 1762 reported babesiosis cases.[52]

When injected into the human bloodstream, the sporozoites of babesia directly invade RBCs. After asexual budding into four merozoites, the parasites perforate the erythrocyte membrane, resulting in hemolysis.[53] They are then free to infect other erythrocytes, and transform into dividing trophozoites (ring forms and tetrads visible on peripheral blood films).[49,53] One to six weeks following inoculation, infected patients develop a flu-like syndrome characterized by fever, fatigue, and malaise.[54] Headache, chills, sweats, myalgia, and arthralgia are frequent complaints. Physical findings may include fever and splenomegaly, and jaundice and pallor may accompany marked extravascular hemolysis. Although most cases are subclinical or mild,[55] severe manifestations, including disseminated intravascular coagulation, respiratory failure, and renal failure, may occur. Immunocompromised or asplenic individuals are typically more severely affected.[49,56]

Transfusion transmission is frequent in endemic areas, leading to infections of those most vulnerable: neonates, the immunocompromised, and the elderly.[57] Although clinical trials are lacking, several case reports and case series suggest that, given the absence of a microvascular sequestration of infection, red cell exchange, whole blood exchange, or red cell exchange followed by plasma exchange, combined with antibiotic therapy, can be beneficial in severe cases of babesiosis with >5% parasitemia.[1,58–60] A single one- to two-volume red cell exchange can reduce the circulating population of parasitized erythrocytes by 85% to 90%.[1] Exchange also appears effective in neonates with severe transfusion-associated babesiosis.[61]

Erythrocytapheresis and therapeutic phlebotomy

Therapeutic phlebotomy or venesection is a procedure that has been performed throughout recorded history. In current clinical practice, therapeutic phlebotomy is an evidence-based intervention for disorders such as polycythemia vera and hemochromatosis.[1] Although erythrocytapheresis has been investigated as a means of more rapid removal of red cell mass and limiting plasma loss, phlebotomy remains the therapeutic mainstay in most settings given its simplicity.

Polycythemia vera

Classified as a bcr/abl-negative classic myeloproliferative neoplasm showing absolute erythrocytosis,[62] it is further characterized by panmyelosis in the marrow and peripheral blood, splenomegaly, hyperviscosity of the blood, thrombosis, and a tendency to evolve into either acute myeloid leukemia or myelofibrosis.[63,64] Over 95% of cases are now known to be associated with an acquired point mutation, V617F, in exon 14 of the Janus kinase 2 (JAK2) gene on chromosome 9p24.[65] The remaining 5% of patients appear to have mutations in exon 12 of JAK2, some of whom may have a more benign phenotype (idiopathic erythrocytosis).[65] A revised World Health Organization (WHO) diagnostic system (Table 34.2) that recognizes the predominance of JAK2 mutations in polycythemia

Table 34.2 Diagnostic criteria for polycythemia vera[62,66].

Major	1. Male: Hgb >18.5 g/dL (Hct 60%); female: 16.5 g/dL (Hct >=56%) or other evidence of increased RBC volume. (Or: >99th percentile for age, sex, and altitude or >2 g/dL sustained rise above patient baseline and >17 g/dL in men and 15 g/dL in females.)
	2. Presence of JAK2 V617F or JAK2 exon 12 functional mutation
Minor	1. Bone marrow with hypercellularity for age and trilineage myeloproliferation
	2. Serum erythropoietin level below laboratory reference range
	3. Endogenous erythroid colony formation in vitro

Diagnosis: Both major and one minor, or first major and two minor.

vera has been widely adopted.[62,66] Setting precise cutoffs for erythrocytosis is challenging. The International Council for Standardization in Haematology recognizes absolute erythrocytosis in an individual whose measured total red cell volume, or *red cell mass*, is more than 25% above the mean predicted value for a person of the same body surface area.[64] This formed the basis for Hb/Hct cutoffs, as absolute erythrocytosis will almost always be present in men with a hematocrit of ≥60% (Hb >=18.5 g/dL) and women with a hematocrit ≥56% (Hb >=16.5 g/dL). But such specific cutoffs for Hb in the WHO criteria are not sensitive enough and have been shown to miss mildly elevated RBC mass in early polycythemia vera.[67] These findings may lead to more nuanced diagnostic cutoffs in the future.

Therapeutic phlebotomy in polycythemia vera

The increased whole blood viscosity that results from the expansion of total red cell volume in patients with polycythemia vera is the underlying basis of the life-threatening prothrombotic state and the headache, fatigue, dyspnea, cyanosis, and other signs and symptoms that characterize the disorder.[66] Aggressive phlebotomy to a hematocrit below 45% in males and below 42–45% in females is indicated for prevention of life-threatening thrombotic complications of polycythemia vera.[66,68] High-risk patients (age >60 years or history of thrombosis) should also be treated with cytoreductive hydroxyurea or, if erythrocytosis is recalcitrant, a second-line agent (e.g., busulfan or interferon-α).[66,68] Low-risk patients (age <60 years, no cardiovascular risk, platelet count <1,000,000/μL) may initially be managed with phlebotomy alone.[66] Low-dose aspirin (100 mg/day) is recommended for all patients without specific contraindications to its use.[66] The pharmaceutical development of JAK2-selective kinase inhibiting agents has shown efficacy in early trials and should influence future management of polycythemia vera.[69]

Erythrocytapheresis in polycythemia vera

According to ASFA, polycythemia vera is a Category I indication for red cell volume reduction by erythrocytapheresis.[1] A retrospective case series of 69 patients with polycythemia vera who underwent 206 isovolemic erythrocytapheresis procedures using 4% albumin as replacement fluid reported reduction of hematocrit from 56.8 ± 5.6% to 41.9 ± 6.6% after removal of 1410 ± 418 mL of red cells.[70] A subset of 21 patients for whom close follow-up data were available maintained a hematocrit of <50% for a median of six months.[70] The volume of red cells to be removed (VR) during an erythrocytapheresis in order to achieve a desired hematocrit can be calculated as (Formula 2):[70,71]

$$VR = \left(\frac{\text{starting HCT} - \text{desired Hct}}{79}\right) \times \left(\begin{array}{c}\text{blood volume}\\(mL/kg)\end{array}\right) \times \left(\begin{array}{c}\text{body weight}\\(kg)\end{array}\right) \quad (2)$$

Thus, for a 70-kg person with a blood volume of 70 mL/kg whose hematocrit is to be lowered from 68% to 55%, the volume of red cells to be removed is calculated as:

$$VR = \left(\frac{68 - 55}{79}\right) \times (70 \text{ mL/kg}) \times (70 \text{ kg}) = 910 \text{ mL of red cells}$$

Additional studies have confirmed that erythrocytapheresis can rapidly decrease hematocrit for extended intervals relative to simple phlebotomy.[72,73] and suggest that automated erythrocytapheresis may have a role for patients with acute thrombotic or microvascular complications, or to avoid perioperative thrombohemorrhagic complications in a patient with an uncontrolled hematocrit who requires urgent surgery.[1,71]

Secondary erythrocytosis

Secondary erythrocytosis includes conditions that result in an elevated total red cell volume but are not clonal disorders of the marrow.[64,66,74] Congenital and acquired causes have been described, and they predominantly involve the regulation or aberrant expression of erythropoietin or abnormalities of the erythropoietin receptor (see Table 34.3).[75,76] The vast majority of cases are hypoxia-stimulated, usually due to chronic lung disease, smoking, or apnea. A diagnostic investigation of a patient with suspected erythrocytosis is performed in order to (1) establish that a true state of erythrocytosis exists (i.e. an elevated total red cell volume), (2) rule out polycythemia vera, and (3) determine the cause of secondary erythrocytosis, thereby leading to clinical management to alleviate the underlying cause.[64,66,74–76]

Therapeutic phlebotomy in secondary erythrocytosis

The role of phlebotomy is less certain in secondary erythrocytosis than in polycythemia vera.[1,76] As suggested by Table 34.3, secondary erythrocytosis is generally an adaptation to the disordered regulation of erythropoietin or to hypoxemia. In some cases, the underlying cause can be treated medically or surgically, and in

Table 34.3 Secondary erythrocytosis[75,76,]

Type	Underlying Cause
Congenital	High oxygen-affinity hemoglobin Bisphosphoglycerate mutase deficiency Erythropoietin receptor mutation Oxygen-sensing pathway mutations (VHL, PHD2, and HIF-2a gene mutations)
Acquired	Hypoxia-stimulated • Cyanotic congenital heart disease • Chronic lung disease • High-altitude habitat • Smoker's erythrocytosis • Carbon monoxide poisoning • Chronic hypoventilation (sleep apnea) • Renal artery stenosis Inappropriate erythropoietin production • Renal cancer • Hepatic cancer • Cerebellar hemangioblastoma • Endocrine tumors • Uterine leiomyoma • Polycystic kidney • Meningioma Drug-mediated • Androgen therapy • "Blood doping" (surreptitious erythropoietin use) Multifactorial etiology • Postrenal transplant erythrocytosis

others the erythrocytosis represents a physiologic adaptation to a chronic condition such as hypoxia but without thrombotic risk.[77] For example, adults with cyanotic congenital heart disease are not considered to be at heightened risk for thrombotic stroke despite mean hematocrits of 57.5% ± 7.2%[78] and do not exhibit symptoms of hyperviscosity until hematocrits reach 65% (in the absence of dehydration or iron deficiency).[79] A program of therapeutic phlebotomy should not be undertaken purely for the sake of achieving a target hematocrit in an asymptomatic individual. Isovolemic phlebotomy, with saline replacement, should be reserved for patients who are neither dehydrated nor iron deficient, and who have moderate symptoms of hyperviscosity (i.e., headache, slow mentation, visual disturbance, tinnitus, dizziness, etc.).[79] Withdrawal of up to a unit of whole blood, replaced by 750 to 1000 mL of isotonic saline, has been recommended for relief of symptoms. Similar recommendations may refer to patients with high oxygen-affinity hemoglobin levels who have symptoms such as dizziness, dyspnea, or angina, which are believed to result, in part, from an expanded total red cell volume.[76] There is again no formal evidence that phlebotomy is beneficial, and a modest target (i.e., a hematocrit <60% achieved with fluid replacement) has been recommended.[76] Likewise, patients with chronic hypoxic lung disease and erythrocytosis or with smoker's erythrocytosis are best managed using medical therapy to deal with their underlying pulmonary disorder. Noncontrolled studies suggest that phlebotomy to a hematocrit of 50% to 52% may improve exercise tolerance, alleviate headache and confusion, and otherwise ameliorate symptoms of hyperviscosity.[76]

Postrenal transplant erythrocytosis, defined as a persistently elevated hematocrit above 51%, occurs spontaneously in 15% to 20% of kidney transplant recipients in the first 8 to 24 months after engraftment.[80–82] One-fourth of cases remit spontaneously within two years of onset, with the balance persisting for up to several years until chronic graft rejection supervenes.[76] The major risk factors are retention of the native kidneys, male gender, smoking, a rejection-free course with a well-functioning graft, and adequate red cell production (without the need for erythropoietin or transfusion) prior to transplant.[80,82] Hyperviscosity symptoms such as malaise, headache, plethora, lethargy, and dizziness are described as common among patients with this condition, and 10% to 30% develop significant thromboembolic complications.[80,82] The pathogenesis appears to be multifactorial, and likely involves an interplay between endogenous erythropoietin production by the retained native kidney, the renin-angiotensin system, androgen secretion, insulin-like growth factors, and cytokines.[80,81] One retrospective series reported 11 thromboembolic events, including transient ischemic attacks and strokes, and venous thromboembolism in 10 of 53 (19%) patients with postrenal transplant erythrocytosis but in none of 49 control cases ($p < 0.001$).[82] This sort of experience has led to an appreciation of the need to control the red cell volume in these patients.[80–82] The mainstay of treatment is angiotensin-converting enzyme inhibition or angiotensin-converting enzyme receptor blockade, sometimes in combination with theophylline, which lowers hemoglobin and hematocrit within eight weeks, with peak effect seen after up to 12 months.[83]

Erythrocytapheresis in secondary erythrocytosis

Automated erythrocytapheresis is seldom recommended for management of secondary erythrocytosis,[71] and its optimum role has not been established, thus requiring individualized decisions.[1] It may be useful in circumstances where isovolemic procedures are called for, such as in cyanotic heart disease.[79] Erythrocytapheresis has not been reported in the management of posttransplant erythrocytosis.

Hereditary hemochromatosis

Hereditary hemochromatosis is an inherited disorder that, untreated, results in iron deposition in, and damage to, the liver, heart, pancreas, and other organs, including bronze pigmentation of the skin.[84,85] Its prevalence is approximately 1:200 among those of European ancestry.[84,86] The most common genetic mutation, accounting for >90% of cases (and almost all cases in persons of Northern European ancestry), is homozygosity for a missense mutation (G845A) in the HFE gene resulting in tyrosine substituted for cysteine (C282Y).[87] HFE C282Y (as well as H63D) decreases hepcidin transcription by stabilizing the ALK3 protein that inhibits transcription.[88] In the absence of a physiological means of body iron excretion, the increased iron uptake resulting from these mutations leads to the slow accumulation of iron in the liver and other organs, and eventual liver failure (via cirrhosis, hepatocellular carcinoma, etc.), diabetes, hypogonadism, hypopituitarism, arthropathy, cardiomyopathy and heart failure, and skin pigmentation.[86,89] A presenting syndrome of asthenia, arthralgia, and abnormal liver function (three A's) has been described as classic for the clinical disease.[85] Because of the central importance of iron loading in the pathogenesis of hereditary hemochromatosis, iron removal by phlebotomy is the mainstay of treatment.[86,89] Diagnostic elements of hereditary hemochromatosis are provided in Table 34.4.

Therapeutic phlebotomy in hereditary hemochromatosis

Therapeutic phlebotomy has been the primary mode of iron reduction in hereditary hemochromatosis for over a half century.[84,86] Phlebotomy therapy should be started in all patients whose serum ferritin level is elevated (Table 34.4) and should not be withheld from the elderly on the basis of age or from iron-loaded patients who have not developed clinical symptoms.[86,87] A common treatment approach is to perform one phlebotomy per week (1 unit or 7 mL/kg of whole blood not to exceed 550 mL per phlebotomy) until the serum ferritin is below 50 ng/mL (although this endpoint is not based on clear-cut evidence).[86,89] Thereafter, it is usually necessary to annually remove 3–4 units of blood to maintain the ferritin between 50 and 100 ng/mL.[86,89]

Table 34.4 Some diagnostic considerations in hereditary hemochromatosis (absent a cause of secondary iron overload)[86,89].

Diagnostic Tool	Factors to Consider
Clinical clues	• Celtic ethnicity • Chronic asthenia • Arthropathy (fourth and fifth metacarpophalangeal joints: "hemochromatosis handshake") • Impotence • Hyperpigmentation • Liver abnormalities (transaminase elevation, hepatomegaly) • Diabetes • Cardiomyopathy
Screening criteria	• Transferrin saturation >45% • Serum ferritin: >200 ng/mL in premenopausal women; >300 ng/mL in men
Diagnostic tests	• Hepatic iron index >1.9 • Hepatic iron concentration >80 (μmol/g dry weight) • Grade 3–4 hepatic iron deposition • HFE gene analysis

Malaise, weakness, fatigability, skin pigmentation, cardiac function, and liver transaminase elevations often improve with treatment, whereas diabetes, cirrhosis, arthropathy, pituitary dysfunction, and hypogonadism almost never improve. Importantly, the risk of hepatocellular carcinoma will persist if cirrhosis was present before the onset of phlebotomy therapy.[85,86]

Erythrocytapheresis in hereditary hemochromatosis

This was first described in Europe, where a German group from Munich reported successful lowering of iron in 14 patients with hemochromatosis, with intervals of 2–11 months between procedures.[10] Their follow-up study[90] described prospective observations on eight patients who were treated with isovolemic erythrocytapheresis (1000 mL removed) every four weeks until serum ferritin fell below 300 ng/mL. Iron depletion, thus defined, was achieved after a mean of 8.5 months, during which a mean of 9.4 liters of red cells were removed in a mean of 8.9 procedures. Subsequent studies have supported these findings, and, based on this rapidity of response and the potential removal of 2–3 times more RBCs per procedure compared to a simple phlebotomy, it has been designated a first-line therapy (Category I) in the ASFA guidelines.[1] Recently, there have been controlled trials comparing the relative efficacy and cost-effectiveness of erythrocytapheresis versus simple phlebotomy.[91,92] The first study compared 500 mL weekly phlebotomies to erythrocytapheresis every two weeks. The authors found that erythrocytapheresis patients demonstrated a more rapid decline and normalization of ferritin; however, this group started with a lower average ferritin. This higher iron load in the phlebotomy group was supported by the fact that threefold more phlebotomies were needed to normalize the serum ferritin level, even though erythrocytapheresis removed only twofold more iron-containing RBCs.[91] Overall, this suggests that an erythrocytapheresis procedure every two weeks and weekly whole blood phlebotomy are equivalent, and this was supported by another randomized control trial that found no significant difference in mean time to iron depletion (ferritin <50).[92] In this study, the mean technician time was increased for the apheresis group,[92] consistent with the added procedural complexity, and thus decisions between the two modalities should probably be determined by patient and institutional preferences related to costs and effort. Intriguingly, although on average two simple phlebotomies remove equivalent iron to one erythrocytapheresis, individuals with larger blood volumes see a greater gain from erythrocytapheresis.[93] This is a consequence of the lack of volume adjustment for simple phlebotomy and suggests that blood-volume-based simple phlebotomies could be an optimal solution in terms of costs and effort.

Therapeutic platelet apheresis

Thrombocytapheresis is a term that describes the selective removal of platelets from a patient, for therapeutic purposes, using a blood-processing (apheresis) device.[1] The 2013 ASFA review of indications for apheresis therapy lists *symptomatic thrombocytosis* as a Category II indication for thrombocytapheresis.[1] This designation refers to primary thrombocytosis, as results from a clonal (myeloproliferative) disorder of the marrow.[94] Thrombocytapheresis for prophylaxis in asymptomatic patients or to lower the platelet count in cases of secondary or reactive thrombocytosis is listed as a Category III (i.e., specific role of the procedure not determined in this condition) indication because published evidence is insufficient to establish when the procedure is of benefit in these

Table 34.5 Some causes of primary (Clonal) and secondary (Reactive) thrombocytosis

Type	Possible Causes
Primary thrombocytosis	Essential thrombocytosis
	Polycythemia vera
	Chronic myelogenous leukemia
	Myelofibrosis
	Myelodysplastic syndrome (5q-)
Secondary thrombocytosis	Acute hemorrhage
	Chronic blood loss with iron deficiency
	Tissue damage or trauma
	Malignancy
	Acute or chronic inflammation
	Acute or chronic infection
	Physical exercise
	Rebound from chemotherapy or immune thrombocytopenic purpura
	Medication

circumstances.[1] Some prominent causes of primary and secondary thrombocytosis are listed in Table 34.5.[94–96]

Secondary thrombocytosis per se does not convey a risk of thromboembolic morbidity absent confounding factors such as malignancy or major surgery.[95,97] Even then, antiplatelet agents should be the first option for treatment.[96] In any case, treatment of the underlying cause is the prime factor in the resolution of secondary thrombocytosis.[94] In fact, given the absence of risk posed by the platelet count in secondary thrombocytosis, the platelet count may be considered a laboratory sign of an underlying condition that should be investigated.[94]

Primary thrombocytosis (essential thrombocythemia)

Thrombocytosis with thromboembolic complications is a feature common to chronic myeloproliferative disorders,[66] of which half are essential thrombocythemia.[95] Thus, the remainder of this discussion will focus on essential thrombocythemia. Both thrombotic and hemorrhagic complications result in patients with essential thrombocythemia.[94] Factors that increase risk of arterial thrombosis include age greater than 60 years; thrombosis history; cardiovascular risk factors such as hypertension, hypercholesterolemia, and diabetes; and JAK2V617F positivity.[98] Interestingly, high platelet counts ($>10^6/\mu L$) were associated with reduced risk of arterial thrombosis, and venous thrombosis was only associated with male gender.[98] The most significant functional consequence of such hyperthrombocytosis is an acquired von Willebrand syndrome (AvWS) that results from the accelerated clearance of hemostatically competent large multimers of von Willebrand factor from the circulation, and which improves with therapeutic reduction of the platelet count.[99,100] There is no evidence in favor of prophylactic apheresis treatment of low-risk, asymptomatic patients, regardless of platelet count, but high-risk and symptomatic patients are treated to lower their platelet count to below 400,000/μL. Low-dose aspirin is a proven treatment in all patients, although AvWS should be screened for in those with extreme thrombocytosis ($>10^6/\mu L$).[66] The United Kingdom Medical Research Council Primary Thrombocythemia 1 Study has established hydroxyurea plus low-dose aspirin as the treatment of choice in high-risk patients.[101] Whereas the rate of first thrombosis in an untreated high-risk population is approximately 26% at two years, the rate decreases to about 4% at two years with hydroxyurea and aspirin.[101]

Therapeutic thrombocytapheresis in primary thrombocytosis

Rapid lowering of an elevated platelet count, using apheresis and/or chemotherapy, is indicated for patients with myeloproliferative disorders who present with clinical syndromes of microvascular thrombosis such as digital or cerebral ischemia.[1] Case series and case reports have reported successful, rapid lowering of the platelet count in symptomatic patients in whom chemotherapy either was not an immediate option or was judged to have an insufficiently rapid effect.[102] Procedures in which 1.5 to 2.0 blood volumes are processed, and crystalloid replacement fluids are used to manage fluid balance, can lower the platelet count by 30% to 60%.[1,102] However, thrombocytapheresis without concomitant chemotherapy is not a practical means for controlling the platelet count beyond the acute setting.[102] Weekly thrombocytapheresis, beginning in the fifth gestational week, has been used in the management of a high-risk pregnant patient with essential thrombocythemia.[103]

Therapeutic white cell apheresis

Hyperleukocytosis (white cell count >100,000/μL) with symptomatic leukostasis is a Category I indication for therapeutic leukocytapheresis.[1] Leukocytapheresis by selective adsorption techniques has shown a disappointing lack of efficacy in trials for idiopathic inflammatory bowel disease.[104,105] For ulcerative colitis, the remission rate was 17% for leukocytapheresis and 11% for the sham control ($p = 0.36$);[104] and for Crohn's disease, the remission rate was 18% for the leukocytapheresis and 19% for the sham control ($p = 0.86$).[105] Currently, ASFA rates immunoadsorption for IBD as a category III indication, except for ulcerative colitis in Japan, which is category II and may be due to the fact that TNFα blockade is not standard therapy in Japan.[1]

Leukocytapheresis for hyperleukocytosis

Hyperleukocytosis is a major risk factor for early mortality, often from pulmonary and/or central nervous system hemorrhage, in adults and children with acute myeloblastic leukemia.[106] It occurs in 5–13% and 12–25% of adult and pediatric AML cases, respectively,[107] The reported incidence in acute lymphoblastic leukemia ranges from 10% to 30%.[107] Mortality rates of 20–40% have been reported.[107] Leukostasis represents end-organ damage due to leukocyte-mediated microvascular occulsion and damage resulting in infarct and hemorrhage. It usually does not occur until white blood cell counts surpass 100,000/μL in acute myelogenous leukemia (AML) and 400,000/μL in acute lymphoblastic leukemia (ALL).[1] Clinical features of leukostasis include respiratory distress, hypoxemia, diffuse interstitial or alveolar infiltrates on chest X-ray, confusion, somnolence, stupor or coma, headache, dizziness, tinnitus, gait instability, or visual disturbances.[107] Physical examination may demonstrate papilledema, dilated retinal veins and/or retinal hemorrhages, cranial nerve defects, or meningeal signs.[107] Metabolic derangements caused by tumor lysis may include hyperkalemia, hyperuricemia, hypocalcemia, and hyperphosphatemia and may result in renal failure and early death. Coagulopathy results from release of lysozomal enzymes from myeloid blasts, disseminated intravascular coagulation, and thrombocytopenia resulting from marrow failure.[107]

A standard treatment approach to hyperleukocytosis includes intravenous hydration and lowering of plasma uric acid using allopurinol or urate oxidase. Hydroxyurea may be prescribed to rapidly lower the total circulating nucleated cell count without precipitating a tumor lysis syndrome.[107] Induction chemotherapy may be used for this purpose but may precipitate tumor lysis syndrome and hemorrhage.[108] The processing of 1.5 to 2.0 blood volumes can reduce the circulating white cell count by up to 60%.[1,109,110] Leukocytapheresis before initiation of definitive induction chemotherapy has been retrospectively reported to lower the leukemic blast count to <100,000/μL in approximately 60% of patients, and to lower the incidence of early death (Day 21 after admission) by half but without an effect on long-term survival.[109–111] However, a recent meta-analysis of 15 studies combining 465 AML patients with hyperleukocytosis found no overall evidence ($p = 0.67$) that leukopheresis reduced acute mortality.[112] Thus, hyperleukocytosis without symptoms is ASFA Category III (individualize decision making). Hyperleukocytosis *with* leukostasis is classified as Category I mainly based on observed reports of rapid reversal of signs and symptoms.[1]

Extracorporeal photochemotherapy

Extracorporeal photochemotherapy (ECP or *photopheresis*) describes a procedure in which circulating mononuclear cells are collected by centrifugal apheresis, exposed to 8-methoxyxpsoralen (8-MOP, a photoactivating agent that intercalates with DNA), and then exposed to ultraviolet A (UVA) light. The treated cells are then reinfused into the patient. A full procedure is completed in approximately 1.5–3 hours.[113] The mechanism of action of ECP is thought to be immunomodulation due to the direct and indirect effects of induced apoptosis in treated cells.[113,114] Although the main effects vary somewhat among diseases, they likely include the generation of tolerogenic dendritic cells, skewing toward anti-inflammatory cytokine production, and increased tolerogenic and regulatory T-cell populations.[113,114] Currently, eythrodermic cutaneous T-cell lymphoma (CTCL) is the only Category I indication for ECP. ASFA has listed the prophylaxis and treatment of heart transplant rejection, cutaneous manifestations of graft-versus-host disease (GVHD), and lung allograft rejection as Category II indications for ECP. There is a growing body of potential applications in transplant rejection as well as in autoimmune diseases for which the ASFA recommendations are generally Category III.[1,115] Some ECP regimens used in the treatment of the Category I and II indications are described in Table 34.6.

Cutaneous T-cell lymphoma (CTCL)
Extracorporeal photochemotherapy in the treatment of cutaneous T-cell lymphoma

The CTCLs are a heterogeneous group of extranodal non-Hodgkin lymphomas of T-cell origin that target the skin.[113] Mycosis

fungoides, the most common form of CTCL, accounts for almost half of all primary cutaneous lymphomas.[113] It is largely a disease of adults (median age 55–60 years at diagnosis) and typically presents as an indolent disorder that progresses slowly over years from patchy skin involvement to infiltrated plaques, tumors, and widespread disease.[113] Whereas localized (e.g., nonerythrodermic) mycosis fungoides is adequately managed with topical therapies, the application of ECP in erythrodermic mycosis fungoides is recommended by ASFA.[1] Whereas limited-stage mycosis fungoides does not shorten life expectancy, advanced-stage disease may be associated with a 10-year disease-specific survival of 20%.[116] Sézary syndrome is defined as a triad of erythroderma, generalized lymphadenopathy, and the presence of neoplastic T cells (Sézary cells) in the skin, lymph nodes, and peripheral blood.[113,116] A retrospective cohort study from Stanford University of 106 patients with erythrodermic mycosis fungoides and Sézary syndrome identified age ≥65 years, clinical Stage IV, and circulating Sézary cells ≥5% of total lymphocytes as independent negative prognostic factors for survival.[117] Median survivals of patients with none, one, or more than one of these adverse prognostic factors were 122 months ($n = 36$), 44 months ($n = 39$), and 18 months ($n = 31$), respectively ($p < 0.005$).[117]

The 1987 report by Edelson *et al.*[118] of a successful pilot trial of ECP, in which 27 of 37 treatment-resistant patients with CTCL experienced an average 64% decrease in cutaneous involvement after 22 ± 10 weeks, led to US Food and Drug Administration (FDA) approval of ECP for treatment of CTCL later that year. Long-term follow-up of the original 29 patients with erythrodermic CTCL from that pilot study[118] reported that median survival of the treated patients was 60.33 months from diagnosis and 47.9 months from the start of ECP. Four of the six patients who achieved complete responses in the original study remained in complete remission.[119] Between 1987 and 2001, 21 studies reported a total of 485 patients treated using ECP.[113,120] Although most patients in these studies had erythrodermic CTCL, most studies did not report the response rates separately for the erythrodermic subjects.[121] In addition, responses were defined as >25% skin clearing in some studies and >50% skin clearing in others, and complete responses were defined as either 75% to 100% skin clearing, >90% skin clearing, or 100% skin clearing.[113] Nonetheless, overall response rates reported in these studies ranged from 31% to 87.5%, and complete response rates ranged from 0% to 54% (20–30% in most studies).[113,120,121] The variability in response rates has been attributed to differences in entry criteria, prior or concurrent therapy, duration between diagnosis and application of ECP, the ECP

Table 34.6 Regimens of extracorporeal photochemotherapy (ECP)

Indication	Treatment
Cutaneous T-cell lymphoma	ECP cycle (2 consecutive days) once or twice a month; continue for 6 months before declaring treatment failure.
Cardiac allograft rejection	Prophylaxis • Month 1 after transplant: ECP day 1 and 2, 5 and 6, 10 and 11, 17 and 18, and 27 and 28 • Months 2 and 3 after transplant: ECP on 2 successive days every 2 weeks • Months 4–6 after transplant: ECP on 2 successive days every 4 weeks
	Acute (moderate) rejection • ECP procedures on 2 consecutive days at weekly episode intervals as needed to resolve rejection as indicated by endomyocardial biopsy
	Recurrent/refractory cellular rejection • ECP on 2 consecutive days weekly for 1 month, then every 2 weeks for 2 months, then monthly for 3 months (total of 22 procedures)
	Chronic rejection • Beginning within 1 month of transplantation: ECP on 2 successive days every 4 weeks for 12 months, every 6 weeks for next 6 months, every 8 weeks during next 6 months
Lung allograft rejection	Brochiolitis obliterans syndrome (BOS) • ECP 2 consecutive days: weekly for 2 months, then every 2 weeks for next 2 months, then monthly for total of 6 months
Chronic graft-versus-host disease	ECP on 2 consecutive days every 1–2 weeks, then consider monthly interval; treat at least 6 months before declaring treatment failure

protocol followed, and the definition of response.[120] Based on the above, ASFA has listed the treatment of erythrodermic CTCL as a Category I indication for ECP.[1]

Cardiac and lung allograft rejection

Between 1990 and 2012, the rate of heart transplantation was fairly constant at 3500–4500 per year, while lung transplants increased more or less linearly from 500 in 1990 to over 3700 in 2012.[122,123] Rejection is still a serious problem for both heart and lung allografts, accounting for approximately 11% of deaths in the first three years after heart transplant, and underlies the majority of graft failures that account for 35% of overall deaths.[122] Similarly for lung allografts, rejection underlies approximately 25% of mortality at five years, when bronchiolitis obliterans syndrome (BOS), the end result of chronic rejection, is included.[123] Immunosuppressive therapy to prevent allograft rejection has included perioperative antilymphocyte antibody (polyclonal antilymphocyte or antithymocyte globulin, OKT3, or IL-2 receptor antibodies), chronic postoperative calcineurin inhibitors (e.g., tacrolimus and cyclosporine), mycophenolate mofetil, sirolimus, and others.[122,123] Because of the association between rejection, graft failure, and death, evidence of rejection should result in adjustment in the immunosuppressive regimen to initially resolve the episode of rejection. For unresponsive cardiac rejection or lung transplant BOS, ECP is an appropriate adjuvant; and these are listed by ASFA as Category II indications for ECP based on the evidence described below.[1]

Extracorporeal photochemotherapy in the treatment of cardiac allograft rejection

Studies in support of ECP for treatment of cardiac allograft rejection focus on the effects of ECP on endomyocardial biopsy findings, rather than on survival or graft function.[120] Two pilot studies have shown evidence that the risk of acute cellular rejection episodes can be decreased by incorporating ECP into the prophylactic immunosuppressive regimen of cardiac allograft recipients without increasing the risk of infection caused by immunosuppression.[124,125] A prospective randomized pilot trial comparing 10 cases receiving ECP and 13 controls treated with only immunosuppression reported that development of panel-reactive antibodies (responsible for chronic antibody-mediated rejection) and coronary artery intimal hyperplasia (a pathogenetic mechanism of graft failure in chronic rejection) are mitigated by the addition of ECP to the posttransplant immunosuppressive regimen for the first two years after transplant surgery.[126] Dall'Amico and colleagues in Padua, Italy, reported a prospective pilot trial in eight patients, with recurrent acute rejection episodes despite immunosuppression, who were treated with two consecutive days of ECP every four weeks for six months.[127] Seven benefited with a reduction in the number and severity of rejection episodes; reduction in daily prednisone, cyclosporine, or azathioprine doses; and improvement on endomyocardial biopsy specimens. Other small case series and case reports have presented corroborating data supporting ECP efficacy.[128]

Extracorporeal photochemotherapy in the treatment of lung allograft rejection

The use of ECP in lung transplant is a promising new avenue,[128] although only retrospective studies have been reported thus far. The first reports of treatment were in 1995 and represented a handful of cases pointing to effective improvement in clinical lung function (FEV$_1$) and histological improvement. A number of small studies followed that generally supported these findings.[128] Only recently have larger studies examining ECP been reported[129–131] encompassing a total 135 patients and supporting a role for ECP in stabilizing lung function (FEV$_1$) with minimal procedural side effects. Although the lack of adequate controls leaves a larger question as to the benefit of ECP compared to regimens that do not include ECP, there is a decrease in donor-specific antibodies in patients treated with ECP compared to controls, akin to ECP for cardiac rejection.[132]

Graft-versus-host disease

GVHD occurs in hematopoietic progenitor cell transplant recipients when T cells of donor origin (either transplanted with, or that develop from, the graft) interact with tissue in the HLA-matched but genetically nonidentical host.[133] Classical acute GVHD develops within 100 days of transplantation, with skin manifestations that vary from an erythematous morbilliform rash to epidermal necrolysis, mucosal inflammation causing diarrhea and abdominal cramping, and abnormalities of liver function tests.[133] GVHD that develops beyond 100 days of transplantation, or persists more than three months, is traditionally referred to as chronic GVHD, and is characterized by an oral, ocular, and mucous membrane sicca syndrome; skin involvement; scleroderma; bronchiolitis obliterans; joint contractures; myofasciitis; esophageal stricture; or other fibrotic complications in various organ systems.[133] The cumulative incidence of acute GVHD is approximately 12% to 75%, and the cumulative incidence of chronic GVHD is approximately 15% to 70% after hematopoietic progenitor cell transplantation, depending on whether the donor–recipient pair are related or unrelated and on whether a myeloablative or nonmyeloablative conditioning regimen was used.[134,135] Accurate diagnosis and staging are important in that recurrent or late-onset acute GVHD may not require prolonged therapy as is required with chronic GVHD, whereas overlap syndromes may require shorter courses of typical treatments for chronic GVHD.[136]

Extracorporeal photochemotherapy in the treatment of GVHD

The application of ECP to the treatment of GVHD has been extensively reviewed.[120,137] Among the larger prospective reports is one from a London group that treated 28 patients who had developed steroid-refractory chronic GVHD following HLA-matched allogeneic marrow or peripheral blood progenitor cell transplant.[138] Among the patients, 27 were classified as having extensive chronic GVHD and 20 had involvement of more than 50% of their skin surface. Patients were given ECP on two consecutive days every two weeks for the first four months, and monthly thereafter. ECP was initiated a median of 34 months (range 10–167) after transplantation and 23 months (range 2–164) from the onset of chronic GVHD. Of the 21 patients with cutaneous involvement who were evaluable, a 25% reduction in skin involvement was noted in eight (38%) after three months and in 10 (48%) after six months, and a statistically nonsignificant improvement in liver function tests was noted.[138] There is only one randomized control study that failed to show significant improvement in the primary outcome, decrease in skin involvement (14.5% for ECP arm vs. 8.5% in control); however, there was significant decrease in steroid usage compared to the control arm.[139] Given the lack of large randomized prospective studies, a meta-analysis was performed combining 18 prospective and retrospective studies of steroid-refractory GVHD with sufficient comparable cases.[137] This meta-analysis found significant efficacy with a complete response rate of 29% (CI 19–42%) along with particularly strong response rates of 74% (CI 60–85%) and 68%

(CI 55–77%) for skin and liver, respectively.[137] Only modest activity was seen for lung or gastrointestinal manifestations. Based on the overall evidence, ASFA considers skin manifestations to be a Category II indication for ECP but does not distinguish chronic from acute in its recommendation.[1]

Specialized therapeutic plasma processing

In its 2013 evidence-based review of apheresis therapies, ASFA lists 14 Category I, II, or III indications for therapeutic immunoadsorption, LDL apheresis, or rheopheresis (a form of double-membrane filtration plasmapheresis, or DFPP).[1] The physiology of non-selective TPE and its indications are addressed in Chapter 33. The following discussion focuses on therapeutic procedures that are designed to remove a specified fraction of the plasma. A pathogenic plasma substance (e.g., a specific autoantibody) is usually present at relatively low levels in the circulation. Thus, selective extraction of pathologic plasma constituents in a way that minimizes the sacrifice of healthy plasma proteins has been proposed as a more efficient treatment of disorders that might otherwise be treated using TPE.[4]

Immunoadsorption apheresis

Immunoadsorption systems employ the principle of affinity chromatography and make use of immobilized sorbents or ligands that have enhanced or specific binding affinity for a specific antigen, antibody, immune complex, or other substance in the patient's circulation.[4,140] Examples include (1) staphylococcal protein A or sheep antihuman immunoglobulin (IgG) for extraction of IgG and immune complexes from the circulation, (2) sheep antihuman low-density lipoprotein (LDL) or apolipoprotein B antibody for extraction of LDL, (3) synthetic blood group substances for removal of ABO isoagglutinins, and (4) DNA for removal of DNA antibody. Although no longer commercially distributed in the United States, two immunoadsorption systems that have received approval from the FDA are the staphylococcal protein A-agarose column (Immunosorba, Fresenius HemoCare, Redmond, WA), and the staphylococcal protein A silica column (Prosorba, Fresenius HemoCare).[141] Protein A is a cell-wall constituent of the Cowan I strain of *Staphylococcus aureus*. Mammalian IgG binds to five homologous regions at its amino terminus, but interaction of protein A with other plasma proteins is insignificant. Processing of 2.5 plasma volumes using a protein A-agarose column resulted in a 97% reduction in IgG1, a 98% reduction in IgG2, a 40% reduction in IgG3, a 77% reduction in IgG4, a 56% reduction in IgM, and a 55% reduction in IgA, whereas plasma levels of albumin, fibrinogen, and antithrombin were reduced by less than 20%.[142] Thus, in principle, plasma adsorption with protein A affinity columns permits the processing of more plasma than does TPE without unacceptable loss of other essential plasma constituents.[140] The use of these devices in a variety of clinical conditions in Europe and Japan has been extensively reviewed.[140,141]

Dilated cardiomyopathy

Dilated cardiomyopathy (DCM) describes a cardiac disorder in which the left ventricle is dilated and exhibits impaired contraction. It may be idiopathic, familial, postviral, alcohol- or drug-induced, or related to other cardiac disease. Both ventricles may be affected. It presents with heart failure, is often progressive, and may be complicated by arrhythmias, thromboembolic events, and sudden death.[143] It is the most frequent antecedent cause of heart transplantation throughout the world.[122] Approximately 60% to 80% of patients with DCM harbor autoantibodies directed against cardiac myosin heavy chain, myocardial β_1-adrenergic receptors, or other cardiac tissue with a predominance of antibodies of the IgG 3 subclass.[144–147]

Immunoadsorption in the treatment of dilated cardiomyopathy

A variety of immunoadsorption (IA) columns, including antihuman polyimmunoglobulin, staphylococcal protein A agarose, β_1-adrenoreceptor antibody peptides, and tryptophan polyvinyl alcohol, have all shown potential efficacy but still await formal comparisons to other therapies.[148] Initially, the potential relevance of heart antibodies to clinical DCM was explored in a pilot study of eight patients with DCM and advanced congestive heart failure who were subjected to a series of four or five IA procedures per week over two weeks using the Therasorb-Ig system.[149] β_1-adrenoreceptor autoantibody levels decreased by an order of magnitude and heart failure symptoms improved in seven of the subjects, but the effect was transient: autoantibodies and symptoms returned to baseline 75 days after completion of IA.[149] In a companion pilot trial, nine patients were subjected to daily IA treatments for five days using Therasorb-Ig.[150] Patients received 35 g of IVIG after the final procedure. Once again, plasma levels of β_1-adrenoreceptor autoantibody were substantially reduced, and significant improvement in hemodynamic parameters (including cardiac output, mean arterial pressure, mean pulmonary arterial pressure, left ventricular filling pressure, and systemic vascular resistance) was demonstrated, thus providing objective preliminary evidence of the clinical benefit of antibody removal by IA.[150] In another randomized trial, 18 patients with DCM and advanced heart failure were randomly assigned to either best medical therapy (control group) or best medical therapy with the addition of IA.[151] During the first course of IA, procedures were performed on three consecutive days, and patients received 0.5 g/kg of IVIG by intravenous infusion. Three subsequent courses of IA, performed on two consecutive days at four-week intervals, were also followed by infusions of IVIG at the same dose. IA was performed using the Therasorb-Ig column. After the first course of IA/IVIG, left ventricular ejection fraction, cardiac index, stroke volume index, and systemic vascular resistance improved significantly in the treatment group, and these changes remained evident after the final series. Improvement in symptoms and functional status paralleled the hemodynamic changes. The control group demonstrated no hemodynamic improvement at the end of the three-month study. β_1-adrenergic receptor antibodies decreased by >80% after the first course of IA but tended to rise between monthly courses of treatment. There have now been multiple trials, case reports, and case series generally supporting improvement.[148]

The vast majority of studies infused intravenous IgG (IVIG), which might solely, or in concert with IA, account for clinical improvement. Unfortunately, trials of treatment with IVIG alone have been equivocal. One trial, in which patients initially received a total of 2 g/kg followed by 0.4 g/kg monthly for five months, demonstrated significant improvement in left ventricular ejection fraction in the treatment group but not the placebo group.[152] A second trial, in which patients received a single course totaling 2 g/kg, demonstrated no effect of IVIG on left ventricular ejection fraction after six or 12 months (although both the treatment and placebo groups showed improvement).[153] One prospective case-control trial was important in that no IVIG replacement was performed for 17 cases receiving IA compared to controls matched for age, body surface area (BSA), duration of symptoms, cardiac function, and New York Heart Association (NYHA) functional class.[154] Specifically, at one year, the IA-treated patients demonstrated significant improvement in NYHA functional class and left ventricular status with 67% improvement in ejection fraction and 14% decrease in the ventricular diameter compared to pretreatment.[154] Controls demonstrated no improvement, and the treated cases demonstrated improved survival at five years compared to controls (82% vs. 42%). Although a single study, it supports the possibility that IA has significant effects irrespective of IVIG. The role for the removal of antibodies is also supported in that patients that respond to IA have stronger negative inotropic antibody activity in vitro.[155] Overall, ASFA does not recommend a singular adsorption modality, and designates DCM a Category II indication for immunoadsorption apheresis.[1]

Familial hypercholesterolemia

Familial hypercholesterolemia (FH), an autosomal dominant disorder, is a major cause of death or early disability resulting from premature atherosclerotic heart and peripheral vascular disease.[156] It is caused by mutations in the LDL receptor, with frequencies of 1:500 for heterozygotes and 1:1,000,000 for homozygotes.[156] Clinical features including xanthomas, xanthelasmas, corneal arcus, and the occurrence of coronary heart disease, stroke, and death are common in the fourth or fifth decade of life.[156] A serum LDL cholesterol level below 100 mg/dL (achieved through diet, lifestyle modification, and 3-hydroxy-3methylglutaryl coenzyme A reductase inhibiting drugs or statins) can lower cardiovascular morbidity and mortality in high-risk patients, but a sizable minority of high-risk patients fail to achieve LDL-cholesterol-lowering goals by this approach.[157]

LDL apheresis

Manual, then automated, plasma exchange was successfully employed as an adjunct to lipid-lowering therapy beginning over 40 years ago. However, the kinetics of restoration of plasma lipid levels and the unwanted lowering of essential plasma proteins (e.g., fibrinogen and albumin) rendered this approach challenging for long-term therapy.[158] The development of apheresis devices that permit a more selective removal of plasma LDL cholesterol and related substances has provided a practical approach to managing statin-resistant patients in conjunction with statins and other medical therapies.[158]

Two apheresis systems for selective removal of LDL cholesterol are FDA-approved for use in the United States. The Liposorber LA-15 system (Kaneka Pharma America, New York, NY) uses dextran sulfate bound to cellulose to selectively extract LDL cholesterol from plasma. In this system, plasma is initially separated from the cellular components of blood by filtration through a disposable semi-permeable polysulfone hollow fiber column, and the separated plasma is then perfused over a disposable adsorption column that contains 150 mL of dextran sulfate. Dextran sulfate has strong affinity for lipoproteins and adsorbs these from the plasma. The H.E.L.P. system (B. Braun Medical, Bethlehem, PA) employs a 0.55-micron hollow fiber column to separate the plasma from the cellular elements of the blood. The plasma is acidified with 0.3 M sodium acetate buffer, and heparin is added to precipitate LDL cholesterol. The LDL cholesterol–heparin precipitate is filtered from the plasma using a 0.45-micron polycarbonate filter, excess heparin is adsorbed from the filtered plasma with a DEAE cellulose membrane filter,

and the filtered plasma is then restored to physiologic pH by bicarbonate hemodialysis.

ASFA has designated FH a Category I indication for LDL apheresis in homozygotes and a Category II indication for LDL apheresis in heterozygotes.[1] The FDA-approved indications include homozygotes with plasma LDL cholesterol >500 mg/dL, and heterozygotes with LDL cholesterol >300 mg/dL (or >200 with known coronary artery disease). A regimen that combines medical therapy with LDL apheresis on a biweekly schedule can effectively lower LDL cholesterol by 60% to 80% in otherwise treatment-resistant patients, improve the physical stigmata of hypercholesterolemia such as xanthomas and xanthelasmas, improve myocardial perfusion and coronary artery patency, and favorably affect other markers of cardiovascular risk (e.g., triglycerides, fibrinogen, homocysteine, C-reactive protein, and adhesion molecules).[1,159–161] More recently, LDL apheresis has been found effective in ameliorating drug-refractory coronary artery disease in patients with Lp(a)-hyperlipoproteinemia.[162,163]

Conclusion

The continued growth of therapeutic apheresis as a treatment option in diverse clinical conditions depends on an understanding of the pathophysiology of the disorders in question and the acquisition of evidence, from properly conducted clinical studies, of the efficacy of apheresis therapies in their management.

Disclaimer

The authors have disclosed no conflicts of interest.

Key References

A full reference list for this chapter is available at: http://www.wiley.com/go/simon/transfusion

1 Schwartz J, Winters JL, Padmanabhan A, et al. Guidelines on the use of therapeutic apheresis in clinical practice-evidence-based approach from the Writing Committee of the American Society for Apheresis: the sixth special issue. *J Clin Apheresis* 2013; **28**(3):145–284.

7 McLeod BC. An approach to evidence-based therapeutic apheresis. *J Clin Apheresis* 2002; **17**(3):124–32.

16 Bunn HF. Pathogenesis and treatment of sickle cell disease. *N Engl J Med* 1997; **337**(11):762–9.

27 Yawn BP, Buchanan GR, Afenyi-Annan AN, et al. Management of sickle cell disease: summary of the 2014 evidence-based report by expert panel members. *JAMA* 2014; **312**(10):1033–48.

40 World Health Organization (WHO). *World malaria report 2010*. Geneva: WHO, 2010.

41 World Health Organization (WHO). *Guidelines for the treatment of malaria*. 2nd ed. Geneva: WHO, 2010.

49 Vannier E, Krause PJ. Human babesiosis. *N Engl J Med* 2012; **366**(25):2397–407.

66 Tefferi A. Polycythemia vera and essential thrombocythemia: 2012 update on diagnosis, risk stratification, and management. *Am J Hematol* 2012; **87**(3):285–93.

67 Silver RT, Chow W, Orazi A, Arles SP, Goldsmith SJ. Evaluation of WHO criteria for diagnosis of polycythemia vera: a prospective analysis. *Blood* 2013; **122**(11):1881–6.

92 Sundic T, Hervig T, Hannisdal S, et al. Erythrocytapheresis compared with whole blood phlebotomy for the treatment of hereditary haemochromatosis. *Blood Transfus Trasfus Sangue* 2014; **12**(Suppl. 1):s84–9.

137 Malik MI, Litzow M, Hogan W, et al. Extracorporeal photopheresis for chronic graft-versus-host disease: a systematic review and meta-analysis. *Blood Res* 2014; **49**(2):100–6.

CHAPTER 35

Hematopoietic growth factors

David J. Kuter

Division of Hematology, Massachusetts General Hospital and Harvard Medical School, Boston, MA, USA

Introduction

Over the past several decades, the major hematopoietic growth factors have been identified, purified, and therapeutic products made. These hematopoietic growth factors affect the growth and differentiation of stem cells and later progenitor cells of all lineages. Several of these molecules play important roles in patient care and are widely used. After a brief review of general principles of hematopoietic growth factor function, this chapter will focus on the clinically relevant hematopoietic growth factors that affect erythroid, myeloid, and megakaryocyte differentiation, specifically erythropoietin (epoetin alfa and darbepoetin alfa), granulocyte colony-stimulating factor (G-CSF; filgrastim, tbo-filgrastim, and pegfilgrastim), granulocyte macrophage colony-stimulating factor (GM-CSF; sargramostim), and thrombopoietin (TPO; romiplostim and eltrombopag). The general biology and clinical use of each will be described as well as their role in transfusion medicine.

General principles of hematopoietic growth factors

Pluripotent stem cells give rise to all of the final differentiated blood cells (Figure 35.1). The molecular differentiation steps for some of these precursor cells have been described and in general involve a random ("stochastic") process in which lineage-specific differentiation occurs at multiple stages. For example, a micro-RNA (miR-150) binds to and downregulates c-Myb, which causes the common erythroid–megakaryocyte precursor to undergo megakaryocytic, not erythroid, differentiation.[1] But the subsequent survival of cells at each differentiation stage is determined by the presence of specific hematopoietic growth factors; if the stage- or lineage-specific hematopoietic growth factor is absent, the cells undergo programmed cell death. For example, erythroid burst-forming cells (BFU-Es) will continue their divisions as long as erythropoietin is present; if absent, BFU-Es undergo programmed cell death.

In this complicated hierarchy of cell division, differentiation, and apoptosis, the hematopoietic growth factors can be generally grouped into those that are early acting, whose circulating levels are not altered and affect multiple lineages (interleukin-3 [IL3], IL6, IL11, GM-CSF, stem cell factor, and TPO), versus those that are late acting, whose levels are modulated and affect single lineages (erythropoietin, G-CSF, macrophage colony-stimulating factor [M-CSF], and TPO). All of these hematopoietic growth factors are active at very low concentrations and work via specific cell surface receptors, thereby promoting the viability of the target cells.

For the clinically relevant hematopoietic growth factors, G-CSF, erythropoietin, M-CSF, and TPO, a number of other general physiological principles should be noted:
- The circulating level of each factor in normal physiology is inversely proportional to the mass of the differentiated cell it regulates; for example, as the hemoglobin, absolute neutrophil count (ANC), monocyte count, and platelet count fall, the respective levels of erythropoietin, G-CSF, M-CSF, and TPO rise.
- The normal physiologic response is usually "log-linear," that is, erythropoietin levels increase exponentially as the hemoglobin declines on a linear scale (Figure 35.2).[2]
- Circulating levels of each factor are determined by the relative rates of its production and metabolism. For erythropoietin, there is a precise mechanism that regulates its production with a rather fixed rate of renal clearance. For TPO and M-CSF, levels are primarily regulated through clearance by the platelet or macrophage, respectively. These cells have very high-affinity receptors for their factor and bind, internalize, and degrade it. There is little effect on the rate of production. Finally, G-CSF is regulated by both production and clearance. Mature neutrophils bind and clear G-CSF, but many other cells (eg, monocytes, endothelial cells) can increase G-CSF production when stimulated. In normal basal physiology, G-CSF production is relatively constant.
- This normal physiologic response may be altered in pathologic states.
  - In anemia of chronic disease, renal erythropoietin production is decreased.[2]
  - In acute infection, there is a marked increase in G-CSF production.
  - In liver failure, TPO production is decreased.[3]
- The clinical effect of pharmacologic administration of a hematopoietic growth factor also operates on an exponential dose–response curve. In a healthy subject, linear increases in any blood cell require an exponentially greater dose of the specific hematopoietic growth factor.[4,5]

Erythroid growth factors

Ever since the initial studies by Paul Carnot in 1906, it has been known that blood contained a "hémopoïétine" that had the ability to

Rossi's Principles of Transfusion Medicine, Fifth Edition. Edited by Toby L. Simon, Jeffrey McCullough, Edward L. Snyder, Bjarte G. Solheim, and Ronald G. Strauss.

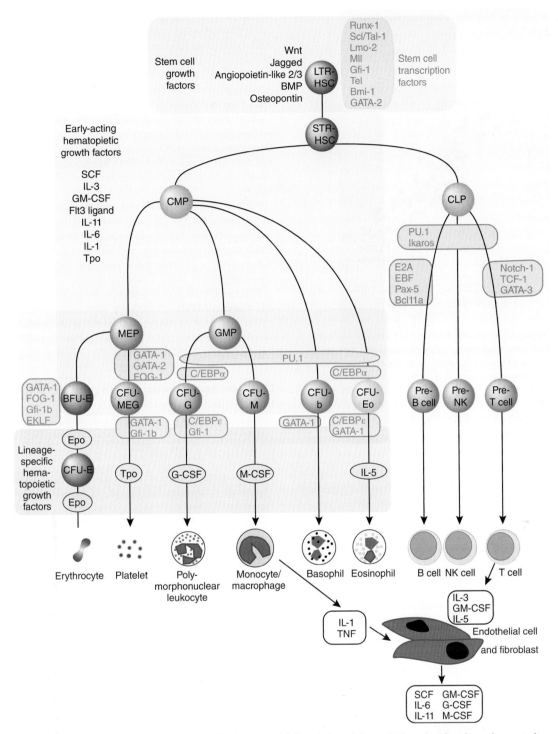

Figure 35.1 Scheme of normal hematopoiesis. The many different stages of differentiation of the myeloid, erythroid, and megakaryocyte lines are illustrated along with their relevant early- and late-acting hematopoietic growth factors. BFU, blast-forming unit; CFU, colony-forming unit; CLP, common lymphoid progenitor; CMP, common myeloid progenitor; Epo, erythropoietin; G-CSF, granulocyte colony-stimulating factor; GM-CSF, granulocyte macrophage colony-stimulating factor; GMP, granulocyte–myeloid progenitor; IL, interleukin; LTR-HSC, long-term repopulating hematopoietic stem cell; M-CSF, monocyte/macrophage colony stimulating factor; MEP, megakaryocyte-erythroid progenitor; SCF, stem cell factor; STR-HSC, short-term repopulating hematopoietic stem cell; TNF, tumor necrosis factor; Tpo, thrombopoietin. Source: Sieff CA, Zon LI. Anatomy and physiology of hematopoiesis. In: Nathan and Oski's Hematology of Infancy and Childhood, 7th ed, Orkin *et al.* (eds.), Elsevier Philadelphia, 2009. Reproduced with permission.

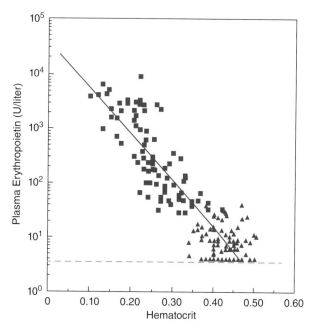

Figure 35.2 Log-linear relationship between EPO level and hematocrit. EPO levels were determined for normal blood donors (triangles) and patients with anemia (squares; those with renal disease, rheumatoid arthritis, or solid tumors were excluded). Dashed line denotes limits of detection for this assay. Note that EPO does not begin to rise until hematocrit falls below ~36, suggesting that other factors (i.e., androgens) account for the higher values. Source: Erslev (1991).[2] Reproduced with permission of Elsevier.

stimulate red cell production.[6,7] Decades after of identifying a factor in the urine that stimulated red cell production,[8] erythropoietin (EPO) was finally purified and a recombinant form was approved by the US Food and Drug Administration (FDA) in 1989.[9,10] EPO was the first hematopoietic growth factor available for clinical use and paved the way for the development of many others.

Structure, function, and physiology
Erythropoietin is made as a 193-amino-acid precursor, of which 27 amino acids are cleaved off to produce a 166-amino-acid form that loses a terminal arg166 to give the final 165-amino-acid (molecular weight [MW] = 30,400 Da) heavily glycosylated (30% carbohydrate) protein. It is made by a single gene (7q22.1) and produced

by interstitial peritubular fibroblasts in the kidney with maybe a small amount being made by the liver. Using an efficient renal sensor of hypoxia (hypoxia inducible factor [HIF]), circulating EPO levels are primarily determined by its rate of transcription. HIF is a dimeric protein made of α and β subunits that binds to a promoter region of the EPO gene and increases its rate of transcription. However, the HIFα subunit undergoes proline hydroxylation in the presence of oxygen and is degraded by the proteasome. So with normoxia, HIFα is rapidly degraded and transcription of the EPO gene reduced; with hypoxia, HIFα survives and increases transcription. EPO has no storage form and once made is immediately secreted into the circulation and cleared by the kidney.

EPO binds to and activates preformed, inactive, dimeric EPO receptors (Figure 35.3) that are present on pronormoblasts, basophilic normoblasts, and polychromatophilic and orthochromatophilic normoblasts, but not on reticulocytes or mature red cells. When EPO is present, these precursor cells do not undergo apoptosis but survive and produce mature red cells.

The usual log-linear relationship between the EPO level and the hematocrit (Figure 35.2) seen in disorders such as iron deficiency is blunted in conditions historically referred to as *anemia of chronic disease* (e.g., diabetes, cancer, renal failure, and inflammation).

Clinically available erythroid growth factors
Epoetin alfa (Epogen, Procrit)
This 165-amino-acid (MW = 30,400 Da) glycosylated protein (Figure 35.3) is made in Chinese hamster ovary (CHO) cells and is available in vials and prefilled syringes in a wide variety of doses. Epoetin alfa is FDA approved for:
- the treatment of anemia due to chronic kidney disease (CKD), including patients on dialysis and not on dialysis, to decrease the need for red blood cell (RBC) transfusion;
- the treatment of anemia in patients with nonmyeloid malignancies where anemia is due to the effect of concomitant myelosuppressive chemotherapy, and upon initiation, there is a minimum of two additional months of planned chemotherapy;
- the treatment of anemia due to zidovudine administered at ≤4200 mg/week in HIV-infected patients with endogenous serum erythropoietin levels of ≤500 IU/mL; and
- reducing the need for allogeneic RBC transfusions among patients with perioperative hemoglobin >10 to ≤13 g/dL who are at high

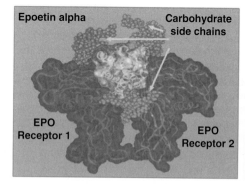
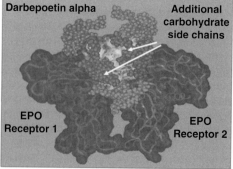

Figure 35.3 Binding of epoetin alfa and darbepoetin alfa to the EPO receptor. Epoetin alfa has three N-linked carbohydrate chains with a maximum of 14 sialic acids. It has a MW of 30,400 Da and is 40% carbohydrate. Darbepoetin alfa has five N-linked carbohydrate chains with a maximum of 22 sialic acids. It has a MW of 39,000 Da and is 51% carbohydrate. Both bind to and activate the preformed dimeric EPO receptor. Source: D. Kuter. Reproduced with permission.

risk for perioperative blood loss from elective, noncardiac, non-vascular surgery and who are not willing to donate autologous blood preoperatively.

The starting dose of epoetin alfa is usually 50 U/kg tiw for renal failure, 100 U/kg tiw for HIV, 150 U/kg tiw for chemotherapy (40,000 units per week has become a standard for oncology patients[11]), and either 300 U/kg daily for 10 days for preoperative anemia with surgery in under three weeks or 600 U/kg weekly for preoperative anemia when surgery is greater than three weeks away. Subsequent doses are adjusted every three to four weeks based upon response. This drug is much more effective when given subcutaneously than IV, with levels rising at two hours, peaking at 18 hours, and with a T1/2 of 8.5 hours.

Darbepoetin alfa (Aranesp)

Darbepoetin alfa was designed from understanding how epoetin alfa is cleared from the circulation. Epoetin alfa has many isoforms due to variations in the number of sialic acids present (Figure 35.3).[12,13] Isoforms with the maximum 14 sialic acids have a prolonged half-life, whereas those with eight have almost no biologic effect. This led to the hypothesis that if the number of sialic acids on epoetin alfa were increased, its T1/2 would be even longer. By creating two additional N-linked glycosylation sites on epoetin alfa, darbepoetin alfa was created and contains a maximum of 22 sialic acids versus the 14 on epoetin alfa (Figure 35.3). Adding these sialic acids minimally reduced binding to the EPO receptor, but markedly increased the T1/2 from 8.5 hours to 25.3 hours, thereby increasing the biologic effect. Darbepoetin alfa (MW = 39,000 Da) is made in CHO cells and is 51% carbohydrate. It comes in vials and prefilled syringes with various doses. It is FDA approved for:

- the treatment of anemia due to chronic kidney disease (CKD), including patients on dialysis and patients not on dialysis; and
- the treatment of anemia in patients with nonmyeloid malignancies where anemia is due to the effect of concomitant myelosuppressive chemotherapy, and upon initiation, there is a minimum of two additional months of planned chemotherapy.

The starting dose for renal failure is of 0.45 mcg/kg weekly; for oncology, either 100 mcg weekly or 200 mcg every two weeks. Doses are subsequently adjusted every four weeks according to response.

Effects and adverse effects of erythopoietin administration

After the administration of epoetin alfa or darbepoetin alfa to healthy individuals, the reticulocyte count starts to rise on day 3 and peaks on day 10, while the hematocrit starts to rise on day 8 and peaks at days 20–25.[14] Importantly, the iron saturation and transferrin begin to fall by day 4 and drop 74% by day 16.[14]

The major side effects of darbepoetin alfa or epoetin alfa administration are listed in Table 35.1. Of these, thrombosis and potential adverse outcomes of cancer patients deserve further detail.

Thrombosis

There is an approximately twofold increased rate of thromboembolism in renal failure and cancer patients receiving these agents. A meta-analysis of 91 trials with 20,102 cancer patients showed that the risk ratio (RR) of thromboembolic complications was increased in patients receiving these drugs compared to controls (RR, 1.52; 95% confidence interval [CI], 1.34–1.74; 57 trials, $N = 15,498$).[15] In a meta-analysis of 27 trials (10,452 patients), chronic kidney disease patients at a higher hemoglobin target (median, 13.0 g/dL; IQR, 12.0–14.0 g/dL)

Table 35.1 Adverse effects of erythroid growth factors

Hypertension: renal failure patients
Seizures: renal failure patients
Allergic reactions: rare
Antibody formation leading to pure red cell aplasia: European formulation: very rare in United States
Thrombosis: twofold increase in all patients
Increased cardiovascular complications and death at Hgb >11: renal failure patients
Decreased survival if target Hgb >12: cancer patients (breast, head-neck, cervical, and lymphoma) on chemotherapy
Decreased survival: cancer patients not receiving chemotherapy

had higher risks for stroke (RR, 1.51; 95% CI, 1.03–2.21), hypertension (RR, 1.67; 95% CI, 1.31–2.12), and vascular access thrombosis (RR, 1.33; 95% CI, 1.16–1.53) compared with those at a lower hemoglobin target (median, 10.1 g/dL; IQR, 9.2–11.0 g/dL). However, there were no statistically significant differences in the risks for mortality (RR, 1.09; 95% CI, 0.99–1.20), serious cardiovascular events (RR, 1.15; 95% CI, 0.98–1.33), or end-stage kidney disease (RR, 1.08; 95% CI, 0.97–1.20).[16]

Tumor progression and cancer mortality

The second major concern with the erythroid growth factors is that they may increase tumor progression and mortality in cancer patients. In one study, head and neck cancer patients treated with erythropoietin to a target hemoglobin of 14 to 15 had worse progression-free survival (RR, 1.62; 95% CI, 1.22–2.14; $p = 0.0008$), loco-regional control (RR 1.69; 95% CI 1.16–2.47; $p = 0.007$), and overall survival (RR 1.39; 95% CI 1.05–1.84; $p = 0.02$) than placebo.[17] However, this study and others reporting similar worsened outcomes[18] were not sufficiently structured or powered to assess cancer progression or survival. In the absence of adequate clinical trials, a massive meta-analysis of cancer patients treated with epoetin alfa or darbepoetin alfa has been conducted of 21,102 subjects in 91 trials.[15] Erythroid growth factors significantly reduced the relative risk of red cell transfusions (RR, 0.65; 95% CI, 0.62–0.68; 70 trials, $N = 16,093$). On average, patients in the erythropoietin arms received one unit less blood than the control group with a suggestion of increased quality of life. However, erythroid growth factors increased mortality during active study (HR, 1.17; 95% CI, 1.06–1.29; 70 trials, $N = 15,935$) and might have decreased overall survival (HR, 1.05; 95% CI, 1.00–1.11; 78 trials, $N = 19,003$). There was no evidence that erythropoietin affected tumor response (RR, 1.02; 95% CI, 0.98–1.06; 15 trials, $N = 5012$).

Clinical use of erythroid growth factors

The erythroid growth factors have been used in a wide range of medical conditions ranging from renal failure to hemochromatosis (Table 35.2).

Chronic renal failure

In patients with chronic renal failure, the use of erythroid growth factors has been shown to increase hematocrit, decreased transfusion needs, and increase quality of life. For most such patients, the hemoglobin target is no higher than 11–12 g/dL.[19] This is based upon clinical studies that showed that patients experienced greater risk for death and serious cardiovascular events with a target hemoglobin of >13 g/dL; those with a target of 11.5–13 g/dL had no better or worse outcomes, but possibly improved quality of life compared to those with a lower hemoglobin level.[16,19]

Table 35.2 Clinical uses of erythroid growth factors

Chronic renal failure
HIV infection
Cancer chemotherapy
Preoperative anemia: hemoglobin 10–13
(Myelodysplastic syndromes [MDS])
(Anemia in rheumatoid arthritis)
(Anemia of chronic disease)
(Anemia in congestive heart failure)
(Treatment of anemia in patients whose religious beliefs forbid transfusion)
(Anemia due to hepatitis C treatment)
(Mobilization of iron in hemochromatosis)
(Improved harvesting of autologous blood)
(Mobilize peripheral blood progenitor cells [PBPCs])
(Neuroprotection—studies in progress)

Uses in parentheses denote lack of FDA approval.

Cancer patients

The use of erythroid growth factors has been shown to decrease the need for red cell transfusions in most populations studied;[11] the exceptions are anemic cancer patients who are not receiving chemotherapy[20] and those with EPO levels >500 IU.[21] Given the concerns over tumor progression and survival, current guidelines[22,23] encourage a thorough discussion of the risks and benefits of these agents before their use in all patients receiving myelosuppressive chemotherapy. Furthermore, these agents are not to be used in cancer patients not receiving myelosuppressive chemotherapy or in those for whom the treatment is expected to be curative. Dosing is not started unless the hemoglobin is <10 g/dL with only the lowest dose being used to avoid transfusions, and treatment is discontinued when chemotherapy ends. It should be remembered that improvement in quality of life reaches a plateau once the hemoglobin rises above 11 g/dL (range, 11–13 g/dL).[24]

HIV infection

Clinical benefit has been demonstrated in anemic (Hct <30) HIV-infected patients with endogenous EPO levels ≤500 IU/mL undergoing treatment with zidovudine at doses ≤4200 mg/week. In a pooled analysis of four trials,[25] 297 AIDS patients treated with zidovudine received either epoetin alfa or placebo for 12 weeks. No benefit was seen in those with EPO levels >500 IU, but in those with lower levels, epoetin alfa therapy decreased the mean number of units of blood transfused per patient compared with placebo (3.2 units vs. 5.3 units, respectively; $p = 0.003$) and increased the mean hematocrit from the baseline level (4.6 vs. 0.5 percentage points, respectively; $p < 0.001$). Overall quality of life improved in patients on epoetin alfa but was not statistically significant ($p = 0.13$).

Preoperative anemia

In patients who are not candidates for autologous blood transfusion, epoetin alfa has been shown to increase the hemoglobin and decrease the need for subsequent allogeneic transfusions when given to patients with hemoglobin between 10 and 13 prior to therapy. In two studies of 461 patients undergoing major orthopedic surgery, 358 received epoetin alfa (100–300 IU/kg sq daily for 15 days [10 days preoperative] or 600 IU/kg weekly for four weeks). The use of allogeneic transfusions was significantly reduced ($p < 0.001$).[26]

An important issue associated with use of erythroid growth factors

The response to erythroid growth factors depends on the availability of adequate reserves of bone marrow and iron. Because the ferritin falls dramatically after administration of EPO,[14,27,28] iron supplementation has been shown to be critical in amplifying the hemoglobin response to erythroid growth factors in chronic kidney disease patients[29] and in cancer chemotherapy patients.[30] In most studies, intravenous iron was superior to oral iron repletion.

Implications for transfusion medicine

The impact of the erythroid growth factors on blood resource utilization has received little attention. With the recent guideline changes for erythroid growth factors in chemotherapy patients, their use has dropped dramatically with an estimate that RBC transfusions will increase 1% nationally.[31] Similar regulatory changes have also reduced the use of these agents in chronic kidney disease and have been accompanied by increased rates of transfusion.[32] These changes have the potential to increase the pressure on available blood supplies.[33]

Although neither epoetin nor darbepoetin act sufficiently rapidly to replace RBC transfusions in acute settings, the newly described sotatercept (ACE-011) may fulfill this role. This recombinant human fusion protein contains the extracellular domain of the human activin receptor IIA, and it binds to and inhibits activin and other members of the transforming growth factor-β (TGF-β) superfamily. Administration of sotatercept to healthy volunteers led to a rapid and sustained increase in hematocrit in phase I clinical trials by an as-of-yet unclear mechanism.[34]

The erythroid growth factors remain the only option for many patients who cannot receive RBC transfusions for religious or medical reasons. Administration of 140 IU/kg epoetin alfa three times a week for three weeks along with oral iron three times a day to 45 Jehovah's Witness patients increased the hemoglobin and allowed all patients to undergo major cardiac procedures without blood transfusion.[35]

Finally, the use of erythroid growth factors has been demonstrated to increase the preoperative collection of RBCs. In a randomized study of 47 patients scheduled for orthopedic surgery, patients received 600 IU/kg or placebo twice a week for 21 days (along with oral iron) during which time up to six units of RBCs were scheduled to be collected. Epoetin alfa–treated patients collected a mean (±SD) of 5.4 ± 0.2 units compared with 4.1 ± 0.2 for the placebo group.[36]

Myeloid growth factors

While deficiencies in RBCs and platelets can be readily treated with transfusion, neutropenia may be a severe, life-threatening disorder that is not readily amenable to transfusion. Although neutrophil transfusions may be arranged, they are neither readily available nor of demonstrated benefit.[37] With the FDA approval of both G-CSF (filgrastim) and GM-CSF (sargramostim) in early 1991, treatment and prevention of neutropenia became a reality.

Structure, function, and physiology

G-CSF is a 174-amino-acid glycosylated protein (MW = 25,000 Da) and is encoded by a single gene (17q21.1). G-CSF is synthesized by macrophages, monocytes, endothelial cells, and fibroblasts, and its production can be vastly increased when other inflammatory molecules (TNFα, IL1, IL3, interferon γ, and IL4) are present. It is made without a storage form and immediately released into the circulation, where it is cleared by neutrophils via their G-CSF receptor (Kd = 65 pM) and less so by the kidney. In the noninfected individual, production is constant, and circulating levels are inversely proportional to the ANC by way of neutrophil clearance. With infection, production is stimulated by inflammatory cytokines.[38] Normal G-CSF levels are <39 ng/L, but rise to a different

Table 35.3 Biological effects of G-CSF and GM-CSF

↑ Demargination of neutrophils
↑ Release of neutrophils, *monocytes*, and *eosinophils* from marrow reserves
↑ Neutrophil, *monocyte*, and *eosinophil* survival
↑ Production of neutrophils, *monocytes*, and *eosinophils*
↓ Motility of phagocytes; ↓ skin window migration
↑ Neutrophil function (↑ of both normal and abnormal neutrophils)
  ↑ Phagocytosis
  ↑ Endocytosis
  ↑ *Destruction of T. cruzi, Mycobacterium avium, Influenza A, Candida*
  ↑ O_2 generation
↑ Mobilization of PBPCs

Italics denote effects seen only with GM-CSF.

extent depending on the type of infection: bacterial, 799 ± 1501 ng/L; viral, 58 ± 34 ng/L; and mycoplasma, 60 ± 33 ng/L.

G-CSF has many biological effects (Table 35.3). For existing neutrophils, it promotes demargination and release from bone marrow reserves and increases neutrophil survival. Neutrophil production is markedly increased, with the maturation time reduced from six days to three days, an increase in "left shift," and often the appearance of Dohle bodies and toxic granulation. Neutrophil motility is altered. Neutrophil function (phagocytosis, O_2^- generation, endomitosis, antibody-dependent cell-mediated cytotoxicity [ADCC], and FcγRI receptors) is increased, an underappreciated effect. Finally, G-CSF mobilizes peripheral progenitor cells. In animals lacking G-CSF,[39] neutrophils are 20–30% of normal, neutrophil precursors are 50% of normal, and there is decreased neutrophil mobilization into the circulation.

Although G-CSF is necessary for the normal production and maturation of myeloid precursors into neutrophils, GM-CSF has no physiologic importance for hematopoiesis. In GM-CSF deficient mice, neutrophils, macrophages, and their precursors are normal but the mice develop pulmonary problems.[40]

GM-CSF is a 127-amino-acid (23,000 Da) glycosylated protein made from a single gene (5q31.1). It is made by T cells, macrophages, monocytes, endothelial cells, and fibroblasts. Significant levels are not detected in the circulation, and amounts of this protein do not vary inversely to the ANC. GM-CSF does not increase in amount during infection, but its production by bone marrow stromal cells may be decreased by interferon 1β. It is normally cleared by the GM-CSF receptor on neutrophils and monocytes, with less than 40% being renally cleared.

The biologic effects of GM-CSF on neutrophil survival, production, and mobility are comparable to those of G-CSF but are extended to eosinophils and monocytes (Table 35.3). In addition to increasing neutrophil function like G-CSF, it also increases the destruction of *Trypanosoma cruzi, Mycobacterium avium*, influenza A, and *Candida*. Unlike G-CSF, GM-CSF can increase the production of TNFα and IL1, which may explain some of its clinical adverse effects.

Clinically relevant myeloid growth factors
Filgrastim (Neupogen)
Filgrastim is a 175-amino-acid protein (MW = 18,800 Da) identical to the native molecule except for an added N-terminal methionine (r-met huG-CSF) and a lack of glycosylation since it is made in *Escherichia coli*. Vials and prefilled syringes of filgrastim are available in doses of 300 and 480 mcg. For most uses, the dose is 5 mcg/kg/day (~230 mcg/m^2/day). Remembering the log-linear dose–response curve for hematopoietic growth factors, one rounds down to the nearest vial or syringe size. Although doses for stem cell mobilization are usually higher, much lower doses (0.4 mcg/kg/day) are often adequate in neutropenic patients with HIV, idiopathic neutropenia, or drug-induced neutropenia. Filgrastim has a T1/2 of 3.5 hours and is metabolized mostly by mature neutrophils and less so by the kidney. Like most hematopoietic growth factors, subcutaneous administration gives a better response than intravenous administration. In chemotherapy patients, filgrastim is usually started 24 hours after the end of chemotherapy and stopped at least 24 hours before the next chemotherapy dose. In chemotherapy patients, prescribing information suggests stopping once the ANC is >10,000, but it is often stopped once the ANC is >2000.

Filgrastim is FDA approved for:
- decreasing the incidence of infection, as manifested by febrile neutropenia, in patients with nonmyeloid malignancies receiving myelosuppressive anticancer drugs associated with a significant incidence of severe neutropenia with fever;
- reducing the time to neutrophil recovery and the duration of fever following induction or consolidation chemotherapy treatment of adults with acute myelogenous leukemia (AML);
- reducing the duration of neutropenia and neutropenia-related clinical sequelae (e.g., febrile neutropenia) in patients with nonmyeloid malignancies undergoing myeloablative chemotherapy followed by marrow transplantation;
- mobilizing hematopoietic progenitor cells into the peripheral blood for collection by leukapheresis;
- chronic administration to reduce the incidence and duration of sequelae of neutropenia (e.g., fever, infections, and oropharyngeal ulcers) in symptomatic patients with congenital neutropenia, cyclic neutropenia, or idiopathic neutropenia; and
- increase survival in patients acutely exposed to myelosuppresive doses of radiation.

Tbo-filgrastim (Granix)
Tbo-filgrastim is a protein identical to filgrastim, but with slightly different concentrations of excipients. Its pharmacokinetics and neutrophil response are identical to filgrastim in clinical trials in chemotherapy, stem cell mobilization, and stem cell transplantation. Although it has been regarded as a "biosimilar,"[41] it has gone through the full FDA approval process just like filgrastim. It is available as 300 and 480 mcg prefilled syringes and used just like filgrastim. It is FDA approved only for reducing the duration of severe neutropenia in patients with nonmyeloid malignancies receiving myelosuppressive anticancer drugs associated with a clinically significant incidence of febrile neutropenia.

Pegfilgrastim (Neulasta)
Pegfilgrastim is a longer acting form of filgrastim produced by adding a 20,000 Da polyethylene glycol (PEG) moiety to the amino-terminus of the filgrastim protein. It has a MW of 39,000 Da and is available only as a 6 mg prefilled syringe that is usually administered every two weeks. Its action is prolonged because it is cleared mostly by neutrophils, not the kidney. Its T1/2 of 33 hours (varies from 15 to 80 hours depending upon the ANC) is at least 10 times longer than that of filgrastim. It is usually given one day after the end of the chemotherapy cycle and is not to be given in the period 14 days before to 24 hours after chemotherapy. Its major attribute is that of convenience; one 6 mg pegfilgrastim dose every two weeks is equivalent to 10–14 daily doses of filgrastim.[42] It is FDA approved only to decrease the incidence of infection, as manifested by febrile neutropenia, in patients with nonmyeloid malignancies receiving myelosuppressive anticancer drugs associated with a clinically significant incidence of febrile neutropenia.

Sargramostim (Leukine)

Sargramostim has a structure identical to that of native GM-CSF except that it has a leucine at amino acid 123. This glycosylated protein is prepared in yeast and has three different molecular forms of 19,500, 16,800, and 15,500 Da. It is available in vials of 250 and 500 mcg with a chemotherapy dose of 250 mcg/m^2/day. It is more effective when given subcutaneously than intravenously and is usually given 24 hours after the end of the chemotherapy and not in the 24 hours before chemotherapy starts. It is recommended that sargramostim be stopped after chemotherapy when the ANC is >10,000, but many stop at lower ANCs. It is FDA approved for:

- use following induction chemotherapy in older adult patients with AML to shorten time to neutrophil recovery and to reduce the incidence of severe and life-threatening infections and infections resulting in death;
- mobilization of hematopoietic progenitor cells into peripheral blood for collection by leukapheresis. Myeloid reconstitution is further accelerated by administration of sargramostim following peripheral blood progenitor cell transplantation;
- acceleration of myeloid recovery in patients with non-Hodgkin's lymphoma (NHL), acute lymphoblastic leukemia (ALL), and Hodgkin's disease undergoing autologous bone marrow transplantation (BMT);
- acceleration of myeloid recovery in patients undergoing allogeneic BMT from HLA-matched related donors; and
- patients who have undergone allogeneic or autologous bone marrow transplantation (BMT) in whom engraftment is delayed or has failed.

Effects and adverse effects of G-CSF and GM-CSF administration

The neutrophil response to the filgrastims and sargramostim in healthy volunteers are comparable in some ways:

- *15–30 minutes*: Neutrophils decrease modestly and then return to baseline, probably due to transient sequestration/margination.
- *1–36 hours*: The neutrophils gradually rise due to de-margination and release from bone marrow stores.
- *>36 hours*: Increased production of neutrophils.

But, in other ways, the filgrastims and sargramostim differ greatly with much of the white blood cell (WBC) response of the latter coming from increases in eosinophils. Most of the GM-CSF effect on neutrophils is to increase their survival,[43] not their production (Table 35.4).

The side effects of the myeloid growth factors are listed in Table 35.5. The three G-CSFs are comparable in terms of their side effects, but GM-CSF has a somewhat expanded repertoire. These commonly include myalgias, but capillary leak syndrome and a *first-dose* phenomenon of hypotension, tachycardia, and dyspnea may be seen at high doses of GM-CSF in the transplant setting. If myeloid growth factors are administered concurrent with chemotherapy or radiation therapy, subsequent neutropenia is usually worsened.

Table 35.4 Effects of G-CSF and GM-CSF on neutrophil kinetics

Neutrophil Production	Normal	GM-CSF	G-CSF
Maximum count (×10^{-6}/mL)	5.2	17.0	35.0
Appearance in peripheral blood (days)	4–7	4.5–6.5	1–2
Peripheral t1/2 (h)	8	48	7.6
Amplification factor	1	1.5	9.4
Extra divisions	0	0.6	3.2

Source: Lord *et al.* (1992).[43] Reproduced with permission of Wiley.

Table 35.5 Adverse effects of myeloid growth factors

Bone pain (15–39% on G-CSF vs. 0–21% on placebo)
Exacerbation of preexisting inflammatory conditions (eczema, psoriasis, and vasculitis)
Allergic reactions at injection sites (rare)
Sweet's syndrome (acute, febrile neutrophilic dermatosis)
Antibody formation (none are neutralizing)
Splenic rupture, acute respiratory distress syndrome, and precipitate sickle cell crisis (all rare)
Capillary leak syndrome
Alveolar hemorrhage and hemoptysis
↑ Risk MDS and AML in patients receiving chemotherapy or with congenital neutropenia
↑ *LDH, uric acid, LAP; ↓ cholesterol*
Myalgias, fever
"First dose phenomenon": rare; hypotension, tachycardia, and dyspnea due to transient pulmonary leukocyte sequestration (very high doses)

Italics denote effects seen only with GM-CSF.

The use of myeloid growth factors in chemotherapy patients may be associated with a small increased risk of treatment-related acute myeloid leukemia or myelodysplasia.[44,45]

Clinical uses of myeloid growth factors

Table 35.6 lists the uses of myeloid growth factors. Most of these have been studied only with G-CSF, but current National Comprehensive Cancer Network (NCCN) guidelines draw no strong distinction yet between GM-CSF and G-CSF.[46]

Chemotherapy-induced neutropenia

Filgrastim, tbo-filgrastim, and pegfilgrastim have all shown marked ability to stimulate neutrophil production and to mitigate chemotherapy-induced neutropenia. In small cell lung cancer patients undergoing chemotherapy,[47] neutropenic fever for all chemotherapy cycles was decreased from 77% with placebo to 40% ($p < 0.001$) with filgrastim; hospital days were shortened from 4.2 to 2.3 for all cycles. Antibiotic use and days with an ANC <500 were also markedly decreased. NCCN guidelines[46] suggest using myeloid growth factors for primary prophylaxis of febrile neutropenia when the expected incidence of such is greater than 20%. Additionally, myeloid growth factors can be considered for primary prophylaxis for patients receiving chemotherapy where

Table 35.6 Clinical Uses of myeloid growth factors

Primary prophylaxis of FN if incidence >20%
Primary prophylaxis considered if FN incidence >10–20% (usually "high-risk" patients)
Primary prophylaxis if FN incidence <10% (rarely)
Secondary prophylaxis of FN to keep dose intensity
All high-risk chemotherapy patients admitted with FN
After allogeneic or autologous stem cell txp
PBPC mobilization
MDS with neutropenia and recurrent infection
AML induction chemotherapy (≥55 years old)
Severe chronic neutropenia
(Drug-induced neutropenia—low dose [0.4–5 µg/kg])
(Aplastic anemia)
(Hairy cell leukemia)
(Acute lymphoblastic leukemia)
(Agranulocytosis)

FN, febrile neutropenia; PBPC, peripheral blood progenitor cells; MDS, myelodysplastic syndrome; AML, acute myeloid leukemia. Uses in parentheses denote lack of FDA approval.

febrile neutropenia risk is 10–20% if patients are high risk[46] (e.g., age >65, prior chemotherapy or radiation therapy, preexisting neutropenia or bone marrow involvement or infection, poor performance status, and/or HIV infection). Prophylactic myeloid growth factors are rarely considered for chemotherapy patients where the rate of febrile neutropenia is expected to be <10%.

In chemotherapy patients experiencing febrile neutropenia in a chemotherapy cycle not supported by myeloid growth factor, subsequent use of myeloid growth factor (secondary prophylaxis) is recommended to maintain dose intensity.

Unless considered high risk, myeloid growth factor treatment is not indicated for chemotherapy patients (not already on myeloid growth factor therapy) who develop severe neutropenia without fever or those currently hospitalized with febrile neutropenia.

Severe chronic neutropenia

The clinical benefit of long-term myeloid growth factor administration for patients with severe congenital neutropenia (including Kostmann syndrome), severe idiopathic neutropenia, or cyclic neutropenia has been well established.[48–50] In a large randomized clinical trial of patients with severe chronic neutropenia, the occurrence of fever, oropharyngeal ulcers, infections, hospitalizations, and antibiotic use were all significantly reduced with filgrastim treatment. The quality of life and activity profiles of patients also improved. The only complication of therapy was the increased risk of developing myelodysplasia and acute leukemia in patients with severe congenital neutropenia.[51,52] This risk appears to be disease specific with substantially lower or no risk for patients with cyclic or idiopathic neutropenia. Those with severe congenital neutropenia need to be monitored with regular white counts, clinical observation, and possibly bone marrow examinations.

Mobilization of peripheral blood progenitor cells

Four to six days after administration of G-CSF, peripheral blood progenitor cells (PBSCs) increase as much as 100-fold. This has allowed for the marked improvement of collection of such cells in patients or donors for stem cell transplant. The basic physiologic principles governing mobilization of PBSCs probably involve breakage of molecular bonds between the adhesive marrow elements, that is, CXCR-4 on the progenitors and stromal-cell-derived factor 1 (SDF-1) on the marrow stromal cells.[53] Administration of G-CSF expands myeloid and progenitor mass, and there is good evidence that the proteases released from neutrophils disrupt key adhesive bonds holding the progenitors in the marrow and allow their mobilization from marrow spaces.[54]

Implications for transfusion medicine

The use of myeloid growth factors to mobilize peripheral blood progenitor cells is a standard transfusion medicine practice. They can also be used to ameliorate drug-induced neutropenia such as that occurring after the administration of IVIG. Widespread use of myeloid growth factors in oncology may reduce the need for hospitalization and antibiotics. Unfortunately, their use to provide neutrophils for transfusion has not met with much success. Indeed, a recent heroic effort was unable to show a significant effect of neutrophil transfusion on the outcomes of infected, neutropenic patients.[37]

Thrombopoietic growth factors

Although James Homer Wright described how bone marrow megakaryocytes produced platelets in 1902,[55] it was not until 1958 that Kelemen proposed that a "thrombopoietin" regulated this process.[56] This last of the major hematopoietic growth factors was not purified until 1994.[57] Initial clinical studies with two types of recombinant TPO (recombinant human TPO [rhTPO] and pegylated recombinant human megakaryocyte growth and development factor [PEG-rhMGDF]) showed they were quite effective in raising the platelet count in healthy subjects[58] and increasing platelet apheresis yields.[59,60] They raised the platelet count nadirs and decreased platelet transfusions after non-myeloablative chemotherapy, but had minimal effect on the recovery of platelets to >20,000 or need for platelet transfusions in patients undergoing leukemia induction chemotherapy or stem cell transplantation.[58] There was a modest platelet count increase when given to myelodysplastic syndrome (MDS) patients. Unfortunately, these studies were terminated when antibodies developed against one of these recombinant molecules (PEG-rhMGDF) that cross-reacted with native TPO and produced thrombocytopenia.[61] Subsequently, two TPO receptor agonists, romiplostim and eltrombopag, were not antigenic and proved to be potent stimulators of platelet production.[62] Both were FDA approved in 2008 for the treatment of immune thrombocytopenia (ITP).

Structure, function, and physiology

TPO is encoded by a single gene (3q27.1) that produces a 332-amino-acid (MW = 95,000 Da) glycoprotein of which the first 153 amino acids are 23% homologous with EPO, and probably 50% similar if conservative amino acid substitutions are considered.[63] This region also contains four cysteine residues like those in EPO and is responsible for binding to the TPO receptor. But, despite these similarities, TPO does not bind the EPO receptor and EPO does not bind the TPO receptor. The rest of the molecule is rich in carbohydrates that increase its half-life.

TPO is the key regulator of platelet production. In mice deficient in both genes for either TPO or the TPO receptor, the platelet count, bone marrow megakaryocytes, and megakaryocyte precursors are 10–15% of normal.[64] These animals also have reduced levels of erythroid and myeloid precursors but with no subsequent anemia or neutropenia.[65]

TPO is made primarily in the liver. Whether its basal rate of production is regulated remains unclear. Multiple studies of animals with ITP or after chemotherapy have shown no increase in the hepatic TPO mRNA levels. However, in a recent study, hepatocytes were found to increase TPO mRNA production after desialyated platelets bound to the Ashwell–Morell receptor.[66] How this affects normal physiology remains unclear at the present time.

TPO levels are inversely related to the rate of platelet production. Once in the circulation, TPO is bound to and cleared by high-affinity platelet TPO receptors leaving a small basal amount of TPO.[67] This primitive normal feedback loop is shared with other hematopoietic growth factors such as M-CSF and G-CSF; there appears to be no specific sensor of the platelet count in the body. In aplastic anemia patients, TPO levels are >2000 pg/mL (normal: 7–99 pg/mL). In animals or humans transfused to platelet counts above normal, TPO is suppressed below basal levels. In patients with hepatic cirrhosis, TPO production is reduced.

TPO has no carrier molecule and works by binding to TPO receptors on target hematopoietic cells. TPO is necessary for the viability of stem cells; humans born without it are thrombocytopenic at birth and eventually become pancytopenic. TPO is necessary for the viability of precursors of all lineages (Figure 35.1) but only amplifies the megakaryocyte lineage by promoting the mitosis of megakaryocyte colony-forming cells, increasing the rate of megakaryocyte endomitosis and maturation, and thereby increasing platelet production (Figure 35.4).

Clinically available thrombopoietic growth factors
Romiplostim (Nplate)

Romiplostim is a TPO receptor agonist composed of an IgG1 heavy chain carrier molecule into which have been inserted four identical 14 amino acid peptides that activate the TPO receptor.[68] This peptide (IEGPTLRQWLAARA) has no sequence homology with TPO but was found to bind and activate the TPO receptor. If dimerized, it was as potent as thrombopoietin in vitro but given its short half-life had minimal activity in vivo. By inserting this peptide into the IgG carrier construct, romiplostim has a T1/2 of ~120 h, three times longer than native TPO.[69] Although romiplostim binds to the TPO receptor with an affinity 25% of that of TPO, it is a very potent activator of platelet production. Romiplostim is available as vials containing 250 or 500 mcg of lyophilized drug. It is administrated as a subcutaneous injection of 1–10 mcg/kg once a week for the treatment of ITP. There is no effect upon white cell or red cell production. Romiplostim is currently FDA approved only for the treatment of thrombocytopenia in patients with chronic ITP who have had an insufficient response to corticosteroids, immunoglobulins, or splenectomy.

Eltrombopag (Promacta, Revolade)

Efforts to identify small molecules that bound and activated the TPO receptor successfully identified a number of compounds. One was subsequently modified to enhance its pharmacological and biological properties, resulting in eltrombopag.[70] Eltrombopag binds the TPO receptor at a transmembrane site distant from where TPO binds. It thereby activates the TPO receptor differently than TPO or romiplostim: JAK and STAT phosphorylation are less, and there is no effect upon the AKT pathway.[71] Nonetheless, eltrombopag increases megakaryocyte growth and maturation to increase platelet production.

Eltrombopag is available as 12.5, 25, 50, 75, or 100 mg tablets. Eltrombopag is primarily metabolized by the liver, and dose adjustments are necessary for patients with reduced metabolism of this drug due to East Asian ancestry or liver dysfunction. It is usually taken orally once a day and distant from calcium-containing compounds or food stuffs that would neutralize its activity if co-administered. Eltrombopag is currently FDA approved for the treatment of:

- thrombocytopenia in adult and pediatric patients 1 year and older with chronic ITP who have had an insufficient response to corticosteroids, immunoglobulins, or splenectomy;
- thrombocytopenia in patients with chronic hepatitis C to allow the initiation and maintenance of interferon-based therapy; and
- patients with severe aplastic anemia who have had an insufficient response to immunosuppressive therapy.

Effects and adverse effects of thrombopoietin administration

After giving a single dose of romiplostim[69] or 10 daily doses of eltrombopag[72] to healthy volunteers, platelet counts begin to rise on day 5, peak at days 10–15, and return to baseline by day 28. Eltrombopag is probably one-eighth as potent as romiplostim:

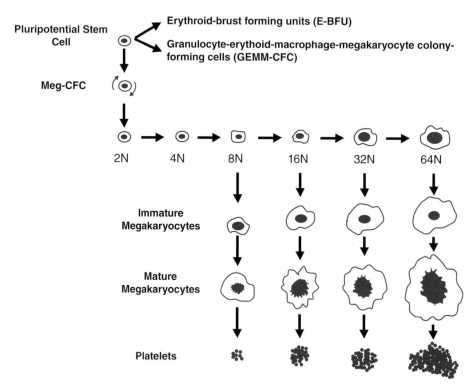

Figure 35.4 Scheme of megakaryocyte maturation from stem cell to mature platelet. Stem cells and megakaryocyte colony-forming cells (Meg-CFCs) undergo mitosis, but at some stage they stop mitosis and undergo endomitosis during which nuclear and cytoplasmic division do not occur, giving rise to polyploid early megakaryocytes that contain 2–16 times the normal diploid (2 N) amount of DNA. The early megakaryocytes then stop endomitosis and mature into morphologically identifiable megakaryocytes and then shed platelets. TPO plays a major role in all but the last process. Source: D. Kuter. Reproduced with permission.

Table 35.7 Adverse effects of thrombopoietic growth factors

Thrombocytosis	Autoantibody formation
Thrombosis	Liver function abnormalities (eltrombopag only)
Increased bone marrow reticulin	Reduction in threshold for platelet activation (romiplostim only)
Stimulation of leukemic blasts	Rebound worsening of thrombocytopenia with discontinuation in ITP patients

at the maximum dose of 75 mg/d, eltrombopag increases the platelet count by about 150,000 above baseline compared with a rise of 1,400,000 for romiplostim. Nonetheless, this difference in potency has not translated into any different response rate for eltrombopag compared to romiplostim in clinical trials. With continued administration of either molecule, peak platelet counts can be maintained indefinitely with no effect on the RBCs or WBCs. The platelets so produced have normal function.

The TPO receptor agonists have not demonstrated any tachyphylaxis or significant long-term complications.[73,74] The potential and real adverse effects are listed in Table 35.7. A few deserve additional comment.

Thrombosis
Although both TPO receptor agonists can significantly increase the platelet count, thrombosis has not been clearly associated with either in placebo-controlled ITP studies. Rather, what has been uncovered is that ITP is itself a prothrombotic disorder[75] whose rate of thrombosis does not appear to be exacerbated by either agent. Compared with placebo treatment, thrombosis was not increased by recombinant TPO treatment in earlier trials in cancer patients. Platelet function studies have shown no increase in platelet activation with either agent despite the finding that romiplostim (but not eltrombopag) reduces the activation threshold for some agonists (eg, ADP) by about 50% in platelet aggregation tests.

Tumor progression and cancer mortality
Unlike the controversy over erythroid growth factors, solid tumor cells lack the TPO receptor.[76] Furthermore, in cancer chemotherapy studies with recombinant thrombopoietins in the 1990s, there is no effect on tumor progression or survival.[58]

Antibody formation
Although antibody formation ended the development of the recombinant TPO molecules, no clinically relevant antibodies have been developed against the TPO receptor agonists. Three patients have developed non-neutralizing antibody against romiplostim, and none have developed antibodies against eltrombopag.

Hepatic toxicity
Eltrombopag is metabolized by the liver, and in one ITP study 13% of patients developed abnormal liver function tests. In general, these were mild and reversible, and did not often require cessation of medication. Intermittent monitoring of liver function tests is recommended for eltrombopag.

Rebound thrombocytopenia
The major concern with TPO receptor agonists occurs in ITP patients in whom the drug is abruptly stopped. Current prescribing information is incorrect and states that either agent be stopped when the platelet count exceeds 400,000. Unfortunately, in 10–20%

of such situations, stopping the drug results in a rebound thrombocytopenia with the platelet count rapidly dropping below prior baseline values 7–10 days later and a markedly increased bleeding risk.[62] Such patients are better treated by a gradual dose reduction over several weeks.

Reticulin fibrosis
Reticulin is a normal component of the bone marrow and may increase in patients with ITP[77] and in those receiving TPO receptor agonists.[78] This reticulin is generally mild, reversible, and clinically silent, and does not portend progression to the disease myelofibrosis. Recent prospective bone marrow studies of ITP patients receiving TPO receptor agonists have shown infrequent increases in reticulin over three years of treatment.[79]

Clinical use of thrombopoietic growth factors
Table 35.8 provides a complete list of conditions that have been treated with thrombopoietic growth factors.

Immune thrombocytopenia
ITP is a disease of increased platelet destruction and inappropriately low platelet production.[80] Although standard therapies such as immunosuppression, rituximab, and splenectomy decrease platelet destruction, thrombopoietic growth factors increase platelet production, thereby mitigating thrombocytopenia. Both TPO receptor agonists increase the platelet count >50,000 in more than 85% of patients, accompanied by reduced bleeding and need for other therapies.[81,82] Long-term use of both molecules is successful[73,74] and may be associated with increased numbers of T-regulatory lymphocytes and occasional disease remission.

Hepatitis C–related thrombocytopenia
Hepatitis C produces two forms of thrombocytopenia that may be difficult to distinguish in any one patient. One is an ITP-like condition that responds to ITP therapies; the second is TPO deficiency due to hepatic injury. Nonetheless, in patients with platelet counts <70,000, antiviral therapy with ribavirin and interferon may be contraindicated. When such patients with a mean baseline platelet count of 55,000 were treated with eltrombopag 75 mg/d for four weeks, the mean platelet count rose to 209,000 compared with 54,000 in those receiving placebo.[83] With continued eltrombopag support, 65% of patients could finish antiviral treatment compared with 6% receiving placebo. In a large phase III study, hepatitis C patients with platelet counts under 100,000 were all treated with eltrombopag and 95% increased their platelet count to over 100,000 by week 9. They were then randomized to continue eltrombopag or receive placebo during the next 24–48 weeks of

Table 35.8 Clinical uses of thrombopoietic growth factors

Chronic ITP	(Liver failure)
Hepatitis C–related thrombocytopenia	(Myosin heavy chain 9–related disease)
Aplastic anemia	(Stem cell mobilization)
Pediatric ITP	(Stem cell transplant, failed engraftment)
(ITP initial therapy)	(Acute leukemia)
(Chemotherapy-induced thrombocytopenia)	(Platelet apheresis)
(Presurgical thrombocytopenia)	(Myelodysplastic syndromes)

Uses in parentheses denote lack of FDA approval.

antiviral treatment.[84] Sustained virologic response was seen in 19–23% of eltrombopag patients compared with 13–15% on placebo ($p < 0.02$), with more patients maintaining a platelet count >50,000 (69–81% vs. 15–23%, respectively).

Aplastic anemia

Although TPO levels are markedly elevated (>2000 pg/mL) in most aplastic anemia patients, eltrombopag produced a platelet count rise in 9/25 patients with a trilineage response in 6/25 patients.[85] In responders, marrow cellularity increased and response was maintained long-term with some coming off treatment.[86] These striking results were not seen in prior studies with recombinant TPO[58] and suggest that eltrombopag may not be working through the TPO receptor.

Presurgical treatment of thrombocytopenic patients

Thrombocytopenia complicates many illness, and such patients are often given aggressive platelet transfusions or even refused needed surgical procedures. Several studies have shown that romiplostim and eltrombopag can increase platelet counts in such patients, reduce bleeding, and allow procedures to be performed. In one study of 17 thrombocytopenic patients treated with romiplostim, all were able to raise their platelet count and undergo surgery with no excessive bleeding and with minimal need for transfusion.[87] In a second study of thrombocytopenic cirrhotic patients being prepped for liver biopsy, platelet transfusion was avoided in 72% of patients receiving eltrombopag compared with 19% of those receiving placebo ($p < 0.001$); there was no difference in bleeding (17% vs. 19%, respectively).[88] However, this study was terminated early because 6/145 eltrombopag patients had portal vein clot versus 1/147 on placebo. The study was weakened by the absence of pretreatment assessment for portal vein clot.

Chemotherapy-induced thrombocytopenia

This remains a major challenge, and there are as yet no completed studies with the TPO receptor agonists. Early studies in patients receiving non-myeloablative chemotherapy for ovarian cancer[89] or lung cancer[90] showed that treatment with rhTPO and PEG-rhMGDF increased the nadir platelet count, decreased the need for platelet transfusions, and allowed chemotherapy to be given on time.[58] However, neither TPO showed benefit in patients receiving myeloablative chemotherapy for acute leukemia induction or for stem cell transplant.

Myelodysplastic syndrome

Thrombocytopenia commonly complicates the care of patients with MDS. In a study of thrombocytopenic (<20,000 or history of bleeding and platelets ≥20,000) low-risk/intermediate-1-risk MDS patients, romiplostim or placebo was administered for 58 weeks. Overall, clinically important bleeding events were not significantly reduced with romiplostim (HR, 0.83; 95% CI, 0.66–1.05; $p = 0.13$), but in those with platelet counts ≥20,000 significant reductions were seen (HR, 0.34; 95% CI, 0.20–0.58; $p < 0.0001$). Romiplostim reduced bleeding events (RR, 0.92) and platelet transfusions (RR, 0.77) and increased platelet response (OR, 15.6). This study was stopped at an interim analysis because of a perceived increase in AML rate (HR, 2.51) with romiplostim, but final analysis showed AML rates of 6% with romiplostim and 4.9% placebo (HR, 1.20; 95% CI, 0.38–3.84) and similar survival rates.

Other thrombopoietic growth factors
Interleukin-11 (Oprelvekin, Neumega)

IL11 is not a normal regulator of platelet production.[91] In mice in which this gene is deleted, all blood counts are normal.[92] But administration of IL11 does increase the platelet count[93] and has been found to reduce the transfusion rate from 96% to 70% in patients who had experienced thrombocytopenia in a prior chemotherapy cycle.[94] Oprelvekin is FDA approved for the prevention of severe thrombocytopenia and the reduction of the need for platelet transfusions following myelosuppressive chemotherapy in adult patients with nonmyeloid malignancies who are at high risk of severe thrombocytopenia. It is not indicated following myeloablative chemotherapy. Unfortunately, oprelvekin has a fairly large number of side effects that make it unwise to recommend for any patient.

Implications for transfusion medicine

This area is still early in its development. TPO receptor agonists clearly decease the use of IVIG and platelet transfusions in ITP patients.[81] They can also reduce or eliminate the need for transfusions in thrombocytopenic patients undergoing major surgery. They have helped a number of Jehovah's Witness patients or those with severe platelet alloimmunization to undergo surgery without platelet transfusion.[87]

The bigger issue is whether TPO receptor agonists can decrease the thrombocytopenia associated with chemotherapy and reduce the need for platelet transfusions. Early data showed that rhTPO reduced the rate of platelet transfusion from 75% to 25% in women being treated for ovarian cancer.[89] It is anticipated that studies with the current TPO receptor agonists will show similar benefit.[95]

Whether TPO receptor agonists will ever play a role in stimulating platelet apheresis donors remains unclear. Prior studies showed that PEG-rhMGDF increased the median platelet count from 248,000 to 602,000, with an increase in median (range) apheresis yield from 3.8×10^{11} ($1.3 \times 10^{11} - 7.9 \times 10^{11}$) to 11.0×10^{11} ($7.1 \times 10^{11} - 18.3 \times 10^{11}$) platelets.[59] Once transfused, these products were hemostatically active and provided a dose-dependent rise in platelet count and increased transfusion-free interval.[96] Such rhTPO mobilized platelets have also been frozen and later transfused into alloimmunized chemotherapy patients.[60]

General conclusions

The hematopoietic growth factors have markedly affected the practice of medicine over the past 30 years. Beginning with erythropoietin and then extended with myeloid growth factors and now with thrombopoietic growth factors, there is an ability to increase specific blood cell production in patients who have anemia, neutropenia, or thrombocytopenia. These molecules are generally safe and effective and with adequate time will raise the blood count. Unfortunately, none is immediately active, and most take days for the onset of activity. None of these will replace the need for transfusion in acute situations of anemia or thrombocytopenia. However, all three offer the opportunity to prevent subsequent transfusion therapy or infection. In some settings, they have been demonstrated to reduce medical care costs.

Key references

A full reference list for this chapter is available at: http://www.wiley.com/go/simon/transfusion

9 Goldwasser E. Erythropoietin: a somewhat personal history. *Perspect Biol Med* 1996; **40**: 18–32.

10 Lin FK, Suggs S, Lin CH, *et al.* Cloning and expression of the human erythropoietin gene. *Proc Natl Acad Sci USA* 1985; **82**: 7580–4.

15 Tonia T, Mettler A, Robert N, *et al.* Erythropoietin or darbepoetin for patients with cancer. *Cochrane Database Syst Rev* 2012; **12**: CD003407.

23 Rizzo JD, Brouwers M, Hurley P, *et al.* American Society of Hematology/American Society of Clinical Oncology clinical practice guideline update on the use of epoetin and darbepoetin in adult patients with cancer. *Blood* 2010; **116**: 4045–59.

46 Crawford J, Armitage J, Balducci L, *et al.* Myeloid growth factors. *J Natl Compr Canc Netw* 2013; **11**: 1266–90.

48 Dale DC, Bonilla MA, Davis MW, *et al.* A randomized controlled phase III trial of recombinant human granulocyte colony-stimulating factor (filgrastim) for treatment of severe chronic neutropenia. *Blood* 1993; **81**: 2496–502.

65 Carver-Moore K, Broxmeyer HE, Luoh SM, *et al.* Low levels of erythroid and myeloid progenitors in thrombopoietin- and c-mpl-deficient mice. *Blood* 1996; **88**: 803–8.

81 Kuter DJ, Rummel M, Boccia R, *et al.* Romiplostim or standard of care in patients with immune thrombocytopenia. *N Engl J Med* 2010; **363**: 1889–99.

90 Fanucchi M, Glaspy J, Crawford J, *et al.* Effects of polyethylene glycol-conjugated recombinant human megakaryocyte growth and development factor on platelet counts after chemotherapy for lung cancer. *N Engl J Med* 1997; **336**: 404–9.

96 Goodnough LT, Kuter DJ, McCullough J, *et al.* Prophylactic platelet transfusions from healthy apheresis platelet donors undergoing treatment with thrombopoietin. *Blood* 2001; **98**: 1346–51.

CHAPTER 36

Hematopoietic stem cells and cord blood

Jeffrey McCullough

Department of Laboratory Medicine and Pathology, University of Minnesota Medical School, Minneapolis, MN, USA

Hematopoietic stem cells

The concept of a common stem cell that would produce all blood elements was first mentioned in the early 1900s. Stem cells are those that can undergo both self-renewal and differentiation[136]. Hematopoietic stem cells (HSCs) are those capable of not only self-renewal but also formation of all lines of blood cells. Thus, the HSC could be referred to as *multipotent*, but when the cell begins to differentiate so that it can produce only one kind of daughter cell, it is referred to as *unipotent*.

In mice, cells capable of producing hematopoietic colony-forming units (CFUs) develop at about seven to eight days of gestation in an animal with a 21-day total gestation. It is not clear exactly where these cells first appear because of the multiple embryonic processes to produce hematopoiesis—both extra-embryonic (yolk sack) and intra-embryonic. Fetal liver becomes a main source of hematopoiesis in the mouse and the human, evolving to the fetal spleen and fetal bone marrow. HSCs can be found in blood throughout fetal life, but it appears that they localize in sites such as spleen, bone marrow, and lymphoid sites such as thymus at different times, suggesting that there is something in fetal development that prepares those sites to accept fetal HSCs at different times.[1]

More than 60 years ago, it was established that lethal doses of whole-body irradiation in mice caused death by hematopoietic failure, but this could be averted by shielding the hematopoietic organs or by transplantation of un-irradiated marrow. This was followed about a decade later by the seminal work of Till and McCulloch.[2] In those early studies, only myeloid lineages developed, and the extent of lineage development was proportional to the number of bone marrow cells transplanted. Subsequent experiments established that lymphoid lineages could also be produced, thus establishing that in the marrow there were single cells capable of not only self-renewal but also differentiation into all hematopoietic cell lines.

It is estimated that humans possessed 2×10^4 pluripotent HSCs, but only a small fraction of these are cycling at any one time, which suggests that there is a huge amplification process. It appears that HSCs are divided into short-term and long-term repopulating cells based on their appearance in circulation following transplantation.[3] HSCs are heterogeneous because some cells may expand locally in the marrow or spleen, or others may seed other sites.

The hematopoietic microenvironment

Because of the high concentration of cells (10^9/mL) in the marrow, there are multiple cell–cell and cell–matrix interactions[137]. This is mimicked in in vitro long-term culture assays in which stroma develops and HSCs can be replaced on the stroma for extended periods. This in vitro environment in some ways resembles the in vivo situation.

Marrow stromal cells

Marrow stromal cells that develop from mesenchymal stem cells are composed of fibroblasts, endothelial cells, CXCL12 abundant reticular (CAR) cells, and osteoblasts, among others. Marrow stromal cells produce a number of cytokines involved in HSC development, provide receptors for the integrins present on HSCs, support interactions involving cell proliferation and cell survival, and produce extracellular matrix components, including collagen, laminin, fibronectin, heparin, hyaluronan, and tenascin. There is a specialized area of the marrow in which HSCs transition into other cell lines. This niche includes mesenchymal cells, perivascular lipocites, endothelial cells, macrophages, and the hematopoietic progenitors.[4] The primary cytokines involved in regulation of stem cell survival, proliferation, and differentiation are briefly described in Table 36.1.

Integrins

Integrins are a family of cell surface adhesion receptors that are involved in two-way communication between a cell and the external environment. Many cell types, including HSCs, must have external contact for survival. In vitro, breaking this adhesion usually leads to apoptosis. However, breaking the cell–matrix interaction in vivo results in mobilization of HSCs, especially by granulocyte colony-stimulating factor (G-CSF) and interleukin-8 (IL8).[4] In addition, integrins are also responsible for adherence to stroma and thus for homing and retention of stem cells in the marrow. Antibodies that interfere with integrin–cell interaction cause release of stem cells into the blood.[5]

Self-renewal and expansion of HSCs

Self-renewal is the distinguishing factor between long-term HSCs and other hematopoietic progenitors. HSCs may undergo "asymmetric" or "symmetric" cell division. In asymmetric division, the dividing cell yields one daughter cell that remains an HSC and a second daughter cell that has lineage commitment. In symmetrical

Rossi's Principles of Transfusion Medicine, Fifth Edition. Edited by Toby L. Simon, Jeffrey McCullough, Edward L. Snyder, Bjarte G. Solheim, and Ronald G. Strauss.

Table 36.1 Cytokines and hormones active on stem cells and progenitors

Cytokine	Principal Activities
IL1	Induces production of other cytokines from many cells; works in synergy with other cytokines on primitive hematopoietic cells
IL2	T-cell growth factor
IL3	Stimulates the growth of multiple myeloid cell types; involved in delayed type hypersensitivity
IL4	Stimulates B-cell growth and modulates the immune response by affecting immunoglobulin class switching
IL5	Eosinophil growth factor; affects mature cell function
IL6	Stimulates B-lymphocyte growth; works in synergy with other cytokines on megakaryocytic progenitors
IL7*	Principal regulator of early lymphocyte growth
IL11	Shares activities with IL11; also affects the gut mucosa
IL15*	Modulates T-lymphocyte activity and stimulates natural killer cell proliferation
IL21	Affects growth and maturation of B, T, and natural killer cells
SCF*	Affects primitive hematopoietic cells of all lineages and the growth of basophils and mast cells
EPO*	Stimulates the proliferation of erythroid progenitors
M-CSF*	Promotes the proliferation of monocytic progenitors
G-CSF	Stimulates growth of neutrophlic progenitors, acts in synergy with IL3 on primitive myeloid cells, and activates mature neutrophils
GM-CSF	Affects granulocyte and macrophage progenitors and activates macrophages
TPO	Affects hematopoietic stem cells and megakaryocytic progenitors

*Primary regulator of the corresponding cell lineage.
Source: Beutler (2010). Genetic principles and molecular biology. In: Kaushansky *et al.*, Eds. Williams hematalogy. 8th ed. Adapted with permission of McGraw-Hill.

Table 36.2 Cells Identified in In Vitro Progenitor Assays

Assay	Progenitors Identified
LT-CIC	HSC
CFU-GEMM	Myeloid, erythroid, megakaryocyte
CFU-GM	Myeloid
CFU-MEG	Megakaryocytes
BFU-E	Erythroid burst-forming units

cell division, the two daughter cells are lineage specific. An important but not well-understood issue is the factors that determine the nature (asymmetric or symmetric) of the cell division. HSCs appear to have an unlimited capacity for proliferation, but there must be controls on the size of the stem cell pool. Biologically, it is important that this be reasonably well controlled in order to maintain the size of the HSC pool but also to generate the needed number of lineage-specific progenitors.

One approach to demonstrating the renewal capacity of HSC is the observation that self-renewal is illustrated by successful serial transplantation of multiple generations of mice. However, the ability to continue effective serial transplantation ultimately begins to decline or is lost, suggesting that these cells do not have an indefinite ability at self-renewal. It appears that HSCs have a relatively high telomerase activity,[6] which may slow the shortening of the telomerase and thus extend the HSC lifespan. However, because of the ultimate loss of ability of self-renewal, other factors—possibly genetic—are probably involved in HSC self-renewal and maintenance of the HSC pool.

As HSCs lose their pluripotency and capacity for self-renewal and become lineage specific, several cell characteristics change. A higher portion of cells are in the cell cycle, and there are changes in their cell surface characteristics. The change to lineage-specific cells is characterized by a downregulation of HSC-associated genes and upregulation of lineage-specific genes.

Lineage commitment

Cells in bone marrow can give rise to all myeloid elements, including granulocytes, red cells, macrophages, megakaryocytes, and all lymphoid elements.[7] There are two current thoughts regarding control of lineage differentiation from the HSC[138]. The *extrinsic control hypothesis* is that a combination of stimuli such as cytokines, extracellular matrix, and others cause the HSC to differentiate along specific lines. In the *intrinsic control hypothesis*,

lineage differentiation is thought to be caused by transcription factors that direct cells toward a specific lineage by either enhancing expression of genes that are involved in that pathway or interfering with genes responsible for self-renewal while interfering with the transcription factors that influence development along other lines. It is not known whether either or both of these approaches are active, and it seems likely that both mechanisms may be involved.[4]

Assays for HSCs and other progenitors

Early studies involved mostly murine systems with detection of different kinds of in vivo colonies resulting from engraftment. Human HSCs can be studied using in vivo assays in NOD (non-obese diabetic) SCID (severe combined immunodeficiency) mice.[8] A number of genetic variants of this mouse model have been developed for different research purposes. For instance, the NOD SCID mouse model has enabled assessment of the proportion of CD34 cells that are HSCs in mobilized peripheral blood or umbilical cord blood (UBC).[9] However, studies in NOD SCID mice are difficult and expensive, and so in vitro culture methods have been developed. These in vitro assays facilitate a study of marrow and cellular subsets by incubation of cells under different conditions and with different growth factors or cytokines.[10] A few assays have been used to attempt to study the multipotent HSCs. The long-term culture initiating cell (LTC-IC) assay is the study of the cell with the capacity to produce hematopoietic cells for months, and the cobblestone area-forming cell (CAFC) assay allows study of multiple hematopoietic cell types. In both of these assays, however, HSCs make up only a fraction of the repopulating cells ultimately found in the marrow.[4] In vitro assays are available to detect myeloid (CFU-GM), megakaryocyte (CFU-Meg), and multipotent progenitor cells (CFU-GEMM) (Table 36.2).

Cell surface phenotype

As the HSC becomes lineage specific, the cell surface changes. Monoclonal antibodies against cell surface proteins have been used extensively to characterize HSCs and maturing forms of blood cells. There are nine antigenic proteins or glycoproteins identified on HSCs (Table 36.3). However, many or most of these proteins found on HSCs are also present on lineage-specific differentiating cells. Thus, it is not feasible to use these surface markers for positive selection and purification of HSCs. Conversely, these cell surface markers can be used for a *negative selection*, which is removal of cells containing markers on more lineage-specific mature blood cells. When cocktails of these antibodies are used, the non-lineage-committed cells are left and these negative-selecting antibodies produce cells termed "*Lin*-negative." More recently, the proposed phenotype of HSCs, the common myeloid progenitor, and the common lymphoid progenitor have been reported (Table 36.4).[4] It appears that the HSC is CD34+ and Thy1 (CD90)+, but negative for CD38− and for all of the other markers that define lineages for

Table 36.3 Protein and glycoproteins on hscs based on murine studies

CD34	Adhesion; cycle arrest
CD90 (Th1)	Adhesion to stroma
CD117 (c-kit receptor)	Cell survival and proliferation
AA4	C1q receptor homolog
Sca-1	Normal stem cell development
CD133	Maintains membrane
CD164	Blood cell homing
CD150	Lymphocyte proliferation receptor
CD110	Thrombopoietin receptors c-Mpl

Source: Kaushansky (2009).[4] Reproduced with permission of Wiley.

T cells, B cells, red cells, granulocytes, monocytes, platelets, and natural killer cells, thus referred to as *Lin−* (Table 36.4).[11,12]

Metabolism of stem cells

Fortunately, HSCs are highly resistant to damage by chemotherapeutic agents, probably because of effective intracellular pumping systems and the high content of aldehyde dehydrogenase to remove drug.[13,14] This process can also be used to identify HSCs because of their low-level retention of fluorescent markers. However, this strategy is not yet clinically effective for the isolation of HSCs. Only about 1% of HSCs enter the cell cycle each day. Stem cell engraftment occurs only with cells that are quiescent in the G_0–G_1 phase; however, this is due for adult HSCs but not for UBC HSCs.[4]

Gene expression

The primitive HSC must be able to undergo self-renewal, differentiation, or apoptosis, and therefore the gene expression profiles of HSCs must include the genes for all of these pathways. As differentiation occurs, the genes associated with that pathway are expressed or upregulated, but the genes for other pathways are not expressed.[15] Increasingly effective approaches to gene analysis have made it possible to find many genes expressed at different stages of hematopoietic development[16] and interestingly revealed that genes supporting self-renewal are shared by cells in different organs.[17] Identification of the proteins (transcription factors) that control the development and maturation of hematopoietic cells is a major area of investigation. There are a number of different transcription factors that determine the lineage and differentiation of HSCs.[4] The Hox group of transcription factors is important in the regulation of HSC self-renewal.[4] The Ikaros and PU1 genes are

Table 36.4 Cell surface markers

HSC	CD34+, CD38−
	Thy-1 (CD90)+
	Lin−
Lymph Precursors	
Common lymph precursor	IL7R+/LIN−/Thy−/Sca^{lo}/kit^{lo}
Bipotent progenitor	CD3+/Thy1+
B cell progenitors	CD3−/NK1.1^t
ProB cell	CD34+/CD10+/CD38+/CD19+/CD20+
PreB cell	CD34−/CD10+/CD38−/CD19/+/CD20+
Immature B cells	CD10+/CD19+/CD20+
Myeloid Precursors	
All lineages	IL7Ra/Lin−/cKit+/Sca1−/CD34+/FcRy^{lo}
	CFU-MIX, BFU-E, CFU-Meg, MEP, CFU-GM,
	CFU-G, CFU-M
	IL7Ra−/Lin−/cKit+/Sca-1−/CD34−/FCRy^{lo}

crucial in the differentiation of HSCs into a lymphoid lineage.[18] Myeloid lineage is controlled primarily by the stem cell leukemia (SLC) gene.[19] Interestingly, the gene acts in reverse, with downregulation of the transcription factor inhibiting myeloid development.

HSCs producing other kinds of cells: HSC plasticity

It has been reported that marrow hematopoietic cells could give rise to brain cells, brain stem cells could give rise to blood, fat cells could give rise to neurons and mesenchymal cells, muscle stem cells could give rise to hematopoietic cells, and various other combinations of tissue could be generated from various other tissues' stem cells.[20] This is referred to as *HSC plasticity*. These reports of cross stem cell differentiation have not been substantiated. The original reports appear to be due to lack "of purifying the populations to homogeneity, populations of cells of apparent phenotypic and functional heterogeneity, and did not mark cells retrovirally or with other genetic markers to follow the fate of clonogenic precursors."[7] Most of these studies have been performed using mixtures of cells in which it is not possible to determine whether there might be other kinds of multipotent progenitor cells in the cell mixture. None of these studies have been performed using single cells, which would be necessary to prove that HSCs have potency for other organs or tissues or have plasticity. Thus, although HSC plasticity is an exciting concept, it has not been substantiated.

Production of hematopoietic progenitors from HSCs

There have been many attempts to expand HSCs in vitro, but none of these has been successful. CD34+ cells can be expanded in vitro, but this marker is also present on a number of other kinds of cells. Considerable effort has been devoted to producing large numbers of myeloid progenitors that could be transfused shortly after stem cell transplantation as a bridge during the period of posttransfusion neutropenia.[21] This has not proven to be clinically practical and is not a strategy in use. However, a new system is being used for this purpose to shorten the time to engraftment of cord blood (discussed further in this chapter). Stimulation with thrombopoietin does generate cells with the megakaryocyte lineage, and considerable work has attempted to produce platelets for transfusion in vitro. The number of HSCs needed to "seed" the production system and the number of hematopoietic growth factors have not made large-scale in vitro platelet production practical. However, a recent report where the genes for thrombopoietin, IL6, and IL11 were used to create self-splicing fusion genes suggested that this could be a promising approach to generate platelets in vitro.[22] Similar attempts have been made to produce red cells in vitro that might be suitable for transfusion.[23] In many ways, this is even more difficult than platelet production because of the huge numbers of red cells needed. It is beyond the scope of this chapter to review all of the various cytokines and growth factors that have been used to attempt to stimulate continued self-renewal or development into a particular lineage to the extent suitable for clinical use.

Mobilization of HSCs

Observations that hematopoietic progenitors were found to increase in the circulation of patients following cytotoxic drug therapy led to the possibility of using that strategy to mobilize hematopoietic stem cells for transplantation.[24,25] Currently G-CSF, granulocyte macrophage colony-stimulating factor (GM-CSF), or circulating steel factor (SLF) alone or in combinations with IL2 and IL3 are used following chemotherapy regimens to mobilize HSCs for collection and transplantation[26–30] (see also Chapter 35). In normal donors, G-CSF is used for HSC mobilization because it has fewer side effects than GM-CSF. PBSC collection is performed 5–7 days after a single dose of G-CSF. It appears that mobilization is due to not only HSC proliferation but also movement of HSCs from intravascular sites such as liver and spleen into the blood circulation. It is possible that one contributing factor is matrix metalloproteinase, which is mobilized and cleaves the binding of HSCs to marrow stroma, thus releasing HSCs into the circulation. Other cytokines such as IL8, integrin alpha 1 and beta 1, c-kit, and several other adhesion and integrin molecules may play a role in either cell proliferation or release from marrow stroma, resulting in migration into the bloodstream.

Collection of HSCs for transplantation
Bone marrow
The bone marrow is the obvious site for collection of HSCs, and this was the mainstay for transplantation for many years. This is a surgical procedure obtaining marrow from the posterior iliac crest in the operating room, usually under general anesthesia. The volume of marrow collected is based on the dose of cells desired for transplant, which in turn is based on the size of the patient. The usual desired dose is $2–5 \times 10^9$/Kg. Because the decision about the volume of marrow to collect must be made during the collection, the decision is based on periodic samples of marrow total nucleated cell count because it is usually not practical to obtain CD34+ counts during the collection time. The volume of marrow collected varies from a few hundred milliliters for small patients to a liter or more for most adults. It is important to puncture multiple bone sites in order to maximize the amount of marrow and minimize the amount of blood collected in order to avoid anemia. If a large volume of marrow is anticipated, the donor can donate autologous blood for replacement.[31] Usually, this is not necessary.

Marrow donation is a low-risk procedure, but there is moderate discomfort for several days post donation,[32] and fatalities have occurred.[33,34] For these reasons, there was great attention to the risks of marrow donation during the establishment of the National Marrow Donor Program in which marrow for transplant is collected from donors unrelated to the patient.[32,35]

Peripheral blood
As it became apparent that chemotherapy resulted in a rebound of HSCs in the blood, techniques were developed to collect these and use them for autologous transplant because it was presumed that there would be few, if any, remaining malignant cells. Autologous transplantation of blood progenitor cells has been used successfully for several diseases. Although this strategy proved effective for autologous transplants, its use for allogeneic transplants was slow due to concerns that the number of T cells in the graft would cause graft-versus-host disease (GVHD), but that this could not be avoided by T depletion due to loss of progenitor cells. However, this has not proven to be the situation, and peripheral blood stem cells (PBSCs) are now used in allogeneic transplantation with results similar to those of bone marrow.[36,37]

In healthy donors, the number of circulating PBSCs is small, and thus several collection procedures would be necessary, making this an impractical way of collecting cells for transplantation. Because G-CSF stimulates release of PBSCs from the marrow, this can be given to donors to increase the PBSCs.[39,40] This yields about $4–5 \times 10^8$ CD34+ cells from one apheresis collection. Since the desired dose of CD34+ cells for transplant is $2.5–5 \times 10^6$ or about 2×10^8 for an average-sized adult, one or two collections provide a suitable dose for transplantation.

The chemokine receptor antagonist Plerixafor was initially studied as potential therapy for HIV because it blocks CXCR4, a chemokine receptor that acts as a co-receptor for certain strains of HIV. This proved ineffective, but it was noticed that the molecule caused release of progenitor cells from the marrow. Initially, plerixafor was used in patients undergoing autologous transplant who had a poor response and inadequate blood stem cell collections, but its use has broadened and it is often now used in combination with GCSF to enhance cell yields, especially in those who have a less optimal response to GCSF.[41]

PBSC collection
PBSCs can be collected using the Fresenius/Kabi Amicus or the Terumo Optia instruments. With the Amicus, there are several cycles of filling and emptying the separation and collection chambers using computer software designed for PBSC collection. The operator determines the number of cycles, cycle volume, flow rate, RBC offset, and interface set point to optimize the collection. The Optia has continuous-flow centrifugation and optical detection technology by performing real-time interface monitoring of the interface position and thickness of separated blood components, interprets interface information using unique optical detection software, and adjusts the pumps and valves to manage the interface position and efficiently remove targeted component.

It appears that there is no difference in the effectiveness of the two instruments in obtaining doses of PBSCs,[42] although the Optia removes PBSCs more efficiently and thus the collection is done in a shorter time.[43] However, the Amicus results in less platelet loss, thus potentially making it preferable for autologous collections because it is desirable to avoid thrombocytopenia in patients recovering from chemotherapy. The Optia has a lower extracorporeal volume, thus making it preferable for small donors.

Migration of HSCs
Because in transplantation the HSCs are infused intravenously, the factors that control migration of these cells to bone marrow or appropriate locations to support their continued renewal and proliferation to generate new cells are of great interest. HSCs migrate to hematopoietic sites in a directed nonrandom manner. For instance, if red cells are infused simultaneously, the HSCs disappear from the circulation almost immediately while red cells continue to circulate. HSC disappearance is similar to that of monocytes and other nucleated cells rapidly leaving the circulation, probably because they have homing receptors. Apparently, HSCs and progenitors reside in the tissue for up to about 36 hours before returning to the blood,[44] but it is not clear whether there is a subpopulation of cells that reenter the bloodstream versus those cells that remain deep in the marrow. During migration of HSCs into marrow, they must cross sinusoids lined with macrophages. However, HSCs are not phagocytized by the macrophages possibly due to an integrin-associated protein, CD47.[45] About 0.5% of marrow niches for HSCs appear to be available at any one moment," and "a large flux of recirculating HSCs likely provides for the continuous replacement of empty HSC niches."[7]

Biology of umbilical cord blood stem cells
The concept of placental and UBC transplantation grew out of interest in using what at the time was medical waste material.[46]

Initially, the interest was to generate new red cells, but this evolved into using the placental HSCs.

Early laboratory studies provided some initial support for the presence of hematopoietic progenitor/stem cells in human UCB,[47–49] with one study suggesting that UCB "might be used as a source of hematopoietic stem cells for the restoration of bone marrow function in humans."[34] Subsequent experiments further established that certain cells within UCB were capable of hematopoietic multilineage differentiation.[50,51] Milton and Norman Ende described the use of several UCB units as a source of HSCs in a "mini"-transplant setting for a 16-year-old boy with leukemia.[52]

When the results were encouraging, the work was extended to mouse studies that established that cord blood could repopulate murine hematopoiesis.[53,54] Actually when cord blood began to be collected, the numbers of cells indicated by progenitor assays were similar to the numbers in marrow successfully engrafted.[54]

A series of experiments led by Professor Harold Broxmeyer established that cord blood contained cells with hematopoietic progenitor capability.[53–55] Firstly, this was established using in vitro colony assays to compare progenitor activity of cord blood with bone marrow, which at the time was the main source of cells for transplantation. The number of nucleated premature cells is less in cord blood than marrow, but progenitor assays suggested that there were equal or more immature cells in cord blood than marrow.[53–55]

In early experience with transplantation, the progenitor content of cord blood was more closely indicative of graft outcome than marrow.[56] UCB has "extensive proliferation capacity. . . . Respond very rapidly to combinations of cytokines . . . have great capacity to engraft/repopulate the hematopoietic systems of mice."[57] There is slower engraftment of neutrophils and platelets from UBC than marrow or blood stem cells, which is thought to be due to the less mature stem cells in UBC.[57] Following more extensive and clinically practical studies that confirmed in vitro functionality post-cryopreservation and thaw,[55] the first related UCB transplant was performed in October 1988.[58] After receiving an HLA-matched sibling UCB unit for the treatment of Fanconi anemia, this patient continues to be healthy in complete hematologic and immunologic donor reconstitution over 20 years later.[59] Since this early success, the use of UCB for hematopoietic reconstitution has increased markedly in both related[60] and unrelated[61–64] settings. UCB is an acceptable alternative to HLA-matched bone marrow for pediatric patients[65,66] and for adults lacking an HLA-matched adult donor.[67,68]

Beyond containing HSCs with higher proliferative and self-renewal capacity,[57,69–71] UCB has additional advantages over bone marrow and PBSCs. Clinical trials have shown a decreased incidence of GVHD, particularly acute disease, despite the lower HLA-matching requirements of UCB.[67,68,72] In vitro and in vivo animal research suggests that these particular attributes of UCB transplantation are due to the naïve immune system of UCB.[73–75] Cord blood stem cell immaturity is indicated by studies of telomeric DNA and immature colony-forming cells.[53] Additionally, transplant candidates with rare HLA types are often successful in finding an acceptably matched unit; search time, in general, is markedly decreased compared to that of other HSC sources, as UCB units are banked and already HLA typed.[76]

Delayed platelet engraftment may be due to low numbers of megakaryocyte progenitors and also delayed megakaryocyte maturation.[57] The volume and number of stem cells in units of UCB for transplant are small, and thus efforts at ex vivo expansion of UCB have been attempted most unsuccessfully. However, current unpublished experience with the aryl hydrocarbon receptor

antagonist[77] has shown encouraging shortening of time to neutrophil engraftment.

UCB also contains endothelial progenitor cells and mesenchymal stem/stromal cells. There is considerable variation in the mesenchymal stem cell content, and some samples of UCB have none. The clinical significance of this variation is not known; however, UCB could become a source of these red cells in the future.

Transplantation of umbilical cord blood stem cells

Cord blood stem cells can establish hematopoiesis in the setting of allogeneic transplantation (see also Chapter 37). Cord blood from sibling donors was initially used for transplant. In a large review, related donor UCB was associated with a lower risk of GVHD, delayed engraftment, and similar survival when UCB and marrow were compared.[78] Early experience with unrelated donor transplants was promising.[79–82] In the largest summary[83] of 861 mostly children with hematologic malignancies who received UCB transplants from unrelated donors, engraftment was related to cell dose and HLA match, and GVHD was associated with HLA disparity. Other reports compared UCB with unrelated bone marrow transplants. Despite greater HLA disparity for UCB transplants, the probability for engraftment, GVHD, and survival were similar for UCB and marrow;[84–87] similar results were reported from Eurocord[75] and from a meta-analysis.[87] Aggregating the experience, UCB and marrow "have different risks and potential advantages, with similar overall survival."[57] The conclusion is that unrelated UCB is a satisfactory stem cell source for adults and children who do not have a matched donor.

Although experience with UCB transplantation is less than that with marrow or blood stem cells, it is estimated that about 30,000 transplants have been performed using UCB.[89] UCB is suitable for diverse populations due to the ability to obtain UCB from diverse donor sources. However, there are several disadvantages to the use of UCB: (1) relatively small numbers of cells, (2) limited numbers of UCB units available, and (3) variability in composition of the UCB unit, although this latter may not be important (discussed further in this chapter). This positive experience led to the National Heart, Lung, and Blood Institute (NHLBI)-funded multicenter Cord Blood Transplant (COBLT) study. This involved establishing several cord blood banks to generate UCB for transplant. The patients were older than two years and with hematologic malignancy. The COBLT results were very encouraging for both adults[90,91] and children.[82] The overall disease-free survival was 49.5% at two years, the incidence of relapse at two years was 19.9%; for Grade II-IV acute GVHD, the rate was 19.5%, and for chronic GVHD it was 20.8%. The CD34+ cell dose was the only one used in transplants for malignant and nonmalignant disease. The advantages of UCB are (1) ready availability, (2) less stringent HLA matching necessary compared with marrow or blood stem cells, (3) possibly reduced GVHD, and (4) potential in making transplantation more available (a characteristic associated with engraftment whether the cell count is on the pre-cryopreservation or postthaw unit).

The small number of cells in many cord blood units limits transplants in adults[76,92] because a minimum dose of 2.5×10^7 nucleated cells/kg is considered the minimum effective dose. Because this relatively low dose of CD34+ cells in UCB limits UCB use in adults, two closely HLA-matched units have been used as a way of increasing the dose. A protocol was developed using two cord blood units, and this approach appeared to be quite successful.[93]

For a more stringent determination, a clinical trial was carried out comparing one and two units of cord blood.[94] Patients were 1–21 years of age and had acute leukemia, chronic myeloid leukemia, or myelodysplastic syndrome. HLA matching for A, B, and DRB1 loci were 4/6, 5/6, and 6/6. One hundred thirteen patients received a single-unit and 111 patients a double unit transplant. The median age was 9.9 years for double-unit and 10.4 years for single-unit transplant patients. Single-unit transplants involved total nucleated cell content of 3.9×10^7, and CD34+ 1.9×10^5 for single-unit and 7.2 TNC and 3.7 CD34+ for double-unit transplants. The one-year overall survival was 65% in double-unit and 73% in single-unit transplants ($p = 0.17$). There were no significant differences in disease-free survival, hematopoietic recovery, or infections. GVHD was higher and platelet recovery longer in the double-unit transplant group. Although the double-unit transplant strategy was not superior, survival in both groups was better than in previous reports.[82] Surprisingly, a lower rate of disease-free survival was associated with better HLA match, and nonwhite race and AML were associated with two-unit transplants. Thus, double-unit cord blood transplants do not provide a survival advantage, and the future of this transplant strategy is not clear.

Umbilical cord blood banking

Background

Once considered biological waste, UCB has since become an important source of HSCs for transplantation. The first UCB bank, established by Professor Harold Broxmeyer, provided UCB for the historic 1988 UCB transplant[59] as well as the successive four HLA-matched sibling transplants.[95] As UCB gained initial acceptance as an HSC source in the related setting, the possibilities for unrelated units became apparent, supporting a rationale for the establishment of unrelated UCB banks. The first unrelated UCB bank was established by Dr. Pablo Rubinstein at the New York Blood Center, New York, New York, in 1992.[83] Banks in Dusseldorf and Milan were initiated shortly thereafter. Recent reports indicate there are greater than 450,000 unrelated units banked worldwide for potential clinical use with well over 30,000 unrelated UCB transplants performed to date.[97] Several private banks have been established worldwide for family use as well; it is uncertain how many units collected and stored by "private" banks have been stored and transplanted.

Use of cord blood as the cell source for hematopoietic cell transplant increased substantially but has been stable or decreasing recently. As any emerging technology, UCB banking has evolved over time to become a more established, standardized program and is now a US Food and Drug Administration (FDA)-licensed product. As part of this evolution, cord blood banking has progressed from the research laboratory through translational research into rather standardized practices. With this progression, considerable experience was obtained with the medical evaluation of the mother, collection procedures, processing procedures, testing for transmissible diseases, and quality control (QC). Current FDA licensing requirements are extensive and complex and are designed to assure the quality and safety of the final product. However, these requirements are extensive, and complex physical facilities are now used to process and store cord blood units. All of these activities and facilities determine the cost that cord blood banks must recover to maintain financial stability. This cost is high, may lead to constraints on the use of cord blood, and may affect its future.

There are public and private cord blood banks. Public banks are operated by nonprofit organizations, and the cord blood is available for transplant to any patient. Matching of donor unit and patient is performed similarly to that for bone marrow and blood stem cells primarily through the National Marrow Donor Program. A private bank collects the cord blood and stores if for a fee for potential future use only by the donor or family member. Those units are not available to the general public.

Recruitment

Recruitment typically begins with physician/midwife education and distribution of informational materials in obstetrics offices or to prenatal classes. Materials about UCB donation include information about the nature of the bank (whether public or private), the cost or lack of cost associated with donation, a list of participating hospitals, the medical uses of UCB, a brief description of UCB collection, the risks of UCB donation to the mother and baby, whether the unit will be available for use by the donating family, and the need for the mother's written permission to collect and store the cord blood for later use in transplant or research. Participating mothers must understand that their blood will be drawn and tested for diseases such as hepatitis and HIV to reduce transmission of disease through the transplantation of their baby's UCB.

Pregnant women may also be solicited for UCB donation by private banks. These banks provide written or video information that is specific to their bank, and the costs to collect and store the UCB.

Consent

Although UCB has historically been considered medical waste, consent must be obtained for its collection, processing, testing, storage, and medical use. Although the UCB actually belongs to the newborn, consent is obtained from the mother because of her availability and because testing of her blood for transmissible diseases is required. Although consent for collection must precede delivery, UCB banks use different approaches in obtaining consent for further processing, testing, and use. A UCB bank may choose to employ a single consent covering all activities. Presented in the prenatal period, a single consent process affords the mother adequate time to seek information and consider her options under low-stress circumstances. Other banks may use a phased consent process,[98] which permits collection and, if the resulting UCB unit meets criteria for banking, to later approach the mother for permission to screen, process, test, and store the unit. This latter approach facilitates collection from mothers who have not previously been introduced to UCB banking as it does not require discussion and comprehension of the full program during labor. Each bank should have a policy that considers the stage of labor and stress of the mother, the amount of pre-counseling that has occurred, and the amount of time available for an adequate discussion.[99] Final judgment regarding the woman's ability to give intralabor consent should rest with the obstetrical staff. Consent from the father is not necessary and does not add to the safety of the UCB.[100]

Donor evaluation

Donor screening and testing for relevant transmissible disease are required for all donors of cells or tissue. The health history is designed to identify exposure to infectious disease and a history of symptoms suggesting genetic disorders, to minimize the potential transmission through transplantation. The medical health history is obtained by interviewing the mother and reviewing her medical record. The father's medical history is not helpful.[100] If not secured prior to delivery, the history must be obtained no later than 48 hours after delivery.[101] The history may be self-administered with follow-up by bank staff, or it can be obtained through direct interview by bank staff or hospital staff who are adequately trained and capable of answering the mother's questions.

The approach of testing the mother should be more effective than testing the infant donor. It is the mother's circulation that nourishes the fetus during pregnancy, and thus her infectious exposures are relevant to determining suitability of the UCB. Maternal conditions at labor and delivery such as fever, prolonged time after rupture of the membranes, or use of antibiotics suggest possible bacterial contamination that could be transmitted through the UCB. However, studies to relate these factors to contaminated UCB have not been published, and they do not seem to be related to transplant complications.[102]

Medical screening includes family genetic history because the infant has not had an opportunity to manifest many inherited diseases. Although first-degree relatives with a history of malignancy or parents who have been treated with chemotherapy may be a concern, there is no evidence that these factors cause transfer of malignancy. UCB used to compensate for deficiencies in specific genetic disorders will be tested for presence of the targeted enzyme before transplant when testing is available.

It is not recommended that Infants be retested or re-examined at 6–12 months of age for the purpose of donor eligibility because of difficulty in locating some families, concern for parental and infant privacy, necessary recordkeeping for family tracing, and cost.

Although these donor-screening processes are extensive, it is possible that they may not add much to the safety or quality of the UCB. We have categorized the quality issues in all cord blood units shipped to the University of Minnesota during 2001–2003 and again in 2011–2013. About 65% of units had one or more quality issues, the most common being medical history or QC with a few issues in documentation and labeling.[102] Of these, only seven (3%) issues were thought to likely affect quality of the UCB. Fewer quality issues were considered likely to be a potential cause of adverse clinical outcomes than in the previous study. The category with the greatest number of deviations with likely potential to affect the quality of the units was *labeling and documentation* (four deviations, 1.6%). In addition, transmissible disease testing accounted for 11% of the issues. This includes units with incomplete or inaccurate documentation and units for which transmissible disease testing was either incomplete or not done according to manufacturers' directions. The number and type of issues were similar in those patients who engrafted and those without engraftment problems, suggesting that most of these quality issues are irrelevant clinically. It appears that considerable time, effort, and thus funds may be used to obtain a detailed medical history that contributes little or nothing to the safety or quality of the cord blood unit.

The cost of collecting, testing, processing, and storing umbilical cord blood is very high, and this may begin to limit cord blood use and constrain some banks, limiting the ability to continue to increase the national bank.

Cord blood collection

The methods of UCB collection are simple and similar to those of whole-blood collection. The collection bags are similar to those used for whole blood, and acid–citrate–dextrose (ACD) is used as the anticoagulant for UCB collection. After delivery, the umbilical cord is clamped, cut, and separated from the infant in a manner that does not interfere with routine delivery practice. UCB can be collected before (*in utero*) or after (*ex utero*) the placenta has been delivered. There are advantages and disadvantages to each method, but neither seems to be better overall.[103] As in whole-blood collection, the venipuncture needle is integral to the bag. After an appropriate umbilical vein is identified, the site is cleansed prior to venipuncture. While the UCB is being collected (a three to five-minute process), it should be gently mixed with the anticoagulant to prevent clotting. The umbilical cord will appear collapsed when the collection is complete. Placing the bag on a laboratory scale during collection allows the collector to monitor the volume and provides an additional means for determining when collection is complete.

Ex utero collection

With *ex utero* collections, the placenta is removed from the delivery suite and transported to a nearby room for the collection. Usually, the placenta is suspended in a device to allow collection of blood by gravity. The placenta and cord are more accessible in the *ex utero* setting, and therefore more manipulation, such as "milking" of the cord, could increase collection volume as long as caution is used to prevent maternal contamination and lysis of cells. Speed is important in this process because the blood begins to clot and the volume and number of cells obtained will be inadequate if the collection is not done quickly.

The cost of dedicated collection personnel may be substantial depending upon the size and organization of the institution. The lack of availability of collectors on all shifts may limit the opportunity for donation. However, because of the standardization with dedicated collectors, *ex utero* collections potentially include less clotting due to inadequate mixing, less bacterial contamination, and fewer labeling errors.[103]

In utero collection

In utero collections are performed by the obstetrician or nurse/midwife after the newborn has been delivered and assessed, and the umbilical cord has been clamped and cut. If the well-being of the newborn and/or mother is in question, the collection is not attempted. If the decision to collect is made, care must be taken to maintain a relatively clean field. Unless a sterile bag or extension set is used, the traditional supplies are not sterile, and inadvertent misplacement could contaminate the surgical field.

The primary advantage of *in utero* collections is the substantially lower cost of collection. As dedicated UCB bank collection personnel are not needed, the cost of collection is limited to collection and shipping supplies. Initial costs and efforts associated with education and training of the physician/midwife collectors must also be considered. However, once the obstetrics practice groups are trained, hands-on experience will improve the quality of collections; in-service and educational sessions can serve as a refresher course as well as a means to demonstrate appreciation of the clinicians' support. A program of continued competency, collection site visits, and regular communication can support quality collections. In addition to the economic advantages, several studies have suggested that higher volume, greater nucleated and CD34+ cell counts, as well as greater numbers of CFUs may be seen with units collected by *in utero* methods.[104,105] As data supporting both methods exist, it follows that UCB can be collected successfully using either an *in utero* or *ex utero* approach.[103]

Donor testing

The decision whether to process and bank a CBU is based on the total nucleated cell count (TNC). The threshold used for several years has been 9×10^9. However, African Americans normally have a lower TNC than Caucasians, and thus a lower proportion of African American CBU may be banked. Because HLA matches are more likely to be found within the patient's ethnic group, the use of Caucasian TNC values may not be ideal. This situation is not standardized among all CBU banks.

Laboratory testing for transmissible diseases is done on maternal blood because it is assumed that infectious disease present in the UCB would have originated from the mother and, thus, the best chance of detecting infectivity would be in a maternal blood sample. Because testing is done on maternal blood, it is necessary to obtain the mother's consent for testing as well as for collection of the UCB.

Screening for hemoglobinopathies is usually done at state health department laboratories. Some UCB banks store units that have sickle cell or alpha thalassemia trait because these units may have unique HLA types needed for transplantation of minority patients. UCB units selected for transplant for a patient with an inherited disease are tested for that specific disease before being used for transplantation.

Processing and storage

UCB processing laboratories use a variety of processing techniques for volume reduction and/or removal of red blood cells. Concern for infusion-related complications (associated with red cell incompatibility, free hemoglobin, and dimethyl sulfoxide [DMSO]) and limited storage capacity lead to processing methods designed to minimize red cell content and the size of the final UCB unit while limiting stem cell loss. Most methods involve centrifugation, sedimentation, and/or filtration for reducing the red cell content and/or plasma volume. Centrifugation for the removal of plasma is the simplest method in terms of cost and degree of manipulation, but does not remove any of the red blood cells. The most common means of reducing red cell content has been the use of sedimenting agents such as hydroxyethyl starch (HES), gelatin, poligeline, and dextran.[106,107] Density separation by layering UCB cells over Percoll or Ficoll Hypaque provides a mononuclear cell–enriched product essentially devoid of red cells.[108] More recently, leukocyte removal filters and semiautomated methods have demonstrated similar *in vitro* cell recoveries to the standard HES method.[106,109] Each of these methods has advantages and disadvantages in terms of cell recovery, red cell removal, processing time, and cost. Cell recovery (nucleated and CD34+), viability, clonogenic function (such as CFUs), and sterility testing (pre- and post-cryopreservation) are typical validation performance measures. Factors such as process time, cost, maximization of storage, and production efficiency (number of UCB units processed per staff per day) are also important.

One of the earliest methods for processing UCB was developed by Rubinstein;[110] modifications of this method are still commonly used today.[111] This process sufficiently reduces red cell content using HES and depletes the units of plasma and anticoagulant to minimize the final product and cryoprotectant volumes.

Long-term preservation

Freezing and storage methods must be robust enough to ensure that the quality of the UCB unit is maintained for many years. The most common means of cryopreservation for UCB, as for bone marrow and peripheral blood, consists of freezing the cells in a cryogenic bag with a cryoprotectant solution of 10% DMSO.[112–114] Slow cooling in a programmable controlled-rate freezing device at a rate of 1 °C/min will result in adequate recovery of CD34+ cells and human progenitor cells.[113,114] Both AABB and FACT (Foundation for the Accreditation of Cellular Therapy) have defined storage limits for cryopreserved UCB to be ≤ -150 °C.[101,115] Once frozen, UCB units are typically transferred to long-term storage into a monitored liquid nitrogen (LN_2) storage container, immersed in liquid at -196 °C. Some banks keep UCB in vapor phase to minimize the potential for cross-contamination. Retention of viabilities and/or proliferative function of UCB cells frozen in liquid phase of LN_2 remains acceptable for many years,[116] and transplantation of UCB stored for more than 10 years has been successful.[117]

To ensure the safety and stability of the stored UCB units, control measures should be established for product security and segregation, storage container monitoring, inventory control, and duration of storage. To ensure that temperature and LN_2 levels are continuously maintained, a monitoring system should be in place with local and remote alarm capabilities.

Quality control testing of cord blood

QC testing is done to assess the safety and potential clinical effectiveness of the UCB. Testing is usually performed prior to initial manipulation and before cryopreservation. Typical QC assays include nucleated cell count, hematocrit, ABO/Rh typing, CD34+ cell enumeration, CFU assay, viability, sterility, and human leukocyte antigen (HLA) for HLA class I and class II antigens, including HLA-A, B and DRB1 loci, with HLA-C and DQB typing recommended.

Shipment

Collection sites may be located some distance from the UCB processing laboratory, and thus short-term preservation and transportation are important. Fresh UCB units may be transported at room temperature or on ice. Although there is a 1% drop in viability for every four hours of transport time for UCB units shipped at ambient temperature,[118] a series of studies has shown that UCB can be preserved in CPD for up to 24 hours prior to processing and retain satisfactory cell recovery and progenitor content.[119–121] A more recent report suggests this could be up to 96 hours at room temperature.[122] Storage at either room temperature or 1–4 °C does not seem to make a large difference, but lower temperature may minimize growth of any contaminating bacteria.

Thawing and transfusion

There are three general approaches to thawing and transfusion: (1) bedside thaw, (2) thaw and dilute, and (3) thaw, dilute, and wash.

Bedside thaw: This is as the term implies and was the original method for preparing CBU for transplant. At least one report suggested that DMSO was toxic to HSCs after thawing.[123] Because stem cell preservation was not well understood, it was felt best to minimize the time between thaw and infusion. This bedside thaw is cumbersome, necessitates a water bath in or near the patient's room, and does not remove any supernatant or cryopreservatives. Reactions were not common due to the small amount of volume of the cord blood unit.[124,125] Cells preserved in DMSO are hypertonic and subject to injury on infusion, but this has not interfered with engraftment.[124,125]

Thaw, dilute, no wash: The *thaw, dilution* and *thaw, dilution, and wash* approaches were added to minimize infusion of the DMSO, PrepaCyte-CB, or dextran used in cryopreservation and cytokines, and to minimize cell debris. In this method, the cord blood unit is thawed in the laboratory and diluted with equal volumes of saline and dextran.[110] This has the advantage of minimizing manipulation of the cord blood unit, limiting cell loss and limiting preparation time.[124,125] This method provides satisfactory engraftment.[126]

Thaw, dilute, and wash: This method is similar to the thaw-and-dilute method in that saline and dextran are added, but then the thawed cord blood unit is centrifuged, the supernatant is removed, and the remaining cells are resuspended in saline and dextran.

In summary, both the dilute and dilute–wash methods use the same solution, but there is loss of some nucleated cells with washing. In our experience,[127] thawing and washing result in TNC loss approaching 20% when compared with pre-freeze counts. The wash step was responsible for nearly half of the cell loss. Postthaw viability decreased by 50–60%, and CFU-GM colonies decreased by 30–40%; however, CD 34+ cells did not decrease at all, and CD34+ viability decreased by only about 10%. Elapsed time post wash resulted in further loss of NCs but no detectable significant changes in CD34+ cell content and viability and/or CFU. These observations along with extensive clinical experience establish that CBU can be diluted with or without subsequent washing and used successfully for transplantation.[126]

Transfusion of UCB

The general approach to transfusing stem cell products applies to the UCB.[128] The general approach and potential adverse reactions are similar to those for other stem cell products.[129] Once a cord blood unit has been thawed and washed, it should be delivered to the patient care unit without delay. Following physician approval for infusion and proper identification procedures, the unit is infused by intravenous drip or syringe push directly into a central venous line without a needle or pump. Some institutions use a standard blood filter at the bedside. If a filter is used in the lab after thaw–wash, a second standard blood filter at the bedside is not needed.

The unit bag and IV tubing should be flushed with sterile saline after the UCB bag empties to maximize cell dose. Sterile saline also may be added directly to the UCB bag if the flow rate becomes unusually slow. As the final volume of an UCB unit is relatively low (roughly 60–100 mL with thaw–wash methods detailed above), infusion is typically completed within 15–30 minutes and preferably within 60 minutes of its receipt on the patient care unit.

The thawed UCB should be transfused as soon as possible. Timely infusion is most likely to become an issue with UCB that has not been washed or diluted because of the possible toxicity of the DMSO. Although Rowley and Anderson concluded that DMSO is not toxic to HSCs at clinically relevant concentrations (i.e., 5% and 10%) at either 4 °C or 37 °C for up to one hour of incubation, they also noted that addition of 1% DMSO to culture dishes suppressed CFU assays.[123] It is important to note that these studies[123] were performed on fresh cells. Studies of the effects of DMSO on HSCs that have been previously cryopreserved are limited. However, some investigators have noted similar suppression of colony formation when thawed UCB samples are not washed and are immediately placed into CFU culture.[130] Thus, the possible functional defect due to DMSO coupled with the occasional need to hold thawed UCB raises the concern for cell injury, particularly when cells are not washed or diluted.

Vital signs should be checked before infusion, immediately after infusion, and one hour after infusion at a minimum. Should an adverse reaction occur, monitoring would be based on the nature of the reaction. The transplant physician and the medical director of the cell therapy laboratory should be notified immediately of an unexpected or moderate to severe reaction. An investigation should be initiated and should include any appropriate laboratory testing (e.g., direct antiglobulin test, red cell antibody titers, Gram stain, or culture). It is important that the UCB bank be notified so that they can review their records and procedures.

Reactions associated with HSC infusion may be very similar to those occasionally seen with blood transfusion (i.e., allergic, hemolytic, febrile, and those due to microbial contamination). However, with combinations of the various processing methods for UCB (e.g., red cell depletion, plasma reduction, and postthaw wash step), some types of these reactions (i.e., those attributed to red cell antigens and plasma proteins) may be less likely to occur. Likewise, if red cell depletion and wash steps are included, the risk of renal failure due to infusion of red cells and free hemoglobin would not be expected as often as with other HSC sources containing red cells. Reactions (e.g., nausea, vomiting, cough, and headache) often attributed to DMSO would be expected to be less common with UCB as well[131,132] because of its smaller volume compared to bone marrow. Bacterial contamination, which occurs with up to 5% of collections,[133] is usually not an issue with banked UCB units, as banks would not routinely include these units in the usable inventory.

UCB infusions are generally very well tolerated; if reactions occur, they are typically mild and readily managed by the healthcare team.[129] However, because the possibility for a severe reaction does exist, this may be minimized by aggressive IV hydration (e.g., 2–6 hours before and six hours after infusion, with diuretics as needed). The general use of prophylactic antiemetics, antipyretics, and antihistamines is recommended as well.

Regulation

The AABB has applied their standard-setting and accreditation expertise to UCB collection, testing, processing, and storage.[134] FACT/NET CORD is a freestanding, nonprofit peer organization established for the specific purpose of establishing standards and accrediting cord blood banks and cellular processing facilities.[135] The activities of both organizations have been very successful and have brought high quality into the UCB activities.

The FDA published guidelines for UCB several years, and it has now determined that UCB banks must be licensed and that all units collected after 2016 must be licensed. Thus, UCB is becoming a standard blood stem cell product. The AABB and NET-CORD will continue to provide valuable standards, education, and accreditation.

Key references

A full reference list for this chapter is available at: http://www.wiley.com/go/simon/transfusion

4 Kaushansky K. Hematopoietic stem cells, progenitors, and cytokines. In: Appelbaum FR, Forman SJ, Negrin RS, Blume KG, Eds. *Thomas' hematopoietic cell transplantation.* 4th ed. Oxford: Wiley-Blackwell; 2009:231–49.

6 Morrison SJ, Prowse KR, Ho P, *et al.* Telomerase activity in hematopoietic cells is associated with self-renewal potential. *Immunity* 1996;5:207–16.

7 Prohaska S, Weissman I. Biology of hematopoietic stem and progenitor cells. In: Appelbaum FR, Forman SJ, Negrin RS, Blume KG, Eds. *Thomas' hematopoietic cell transplantation.* 4th ed. Oxford: Wiley-Blackwell; 2009:36–63.

9   Tanavde VM, Malehorn MT, Lumkul R, *et al.* Human stem-progenitor cells from neonatal cord blood have greater hematopoietic expansion capacity than those from mobilized adult blood. *Exp Hematol* 2002;**30**:816–23.

16 Phillips RL, Ernst RE, Brunk B, *et al.* The genetic program of hematopoietic stem cells. *Science* 2000;**288**:1635–40.

55 Broxmeyer HE, Douglas GW, Hangoc G, *et al.* Human umbilical cord blood as a potential source of transplantable hematopoietic stem/progenitor cells. *Proc Natl Acad Sci USA* 1989;**86**:3828–32.

89 Ballen KK, Gluckman E, Broxmeyer HE. Umbilical cord blood transplantation: the first 25 years and beyond. *Blood* 2013;**122**:491–8.

110 Rubinstein P, Dobrila L, Rosenfield RE, *et al.* Processing and cryopreservation of placental/umbilical cord blood for unrelated bone marrow reconstitution. *Proc Natl Acad Sci USA* 1995;**92**:10119–22.

136 Eaves CJ. Hematopoietic stem cells: concepts, definitions, and the new reality. *Blood* 2015;**125**(17):2605–2613.

137 Boulais PE, Frenette PS. Making sense of hematopoietic stem cell niches. *Blood* 2015;**125**(17):681–2629.

138 Gottgens B. Regulatory network control of blood stem cells. *Blood* 2015; **125**(17):2614–2620.

CHAPTER 37

Hematopoietic stem cell transplantation

Sameh Gaballa,[1] Amin Alousi,[2] Sergio Giralt,[3] & Richard Champlin[2]

[1]Division of Hematological Malignancies and Bone Marrow Transplantation, Thomas Jefferson University, Philadelphia, PA, USA
[2]Department of Stem Cell Transplantation and Cellular Therapy, The University of Texas MD Anderson Cancer Center, Houston, TX, USA
[3]Weill Cornell Medical College Chief, Adult BMT Service, Memorial Sloan Kettering Cancer Center, New York, NY, USA

In 1957, Thomas and colleagues published the first attempts at bone marrow transplantation as treatment for advanced malignancies after receiving supra lethal doses of chemo- or radiotherapy.[1] For the next decade, this therapy was limited to patients with terminal leukemia or severe marrow failure resulting from radiation exposure or disease. Success was rare with almost all of these early patients dying from complications of toxicity of high-dose therapy, graft failure, graft-versus-host disease (GVHD), infections, or relapse of their primary disease. These early studies established the principles that allowed hematopoietic transplantation to develop as an effective treatment modality for a broad range of hematologic, immune, metabolic, and malignant diseases.[2,3] In 2013, the Worldwide Network for Blood and Marrow Transplantation announced that the world's 1 millionth blood stem cell transplant was performed. This chapter provides a brief overview of hematopoietic stem cell transplantation (HSCT), including the types of transplants, key procedural elements, donor sources, disease indications, and potential complications.

There are three major forms of HSCT performed clinically: (1) autologous transplantation, in which a patient serves as a self-donor; (2) syngeneic transplantation, where the donor is a genetically identical twin; and (3) allogeneic transplantation from another person. Most hematopoietic transplants are performed as treatment for malignancies. Marrow transplantation was initially conceived as a means for providing hematopoietic recovery following the administration of dose-intensive myeloablative chemo- and radiotherapy. For autologous and syngeneic transplants, the therapeutic role remains regeneration of hematopoiesis following high-dose therapies. In allogeneic transplants, the infused cells also produce an additional donor immune-mediated response against the host malignancy, a phenomenon referred to as *graft-versus-tumor* (GVT) effect. Numerous lines of evidence support the therapeutic potential in the GVT effect mediated by the donor lymphocytes,[4–11] including:

- Relapse is lower in allogeneic transplants when compared to autologous or syngeneic transplants.
- T-lymphocyte-depleted transplants have a higher incidence of relapse in many malignancies when compared to T-lymphocyte-replete transplants.
- Patients with GVHD have a lower risk of malignancy relapse.
- There is a delayed clearance of minimal residual disease following allogeneic transplantation beyond the timeframe in which it could be attributed to cytotoxic therapy administered with the conditioning regimen.

- Induction of remission occurs following withdrawal of immunosuppression after transplantation in a minority of cases.
- Induction of remission occurs following infusion of donor lymphocytes.

Although a GVT benefit does not occur with autologous transplants, these grafts are associated with less risk because the infused cells will not be immunologically rejected or mediate GVHD. In comparison, allogeneic transplants have a greater risk of complications because of the potential for graft rejection, GVHD, and more delayed immune reconstitution.

Autologous hematopoietic stem cell transplantation

Autologous transplantation is a strategy in which high-dose chemotherapy is administered to patients with a malignancy known to be dose-responsive. In order to receive an autologous HSCT, the patient must first undergo collection of hematopoietic stem cells (HSCs) from the bone marrow or peripheral blood, followed by cryopreservation and storage. Once marrow or peripheral blood progenitor cells (PBPCs) are successfully collected, the patient can receive intensive myeloablative chemotherapy and/or radiotherapy, followed by reinfusion of the previously cryopreserved autologous HSCs to restore hematopoiesis. This procedure is relatively safe with a low risk of treatment-related mortality. There is no specific age cutoff for undergoing autologous HSCT, and patients well into their seventh and eighth decades of life safely undergo the therapy.[12] Specific disease indications and complications are discussed later in the chapter.

Progenitor cell collection

The resting marrow contains both HSCs and hematopoietic progenitor cells (HPCs). HSCs are defined as clonal precursor cells that are capable of self-renewal as well as giving rise to differentiated progeny restoring hematopoiesis and immunity. HPCs lack the ability for self-renewal but have the ability to differentiate and proliferate.[13] This chapter collectively refers to these cells as HPCs, which can be identified by the cell expression of CD34 and Thy-1 and the absence of Lin and CD38 cell markers.[14,15]

Selection of stem cell source

Historically, HSCs capable of reconstituting hematopoiesis were collected through harvesting the marrow via multiple aspirations.

Rossi's Principles of Transfusion Medicine, Fifth Edition. Edited by Toby L. Simon, Jeffrey McCullough, Edward L. Snyder, Bjarte G. Solheim, and Ronald G. Strauss.

More commonly today, HSCs are collected from the peripheral blood by leukapheresis, termed *peripheral blood progenitor cells* (PBPCs). Few HSCs are present in the peripheral blood. The levels of circulating hematopoietic stem and progenitor cells increase after treatment with hematopoietic growth factors such as granulocyte colony-stimulating factor (G-CSF), a process termed *stem cell mobilization*. HSCs are also mobilized during recovery after cytoreductive chemotherapy (chemomobilization).[16] More recently, a CXC chemokine receptor 4 (CXCR4) antagonist (Plerixafor) has been shown to synergistically mobilize CD34-positive cells into the peripheral blood. Plerixafor is commonly used in combination with G-CSF to increase the yield of CD34 stem cells collected from the peripheral blood. This approach with hematopoietic growth factors is used for collecting HPCs both for autologous transplantation and also from normal donors for allogeneic transplantation. HPCs naturally increase during the recovery from many kinds of chemotherapy, and chemomobilization is often performed to collect PBPCs for autologous HSCT. Chemomobilization strategies generally result in a higher yield of HPCs when compared to use of hematopoietic growth factors alone.[17,18]

PBPC transplants have now largely replaced marrow for autologous transplantation because of the ease and safety of collection (sparing the need for general anesthesia) of the procedure. In addition, PBPC transplantation results in quicker recovery of granulocytes and platelets compared to marrow transplantation.[19] The tempo of hematologic recovery depends on the cell dose of CD34-positive cells infused.[20] Most centers require at least 2×10^6 CD34+ cells/kg body weight, and optimal recovery occurs with infusion of $\geq 5 \times 10^6$ CD34+ cells/kg.

Cryopreservation

After their collection, HSCs can be cryopreserved. The cells can safely be stored for extended periods of time and thawed immediately prior to infusing the patient. To avoid damage to the cells, a cryoprotective agent is needed such as dimethyl sulfoxide (DMSO). Adverse reactions from infusion of the cryopreserved stem cells are usually mild infusion reactions such as hypotension, skin flushing, dyspnea, abdominal cramping, nausea, or diarrhea, and are triggered by histamine release by DMSO. Thus, patients should be adequately pre-medicated with antihistaminic medications prior to the infusion. If a large volume of stem cells will be infused, then the infusion can be separated into two days to avoid the complications of infusion of excessive amounts of DMSO. Rarely, some patients can be allergic to DMSO and develop anaphylactic reactions during the administration of the thawed cells.[21]

Preparative regimens for autologous HSCT

The combination of chemo-, radio-, and biologic therapies given prior to HSCT is referred to as the *preparative* (or *conditioning*) *regimen*. The sole role of the preparative regimen in the autologous transplant setting is eradication of any residual cancer. High-dose therapy is employed to overcome tumor resistance. The doses of total body radiation and many chemotherapy drugs are limited by myelosuppression, and their dose can be markedly increased if followed by HSCT to restore hematopoiesis. Combination regimens are generally based on the principles of minimizing overlapping toxicity and mechanisms of resistance. Dose escalation achievable with the combination regimens is usually less than with each drug alone. Candidate drugs for incorporation into preparative regimens are those agents with a steep dose–response curve and myelosuppression as their dose-limiting toxicity. Dose escalation is not feasible when extramedullary toxicity occurs at the same or lower dose levels as myelosuppression. For this reason, alkylating agents such as busulfan, melphalan, or nitrosoureas are commonly employed. Conversely, Adriamycin (doxorubicin) is seldom used because the mucositis and cardiac toxicity associated with dose escalation of this drug cannot be overcome by the use of HPCs.

Prior to HSCT, patients must undergo a detailed evaluation to assess any organ dysfunction that might preclude administration of high-dose chemotherapy. This includes adequate pulmonary, cardiac, liver, and renal functions to avoid organ toxicity from high-dose chemotherapy.

The chemotherapeutic drugs used in the preparative regimen should be effective in treating the underlying malignancy and demonstrate improved efficacy at higher doses. For example, melphalan is effective in treating multiple myeloma at standard doses and is therefore used in much higher doses when used as a preparative regimen. Nonmyelosuppressive agents may be incorporated if they provide synergistic cytotoxicity. For example, preparative regimens for CD20-positive B-cell lymphomas commonly incorporate rituximab due to its synergism with alkylating agent-based chemotherapy.[22,23]

Allogeneic hematopoietic transplantation

Historically, most allografts used marrow cells obtained from a human leukocyte antigen (HLA)-matched sibling. Given that average family size continues to shrink in the Western world, only about 20% of patients have a matched sibling donor.[24] Alternative donor sources include volunteer unrelated donors, mismatched family members, and cord blood.

Compatibility for HLA is the strongest predictor for the occurrence of graft rejection and severe GVHD.[25,26] HLA is the human major histocompatibility complex (MHC); it is located at p21.3 on the short arm of chromosome 6. These genes have been subdivided into class I loci, which include HLA-A, -B, and -C, and class II loci, which include HLA-DR, DQ, and -DP. Matching at HLA-A, B, C, and DRB1 has been confirmed to have a major impact on outcomes of related and unrelated donor transplants.[25,26] In its strictest sense, HLA identity means that the donor and recipient are genetically matched for all HLA loci. HLA genotypically identical siblings inherit the same MHC haplotypes and, therefore, are also identical for other non-HLA genes and polymorphisms encoded on chromosome 6. In HLA-matched transplants, GVHD is felt to result from mismatching of poorly defined minor histocompatibility antigens. The only easily identified minor histocompatibility antigen is the HY antigen.[27,28] The chance of mismatching for these minor antigens should increase with increasing distance in the relationship between donor and recipient.[29] Unrelated donors are phenotypically matched to patients for class I and II alleles, but are expected to be less likely than relatives to match for non-HLA (minor) histocompatibility antigens; HLA-matched unrelated donor transplants do have a somewhat higher risk of acute GVHD than matched sibling transplants.

Historically, HLA typing was performed by serologic typing using selected HLA-specific antisera to identify HLA antigens.[30] This has been replaced by molecular typing methodologies, including sequencing of the HLA loci. Sequence-based HLA typing is the most precise technique available.[31] High-resolution molecular methods accurately define HLA alleles. Allele-level HLA matching has had a profound impact, reducing the risks of rejection, GVHD, and transplant-related mortality with unrelated allogeneic transplantation.[32–34] In most recent studies, results of HLA-matched unrelated donor transplants have similar survival rates as transplants from matched sibling donors, although the risk of acute GVHD remains somewhat higher.[35]

Donor selection

Efforts to identify a donor should be carried out as soon as a patient is considered as a possible candidate for HSCT. All potential sibling donors should get typed first, and if no compatible donors are identified, an unrelated donor search should be performed. Registries containing HLA-typed potential adult donors were created to facilitate this process. The first large registry was the Anthony Nolan Trust in the United Kingdom, and the largest of these registries is the National Marrow Donor Program (NMDP) in the United States. A well-matched donor is identical for HLA-A, B, C, and DRB1 loci. There are approximately 24 million individuals registered in unrelated donor registries worldwide. The frequency of unrelated donor transplant is becoming more common, and allogeneic transplants from unrelated donors surpassed the number of allogeneic transplants from related donors after 2006; the gap between these two types of approaches continues to widen annually (Figure 37.1).[36] Due to linkage disequilibrium, there is a different frequency of HLA haplotypes in each racial and ethnic group; patients are most likely to match an unrelated donor from the same ethnic origin. Because most registries are in Europe or North America, over half of Caucasians of European descent can find an unrelated donor match, whereas less than 30% of other racial groups will have an HLA-matched unrelated donor.[37]

Donor source

Allogeneic HSCT initially used bone marrow as the stem cell source. Since the early 1990s, the use of PBPCs has become increasingly common and now constitutes the most common HPC source. Use of PBPCs has shortened the duration of absolute neutropenia and thrombocytopenia compared to bone marrow by approximately 4–8 days.[38] Donor T cells are found in much higher concentration in PBPC grafts and help to facilitate engraftment, especially after less dose-intense preparative regimens. The presence of higher numbers of T cells initially raised the concern for greater frequency and severity of GVHD; however, most studies have shown that the risk of severe acute GVHD using PBPC grafts is not substantially greater than with marrow grafts.[39] Recently however, a recent phase III trial

and a meta-analysis found a higher incidence of chronic GVHD and no improvement in survival using PBPC versus marrow grafts.[19,38] Based on these data, many investigators recommend using bone marrow rather than PBPCs for unrelated donor allogeneic HSCT.

Alternative donor sources

Only a fraction of patients will have a fully matched unrelated donor identified despite the growing number of typed volunteers on worldwide registries. Alternative donor sources of hematopoietic cells for transplantation include umbilical cord blood (UCB) transplants and haploidentical related donors.

Umbilical cord blood source

UCB is a rich source of hematopoietic stem cells. Sufficient cells can be collected from the placenta after childbirth to perform hematopoietic transplantation. A worldwide system of cord blood banks has been established to collect and cryopreserve cord blood units and provide them for transplantation. Over 100,000 cord blood units are now available. Cord blood lymphocytes are immunologically immature and less likely to induce GVHD than cells from adult donors. UCB transplants have increased the available donor pool because less stringent HLA compatibility is required between the donor and recipient. Although unrelated adult donors are matched using high-resolution HLA typing at HLA-A, -B, -C and –DRB1, cord blood units are selected using lower resolution HLA typing (antigen level) for at least four of the six HLA-A, -B, and DR loci.[40] In addition, UCB has shortened the time it takes to secure a donor, because the cells are readily available and do not require delays in the collection process. In one study, the median time from search to clearance of an unrelated donor was 49 days; securing UCB units took just 13.5 days.[37,41] This is particularly important when a stem cell transplant is urgently needed. Retrospective studies in adults have confirmed a low rate of acute GVHD when comparing one-antigen and two-antigen mismatch UCB transplants to one-antigen mismatch unrelated marrow recipients, but most have demonstrated inferior outcomes when compared with matched unrelated donor recipients. In one of the largest registry trials, chronic GVHD in the cord blood group was lower (HR, 0.38; $p = 0.001$) and transplant-related mortality (TRM) was similar between cord blood and HLA-mismatched peripheral blood or bone marrow grafts, but TRM was higher in cord blood compared to fully matched grafts.[42]

Transplant Recipints in the United States, by Transplant and Donor Type

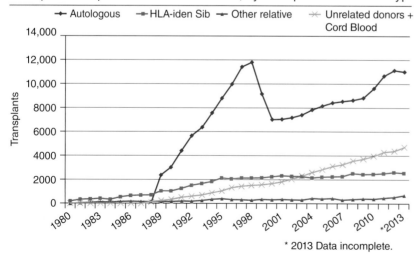

Figure 37.1 The number of autologous transplants in the United States has steadily increased since 2000, mainly for treatment of plasma cell and lymphoproliferative disorders. Allogeneic transplants from unrelated donors surpassed the number of allogeneic transplants from related donors after 2006. Source: Pasquini MC, Wang Z. Current use and outcome of hematopoietic stem cell transplantation: CIBMTR Summary Slides, 2013. http://www.cibmtr.org. Reproduced with permission of the CIBMTR.

* 2013 Data incomplete.

Another retrospective study in patients with high-risk ALL found similar overall survival, TRM, and relapse risk in cord blood compared to 7–8/8 HLA-matched peripheral blood or bone marrow sources.[43] Many recent studies report similar outcomes of cord blood transplants with 8 of 8 matched unrelated donor transplants.[44] Improved survival in cord blood transplants occurs with higher cell doses and better HLA matching.[45]

One of the limitations of cord blood transplantation is slow engraftment, high graft rejection rates, and delayed immune reconstitution leading to high infectious complications and non-relapse mortality.[42,44,46,47] The stem cell dose in cord blood grafts is usually small for adult patients leading to delayed engraftment and high graft rejection rates. One way to avoid this is using two cord blood units for adult patients. A recent analysis showed comparable clinical outcomes when using a double cord blood unit or an adequately dosed single cord blood unit as the stem cell source.[48] Ultimately, one donor cord blood source will dominate in the vast majority of patients. The factors leading to which cord blood unit dominates are not well understood at the present time.[49,50]

One major challenge for cord blood transplant is slow immune recovery. This predisposes patients to infectious complications early after transplant and high nonrelapse mortality. Whereas B-cell recovery starts 3–4 months after cord blood transplantation, T cell recovery is substantially prolonged and can remain low for six months, reaching near normal values after one year.[51] Moreover, T cells can remain dysfunctional, and some patients fail to recovery adequate thymic function in contrast to other allogeneic stem cell recipients.[52] This leads to high susceptibility to viral, bacterial, and fungal infections with a high rate of infection-related deaths.[50,53] Nonetheless, UCB transplants are a feasible option for adults who do not have a related or unrelated matched donor, and strategies for improving engraftment are an active area of research.

Haploidentical transplants
Haploidentical transplants offer another option when a matched sibling or unrelated donor cannot be identified. The advantage of these transplants is that parents, children, or half-matched siblings can serve as a donor and are thus rapidly available with a very short wait time. Major advances have been made during the last decade in the field of haploidentical transplantation. Historically, haploidentical transplants using unmanipulated grafts were associated with unacceptably high GVHD rates and poor outcomes.[54–56] Initial approaches to avoid severe GVHD involved removal of T cells (T-cell depletion), and indeed with this approach GVHD rates were controlled. However, this came at the expense of slow cell-mediated immune recovery, thus leading to high nonrelapse mortality from infectious complications, particularly in adult recipients.[57–59] The rates of graft rejection were also high with T-cell depletion given the susceptibility of the incoming CD34+ stem cells that are targeted by remaining recipient T cells that survived the conditioning regimen.[60] Subsequently, the Perugia group demonstrated that the rates of graft rejection can be lowered with using a higher dose of CD34+ stem cells or a "mega CD34+ stem cell dose," typically >10^7 CD34+ cells per kilogram of recipient body weight, but immune recovery remained slow given the lack of T cells in the graft.[61,62] Novel approaches, including selective depletion of alpha and beta T cells (which retains other lymphoid populations) and infusion of T-regulatory cells, have improved results in preliminary studies.[63]

Recently, investigators at Johns Hopkins University introduced the concept of *post-transplant* cyclophosphamide using a T-cell *replete* graft.[64] Following the transplant, the donor alloreactive T-cells proliferate, whereas non-alloreactive cells remain quiescent. The cyclophosphamide is given on days 3 and 4 post transplant, selectively eliminating the alloreactive cells and leaving behind non-alloreactive T cells to contribute to immune reconstitution. Hematopoietic stem cells and T-regulatory cells are retained because they are resistant to cyclophosphamide given their high content of aldehyde dehydrogenase.[65,66] This approach leads to rapid immune recovery with low incidence of GVHD and infectious complications. Several retrospective studies have shown that clinical outcomes using haploidentical donors are now similar to those of matched unrelated donors.[67] The field of haploidentical transplantation continues to rapidly grow, and several ongoing trials are currently investigating different conditioning regimens and other measures to further reduce GVHD incidence. Controlled trials are needed to compare alternative sources of hematopoietic cells for transplantation in patients who lack a matched sibling donor.

Preparative regimens for allogeneic HSCT
In allogeneic transplantation, the preparative regimen serves two main purposes: eradicating the underlying malignancy and inducing a state of immune tolerance to allow for the donor cells to engraft and expand. Generally speaking, efforts to decrease relapse through intensification of the preparative regimen have come at the expense of increased treatment-related mortality. As in autologous transplantation, there is no one standard preparative regimen in the setting of allogeneic transplantation. Allogeneic transplant conditioning regimens can generally be divided into chemotherapy-based protocols or total body irradiation (TBI)-based protocols.

TBI provides both immunosuppressive and myeloablative effects. The use of fractionated regimens and organ shielding has lowered the toxicity.[68–71] Most modern regimens deliver a total dose of 1000 cGy to 1500 cGy using a variety of fractionation schedules. Although there is some evidence that further escalation of the total dose of TBI is more effective at preventing relapse, these benefits have been offset by increased nonrelapse mortality.[72,73] TBI is most often combined with high-dose cyclophosphamide (Cy), a potent immunosuppressive agent. Other chemotherapy regimens with demonstrated efficacy in conjunction with TBI include etoposide either alone or together with Cy. TBI-based regimens are still commonly used in all disease states; however, it remains the most favored transplant regimen for patients with acute lymphoid leukemia.[74,75] Although efficacious, TBI is associated with a number of short- and long-term complications, including secondary malignancies, cataracts, and endocrine dysfunction.

The creation of non-TBI-containing regimens was developed with a goal to decrease toxicity. The most extensively studied regimen involved busulfan (Bu) and cyclophosphamide[76] and was later modified by Tutschka.[77] This regimen remains in wide use today for various malignancies in both allogeneic and autologous transplantation. Recently, two recent large registry studies from Europe and the United States showed either similar outcomes or better outcomes using intravenous (IV) busulfan versus TBI.[78,79] Recent modifications to the BuCy2 regimen with pharmacokinetic (PK)-guided dosing of Bu and/or an IV formulation probably eliminate any small advantage in the TBI-Cy regimen that has thus far been inconsistently demonstrated.

The dose-limiting side effect of oral Bu is hepatotoxicity with veno-occlusive disease (VOD) of the liver. The introduction of an intravenous formulation of busulfan avoids the problem of erratic absorption of the oral drug, and has improved the safety and effectiveness of busulfan-containing preparative regimens. IV Bu bypasses the haptic first-pass metabolism, making it less hepatotoxic.

Additional modifications to the BuCy regimen have stemmed from reports determining that Cy and its metabolites contribute not only to the development of hemorrhagic cystitis after transplantation but also to the liver toxicity of the preparative regimen.[80] Fludarabine has replaced Cy in many regimens. The combination of fludarabine and Bu has produced high rates of engraftment with low nonrelapse mortality.[81–83] Although in one randomized study, Bu-Cy was found to be superior to busulfan fludarabine,[84] in this study the Bu-Flu group had poorer results than generally achieved. A large retrospective review showed similar results of Bu-Flu and Bu-Cy.[85]

Reduced-intensity conditioning regimens

Traditionally, allogeneic transplantation has been limited to younger patients because of toxicity related to the intensive myeloablative conditioning regimens. Unfortunately, hematologic malignancies are most common in older adults. Nonmyeloablative and reduced intensity regimens were developed as less toxic alternative conditioning regimens for older or medically infirm patients who could not tolerate myeloablative regimens. The goal of reduced-intensity conditioning regimens is to employ lower doses of chemo- or radiotherapy to allow for engraftment and rely on the GVT effect to prevent relapse. There is no one standard reduced-intensity regimen, with commonly used regimens differing in the degree of intensity administered. Some regimens employ the same agents used in full-intensity regimens, but at reduced doses. On the other end of the spectrum are nonmyeloablative regimens that are immunosuppressive to allow engraftment and GVT, but provide minimal direct cytoreduction of the malignancy.[86] Agreed-upon definitions of reduced-intensity regimens as well as commonly used agents are listed in Table 37.1 [87] and Table 37.2.[88] Reduced-intensity and nonmyeloablative transplants have produced similar disease-free survival as myeloablative regimens; a higher rate of relapse is offset by less treatment-related

Table 37.1 Examples of reduced-intensity conditioning regimens

1. Total body irradiation at doses ≤500 cGy
2. Total busulfan dose ≤9 mg/kg
3. Total melphalan dose ≤40 mg/m^2
4. Regimen includes a purine analog—fludarabine, cladribine, or pentostatin

Table 37.2 Most commonly used reduced-intensity conditioning regimens

1. Low-dose total body irradiation (200 cGy) ± fludarabine
2. Busulfan + fludarabine ± others
3. Fludarabine + cyclophosphamide ± others
4. Fludarabine + melphalan ± others
5. Fludarabine + others

mortality.[89] Reduced-intensity regimens are most effective in diseases that are highly sensitive to GVT effects, particularly indolent lymphoid malignancies.[90] A recent randomized study by the Blood and Marrow Transplant Clinical Trials Network comparing myeloablative versus reduced-intensity conditioning in adults with AML was stopped early due to better results in the myeloablative arm; no further information is currently available.

Indications for hematopoietic transplants

The current disease indications for autologous and allogeneic transplants are summarized in Figure 37.2 based on data reported to the Center for International Blood and Marrow Transplant Research (CIBMTR). Multiple myeloma and lymphomas are the most common indications for autologous stem cell transplants. Leukemia and myeloid malignancies are the most common indications for allogeneic transplants; acute myelogenous leukemia (AML), acute lymphoid leukemia (ALL), myelodysplastic syndromes

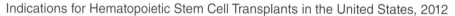

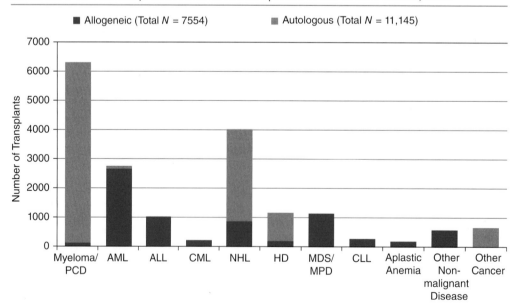

Indications for Hematopoietic Stem Cell Transplants in the United States, 2012

Figure 37.2 The most common indications for HSCT in the United States in 2011 were multiple myeloma/plasma cell dyscrasias (PCD) and lymphoma, accounting for 58% of all HSCTs. Multiple myeloma continues to be the most common indication for autologous transplantation, and acute myeloid leukemia for allogeneic transplantation. Source: Pasquini MC, Wang Z. Current use and outcome of hematopoietic stem cell transplantation: CIBMTR Summary Slides, 2013. http://www.cibmtr.org. Reproduced with permission of the CIBMTR.

Trends in Transplants by Transplant Type and Recipient Age*

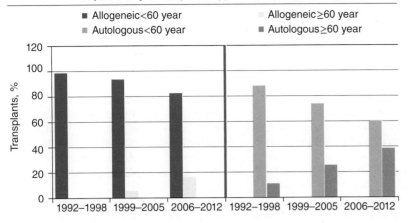

* Transplants for AML, ALL, NHL, Hodgkin disease, and multiple myeloma.

Figure 37.3 Expanding the number of years demonstrates a better picture of the change in demographics among transplant recipients. Improvements in supportive care, patient and donor selection, and use of reduced-intensity conditioning regimens for allogeneic transplants are the major contributors to this trend. Source: Pasquini MC, Wang Z. Current use and outcome of hematopoietic stem cell transplantation: CIBMTR Summary Slides, 2013. http://www.cibmtr.org. Reproduced with permission of the CIBMTR.

(MDS), and myeloproliferative disorders (MPN). The indications for transplantation have changed over time (e.g., CML is no longer the most commonly transplanted hematologic malignancy because of the advent of imatinib and other tyrosine kinase inhibitors). Likewise, the average age of transplant recipients has increased over time. The proportion of patients receiving allografts over the age of 50 years is currently approaching 35% (Figure 37.3). Paralleling the increasing age of recipients has been the use of less intense conditioning regimens, which harness the immunological graft-versus-malignancy effect and thus have lower toxicity than myeloablative conditioning regimens (Figure 37.4).[86,91–93] Allogeneic hematopoietic transplants are used for nonmalignant diseases of hematopoietic and immune cells. The most common nonmalignant indications include aplastic anemia and other bone marrow failure states, hemoglobinopathies, severe combined immune deficiency, and metabolic disorders involving hematopoietic cells.

Numerous recipient factors determine the outcome following transplantation; these include the disease stage at transplantation, recipient age, performance status, and presence of comorbidities.[94] All potential transplant recipients undergo an extensive pre-transplant evaluation that usually includes a complete history and physical examination in addition to evaluation of cardiac, pulmonary, hepatic, and renal function. Patients require adequate general medical condition and organ function. The decision to undertake transplantation depends on a careful assessment and discussion of the risks and benefits of the procedure when contrasted with the natural history of the disease.

Potential complications of dose-intensive therapy followed by HSCT

The potential risks resulting from high dose chemoradiotherapy and blood and marrow transplantation are numerous and include toxicity from the preparative regimen, infections resulting from granulocytopenia or post-transplant immunodeficiency, hemorrhage caused by thrombocytopenia and tissue toxicity, and, in the case of allogeneic transplants, transplant rejection and GVHD. The creation of better supportive medications has minimized many of the acute toxicities associated with high-dose chemoradiotherapy regimens.

Myelosuppression

Shortly after infusion, HPCs migrate to sites in the lungs, liver, spleen, and marrow. For most patients, some degree of marrow cellularity can be demonstrated within 14 days of transplantation. Neutrophil and platelet engraftment is defined as being the first of three consecutive days in which the absolute neutrophil count is >500/μL and the platelet count is >20,000/μL (without transfusion support), respectively. This generally occurs 14 to 24 days after stem cell infusion, with longer time to engraftment in cord blood transplants. Before engraftment, patients require aggressive hematologic support with transfusion of platelets and red cells. Blood components must be irradiated to minimize the possibility of graft-versus host reactions mediated by blood donor T cells.[95] Growth factors may be used to shorten the duration of aplasia without increasing the risk of GVHD or relapse.[96,97] In the allogeneic setting, engraftment of donor cells can be documented by the use of molecular tests

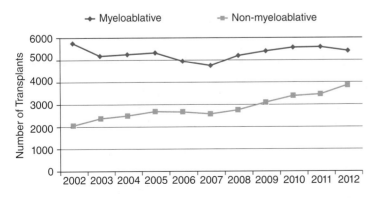

Figure 37.4 The number of transplants using reduced-intensity conditioning has steadily increased in the last decade, mainly for patients aged 50 years and older. In 2011, 66% of all transplants with reduced-intensity conditioning were performed in patients 50 years and older. Source: Pasquini MC, Wang Z. Current use and outcome of hematopoietic stem cell transplantation: CIBMTR Summary Slides, 2013. http://www.cibmtr.org. Reproduced with permission of the CIBMTR.

such as DNA restriction fragment length polymorphisms, or by polymerase chain reaction of microsatellite regions demonstrating a donor pattern. Following successful transplantation, cells of the recipient's reconstituted hematologic and immunologic systems are derived primarily from the donor's blood or marrow, although in some cases mixed chimerism occurs in which both donor- and recipient-derived cells are present in the recipient's circulation and marrow.

Graft failure

The failure to recover hematologic function or the loss of marrow function after initial reconstitution constitutes graft failure. Graft failure is an unusual event for autologous transplant recipients but can occur in 5% to 11% of HLA-identical allogeneic recipients.[98] Graft failure generally takes place within 60 days of transplantation, although late graft failure has been known to occur.[99] Several factors are known to increase the risk of graft failure in allogeneic transplantation, including a low nucleated cell count infused, increasing HLA disparity between donor and host, T-cell depleted grafts, and inadequate immunosuppression of the host.[100] Historical graft failure rates were as high as 35% in patients undergoing transplantation for aplastic anemia, which was felt to be caused in large part by alloimmunization from prior transfusions. This has now been reduced to <10% for patients with aplastic anemia through the minimizing of pre-transplant transfusions and administration of leukocyte-reduced, irradiated blood components.[101] Evidence now exists implicating host T cells as the mediators of an active host immune response against minor alloantigens expressed by the donor cells. On the basis of this understanding, several strategies to further eliminate or inactivate host T cells have evolved, including the use of additional or increased-intensity immunosuppressive agents such as fludarabine or the elimination of host T cells through the use of antithymocyte globulin (ATG) or anti-CD52.[102–105] In contrast, in the haploidentical transplant setting, recipient HLA-specific antidonor antibodies have been implicated in graft rejection, and every effort should be made to avoid selecting donors whom the recipient has anti-HLA antibodies against.[106,107] Treatment of graft failure depends on whether donor cells can be detected in the patient's marrow. If present, a repeat infusion of donor cells can be attempted with or without further conditioning. When no donor hematopoietic cells are detected, a second conditioning regimen may be administered followed by donor stem cells; however, outcomes in this setting are extremely poor.[108,109]

Graft-versus-host disease

GVHD represents one of the most frequent complications of allogeneic transplantation and has been the major barrier to wide-scale application of this therapy. GVHD results from the recognition of host tissues as foreign by donor immunocompetent cells. The syndrome of GVHD involves alloreactivity superimposed on the toxicity of the preparative regimen and amplified by inflammatory cytokines.[110,111] The incidence increases with greater HLA disparity between the donor and host. A fundamental problem for allogeneic transplantation is the close association between this complication and the derived benefit resulting from a GVT effect. Both GVHD and GVT effect are mediated by donor T cells with both being reduced when T cells are depleted from the infused graft (referred to as *T-cell-depleted transplants*). Identifying and separating the target antigens resulting in GVHD and GVT effect are active areas of research that may one day result in maximizing the therapeutic potential of this modality while eliminating this frequent obstacle.

Two forms of GVHD are commonly distinguished: acute and chronic. Historically, acute GVHD was defined as occurring within the first 100 days of transplant, and chronic GVHD was defined as occurring after the 100-day mark. It is now clear that this time point was an artificial one, and clinical manifestation and histologic findings are now the sole factors used in defining these distinct entities.[112]

The incidence of acute GVHD varies from 20% to 70%, depending upon the intensity of the conditioning regimen, the extent of histocompatibility differences with the donor, the age of the recipient, and the stage of primary disease.[113–115] Acute GVHD is graded clinically using a standardized system that takes into account clinical changes in the primarily affected organs: skin, liver, and gastrointestinal tract. This grading system allows for quantitative estimates of disease severity, transplant-related mortality, and response to therapy with scoring consisting of Grades I to IV (Table 37.3).[116,117] These clinical findings are usually confirmed by pathologic changes in the affected organs, although the pathologic findings do not change the grading or staging of the disease. Recently, biomarkers predictive of GVHD severity and mortality have been reported.[118–120]

Corticosteroids remain the standard initial treatment, but even with prompt initiation of such therapy, the treatment is suboptimal. Fewer than 50% of patients with acute GVHD have a durable response after initial therapy; most patients require secondary

Table 37.3 Grading and Staging of Acute GVHD

Organ	Skin	Liver	Gut
Individual Organ Staging			
Stage	BSA (%)	Bilirubin (mg/dL)	Diarrhea volume (mL/day)
1	Rash <25	2–2.9	500–1000 or biopsy–proven upper GI involvement
2	Rash 25–50	3–6	1000–1500
3	Rash >50	6.1 to 15	1500–2000
4	Generalized erythroderma with bullae	>15	>2000 OR severe abdominal pain OR ileus
Consensus Grading			
I	Stage 1–2	None	None
II	Stage 3	Stage 1	Stage 1
III	–	Stage 2–3	Stage 2–4
IV	Stage 4	Stage 4	–
International Bone Marrow Transplant Registry (IBMTR) grading system			
A	Stage 1	None	None
B	Stage 2	Stage 1 or 2	Stage 1 or 2
C	Stage 3	Stage 3	Stage 3
D	Stage 4	Stage 4	Stage 4

treatment.[121,122] Moreover, the outcome for patients with steroid-refractory GVHD is poor, with a mortality rate of 70%; at this time, no therapy has been shown to affect survival.[123] The causes of death among patients with advanced GVHD include organ failure and infections related to poor immune reconstitution. For these reasons, improving post-transplant immunosuppressive therapy (GVHD) prophylaxis has been the preferred strategy.

The prophylactic use of cyclosporine (CSA) and methotrexate (MTX) is effective prophylaxis to reduce the risk of acute GVHD and improve survival.[124] The addition of prednisone to CSA and MTX has been shown not to add additional benefit.[125] Tacrolimus is a macrolide lactone that closely resembles CSA in mechanism of action, spectrum of toxicities, and pharmacologic interactions. In a randomized study,[126] the prophylactic regimen of tacrolimus and MTX was demonstrated to reduce Grade II–IV acute GVHD when compared to CSA and MTX. However, overall survival was not improved. Most allogeneic transplants receive either tacrolimus or cyclosporine for 3–6 months post transplant as GVHD prophylaxis. At the M.D. Anderson Cancer Center, a modification of the tacrolimus–MTX regimen using "mini-dose MTX" was found to be as effective as full-dose therapy with less toxicity.[127]

ATG has also been used in the prophylactic setting.[128,129] In patients with aplastic anemia who underwent transplantation using a Cy and ATG conditioning regimen, low rates of acute GVHD (15%) and chronic GVHD (34%) were reported, and a significant survival benefit at three years was identified for patients receiving this regimen when compared with historical controls who received Cy alone (92% vs. 72%).[130] ATG has been shown to reduce chronic GVHD without adversely affecting other transplant outcomes with myeloablative transplants.[129] ATG treatment was associated with a higher risk of malignancy relapse in a recent CIBMTR study in recipients of reduced-intensity conditioning, presumably adversely affecting GVT effects.[131]

T-cell depletion before marrow infusion, an alternative approach to prevent GVHD is to physically deplete T lymphocytes from the transplant,[132] has been shown to effectively reduce the incidence and severity of GVHD; however, it also results in increased graft rejection, infectious complications, and relapse rates in a disease specific manner.[7,133] Selective T-cell subset depletion and "add-back" of allo-depleted T cells are strategies that may be effective for reducing the risk of acute GVHD while preserving the GVT effect.[134–137] For example, some strategies involve selective depletion of CD45RA+ T cells, which are naïve T cells thought to play a major role in GVHD in some mouse models.[138–140] Likewise, others are investigating graft manipulation to deplete the alpha and beta T cells. This approach preserves only the gamma and delta T-cell subsets that are known to possess innate and adaptive immune response without a major role in GVHD.[141,142] Chronic GVHD shares many features with various autoimmune disorders, including autoantibodies and disease manifestations that are similar to those of such disorders as sicca syndrome and scleroderma. The manifestations of chronic GVHD are extensive with nearly every organ potentially affected.[112] The consequences for affected patients can be profound, with its presence or absence being the most significant determinant of long-term outcome and quality of life following allogeneic HSCT.[143–145] Approximately 60% to 70% of patients who receive an allogeneic transplant are affected to some degree by chronic GVHD.[146] Despite progress in other areas of this field, our understanding of this entity is limited; therefore, advancements in the prevention and treatment of chronic GVHD have been sparse.

Organ toxicity

Hepatic veno-occlusive disease (VOD)

Hepatic VOD, also referred to as *sinusoidal obstruction syndrome*, is a complication of both allogeneic and autologous transplant as well as occasionally chemotherapy regimens in the non-transplant setting. The process occurs as a result of direct injury to the hepatic venous endothelium. The syndrome is characterized by the constellation of signs and symptoms consisting of tender hepatomegaly, jaundice, weight gain, and ascites.[147] The incidence of this syndrome has varied among reports and has ranged from 5% to 50% of all allogeneic and autologous transplants.[148,149] These studies suggest VOD is life-threatening in roughly one-quarter of cases. Risk factors include preexisting liver disease, high-intensity conditioning regimens, prior chemotherapy regimens, and mismatched or unrelated donor transplants.[149] Defibrotide is currently approved in Europe for the treatment of severe VOD and is available in the United States via an expanded-access protocol.[150,151]

Lung

Myriad pulmonary complications can occur in patients following autologous and allogeneic transplantation. Most of these complications are a result of acute or delayed complications of the conditioning regimen and previous treatments. It is important to distinguish these entities from an infectious etiology. Direct toxicity can result from the conditioning regimen, including carmustine induced pulmonary toxicity and radiation-induced lung injury. Diffuse alveolar hemorrhage (DAH) may occur in the immediate post-transplant period during pancytopenia. One study found a strong association between DAH and previous thoracic irradiation, whereas no association was found between the presence of thrombocytopenia, coagulopathy, or neutropenia.[152] Idiopathic pneumonia syndrome may occur following allogeneic transplant. It is described as a diffuse, noninfectious pneumonia that in animal models appears to be an immune-mediated process in part induced by the toxicity of the conditioning regimen.[153–155] Bronchiolitis obliterans is a pulmonary manifestation of chronic GVHD.[112,156,157] There is evidence to suggest that the occurrence of bronchiolitis obliterans after allogeneic HSCT can be triggered by some lung infections, particularly viral infections.[158]

Infections

Patients undergoing autologous and allogeneic transplants are at risk for a variety of infections as a result of the myelosuppression induced by the chemo- and radiotherapies employed during conditioning, delayed immune reconstitution following myeloablative therapy, and, in the case of allogeneic transplantation, immunosuppression used to prevent and treat GVHD as well as GVHD itself.[159] Risk for infection is generally divided into three phases: Phase I, the period following the preparative regimen while awaiting engraftment; Phase II, following engraftment and up to day 100; and Phase III, from day 100 to months and year(s) following transplantation (Figure 37.5) . Infectious risks for each of the three periods varies, respectively, depending on the degree of tissue toxicity and length of neutropenia following the preparative period, the presence of acute GVHD, and the presence of chronic GVHD. Based on the high risk and associated morbidity resulting from bacterial, fungal, and viral pathogens, several prophylactic and surveillance strategies have been developed for patients undergoing transplantation.

Bacterial, fungal, and herpes simplex virus (HSV) infections pose the greatest risk for patients during the pre-engraftment period. In addition to conditioning-induced myelosuppression, patients often

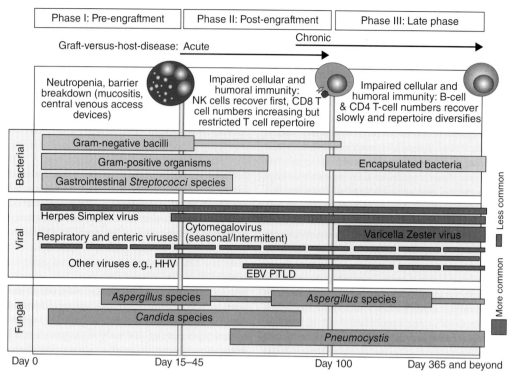

Figure 37.5 Phases of opportunistic infections among allogeneic HCT recipients.[159] EBV, Epstein–Barr virus; HHV6, human herpesvirus 6; PTLD, post-transplant lymphoproliferative disease. Reprinted from "Guidelines for preventing infectious complications among hematopoietic cell transplantation recipients: a global perspective", Tomblyn M et. al, Biology of Blood and Marrow Transplantation; Volume 15, pages1143–1238, Copyright 2009, with permission from Elsevier.

have impaired primary immunity as a result of indwelling catheters and tissue toxicity (mucositis, gastroenteritis, etc.). Bacterial prophylaxis with a quinolone antibiotic is often employed in an effort to suppress intestinal flora and prevent serious Gram-negative infections, typically till recovery of neutrophil count; it is endorsed by guidelines, including those of the Infectious Disease Society of America (IDSA).[160–162] The prompt administration of broad-spectrum antibiotics following a neutropenic febrile event is of paramount importance in preventing morbidity of bacterial infections. Administration of antibiotic prophylaxis with a quinolone antibiotic is also recommended in patients who are actively being treated for GVHD.[160]

In a randomized study,[163] the prophylactic use of fluconazole has been shown to reduce the incidence of systemic and superficial fungal infections. Fluconazole has not, however, been shown to affect the incidence of infections with resistant organisms such as *Candida krusei* or *Candida glabrata* and invasive mold infections. Prophylaxis against other invasive fungal infections such as *Aspergillus* species is an area of debate, with some studies supporting the use of newer azole agents such as posaconazole[164] or echinocandins.[165] Posaconazole and voriconazole have greater activity against molds than fluconazole, and have been advocated for patients at high risk for these infection.[166,167] Patients receiving therapy for GVHD should also receive antifungal prophylaxis.[164]

HSV reactivation is seen commonly in seropositive patients during the first six weeks after transplantation unless prophylaxis is administered. Acyclovir prophylaxis has been shown to prevent reactivation, reduce morbidity, and lower the incidence of antibiotic resistance and is routinely administered.[168,169] Patients in whom

HSV reactivation occurs should be treated with acyclovir or valacyclovir. For patients who develop resistance after multiple episodes of HSV reactivation, foscarnet may be required.[160,170,171]

Prophylaxis against *Pneumocystis carinii* (PCP) is recommended following engraftment and continued for a minimum of six months following transplantation or while taking immunosuppressive drugs. Trimethoprim–sulfamethoxazole is the agent of choice for PCP prophylaxis given that it has the lowest breakthrough rate.[172] Various other agents have been used, including dapsone and aerosolized pentamidine.[173,174]

Cytomegalovirus (CMV) infections were once a common and fatal occurrence in the first three months following marrow transplantation. The routine prophylactic use of ganciclovir has largely eliminated CMV disease after transplantation. Randomized studies have clearly demonstrated efficacy in reducing the incidence of CMV disease by the prophylactic treatment of all CMV-seropositive patients.[175] However, this strategy is problematic in that many patients will require discontinuation of therapy because of the development of neutropenia, which places the patients at increased risk for other infections. The creation of highly sensitive tests capable of detecting CMV reactivation before overt CMV disease has allowed for an alternative strategy to routine prophylaxis. These tests include direct detection of CMV pp65 antigen in peripheral blood leukocytes[176] and detection of CMV DNA in leukocytes, plasma, or serum.[177] Preemptive therapy when reactivation is first detected has been shown to result in similar rates of CMV-related death and survival when compared with universal ganciclovir prophylaxis starting at the time of engraftment. Patients receiving routine prophylaxis experienced less CMV disease in the first 100 days after transplantation; however, this benefit was offset by a higher rate of invasive fungal infections and late CMV disease.[176] Thus, current recommendations support either approach for patients at risk for CMV disease (i.e., all CMV-seropositive recipients and seronegative recipients with seropositive donors). For CMV-seronegative patients with CMV-seronegative donors, the use of CMV-seronegative or leukocyte-reduced blood components are effective in preventing primary infections.[178] There are new promising investigational agents under development for prevention and treatment of CMV, including letermovir, brincidofovir (CMX001), and maribavir.[179–181] Moreover, adoptive transfer of virus-specific T cells specific against CMV and other viruses is also a promising approach that is currently being evaluated in clinical trials.[182]

Viral infections continue to pose significant challenges to clinicians managing post-transplant patients. In addition to community respiratory viruses, intestinal viruses are easily transmitted through person-to-person contact and have been associated with increased morbidity and mortality. Because of a lack of specific therapies for these agents, the focus must be on appropriate isolation of patients and the prevention of person-to-person transmission.

Long-term complications of high-dose therapies

Several long-term complications occur following HSCT, requiring patients to maintain regular office visits and practitioners familiar with post-transplant follow-up guidelines to monitor patient progress. Regular eye screening for cataracts is required, especially for those who received a TBI-containing regimen or steroids for the treatment of GVHD.[183] Several endocrine complications occur, including hypothyroidism, stunted growth and development (in pediatric patients), and premature gonad failure or sterility.[184] Patients who have undergone autologous HSCT are at increased risk for treatment related MDS and AML, especially if they were subject to prior radiation (especially to the pelvis), were heavily pretreated, were slow PBPC mobilizers, or were subject to TBI-containing conditioning regimens.[185,186] Both autologous and allograft recipients are at higher risk for additional secondary cancers, especially bone, head, neck, and connective tissue malignancies.[187–189]

Disease indications

Autologous HSCT is effective for diseases that are known to have better responses to higher doses of chemotherapy. Allogeneic transplants can confer a potent immune-mediated graft-versus malignancy effect, but they have a higher risk of complications, including graft rejection, GVHD, and infections, due to more severe post-transplant immune deficiency. For each diagnosis, treatment recommendations are made depending on the results with conventional chemotherapy, high-dose chemotherapy with autologous hematopoietic transplantation, or allogeneic transplantation.

Given that allogeneic transplantation is a risky procedure, it is usually reserved for intermediate to high-risk diseases known to have poor outcomes with conventional non-transplant therapy options and autologous transplants. Hematopoietic transplantation is generally not effective in patients with chemotherapy refractory disease or debilitated patients who are at high risk for complications. The American Society for Blood and Marrow Transplantation has published evidence-based reviews regarding the role of autologous and allogeneic HCT for the major hematologic malignancies.[190] This section summarizes the current indications for HSCT in different malignancies.

Acute myeloid leukemia

AML is the most common indication for allogeneic transplantation (Figure 37.2). Autologous HSCT in patients with AML remains investigational.[191,192] Allogeneic HSCT is indicated for patients with AML in first complete remission (CR) with intermediate or high-risk features[193] or for patients with primary induction failure or after relapse.

Treatment decisions pertaining to post induction therapy are centered on disease risk for relapse as determined by cytogenetic and molecular data. During the last decade, significant progress has been made in risk-stratifying patients based on their cytogenetic and molecular prognostic factors.[194,195] Patients with favorable cytogenetic abnormalities such as t(8;21), inv 16, or t(15;17) should not be offered HSCT in first remission given that HSCT has not been shown to improve outcomes compared to chemotherapy alone.[196,197] Some studies also suggest using standard-dose chemotherapy for patients with other favorable molecular abnormalities, such as NPM1 or CEBPA mutations without a FLT3 mutation.[198–200] Suitable candidates for allogeneic HSCT include patients with intermediate risk and all poor-risk candidates such as patients with FLT3 internal tandem duplication, complex cytogenetics, monosomy 5 or 7, and secondary AML, the latter preferably while in first CR.[201] Likewise, patients in first relapse or second remission should also be offered an allogeneic transplant regardless of their original cytogenetics, provided that they have a suitable donor, as chemotherapy alone would be unlikely to result in a durable remission. Although the likelihood of success with allogeneic transplantation is substantially lower for this group of patients when compared to those in first CR, no other therapy is known to offer long-term cures.[202] Reduced-intensity conditioning regimens have allowed older adults up to age 75 years to undergo allogeneic transplantation with acceptable treatment-related mortality and with disease-free survival superior to that of standard chemotherapy.[203] This is extremely pertinent for a disease that has an average age of onset in the seventh decade of life.

Myelodysplastic syndromes

Allogeneic HSCT represents an effective treatment strategy in some patients with myelodysplastic syndromes.[204,205] Several prognostic indices, such as the IPSS and World Health Organization prognostic indices, help risk-stratify MDS into low-, intermediate-, and high risk groups.[206,207] Allogeneic HSCT is not recommended for patients with stable low-grade MDS who may have a long natural history with current standard therapies.[208] However, allogeneic HSCT is indicated for patients with intermediate-2 and high-risk features by the IPSS scale or those with therapy-related MDS.[209,210] Allogeneic HSCT is also effective for patients with intermediate-1 disease, particularly those who are not responding to alternative treatments.[211] Given that MDS occurs more frequently in older patients, the use of reduced-intensity conditioning has extended allogeneic HSCT to a substantial fraction of older patients with MDS, leading to durable disease-free survival rates.[93]

Myeloproliferative disorders

Myeloproliferative syndromes are a clonal disorder of hematopoietic cells. Allogeneic HSCT is an established potential curative treatment for a selected group of patients with these disorders. This includes patients with high-risk disease who are unlikely to have a prolonged overall survival with currently available therapies. Prognostic factors have been determined to help identify high-risk patients who would be best treated with allogeneic HSCT.[212–214]

This includes patients with de novo myelofibrosis or secondary myelofibrosis in patients with polycythemia vera and essential thrombocythemia.

Acute lymphocytic leukemia

Conventional chemotherapy offers prolonged remission and even a cure for most children and many adults. In children, allogeneic HSCT is generally reserved only for those with high-risk ALL, such as Philadelphia (Ph) chromosome–positive disease, MLL-mutated disease, and those in second remission.[215–217] However, in adults, there is controversy regarding which patients should receive an allogeneic transplant for ALL in first CR. Allogeneic HSCT is indicated in high-risk adult patients in first remission such as patients with t(4:15), Ph-positive disease, or those with MLL mutation.[218–222] Adult patients with relapsed ALL or those who fail to achieve remission with initial chemotherapy should also undergo allogeneic HSCT after achieving remission with salvage chemotherapy.[223] Successful results of marrow transplants in first remission for these patients range from 30% to 60%, depending on patient age and donor type. The GVL effect may be less in ALL than is observed in CML or more indolent malignancies. The rarity of allogeneic donor lymphocyte infusion inducing remission for relapses after allogeneic transplantation supports this observation.[224] Patients with active leptomeningeal leukemia should have this complication treated before transplantation, because few marrow transplant preparative regimens have agents that cross the blood–brain barrier. Most recently, a 90% complete remission rate was achieved in high-risk patients with relapsed or refractory ALL who received genetically modified autologous T cells expressing a chimeric antigen receptor (CAR-T cells) enabling them to recognize and kill all CD19-expressing cells, including CD19-expressing ALL cells.[225] This represents a major advance in the field, and more clinical data are expected to come over the next few years.

Chronic myeloid leukemia

Before the advent of tyrosine kinase inhibitors (TKIs) such as imatinib, CML was the most common disease treated with allogeneic hematopoietic transplantation. There are currently several generations of TKIs that are effective in CML, and allogeneic transplantation is currently reserved only for patients who fail to respond to TKI therapy.[226,227] In patients who relapse post allogeneic HSCT, donor lymphocyte infusions have been shown to be effective in inducing durable remissions.[228–230]

Multiple myeloma

Multiple myeloma currently represents the most common indication for autologous HSCT. It is relatively safe and can be performed in elderly patients who are in a good general medical condition.[231] This approach is associated with high CR rates, which is a primary determinant of long-term survival, but it remains noncurative for the majority of patients.[232,233] High-dose melphalan at a dose of 200 mg/m^2 is associated with better complete remission rates, event-free survival, and overall survival compared to chemotherapy alone.[234,235] There is some controversy whether to perform autologous HSCT to consolidate the initial response to chemotherapy or delay it after first relapse. There is also some controversy whether to perform a second planned autologous HSCT (tandem transplant) given conflicting results from randomized trials.[236–238] Most recently, tandem autologous HSCT was shown to improve progression-free and overall survival compared to melphalan, lenalidomide, and dexamethasone consolidation therapy in a well-designed

multicenter trial.[239] The question if transplant is still more efficacious than a combination of proteasome inhibitor (e.g., bortezomib) and an immunomodulator (e.g., lenalidomide) still remains unanswered and is the focus of an ongoing clinical trial (NCT01208662, Clinicaltrials.gov). Maintenance therapy with post-transplant lenalidomide is also associated with better progression-free survival, especially in patients who do not achieve at least a very good partial response after transplant.[240] However, it is associated with bone marrow suppression and a small increase in secondary malignancies, and more information with longer follow-up time is needed to evaluate the potential benefits and long-term toxicities.[241] Allogeneic transplantation is also being investigated in myeloma as a potentially curative therapy. However, there is a higher risk of treatment-related mortality with allogeneic transplants compared with autologous HSCT, and its use is generally not recommended outside of a clinical trial.[242] Another approach is to perform "debulking" with an autologous transplant followed by a non-myeloablative allogeneic transplant. However, most studies have not demonstrated a benefit of the autologous–allogeneic tandem transplant, and it is not generally recommended as an initial therapy for multiple myeloma except in the context of a clinical trial.[243,244]

Amyloidosis

AL amyloidosis constitutes a plasma cell dyscrasia, and high-dose melphalan with autologous HSCT can induce complete remissions and arrest progression of amyloid deposition, even in patients over 65 years of age.[245–247] However, many patients with AL amyloidosis are diagnosed late in their disease course and may be highly debilitated. Patients with severe cardiac involvement are at high risk for treatment-related mortality.

Chronic lymphocytic leukemia

There is a strong graft-versus-leukemia effect in CLL, and non-myeloablative regimens are effective.[248,249] Allogeneic HSCT is recommended for patients with Richter's transformation who have extremely poor prognosis with chemotherapy alone.[250] Although allogeneic HSCT is an effective treatment for CLL, its role will have to be redefined given the recent introduction of targeted therapies that are effective and less toxic than allogeneic HSCT, including the Bruton's tyrosine kinase inhibitor, ibrutinib, and the phosphatidylinositol-3-kinase delta (PI3 Kδ) inhibitor, idelalisib.[251,252] Cellular therapy with CAR-T cells targeting CD19 is also a promising approach in the treatment of refractory CLL.[253]

Lymphoma

Diffuse large-cell non-Hodgkin's lymphoma (DLBCL)

High-dose therapy followed by autologous HSCT is considered standard treatment for patients with diffuse large-cell lymphoma who fail to achieve remission following initial therapy, or subsequently relapse after an initial remission with chemosensitive disease. The Parma study was a randomized trial comparing standard salvage chemotherapy in first relapse for large-cell lymphoma to standard chemotherapy plus autologous HSCT.[254] This trial demonstrated a definitive advantage for patients receiving an autologous transplant. The best results are seen in patients who achieve a negative positron emission tomography (PET) scan at the time of the transplant.[255,256] In addition, conditioning regimens and the incorporation of the CD20 monoclonal antibody, rituximab, into chemo-mobilization have been shown to improve outcomes.[22

Autologous and allogeneic HSCT have similar results for treatment of lymphoblastic lymphoma.[257,258] However, allogeneic HSCT can be considered for a subgroup of high-risk patients such as those who have a very short duration of remission (<1 year) or those relapsing after an autograft provided they are transplant eligible and have a suitable donor, but this remains controversial.[259–264]

Hodgkin's disease

Autologous HSCT is the accepted treatment for patients with chemo-sensitive relapsed or primary refractory Hodgkin disease.[265] Patients who achieve a second CR following salvage treatment have the best outcomes with this approach, with over 50% of patients achieving a long-term cure. There have been no randomized studies comparing TBI-containing to chemotherapy-alone conditioning regimens, but generally radiation-based regimens are avoided in those patients who have previously received radiation therapy. Allogeneic HSCT is a reasonable option that can induce durable CRs in selected patients with high-risk recurrent disease or with chemosensitive relapse after autologous stem cell transplantation.[266–268]

Follicular lymphoma

The use of either autologous or allogeneic HSCT in follicular lymphoma is controversial and the subject of ongoing clinical trials. High-dose therapy and autologous stem cell transplantation can also produce long-term remissions in patients with low-grade lymphoma.[235,269–271] Ex vivo purging can reduce the amount of malignant cells in the autograft.[272,273] The use of autologous or allogeneic HSCT is usually reserved to patients with aggressive disease that is refractory to immuno-chemotherapy. However, the optimal timing to perform HSCT in follicular lymphoma is unknown. Given the strong graft-versus-lymphoma effect in follicular lymphoma, allogeneic HSCT is usually effective in advanced follicular lymphomas, particularly with chemosensitive disease. In that setting, nonmyeloablative regimens are safe and effective with low transplant-related mortality rates.[274,275]

Mantle cell lymphoma

Several trials have shown that autologous stem cell transplantation is an effective consolidation strategy for patients with mantle cell lymphoma in first remission.[276–281] However, for patients with relapsed or refractory disease, allogeneic transplants are more effective.[264,274,282–285] Advances using reduced-intensity conditioning regimens, which rely more on the graft-versus lymphoma effect, have reduced treatment-related mortality and improved outcomes in patients with relapsed or refractory mantle cell lymphoma.[285]

T-cell and natural killer (NK) cell lymphoma

With the exception of Alk+ve anaplastic large-cell lymphoma (ALCL), most T-cell and NK-cell lymphomas generally have a poor prognosis with chemotherapy alone.[286] Thus, except for Alk+ve ALCL, autologous transplants are generally recommended for treatment of T- and NK-cell lymphomas to consolidate initial remission or treatment of relapse.[287,288] Allogeneic transplants have a role in selected patients with advanced T-cell and NK-cell lymphomas.[289]

Solid tumors

Given that some solid tumors have a steep dose response to chemotherapy or radiotherapy, using high-dose chemotherapy followed by autologous transplantation is a feasible option. The most common indications for autologous transplants in solid tumors are currently in advanced germ cell tumors, and these transplants can produce durable remissions in patients with advanced disease.[290–295]

Breast cancer was once the most common indication for high-dose chemotherapy followed by autologous HSCT. However, a series of randomized trials failed to demonstrate an improvement in long-term progression-free or overall survival in patients with high-risk[296,297] or metastatic breast cancer.[298] Apart from participation in a clinical trial, this approach is no longer justified.

Future directions

Hematopoietic transplantation is a definitive modality of treatment for a broad range of hematologic, immune, metabolic, and malignant diseases. The field has advanced so that this therapy can now be offered to more patients with less risk for acute and long-term toxicity. HSCT has become progressively safer with a lower risk of nonrelapse mortality. Incorporation of molecularly targeted therapies and recent advances in cellular immunotherapies, including chimeric antigen receptor T cells and NK cells, are emerging promising therapies to reduce the risk of recurrent malignancy. New strategies for harnessing the immunotherapeutic potential of a GVL effect while reducing the risk of GVHD will make allogeneic transplantation a more widely applied modality.

Key references

A full reference list for this chapter is available at: http://www.wiley.com/go/simon/transfusion

2 Thomas ED, Storb R, Clift RA, et al. Bone-marrow transplantation. *N Eng J Med*. 1975;**292**:832–43.

3 Thomas ED. Bone marrow transplantation for malignant disease. *J Clin Oncol* 1983;**1**:517

14 Weissman IL. Translating stem and progenitor cell biology to the clinic: barriers and opportunities. *Science* 2000;**287**:1442–6.

CHAPTER 38

Gene therapy applications to transfusion medicine

Eric A. Gehrie, Alexey Bersenev, Emanuela Bruscia, Diane Krause, & Wade L. Schulz

Department of Laboratory Medicine, Yale School of Medicine, Yale University; and Blood Bank, Yale-New Haven Hospital, New Haven, CT, USA

Introduction

The delivery of genetic material into a patient's cells as a medical therapy is referred to as *gene therapy*. The specific manner by which gene therapy is performed varies significantly based on the disease being treated, the amount of genetic material to insert, the target cells, and the route of administration. In the last several years, the number of worldwide clinical trials for cellular therapy, including gene-modified cells, has increased from approximately 151 in 2011 up to 373 in 2014.[1] On the other hand, the total number of gene therapy clinical trials registered worldwide progressively increased from just one in 1989 to 120 in 2013.[2]

Traditionally, transfusion medicine has only been able to provide supportive therapy for patients with inherited hematologic diseases, rather than a curative treatment. For example, chronic transfusion can be used to treat anemia associated with sickle cell disease (SCD) or thalassemia, and the administration of clotting factor concentrates can be used to treat or prevent hemorrhage in patients with hemophilia. However, in the future, novel therapies directed at the genetic basis of these diseases may reduce, or even prevent, the need for such patients to require chronic supportive therapy. The focus of this chapter will be on the possible applications of gene therapy to transfusion medicine.

Gene therapy and transfusion medicine

Gene therapy falls within the purview of transfusion medicine when it requires the infusion of either gene-modified cells or direct administration of vectors that contain the therapeutic genetic material. In addition, transfusion medicine physicians will surely be impacted by gene therapies used to treat diseases that are currently managed with transfusion or factor infusion. For example, hemophilia B, a disease in which patients lack expression of functional clotting factor IX, has been successfully treated with gene therapy in small, early-phase clinical trials.[3] Gene therapy also shows promise as a possible treatment for sickle cell anemia and hemophilia A.[4,5]

Three major considerations for the design of a gene therapy strategy are: which gene to insert, which vector to use, and how to administer the vector. Because hematopoietic stem cells can be mobilized, modified, and reinfused to patients, many hematologic disorders are uniquely suited to gene therapy. At the same time,

hematological disorders also pose several unique challenges. This is due to the difficulty of delivering the often large genes required to treat hematologic disease and the risk of malignancy from gene insertion. Yet another challenge is to isolate hematopoietic cells in suitable quantities for transduction–transfection and to support them ex vivo in culture.

Gene selection and targeted insertion

Based on the disease to be treated, the gene that will be inserted can have a variety of attributes. The gene can provide a functional form of a missing or defective gene, it can augment a dysfunctional gene, or it can regulate cell survival. Ideal vectors should be designed to affect specific target cells. In the last few years, the importance of controlling where a gene therapy vector integrates into the genome has become clearer. For example, in the case of gene therapy trials in X-linked immunodeficiency, the retroviral vectors integrated into the genome at sites that activated proto-oncogenes, subsequently causing leukemia in treated patients.[6] In addition, a gene therapy trial for hemophilia B was stopped after the viral vector was detected in a subject's semen, raising concern that a therapeutic gene could be inherited by a subject's future offspring.[7]

Gene therapy administration

Gene therapy vectors can be delivered to cells ex vivo and then returned to the patient. Alternatively, nonviral and replication-incompetent viral vectors can be directly administered to the patient for transduction of target cells in vivo. There are several benefits to the ex vivo approach, in particular that transduced cells can be selected prior to reinfusion (see Table 38.1).[8] The ex vivo approach also minimizes infection of nontarget cells, significantly decreases the potential risks of exposing the patient to large amounts of viral vector, and allows for the insertion of an additional gene that could be activated to destroy the designed cell, if necessary. On the other hand, direct administration of vectors to the patient overcomes the difficulty of maintaining fully functional cells during ex vivo culture. Because there are risks associated with transgene expression in unintended host cells, it is critical that a vector administered in vivo has target specificity or minimal toxicity if expressed by cell types other than the intended target.

Rossi's Principles of Transfusion Medicine, Fifth Edition. Edited by Toby L. Simon, Jeffrey McCullough, Edward L. Snyder, Bjarte G. Solheim, and Ronald G. Strauss.
© 2016 John Wiley & Sons, Ltd. Published 2016 by John Wiley & Sons, Ltd.

Table 38.1 Advantages and disadvantages of different modes of vector administration

Manner of Vector Administration	Ex Vivo	In Vivo
Possible advantages	• Ability to select transduced cells prior to reinfusion • Minimizes infection of nontarget cells • Exposes patient to smaller dose of viral vector • Ability to insert a suicide gene to inactivate a therapeutic gene	• No need to maintain ex vivo fully functional cells that can engraft long-term after administration to the patient
Possible disadvantages	• Can be technically difficult to maintain and transduce fully functional cells ex vivo	• Exposes patient to larger dose of viral vector • Vector may unforeseen effects on unintended target cells • Immune system may target the vector for destruction

Table 38.2 Common viruses that have been modified for gene therapy research

Family/Subfamily and Characteristics	Specific Virus
Retroviruses (single-stranded RNA, with maximal insert size of approx. 8 kb) Oncoviruses	Murine leukemia virus Spleen necrosis virus Rous sarcoma virus Avian leukocytosis virus
Lentiviruses	Human immunodeficiency virus, type 1 Human immunodeficiency virus, type 2
Spumaviruses	Foamy virus
Adenoviruses (double-stranded DNA, with maximal insert size of approx. 8 kb for first generation; up to 37 kb for new generation)	Adenovirus, type 5
Adeno-associated virus (single-stranded DNA with maximal insert size of approx. 5 kb)	Adeno-associated virus, type 2

Vector selection

The ideal vector should have no toxicity, lead to minimal inflammation, and have a large gene carrying capacity. In addition, vectors should be able to target specific cell types and genetic integration sites within the host. Other factors to consider are whether gene expression needs to be inducible and if lifelong expression is necessary. Unfortunately, a single vector that achieves all of these goals is not yet available. However, based on the above needs, a suitable vector can often be selected. Many research laboratories are developing strategies to optimize current vectors to meet the criteria for an ideal vector. Three of the most well-established viral vector systems for clinical trials are retroviruses, adenoviruses, and adeno-associated viruses. (Note that the use of lentiviral vectors, which are a subtype of retroviruses, is covered in Chapter 41, "Adoptive Immunotherapy.") Table 38.2 summarizes the salient features of these viral vectors. Nonviral techniques that are under development for gene therapy are discussed in the following sections as well.[9]

Virus inactivation

For safety reasons, all viral vectors for gene therapy must be incapable of replication in the human host. For example, replication-incompetent retroviruses (RIRs) are produced by removal of the *gag*, *pol*, and *env* genes. Before viral vectors can be used in clinical trials, each batch must be tested extensively to ensure that no replication-competent particles are present.

Risks

The major risks associated with viral vector–based gene therapy are the generation of replication-competent viruses and gene integration that could lead to the activation of oncogenes or loss of function of tumor suppressor genes.

Replication-competent viruses

Replication-competent viruses develop either by recombination of the constituent parts of the vector system with endogenous viral sequences in the vector packaging cell lines or by activation of endogenous proviral sequences. The significant risks of retroviral reactivation for gene therapy were elucidated when primate studies were initially performed. In these studies, CD34-selected primate marrow cells were infected with replication-incompetent virus from packaging cell lines. There were, however, some replication-competent viruses that had not been detected by existing assays. Upon infusion, three of eight primates subsequently developed lymphomas containing the active, rearranged retrovirus.[10] As mentioned, investigators are optimizing safety by creating replication-incompetent vectors, and minimizing the regions of homology between the vectors and packaging cell lines. Currently, clinical trials require stringent testing to guarantee that the retroviral vector to be used in humans is entirely replication incompetent.

Genotoxicity (insertional mutagenesis)

Genotoxicity occurs when genetic material is inserted in proximity to a proto-oncogene or disrupts expression of a tumor suppressor gene. The presence of the strong viral promoter near a proto-oncogene can lead to transcriptional activation of the gene. This has led to the development of malignancy in patients enrolled in a clinical trial for X-linked immunodeficiency.[6,11–13] Unfortunately, no strategies are currently available for site-directed insertion of the genetic payload. In addition, insertion of a transgene into a portion of the genomic DNA that is essential to cell survival can lead to disruption of critical cell processes, resulting in cell death.

Nonviral gene therapy vectors

Nonviral vectors for gene therapy are also undergoing intensive investigation.[14] Unlike viral vectors, nonviral methods do not need to overcome the extensive immune mechanisms that inhibit transduction in vivo. There is also no risk of replication-competent forms of the vector. These methods include DNA microinjection or chemical transfection of episomal or other exogenous DNA.

Gene editing

Various gene-editing approaches such as transcription activator–like effector nucleases (TALENs), zinc finger nucleases (ZFNs), and clustered regularly interspaced short palindromic repeats (CRISPRs) have been described.[15] All three of these technologies can be used to disrupt, add, or correct genes in animal cells.[15] Unlike gene therapy vectors, which insert genetic information into a patient's genome, TALENs, ZFNs, and CRISPRs actually correct mutations in the patient's DNA.

Studies that have assessed the possible application of gene-editing techniques to hemoglobinopathies are discussed in the "Transfusion-Medicine Related Gene Therapy Trials" section, below. Notably, gene-editing approaches have also shown promise for other conditions. For example, a trial of HIV patients treated with autologous T cells that were engineered to have dysfunctional CCR5 genes by a ZFN was recently reported.[16] Although one of the 12 patients in the trial had a transfusion reaction to the infusion of T cells, the study found that infusion of these engineered cells appeared to be safe.[16] Long-term monitoring of study participants is needed to confirm the safety of this approach.

Transfusion-medicine related gene therapy trials

Hemophilia B

Hemophilia B is an X-linked genetic disease that results in bleeding due to reduced or absent activity of factor IX, a serine protease synthesized in the liver. Patients with mild hemophilia B have between 6% and 49% of normal factor IX activity, and may never be diagnosed unless they undergo a major trauma or surgery. Moderate hemophilia B is classified as factor IX activity between 1% and 5% of normal. Patients with moderate hemophilia B may have spontaneous bleeding or prolonged or major bleeding after injuries. Severe hemophilia B is diagnosed when <1% of normal factor IX is detectable in the blood and can result in debilitating, spontaneous bleeding episodes. At present, bleeding prevention in hemophilia B is accomplished via administration of source plasma–derived or, ideally, recombinant factor IX concentrates. Many patients with severe disease require frequent infusions of factor IX to prevent spontaneous bleeding episodes.

Severe hemophilia B is an attractive target for gene therapy because even a small increase in endogenous factor IX activity could reduce dependence on factor IX infusions and prevent spontaneous bleeding episodes. In the late 1990s, researchers using various animal models of hemophilia B found that a gene therapy technique using an adeno-associated virus (AAV) vector could be used to induce sustained circulation of factor IX.[17,18] Shortly thereafter, a human trial established that administration of an AAV vector to human subjects was safe.[19] A subsequent study of seven patients with severe hemophilia B showed that treatment with a recombinant AAV vector (rAAV-hAAT-F.IX) led to only transient elevations in circulating factor IX.[20] Because the reduction in factor IX activity was associated with an increase in transaminases, the study authors concluded that it was immune-mediated destruction of transduced hepatocytes expressing the AAV capsid may have occurred. In contrast to animal models, humans are frequently infected by AAV during childhood. This may explain why animals were capable of a sustained response to AAV-mediated gene therapy while humans generated a secondary immune response that led to the destruction of transduced hepatocytes. However, a more recent trial of 10 patients with severe hemophilia B treated with a different AAV vector (scAAV2/8-LP1-hFIXco) demonstrated a sustained, dose-dependent increase in factor IX activity.[3,21] After a median of 3.2 years of follow-up, these patients have required fewer factor IX infusions, have had fewer bleeding episodes, and have not had significant treatment-related toxicity. The authors of the study estimate that, in addition to the benefits to the patients, the gene therapy treatment has saved $2.5 million in factor IX injections to these 10 patients.[3]

There are three clinical trials (all phase 1 or phase 1/2) of AAV vector–mediated gene therapy for hemophilia B registered with ClinicalTrials.gov. All three trials (NCT979238, NCT01620801, and NCT01687608) are recruiting patients. Projected primary completion dates for these trials range from June 2015 to November 2019. The results of these trials will likely determine the fate of AAV vector–mediated gene therapy as a treatment for hemophilia B.

Hemophilia A

Hemophilia A is caused by a deficiency in factor VIII, which is the only clotting factor synthesized by endothelium (rather than the liver). Similar to hemophilia B, patients with hemophilia A are stratified into mild (6–49% of normal factor VIII activity), moderate (1–5% of normal factor VIII activity), and severe (<1% of normal factor VIII activity) categories based on their level of circulating factor VIII. Also similar to factor IX deficiencies, even a small increase in factor VIII activity would be expected to protect patients from bleeding episodes. Therefore, hemophilia A is another appealing target for gene therapy.

However, unlike factor IX, factor VIII is difficult to efficiently express in vitro. Attempts to induce cultured cells to produce factor VIII can result in the production of misfolded factor VIII protein, which can, in turn, activate the unfolded protein response and trigger apoptosis of the cells. Secondly, the gene that encodes factor VIII is significantly larger than that of factor IX, and, in the absence of complex laboratory manipulations, is too large to fit into the AAV vector.[22] Finally, patients with hemophilia A are more likely to develop circulating inhibitors to factor VIII, making long-term expression of the transduced gene product difficult. For these reasons, gene therapy for hemophilia A lags behind gene therapy for hemophilia B. At least one group has published plans for a clinical trial of an AAV vector–mediated approach to hemophilia A therapy as early as 2015.[22] At present, no gene therapy trials for hemophilia A are registered with ClinicalTrials.gov.

Attempts to use other vectors for the treatment of hemophilia have shown promise, but advancement beyond the preclinical stage has been elusive. Over a decade ago, Roth *et al.* showed that skin-derived fibroblasts could be transfected with the factor VIII gene without the use of a viral vector.[23] When these fibroblasts were injected into the omentum of patients with hemophilia A, some patients experienced less bleeding and had increased factor VIII activity levels. Later studies demonstrated that infusion of a retroviral vector containing the factor VIII gene with a deleted β-domain resulted in a temporary increase of circulating factor VIII in more than half of participants.[5] More recently, Du *et al.* reported that long-term bleeding prophylaxis can be accomplished by inducing factor VIII expression in blood cells, including platelets, using a lentiviral vector to modify gene expression in hematopoietic progenitor cells in a canine model of hemophilia A.[24] Gene therapy to induce platelet-specific expression of factor VIII could one day be used to treat human hemophilia A in patients with factor VIII antibodies (inhibitors).[25] Hopefully, these preclinical and stage I trials will continue to show promise.

Hemoglobinopathies

Hemoglobinopathies such as SCD and thalassemia are some of the most common single-gene defects worldwide. SCD affects approximately 275,000 and β-thalassemia affects approximately 56,000 newborns every year.[26] The current treatment for these diseases is primarily supportive therapy, which includes chronic transfusion for the management of anemia. However, this approach comes with several consequences, including alloimmunization, iron overload, and splenomegaly.[27] While hematopoietic stem cell transplantation is an option as a definitive therapy, very few patients have suitable matched sibling donors, and there is a significant chance of adverse outcomes, including graft-versus-host disease and graft failure.[28] Alternative therapies that lead to decreased reliance on transfusion and other supportive therapies would likely be beneficial to patient outcomes.

Much like hemophilia, the hemoglobinopathies are attractive targets for gene therapy. However, these diseases have been more difficult to treat with this approach as they require large genetic sequences with stable, long-term expression to be effective.[4] In addition, they require a high level of gene expression for correction, which is difficult to achieve with traditional vectors.[4] As of this writing, no approved gene therapies are currently available for the treatment of SCD.[29] Mouse models of SCD have demonstrated that lentiviral vectors carrying an antisickling globin are able to persistently express the globin gene at levels high enough for symptomatic correction.[30] In addition, approaches that use the γ-globin gene with a β-globin promoter, to ensure expression in adults, have been promising in mouse models,[31] and an SCD gene therapy trial recently began enrolling patients.[4]

Clinical trials for the treatment of β-thalassemia with gene therapy have progressed more quickly. Several trials have enrolled patients in phase 1/2 trials in several centers across the United States, but long-term patient outcomes have yet to be reported.[28] A single patient with β^E/β^0-thalassemia, without an HLA-matched hematopoietic stem cell donor, has been reported to have achieved transfusion independence three years after lentiviral β-globin gene transfer.[32]

Other novel approaches to hemoglobinopathies use a gene-editing technique. Although these are not yet available in clinical trials, early studies using induced pluripotent stem cells have shown that TALENs and CRISPRs can be used to correct mutations causing β-thalassemia[33,34] and CRISPRs and ZFNs can be used to correct the SCD mutation.[35,36] Similarly, TALENs have been reported to correct mutations causing α-thalassemia major in induced pluripotent stem cells.[37] With the promising results so far, it is hoped that gene therapies for the hemoglobinopathies will continue to progress quickly through clinical trials.

Wiscott–Aldrich syndrome (WAS)

WAS is a rare, X-linked immune deficiency caused by mutations in the WAS gene. Patients classically present with thrombocytopenia (with small platelets), susceptibility to infections, and eczema.[38]

Affected patients also have an increased risk for the development of autoimmune diseases and cancer.[38] Patients are typically treated with a stem cell transplant, if an HLA-matched donor is available. Patients with WAS may come to the attention of the transfusion service as a result of bleeding in the context of thrombocytopenia.

A phase I/II clinical trial of three pediatric patients with WAS, who lacked an HLA-matched donor or were otherwise ineligible for stem cell transplant, was recently reported.[39] In this trial, autologous CD34+ cells were transduced with a normal WAS gene ex vivo using a lentiviral vector. When the engineered hematopoietic stem cells were infused, they engrafted successfully. The patients went on to demonstrate improvements in hemostasis and immunity.[39] Encouragingly, a similar approach using a lentiviral vector to engineer hematopoietic stem cells for treatment of children with metachromatic leukodystrophy also showed success without apparent evidence of genotoxicity.[40] Although long-term safety monitoring is needed, the results of these trials are promising for patients without HLA-matched stem cell donors suffering from WAS or other diseases.

Summary

Gene therapy continues to offer much promise for the treatment of genetic and acquired diseases. Transfusion medicine laboratories are currently involved in clinical gene therapy trials and, in the future, if these therapeutic modalities are approved, will likely oversee what may be "routine" administration of gene therapy vectors and vector-infected cells.

Disclaimer

The authors have disclosed no conflicts of interest.

Key references

A full reference list for this chapter is available at: http://www.wiley.com/go/simon/transfusion

3 Nathwani AC, Reiss UM, Tuddenham EGD, et al. Long-term safety and efficacy of factor IX gene therapy in hemophilia B. *N Engl J Med* 2014;**371**:1994–2004.

21 Nathwani AC, Tuddenham EGD, Rangarajan S, et al. Adenovirus-associated virus vector-mediated gene transfer in hemophilia B. *N Engl J Med* 2011;**365**:2357–65.

23 Roth DA, Tawa NE, O'Brien JM, et al. Nonviral transfer of the gene encoding coagulation factor VIII in patients with severe hemophilia A. *N Engl J Med* 2001;**344**:1735–42.

34 Xie F, Ye L, Chang JC, et al. Seamless gene correction of β-thalassemia mutations in patient-specific iPSCs using CRISPR/Cas9 and piggyback. *Genome Res* 2014;**24**:1526–33.

35 Huang X, Wang Y, Yan W, et al. Production of gene-corrected adult beta globulin protein in human erythrocytes differentiated from patient iPSCs after genome editing of the sickle point mutation. *Stem Cells* 2015. doi: 10.1002/stem.1969

CHAPTER 39

HLA antigens and alleles

Christian Naper and Bjarte G. Solheim

Institute of Immunology, Oslo University Hospital–Rikshospitalet and University of Oslo, Oslo, Norway

The existence of white cell antigens independent of red cell genetic systems was suggested as early as 1952. In 1958, Jan Dausset[2,3] detected, in a patient who had undergone multiple transfusions, the first leukocyte antibody (toward MAC, or human leukocyte antigen A2 [HLA-A2]). This discovery was followed in 1958 by independent studies on similar antibodies in postpartum serum, reported by van Rood et al.[4] and Payne and Rolfs.[5] These antibodies originally were thought to be autoimmune in nature or to be isoantibodies responsible for febrile (nonhemolytic) transfusion reactions. Early in 1960, Brunning et al.[6] found that these antibodies could be used to detect several diallelic genetic systems present on the cells of most tissues. Until 1964, advances in HLA typing were hampered by inconsistent and nonspecific leukoagglutination testing methods. This status changed with the development of the microlymphocytotoxicity assay by Terasaki and McClelland.[7,8] In a slightly modified form, this test continued to be the standard for clinical HLA typing until the widespread adoption of nucleic-acid-based methods in the 1990s.

In 1964, the first International Histocompatibility Workshop was held. Since then, 15 workshops have been held at 2- to 4-year intervals. These workshops are designed to confirm scientific findings, to develop unifying concepts regarding the major histocompatibility complex (MHC), and to upgrade existing HLA nomenclature. Table 39.1 presents an overview of the workshops, the year, and their major themes. In the third workshop (1967), it was established that the HLA antigens belonged to the same genetic system,[9] and the term HL-A, coined from the Hu leukocyte system of Dausset et al.[10] and the LA system of Payne et al.,[11] was assigned to identify this system. By 1970, it was established through skin-grafting studies with human subjects, particularly families with HLA-identical siblings, that these antigens were important in organ transplantation.[12] In 1973, it became clear from results of one-way mixed leukocyte cultures with homozygous testing cells that other genetic polymorphisms existed within the MHC.[13] Also by 1973, the remarkable association of HLA with certain diseases became apparent.[14,15] In the late 1970s, HLA-D (defined by mixed leukocyte culture) antigens were established,[16] serologically detected antigens on B lymphocytes (HLA-DR [D-related]) were found to be closely related to the HLA-D antigenic products,[17,18] and the existence of the HLA-C locus was confirmed.[19]

From 1980 to 1987, advances in biochemistry, molecular biology, and the development of monoclonal antibodies to the MHC antigenic product markedly expanded knowledge about the MHC. Workshops during this time confirmed the existence of the DQ and DP loci[20,21] and focused on increasingly refined methods for identifying the burgeoning number of HLA alleles and correlation of the serologic, biochemical, and molecular biologic findings related to the MHC. In the 1996 and subsequent four workshops, a primary focus was the use of powerful genomic technology to identify the almost 14,000 MHC alleles now known to exist in human populations around the world.

Major histocompatibility complex

The Class I, II, and III genes of the MHC lie in a 4-megabase region of chromosome 6 (8 megabases if one includes the more telomeric Class I–related gene HFE and the butyrophilin family of genes).[22]

The telomeric 2000 kb of the MHC contains a number of genes, including those encoding the Class I antigens (Figure 39.1). The Class I HLA-A, -B, and -C genes reside in this region, as do the nonclassical MHC-Ib genes HLA-E, -F, and -G. HLA-E, -F, and -G are expressed at lower levels than are the classical genes; do not have the extensive polymorphism of the HLA-A, -B, and -C genes; and appear to have more limited functions in the immune system. Between the HLA-B locus and the tumor necrosis factor loci described later resides the MHC Class I chain-related genes MICA and MICB that encode variants of Class I proteins. They display extensive polymorphism and encode proteins that interact with the activating NKG2D receptor on T cells and NK cells.[23] Finally, the HFE gene responsible for genetic hemochromatosis lies approximately 4.3 megabases telomeric to HLA-A.[24]

Centromeric of the HLA-B locus of the Class I region is a 1-megabase segment traditionally called the Class III region (Figure 39.1).[22] This region has a dense and diverse array of genes, many with as yet unknown functions. Some of these Class III genes encode proteins with functions in innate immunity and inflammation. This region includes the complement components C2, Bf (factor B protein of the alternate pathway of complement activation), and C4. In most persons, the C4 locus is duplicated as C4A and C4B, each encoding a functional, somewhat biochemically different, molecule. Members of the tumor necrosis family also

Unfortunately Dr. Thomas Williams, the original author of this chapter, got seriously ill at the end of 2014 and passed away early in 2015 before having revised his chapter. The current chapter is an updated and slightly revised version of Dr. Williams' chapter from the 4th edition of *Rossi's Principles of Transfusion Medicine*.

Table 39.1 Historical overview of international histocompatibility workshops

International Workshops	Year	Major Theme
I	1964	Comparison of serologic techniques
II	1965	Standardized techniques and nomenclature
III	1967	One major genetic system named HL-A
IV	1970	International antisera analysis
V	1972	Population differences for HLA
VI	1975	Identification of D(DR) locus by cellular techniques; HLA-C locus confirmed
VII	1977	Serologic detection of DR antigens
VIII	1980	Compendium of HLA antigen frequencies
IX	1984	Introduction of RFLP molecular techniques; DQ/DP loci confirmed
X	1987	Standardization and application of RFLP; introduction of PCR/SSOPH typing
XI	1991	Standardization and application of PCR/SSOPH HLA Class II typing to transplantation, disease association, and population genetics
XII	1996	Analysis of Class I and Class II alleles by means of DNA sequencing
XIII	2002	Definition of extent of Class I and II gene variation and application to typing of volunteer donors
XIV	2005	Genomics and immune responses
XV	2008	Applications in clinical medicine, anthropology, etc.; new HLA nomenclature
XVI	2012	Global distribution of KIR genes and ligands; MICA antibodies, HLA IgA antibodies; next-generation sequencing

RFLP, restriction fragment length polymorphism; PCR, polymerase chain reaction; SSOPH, sequence-specific oligonucleotide probe hybridization.

lie within the Class III region. Other genes within the Class III region, such as those encoding 21-hydroxylase enzymes involved in steroid metabolism, have no direct link to immunity. Although linkage to specific HLA alleles may be helpful in assessing 21-hydroxlase deficiency associated with congenital adrenal hyperplasia, direct genotyping is now possible.

The Class II gene loci occupy approximately 1 megabase of DNA centromeric to the Class III region (Figure 39.1).[22] Within this region are 18 closely linked loci that code for the α and β chains of the Class II antigenic proteins. Proceeding from the telomeric to the centromeric boundaries of the region, the first gene cluster is composed of several β-chain loci and one α-chain locus that encode the HLA-DR antigens. The DRB1 locus is responsible for the DR1 to DR18 specificities, whereas the DRB3, DRB4, and DRB5 loci are responsible for the DR52, DR53, and DR51 specificities,

respectively. Each DR specificity is formed by a heterodimer encoded by DRB1, 3, 4, or 5 and the DRA locus. Centromeric to the DRB genes are the DQ genes (Figure 39.1). The DQA1 and DQB1 loci encode the HLA-DQ specificities. Near the centromeric end of the MHC, the genes DPA1 and DPB1 encode the HLA-DP specificities. The Class II region also contains several pseudogenes related to the genes encoding the DR, DQ, and DP antigens, with errors preventing successful transcription and translation. Other genes with important accessory functions to Class I and II antigen presentation are present in the Class II region. The LMP2 and LMP7 genes, the TAP1 and TAP2 genes, and the tapasin gene encode proteins that participate in protein degradation and peptide transport and loading in the Class I system.[25] The HLA-DM and HLA-DO loci encode proteins involved in peptide loading in the Class II system.

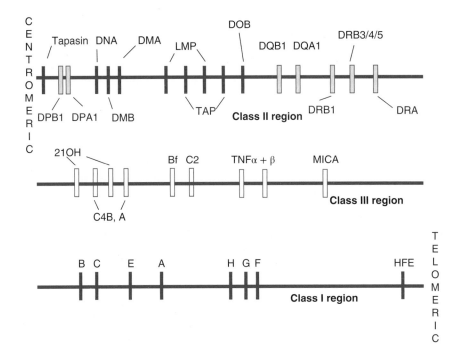

Figure 39.1 Selected genes in the major histocompatibility region on human chromosome 6 in the Class I, II, and III regions. Distances between loci are not drawn to scale. For exact gene locations, see http://www.sanger.ac.uk/HGP/Chr6/MHC.shtml.

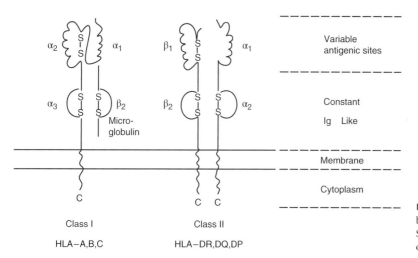

Figure 39.2 Simplified illustration shows the biochemical structure of Class I and II antigens. Source: Strominger *et al.* (1985).[27] Reproduced with permission of Elsevier.

Class I and II antigens and their function

The structure, tissue distribution, and function of the glycoprotein antigenic products of the Class I and Class II genes of the MHC differ considerably. Both Class I and Class II antigens are heterodimeric, having three to four extracellular domains in addition to transmembrane and intracytoplasmic regions (Figure 39.2).[26] Class I antigens are composed of a 45,000-D α heavy chain encoded by the HLA-A, -B, and -C gene loci non-covalently bound to a non-polymorphic 12,000-D light chain, β_2-microglobulin, encoded by a gene locus on chromosome 15. β_2-microglobulin stabilizes the Class I complex. The α chain is a transmembrane protein, whereas β_2-microglobulin is extracellular and bound to the α_3 domain. Domains α_1 and α_2 contain variable amino acid sequences and thus represent the antigenic sites. The α_3 domain has constant sequences homologous to the constant regions of immunoglobulin proteins. The α_3 domain of the heavy chain and β_2-microglobulin are noncovalently associated with each other near the cell membrane. The α_1 and α_2 domains sit on top of them to form a peptide antigen-binding cleft with a floor of eight flat β sheets bound on the sides by two long α helixes, as illustrated in Figure 39.3. Most of the polymorphic amino acid changes of the Class I histocompatibility antigen differences are associated with the floor or sides of this pocket, although some map to other domains.[28,29]

Class II antigens are composed of a 33,000-D α chain non-covalently associated with a 28,000-D β chain (Figure 39.2). The α chain is encoded by the A gene loci and the β chain by the B gene loci in the HLA-D region of the MHC. For example, the DQ antigen α and β chains are encoded by the DQA1 and DQB1 genes,

respectively. The α_1 and β_1 domains are variable and form an antigen-binding groove similar to that described earlier.[30] The α_2 and β_2 domains are relatively constant with immunoglobulin-like homology.

Class I antigens have a universal tissue distribution as plasma membrane proteins of all nucleated cells and platelets. Class II antigens have a limited tissue distribution primarily on antigen-presenting cells such as B lymphocytes, macrophages, and dendritic cells, although they can be induced in several cell types, including endothelial cells.

Class I and II molecules acquire self and nonself peptides in their binding cleft and display them on the plasma membrane of cells for recognition by the T-cell antigen receptor.[25] In the normal state, T cells that bind with high affinity to self peptides in the context of an individual's Class I and II molecules are either deleted or suppressed by a variety of mechanisms to prevent autoimmune disorders. However, peptides derived from viruses, bacteria, and some parasites presented by the Class I and Class II molecules to T-cell antigen receptors evoke an immune response. Class I molecules primarily acquire 8- to 10-amino-acid peptides generated by means of degradation of cytoplasmic proteins in the proteosome system. Class I antigens function as MHC restriction elements in the destruction of virus-infected target cells and present peptides to CD8 cytotoxic T cells. Class II molecules bind 13- to 25-amino-acid peptides of exogenous and endogenous origin degraded within the endosomal system. Class II antigens are MHC restriction elements that augment the sensitizing limb of the immune response and present peptides to CD4 helper T cells. Activation of CD8 and CD4 T cells then results in a program of cell division and differentiation resulting in cellular and humoral immune responses.[25]

Nomenclature and polymorphism of the HLA system

Table 39.2 illustrates the HLA gene loci, the variable polypeptide chains, the number of related serologic specificities, and the number of alleles within each specificity. In the Class I region, the HLA-A, -B, and -C loci are all highly polymorphic with 2800 to 4100 known alleles.[31] Multiple alleles are present within most of the known serotypes. For example, the A2 serotype has more than 700 alleles. In the Class II region, the HLA-DRA locus is almost monomorphic, whereas DRB1 is highly polymorphic, with more than 1800 known alleles. The DQA1 and DQB1 genes and the DPA1 and DPB1 loci demonstrate similar but less extensive polymorphism. The DQA1,

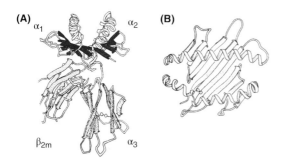

Figure 39.3 (A) Side view of Class I antigen molecule. (B) View of the antigen-binding pocket looking down toward the cell membrane. Source: Bjorkman *et al.* (1987).[28] Reproduced with permission of Nature Publishing.

Table 39.2 HLA nomenclature

Genetic Locus	Encoded Polypeptide	Antigen or Associated Specificity	Alleles	Number of Known Alleles/Polypeptides
HLA-A	α	A1 to A80	A*01:01 to *80:03	3285/2313
HLA-B	α	B5 to B82	B*07:02 to *83:01	4077/3011
HLA-C	α	Cw1 to Cw10	C*01:02 to *18:09	2801/1985
DRA	α		DRA*01:01 to *01:02	7/2
DRB1	β1	DR1 to DR18	DRB1*01:01 to *16:37	1825/1335
DQA1	α		DQA1*01:01 to *06:02	54/32
DQB1	β1	DQ1 to DQ9	DQB1*02:01 to *06:197	876/595
DPA1	α1		DPA1*01:03 to *04:01	42/21
DPB1	β1	DPw1 to DPw6	DPB1*01:01 to *497:01	587/480

The number of polypeptides known for each locus reflects unique amino acid sequences encoded by a larger number of alleles that may differ only by silent polymorphisms.

DPA1, and DPB1 allelic variation can be detected with DNA typing but not with serologic testing.[32] The HLA system is the most polymorphic genetic system known to exist in humans. The number of different phenotypes possible from all combinations of these HLA alleles is greater than the global population. Fortunately, linkage disequilibrium in all human populations results in great overrepresentation of certain haplotypes, which makes finding HLA-identical individuals within a population for purposes such as unrelated stem cell transplantation possible.

Exons in which most of the polymorphism in the Class I (exons 2 and 3) and Class II (exon 2) genes occurs encode the α_1 and α_2 and the α_1 and β_1 domains, respectively, which interact with bound peptides.[31] New alleles appear to emerge at a fairly high rate and become fixed in populations, in theory, if they provide a selective advantage in presenting peptides from infectious organisms. New alleles are generated by means of point mutation, recombination, and gene conversion-like events.[31,32]

The nomenclature of the HLA system is established by an international committee sponsored by the World Health Organization and is updated frequently.[33,34] Table 39.2 shows the general scheme for designating HLA antigens and alleles. Each serologic specificity is prefixed by the genetic system designation HLA-, followed by a letter denoting the encoded antigen (e.g., A, B, C, DR, or DQ). This letter is followed by a digit indicating specificity.[33] For example, the A locus encodes the specificities HLA-A1 through A80; the B locus, HLA-B5 through B82; the C locus, HLA-Cw1 through Cw10; the DRA and DRB1 loci, HLA-DR1 through DR18; and the DQB1 and DQA1 loci, HLA-DQ1 through DQ9.

The nomenclature of the HLA system was first established with serologic data. Molecular data were introduced later according to the precise DNA sequences of each allele. The existing nomenclature had to be modified to accommodate this information. This modification is shown in Table 39.2. For Class I alleles, because only the α chain is variable, the molecular designation is the system (HLA-), the locus (A, B, or C), an asterisk (∗), followed by up to four sets of digits separated by colons. All alleles receive at least a four-digit name, which corresponds to the first two sets of digits; longer names are assigned when necessary. The first set of digits corresponds to the serologic specificity; for example, HLA-A*03:01 is the first molecular allele of the HLA-A3 serologic specificity, and HLA-A*03:02 is the second. In the Class II region, because both the α and β chains can be variable, the locus designation must include the polypeptide chain responsible for the allele. For example, Class II, HLA-DRB1*15:01 is interpreted as HLA system, DR locus, β1 polypeptide chain (B1), DR15 serologic specificity (15 after the asterisk), first molecular allele (01). For molecular alleles that have no serologic equivalents, alleles are sequentially numbered; for

example, HLA-DQA1*01:01 is the first molecular allele of the α_1 polypeptide chain of the DQ. The third and fourth sets of digits are employed to designate alleles with silent polymorphisms or with variation occurring outside exons.

Identification of HLA antigens and alleles

The detection of HLA antigens and alleles is generally accomplished with three basic methods (Table 39.3). The microlymphocytotoxicity assay developed by Terasaki and McClelland[7] of peripheral blood lymphocytes isolated from whole blood has been the standard test for the serologic detection of HLA-A, -B, and -C antigens. This is a complement-dependent test in which the addition of rabbit serum to HLA antibodies fixed to the lymphocyte membrane causes cell death. The endpoint is leakage or retention of fluorescent dyes from lymphocytes with damaged or intact cell membranes, respectively. Modifications of this test, primarily an increase in incubation time and isolation of B lymphocytes from peripheral blood, allow typing for the HLA-DR and -DQ antigens.[17]

Variations of the mixed leukocyte reaction (Table 39.3) with homozygous testing cells, primed lymphocytes, or T-cell clones were the primary methods for detecting HLA-D(R), -DQ, and -DP antigens.[35–37] These methods have now been replaced by nucleic-acid-based techniques.

The application of molecular genetic technology to the field of histocompatibility has led to an unprecedented expansion in knowledge of the MHC at the molecular level. DNA sequences have been obtained for HLA genes and alleles in a variety of populations worldwide.[33] These sequence data have been useful for several reasons.

Table 39.3 Detection of HLA antigens and alleles

Serologic Methods
- HLA-A, -B, and -C: microlymphocytotoxicity test
- HLA-DR and DQ: modified microlymphocytotoxicity test, B-cell-enriched lymphocytes

Cellular Methods
- HLA-D(R) and DQ: one-way mixed lymphocyte reaction (MLR) with
  - Homozygous testing cells
  - Primed lymphocytes (PLT)
  - Cloned T cells
- HLA-DP: MLR in PLT or with T-cell clones

Nucleic-Acid-Based Methods for Class I and II Allele Identification
- Sequence-specific oligonucleotide probe hybridization analysis
- Sequence-specific primer polymerase chain reaction
- Sequence based typing
- Next-generation sequencing

- They have revealed the underlying DNA sequence variations among individuals (and, therefore, amino acid variations) responsible for the antigenic differences in HLA molecules detectable with traditional serologic and cellular HLA testing.
- They have made apparent the fact that results of serologic HLA tests define only broad groups of Class I and Class II alleles. Numerous subgroups of alleles distinguishable by sequence differences are present within these broad serologic groups. The result is a very large number of known alleles.[38]
- Sequence data have allowed detailed definition of the genetic basis of the HLA-mediated disease associations described later in this chapter.
- Knowledge of the DNA sequences of HLA alleles has facilitated the change from serologic and cellular methods to nucleic-acid-based methods.

Several methods have been developed to identify Class I and II alleles. These range from restriction fragment length polymorphism assays to direct DNA sequencing (Table 39.3). Most laboratories have replaced or complemented serologic typing with DNA-based typing methods for several reasons. Precise identification of alleles not possible by serologic means is clinically important in unrelated stem cell transplantation, as discussed later in the chapter. Secondly, nucleic-acid-based typing can help resolve serologic typings compromised by cross-reactivity or complicated by clinical states resulting in pancytopenia or poor expression of HLA antigens on lymphocyte membranes. Thirdly, even in the best circumstances, serologic typing may not be accurate, especially in ethnic groups with great diversity at loci such as HLA-B.[39]

Sequence-specific oligonucleotide probe hybridization

Relevant regions of the Class I and Class II genes are amplified from genomic DNA by means of the polymerase chain reaction (PCR) with two oligonucleotide primers that anneal to 5' and 3' flanking regions that are conserved (are identical) among individuals. Care must be taken in choosing primers to find ones that are locus-specific (e.g., amplify HLA-A but not the related HLA-B locus), that amplify all known alleles at a locus, and that result in roughly equal amplification of the two alleles in a heterozygous individual. After the PCR, the amplified DNA is generally interrogated with allele-specific DNA probes attached to solid supports. Identification of the individual alleles is accomplished by means of hybridization of the PCR products with a series of fluorescently labeled sequence-specific oligonucleotide probes.[40,41] Probes are chosen to anneal to amplified regions of the Class I and II genes that vary from allele to allele. Probes with nucleotide sequences perfectly complementary to the amplified DNA hybridize specifically to the PCR product target and can be detected via fluorescence. With careful control of stringency conditions of hybridization and washing, these probes can detect single-base-pair differences. Alleles are assigned on the basis of panels of positive and negative hybridization reactions with oligonucleotides specific for a particular allele or sequence. Sequence-specific oligonucleotide probe hybridization (SSOPH) typing is complex because it requires a substantial number of oligonucleotide probes to detect and differentiate among the large number of known Class I and II alleles. However, the development of multiplexed methods for SSOPH employing fluorescent microspheres with attached allele-specific probes has greatly improved the ease of use and efficiency of this method and made it a leading means for HLA typing in many laboratories.[42]

Sequence-specific primer polymerase chain reaction

PCR primers are designed so that their 3'-most one or two nucleotides are complementary to base positions within Class I and II genes that differ for different alleles.[43] Sequence-specific primers with 3' ends that anneal perfectly to sequences present in a particular allele or allele subgroup result in productive DNA amplification. Other alleles or allele subgroups are not amplified. Gel electrophoresis can then be used to detect the presence or absence of PCR products of the appropriate size, and hybridization assays are avoided. Sequence-specific PCR is most useful for medium-resolution HLA typing and for initial quick identification of broad antigen groups, such as DR52. Then, SSOPH or DNA sequencing can be used to define microvariants of these specificities, if necessary. Sequence-specific PCR requires 100 or more simultaneously performed PCR assays per patient to identify HLA-A, -B, and -DRB1 allele groups at serologically equivalent resolution. The method requires optimization to avoid failed amplification reactions in each run.

Sequence-based typing

Sequence-based typing has the advantage of requiring only a limited number of primers for the PCR for each HLA locus. There is no need for a series of detecting oligonucleotide probes for each allele. Polymerase chain reaction products are prepared that will encompass the relevant polymorphic positions within the Class I or II gene to be sequenced. Sequencing primers are annealed to the PCR products to generate sequencing ladders that are separated on a high-resolution gel. Any known or previously unknown allele in the population can be identified by means of inspection of the DNA sequence or electropherogram. Electropherograms must be of high quality for accurate detection of heterozygous positions in the sequenced PCR products. The development of high-throughput automated fluorescent DNA-sequencing machines, analysis software, and capillary electrophoresis systems has made this method less cumbersome. Direct sequencing for HLA typing yields unparalleled precision in allele identification. As the number of known Class I and II alleles continues to escalate, the SSOPH and sequence-specific PCR methods have become increasingly complex, making direct sequencing an increasingly attractive method for laboratories.[44,45]

Next-generation sequencing

Several new technology platforms have been developed in the last decade. They produce massive amounts of sequencing data (millions of bases) per run. A major advantage is that the sequences are generated from single molecules. Therefore, there are no complications with heterozygous positions in the sequences. This technology is capable of giving highly accurate full-length gene sequences, including the correct phase of exons. Processing this huge amount of data, however, requires specialized software. Tissue-typing laboratories are now starting to implement this technology.[46]

Choice of HLA typing method

Several factors influence the decision to use one HLA typing method over another. Sequence-specific PCR and reverse SSOPH can be performed in a time (2 to 5 hours) appropriate for clinical situations such as renal transplantation with deceased donors. DNA sequencing is a reasonable approach for situations such as unrelated stem cell transplantation in which allele-level HLA matching of donors and recipients is desired and turnaround times of a few days to a week are acceptable.

Genotypes, phenotypes, and haplotypes

HLA antigens are expressed codominantly. The phenotype of expressed antigens for any given person is not equivalent to the genotype. Because HLA genes are closely linked on chromosome 6, they are inherited in units known as *haplotypes*. Each sibling of a family inherits one of two HLA haplotypes from each parent.

Figure 39.4 illustrates the segregation of haplotypes in a family of seven, focusing on the A, B, Cw, and DR serologic specificities. Analysis of the data for a single individual does not allow assignment of the serologic types present to a specific paternally or maternally derived chromosome; that is, the typing data are unphased. Thus, one cannot be certain whether the DR7 in sibling 3 is present on a chromosome carrying B8 or B13. However, analysis of the typing data for the entire family and the transmission of specificities to the children make it possible to phase each of the pairs of parental chromosomes and to determine haplotypes. For example, one of the paternal chromosome-6 pairs, haplotype [a], contains HLA-A1, Cw4, B35, and DR1; the other paternal chromosome, haplotype [b], includes HLA-A3, Cw7, B8, and DR7. Similarly, the maternal chromosome-6 pairs can be separated as haplotypes [c] and [d]. Each child in this family inherits [a] or [b] from the father and [c] or [d] from the mother. Each child differs from each parent by one HLA haplotype. Because there can be only four parental haplotypes, the chances are 1 in 4 that the siblings will have the same paternal-maternal haplotypes (are HLA-identical), 1 in 2 that siblings will differ by one haplotype, and 1 in 4 that they will differ by two haplotypes. For example, siblings 4 and 5 are HLA-identical, and sibling 4 shares one haplotype with siblings 2 and 3 but no haplotypes with sibling 1. Because siblings 4 and 5 are genetically identical with regard to the MHC, their lymphocytes will not react in mixed leukocyte culture.

The difference between phenotypes and genotypes can be clarified even further with sibling 4 (Figure 39.4) as an example. If family data were not available, this sibling's phenotype would be written as HLA-A3, A24; Cw2, Cw7; B8, B27; DR4, DR7. This implies lack of family data that would allow assignment of the A, C, B, and DR combinations to the appropriate haplotypes. With family data available, however, the genotype is written HLA-A3, Cw7, B8, DR7/A24, Cw2, B27, DR4. The slash in this statement clearly defines the two haplotypes inherited by this child.

Although HLA gene loci are closely linked, there is a low frequency of recombination during meiosis. The crossover rate is approximately 0.8% between the A and B loci and approximately 0.5% between the B and DR loci. For example, 1 of every 200 families exhibits recombination between the B and DR genes.

HLA allele and haplotype frequencies exhibit ethnic variation. Some alleles and haplotypes are widely distributed around the globe, and others are almost exclusively within a particular ethnic group. In population studies, the phenomenon of linkage disequilibrium is apparent in all groups. This term indicates that in randomly mating populations, the haplotype frequency for two or more linked gene loci is significantly higher than would be expected by chance alone. The expected frequency is obtained from the product of the gene frequencies of the involved genes. For example, among persons of European ancestry, the observed A1, B8 haplotype frequency (7.0%) is approximately 4.4 times greater than the expected haplotype frequency (1.6%). These excess haplotype frequencies may exist for a variety of reasons, including high prevalence in the founders of a population and selective pressure from infectious organisms.[47]

Medical and biologic significance of HLA

The HLA system plays a role in several areas of biomedical significance, including the following:

- Antigen presentation;
- Association with certain diseases;
- Organ and stem cell transplantation;
- Platelet transfusion; and
- Population genetics and anthropology.

Tracing the appearance of novel HLA alleles in populations and comparing the frequencies of alleles among populations to gain information about human origins and migration in anthropologic and evolutionary studies is a fascinating field of inquiry but beyond

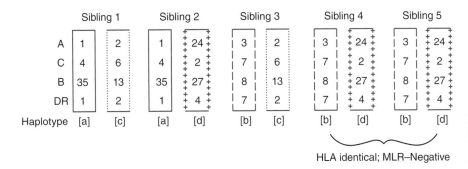

Figure 39.4 HLA-A, -B, -C, and -DR antigens segregating as haplotypes in a family. The data reflect the genotypes of each family member as well as the parental haplotypes.

the scope of this chapter.[48] The extensive polymorphism of the HLA loci has been exploited for many years in identity testing; however, the use of microsatellite loci for this purpose has supplanted the use of HLA loci. The role of HLA Class I typing to support platelet transfusion is described in Chapter 20.

Transplantation

Transplantation poses a special problem in medicine because the extreme polymorphism of the HLA loci makes it unlikely that an unrelated donor of cells, tissues, or organs will be matched at an allele level or at a serologic level with a recipient without a concerted effort to identify matched donors and recipients. One solution is to identify an HLA-identical sibling, but many potential transplant recipients do not have access to these donors. For organ transplantation, powerful immunosuppressant drugs have made transplantation feasible with mismatched living and cadaveric donors and recipients. However, better HLA-A, -B, and -DR matching at a serologic level generally increases the half-life of the transplanted organ and decreases overall morbidity.[49] Thus, deceased donor kidneys are shared on a national and regional basis with waiting recipients who have end-stage renal failure and no mismatches.[50]

Finding well-matched donors of hematopoietic stem cells if there are no HLA-identical siblings is facilitated by resources such as the National Marrow Donor Program, which has enrolled several million potential donors with known HLA types.[51] The goal for unrelated stem cell donation is increasingly allele-level matches for HLA-A, -B, -C, -DRB1, -DQB1 and -DPB1, although the level of mismatching permissable is incompletely understood. Subtle allelic mismatches between stem cell donors and recipients appear to increase the risk of severe graft-versus-host disease and decrease overall survival.[52,53] The use of umbilical cord blood stem cells and the depletion of T cells from transplanted cells may allow greater donor–recipient mismatches.[54,55] Retrospective studies are continuing to assess in a definitive manner the level of matching necessary for successful stem cell transplantation.[56] Hematopoietic stem cell transplantation is discussed in Chapters 36 and 37.

There are two major mechanisms by which Class I and II donor–recipient mismatches may adversely affect transplantation: production of HLA antibodies and cell-mediated rejection. Transplant recipients become sensitized or produce antibodies directed against Class I and Class II specificities through several routes. Exposure to fetal HLA molecules encoded by paternal haplotypes during pregnancy, especially multiple pregnancies, can lead to the presence of long-lasting, high-titer HLA antibodies. Similarly, mismatched HLA antigens from previous organ donors and donors of transfused blood components can lead to sensitization. The presence of recipient preformed HLA antibodies may lead to hyperacute rejection of a donor organ bearing the relevant HLA specificities.[26] Therefore, laboratories maintain serum-screening programs to detect and identify HLA antibodies in waiting recipients so that inappropriate donors can be avoided. Immediately before transplantation, crossmatches to detect donor-directed HLA antibodies are performed between donor lymphocytes and recipient serum by means of the microcytotoxicity assays described in this chapter or more sensitive flow cytometric technology.[57]

Donor HLA antigens mismatched with recipient HLA antigens can elicit a strong cell-mediated immune response. As many as 10% of a recipient's T cells are able to recognize and respond to donor-mismatched HLA antigen.[58] These responses contribute to acute rejection in organ transplantation and graft-versus-host disease in stem cell transplantation. HLA matching and immunosuppressive therapy help to mitigate this problem.

Disease association

The association of certain HLA alleles and their encoded antigens with particular diseases, especially autoimmune disorders, has been known for some time. In more than 40 disorders, there is significant deviation in the frequency of HLA antigens from that of healthy controls (Table 39.4).[59] In general, HLA-associated diseases have certain common features. They are known or suspected to have an inherited component, usually have autoimmune features, and display a clinical course often featuring repeated acute relapses followed by remission. For most HLA-associated diseases, the etiologic factor is unknown and the pathophysiologic mechanism is incompletely understood. One hypothesis for the link between HLA antigens and disease suggests that a necessary but not sufficient requirement for disease development is the differential ability of a Class I or II heterodimer encoded by a specific allele to present autoantigens to the T-cell receptor.

Two of the strongest HLA associations are the $DQB1^*06:02$ allele with narcolepsy[60] and B^*27 alleles with ankylosing spondylitis.[59] Almost all patients with narcolepsy have the associated alleles; approximately 90% of patients with ankylosing spondylitis have the associated alleles. In populations without these disorders, the frequencies of $DQB1^*06:02$ (25% to 30%) and of the B^*27 group (5% to 10%) are substantial but do not approach the frequencies among

Table 39.4 Selected diseases associated with HLA alleles

Disorder	HLA Linkage	Comments
Class I and II Associations		
Ankylosing spondylitis	B^*27 alleles	Absence of B^*27 may be useful in ruling out diagnosis of ankylosing spondylitis.
Narcolepsy	$DQB1^*06:02$	DQB1 locus or linked loci and alterations in hypocretin or orexin peptides/receptors contribute to narcolepsy.
Celiac disease	$DQ2.5$, $DQ2.2$, and $DQ8$	The absence of DQB1*02 is a strong negative predictor of disease.
Type 1 diabetes mellitus	$DRB1^*03/^*04$, $DQB1^*02$, and ^{*03} alleles	Presence of $DRB1^*03/^*04$ confers a 25-fold relative risk.
Rheumatoid arthritis	$DRB1^*04$ alleles sharing epitope encoded by codons 67–74	May be most useful in predicting severity of disease.
Latency period before onset of AIDS	Multiple loci and alleles	Latency period shortened by homozygosity at loci and modified by multiple susceptibility and resistance alleles.
Abacavir hypersensitivity	$B^*57:01$	Abacavir hypersensitivity is largely a result of inheritance of $B^*57:01$.
Mutation of Nonimmune Response Genes within the MHC		
21-Hydroxlase deficiency	Diagnosis by direct CYP21 genotyping	Linked to cosegregating HLA haplotypes in families.
Complement component 2 (C2) deficiency	Diagnosis by assessment of complement levels	
Hemochromatosis	Diagnosis by direct HFE genotyping	HFE is a Class I–related gene at the telomeric end of the MHC.

persons with these disorders. Thus, the antigens involved are not unique to narcolepsy and ankylosing spondylitis but are overrepresented among affected persons. Approximately 3% of persons with a B^*27 allele have ankylosing spondylitis, a risk approximately 100-fold greater than that among persons without B^*27. Results of HLA testing that show the absence of $DQB1^*06:02$ or B^*27 alleles are useful to help rule out a diagnosis of narcolepsy or ankylosing spondylitis for a patient. Results that show the presence of these alleles are less useful because of the prevalence of these alleles in the general population.

Celiac disease[61] occurs almost exclusively in individuals that express HLA-DQ2.5, -DQ2.2, or -DQ8. Ninety percent of the patients express the DQ2.5 heterodimer (DQA1*05, DQB1*02). Five percent of the patients express DQ2.2 (DQA1*02:01, DQB1*02:02), and 5% express DQ8 (DQA1*03, DQB1*03:02). The α and β chains of DQ2.5 may be encoded by the same chromosome (*cis* configuration) or different chromosomes (*trans* configuration).[62] Most commonly, it is encoded in *cis* by the DR3–DQ2 (DQB1*02:01–DQA1*05:01–DRB1*03:01) haplotype, but may also be encoded in *trans* by the DR5–DQ7 (DQB1*03:01–DQA1*05:05–DRB1*11/12) and DR7–DQ2 (DQB1*02:02–DQA1*02:01–DRB1*07) haplotypes.[63]

The association of HLA antigens with most other autoimmune disorders usually does not carry the high relative risk that narcolepsy, ankylosing spondylitis, and celiac disease do. Although these HLA associations are generally less useful in diagnosis, they provide important insights into the pathophysiologic mechanism of these diseases and may help assess prognosis. For example, approximately 95% of patients with type 1 diabetes mellitus (formerly known as insulin-dependent diabetes mellitus) have either the $DRB1^*03$ or the $DRB1^*04$ allele or both.[64] Patients heterozygous for $DRB1^*03/^*04$ have a relative risk for type 1 diabetes mellitus three to six times greater than that of patients with $DRB1^*03$ or $DRB1^*04$ alone or in combination with another $DRB1$ allele. Susceptibility to type 1 diabetes mellitus appears to be linked to haplotypes containing $DRB1^*03$ or $DRB1^*04$ with $DQB1^*02$ and $DQB1^*03$ alleles.

Many persons with rheumatoid arthritis have inherited $DRB1^*04$ alleles encoding a common epitope. Heterozygosity and homozygosity for alleles encoding this epitope may be predictive of a more severe course of arthritis. Thus, allele identification may be helpful in assessing prognosis.[65]

A number of studies have been performed in an attempt to define specific HLA alleles that confer susceptibility or resistance to AIDS (Table 39.4).[66,67] There appear to be HLA alleles that interact with other genetic and environmental factors to influence the outcome of this multifactorial disease. However, results may vary somewhat among studies given the complexity of AIDS, differences in the ethnicity of the populations studied, and the subtypes of the human immunodeficiency virus type 1 involved. Recently, hypersensitivity to the antiretroviral drug abacavir was linked to the presence of $HLA-B^*57:01$ in treated patients.[68,69] Near complete elimination of hypersensitivity morbidity was achieved by first screening patients to exclude the 5% to 10% with $B^*57:01$ from exposure to this agent. In this example, HLA allele identification serves as a pharmacogenomic test to stratify a patient population for targeted therapy.

Because the MHC contains genes with no obvious role in immune system function, some diseases caused by point mutation or deletion of genes in this region cause disorders not directly related to immunity. However, because of linkage disequilibrium, overrepresentation of specific Class I or Class II antigens may occur in these disorders. Congenital adrenal hyperplasia is caused by mutations in the MHC Class III region genes encoding 21-hydroxylase.[70] Although linkage to specific HLA alleles is present in persons with congenital adrenal hyperplasia, direct genotyping is generally preferable for diagnostic purposes. Similarly, genetic hemochromatosis is caused by mutations in the HFE gene telomeric to the HLA-A locus.[24] Although the presence of A^*03 confers several-fold excess risk of hemochromatosis, the most direct route to genetic diagnosis is HFE genotyping.

Summary

The HLA loci on chromosome 6 are composed of a series of Class I and II genes that display a degree of naturally occurring polymorphism unmatched within the rest of the human genome. This polymorphism appears to be maintained to ensure appropriate responses to the infectious organisms encountered by global human populations. The crucial role of the Class I and II molecules is to bind the degradation products of proteins and present them to T-cell antigen receptors for recognition as endogenous or foreign peptides. MHC polymorphism has several consequences in medicine and biology beyond the normal immune response: (1) MHC genetic variation can be exploited as a tool for anthropologic study of human migration and development; (2) specific HLA alleles are associated with a propensity to development of particular disease entities, especially autoimmune disorders; and (3) the challenge of finding HLA-matched donors and recipients presents special problems in stem cell and organ transplantation.

Disclaimer

The authors have disclosed no conflicts of interest.

Key references

A full reference list for this chapter is available at: http://www.wiley.com/go/simon/transfusion

1 Complete human MHC sequence. Cambridge, UK: Wellcome Trust Sanger Institute, 2001. http://www.sanger.ac.uk/HGP/Chr6/MHC.shtml

21 Bodmer WF. The HLA system, 1994. In: Albert ED, Baur MP, Mayr WR, eds *Histocompatibility testing 1984*. Berlin: Springer-Verlag, 1984:11–22.

27 Strominger JL. Human histocompatibility antigens: genes and proteins. In: Pernis B, Vogel HJ, eds *Cell biology of the major histocompatibility complex*. New York: Academic Press, 1985:17–24.

28 Bjorkman PJ, Saper MA, Samraoui B, *et al.* Structure of the human Class I histocompatibility antigen, HLA-A2. *Nature* 1987;**329**:506–12.

29 Bjorkman PJ, Saper MA, Samraoui B, *et al.* The foreign antigen binding site and T cell recognition regions of Class I histocompatibility antigens. *Nature* 1987;**329**:512–18.

30 Brown JH, Jardetzky TS, Gorga JC, *et al.* The three-dimensional structure of the human Class II histocompatibility antigen HLADR1. *Nature* 1993;**364**:33–9.

58 Murphy KM, Travers P, Walport M. Antigen presentation to T lymphocytes. In: *Janeway's immunobiology*. 8th ed. New York: Garland Science, 2012:201–237.

60 Pelin Z, Guilleminault C, Risch N, *et al.* HLA-DQB1*0602 homozygosity increases relative risk for narcolepsy but not disease severity in two ethnic groups. US Modafinil in Narcolepsy Multicenter Study Group. *Tissue Antigens* 1998;**51**:96–100.

63 Megiorni F, Pizzuti A. *HLA-DQA1* and *HLA-DQB1* in Celiac disease predisposition: practical implications of the HLA molecular typing. *J Biomed Sci* 2012;**19**:88.

CHAPTER 40

Tissue banking

Ralph M. Powers[1] & Jeanne V. Linden[2]

[1]Institute of Regenerative Medicine, LifeNet Health, Virginia Beach, VA, USA

[2]Blood and Tissue Resources, Wadsworth Center, New York State Department of Health, Albany, NY, USA

In the United States, organ and tissue procurement has been organized in such a way so as to maximize availability in an efficient fashion that is fair to both donor and recipient. There is a growing cooperation between organ procurement organizations (OPOs) and tissue recovery organizations to facilitate meeting the requirements of both organ and tissue procurement. Successful tissue preservation has encouraged the use of bone and soft tissue grafts, cardiovascular tissue, and skin in the clinical setting. Semen cryobanking has been practiced for many years, and the demand for embryo banking services has greatly increased recently as assisted reproductive procedures have become more diverse and much more widely available. As technology in this area continues to improve, hospital transfusion services may play an increasingly important role in coordinating, supporting, and directing transplantation and transplant-related interventions.

Growth of tissue banking

Each year, hundreds of thousands of patients benefit from donated bone, cartilage, ligament, and tendon used to reconstruct and rehabilitate joints and other bony structures; corneas to restore sight; skin to treat burns and wounds and reconstruct soft tissues; veins and great vessels to restore blood flow; heart valves to restore cardiac function; and reproductive tissue to treat infertility. In addition to whole grafts and sections, bone, in particular, can be machined into specialized allografts. It can also be ground and further treated to become demineralized bone matrix (DBM), which is available as a ground powder or as combination forms such as gels, pastes, strips, and even moldable grafts designed to avoid migration in specific applications. Myriad types of tissues are transplanted in a variety of medical and dental specialties for diverse clinical applications (Table 40.1).[1] The most commonly transplanted allografts are bone, musculoskeletal soft tissue, and corneas.

The total number and range of tissues collected, processed, and transplanted in the United States are difficult to determine, in the absence of a national reporting system. Organ statistics, in contrast, are readily available through a number of organizations (donatelife.net and UNOS.org). In 1999, tissue banks accredited by the American Association of Tissue Banks (AATB) distributed approximately 750,000 allografts for transplantation. By 2003, the figure had more than doubled. By 2007, more tissue banks became accredited and the figure had nearly tripled.[2] The quantity of musculoskeletal (bone and soft tissue) allografts distributed annually is greater than 2,000,000 units.[2] A focused survey revealed this number had increase by at least 10% during 2012 (personal communication, Scott Brubaker, Senior Vice President, Policy, the AATB). Skin is distributed at the rate of about 30,000 square feet annually. Distribution of cryopreserved allograft heart valves is now estimated at >6000 annually.[3] Cornea transplants numbered >72,000 in 2013.[4]

In addition to such tissues from deceased donors, many tissues for clinical use are derived from living donors, including semen and oocytes for use in artificial insemination and assisted reproductive technology procedures as well as dermis for various soft tissue reconstruction procedures. In 2005, New York State–licensed semen banks located throughout the United States processed 27,118 ejaculates from 962 semen donors. In addition, semen from 16,347 client depositors was collected and cryopreserved for later use by the client depositor's wife or other "intimate partner" (New York State Department of Health, unpublished data, 2005). Donor oocytes were used in approximately 13% of all assisted reproductive technology cycles carried out in the United States in 2012.[5] Tissue from living donors is also considered by some to include human milk to nourish low-birthweight, premature infants. The Human Milk Banking Association of North America reports the existence of 16 active member banks.[6] The US Food and Drug Administration (FDA), however, does not subject human milk to regulations that apply to human allograft tissue.

Because no comprehensive national usage figures are available, it is difficult to determine the rate of increase in the demand for tissues. However, novel uses for tissue in transplantation have emerged that had not been envisioned even a few years ago. Amniotic membrane is transplanted to correct epithelial eye and soft tissue defects (e.g., ulcers); bioengineered skin allografts are used for wound healing; and nerve tissue is transplanted to serve as a conduit for nerve regeneration in damaged limbs. In late 1998, the medical world was fascinated by the first hand transplant surgery; there have been at least 65 worldwide since.[7] The world's first face transplant procedure was performed in November 2005. Since then, more than 20 patients have received full or partial face transplants at institutions around the world.[8] In the future, human pluripotent progenitor cells from embryos may be used in the treatment of a variety of diseases considered incurable at this time (Parkinson, diabetes, and spinal cord injuries as examples).

Rossi's Principles of Transfusion Medicine, Fifth Edition. Edited by Toby L. Simon, Jeffrey McCullough, Edward L. Snyder, Bjarte G. Solheim, and Ronald G. Strauss.
© 2016 John Wiley & Sons, Ltd. Published 2016 by John Wiley & Sons, Ltd.

Table 40.1 Some common human allograft applications, by specialty

Specialty	Procedure/Application	Allograft Types Used
General orthopedics	Trauma/fracture repair; osseous defect repair; acetabular repair; total joint revision/arthroplasty	Femoral head; femoral condyle; whole, proximal, or distal bone shaft (femur, tibia, humerus); hemi-pelvis; cancellous bone; corticocancellous bone; cortical strut/screw/pin; bi-cortical strip; tri-cortical wedge; whole joint* (knee, ankle, shoulder, elbow); osteoarticular graft*; osteochondral graft*; DBM; osteobiologics
Sports medicine	Tendon, anterior cruciate ligament, posterior cruciate ligament, other knee ligament repair; meniscus repair/replacement; osteochondral defects; rotator cuff repair; ankle/tendon ligament repair; hand/wrist repair	Patellar ligament; Achilles tendon; tibialis tendon; semitendinosus tendon; gracilis tendon; peroneus longus tendon; fascia lata; rotator cuff; meniscus; meniscus w/tibial plateau; osteochondral plug*; femoral hemi-condyle*; acellular dermal matrix
Craniofacial/ maxillofacial	Cranial reconstruction; maxillary/mandibular reconstruction; facial palsy repair	Mandible; dura mater*; pericardium; fascia lata; acellular dermal matrix; bi-cortical strip; tri-cortical wedge; DBM; osteobiologics; sclera
Dental	Alveolar ridge augmentation for dental implant placement; onlay grafting; sinus elevations/augmentation; socket/ridge preservation; intrabony defect repair	DBM; osteobiologics; sclera; acellular dermal matrix; particulate and structural cortical and cancellous grafts and combinations
Ophthalmology	Postcataract corneal edema repair; Fuchs dystrophy repair; glaucoma drainage valve implantation; corneo-scleral fistula repair; keratoconus correction; phaco burn repair; orbital reconstruction following enucleation; eyelid ectropion repair; eyelid reconstruction	Cornea*; sclera*; pericardium
Neurosurgical	Cervical/lumbar interbody fusion; intermedullary rod placement; dura replacement	Dura mater*; fascia lata; pericardium; cancellous bone; corticocancellous bone; cortical strut; bi-cortical strip; various machined and constructed proprietary bone forms*; amniotic membrane*; acellular dermal matrix
Burn treatment	Wound covering†	Fresh skin*; cryopreserved skin*; freeze-dried skin*; acellular dermal matrix; amniotic membrane*
General surgery	Urologic incontinence procedure; pelvic floor reconstruction; herniorrhaphy; breast reconstruction	Fascia lata; pericardium; lyophilized skin*; acellular dermal matrix
Cardiac	Congenital anomaly repair (both valve and outflow tract major vessel repair/replacement†); cardiac valve and vessel repair/replacement; major vessel blood "shunting" procedures	Aortic valve*; pulmonary valve*; various conduit-use-only grafts* from the ascending aorta or thoracic aorta or from the pulmonary artery trunk or its branches
Vascular	Vaso-occlusive disease (peripheral, abdominal, thoracic); cardiac artery bypass grafting; arteriovenous shunt insertion; muscle-flap or organ transplant vascular bed extensions; replacement of infected prosthetic devices	Greater saphenous vein*; aorto-iliac artery*; iliac vein*; iliac artery*; femoral vein*; femoral artery*

* Not sterilized.
† Can be life-saving.
DBM, demineralized bone matrix.
Source: Eisenbrey *et al.* (2008).[1] Reproduced with permission of American Association of Blood Banks.

Tissue donation

Living donors

The tissue most commonly donated by living donors is blood, the primary subject of this book, but living donors also provide other tissues. Tissue donation by a living person generally is limited to renewable tissue, such as gametes, extraembryonic tissue, and milk. Except for autografts, which can be expanded by culturing for use on burned patients, skin is usually recovered from deceased donors. Cartilage can also be cultured for autologous transplant in knee repair. Bone can be obtained from living donors in the form of a femoral head, or a tibial plateau that is removed and would otherwise be discarded (e.g., a total hip or knee replacement with a prostheses). Outside the United States, such surgical bone banking remains a significant source of bone grafts in many countries.

Deceased donors

In contrast to organ donors, tissue donors (excluding living donors, of course) need no functioning circulation. Tissues such as bone, eyes, and skin can generally be collected up to 24 hours after cessation of the donor's cardiac and respiratory functions, depending on the temperature and environment in which the donor body is stored. Tissues such as bone and skin can be donated by deceased organ donors (a standard criterion for organ donors in the United States is brain death), but more commonly, tissues are donated by other hospitalized patients who have been judged deceased by both cardiorespiratory and neurologic criteria. Tissue procurement

practices have become more effective as a result of increased cooperation between tissue banks and OPOs, through routine referral requirements.[9] Referrals to eye banks are also made through OPOs.

The availability of tissues for transplantation depends on strong public support, the presence of laws that clear legal barriers to donation and that authorize consent (authorization) before death (through such means as driver's licenses, donor registries, and advance directives), and the availability of health professionals trained in how to approach the next of kin or other authorizing person on the subject of donation. (The next of kin is/are usually a deceased person's closest relative[s], as determined by a hierarchy specified in state law as defined by the Uniform Anatomical Gift Act.)

In the late 1980s, most states enacted "required request" laws that sought to increase the supply of organs and tissues by requiring that hospital personnel request permission of the next of kin for organ and tissue donation at the time of a patient's death (if the prospective donor was medically eligible). Following findings that families were more likely to consent to donation if approached by requesters who had received training in the most effective ways to present donation opportunities, some states amended these laws to require referral of all deaths to an OPO or designated tissue bank, whose specially trained requesters would then ask for consent. Federal routine referral requirements were implemented by the Health Care Financing Administration (now the Centers for Medicare and Medicaid Services) in Hospital Conditions of Participation for

Organ, Tissues, and Eye Donation, which became effective August 21, 1998.[9] These rules mandate, as a condition of Medicaid and Medicare reimbursement, that all hospitals establish formal relationships with an OPO in the service area, with a tissue bank, and with an eye bank. Further, the rules require that hospital personnel notify OPOs of all deaths and imminent deaths so that potential donors are identified, and so that the next of kin will be approached about donation, when appropriate. Under routine referral, the costs associated with around-the-clock reporting of deaths and imminent deaths are proving to be high in certain areas, although the cost to OPOs is shared by Medicare and the transplanting hospitals through "standard acquisition charges" applied to individual organs transplanted. Uniform Anatomical Gift Laws were developed to standardize state requirements for first party consent, requesting personnel, and recovery. A 2006 revised version, which expanded definitions, clarified roles, and enhanced focus on personal autonomy, has been enacted in nearly every state (see http://uniformlaws.org). The National Association of Attorneys General adopted a resolution in 2010 in support of respecting and upholding the decisions made by persons who elect to be organ, eye, and tissue donors.[10]

Organization of tissue banking in the United States

Unlike the organ procurement and sharing system, tissue banking is not formally organized based on geography. There are approximately 21 independent tissue banks that process conventional musculoskeletal tissue, four that process cardiovascular tissue, and 14 that process skin. Although most are not-for-profit, a few for-profit companies process human tissue for transplantation. Processors usually independently perform donor eligibility assessment and laboratory testing, even if the tissue bank that recovered the tissue had already performed such steps. There are approximately 80 not-for-profit eye banks accredited by the Eye Bank Association of America (EBAA; see http://www.restoresight.org). Almost all cornea allografts are provided by these eye banks. Blood centers with expertise in donor recruitment, donor eligibility determination, cell cryopreservation, and compliance with standards and regulations are good candidates to undertake tissue banking services. A few blood centers have taken on the challenge of providing comprehensive tissue bank services, and they recover, process, store, and distribute tissues.

Procedures to achieve allograft safety and efficacy are guided by national professional standards set by such organizations as AATB,[11] EBAA,[12] and the American Society for Reproductive Medicine.[13] The FDA and some states have regulatory and licensure requirements (see the "Oversight" section).

Tissue transplant-transmissible diseases and their prevention

Transmissible diseases

Despite a careful donor selection process, the risk of donor-to-recipient transmission of viral, bacterial, fungal, and prion diseases cannot be eliminated (Table 40.2).[14,15] In one well-publicized case, 48 organ or tissue recipients received an organ or tissue from a single donor who, although he had no apparent risk for HIV infection according to medical history, proved to have been recently infected with HIV and in the window period before HIV-1 antibody could be detected by the assays in use at the time (October 1985).[14] All four organ recipients became infected with HIV, but the

Table 40.2 Infectious diseases reported to have been transmitted by deceased donor allografts

Allografts	Infectious Disease
Bone	Hepatitis C
	Hepatitis, unspecified type
	Human immunodeficiency virus type 1
	Bacteria
	Tuberculosis
	Fungus
Cornea	Hepatitis B
	Rabies
	Creutzfeldt–Jakob disease
	Cytomegalovirus (?)
	Bacteria
	Fungus
Dura mater	Creutzfeldt–Jakob disease
Heart valve	Hepatitis B
	Tuberculosis
	Fungus
Skin	Bacteria
	Cytomegalovirus (?)
	Human immunodeficiency virus type 1 (?)
Pericardium	Creutzfeldt–Jakob disease
	Bacteria
Pancreatic islet	Bacteria

Source: Adapted from Eastlund.[15]

majority of tissue recipients did not. Whole unprocessed frozen bone did transmit HIV to three recipients, whereas bone from which the marrow had been removed did not; transplanted corneas, lyophilized soft tissue, and γ-irradiated dura mater also did not transmit the virus. This case additionally served to highlight vulnerabilities associated with inadequate disposition records, given that six recipients could not be identified from hospital records. In 2002, before routine implementation of hepatitis C virus (HCV) nucleic acid testing (NAT) for tissue donors, tissue from a man with no identifiable infectious disease risk by history or physical examination, and a negative test for anti-HCV, was found to have transmitted HCV to recipients.[16] All organ recipients who could subsequently be tested were found to be infected with HCV. Among 32 tissue recipients, five probable cases occurred: one of two saphenous vein recipients, one of three tendon recipients, and three of three recipients of tendon with bone allografts. No cases occurred in recipients of skin, cornea, or irradiated bone. All eight recipients whose infection was linked to the transplant were determined to be infected with the same HCV genotype. The current risk of viral transmission is thought to be exceedingly low[17,18] as a result of stringent donor selection, testing strategies, and processing methods now in use that reduce the risk for tissues not requiring viable cells.

West Nile virus transmission linked to breastfeeding of a woman's own infant, to organ transplantation, and to blood transfusion have been reported,[19] but transmission through donor tissue has not been observed. Chagas' disease has been linked to transplantation of organs but transmission of parasitic diseases through vascular tissue allografts (considered likely to be possible) has not been reported.[20,21] Although vessel grafts associated with organ transplantation, in which arteries or veins from a different donor may be used if the donor and/or recipient vessels are damaged or insufficient, are not considered tissue by the FDA, such grafts caused documented transmission of rabies to two recipients in 2004.[22] Transmission of malignancy via tissue transplantation has not been reported, but is thought to be possible. Infectious diseases can also be transmitted through transplantation of tissue from living donors. Cases are well documented in the semen banking arena with a variety of agents and diseases having been transmitted to semen recipients. Human immunodeficiency virus, type 1 (HIV-1) has been transmitted both by unrelated donors and from husband to wife. This virus has the greatest number of reports of transmission. Hepatitis B virus (HBV), gonorrhea, *Ureaplasma urealyticum*, *Mycoplasma hominis*, *Trichomonas vaginalis*, *Chlamydia trachomatis*, group B *Streptococcus*, and herpes simplex virus type 2 (HSV-2) have also been reported. Transmission of HCV and human T-cell lymphotropic virus, type 1 (HTLV-1) is likely, and transmission of cytomegalovirus, human papilloma virus, and syphilis is a possibility.[23]

In addition, transmission has occurred with the use of bone removed during surgery, such as a femoral head collected during hip arthroplasty.[15]

Transmission of bacteria is a known risk of tissue transplantation. Bacteria can be present in the donor, either as a normal occurrence or as the result of a disease process or medical intervention.[15] Resuscitation efforts can increase the dispersion of such organisms. In addition, agonal bacteremia is a well-known process whereby endogenous bacteria, such as normal intestinal flora, begin to disperse throughout the body after cessation of cardiopulmonary functions, as the putrefaction process begins. This process is accelerated in persons with sepsis, rhabdomyolysis, or a cocaine overdose before death.[15] Bacteria can be introduced during tissue recovery; during processing, whether through cross contamination, insufficient aseptic technique, or contaminated chemicals or solutions; or even during packaging. Some tissues, including ocular tissue, skin, and semen, are inherently not sterile even if collected aseptically; fortunately, the contaminants are primarily skin contaminants with low virulence in most recipients, and are susceptible to standard antibiotics.

At particular risk for transmission of bacteria are the articular cartilage allografts used in knee surgery, because these cannot be subjected to extensive processing if their mechanical properties and chondrocyte viability are to be preserved (note, however, that the latter has not been proven to be essential). In 2001, a 23-year-old man was found to have died from *Clostridium sordellii* sepsis following receipt of a femoral condyle allograft. An extensive investigation identified 14 patients who had received allografts between 1998 and 2002 and who developed postoperative infections with *Clostridium* species.[15,24] The tissues were derived from nine donors, but all were prepared by the same processor, and investigation identified several factors that could have contributed to the infections. Although the tissues were cultured, they had already been suspended in antimicrobial solutions, likely leading to false-negative results. Additionally, for two of the donors, including the donor of the tissue that was implicated in the fatal case, the interval between death and refrigeration of the body (19 hours for the donor in the fatal case) exceeded the industry's voluntary standards at the time of 15 hours maximum without refrigeration of the deceased donor. This likely permitted excessive bacterial proliferation prior to tissue recovery. In addition, tissue was processed aseptically without the use of terminal sterilization, and the processing methods used had not been validated. Human error can also lead to release of contaminated tissues. In one case, a technician failed to follow standard procedures, resulting in release of tissue labeled as having been subjected to irradiation when, in fact, no irradiation had occurred.[25] However, a wound infection in a tissue recipient, or even disseminated bacteremia, does not necessarily implicate the donor tissue. Site infections are a well-known risk of many surgical procedures and can result from the use of contaminated solutions or equipment insufficiently sterilized between procedures.[26]

Risk reduction procedures

After death has been declared and authorization for donation has been given, the process of determining the suitability of the potential deceased donor begins. The risk of disease transmission is minimized by collection and careful review of (1) information obtained during interviews with family member(s) or other knowledgeable historian(s) and healthcare providers; (2) available medical records; (3) findings of a physical assessment; (4) results of an autopsy, if performed; and (5) results of blood tests for infectious disease markers. Procedures for processing and, in some cases, sterilizing tissues also contribute to tissue safety.

Donor history screening

Evaluation of the health and behavioral risk history of the prospective donor is an important step in establishing the suitability of tissues for transplantation and preventing the transmission of infectious diseases. Family members may be able to provide reliable medical and behavior information, but friends and associates may provide relevant information not known to family members, especially the legal next of kin. Medical personnel may also be aware of significant medical and risk information. General donor eligibility criteria include the absence of systemic infection or any infectious or malignant disease transmissible by tissues and of behavioral risks for HIV infection or viral hepatitis. Malignancy generally disqualifies the donor, unless the malignancy is nonmetastatic or not known to metastasize to the tissue to be recovered (e.g., virtually no cancer is known to metastasize to the eye or skin), and there is no suspicion of direct regional spread. The donor history screening is specifically designed to reject those at high risk for viral hepatitis or HIV (e.g., nonmedical injected drug users, men who have had sex with another man in the past five years, persons who exchanged sex for money or drugs, persons with hemophilia or related clotting disorders, and persons with recent significant incarceration or with symptoms suggestive of a current viral infection).[11]

Beyond the general selection criteria for donors, there are specific eligibility criteria for each tissue type, to facilitate selection of tissues that will function adequately, as well as those that will not transmit disease. For bone and soft tissue, these include such factors as: donor age, for bone that is intended to be used for weight-bearing functions; no evidence of significant metabolic bone disease or a connective tissue disorder; and no exposure to toxic substances that could accumulate in the tissue to be recovered. Donors of cardiac tissues are screened for a history of significant valvular disease or cardiac infection, and vascular donors may be determined ineligible if there is a history of diabetes, vasculitis, varicose veins, or significant atherosclerosis. Cardiac and vascular tissue donations are also limited by age restrictions per AATB standards and individual tissue bank policy. When skin is recovered, areas of skin exhibiting signs of a skin infection, or where a rash, nevus, or tattoo is present, are avoided. Cornea donors cannot have a history of refractive corneal procedures, such as radial keratotomy. Also per EBAA and AATB standards, tissue recovery sites in deceased donors are evaluated for trauma and infection and tissue should not be recovered from sites found to be damaged or contaminated. Donors of reproductive cells or tissues are screened for evidence or risk of inheritable diseases, and there are age restrictions. Extraembryonic tissue such as amnion and umbilical vein require the delivery to be full term; meconium staining of amniotic fluid is not acceptable, and there can be no current pelvic or vaginal infection in the mother. Consent is obtained from both parents.

In an effort to improve the efficacy and uniformity of the donor history acquisition process, a multiorganizational project team was established to develop a standardized donor history questionnaire and materials, modeled after the acceptable full-length donor history questionnaire and accompanying materials for blood donors. The project team included members from the AATB, Association of Organ Procurement Organizations, EBAA, NATCO (formerly the North American Transplant Coordinators Organization), Centers for Disease Control and Prevention (CDC), FDA, Health Resources Services Administration (HRSA), United Network for Organ Sharing (UNOS), and Health Canada. The goal was to eliminate questions that do not contribute significant information, and to develop simple and concise questions that employ terminology easily understood by the lay public. The effort produced a standardized form to serve as a guide for donor history information collection by tissue banks. Use of the form is not intended to be mandatory, but is designed to facilitate effective history collection, in compliance with regulatory and professional standards requirements and is highly recommended. The "Donor Risk Assessment Interview" form was made available by the AATB in 2012.

Donor physical assessment

The physical assessment seeks evidence that is consistent with risk for infectious diseases that would disqualify the donor. Such findings include unexplained jaundice or icterus; enlarged lymph nodes; unexplained white lesions in the oral cavity; blue or purple spots on the skin (possible Kaposi sarcoma); signs of nonmedical injected drug use; unexplained hepatomegaly; genital lesions consistent with a sexually transmissible disease; signs of systemic infection (generalized rash or petechiae); tattoos, piercing, or other body art that appears recent; trauma to intended recovery sites; corneal scarring; and a rash, a scab, or a lesion that is suspicious for vaccinia. The physical assessment is fully documented so that it can be reviewed, along with medical/social/behavioral history, medical records, and records of an autopsy (if performed). AATB offers a sample tissue donor physical assessment form and instructions for its use (see http://www.aatb.org/Guidance-Documents), to facilitate the performance and documentation of this assessment in a thorough manner by tissue banks.

Tissue recovery

Tissues are collected aseptically in an operating room, an autopsy room, or other suitable location where aseptic procedures can be performed. AATB standards require control of recovery site parameters including size/space, location, traffic, lighting, plumbing/drainage, ventilation, cleanliness of the room and furniture surfaces, absence of pests, absence of other activities occurring simultaneously, freedom from sources of contamination, and capacity to permit proper handling of contaminated equipment and disposal of biohazardous waste. In addition, all working surfaces must be disinfected. Following a surgical scrub, the person performing the recovery dons proper attire (gown and gloves). Body preparation, including shaving body hair, cleansing the skin with antimicrobial agent(s), and surgical draping of the body, is performed consistent with aseptic technique. Using aseptic technique, recovery of tissue is sequenced, and well-defined zone recovery methods are employed. Recommended recovery methods are described in AATB's Guidance Document, "Prevention of Contamination and Cross-contamination at Recovery: Practices and Culture Results" (http://www.aatb.org/Guidance-Documents). Generally, recovered tissues are not processed at the time of recovery. Tissues are often cultured at recovery, then individually packaged in sterile wraps,

labeled with a unique donor identifier, placed on wet ice, and sent without delay to tissue banks that will process them. Following donation, the donor body is usually reconstructed to permit normal funeral arrangements and viewing. The organ/tissue donor coordinator's responsibilities continue after the transplant procedure, in that a letter of appreciation may be sent to the next of kin, giving general information about the use of the donated organs and tissues. This communication serves as a liaison between the donor's family and the organ/tissue procurement agency. Later, contact may be reestablished to assist in amelioration of grief and bereavement. However, some donor families specifically request that there be no postdonation communication. AATB standards require formal establishment of donor family services. AATB has published a guidance document, "Providing Service to Tissue Donor Families," which describes support that should be offered (http://www.aatb.org/Guidance-Documents).

Infectious disease testing

Infectious disease marker testing includes HIV-1 and HIV-2 antibodies, HCV antibody, hepatitis B surface antigen (HBsAg), and syphilis. In addition, nucleic acid testing (NAT) is performed for HIV-1 and HCV. Tissue banks also screen donors for antibodies to hepatitis B core antigen (anti-HBc), which, although a confirmatory test is not available, may indicate HBV infection even when HBsAg is not detectable. Tissue banks may perform HBV by NAT. Whenever possible, infectious disease marker testing is performed on pretransfusion/preinfusion blood samples to avoid false-negative results caused by hemodilution in the event that transfusions and/or infusions had been given shortly before the time of death.[27] In the case of posttransfusion/infusion specimens, algorithms for determining the extent of plasma dilution are available.[11] Testing of postmortem (postasystole) blood specimens may be complicated by hemolysis or the presence of sediment, which can cause false-positive results in some HBsAg enzyme immunoassays (EIAs) and false-negative results in some HIV, HBV, and HCV NAT assays.[17] The tests for HIV and hepatitis must have been validated for use with postmortem specimens and approved by the FDA for use in tissue donor screening (www.fda.gov/cber/products/testkits.htm). When practical, tissue from living donors, such as semen donors, is preserved and quarantined until the donor is retested for HIV and hepatitis viruses in order to rule out seroconversion during the period of storage. Additionally, both semen and oocyte donors must be found negative for *Neisseria gonorrhea* and *C. trachomatis* and are usually tested for carriage of one or more genetic disorder, as indicated by donor racial and ethnic background. Donors may also undergo specific testing for rare genetic disorders if the recipient couple seeks a donor known to be negative for a particular gene mutation.

Tissue sterilization

Tissue sterilization is defined as the killing or elimination of all microorganisms from allograft tissue, whereas disinfection refers to the removal of microbial contamination. The Association for the Advancement of Medical Instrumentation (AAMI), a standard-setting organization for the medical instrumentation and technology industry, defines Sterility Assurance Level (SAL) as the probability that an individual device, dose, or unit is nonsterile (i.e., one or more viable microorganisms being present) after it has been exposed to a validated sterilization process. While absolute sterility theoretically would represent an absence of any pathogen, SAL is generally applied only to the level of possible contamination with bacteria or parasites. In contrast to log reduction of viruses determined in assessments of virus reduction methods, SAL is an absolute determined by the ability of the method to eradicate or reduce microorganisms, the susceptibility of organisms that may be present to the sterilization method applied, and the maximal bioburden that could occur in the initial material. For example, a SAL of 10^{-6} means that there is less than a 1 in 1,000,000 chance of a viable microorganism remaining after the sterilization procedure. The FDA requires that medical devices be sterilized using a method validated to achieve a SAL of 10^{-6}. A medical device derived from or that includes a biological product component must also meet a SAL of 10^{-6} if it is to be labeled sterile. A SAL of 10^{-3}, or a 1 in 1000 chance of a viable microorganism being present, is a more achievable goal selected by some processors for aseptically processed tissues if the processor has been unable to validate their process to the more stringent SAL of 10^{-6} level or if the tissues are unable to withstand the harsh treatment needed to achieve a more restrictive SAL without an impairment of tissue function. Such tissues may not then be labeled as sterile.

The complex physical structures and density of musculoskeletal tissues pose challenges for adequate penetration of antimicrobial agents to eradicate microorganisms. Allografts will not tolerate methods usually applied to metal and plastic medical devices because such treatment would impair the mechanical and biologic properties necessary for clinical utility. As an alternative, sterilization of tissues has been accomplished by several methods, including heat, chemicals, ethylene oxide gas, supercritical CO_2, and gamma or electron beam irradiation. However, not all sterilants have adequate tissue penetration. This is particularly the case for gases and liquids. The initial bioburden, which may be high in some tissues, must be considered. Some tissues are treated with antibiotics in vitro before storage, but this treatment decontaminates only the surface and may be effective against bacteria only.

A variety of methods, including chemical treatments and irradiation, have been used to reduce or eliminate pathogens in tissue intended for transplantation. The introduction of bone sterilization by ethylene oxide gas simplified bone processing and facilitated the widespread use of sterilized air-dried and lyophilized bone products.[28] The effects of ethylene oxide treatment on the biomechanical and osteoinductive capacity of bone allografts have been questioned, although animal studies have yielded inconsistent results.[29-31] These concerns, combined with those regarding the carcinogenic potential of ethylene oxide and its breakdown products, have largely led to abandonment of this method in the United States and the United Kingdom.

First introduced over 40 years ago, γ-irradiation of bone is still used widely, usually employing a cobalt-60 source. The γ-rays penetrate bone effectively and work by generating free radicals, which may have adverse effects on collagen and limit utility in soft tissues unless performed in a controlled dose fashion at ultra-low temperature. The minimal bacteriocidal level of γ-irradiation is 10 to 20 kGy (1 kGy = 100,000 rad). Uncontrolled human studies have shown irradiated, calcified, and demineralized bone grafts to be clinically effective.[32,33] Numerous studies have shown that mineralized bone allografts irradiated at 25 to 30 kGy are also clinically effective, with success rates of 85% to 91% reported.[34,35] In controlled studies, the clinical effectiveness of bone allografts subjected to 25 kGy irradiation was comparable to that of nonirradiated bone grafts,[36] although doses exceeding 25 kGy for cortical bone and 60 kGy for cancellous bone have been found to induce cross-linking of collagen and to impair mechanical function in a dose-dependent

fashion.[37] There is in vitro evidence that high irradiation reduces osteoclast activity and increases osteoblast apoptosis, and that residual bacterial products induce inflammatory bone resorption following macrophage inactivation.[37] However, the clinical significance of these findings has not been established. Newer processes employing radioprotectants have preserved bone allograft integrity when doses ≥25 kGy are applied and controlled-dose methods permit successful irradiation at lower doses (see proprietary chemical sterilization methods to follow). Irradiated demineralized bone has active osteoinductive activity and has been effective in nonstructural clinical applications.

Concerns about pathogen transmission and the limitations of irradiation, especially for soft tissues, have prompted improvements in sterilization methods and in the validation of these methods. A number of proprietary chemical–based processing methods have been developed with aims of effectively penetrating tissues and reducing, killing, or inactivating microorganisms and viruses without unacceptable adverse effects on the tissue's biomechanical properties. Additionally, for use in transplantation, the agents must either be able to be effectively removed or be nontoxic. All methods in current use are applied only to tissue from donors who have met stringent criteria for medical history and behavioral risk assessment as well as negative results on infectious disease marker testing.[11] Some popular methods used are described in this section.

The Tutoplast process (Tutogen Medical, Gainesville, FL) was the first process to sterilize and preserve tissue without affecting biological or mechanical properties. The process has been in use for over 30 years, for a variety of hard and soft tissues, including bone, fascia lata, pericardium, skin, amniotic membrane, and sclera. Initially, lipids are removed in an ultrasonic acetone bath that also inactivates enveloped viruses and reduces prion activity. Bacteria are destroyed using alternating hyperosmotic saline and purified waterbaths that also wash out cellular debris. Soluble proteins, nonenveloped viruses, and bacterial spores are destroyed in multiple hydrogen peroxide baths, and a 1N sodium hydroxide treatment further reduces prion infectivity by 6 logs. A final acetone wash removes any residual prions and inactivates any remaining enveloped viruses. Vacuum extraction dehydrates the tissue before the grafts are shaped and then double-barrier packaged. Terminal sterilization using low-dose γ-irradiation yields a SAL of 10^{-6}.

The Allowash XG process (LifeNet Health, Virginia Beach, VA) employs six steps: (1) bioburden control, (2) bioburden assessment, (3) minimization of contamination during processing, (4) rigorous cleaning, (5) disinfection steps, and (6) a final step of low-temperature, controlled-dose γ-irradiation. The process has been validated to achieve a SAL of 10^{-6}.

The BioCleanse process (Regeneration Technologies, Alachua, FL) employs low-temperature addition of chemical sterilants, such as hydrogen peroxide and isopropyl alcohol, which permeate the tissue's inner matrix, followed by pressure variations intended to drive the sterilants into and out of the tissue. Regeneration Technologies reports a SAL of 10^{-6} for soft tissues without adverse effects on the initial allograft mechanical properties.

The Clearant process (Clearant, Los Angeles, CA) is designed to avoid the negative effects of γ-irradiation through addition of free radical scavengers, employing dimethylsulfoxide (DMSO) and propylene glycol as pretreatment radioprotectants. Although the process subjects tissue to 50 kGy of radiation and achieves a SAL of 10^{-6} for bacteria, fungi, yeast, and spores, the tissue's biomechanical properties are retained.

The Musculoskeletal Transplant Foundation (Edison, NJ) uses a series of chemicals, including nonionic detergents, hydrogen peroxide, and alcohol, to treat cortical and cancellous bone grafts. For soft tissues, such as bone-patellar tendon allografts, an antibiotic mixture containing gentamicin, amphotericin B, and primaxin is added, and then washed out to a nondetectable concentration. The Musculoskeletal Transplant Foundation claims a SAL of 10^{-3} for its products. Incoming tissues whose bioburden exceeds prescribed parameters are pretreated with low-dose γ-irradiation.

NovaSterilis (Lansing, NY) has developed a sterilization technique that uses supercritical carbon dioxide at low temperatures and relatively low pressures, resulting in transient acidification, which is lethal to bacteria and viruses, with good penetration reported. However, this technique only recently became available for clinically available allografts, and data on clinical efficacy and retention of allograft mechanical properties are limited.

General principles of tissue preservation and clinical use

Except for bone, which is usually lyophilized (freeze dried), the most common method of storing processed tissues is at cold temperatures, either by refrigeration or by freezing (Table 40.3).[11,38] For short-term storage, refrigeration at about 4°C often suffices, whereas long-term storage usually requires a frozen state. Several types of tissues can be preserved by multiple methods. Bone, dura mater, and amnion can be effectively cryopreserved or lyophilized. Much of the lyophilized and cryopreserved human tissue used in transplantation is intended to serve a structural purpose and maintenance of cell viability is not necessary. Tissues of this type, which include dermis, are composed of an extracellular matrix (such as collagen) with few or no viable cells present to support the matrix after transplantation, although they can contribute growth factors to facilitate remodeling. Even when the processing method used is intended to preserve cell viability, the donor cells will die following transplantation. The extracellular matrix, whether transplanted containing viable cells or devoid of them, is repopulated through the ingrowth of metabolically active recipient cells. More gradually, depending in part on the size and type of the allograft implanted, remodeling occurs, and the transplanted structure may eventually be entirely replaced by host cells.[39] The transplantation of allograft heart valves and cardiac conduit tissues provided in an

acellular matrix form is being studied to determine the rate and extent of repopulation with recipient cells.[40]

In some tissues, such as cornea, a single layer of viable donor cells is important, and this requirement necessitates maintenance of the tissue in culture medium at refrigerated temperature.[41] Other human tissues, such as marrow, skin, and gametes, are stored by either refrigeration or cryopreservation. In the latter, a controlled-rate freezing process and a cryoprotectant remove water from the cells while maintaining viability. The usefulness of tissues requiring posttransplantation cell viability depends on their maintenance of not only metabolic activity, but also capacity to synthesize protein, proliferate, or differentiate.

Bone

Bone allografts have many uses, including provision of acetabular and proximal femoral support for replacement of failed prosthetic hip joints, packing of benign bone cysts, fusion of the cervical or lumbar spine to correct disk disease or scoliosis, restoration of alveolar bone in periodontal pockets, reconstruction of maxillofacial deficits, and replacement of bone that has been resected because of a bone malignancy, such as osteosarcoma (see Table 40.1). The last procedure is accomplished with large osteochondral allografts that permit tumor resection and achievement of a cure without limb amputation.

Historically, bone allografts have been prepared by cutting a larger graft using simple techniques. Today's technology allows the cutting, machining, and piecing together of allografts via precision instrumentation, and has resulted in stronger and more versatile grafts that can withstand the challenges of new surgical techniques. Linear grooves, notches, or crosshatchings may be incised into bone surfaces to make the bone graft less likely to slip or become dislodged after placement. Many bone allografts, especially those used in neurosurgical applications, are now placed using precision instrumentation that not only ensures exact placement, but also enhances stability. Allografts can be cut or shaped to precise angles that accommodate, for instance, lordosis of the cervical and lumbar spine. Advanced processing methods are being developed to improve availability while retaining or improving function.

Fresh autograft can be taken from the patient's own iliac crest during surgery, but this practice is becoming less common.[39] Fresh bone autograft is preferred by some surgeons, but preserved allografts are practical and accepted alternatives that approximate the

Table 40.3 Human tissue storage conditions and duration

Human Tissue	Storage Condition*	Temperature (°C)
Musculoskeletal	Frozen, (*Cryopreserved and non-cryopreserved*) long term	−40 °C or colder
	Frozen, (*cryopreserved and non-cryopreserved*) temporary storage for 6 months or less	−40 to −20 °C
	Refrigerated, short term	1–10 °C
	Lyophilized, long term	Ambient temperature**
Skin	Frozen, short term	−40 °C or colder
	Refrigerated, long term	1–10 °C
	Lyophilized, long term	Ambient temperature**
Cornea	Refrigerated, short term (defined by method)	2–8 °C
Semen	Frozen, long term	Liquid nitrogen (liquid or vapor phase
Cardiac, vascular	Frozen, *cryopreserved*	−100 °C or colder
Dura mater	Lyophilized, long term	Ambient temperature**

* Or as defined and validated by the processor.

** Ambient temperature monitoring not required for lyophilized tissue.

Source: Adapted with permission from Dock *et al.*[11] and Trainor.[38]

results obtained with fresh bone autograft.[47] In some patients, an autograft is not an option because sufficient high-quality bone is not available. In addition, the use of bone allografts reduces operating room time and the number of operative sites, leading to reduced morbidity and lower cost. The use of bone allograft does carry the risk of donor-to-recipient transmission of infectious disease,[15] although this risk is minimized through careful donor selection and testing, and disinfection and sterilization of tissue during processing as described earlier.

Frozen bone

Frozen bone, collected under aseptic conditions and then frozen or cryopreserved, is available in a wide variety of shapes and sizes from deceased donors, or as a femoral head or tibial plateau obtained from a living donor undergoing total joint replacement in an operating room (now an uncommon practice in the United States, but continuing in Canada, Australia, and Europe). This frozen bone is largely free of bacteria, but it does carry the risk of viral transmission. Diseases known to have been transmitted by unprocessed bone include HIV infection, conditions associated with HTLV, tuberculosis, and hepatitis.[15]

Frozen bone can cause alloimmunization from exposure to antigens on the attached connective tissues, marrow, and blood, although such alloimmunization apparently does not affect the graft's efficacy. Detailed reviews addressing the role of histocompatibility and the immune response in bone allograft transplantation have been published.[42] Antibodies to histocompatibility antigens,[43,44] blood group antigens,[45,46] and bone matrix proteins have been induced by transplanted frozen bone. In order to avoid Rh alloimmunization, bone from an Rh-negative donor is usually selected when using bone that has not been processed to remove red cells and the recipient is an Rh-negative female of childbearing potential.

Bone that otherwise would be discarded can be collected from living donors during surgical procedures (total hip or knee replacements with prostheses). The eligibility of a volunteer living donor is determined by a careful health history review, a directed physical examination if indicated, and donor testing for anti-HIV-1 and -2, HIV-1 NAT, HBsAg, anti-HBc (total), anti-HTLV-I/II, anti-HCV, HCV NAT, and syphilis.[11] In some countries, if NAT assays are not performed, the donated tissue is quarantined, and the living donor is retested six months later for infectious disease markers. This quarantine and retesting process is intended to eliminate donors who were in the early stage of viral infection but were antibody negative at the time of donation (in the window period). A follow-up anti-HBc test may detect donors who had been infected with HBV shortly before donating but who no longer have detectable HBsAg. Generally, culturing for bacteria is performed on each bone to be fresh frozen or on each batch/lot of cryopreserved bone.

Allograft bone is further prepared by removal of extraneous tissue; it is then packaged, and immediately either shipped to the processing tissue bank on wet ice or sent to freezer storage at −40 °C or colder. Frozen bone allografts are available as whole bones or cut into usable shapes and sizes. Frozen bone can generally be stored up to 5 years at −40 °C or colder, but the maximal storage duration and expiration date may vary based on processing and storage methods, as validated by the tissue bank. There is no evidence that the biomechanical or osteoinductive properties decline during frozen storage. However, in the absence of cryopreservation, frozen bone does not maintain cellular viability. Thus, frozen bone is used for structural support that depends on an intact calcified extracellular matrix or is used as filler to promote new bone formation.

Lyophilized bone

Following aseptic recovery, deceased donor bone can be placed on ice for transport to storage in a freezer and maintained frozen at −40 °C or colder, and then can later be sent to a tissue processor with dry ice as a refrigerant. Alternatively, immediately after recovery, the tissue can be placed on wet ice and expedited directly to the processing tissue bank where, within 72 hours of recovery, it is frozen at −40 °C or colder until processing. Such processing includes removal of surface tissues and internal fat, blood, and marrow by means of mechanical agitation, high-pressure water jets, or alcohol soaks. It can also include detergents or other solutions as part of a proprietary process. Then the bone is milled into clinically useful shapes and sizes. This may include computer-guided milling and use of assemblies that result in complex mechanical structures. Conventional allografts include corticocancellous strips, wedges, and dowels; cortical struts and rings; and cancellous and cortico-cancellous cubes and chips. Bone can also be ground into a powder and be available as DBM and products that include it. DBM, which is also known as demineralized freeze-dried bone allograft, is derived from cortical bone and is available in combination products in the form of gels, pastes, putties, and flexible strips or sheets. DBM itself may be obtained in specific granule or particle sizes, as a powder, or in entangled, twisted fiber configurations. DBM primarily provides growth factors, but accompanying collagen can help play a structural role as a scaffold for future bone growth. The combining of DBM with approved polymer carriers results in moldable grafts that are user friendly for the surgeon, do not migrate after placement, and whose bone content does not dissolve following transplantation. Such grafts can readily be applied to completely fill bony defects and to act as a scaffold for ingrowth of the recipient's own cells, or they can be used to enhance other structural repair devices, such as dental implants, vertebral body spacers and cages, or support devices such as rods, screws, and plates.[1]

The bone allografts are lyophilized to a residual moisture content of <6% or 8% (depending on measurement method) and packaged into jars, peel packs or "boat" packaging. Routine quality control testing of bone is designed to monitor safety, rather than potency or efficacy. Sterility is assessed by the testing of samples of each batch, or by another acceptable method. If a robust validated sterilization process is used, sterility may need to be assessed only at established intervals, such as quarterly. Potency can be evaluated by using assays for osteoinductive capacity and biomechanical properties, but these analyses usually are conducted only when there is a change in the production process. Lyophilized bone is brittle unless fully rehydrated before use. Lyophilized bone can usually be stored at ambient temperature for up to five years if the graft's package integrity and its vacuum are maintained, depending on validation performed by the tissue processor.

While the purpose of lyophilization is to allow for convenience, other preservation methods exist that also allow for ambient temperature storage of grafts. Some tissues can be dehydrated via chemicals (such as acetone), some kept in saline (e.g., costal cartilage), and some are packaged with a humectant (such as glycerol). The last two examples are considered prehydrated and are "ready to use" off the shelf. Expiration dates for all of these alternate methods are established by validation of the packaging by the tissue processor.

Bone collected aseptically in an operating room and processed aseptically can be lyophilized without use of a sterilant. Because the bone, theoretically, is bacteria-free, final sterilization with γ-irradiation may not be necessary. Although the bone should be free of bacteria, it still has the potential to transmit disease. Despite this risk, some physicians have preferred aseptically processed, nonsterilized lyophilized bone because it was thought to have better osteoinductive capacity than sterilized bone. However, controlled-dose low-temperature radiation has been found to have no significant effect on osteoinductive capacity.[47]

Ear ossicles

Ear ossicles are used as a special kind of bone graft to correct selected cases of deafness in which the patient's own ossicles have suffered congenital, traumatic, or postinfectious damage.[48] Ear ossicles are procured by removal of the temporal bone en bloc or as a core with a bone-plug cutter. The temporal bone can be stored temporarily, for months if frozen, or up to two weeks if preserved in formalin; the tympanic membrane and ossicular chain are then dissected. Ossicles have been stored for up to two months in cialit (an organomercuric compound), and for up to one year at room temperature in buffered formaldehyde. Alternatively, ossicles are dissected at the time of collection, lyophilized, and then sterilized by γ-irradiation. Lyophilized ossicles can be stored at ambient temperature for up to five years.

Connective tissue
Cartilage and meniscus

Human cartilage can be transplanted at weight-bearing or non-weight-bearing sites. For non-weight-bearing uses such as nasal reconstruction and mandibular or orbital rim augmentation, the graft provides structural support and need not be viable. Costal cartilage can be recovered for this use. The cartilage can be sterilized by γ-irradiation and stored in saline at refrigerated temperatures, or it can be lyophilized and stored at ambient temperature.

Articular cartilage can be transplanted to weight-bearing articular surfaces to replace focal cartilage defects caused by trauma or degenerative disease, particularly in the knee. Cartilage in an osteochondral or osteoarticular allograft can be obtained as a femoral hemicondyle, a tibial plateau or fragment, or a measured segment removed with a template cutter that can be press fitted into a similarly cut area in the recipient. Osteochondral allografts avoid autograft site morbidity and are advantageous when the focal articular cartilage defects being repaired are large (>2.5 cm).[49] It has been assumed that, in weight-bearing applications, chondrocytes must survive the collection and preservation process and remain viable, producing normal cartilage matrix to maintain mechanical properties. It appears that chondrocytes deep within the cartilage matrix resist cell-mediated immune responses by the recipient and, if kept viable during storage, are able to survive after transplantation. Cartilage grafts from histo-incompatible donors, stored <24 hours at 4 °C, have survived for as long as seven years after transplantation, if the grafts developed a sound union and if conditions for correct biomechanical functioning were present.[50] Articular cartilage collected in a sterile manner can be stored at 4 °C in saline or electrolyte solutions with or without 10% fetal (bovine) calf serum and antibiotics.[51] Screening procedures are now in place to reduce the risk of source animals that may have bovine spongiform encephalopathy (BSE). Osteoarticular and osteochondral allografts can be stored refrigerated for up to 28 days with successful clinical outcomes. If such grafts have been cryopreserved, expiry for these allografts can be extended to one year.

The use of a large osteochondral allograft, such as the femur with the articular cartilage attached, is thought to require preservation of cartilage viability in order to maintain biomechanical properties. To accomplish this, grafts have been stored at refrigerated temperatures in electrolyte solutions for up to one month, or have been frozen in 10% glycerol or 15% DMSO and stored at −70 °C or colder.[52] Following transplantation in humans and animals, the surface of the articular cartilage allograft undergoes degenerative changes within a few years. These grafts carry the same risk of disease transmission as other fresh tissue allografts.

Menisci are C-shaped disks of fibrocartilage interposed between the femoral condyle and tibia. The presence and integrity of the meniscus are essential for knee mechanics and biochemical functions. Loss or disruption of the meniscus is associated with pain, joint laxity, and degenerative arthritis. Meniscal transplantation has been proposed as a method of providing a biologically and biomechanically acceptable structure to replace a damaged or removed meniscus, with a goal of relieving pain, decreasing stress on the anterior cruciate ligament, and preventing late arthritis, although evidence of allograft tissue being chondroprotective is lacking. Although there have been unpublished reports of successful transplantation of menisci stored <24 hours at 4 °C, fresh menisci are not usually available. Cryopreserved menisci are used successfully, with good outcomes (including reduced pain and increased knee function) reported.[53,54]

Tendon and ligament

The knee is the joint most frequently involved in sports-related injury. Arthroscopic methods for replacing the anterior or posterior cruciate ligaments with autografts, allografts, or artificial tendons and ligaments are frequently used. Despite the attendant need for sacrifice or weakening of normal structures, the use of autografts appears to have a high success rate and low incidence of complications. However, allografts may be indicated for multiple ligament knee injuries, anterior cruciate ligament revisions, or posterior cruciate ligament reconstruction, and when extensor mechanisms are impaired (as with previous tendon tears). It is also sometimes preferable to avoid the morbidity associated with autograft. In addition, there are occasions when sources of adequate autograft tissue are not available.[55] Allografts used to replace the injured anterior cruciate ligament are usually derived from deceased donor patellar ligaments, tendons of the leg (e.g., tibialis, semitendinosus, gracilis, and peroneus longus), or Achilles tendons. Ligament and tendon allografts are usually stored frozen, but some are stored lyophilized. In vitro biomechanical properties of tendons do not seem to be greatly affected by freezing, lyophilizing, or ethylene oxide sterilization.[56] However, many surgeons eschew lyophilized tendon allografts because of experiences with clinical failure. Frozen tendon allografts are commonly sterilized by γ-irradiation, although this can reduce their mechanical strength, particularly if performed at room temperature or if the dose exceeds 20 kGy.[57] There is no evidence that maintenance of cellular viability during processing and storage is important to clinical effectiveness. The effect of irradiation on the biomechanical properties of human tissue has been explored extensively, with inconsistent results. This is probably because the studies failed to use uniform irradiation methods and comparable study designs. A key study found a difference in average stress at failure between nonirradiated and γ-irradiated tendons; that difference is likely a consequence of the free radicals generated, which can cause minor crosslinking of collagen fibers and alteration of the tendon's material properties.[58] In order to eliminate the potential for elongation of irradiated grafts after implantation, the authors encouraged pretensioning of grafts before insertion.

Fascia lata

The fascia lata is a broad fibrous membrane surrounding the thigh muscles. The thick lateral portion acts as a flattened tendon, and its muscular insertions helping to maintain the trunk in an erect posture. Fascia lata can be removed and transplanted as an autograft or allograft. As an allograft, fascia lata has been used to suspend the upper eyelid to correct ptosis, as a covering for bone grafts in dental surgery, to replace injured anterior cruciate ligaments, to provide support for bladder suspension, and to repair ankle, hip, and shoulder suspensions (e.g., repair of a ruptured shoulder rotator cuff). Fascia lata usually is preserved by lyophilization, resulting in a residual moisture of <6% or 8% (depending on measurement method), the graft is then sterilized by γ-irradiation and stored for up to five years at ambient temperature. After rehydration, the graft's biomechanical properties equal those of fresh frozen fascia lata. The use of fascia lata has become less popular because of the availability of alternative products, such as decellularized skin.

Dura mater

Dura mater is the outermost, toughest, and most fibrous of the three meningeal membranes covering the brain and spinal cord. The intracranial portion is collected, processed, stored, and distributed for several clinical applications; the most common use is the closure of dural defects caused by resection of tumor or the repair of traumatic injury. Human dura allograft is most commonly preserved by lyophilization. Ethylene oxide and γ-irradiation are effective in preventing transmission of viruses and bacteria; however, Creutzfeldt–Jakob disease (CJD) has been transmitted by dura mater treated by these methods. Following findings by Brown and coworkers,[59,60] in 1986 The Committee on Health Care Issues of the American Neurological Association recommended using 1N NaOH for one hour or steam autoclaving for one hour at 132 °C as standard sterilization procedures for CJD-infected tissue or contaminated materials. Donors with a history of clinical dementia or other central nervous system disorders are not accepted as donors. Lyophilization and sterilization treatments do not lessen the effectiveness of dura mater allografts. Reconstituted freeze-dried dura mater is thick and strong, holds suture well, and is incorporated into normal surrounding tissue without rejection. Because of the risks and resulting decreased demand, dura mater is currently processed in the United States by only one tissue bank.

Skin

Human skin allograft is the dressing of choice for temporary grafting onto deep burn wounds whenever sufficient amounts of autograft skin are unavailable. Early excision of burned tissue and covering of the wound with deceased donor skin allograft has shortened hospitalization and decreased mortality more than has any other treatment.[61] A skin allograft provides temporary coverage and acts as a barrier against loss of water, electrolytes, protein, and heat. It reduces opportunities for the invasion of bacteria and speeds re-epithelialization. Skin allografts are replaced periodically until the patient's vascular bed is reestablished. Skin allografts also are used for unhealed skin defects (decubitus ulcers, autograft skin sites, pedicle flap sites, and traumatically denuded areas). Although skin has historically been used only as a covering, decellularized (mechanically and chemically treated) skin offers the opportunities for use of a collagen matrix that can be implanted and be remodeled within the site with the recipient's own cells. It is used for such applications as bladder suspension surgery, tendon repair, post-mastectomy breast reconstruction, oral reconstruction, and repair of large defects, such as postoperative hernias and dehisced wounds. In an analogous fashion, Taylor and colleagues[40] have used perfusion-decellularized cardiac tissue matrix in an attempt to develop a bioartificial heart.

After collection, fresh skin can be stored in medium at 1 to 10 °C for up to 14 days,[11] but fresh skin is seldom used today. Skin also can be frozen using a method that retains cell viability, in order to improve availability. Because cell viability declines during refrigerated storage, results are best when cryopreservation is performed within 2 to 3 days after recovery. Cryopreserved skin can be prepared as strips (often 3-inch by 8-inch sections), either unmeshed or meshed (most commonly with a 1:1.5 expansion ratio, which triples the area that can be covered). The skin is then covered in fine-mesh gauze and laid flat, packaged, and then cryopreserved with glycerol or DMSO at a concentration of 10% or 15% as a cryoprotectant. Cryogenic damage is minimized by controlling the rate of freezing to between −1 and −5 °C/minute. Many tissue banks use a "heat sink" freezing method, rather than one that employs computer-controlled freezing chambers. Heat sinks involve aluminum plates combined with styrofoam-insulated boxes; these are placed directly into a −70 °C mechanical freezer. This simple process provides a slow, controlled freezing rate that is acceptable for skin and that also maintains cellular viability.[62] AATB standards permit frozen storage in a mechanical freezer at −40 °C or colder, in the vapor phase of liquid nitrogen, or submerged in liquid nitrogen.[11] The maximal allowable storage period in the frozen state during which viability and structural integrity are maintained has not been determined. Cryopreserved skin allograft usually is transported from the tissue bank to the hospital with dry ice in order to maintain a frozen environment until use.

Skin for use in burn applications generally is not preserved by lyophilization because this method decreases clinical efficacy. However, lyophilized skin is sometimes used by oral surgeons to cover oral mucous membrane defects and to speed re-epithelialization. Lyophilized (and prehydrated) acellular dermal matrix is also available, in several thicknesses for different applications, and can serve as a natural biological matrix for soft tissue augmentation in soft tissue defects and in periodontal peri-implant soft tissue management. Following hydration, lyophilized skin has multidirectional strength and can adapt to surface contours, and it then is resorbed over 4–6 months, depending on the site, defect size, patient age and health status, and the biomechanical load on the graft. Depending on processing method and packaging configuration, lyophylized skin can be stored as long as five years at ambient temperature or it may require refrigeration.

Ocular tissue

Cornea is one of the most frequently transplanted tissues; >46,000 corneas were transplanted in the United States in 2013. Corneal transplantation has become highly effective because of improvements in suture materials, surgical instruments and techniques, and medications to prevent and reverse rejection. It is considered a standard therapy for a variety of conditions. However, early in this century, demand decreased because of improvements in cataract surgery techniques compared with those in use in the 1990s, during which time use for complications of cataract surgery had supplanted keratoconus as the leading indication. In the last 10 years, there has been a paradigm shift from full thickness keratoplasty to selective keratoplasty, where only the diseased layers of the cornea are replaced. One such selective keratoplasty techniques is Descemet's stripping endothelial keratoplasty (DSEK), which transplants only the innermost portion of the cornea; the tissue adheres to the host cornea with the use of an air bubble. The benefits of this technique are a smaller, stronger wound with minimal disruption of the interior curvature of the cornea, resulting in faster recovery improved visual acuity, as well as a reduction in the occurrence of adverse effects such as graft rejection and vision threatening intraoperative and postoperative complications. As a consequence, DSEK for Fuchs endothelial dystrophy has become the preferred surgical therapy at much earlier stages of the disease, resulting in a resurgence of demand for cornea allografts. Currently the most common indications for corneal transplantation are keratoconus, Fuchs dystrophy, post–cataract surgery corneal edema, and corneal regrafting. Donor cells in the avascular full-thickness cornea graft enjoy long-term survival without the aid of histocompatibility matching because the recipient site is also almost completely avascular. Because of the avascularity of the cornea, routine immunosuppression is accomplished with topical corticosteroids. However, systemic immunosuppression may be used in conjunction with topical agents for high-risk cases. Some experts believe that the failure rate of 5% to 10% might be improved by HLA matching; recipients known to be sensitized to HLA antigens have rejection rates higher than nonsensitized recipients.[63] The possibility of alloimmunization is of particular concern in patients who are undergoing repeat grafting procedures because of graft failure or who have ocular infections, as the corneal rim may become quite vascularized. Sclera may be used in the repair of ocular defects, in orbital reconstruction following enucleation, and in some dental applications.[64]

Ocular tissue can be recovered by enucleation or by in situ excision of the cornea, with a rim of sclera. It is preferable that recovery be performed within 10 hours after death. The oldest method of storage for whole globes was at 4 °C in a moist chamber; this method appeared to maintain viable endothelial cells sufficient for graft efficacy for as long as 48 hours after recovery. Because it yields improved viability, a more common method today is storage of the cornea, with attached rim of sclera, at 4 °C in a modified tissue culture medium, based on that developed in 1974 by McCarey and Kaufman.[65] One example commonly used is Optisol-GS (Bausch & Lomb, Irvine, CA), which contains dextran (as an osmotic agent), chondroitin sulfate, gentamicin, and streptomycin. Storage of corneas in the medium, at 2 to 8 °C, can maintain endothelial viability for as long as 14 days, and can maintain functional integrity for eutopic graft applications not requiring visual acuity for even longer storage periods.[66] Grafts are usually used within seven days. Although they have been treated with antibiotics, allograft corneas are not considered sterile. Organ culture stored corneas may be used internationally (particularly in the European Union), but US banks do not use this method. Rarely, corneas are frozen with cryoprotectants. Sclera is usually preserved in ≥70% ethyl alcohol; such a method yields a shelf-life as long as two years.

Cardiac and vascular tissue

Cardiac and vascular tissue includes heart valves, patches, nonvalved outflow tract arteries and vessels that can be used as conduits. Donor medical history requirements differ, so AATB has established separate standards for cardiac tissues and for vascular tissues.[11] Since their introduction nearly five decades ago, human heart valve allografts have been shown to be an alternative for patients needing heart valve replacement for whom mechanical and xenograft valves are contraindicated. Human heart valve allografts do not require recipient anticoagulation, have a lower incidence of thromboembolism, and appear relatively resistant to infection. After valve

allograft transplantation, donor endothelium is not maintained, but donor fibroblasts may remain for an undetermined period. Because anticoagulation is unnecessary, human valve allografts are the graft of choice for children, females of childbearing potential, and patients with cardiac infection in the aortic root. The use of allograft valves has been slowed, however, because implantation is more technically difficult compared to modern versions of stented prosthetic valves. In addition, their availability is limited, especially for pediatric use. Additionally, clinical results with transplantation of xenograft tissue valves have improved, although these are not available in the small sizes required by many pediatric patients.

Technical impediments have made it impossible to successfully produce man-made (either completely artificial or modified xenograft) replacement heart valves for use in neonates and other pediatric patients who require very small grafts. Only donated human heart valves from newborns or small children offer unobstructed blood flow through such a small annulus. Also, the tissue's pliability renders human allografts adaptable to the ingenuity of cardiothoracic surgeons who repair congenital defects by using allografts to replace underdeveloped or otherwise defective valves or outflow tracts, or to construct valves and tracts that may be absent.[67] Complex repairs may need to be staged over many years or may be only palliative. Demand for clinical use of nonvalved conduit sections of cardiac allografts (mostly from the main pulmonary artery and/or its branches) has shown superior results in use as treatment of defects of the right ventricular outflow tract.[68] On a global scale, availability of cryopreserved pediatric allograft heart valves has historically been low and unable to meet demand.

To obtain cardiac allografts, hearts are recovered aseptically, immersed in a sterile isotonic solution within a sterile container, placed on wet ice, and transported expeditiously to a tissue processing facility. The pulmonic and aortic valves, along with their intact outflow tracts and/or small pieces of these conduits, are dissected free of the heart within 48 hours of donor asystole, and then placed in tissue culture medium amended with a low-dose antibiotic cocktail. Studies demonstrate that cryopreservation of heart valves allow successful banking of valves of various sizes and types while retaining the intact matrix and having a low clinical incidence of valve degeneration, rupture, leaflet perforation, and valve-related death. For these reasons, human heart valves generally are cryopreserved,[69] with a method that includes an initial exposure to antibiotic solutions for 12 to 24 hours. Cryopreservation then follows, using a 10% DMSO solution tissue culture medium that often is amended with 10% fetal calf serum. Freezing is accomplished using a computer-assisted controlled rate of −1 °C/minute to −40 °C. Valves generally are stored in the vapor phase of liquid nitrogen. Theoretically, heart valves can be stored indefinitely in liquid nitrogen, although the nature of any deterioration during storage is not well characterized. The viability of cryopreserved connective tissue matrix cells is maintained, but at a lower level than that of fresh valves, and endothelial viability is lost. In addition, noncellular matrix elements are maintained.

The aorta and iliac arteries can be preserved using the same methods applied to heart valves. Frequently, the aortic arch is preserved with the aortic valve intact; such grafts are intended for transplantation as a valved conduit. Preservation and storage methods are similar to those for valves. Synthetic grafts are often the graft of choice, but such grafts may be less effective in an infected field. Aortoiliac arteries are used successfully as conduits in mycotic aneurysm repairs, when synthetic grafts have become infected, and for aortoenteric fistulas in an infected field.[70]

Arterial or venous segments of vascular organs may be recovered in order to provide a source of vascular "conduits" for use in organ transplants when the organ's attached vessels are damaged or inadequate. Vascular conduits that have been recovered and transplanted under these conditions are not considered tissues under the FDA's human cells, tissues, or cellular or tissue-based products (HCT/Ps) rules, but they are regulated as organs under 42 CFR Part 121. Donor screening and testing, as well as labeling and storage requirements, are identical to those for donor organs specified in a federal contract with the Organ Procurement and Transplantation Network.

Autograft veins are used in cardiac and peripheral vascular bypass graft procedures whenever it is possible, but veins from deceased donors that have been recovered under aseptic conditions may be used for revascularization when autologous vein grafts are not available. Cryopreservation of allograft vessels is similar to that of cardiac allografts. Well-established tissue bank procedures are designed to retain venous endothelial cells during recovery, processing, and preservation, but these cells are rapidly sloughed off the lumen after the vein is transplanted into the high-pressure arterial system. Retention of endothelial cells during recovery and processing does aid, however, in reduction of the risk of thrombosis or failure after implantation through protection of the integrity of the vessel's basement membrane and acellular matrix.[67]

Although not proven to be necessary for successful clinical outcome or to prevent alloimmunization, ABO- and Rh-compatible allograft valves and vessel conduits are usually requested. One recent case series, involving limb salvage utilizing allograft saphenous veins, showed significantly better results in cases with ABO blood type compatibility.[71] Some studies have shown that the use of these tissue allografts carry a risk of HLA antigen sensitization.[72]

Peripheral nerve

Fresh autografts of peripheral sensory nerves are used in nerve repair, but this practice is hampered by collection morbidity and resulting limitations on the amount of autologous nerve tissue that can be made available. Although allografts ideally might repair peripheral nerve defects without requiring the sacrifice of the patient's own nerve, frozen, irradiated, and lyophilized allografts have not functioned well. New animal studies using nerve allografts cold-preserved for seven weeks have shown promising results, as have cultured Schwann cells added into synthetic conduits.[73] Axogen, Inc. (Alachua, FL), has developed a thermally acellularized nerve allograft scaffold called Avance that is treated with chondroitinase in order to degrade chondroitin sulfate proteoglycan. Such grafts have been shown to inhibit both aberrant growth and retrograde regeneration in the absence of any immunosuppressive therapy. Animal studies employing such an approach demonstrated enhancement of nerve regeneration. The first human Avance nerve allograft was implanted in 2007 into a 38-year-old man who had suffered a traumatic facial nerve injury; a single nerve allograft was used to connect the severed facial nerve root to three nerve branches. The surgeons informally reported that the graft's handling characteristics were superior to those of autograft tissue.

Parathyroid

Hypercalcemia, kidney stones, and other complications associated with hyperparathyroidism can be treated by surgical removal of the parathyroids. Hyperparathyroidism often is caused by a single parathyroid adenoma, but in 10% of cases, generalized parathyroid hyperplasia is found, rendering the removal of all four parathyroids necessary. Postoperatively, the lack of parathyroid hormone can result in permanent hypocalcemia in 5% of patients. To prevent this outcome, autotransplantation of a small amount of parathyroid tissue is performed during total parathyroidectomy in order to provide a controlled source of parathyroid hormone.[74] Cases of parathyroid cell allotransplanation have been reported, with durable results in selected cases where the recipient was being immunosuppressed to prevent rejection.[75]

The parathyroid tissue is placed in the sternocleidomastoid muscle, flexor muscle groups, or subcutaneous tissue of the forearm. The remaining parathyroid tissue can be divided, placed in vials containing chilled tissue culture medium, and then cryopreserved using autologous serum, RPMI, and DMSO. The excess tissue then can be frozen under controlled conditions and stored in liquid nitrogen at $-196\,°C$.[76,77] Frozen parathyroid autograft can be retrieved for subsequent use if the tissue implanted at the time that the parathyroid was resected proves to be insufficient, fails to function, or becomes infected. Cryopreservation of parathyroid tissue maintains cell viability and graft function. This is illustrated by postimplant amelioration of hypocalcemia and sustained elevation of parathyroid hormone in the venous effluent of the grafted forearm compared with that of the nongrafted forearm.[78] Postthaw viability can also be demonstrated in vitro by the suppression of parathyroid hormone secretion by the addition of increasing calcium concentrations.[79] The maximal duration of cryopreserved parathyroid tissue storage has not been determined.

Reproductive tissue
Semen

Assisted reproductive technology procedures and artificial insemination of a female with her partner's previously stored semen or with donor semen are established therapies for the clinical management of infertility or when a woman does not have a male partner. Cryopreserved semen can be stored by a man, termed a *client depositor*, who may become sterile as a consequence of therapy for testicular malignancy or for another reason, for later use with his wife or other "intimate partner," or even with a gestational carrier. Sperm can even be collected postmortem, but such a practice poses ethical issues regarding the lack of consent. According to the FDA, there are approximately 706 registered establishments that provided cryopreserved semen storage in the United States in 2015. The vast majority of these sites are fertility clinics that process and store semen for their patients' own use with their partner. Each ejaculate can be separated into several vials or straws for separate storage that can be retrieved and thawed for use when needed.

Semen banks, or sperm banks, usually offer a library of donors from whom donated frozen semen specimens are available. According to a survey conducted by the American Association of Tissue Banks in 2014, there were 26 sperm banks in the United States that offered, as their main business, donor sperm for use by patients in need of donor sperm. The offering of a selection of donors facilitates the matching of donor's hair and eye color, race, and other genetically determined characteristics with those of the intended father or co-parent or with those of both parents. These donors are usually "anonymous"; such a donor's identity is known only to a few of the semen bank staff. However, some semen banks offer a program through which some donors have agreed to disclose their identities when offspring reach the age of 18 or, sometimes, even before use of the semen. Sexually transmitted diseases, including HIV infection, can be transmitted by donor semen to women undergoing artificial insemination.[23,80,81] Cryopreservation permits extended storage and the retesting of donors at least 6 months after the donation of specimens to be released. This process is intended to prevent use of semen donated by a recently infected man, before development of detectable antibody or viral nucleic acid (during the "window period"). Other diseases and organisms transmissible by donor semen include hepatitis B, gonorrhea, *U. urealyticum*, *M. hominis*, *T. vaginalis*, and *C. trachomatis*. Transmission of HTLV-I, syphilis, HCV, and human papillomavirus may also be possible.[23]

The basic practices and techniques of semen cryopreservation have changed little since the cryopreservative glycerol was discovered accidentally by Polge and coworkers[82] in 1949. Glycerol remains the standard cryoprotectant, with storage in liquid nitrogen. Freezing methods in use have been designed to control the rate of temperature decline, and to prevent thermal shock by cooling the semen, slowly, in air or in a waterbath, to 5 °C before initiation of the actual freezing process. This takes place in the vapor phase of liquid nitrogen, or in a programmable controlled-rate freezing device. After freezing, semen can be stored in the liquid phase of liquid nitrogen indefinitely. The longest period of semen cryo-storage, followed by documented birth of healthy offspring, is 40 years.[83]

Although a defective pregnancy as a result of sperm injury during the freezing–thawing process is a theoretic concern, such an effect has not been demonstrated. Cryopreservation of semen does not influence the frequency of abortions or multiple births, or the infant's gender, body size, or intelligence.[84] In fact, there is some evidence that indicates that favorable outcomes of cryopreserved semen actually might exceed that of fresh semen. One study reported finding birth defects in 0.7% of offspring and spontaneous abortion of 7.7% of pregnancies achieved using cryopreserved semen, whereas in the general population the frequency of birth defects is 6% and the frequency of spontaneous abortion is 10% to 18% of pregnancies.[85]

Oocytes and embryos

Since the birth of Louise Brown, the world's first "test tube baby," on July 25, 1978, there has been an explosion in the use of assisted reproductive technologies, such that several techniques have been accepted as standard medical therapy. According to the Centers for Disease Control and Prevention's 2012 National ART Success Rates report, there are at least 456 assisted reproductive technology programs in the United States.[5] Although the technology to freeze unfertilized oocytes reliably only recently moved from the research setting, embryos are routinely cryopreserved. In 2012, these programs performed nearly 135,000 embryo transfers. Among embryos created using nondonor oocytes, 69% were employed fresh, while 31% had been frozen. Many of those embryos were created using donor semen and/or donor oocytes. Donor oocytes were used in approximately 13% of embryo transfers carried out in the United States in 2012.[5] Many of these were embryos created for recipients >35 years of age, using an oocyte donor much younger than the recipient. Embryo transfer success rates have been shown to be influenced far more by the age of the oocyte source than by the age of the uterus into which embryos are transferred. Medical history and infectious disease testing requirements similar to those for semen donors apply, although a quarantine period and retesting are not required.

Extraembryonic tissue preservation and transplantation

Extraembryonic tissues that have been used occasionally for transplantation include the amnion and the umbilical vein. Fetal amnion, which is the smooth, slippery, glistening membrane lining the fluid-filled space surrounding the fetus, has been used as a covering for nonhealing chronic leg ulcers, burns, and raw surfaces following mastectomy, and in major oral cavity reconstruction and vaginoplasty. Amnion also has been used as a pelvic peritoneum substitute following pelvic exenteration and as a source of replacement enzymes for infants with inborn errors of metabolism.[86] Most of the fetal amnion is covered on the maternal side by the chorion, a slightly roughened membrane. Amnion is sterilely collected during cesarean section. The amnion's epithelium and basement membrane can be separated by blunt dissection from the underlying chorion immediately after collection or after temporary storage. The amnion is then cryopreserved or lyophilized. Human umbilical vein allografts previously were used occasionally as vascular substitutes to provide venous access for hemodialysis or as an arterial bypass graft, but such allografts proved to be inferior to saphenous vein autografts. Such umbilical vein grafts are no longer available, following application of FDA device manufacturing requirements to their recovery and processing.

Donor–recipient matching

For most tissues, donor–recipient HLA matching is not necessary and is rarely done. Tissues such as bone, fascia, tendon, cartilage, and dura mater are not preserved or transplanted in a viable state; rather, they serve as a support or matrix that the recipient's own cells can enter and gradually replace. Immunologic rejection, therefore, is not a significant concern, and matching of blood group or HLA antigens is considered unnecessary. There are exceptions, however. Immunologic rejection can occur in patients who have received a repeat cornea graft; therefore, efforts are made to use HLA-matched corneas in these patients.[87] HLA sensitization has also been reported in recipients of vascular allografts or allograft heart valves.[88]

The ABO antigens are a significant consideration in transplantation because they constitute very strong histocompatibility antigens. Because they are expressed on vascular endothelium, major ABO mismatching can cause rapid graft rejection resulting from endothelial damage by ABO antibodies and subsequent widespread thrombosis within the graft. Therefore, ABO matching is important to the success of vascularized organ grafts (i.e., kidney, heart, liver, and pancreas). ABO matching is not important for a successful outcome when using most tissue grafts (i.e., fascia, bone, heart valves, skin, and cornea). However, hypersensitivity to antigens expressed by fresh or cryopreserved donor tissue is a rare occurrence and appears to be dependent on an undetermined unusual immune response by the recipient.

Alloimmunization to RhD, Fy^a, and Jk^b red cell antigens following transplantation of frozen unprocessed bone has been reported.[45,46] Consequently, frozen unprocessed bone allografts usually are matched with the donor for the D antigen if the recipient is a female of childbearing potential, in addition to being matched for ABO group.

Transfusion service support of tissue transplantation

Hospital transfusion services have been greatly affected by transplantation, and have encountered new and increased demands for services. They are involved in transplantation in several ways, including (1) providing traditional blood components; (2) providing new or special blood components; (3) taking responsibility for tissue acquisition, storage, distribution, and tracking; and (4) providing specialized services. For organ transplants, the major demand is for traditional blood components, although special preparation may be required.

FDA regulations pertaining to tissue (see below) cover donor selection and testing, tissue recovery, processing, storage, labeling, and distribution to the "consignee" (21 CFR Part 1271). The consignee can be a distributor, a surgeon in a hospital operating room, a dentist in his or her office, or a designated individual or department in a hospital or other healthcare institution. Tissue "banks" that are located in hospitals are not regulated by the FDA if they serve only to store and dispense tissues provided by comprehensive tissue banks or distributors. A hospital tissue service can be centralized in a support area for the operating suite, hospital central supply service, or hospital transfusion service.

Alternatively, tissues can be handled using a decentralized system and be ordered, received, and stored by each functional area of the hospital in which they are used. However, in the absence of centralization, records of storage and recipient identification may be inadequate. In one case involving an HIV-infected donor, the recipients of five of the tissues could not be identified from hospital records. Other examples of inadequate traceability exist.[89] The Joint Commission standard[90] on recordkeeping and traceability of tissues, College of American Pathologists Transfusion Medicine Checklist,[91] and AABB *Standards for Blood Banks and Transfusion Services*[92] require that the institutions' records permit tracing of any tissue from the donor or source facility to all recipients or other final tissue disposition. However, New York State is the only government regulatory agency that requires tracking of tissues to the recipients with records kept separate from patient charts.

The hospital transfusion service has the capacity, experience, and skills to act as a central depot and distribution point for all human tissue and to ensure that storage, issuance, and disposition records are maintained. Functions include allograft selection; vendor qualification and price negotiation; receipt of tissues, including inspection and accessioning; proper storage; inventory control; issuance; and recordkeeping, which must ensure traceability to recipient or other disposition.[93] Recordkeeping, especially if barcodes are used in the laboratory, is complicated by the fact that barcodes are not yet standardized among tissue banks, although adoption of ISBT 128 labeling standards has been suggested.[94] An additional challenge is that some tissues are produced in lots or batches, so each individual unit may not carry a unique identifier. Effective development of such tissue storage and distribution services takes time and relies on good relationships and communications with both operating room staff who will handle tissues and the surgeons who use them.[93]

A transfusion service operating as a central tissue repository and dispensing service may also be called upon to manage autologous tissues, such as calvaria (skull bone flaps), bone, skin, and parathyroid gland. Such tissues may require preparation and packaging before storage. Testing is not required, but careful labeling and recordkeeping are essential. Such tissues may ultimately be reimplanted in the original location (e.g., calvaria) or in a heterotopic location (e.g., limbs for parathyroid gland). It is prudent to establish time limits for storage either on an individual basis as specified by the surgeon or on a generalized basis, because stored tissues may not be claimed if the tissue was not needed because the patient died or for other reasons. The tissue dispensing service may also be called upon to package tissues in an appropriate, qualified, properly labeled transport container for transport to another institution.[93]

Reimbursement

Reimbursement for tissue transplantation is similar to that for blood transfusion. The tissue bank recovers expenses through a service fee (per tissue) billed to the hospital. This service fee includes such costs as services rendered by the organ/tissue recovery agency; recovery supplies and logistical support of the recovery agent that may be provided by the tissue processor; the tissue processor's operating costs associated with processing, storage, and distribution, as well as research and development; and overhead costs incurred with support of all operations. Healthcare insurance carriers reimburse hospitals for most tissue service fees. Current procedural terminology codes specific to allograft transplantation procedures are available and used routinely.

Oversight

With the rapid growth of all areas of tissue banking, there has been an increasing need for accountability and for measures that ensure that safe, quality tissues are available for clinical use. Quality improvement can be effected through voluntary standards, and most tissue banks have incorporated the achievement of high standards into their goals. The AATB has established comprehensive standards for donor screening, recovery and processing of musculoskeletal, cardiac, vascular, and skin tissues, and reproductive cells.[11] Additionally, the standards contain institutional requirements; descriptions of required functional components of a tissue bank; requirements for construction and management of records and development of procedures; requirements for informed consent, tissue labeling, storage, and release; expectations for handling adverse outcomes, investigations, and tissue recalls; requirements for establishment of a quality program; specifications for equipment and facilities; and guidelines for tissue dispensing services and tissue distribution intermediaries. AATB's *Standards for Tissue Banking* are consulted not only by tissue bankers, but also by end-user healthcare facilities, other standard-setting organizations, and regulators worldwide. In 2015, 124 tissue banks in North America held AATB accreditation. Best practice for checking a tissue bank's accreditation status is to perform an accredited bank search on the AATB website (www.aatb.org).

AABB *Standards for Blood Banks and Transfusion Services*[92] address tissue inspection, handling, storage, preparation and dispensing, handling adverse events, and recordkeeping, which must provide traceability to each recipient or other disposition. The Joint Commission has standards for storage and issuance of tissue for hospitals and ambulatory surgery centers. These standards apply to bone, tendon, fascia, and cartilage, as well as cellular tissues of both human and animal (xenograft) origin. The standards address key functions, including the need to develop procedures for tissue acquisition and storage, recordkeeping and tracking, and follow-up of adverse events and suspected allograft-caused infections, which must be reported to the tissue bank from which the tissue was obtained. Similar to federal regulations and AATB *Standards*, the minimal record retention period is specified to be 10 years from the date of transplantation, distribution, other disposition, or expiration, whichever is latest. The College of American Pathologists' Laboratory Accreditation Program's Transfusion Medicine Checklist includes several questions on storage and issuance of tissues, including accountability; procedures for proper storage, handling, in accordance with the source facility's directions; procedures for investigating recipient infections and adverse events, and handling lookback notifications from a supplier; and recordkeeping, which allow for tracking from donor to recipient and vice versa.

FDA authority to create and "enforce regulations necessary to prevent the introduction, transmission, or spread of communicable diseases between the States or from foreign countries into the States" under section 361(a) of the US Public Health Service Act (42 USC 264) applies to human tissue intended for transplantation. Formal enforcement policy and regulations did not exist until December 14, 1993 (codified in 21 CFR Parts 16 and 1270), when the "Interim Rule: Human Tissue Intended for Transplantation," which required donor screening, infectious disease testing and recordkeeping "to prevent transmission of infectious diseases through human tissue used in transplantation," was adopted in response to reports of HIV transmission by human tissue and of potentially unsafe bone imported into the United States.[95]

These regulations were supplanted by a series of federal regulations, published in stages, first announced in the Proposed Approach to the Regulation of Cellular and Tissue-Based Products in March 1997.[96] A final rule, "Human Cells, Tissues, and Cellular and Tissue-Based Products: Establishment Registration and Listing," published in January 2001, required organizations that are engaged in tissue recovery, donor qualification, tissue processing, and/or tissue-related laboratory testing to register as a tissue establishment with the FDA. The rule (21 CFR Part 1271) became effective for all tissue banks on March 29, 2004.

A final rule, "Eligibility Determination for Donors of Human Cells, Tissues, and Cellular and Tissue-Based Products," published May 25, 2004, set forth donor eligibility requirements, including health history screening and laboratory testing. Another final rule, "Current Good Tissue Practice for Human Cell, Tissue and Cellular and Tissue-Based Product Establishments; Inspection and Enforcement," published on November 24, 2004, established elements of good tissue practice, analogous to good manufacturing practice for blood banks. Both rules became effective May 25, 2005 (see 21 CFR Parts 1270 and 1271).

In addition to requirements for establishment registration, donor eligibility screening and testing, and good tissue practice, the regulations set forth requirements for adverse reaction reporting and also define inspection and recall authority. To improve tissue safety and surveillance, the FDA Current Good Tissue Practice Rule, effective May 25, 2005, requires that tissue establishments report infectious adverse events after allograft transplantation to the FDA through its MedWatch adverse event reporting system. More than half of the reports filed by tissue banks have been flagged to indicate possible recall of tissue(s). Of these flagged reports, the majority pertained to acceptance of ineligible donors for whom one or more components of the donor qualification process was not performed or was insufficiently documented. The FDA also encourages healthcare professionals, patients, and consumers to voluntarily report tissue adverse reactions through the MedWatch system (see http://www.fda.gov/Safety/MedWatch). There is an effort to develop the Transplantation Transmission Sentinel Network, which is intended to facilitate recognition of adverse events associated with transplanted allografts. The system is being developed by UNOS in collaboration with several stakeholders, including the AATB, EBAA, Association of Organ Procurement Organizations, American Academy of Orthopaedic Surgeons, American Orthopaedic Society for Sports Medicine, Society of Thoracic Surgeons, Health Resources Services Administration, and FDA.[97]

Acknowledgments

The authors thank W. Brent Hazelrigg, Michelle Rhee, Patricia Dahl, Mark Moore, Perry Lange, and Scott Brubaker for their technical advice.

Disclaimer

The authors have disclosed no conflicts of interest.

Key References

A full reference list for this chapter is available at: http://www.wiley.com/go/simon/transfusion

1 Eisenbrey AB, Eastlund T, Gottschall JL, Eds. *Hospital tissue management: a practitioner's handbook.* Bethesda, MD: AABB, 2008.

5 Centers for Disease Control and Prevention; American Society for Reproductive Medicine; Society for Assisted Reproductive Technology. 2005 Assisted reproductive technology success rates: national summary and fertility clinic reports. Atlanta, GA: Centers for Disease Control and Prevention, 2007.

9 Health Care Financing Administration. 42 CFR Part 482. Final rule. Medicare and Medicaid programs: Hospital conditions of participation: identification of potential organ, tissue and eye donors and transplant hospitals provision of transplant-related data. *Fed Regist* 1998;**63**:33856–75.

11 Dock NL, Osborne JC, Brubaker S, ed. *American Association of Tissue Banks: standards for tissue banking.* 13th ed. McLean, VA: AATB, 2012.

12 Eye Bank Association of America. *Medical standards.* Washington, DC: Eye Bank Association of America, 2013.

13 The American Society for Reproductive Medicine. *Guidelines for gamete and embryo donation.* Birmingham, AL: The American Society for Reproductive Medicine, 2006.

15 Eastlund T, Warwick, RM. Diseases transmitted by transplantation of tissue and cell allografts. In: Warwick RM, Brubaker SA, Eds. *Tissue and cell clinical use: an essential guide.* Oxford: Wiley-Blackwell, 2012:72–113.

89 Brubaker SA, Wilson D. Coding and traceability: cells and tissues in North America. *Cell Tissue Banking* 2010;**11** (4):379–89.

CHAPTER 41

Adoptive immunotherapy

Sarah M. Drawz,[1] Jeffrey S. Miller,[2] & David H. McKenna[1]

[1]Department of Laboratory Medicine and Pathology, University of Minnesota Medical School, Minneapolis, MN, USA
[2]Blood and Marrow Transplant Program, University of Minnesota, Minneapolis, MN, USA

Introduction

Immunotherapy may be in the form of cellular therapy, antibodies, cytokines, or other modalities that induce, enhance, suppress or release suppression of the immune system response. *Adoptive immunotherapy* typically refers to a cellular infusion product, the focus of this chapter. For these cell therapies, the donor may be autologous or allogeneic, and the product may be minimally manipulated (e.g., donor lymphocyte infusion) or the result of a complex isolation and expansion culture (e.g., regulatory T cells). This chapter addresses the four main cellular therapies in adoptive immunotherapy—T cells, dendritic cells (DCs), natural killer (NK) cells, and mesenchymal stem or stromal cells (MSCs)—and their clinical applications.

T-cell immunotherapy

Introduction

More subsets of T cells have been examined for their antitumor and antiviral capabilities than any other immune cell type. T cells are natural inspectors—circulating through tissues via blood and lymphatics looking for threatening signals. Their cell–cell interactions are mediated initially by recognition of peptide antigens presented to naïve T cells by major histocompatibility complex (MHC) molecules. With the appropriate co-stimulation, a naïve cell will be activated to proliferate into effector- and memory-type T cells. After successive exposures to the given antigen, these differentiated T cells are capable of orchestrating a specific immune response including direct cytotoxicity, cytokine production, and appropriate immune regulation. This natural killing ability was recognized as potentially transferrable over 50 years ago in mouse foreign tumor studies.[1] Since that time, increased knowledge of T-cell biology and subset function and technical progress with expansion and manufacture have improved the success and breadth of in vivo studies. The goal of adoptive T-cell immunotherapy is to introduce an antigen-specific arsenal to combat neoplastic or virally infected cells. Broadly speaking, immunotherapeutic T cells may be introduced without manipulation (nonspecific T cells) or following antigen exposure (antigen-specific), genetic engineering, or other modifications through culture conditions. In this section, we will provide an overview of the manufacturing of various types of T cells, as they have been applied to treat infections and cancer.

T-cell therapy for viral infections

Recipients of hematopoietic cell transplants (HCTs) often lose the bulk of their cell-mediated immunity and become susceptible to viral infections that carry high morbidity and mortality. These patients are at particular risk for reactivation of cytomegalovirus (CMV) leading to enteritis and pneumonia, Epstein–Barr virus (EBV) causing posttransplant lymphoproliferative disease (PTLD), and adenovirus-associated enteritis, hepatitis, hemorrhagic cystitis, and pneumonia.[2] Effective antiviral agents and anti-B-cell CD20-mediated therapy have improved many of these complications, but negative side effects and treatment failures are still too common. In contrast to tumor cells, presentation of antigens from virally infected cells is strong and specific. Capitalizing on these properties has led to effective ex vivo cytotoxic T-cell (CTL) expansion and transfer following stimulation of antigen-presenting cells (APCs) with viral particles. Although most models focus on the herpes viruses, CMV and EBV, and adenovirus, additional preclinical work suggests the strategies may have a role in multiviral immunotherapy for additional post-HCT viral threats. Importantly, the rates of graft-versus-host disease (GVHD) have not been significantly increased in recipients of CTL therapies.

Cytomegalovirus

The first reports of viral-specific therapy employed autologous fibroblasts as APCs for stimulation and expansion of sibling donor CD8+ T cells pulsed with CMV.[3,4] The CMV-specific CD8+ population was infused into recipients of matched sibling donor grafts, who showed no adverse effects and successful reconstitution of CD8-mediated immunity for at least eight weeks. Longer term maintenance of the response, however, was only seen with development of a CD4+-specific response. These early manufacturing processes involved live virus and prolonged exposure, and subsequent groups worked to improve on these inefficiencies. Approaches using CMV lysate and a CMV-infected human lung fibroblast line as stimulants for polyclonal CTLs have improved manufacturing time and demonstrated efficacy in patients recovering from refractory CMV disease and in preventing the development of disease following first CMV positivity, respectively.[5,6] Interestingly, the response to transfer of only CD4+ CMV-specific T cells seems not as able to prevent CMV disease,[7] suggesting that a polyclonal population of both CD4+ and CD8+ may be important for the improved protection.[8]

Rossi's Principles of Transfusion Medicine, Fifth Edition. Edited by Toby L. Simon, Jeffrey McCullough, Edward L. Snyder, Bjarte G. Solheim, and Ronald G. Strauss.
© 2016 John Wiley & Sons, Ltd. Published 2016 by John Wiley & Sons, Ltd.

Additional manufacturing approaches include retroviral transfer of CMV-specific T-cell receptors (TCRs) for HLA-matched immunotherapy in HCT recipients from CMV-negative donors.[9] Multimer-based selection of antigen-specific T cells has also been applied to CMV reactivation disease.[10,11] In these assays, reactive T cells are enriched from a donor population using peptide multimers bound to magnetic particles. Although initial clinical study results are promising, the strategy requires a high donor blood volume as well as HLA matching and a high baseline frequency of viral-specific T cells.

Epstein–Barr Virus

EBV is responsible for a variety of B- and T-cell malignancies, all of which are associated with latent viral infections.[12,13] Three types of latent infections have been described, and each has a characteristic protein expression pattern: latency type I expresses primarily EBV nuclear antigen I (EBNA1), latency type II is associated with EBNA I and latent membrane proteins 1 and 2 (LMP1 and LMP2), and latency type III expresses all known latency proteins. Each latency type is associated with a different disease(s). For example, latency type III proteins are expressed in lymphoproliferative diseases of the immune compromised (PTLD), latency type II proteins in immune-competent diseases (e.g., nasopharyngeal carcinoma and Hodgkin's lymphoma), and latency type I proteins are seen in EBV-positive Burkitt's lymphoma.[14] This molecular understanding has helped facilitate successful EBV immunotherapy approaches for over a decade. Latency type III EBV-specific T cells can be generated by repeated stimulation from irradiated lymphoblastoid cell lines (LCLs) produced from donor peripheral blood mononuclear cells infected with a laboratory EBV strain.[15,16] Multiple clinical studies have demonstrated the efficacy of this protocol for both prophylaxis and sustained remission in more than 70% of post-HCT EBV-associated PTLDs.[17–19] Failures in the cohorts treated for overt lymphoma were tied to both antigenic differences between the laboratory versus patient's EBV strain and mismatches of HLA between recipient and donor CTLs. These studies underscore the importance of creating donor cells with either, or both, broad specificity and patient-specific HLA matches.[8]

Protein expression of latency type II is associated with EBV diseases of the immune competent, and it generates fewer and weaker immunogenic targets than latency type III proteins. Despite these inherent challenges, clinical trials employing CTLs directed toward the latency type II proteins have met modest success in patients with nasopharyngeal carcinoma and Hodgkin's disease.[20,21] Generally, however, sustained responses are limited to those patients with lower tumor burden, whereas patients with high disease load have seen less benefit from monotherapy with CTLs. A recently published trial sought to increase the frequency of the EBV-type II specific T cells in a manufactured donor product by stimulating with both LCLs and DCs transduced with adenoviral vectors expressing LMP1 and LMP2.[22] In 28 of 29 high-risk or multiple-relapse patients in remission from Hodgkin's or non-Hodgkin's lymphoma, infusion of these enriched autologous CTLs as adjuvant therapy led to sustained remission for a median of three years. Responses were also seen in 13 of 21 additional patients with relapsed or resistant disease at the time of CTL infusion.

The latency type I protein EBNA1 is poorly processed by MHC class I and was thought until recently to evade T-cell recognition.[23] The identification of EBNA1-specific T cells in patients with PTLD and successful ex vivo expansion argue for reexamination of this effector cell type as an immunotherapy target.[24]

In contrast to the lymphomas that arise from donor cells following HCT, solid organ transplant patients tend to develop lymphoma derived from recipient cells. Furthermore, solid organ donor lymphocytes are often not available or HLA matched. Thus, studies of solid organ recipients involve the manufacture of autologous CTLs from the patient's own peripheral blood. Although this strategy has been safe and effective for prophylaxis and treatment,[25,26] the immunity is less persistent than that seen in HCT patients, likely due to the long-term immunosuppressive treatment these patients require.

Adenovirus

Like EBV and CMV, systemic adenoviral infections are a significant source of serious complications in immune-compromised patients. Viral-specific allogeneic CTL infusions have been tested in pediatric HCT patients, using populations expanded with viral antigen challenge and enriched for stimulated cells by anti-interferon-γ (IFNγ) magnetic bead selection.[27,28] The infusions have a good safety profile and facilitated clearance in a majority of patients; however, adenovirus-specific T-cell in vivo expansion depended on active viremia. Use of 15-mer conserved regions of highly immunogenic polypeptides as in vivo stimulators has been explored with promising initial clinical studies.[29]

In contrast to EBV and CMV, only a minority of healthy donors have adenovirus-specific T cells, presenting a challenge for source availability. In a manner similar to that discussed for CMV-negative donors, transfecting naïve T cells with adenovirus-specific TCRs may prove to be a productive strategy. Positive in vitro results have recently been published applying this technology to TCR-transfected γ/δ subset T cells, which are not alloreactive and thus can be used in mismatched donor–recipient pairs.[30]

Multivirus and other emerging approaches

Expanded viral coverage has been achieved from CMV-positive donors using monocytes and EBV-LCLs transfected with adenoviral vectors expressing CMV antigens, producing a single culture of CMV-, EBV-, and adenovirus-specific CTLs. Infusion of these trivirus-specific cells provided immune reconstitutions for CMV and EBV, but response to adenovirus only in the context of reactivation or active infection.[31] Comparable results were observed in patients receiving CMV-negative donor bivirus-specific CTLs.[27] However, these approaches mandate stringent regulatory oversight due to genetic engineering, and an attractive alternative has been developed using the professional antigen-presenting DC.[32] This system produces polyclonal CD4+ and CD8+ CTLs specific for 15 antigens from seven viruses: EBV, CMV, adenovirus, BK, human herpes virus-6 (HHV-6), respiratory syncytial virus (RSV), and influenza. Furthermore, the manufacturing period of seven to 14 days is a significant improvement over the conventional three to four weeks (or longer) required for the existing viral methodologies. The addition of prosurvival cytokines interleukin-4 (IL4) and IL7 produced exponential expansion of virus-specific CTLs. These heptavirus-specific CTLs would be the first CTL immunotherapy for BK, HHV-6, and RSV, and in vivo results are eagerly anticipated.

Also relevant will be the application of this multivirus system for producing virus-specific T cells from CMV-naïve donors. Usually, the most severe posttransplant infections are those that arise in recipients of naïve donors. The banking of "third-party" virus-immune T-cell lines with common HLA polymorphisms has been explored for EBV, CMV, and adenovirus.[17,33,34] Generally, the results of these studies have shown significant rates of remission for patients with active infections, although of lower magnitude than traditional specific donor-derived CTLs. Of note, the risk of alloreactivity does not appear to have increased, with one case-reported exception of bystander-induced liver GVHD.[35] Criteria for selecting the best matched third-party line have yet to be defined.

IFNγ capture is a promising emerging selection strategy. Donor T cells are challenged with viral-specific antigens, and the activated IFNγ-secreting subset is isolated. Advantages of this approach include shortened manufacturing times and no HLA restriction. CMV-,[36,37] EBV-,[38,39] and adenovirus-specific[28] CTLs have been tested in patients with active disease, with response rates of at least 83%, 50%, and 44%, respectively. Further work exploring the best stimulating antigens and culture times for lower frequency viruses remains to be seen.

T-cell therapy for cancer

The topic of T cells for cancer therapy is a rapidly expanding field, and already encompasses enough important studies to fill its own chapter. Herein, we will highlight each of the major types of T-cell therapies, including tumor-specific T cells, tumor-nonspecific T cells in donor lymphocyte infusions (DLIs), selected tumor-infiltrating lymphocytes (TILs), and genetically modified T cells. Readers are referred to excellent recent reviews for more coverage of each approach.[40–42]

Donor lymphocyte infusions

Allogeneic HCT as treatment for hematopoietic cancers is itself a form of highly effective immunotherapy that has been recognized since the 1950s. Even before mechanisms were well understood, the indirect relationship between GVHD and leukemia relapse become clear.[14] T cells were soon implicated for their roles in both processes, as T-cell depletion improved GVHD complications but led to higher relapse rates.[43] T cells are essential for controlling tumor cells that survive any preparative regimen (i.e., the graft-versus-leukemia [GVL] effect), but the difficulty is balancing this benefit while preventing severe GVHD.[44,45] These discoveries led to a number of strategies to enhance the limited effect of DLI in non-CML transplantation protocols, where outcomes have been inferior. Higher doses of DLI, combined with lymphodepleting chemotherapy as well as unrelated donors, have been associated with increased GVHD risk, which limits efficacy.[46]

Specific CD4, CD8, and γ/δ T-cell subsets continue to be explored as immunotherapeutic agents.[38,44] For example, the generation of CD4+ T helper 2 (Th2) cells through ex vivo IL4 and IL2 stimulation and infusion into T cell–replete allogeneic HCT patients led to accelerated lymphocyte reconstitution and increased inflammatory cytokine pathways without elevations in GVHD.[47] Another clinical trial recently infused rapamycin-resistant donor CD4+ Th2/T helper 1 (Th1) cells after matched-sibling low-intensity-regimen HCT for refractory hematologic disease.[48] Recipients had preferential and rapid immune reconstitution with the CD4+ Th2/Th1 cells, demonstrating the possibilities of achieving donor immunity (and thus GVL) with reduced-intensity preparative regimens. Acceptable GVHD rates were observed, making this platform an attractive candidate for future comparative efficacy studies.

Overall, DLIs have helped transplant patients overcome relapses of leukemia and low-grade lymphoma with rates of success ranging from 70–80% in chronic myeloid leukemia to 15–45% in acute myeloid leukemia (AML), 40–60% in multiple myeloma, 60% in low-grade lymphomas (including Hodgkin), but only 5% in acute

lymphoblastic leukemia.[49] The varying response rates and durations continue to be areas of active research, but likely relate to regulation of T-cell recognition molecules, pace of disease, and tumor antigen phenotypes.

Tumor-infiltrating lymphocytes

Many tumors are infiltrated by reactive T cells in vivo, and although these T cells have specific antitumor activity, they can fail to control tumor growth.[40] Emerging evidence suggests that these TILs are suppressed by upregulation of a variety of proteins.[50] Removing these TILs from the in vivo environment can facilitate activation and expansion. Additionally, host lymphodepletion and chemoradiotherapy prior to TIL transfer significantly enhance engraftment and efficacy of the transferred cells.[51] Subsequent reinfusion of this tumor-specific population has led to measurable responses in patients with metastatic melanoma, ranging from 49% to 72% depending on the preconditioning regimen.[52] Whereas the three- and five-year survival rates were only 36% and 29%, respectively, those patients who initially achieved complete tumor regression had rates of 100% and 93%. Other groups have reproduced these findings with initial response rates closer to 50%.[53] Efforts to extend this application to epithelial tumors have been generally unsuccessful. One theory suggests that the high number of mutations in melanomas makes this tumor well suited for T-cell-mediated therapy, whereas tumors predominated by epigenetic changes may be less immunogenic and thus less responsive to T-cell-mediated therapy.[40,54,55]

A recent exception to TILs' melanoma-limited efficacy is the durable response seen in a patient with cholangiocarcinoma.[56] Whole-exome sequencing of extracted TILs revealed a population of CD4+ Th1 cells that recognized a *HER2* mutation expressed by the patient's metastatic epithelial cancer. Infusion of ex vivo–expanded TILs enriched for this mutation-specific population led to disease stabilization and regression in a dose-dependent manner. This study underscores the concept that T cells, given the right microenvironment, stimulation, dose, and specificity, are effective tumor eradication tools. As our knowledge and ability to obtain detailed genetic information continue to increase, T cells are positioned as excellent targets for ex vivo engineering specificity, as addressed further in this chapter.

Genetically engineered T cells

T cells can be genetically modified for cancer immunotherapy via two primary approaches: (1) gene-modified TCRs in which an antigen receptor specific for a target antigen is introduced, typically by retroviruses or lentiviruses; and (2) chimeric antigen receptors (CARs), which link a single-chain variable fragment (scFv) domain of an antibody to a TCR intracellular domain that activates the T cell.[57] CARs are HLA independent but generally have lower sensitivity, whereas TCRs can recognize intracellular proteins in addition to cell surface antigens but are susceptible to resistance by HLA downregulation.[58] This is a rapidly growing sector of biotechnology; a September 2013 meeting of the Office of Biotechnology Activities at the National Institutes of Health reported 111 registered protocols for the two approaches combined, with 90% of the TCR trials targeting solid tumors and 50% of the CAR trials focusing on hematologic cancers.[57]

Gene-modified TCRs

One of the first studies of TCRs in human trials engineered T-cell expression of the melanoma antigen recognized by T cells 1

(MART-1). Tansfer of these cells into 15 patients with metastatic melanoma resulted in high levels of engraftment (>10% of peripheral blood lymphocytes) for at least two months post infusion, and for one year in two patients who experienced regression of metastatic lesions.[59] Within several years, the applications extended beyond melanoma. Cancer-testis antigens (CTAs) are genes whose overexpression has been demonstrated in many carcinomas, hematologic malignancies, melanoma, and testicular cancers.[60] Transfer of T cells engineered with the CTA NY-ESO-1 provided tumor regression in four of six patients with synovial cell sarcoma and five of 11 patients with melanoma with NY-ESO-1-expressing tumors.[61] A current clinical trial of transduced TCRs targets the Wilm's tumor-1 antigen found at high levels on leukemic cells (NTC01621724).

Chimeric antigen receptors

First-generation CARs linked the scFv to the CD3z chain, a signal-transduction component of the T-cell antigen receptor.[58] The B-cell antigens CD19 and CD20 are the most common antibody targets for CAR hematologic protocols. These B-cell-specific CARs are designed to eradicate the neoplastic populations in B-cell lymphomas and leukemias and, by nature of CD19 and CD20 expression, also the nonneoplastic B cells. Although these early trials with anti-CD19 and anti-CD20 CARs were safe, efficacy was limited and detection of the transferred CTLs was short-lived (24 hours to 7 days).[62] This poor persistence was thought secondary to the absence of costimulation, and thus second-generation CARs incorporated dual signaling molecules such as CD28, 4-1BB, and OX-40.[63]

Indeed, direct comparisons of first- and second-generation CARs revealed improved expansion and persistence for those CTLs engineered with CD28 costimulation.[64] Clinical trials of these second-generation CARs have been directed toward CD19 in chronic lymphoid leukemia (CLL)[65] and pediatric,[66] adult,[67] and relapsed B-cell acute lymphoblastic leukemia (B-ALL).[68–70] The results differ somewhat by disease. Patients with bulky CLL showed mixed responses in lymphadenopathy,[69] whereas 88% (14 of 16) to 100% (5 of 5) of relapsed B-ALL adults achieved complete molecular remission.[68–70] Of two pediatric B-ALL patients, both obtained complete remission with high levels of circulating CTLs, although they also experienced cytokine-release syndrome and B-cell aplasia.[66] One of these patients remained in remission at 11 months, whereas the other relapsed after two months with blast cells that no longer expressed CD19. Although these results suggest that autologous CAR-expressing T cells have the potential to induce rapid remission and provide a bridge to curative transplant, the emergence of tumor cells with antigen evasion may mandate targeting multiple molecules.

Third-generation CARs add a second costimulatory domain. Early clinical trials with CD20-specific CARs coupled to CD28 and 4-1BB produced modest antitumor activity with relatively low circulating CTLs at one year.[71] Interestingly, this protocol used electroporated DNA plasmids, as opposed to the retroviral vectors or transposons used in other work, and proved not to be as effective for transformation.

Solid tumor studies have designed CARs with both virus- and non-virus-specific T cells. Three of 11 patients with active neuroblastoma achieved remission with EBV-specific CTLs and activated T cells expressing CARs directed to diasialoganglioside GD2 expressed on human neuroblastoma cells.[72] Persistence of these populations six weeks beyond infusion was associated with superior clinical outcome, and both were detectable up to 96 weeks post infusion.[73] The duration of persistence was concordant with the percentage of CD4$^+$ cells and central memory cells (CD45RO$^+$

CD62L$^+$) in the infused product. Preclinical and clinical trials exploring the efficacy of CARs targeting HER2/neu for sarcoma, glioblastoma, ovarian and breast cancer, and human prostate-specific membrane antigen are showing promising results.[57,74,75]

Regulatory T cells

Immunotherapy with an additional CD4$^+$ subset, the regulatory T cells (Tregs), has been explored to take advantage of their role in suppressing immune system activation and promoting tolerance.[76,77] Specifically, Tregs have been targeted for depletion and inactivation because they can effectively limit the expansion of tumor-specific T cells.[78] The best Treg receptor(s) target for depletion is an area of active research; early clinical studies of CD25 blockade have shown mixed results for enhancement of antitumor activity in patients with metastatic melanoma and breast cancer.[79,80]

Interestingly, the majority of Treg cancer applications take a different approach than the direct antitumor effects sought with other lymphocyte subsets. Tregs can promote the immune tolerance that is essential to both solid organ transplant and HCT, with the latter showing promising clinical trial results. Infusion of CD25$^+$ Tregs harvested from partially HLA-matched human umbilical cord blood and expanded ex vivo with anti-CD3/CD28 and recombinant human IL2 reduced the incidence of GVHD in 23 HCT patients, as compared to 108 controls.[81] Adult expanded Tregs from HCT HLA-haploidentical donors have also helped reduce chronic GVHD in high-risk acute leukemia patients.[82] Additional trials of adoptive Treg therapy are currently underway (e.g., NCT02091232 examining Treg infusions in kidney transplant recipients and NCT00602693 examining Treg infusion after umbilical cord blood transplant in patients with advanced hematologic cancer).

Dendritic cell immunotherapy

Introduction

DCs, named for their tree-like cytoplasmic projections, are innate hematopoietic cells that reside in all body tissues, including the lymph tissue.[83] Via environmental surveillance, DCs capture protein antigens and present them as peptides in both MHC class I and II molecules (as well as lipid antigens in nonclassical MHCs).[84] Through these DC-initiated interactions, naïve T cells are differentiated into antigen-specific and effector T cells, Th cells can be expanded, and B cells stimulated. Innate immune cells such as NK cells and mast cells are also receptive to DC interaction. Some DC subsets, such as immature DCs in peripheral tissues, can present self-antigens and induce immune tolerance through T-cell depletion or activation of regulatory and suppressor T cells. As such, DCs orchestrate tolerance and immune defense bridging the innate and adaptive immune systems. Animal models have shown that DCs generate tumor-specific cytotoxic T cells by capturing and presenting tumor antigens to lymph-node-draining T cells.[85] These versatile properties make DCs extremely attractive targets for immunotherapy strategies.

Unmanipulated DCs in the tumor environment

DCs are known to infiltrate the tumor microenvironment, picking up antigens from tumor cells.[86] Both protumor and antitumor responses are generated by DC interactions, ranging from promoting phagocytosis of dying tumor cells[87] to angiogenesis and preventing activation of tumor-specific T cells by interrupting antigen processing.[88,89] Improved understanding for these opposing activation pathways could lead to valuable immunotherapy approaches. Direct DC-dependent tumor cytotoxicity has been described in basal cell carcinoma treated with the toll-like receptor 7 agonist imiquimod.[90]

Ex vivo–engineered DC vaccines

Ex vivo–generated DC vaccines have been used with varied levels of success for treatment of multiple myeloma, colon cancer, renal cancer, prostate cancer, and advanced-stage melanoma.[84] DCs are generally derived from hematopoietic progenitor cells or monocytes with cytokine cocktails, the exact nature of which can yield improved antitumor activity.[86] DC culturing ex vivo helps avoid some of the functional deficiencies and tumor tolerance observed with DCs developed in the tumor microenvironment.[91] The selection of the antigen for DC processing is also crucial to immunogenicity. DC loading with nonmutated self-antigens can lead to negative selection due to high-avidity self-antigens, and using unique mutated tumor antigens will require highly patient-specific vaccine formulations.[92]

An alternative to single antigen loading is fusing autologous DCs with patient-derived whole tumor cells as an antigen source via electrofusion or polyethylene glycol.[93–95] Processed antigens are presented in both MHC class I and II, generating both CD4- and CD8-specific responses. These preparations show increased in vitro tumor killing compared to T cells stimulated by DCs pulsed with tumor lysate or apoptotic bodies.[96] Early clinical studies in patients with renal cell and breast cancer demonstrated the excellent safety profile of the DC–tumor cell fusion vaccines, as well as their ability to expand tumor-specific T cells.[97] More recent studies have shown significant clinical success with DC–myeloma cell hybridomas in the period following autologous stem cell transplant leading to the expansion of CD4$^+$ and CD8$^+$ myeloma-specific T cells. Seventy-eight percent of the phase II study patients achieved a best response of complete response (CR) or very good partial response, and 47% achieved a CR or near CR.[94]

Understanding why some patients experience objective tumor regression and others appear tolerant to the vaccines will require continued investigation of the basics of DC immunology and signaling. Overall, this approach is viewed with optimism as a series of phase II and III clinical trials, in addition to those for multiple myeloma, have shown encouraging outcomes including prolonged survival for ex vivo–generated DC vaccines in metastatic melanoma, prostate cancer, and follicular lymphoma.[94,98–100] One of these vaccines, sipuleucel-T, is currently approved by the US Food and Drug Administration for metastatic prostate cancer (www.fda.gov).

In vivo–engineered DC vaccines

DC targeting is a vaccine approach that conjugates a DC receptor antibody with a specific antigen. These chimeric proteins, when delivered in vivo and exposed to the appropriate DC maturation signals, produce robust antigen-specific CD4 and CD8 T-cell subsets.[101] These studies have been performed primarily in murine models, but offer promise for clinical extension. Of note, this targeted approach has shed light onto the functions of specific DC subsets. For example, CD8$^+$ DCs expressing the surface protein CD205 present antigen via MHC class I and II, whereas CD8$^-$ DCs that respond to antibody 33D1 are MHC class II restricted.[102] This knowledge about DC subsets is likely to prove useful for generating T-cell responses through multiple pathways.

In addition to presenting specific antigen, these antibody-conjugated proteins can be designed to interact with activating receptors. Herein is another illustration of the importance of understanding DC-signaling pathways, as activation signals may promote DCs' role in control of either immune tolerance or clearance. Fundamental work in this area has shown that activation of dendritic cell asialoglycoprotein receptor (DCASGPR) promotes DC release of IL10, differentiating T cells into suppressor types and possibly downregulating tumor-specific T cells. Although one can envision potential applications for DCASGPR targeting in autoimmune diseases, careful and specific work is needed to find a similar approach to enhance antitumor activity.[103]

Artificial APCs

As discussed above, the applications of natural DCs are limited by an incomplete understanding of the activating and suppressive in vivo signaling pathways. Furthermore, collection, culturing, and stimulation of autologous DCs ex vivo have been challenging and often yield mixed-quality product.[104] For these reasons, artificial antigen-presenting cells (aAPCs) have been developed to garner better control of antigen presentation and cell surface receptor signaling in the setting of ex vivo T-cell stimulation. The majority of work on aAPCs to date has targeted the induction of CD8$^+$ T cells through the MHC I pathway to access the direct cytotoxic capabilities of this cell set. The choice of material ranges widely in composition, shape, and size, including 5 µm polystyrene latex microbeads, 200–400 nm "nanoworms," and 100 µm liposomes.[105] Another goal for this strategy is true "off-the-shelf" use, where aAPCs could be directly injected without an ex vivo T-cell co-culturing or expansion. These applications are understandably more complicated; however, murine models have been useful to refine the safety and efficacy of various antigens and synthetic designs (with properties such as size, flexibility, and biodistribution being paramount). Dextran-coated iron oxide magnetic particles (50–100 nm) and dextran-coated quantum dots (30 nm) demonstrated promising in vivo murine tumor growth suppression.[106] Despite the formidable challenges inherent in these synthetic approaches, the early work is promising and certainly worth attention for the future of cancer immunotherapy.

NK cell immunotherapy

Introduction

NK cells are lymphocytes of the innate immune system responsible for surveillance of malignant transformation or infection. They become educated and acquire function by interaction with MHC class I molecules. In the clinic, haploidentical NK cells can be adoptively transferred to treat cancer. Persistence and in vivo expansion of NK cells depend on lymphodepleting chemotherapy to make space, eliminating suppressor cells, and releasing endogenous IL15. In vivo expansion is also enhanced by cytokine administration of IL2 or IL15. It is believed that IL15 may be superior because IL2 has the downside of stimulating CD25^{hi} Tregs. Recent developments of specific NK-cell engagers may help address the limitations of NK cell therapy, including the complexity of exporting cell therapies and lack of specificity.

NK cell biology

In the early 1970s, a new class of lymphocytes, called *NK cells*, was discovered based on their ability to kill target cells without prior sensitization. These lymphocytes from athymic nude mice were highly reactive against syngeneic and allogeneic tumors in a ^{51}Cr release cytotoxicity assay, and antitumor reactivity was not T-cell dependent.[107,108] It is now known that malignant and viral transformed cells may lose expression of MHC class I in a process of "loss of self" and as a result become "susceptible" to NK cell killing.[109–111] NK cells are educated to acquire function by interaction with MHC class I molecules. They are capable of direct cell–cell mediated killing and cytokine production, and both are important in their antitumor activity.[112–114] New data demonstrate that NK cells can be long-lived and remember past exposures, such as CMV challenge, and thus have adaptive properties.[115–118]

NK cell tolerance

Until the discovery of NK cell receptors that recognize class I MHC (killer immunoglobulin-like receptors [KIRs] and the lectin NKG2 receptors representing the main families), it was assumed that NK cells kill targets in an MHC-unrestricted fashion.[119] Karre and Ljunggren overturned this belief in 1985 with their discovery that NK cell killing is directed to targets with "missing self."[120] Inhibitory KIR and NKG2A recognize classical class I MHC or nonclassical HLA-E, respectively, to prevent lysis and thereby induce NK cell tolerance. Both of these receptor families contain activating receptors and thus engender even greater complexity.[121] Although activating KIR2DS1 can recognize HLA-C2[122] and KIR2DS2 recognizes HLA-A11[123] ligands of many activating KIRs are unknown. Like NKG2A, NKG2C can bind to HLA-E.[124] Notably, NKG2C is an activating receptor of particular importance that is induced by CMV infection.[125,126]

NK cell education and licensing

Specific subsets of NK cells bearing HLA class I–recognizing inhibitory receptors acquire function via interactions with their cognate ligands.[127,128] For example, KIR3DL1$^+$ NK cells from individuals bearing the corresponding HLA-Bw4 ligand exhibit maximal function in response to missing self, whereas KIR3DL1$^+$ NK cells from individuals who are homozygous for HLA-Bw6 are hyporesponsive. Immature NK cells that lack receptors for HLA molecules cannot be educated until they begin to express self-recognizing inhibitory KIR or NKG2A.[129]

Adaptive NK cells

The novel concept of NK cell memory has emerged over the past several years with the identification of subsets of NK cells in mice that mount heightened secondary responses in an antigen-specific fashion in models of delayed-type hypersensitivity reactions,[130] immunization,[131] and mouse CMV infection.[132,133] The only known equivalent human cells are CD57$^+$NKG2C$^+$ NK cells that expand specifically in response to human CMV.[116,125,126] However, NKG2C is not the receptor for human CMV (unlike Ly49H in murine NK cells that binds CMV m157).[134] Analogous cells have been identified in humans after transplantation.[125,126] Whether these NK cells possess all of the attributes ascribed to classical memory T and B cells or whether they are "memory-like" is still a matter of debate and terminology. However, it is clear that subsets of NK cells adapt specifically to CMV.

Activating receptors and cytokines

Under normal homeostatic conditions, a balance of activating and inhibitory signals tightly control NK cell function. Activating NK cell receptors include natural cytotoxicity receptors NKp30, NKp44, and NK46; and others such as NKG2D and DNAM-1 that are constitutively expressed on all NK cells.[135,136] Activating receptors recognize stress-induced molecules, HLA class 1–related MICA and MICB, class I–like CMV-homologous ULBP proteins, and ligands CD155 (PVR) and CD112 (Nectin-2).[137] Tumors vary in these activating ligands they express. In vitro, NK cells can mediate the direct killing of freshly isolated human tumor cells from AML, acute lymphoblastic leukemia, multiple myeloma, neuroblastoma, and ovarian, colon, renal cell, and gastric carcinomas.[138,139] NK cells can also be activated or primed directly by cytokines. After incubating NK cells with cytokines, in particular IL2, IL12, IL18, or IL15, NK cells acquire the capacity to lyse a broad array of fresh and cultured tumor targets not normally sensitive to NK lysis.[140] Furthermore, cytokine-activated NK cells are synergistic with monoclonal antibodies against resistant cell lines in vitro and in mouse xenograft models.

Autologous NK cells in therapy of cancer

The initial application of autologous therapy was in the form of lymphokine-activated killer (LAK) cell therapy to treat cancer as pioneered at the National Cancer Institute (NCI) in the 1980s.[141] These LAK cells contained mixtures of T and NK cells activated with IL2, and several models suggest that the smaller population of NK cells may account for most of the antitumor activity. The importance of these early clinical observations taught us that (1) high-dose IL2 used in vivo with the aim of activating lymphocytes has significant toxicity in the form of severe capillary leak syndrome; (2) low-dose subcutaneous IL2 with and without autologous LAK cells lessens toxicity; and (3) mixed populations of lymphocytes have limited but some antitumor activity.

In three clinical trials at the University of Minnesota, we tested use of ex vivo IL2-activated autologous NK cells followed by daily subcutaneous IL2 in patients with a variety of malignancies, including non-Hodgkin's lymphoma and renal cell carcinoma.[142] Therapy was safe, but autologous NK cells failed to demonstrate sufficient efficacy. We hypothesized that this was a result of autologous NK cells being inhibited by self-MHC. Based on knowledge of inhibitory KIRs and rules of NK licensing, we and others began to investigate the possibility of using allogeneic NK cells based on the premise that they would provide a higher frequency of NK cells that would not be inhibited by self-HLA.

Allogeneic NK cells in therapy of cancer

In clinical trials using allogeneic T cell–depleted HCT from haploidentical donors in patients with AML, Rugierri et al. showed that NK cell cytotoxicity is enhanced if a KIR–HLA class I mismatch occurs. Remarkably, the potent antileukemia responses delivered by allogeneic donor-derived NK cells were not associated with GVHD.[143,144] These observations lead us to hypothesize that mature haploidentical NK cells alone without stem cell transplantation can have antitumor responses in AML.

In a trial involving patients with refractory acute myelogenous leukemia, we used a lymphodepleting regimen with high-dose cyclophosphamide (60 mg/kg/day × 2) followed by IV fludarabine 25 mg/m^2/day × 5 days chemotherapy (Hi-Cy/Flu) followed by infusion of adoptively transferred HLA-haploidentical NK cells.[145] IL2 was administered daily (1.75 million units/m^2) for 14 days (subsequently modified to 6 higher doses [10 million units without m^2 correction] for 2 weeks). Administration of the regimen uniformly resulted in lymphopenia and marrow suppression. A marked increase in IL15 concentration (up to 100 pg/dl) was detected in patients receiving Hi-Cy/Flu. Data suggest that decreasing numbers of mature lymphocytes, which utilize IL15, will result in elevated plasma IL15 concentrations. We also found that 26% of poor-prognosis AML patients achieved complete hematologic remission after NK cell adoptive transfer. The apheresis product was CD3 depleted and activated with IL2 in vitro. Cell processing resulted in a significant reduction of T cells in all products, decreasing from 60% in the apheresis product to 1% after CD3 depletion, yielding a final T cell dose of $1.5 \pm 0.3 \times 10^5$ cells/kg. There was an average of 40-fold fewer T cells than NK cells. Other components of the final product included monocytes (27%) and B lymphocytes (14%). All patients received subcutaneous IL2 after infusions. Ten percent of the subjects in this trial met criteria for successful NK cell expansion, defined as >100 NK cell/μL blood in peripheral blood at day 14 after NK cell infusion.

In subsequent applications of donor NK cell infusions to treat non-Hodgkin's lymphoma, breast cancer, and ovarian cancer, we and others have found that host regulatory T cells (Tregs) are resistant to cytotoxic therapy and expand rapidly when IL2 is administered after NK cell infusion.[146,147] Tregs are phenotypically distinct $CD4^+CD25^+Foxp3^+$ immunosuppressive lymphocytes residing in lymphoid organs and peripheral blood. In two subsequent clinical trials, we treated 23 additional patients with Hi-Cy/Flu lymphodepleting chemotherapy. Fifteen patients also received IL2 diphtheria toxin (IL2DT), a recombinant cytotoxic fusion protein composed of the amino acid sequences for diphtheria toxin followed by truncated amino acid sequences for IL2. We hypothesized that IL2DT would selectively deplete IL2 receptor ($CD25^+$) expressing cells, including Tregs. Among the 15 patients treated with this regimen, 10 had detectable donor NK cells at day 7 (median 68% donor DNA). At day 14, 27% had successfully expanded NK cells in vivo, with median absolute donor-derived NK cell counts of 1000 cells/μL blood. These results improved upon our previous rate of 10% in vivo NK cell expansion observed with the same regimen but without Treg depletion. The absence of a Treg population at either day 7 or day 14 correlated with an in vivo NK cell expansion at day 14. Augmented lymphocyte and Treg depletion with IL2DT resulted in 53% patients attaining CR, significantly better compared to strategies without IL2DT (CR rate, 10%; $p = 0.02$). These outcomes suggest that the NK cells themselves played a role in the antileukemia response above the high-dose chemotherapy preparative regimen. Patients achieving remission also had a significantly higher proportion of circulating donor NK cells, further suggesting that persistence and expansion are required to observe clinical efficacy.

Donor NK cell products

Three different processing methods were used to prepare NK cell products for infusion in AML trials. These included CD3 depletion alone (32 patients), CD3 depletion followed by CD56 selection (10 patients), and single-step CD3/CD19 depletion (15 patients). $CD19^+$ B-cell depletion was added after we observed severe hemolytic anemia mediated by NK cell donor passenger B lymphocytes as well as EBV lymphoproliferative disease events.[148] Importantly, we observed that the process of CD56 selection resulted in threefold fewer NK cells per product compared to CD3 depletion alone. All clinical products were highly cytotoxic against K562 targets. The highest NK cell doses (mean 26×10^6 NK cells/kg) were obtained with the CD3/CD19 depletion method, due to the reduced cell loss

with the single negative selection step and extended five-hour apheresis collection time.

Future perspectives and preclinical strategies

Several tumor-targeted antibody strategies have been proposed to enhance NK cell activity or targeting. These approaches are intended to interrupt NK cell inhibition, provide costimulation, or enhance targeting through CD16. Each of these strategies has the potential to augment the therapeutic benefit of NK cells and to broaden the impact of their use beyond hematologic malignancies.

The Fc receptor CD16 is present on most peripheral blood NK cells. Upon recognition of antibody-coated tumor cells, CD16 delivers potent activating signals to NK cells, leading to target elimination through direct killing and cytokine production. Our group recently demonstrated that activated NK cells lose Fc receptor gamma (CD16) and homing receptor CD62L that is clipped by disintegrin and metalloprotease-17 (ADAM17).[149] Inhibition of ADAM17 enhanced CD16-mediated NK cell function by preserving CD16 on the NK cell surface, and thus increased killing of rituximab-coated lymphoma cells. In addition, ADAM family enzymes are highly expressed in lymphoma tumor stroma. Lymphoma-associated stress ligands (e.g., ULB, MICa, MICb, and B7-H6) are also ADAM17 protease targets.[150] These findings demonstrate that novel therapeutic targets such as ADAM17 can be explored clinically to augment the efficacy of monoclonal antibody-dependent NK cell tumor cell killing.

In addition to monoclonal antibodies, we at the University of Minnesota have focused on a platform using bispecific killer engagers (BiKEs) constructed with a single-chain Fv against CD16 and a single-chain Fv against a tumor-associated antigen.[151,152] Using CD16 × 19 BiKEs and a trispecific CD16 × 19 × 22 (TriKE), we have shown that CD16 signaling is potent and delivers a different signal compared with natural recognition of rituximab, especially in regard to cytokine production. One advantage to the BiKE and TriKE platform is its flexibility and ease of production. We have recently developed a CD16 × 33 BiKE to target myeloid malignancies (AML and myelodysplastic syndrome). One of the most remarkable properties of this drug is its potent signaling. In refractory AML, we found that CD16 × 33 BiKE overcomes inhibitory KIR signaling, leading to potent killing and production of cytokines by NK cells.[151] Interestingly, ADAM17 inhibition enhances CD16 × 33 BiKE responses against primary AML targets. These immunotherapeutics will be developed for clinical testing for hematologic malignancies and will allow for NK cells activation via CD16 while approximating NK cells in direct contact with targeted tumor cells. Lastly, IL15 is in phase I/II clinical trials to support allogeneic NK cell adoptive transfer without Treg stimulation.

Mesenchymal stromal cell immunotherapy

Introduction

MSCs were first described in 1968 by Friedenstein et al. as bone marrow–derived, adherent, fibroblast-like cells capable of differentiation to bone.[153] Since then, MSCs have been isolated from a variety of tissue sources, including umbilical cord blood, Wharton's jelly, and adipose tissue,[154] and an abundance of studies exploring a wide array of potential clinical utilities have been undertaken. In an initial effort to better characterize MSCs, Dominici et al. determined minimal criteria for defining these cells.[155] Subsequent work has moved characterization forward; however, there is still a need for further efforts.[156] Clinical applications of MSCs can be categorized, with some overlap, into regenerative medicine and immunomodulation or immuno-therapy.[157] The focus here is on immunomodulation and immunotherapy.

Clinical applications

Basic research has suggested several possible mechanisms of action, including the ability of MSCs to home to injured tissue and to secrete bioactive molecules to stimulate recovery/repair and inhibit additional inflammation. Additionally, many studies have shown MSCs to lack immunogenicity, to essentially be immune-privileged, and to be capable of immunomodulatory functions. Figure 41.1 provides an overview of some of the interactions of MSCs with the immune system.[157]

Because of these apparent unique qualities of MSCs, the targets for treatment have included diseases or conditions such as multiple sclerosis, amyotrophic lateral sclerosis, systemic lupus erythematosus, Crohn's disease, and organ transplantation.[157] The first trial with MSCs was published in 1995, a phase I study for safety and feasibility of autologous MSC manufacturing and infusion into 15 hematology–oncology patients.[158] Follow-up studies showed encouraging results, particularly with GVHD.[159,160] Subsequent negative results from one study in particular led to much debate in the field with discussions focusing on potential issues such

as donor variance, culture expansion, immunogenicity, and cryopreservation.[161]

Future Directions

Over 200 MSC trials are registered with Clinicaltrials.gov showing progress and interest in this strategy.[157] Most of these studies are phase I/II, but several phase III trials have been initiated. Roughly half of the trials use marrow as the starting material for manufacturing MSCs. Umbilical cord blood (UCB) and adipose tissue account for 29% of trials, and several other sources make up the remainder. It remains to be determined which source is best, and it may be that a certain source is better for a given application. In the case of marrow, donor age has been shown to affect MSC quality and quantity.[162] The importance of age is further exemplified by studies indicating a 2-log greater number of MSCs in UCB as compared to adult marrow.[163] In addition to different sources of starting material, studies have involved both autologous and allogeneic (related and unrelated) donations. In trials involving allogeneic donors, the concept of the "qualified" donor has surfaced.[161] As our understanding of MSCs advances, the need for a more robustly characterized, or "qualified," donor may be appreciated.

Although MSCs have been used clinically for several years, there remains a great need for a better understanding of the contributions and impact of the various aspects of culture. There is variation in initial processing (e.g., direct plating and density gradient), type of

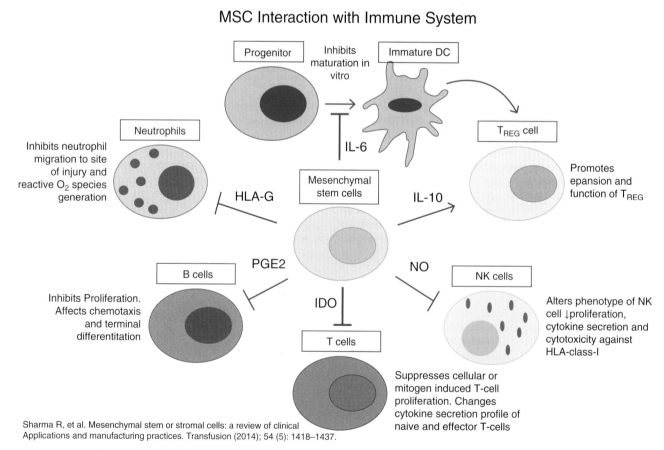

MSC Interaction with Immune System

Sharma R, et al. Mesenchymal stem or stromal cells: a review of clinical
Applications and manufacturing practices. Transfusion (2014); 54 (5): 1418–1437.

Figure 41.1 Mesenchymal stromal cell (MSC) interaction with immune system. Source: Sharma *et al.* (2014).[157] Reproduced with permission of Wiley.

medium (e.g., alpha-minimal essential medium and Dulbecco's modified Eagle's medium), additives (e.g., fetal bovine serum, human AB serum, platelet lysate, and growth factors), seeding densities, length of culture and number of passages, and other culture-related variables (e.g., oxygen tension). Additionally, cryo-preservation continues to be largely based upon experience with hematopoietic stem cells, and thus is not optimized for MSCs.[164] Optimization is further hampered by lack of details on manufacturing in clinical reports.

Although much attention should be given to optimization of methods, it is too early in therapeutic development to propose standardization of manufacturing. Standardization is a goal of preclinical development and clinical manufacturing for any trial. However, for MSCs, it is important to balance standardization against the need for further knowledge and innovation on what cell types and functions are most efficacious.[165,166] MSCs have been shown to be safe and well tolerated, and several studies point toward efficacy in the immunomodulation/immunotherapy application, making the future appear bright for this cell type.

Conclusions

Several adoptive immunotherapies have shown considerable promise in the clinical arena, and the applications have expanded substantially in recent years. Early studies involved nonspecific T cells and lymphokine-activated killer cells, but subsequent studies have applied the knowledge gained in cell biology and immunology to exploit or harness the function of various subsets of T cells, DCs, NK cells, and MSCs. Advances in technology have further enhanced our ability to bring the next generation of cellular immunotherapies into the clinic. As we continue to gain insight into immune mechanisms and develop creative and robust manufacturing methods, there is enthusiasm for the future of adoptive immunotherapy, but challenges remain including cost and exportability.

Key references

A full reference list for this chapter is available at: http://www.wiley.com/go/simon/transfusion

32 Gerdemann U, Keirnan JM, Katari UL, *et al.* Rapidly generated multivirus-specific cytotoxic T lymphocytes for the prophylaxis and treatment of viral infections. *Mol Ther* 2012;**20** (8):1622–32.

65 Porter DL, Levine BL, Kalos M, Bagg A, June CH. Chimeric antigen receptor-modified T cells in chronic lymphoid leukemia. *N Engl J Med* 2011; **365** (8):725–33.

81 Brunstein CG, Miller JS, Cao Q, *et al.* Infusion of ex vivo expanded T regulatory cells in adults transplanted with umbilical cord blood: safety profile and detection kinetics. *Blood* 2011;**117** (3):1061–70.

94 Rosenblatt J, Avivi I, Vasir B, *et al.* Vaccination with dendritic cell/tumor fusions following autologous stem cell transplant induces immunologic and clinical responses in multiple myeloma patients. *Clin Cancer Res* 2013;**19** (13):3640–8.

116 Foley B, Cooley S, Verneris MR, *et al.* Human cytomegalovirus (CMV)-induced memory-like NKG2C(+) NK cells are transplantable and expand in vivo in response to recipient CMV antigen. *J Immunol* 2012;**189** (10):5082–8.

142 Burns LJ, Weisdorf DJ, DeFor TE, *et al.* IL-2-based immunotherapy after autologous transplantation for lymphoma and breast cancer induces immune activation and cytokine release: a phase I/II trial. *Bone Marrow Transplant* 2003;**32** (2):177–86.

146 Bachanova V, Burns LJ, McKenna DH, *et al.* Allogeneic natural killer cells for refractory lymphoma. *Cancer Immunol Immunother* 2010;**59** (11):1739–44.

151 Wiernik A, Foley B, Zhang B, *et al.* Targeting natural killer cells to acute myeloid leukemia in vitro with a CD16 x 33 bispecific killer cell engager and ADAM17 inhibition. *Clin Cancer Res* 2013;**19** (14):3844–55.

160 Le Blanc K, Frassoni F, Ball L, *et al.* Mesenchymal stem cells for treatment of steroid-resistant, severe, acute graft-versus-host disease: a phase II study. *Lancet* 2008;**371** (9624):1579–86.

161 Galipeau J. The mesenchymal stromal cells dilemma: does a negative phase III trial of random donor mesenchymal stromal cells in steroid-resistant graft-versus-host disease represent a death knell or a bump in the road? *Cytotherapy* 2013;**15** (1):2–8.

CHAPTER 42

Tissue engineering and regenerative medicine

Sumati Sundaram, Joshua Siewert, Jenna Balestrini, Ashley Gard, Kevin Boehm, Elise Wilcox, & Laura Niklason

Department of Biomedical Engineering, Yale University, Department of Anesthesiology, Yale School of Medicine, Yale University, New Haven, CT, USA

The fields of tissue engineering and regenerative medicine have evolved into a unified discipline with an interdisciplinary approach being a large part of the merger. The first use of the term tissue engineering in the public domain was at the proceedings of the Granlibakken workshop in 1985:[1] "Tissue engineering is the application of principles and methods of engineering and life sciences toward fundamental understanding of structure–function relationships in normal and pathological mammalian tissues and the development of biological substitutes to restore, maintain, or improve tissue function." This was a broad definition that focused on the incorporation of living cells into acellular, related structures as a source for tissue replacements. In addition to providing a definition of tissue engineering, the basic components necessary to create a tissue-engineered product were identified. These components included a cell source, a method to induce specific tissue growth, and a biomaterial to act as a scaffold.[2] The principles of tissue engineering have been translated to clinical applications with the US Food and Drug Administration (FDA) approval of products in the areas of skin substitutes, bone formation, and cartilage. Tissue engineering has the potential to revolutionize medical care by replacing diseased or damaged tissue without the use of conventional organ or tissue transplantation.

Overview of tissue engineering

A cell source or method that can be used for all cell lineages and has the required characteristics to make it safe, reproducible, and without any immunologic rejection has not been developed. The options for a cell source are primary autologous, allogeneic, xenogeneic, or stem cells. Cells can be cultured with low rates of bacterial contamination through the use of antibiotics and sterile technique. However, concerns about xenogeneic contamination remain if feeder cells or sera from other species are used in the cell culture conditions. An alternative to primary tissue is to induce progenitor cells to differentiate into a specific cell type. Difficulties associated with the usage of primary tissue often include the need for an operative procedure, inability to obtain sufficient normal cells, inability of cells to proliferate, and the presence of cells with the same genetic predisposition for development of a disease. Another complication of primary cell sources is the need to efficiently isolate a specific cell lineage with low contamination rates from other cell types. Cell sorting methods, such as magnetic or fluorescent cell

sorting, provide a reliable method if the cell type has specific membrane proteins with known antibodies.

Stem cell sources

Stem cells are an attractive cell source for tissue-engineering applications. Adult stem cells or human embryonic stem cells (hESCs) each offer their own set of advantages and challenges. Adult stem cells can typically be harvested by less invasive procedures from marrow, fat, or skin. Because these cells are autologous, no immunosuppressive medications are needed when the tissue is implanted in the donor. Purification difficulties and a reduced differentiation potential of adult stem cells as compared to embryonic cells, however, prevent use of these cells for all applications. Adult stem cells do not involve human embryos or any of the ethical controversies related to the collection of embryonic cells. The potential use of embryonic stem cells had created a national debate over ethical issues, because an embryo must be destroyed to harvest the cells. However, with the availability of induced pluripotent stem cells, such issues can be avoided, and therefore we now have access to personalized cell sources. This is a major technical advance and has the potential to transform the field of regenerative medicine.

Scaffolds

A scaffold should enable the creation of a three-dimensional (3D) formation of tissue in vitro and in vivo. Properties for the ideal tissue-engineered scaffold are the support of cell attachment, ability for the cells to proliferate and differentiate, allowance for diffusion of nutrients and waste, and ability to simulate mechanical properties found in vivo.[3] Biomaterials can be categorized as synthetic polymers, natural materials, or inorganic matter; they can also be classified as being biodegradable or permanent.[4]

The preference for tissue-engineered scaffolds has been on biodegradable natural materials and polymers. Natural materials include collagen, gelatin, fibrinogen, dextran, glycosaminoglycans, and chitin. Examples of biodegradable synthetic polymers are polylactic acid (PLA), polyglycolic acid (PGA), and polycaprolactone (PCL). The properties of natural materials are their similarity to the native biologic environment, minimal toxicity, and degradation by natural enzymes.[4] The limitations of natural materials include batch-to-batch variability from different animal sources, and potential immunologic reactions if materials are of xenogeneic origin. The most commonly used FDA-approved biodegradable

Rossi's Principles of Transfusion Medicine, Fifth Edition. Edited by Toby L. Simon, Jeffrey McCullough, Edward L. Snyder, Bjarte G. Solheim, and Ronald G. Strauss.
© 2016 John Wiley & Sons, Ltd. Published 2016 by John Wiley & Sons, Ltd.

synthetic polymers are PGA and PLA. These synthetic polymers are degraded by hydrolysis. Copolymers of PGA and PLA can be designed in specific ratios to match the degradation process for the individual tissue requirements.[4]

Scaffold fabrication techniques provide a variety of methods to form a structure, alter the mechanical properties, and change the degradation rates. Fibers can be woven or knitted to form structures with controlled pore sizes.[5] The molecules self-assemble under the appropriate conditions. Natural materials, such as components in the extracellular matrix (ECM), often are capable of forming scaffolds by self-assembly.[5] Solvent casting and particulate leaching techniques involve dissolving a polymer in a solvent, and then casting into a mold filled with a porogen (e.g., sodium chloride or gelatin). Gas foaming is a process wherein a polymer is prepared by compression molding, or where the gas, for instance CO_2, is dissolved into the polymer melt. The structure is exposed to high pressure CO_2; then, as the pressure is reduced, pores remain when the CO_2 evacuates.[3] Electrospinning is a method in which a polymer forms nanofibers as an electrified jet is deposited on a metallic collector.[3]

Skin tissue engineering

Over the last several years, there have been several advancements in the development of tissue-engineered skin. Clinical applications of skin substitutes primarily include burn injuries and chronic wounds. In the United States alone, there are almost 4000 deaths from fire and burns and approximately 40,000 hospitalizations per year to treat burn injuries.[1] Alternatively, chronic wounds that require skin substitutes are caused by arterial occlusive disease, venous disease, and pressure ulcers. These wounds affect approximately 500,000 people in the United States annually.[2] Although the need for skin substitutes in this group is less acute than in the burn group, the morbidity as a result of these chronic wounds remains significant. For patients with nonhealing lower leg ulcers, such wounds can render amputation necessary.

Structure and function

The structural components of skin include a surface epidermis and deeper layer of connective tissue (the dermis). The epidermis is primarily composed of keratinocytes—cells responsible for the barrier function and strength of the epidermis. The connective tissue layer of the dermis contains fibroblasts, adipose cells, blood vessels, mast cells, nerve endings, hair follicles, and glands. The main components of the connective tissue matrix are collagen, elastin, reticulin, and glycoslyaminoglycans (GAGs). The skin functions to provide a barrier between the body and the external environment, and also provides sensation, temperature regulation, and vitamin D production. The most important function of the skin as related to skin substitutes is for the epidermis to restore the skin barrier.

The origins of the entire field of tissue engineering are often attributed to the creation of skin substitutes. Early pioneering work in this field was performed in the 1980s, where in researchers developed a bilayer artificial skin substitute with a temporary silastic epidermis, and also a collagen dermis that could support the growth of dermal fibroblasts from the wound bed.[3] Other investigators developed similar methods using allogeneic keratinocytes with a collagen gel or on PGA mesh.[4] The first skin substitutes were approved by the FDA in the late 1990s for applications in venous leg ulcers and for temporary covering of partial-thickness burns.

Design goals for skin substitutes

The primary function of an epidermal layer is to provide a barrier function to prevent fluid losses and to inhibit infection. An ideal skin substitute will (1) permanently heal into the wound bed to replace the dermal and epidermal layers in a timely manner, (2) produce a cosmetically desirable result, (3) have minimal risk of infection or immunologic rejection, (4) be cost-effective, (5) be easily handled by doctors and surgeons, and (6) be readily accessible (off the shelf). The "gold standard" for covering large burn wounds is an autologous split-thickness skin graft. Autologous skin grafts permanently heal into the wound bed, contain an epidermal and dermal component, and have no risk of immunorejection. Procuring these grafts is, however, painful and expensive, and results in scarring at the donor retrieval site. Skin substitutes are a viable alternative to autografts because they are readily available, do not require donor site harvest, and allow for better healing than dressing changes alone. Most skin substitutes do not directly heal into the wound; rather, they promote healing by stimulating cytokines and growth factors in the wound bed to recruit and direct host cells to repair the wound site.[5]

Early alternatives to the standard of autologous skin grafts were allogeneic skin grafts and porcine xenogeneic skin grafts. Allogeneic skin grafts have been the preferred material for temporary coverage as a skin substitute over xenografts. The beneficial properties of the allogeneic skin graft are that it prevents desiccation of the wound, minimizes fluid loss, has a dermal component, and stimulates repair of the wound bed for eventual placement of an autograft.[6] Porcine skin grafts are temporary skin grafts that have similar properties to allogeneic skin grafts, with the addition of being more readily available and affordable. Because allogeneic and xenogeneic grafts do not incorporate into the wound, these grafts carry the potential risk of infection and eventual immunorejection.[6]

Acellular skin substitutes

The group of acellular skin substitutes includes Biobrane, Allo-Derm, and Integra. Biobrane (UDL Laboratories, Rockford, IL) is a synthetic bilaminate skin substitute that was introduced in 1979. The outer layer is silicon rubber, while a secondary layer consists of a nylon mesh that is covalently bound to Type I porcine collagen. The outer layer silicon pore size allows for drainage of exudate and permeability to topical antibiotics, but the small pore size acts as a barrier to bacterial invasion. Additional properties of Biobrane are adherence to clean wounds, stimulation of ingrowth of cells from the wound bed, ease of application, and a shelf life of at least three years. Biobrane may be used for superficial partial-thickness burns, over a meshed autograft, and in donor sites. Biobrane has demonstrated a reduced time to re-epithelialization when compared to traditional therapy of topical antibiotics and dressing changes for burn injuries.

AlloDerm™ (LifeCell, Branchburg, NJ) is a dermal skin substitute that removes epithelial cells from harvested human skin to leave an acellular dermal matrix. AlloDerm is approved for treatment of partial to full-thickness burns and chronic wounds. AlloDerm has similar properties to allogeneic grafts, except the immunologic response is reduced because of the processing of the tissue.[7] The clinical use of AlloDerm for partial-thickness or full-thickness burns is similar to that of the dermal component, but an ultra-thin autograft is needed over the AlloDerm. The advantage of the ultra-thin autograft is that it reduces the morbidity or loss of donor site grafts, due in particular to scar formation. It has been shown that an acellular allograft with a thin autograft produces equivalent healing rates at 14 days in comparison to split-thickness skin grafts.[7] Further case studies have demonstrated high success rates of AlloDerm with a split-thickness autograft.[8]

Integra (Integra Life Sciences, Plainsboro, NJ) is a bilayer skin substitute that was approved in 1996 for use in partial-thickness and full-thickness burns. The dermal component is a biodegradable collagen-chondroiten-6-sulfate matrix with an epidermal layer that is a thin silicone elastomer. The thin silicone layer acts as a barrier to bacteria and controls moisture loss. The dermal component encourages the adherence and growth of the wound bed. After two to three weeks when a neodermis has formed, the thin silicone layer is removed and then covered with a thin autograft.

Allogeneic skin substitutes

Current FDA-approved allogeneic skin substitutes include Apligraf, Dermagraft, and Orcel. Apligraf (Organogenesis, Canton, MA) is a bilayer structure with Type I collagen gel and allogeneic fibroblasts that form a dermal equivalent, onto which allogeneic keratinocytes are seeded to provide an epidermal layer. Dermagraft (Organogenesis, Canton, MA) is a single layer skin substitute using allogeneic fibroblasts cultured onto a bioresorbable glycolic acid scaffold. Orcel (Forticell Bioscience, New York, NY) is a bilayer material with fibroblasts cultured in a porous sponge as the dermal layer with keratinocytes seeded on the nonporous side of the matrix. Although the fresh form of Orcel is available, a cryopreserved formulation is in clinical trials. The mechanism of wound healing for these skin substitutes is not clearly understood, but they seem to stimulate epithelialization by the fibroblasts' release of growth factors and ECM to provide recruitment of endogenous cells.[9] Allogeneic fibroblasts themselves likely contribute a temporary response to wound healing, because at four weeks after treatment, only two of 10 patients had Apligraf DNA in the wound site.[10] Apligraf, Dermagraft, and Orcel have all shown improved rate of wound closure when used for chronic ulcers in comparison to conservative treatment with dressing changes.[11,12] The primary application the allogeneic skin substitutes is in the treatment of chronic ulcers or acute wounds, with limited use for partial-thickness or full-thickness burn injuries. Currently available skin substitutes are listed in Table 42.1.

Autologous skin substitutes

Generally, cultured epidermal autografts have been disappointing for several reasons: They are fragile, require extended culture time, and ultimately require a dermal layer for survival and funtion. Epicel is the only FDA-approved cultured epidermal autograft. Epicel (Genzyme, Cambridge, MA) is made of cultured autologous keratinocytes harvested from the patient. Although the effectiveness of Epicel is still under investigation, the product is currently used for the treatment of patients with deep dermal or full-thickness burns over 30% of the total body surface. The current skin substitutes constituted the first step in using tissue-engineered products for clinical applications. These skin substitutes have demonstrated some of the potential successes and challenges that remain in creating an ideal tissue-engineered equivalent. The limitations of the existing materials are related to the allogeneic cells that seem to function by recruiting host cells for wound healing instead of primarily contributing to wound healing. Cultured epidermal autograft techniques are not suitable for widespread application because only the epidermis can be created, without a true bilayer structure.

The future of skin substitutes may incorporate adult mesenchymal stem cells (MSCs) and gene therapy strategies for optimization. The design of a tissue-engineered skin graft could contain autogenous cells in a bilayer structure with a dermal and epidermal component. The use of marrow MSCs cultured with autogenous dermal fibroblasts may enhance epidermal regeneration.[13] Gene therapy can be used to upregulate the delivery of growth factors or cytokines to expedite the regenerative process. In animal models, gene delivery with epidermal growth factor has been shown to dramatically accelerate healing.[14] However, for wound healing, the upregulation of growth factors should be transient, because continued gene expression might result in adverse effects. Additionally, there has been interested in developing electrospun scaffolds to better replicate nanotopographical features of skin. Early work with electrospun scaffolds of silk fibroin and collagen nanofibers have shown improved early-stage healing compared to controls.[15,16] The advancement of skin substitutes and a better understanding of the biology of wound healing will likely lead to the development of rationally based designs to specifically treat the pathology of the wound.

Table 42.1 Clinical skin substitutes

Reference	Skin Substitute	Application	Result (Time to Healing)
Kumar[17]/Barrett[18]	Silver sulfadiazine	Pediatric partial-thickness burn	11.2–16.1 days
Kumar[17]/Wood F[19]	Biobrane	Pediatric partial-thickness burn donor site	9.5–9.7 days
Callcut[8]/Jansen LA[20]	AlloDerm over split-thickness skin graft	Deep partial or full-thickness burn	26/27 graft take
Veves[12]/DiDomenico[21]	Apligraf	Chronic ulcers	Heal % at 12 weeks: Apligraf, 56% Dressing, 38%
Blight[22]/Still[23]/Clugson[24]	Culture epithelial autograft	Full-thickness burn	Heal %: 15–80%
Purdue[25]/Harding K[26]	Dermagraft	Full-thickness burn—temporary coverage; diabetic foot ulcers	95% take Heal % at 12 weeks: Dermagraft, 30% Dressing, 18%
Heimbach[27]/Lagus H[28]	Integra	Full-thickness or deep partial-thickness burn	Take Integra: 76% Take epidermal graft: 88%
Still[23]	Orcel	Donor site; venous ulcer	13.2 days Heal % at 12 weeks: Orcel, 59% Dressing, 36%
Reinwald[29]/Green[30]	Epicel	Deep dermal or full-thickness burns	N/A

Blood vessel tissue engineering

Cardiovascular disease is the leading cause of mortality in the United States.[31] More than 500,000 coronary bypass artery graft procedures are performed annually in the United States, and peripheral disease results in more than 100,000 amputations each year.[32] The therapeutic modalities to treat cardiovascular disease are medical treatments, catheter-based interventional procedures, and surgical procedures. The medical treatments focus on disease modification by treating conditions that lead to cardiovascular disease such as management of hypertension, hyperlipidemia, and diabetes, and cessation of smoking. The interventional procedures such as angioplasty, stents, or thrombolytic therapy offer a less invasive treatment than does surgery for patients with occlusive vessel disease. The surgical options for vascular disease are bypass surgery, endarterectomy, or open thrombectomy.

The currently available conduits for bypass procedures include autologous artery or vein, prosthetic material, and cadaveric vein. Autologous tissue provides the best outcome; however, autologous tissue in many patients may not be available or may not be suitable[33]. Prosthetic materials, such as polytetrafluoroethylene (PTFE) and Dacron, perform well for large-diameter arteries in peripheral vascular disease.[34] In contrast, no prosthetic material is well-suited for small-diameter (less than 6 mm) applications. Another growing area of need for bypass procedures is hemodialysis—more than 250,000 patients require chronic hemodialysis access and frequent graft replacement.[35] Tissue engineering technology has the potential to generate engineered arterial grafts for multiple applications in cardiovascular surgical therapy.

Structure and function

A blood vessel is composed of the intima, media, and the adventitia.[36] The intima contains the endothelium, lamina propria, and the internal elastic lamina. The media contains the smooth muscles arranged concentrically, elastin and collagen fibers, and the external elastic lamina. The adventitia contains connective tissue, fibroblasts, vasa vasorum, and nerve cells. Arterial blood vessels are classified as elastic arteries, muscular arteries, and arterioles. The large elastic arteries have higher elastin content and fewer smooth muscle cells (SMCs) relative to diameter than other vessel types. Muscular arteries contain a greater number of SMCs in proportion to their diameter, and the adventitia is composed of a thicker layer of connective tissue in comparison to the elastic arteries. The arterioles consist of a thin layer of smooth muscle and range from 40 microns to 9 microns in diameter.[36]

Design goals for a tissue-engineered vessel

The primary design goal of a tissue-engineered blood vessel is to create a graft that will maintain patency in small-diameter applications (e.g., 2 to 6 mm). The desirable features of the tissue-engineered vessel are a patency rate comparable to autologous vein, similar mechanical properties to a native artery or vein, minimal immunologic or infective risk, a reasonable time to produce the grafts, and cost effectiveness. The reported five-year patency rates using autologous vein grafts for below-the-knee applications are 50% to 76%.[37] However, the patency rates for below-the-knee bypass with PTFE have a two-year patency rate of 30% and only 18% after five years.[38,39] Synthetic blood vessel prosthetics such as Dacron and PTFE are inherently thrombogenic,[40] and present increased rates of infections that often lead to life threatening complications.[41] Over the past 10 years, the patency of ePTFE grafts has been substantially improved (~65 to 70%) with the help of heparin or endothelial cell (EC) coatings.[42] However, these graft materials are nondegradable and do not remodel in vivo.

Over the past two decades, several tissue-engineering approaches have shown substantial success and have progressed toward clinical trials. These include in vitro approaches in which TEVGs are cultured using living cells, scaffolds, and bioreactors.[43,44] Another major approach is in situ vascular engineering where in graft scaffolds are engineered, and take advantage of the host cells to regenerate a vessel, thus reducing any in vitro culture times.[45]

Cell source

The predominant cell types that form a vessel are fibroblasts, SMCs, and ECs. Both fibroblasts[46] and SMCs[43] have been utilized extensively to create TEVGs, while ECs are utilized to create a non-thrombogenic environment in the lumen. Because human SMCs and ECs have limited growth potential and often exhibit senescence,[47] recent studies have focused on the use of stem cells for vascular tissue engineering. Adult stem cells such as bone marrow MSCs[48] and muscle-derived stem cells[49] as well as embryonic stem cells (ESCs)[50] and human induced pluripotent stem cells (hiPSCs)[51,52] have been shown to differentiate into ECs[53] and SMCs. Research on using ESCs and iPSCs for vascular tissue engineering is still at an early phase.[54-58] A recent report in 2014 demonstrated the utility of hiPSCs for growing TEVGs with good mechanical strength (burst pressure ~800 mmHg);[59] however, the performance of these TEVGs has yet to be tested in vivo.

Substantial data from clinical trials and other studies highlight the importance of a functional endothelium for small-diameter grafts. Without an endothelial coating, there is a significantly higher rate of thrombosis for small-diameter vascular grafts.[60] Non-thrombogenicity can be achieved by seeding endothelial cells on the luminal surfaces or by modifying the lumen with inhibitors of thrombosis. Options for obtaining endothelial cells from a recipient patient are to use primary vascular endothelial cells, or to isolate progenitor endothelial cells (EPCs) from the marrow or the peripheral blood. The limitations to using a primary endothelial cell source are that it requires an operation to harvest a vein, derived endothelium is venous rather than arterial, and that they will have been exposed to potential disease processes. Additionally, expansion of ECs to relevant numbers for clinical use remains challenging. EPCs have high proliferative capacity, are capable of clonal expansion, and can differentiate into endothelial cells.[61] EPCs isolated from the peripheral blood mononuclear fraction are positive for CD34, vascular endothelial growth factor receptor-2 (VEGFR-2) and CD31, although the exact characteristics remain to be defined. As an alternative, groups have focused on coating the lumen with anticoagulants such as heparin[62] or cell recruitment factors such as SDF1.[63]

Scaffold

There are several approaches to developing a scaffold for tissue-engineered vessels. One approach is to use cells to form an ECM without a synthetic scaffold, and the other approach is to use synthetic polymers or natural materials to form the cell culture scaffold. In the first approach, L'Heureux and colleagues cultured sheets of fibroblasts or SMCs and wrapped the sheets around a mandrel (scaffold) in several layers to form a tubular structure.[44] The burst pressure, compliance, and wall thickness were all similar to native arteries.[44] The biomimetic system developed by Niklason and colleagues for small-diameter vessels calls for placing aortic

SMCs on a PGA scaffold under pulsatile flow for eight weeks.[43] The PGA scaffold degrades, and the resulting vessel is composed primarily of smooth muscle cells and collagen. The tissue-engineered vessel does exhibit contractile properties, although at 20% that of native vessels. The mechanical properties demonstrate burst pressure and compliance similar to native vessels.[43] Other approaches use a collagen gel that is coated with a microporous polyurethane film.[64] The collagen gel is compressed to remove water, and then wrapped with the polyurethane film. The compliance of such constructs in the higher strain range is similar to native arteries. Tranquillo and coworkers have demonstrated substantial success with fibrin gels for growing TEVGs with burst pressure of 4000 mmHg and compliance similar to that of native femoral artery.[65] A combination method evaluated in animal models has been to decellularize a native vessel and then to seed this with endothelial cells.[66] There is evidence to suggest that decellularization invokes minimal immunologic reaction, in comparison to cryopreserved vessels, which lead to moderate immunologic reaction.[67] The tissue-engineered graft developed by Shin'oka et al. was designed for low-pressure venous systems, using a copolymer lactide and ε-caprolactone 1:1 scaffold.[68] The graft is seeded with marrow cells at the time of operation and then sprayed with fibrin sealant, after which the graft is implanted.

Bioreactor design

The two most successful bioreactor designs for tissue-engineered vessels are to wrap sheets of fibroblasts around a mandrel or to use a flow bioreactor system to culture a vessel from smooth muscle cells. The first method involves obtaining a skin biopsy to culture fibroblasts.[44] The fibroblasts are grown in sheets, and the first sheet is wrapped around a mandrel to form a tubular structure. The inner sheet is dehydrated to form an acellular inner membrane. Additional sheets of living cells are then placed around the inner membrane, and the tissue remains in culture to mature. The last step of this process involves obtaining endothelial cells harvested from saphenous vein to coat the luminal surface of the graft. The entire process takes approximately 28 weeks to form a vessel for implantation. The second technique is to obtain smooth muscle

from a vessel biopsy, and to seed the smooth muscle on a biodegradable PGA scaffold.[43] The scaffold with the cells remains static for one week to allow for attachment, and then the construct is exposed to pulsatile flow for seven to eight weeks. The luminal side of the graft can be seeded with endothelial cells. This process takes around 10 weeks total to create a vessel for implantation.

Preclinical and clinical data

Table 42.2 lists some of the important animal models that have combined a cell source with a scaffold to produce a functional vascular graft. Apart from these preclinical studies, a few approaches have also reached clinical testing.[69–72] Most notable successes to date have been demonstrated using the cell-seeded polymer scaffolds utilized by Shin'oka et al. In the first study in 2001, TEVGs were prepared using poly-E-caprolactone and poly-L-lactic acid, reinforced with PGA and seeded with cells from the patient.[45] In a subsequent larger study, a cohort of 25 patients was treated with biodegradable TEVGs.[73] Studies focused on understanding the mechanism of vessel regeneration using cell-seeded scaffolds in animal models have found substantial involvement of the body's intrinsic regenerative capabilities over the cells seeded in the grafts.[74] Clinical outcomes using off-the-shelf TEVGs are yet to come, although several studies are currently ongoing.

Future of vascular tissue engineering

Tissue-engineered vessels appear to be the next generation of small-diameter bypass grafts, addressing the growing need for alternative materials for small-caliber arterial replacement. The field of vascular tissue engineering has demonstrated proof-of-principle methods with various scaffolds and cell sources that are now ready to emerge in the clinical arena. Historically, tissue-engineered grafts need some amount of culture time ranging from few weeks to few months. However, with the recent improvement in TEVG technology leading to off-the-shelf grafts,[72,75,78] the wait time will be negligible. New technology using tissue-engineered grafts will likely be more expensive than the current prosthetic materials. However, the increase in cost for a tissue-engineered graft could be justified when considering reduced cost of chronic wound management,

Table 42.2 Selected animal models that have produced a functional vascular graft

Reference	Model	Cell Source	Scaffold	Outcome
Shin'oka:[68] cell-seeded scaffold (low pressure)	Human tube graft cavopulmonary connection (n = 23)	Endothelial cells—marrow	Polylactide/caprolactone-einforced PGA mesh	Follow-up: median 16.7 months
	Sheet graft patch (n = 19)			Patency: 100% No complications
L'Heureux[46] – cell sheet based	Canine aortic graft	Fibroblasts	Fibroblast sheet	Rat: patency 85% at 90–225 days
	Rat aortic graft (n = 27) Primate aortic graft (n = 3)	Endothelial cell—primary cells		Primate: all patent at 6–8 weeks
Niklason:[75] cell-seeded scaffold (high pressure)	Canine Carotid artery bypass Canine coronary artery bypass Baboon AV model (n = 9)	Human SMCs	Tissue-engineered SMCs over PGA mesh, then decellularized	Canine—patency 5/6. Follow-up up to 1 year Baboon—patency 2/2 at 1 month, 2/3 at 3 months, 3/3 at 6 months
Tranquillo:[65] cell seeded fibrin gels	Sheep femoral artery (n = 9)	Fibroblasts	Fibroblast seeded fibrin gels then decellularized	100% patent at 24 weeks
Cho[76]	Canine carotid (n = 6)	Endothelial—marrow SMC—marrow	Decellularized canine carotid	100% patent for 8 weeks
Matsuda[77]	Canine (n = 12)	Endothelial—peripheral blood	Collagen mesh reinforced with polyurethane film	11/12 patent for up to 3 months

PGA, polyglycolic acid; SMC, smooth muscle cell.

multiple surgical procedures with ineffective material, and reduction in patient morbidity. With several different approaches in ongoing clinical trials, there exists a real possibility that morbidity and mortality of cardiovascular disease can be dramatically reduced in the near future.

Bone tissue engineering

Bone tissue regeneration is a potential clinical treatment to replace loss of skeletal function for orthopedic and oral-maxillary applications. With the worldwide incidence of bone disorders and conditions on the rise, particularly in aging populations faced with obesity and physical inactivity, there is a great demand for bone replacement materials.[79] The most common needs for replacement arise from trauma, pain, functional and structural problems, benign and malignant tumors, infection, congenital skeletal disorders, and a broad range of diseases.[80,81] Current bone replacement materials are derived from autologous bone, allogeneic bone, demineralized bone matrices, and synthetic biomaterials. The design and development of functional bone tissues are based on our understanding of bone structure, bone mechanics, and tissue formation. In order for engineered bone tissue to be considered functional, it must be fully integrated with the neighboring host bone and capable of performing the essential functions of the native bone.[79]

Historically, the gold standard of treatment in bone tissue regeneration has been the autologous bone graft.[82–84] The advantages of autologous bone grafts are due to the tissue's inherent osteoconductive and osteoinductive properties, native osteogenic cells, and structural integrity. The robust osteogenic capabilities of these tissues are highlighted by their ability to recruit additional native host mesenchymal cells into the graft through stimulation by osteoinductive factors, such as bone morphogenic proteins (BMPs).[79,83,85,86] Despite the advantages of autologous tissue being immune-compatible and the provisions of bone cells and matrix for osteogenesis, there are several shortcomings. The use of autografts is limited by the morbidity associated with the donor sites (e.g., iliac crest and fibula), and this morbidity increases with the amount of transplanted bone.[87] After the procedure, approximately 20% or more of patients experience complication(s) and have significant pain at the donor site.[88–92]

An alternative to autologous bone grafting is allogeneic bone grafts, which are available as fresh, frozen, or freeze-dried.[91] The advantages of allogeneic bone tissue include its osteoconductive and osteoinductive potential, absence of donor site morbidity, and range of available geometries and sizes.[93] Even though allografts overcome some of the complications posed by autografts, there are serious disadvantages due to their high immunogenic potential, the risk of viral transmission to the recipient, and heterogeneity of the donor population.[79,90] Unfortunately, some attempts to reduce these risks (e.g., irradiation or freeze-drying) have been met with reduction of osteoinductivity, osteogenic properties, and bone healing; decreased vascularization; and alterations in the biomechanical properties of the processed allogeneic bone tissue.[83,84,90] Even with the above complications, allogeneic bone seems to be comparable to autologous bone for smaller defects, such as bone chips in a distal radial fracture or for use in a cervical fusion.[83,91] Rates of graft subsidence, arthrodesis, fusion, and collapse are quite similar between allografts and autografts.[91]

Due to the substantial costs associated with auto- and allografts and the fact that the bone grafting market has greater demand than

supply, biologic and synthetic substitutes have developed as an alternative to the conventional use of autologous and allogeneic bone grafts.[79] Examples of these substitutes include demineralized bone scaffolds deriving from allogeneic or xenogeneic sources and ceramic- or polymer-based synthetics.[93,94] Often deemed a superior approach for repairing bone defects, these natural and synthetic bone substitutes are immunological compatible because they do not transmit allogeneic or xenogeneic material to the recipient and can be customized with the recipient's own cells. Acrylate bone cements, and cementless alternatives such as hydroxyapatite (HA)-coated prosthesis[95–98] and HA-based pastes,[99,100] are alternative biomaterials that have been introduced for fixation or repair of various bone defects.

Structure and function

Bone has the ability to perform a wide array of functions and respond to myriad physical, metabolic, and endocrine stimuli.[79] Most notably, bone provides load-bearing capabilities, bodily locomotion, and protection of vital organs and regulates entrapment of dangerous metals, electrolyte storage homeostasis, and aspects of hematopoiesis. The dynamic and diverse nature of bone, both structurally and functionally, permits the tissue to undergo a constant cycle of resorption and renewal in order to adapt to the chemical and mechanical demands of the tissue. Influenced by distinct loading conditions, bones can be compact or trabecular and range in mechanical strength and modulus.

Bones are composed of extracellular bone matrix and bone cells that form the shape of long, short, flat, or irregular bones.[79,101] The bone matrix consists of an organic component of collagen type-1 and proteoglycans, and a mineralized inorganic component that is a calcium phosphate crystal called *hydroxyapatite*. This tough yet flexible fiber-composite is essential to the compressive strength and high fracture toughness of bone. Surrounded by the matrix are the four primary types of bone cells: osteoprogenitor cells, osteoblasts, osteoclasts, and osteocytes.[102] These cells continually remodel bone matrix to accommodate growth and structural reshaping in response to varying loading stresses. Osteoprogenitor cells reside in the marrow, periosteum, and bone canals and eventually migrate, proliferate, and differentiate into osteoblasts. Osteoblasts are bone cells that produce collagen and proteoglycans, and thus form bone. Osteoclasts are the cells responsible for the breakdown of bone by producing an acidic environment that causes decalcification of the bone matrix. These cells are found on the growth surfaces of bone. Osteocytes are osteoblasts that are surrounded by matrix. Some of the many roles of osteocytes include sensing mechanical stress on bone, secreting growth factors that stimulate osteoblasts, and transferring minerals from bone interior to its growth surfaces. The interaction of bone cells with hormones regulates the homeostasis of calcium and phosphate in the blood.

Scaffold

The structure of the scaffold for bone regeneration is related to the function of bone. A 3D bone scaffold must provide a suitable environment for osteogenic cell migration, proliferation, and differentiation and promote new bone formation. Thus, a bone scaffold should be osteoconductive, osteoinductive, and osseointegrative. It must also generate appropriate mechanical strength and stability, stimulate vascularization for nutrients/waste exchange, slowly degrade into nontoxic products with increasing cellular infiltration, and be biocompatible, permeable, and porous in structure.[103]

Given the many intended roles for bone scaffolds, each scaffold must be optimized for its intended function. For example, the different requirements for the strength of long bones and for the flexibility of craniofacial bones require the development of unique scaffolds for each of these applications. This is because mismatched mechanical properties of bone tissue can lead to stress disparities between tissues and possibly failure of the engineered tissue. Careful consideration of the composition and macro- and microstructure of the scaffold is needed since the physical (i.e., topographical and mechanical) and (bio)chemical properties of the scaffold serve to influence the behavior and function of resident or infiltrating cells and the release of signaling molecules.[104] As an example, scaffold porosity and pore size are important factors in bioactivity, affecting cell adhesion, growth, and migration; the exchange of nutrients and waste products; and vascularization. Fibrous scaffolds exhibiting porosity greater than 50% and approximately 500 μm sized pores permit enhanced scaffold vascularization.[104]

The wide range of biomaterial scaffolds used for bone tissue engineering can be made using natural, synthetic, or suitable composites materials.[103,105] Natural substitutes include demineralized bone matrix, biological polymers matrices such as collagen I and hyaluronic acid, and inorganic ceramic materials such as HA and tricalcium phosphate (TCP), which provide bio-mimetic environments for bone cells.[93] HA and TCP are calcium phosphate compounds that are the primary components of bone matrix.[101] As scaffolds, HA and TCP offer a high degree of biocompatibility, robust osteoconductivity, and slow degradation, although HA is more inert and has higher mechanical strength than TCP.[106] Because they are porous materials, HA and TCP allow ingrowth of bone and vascular cells.[107–109] HA and TCP implants are known to be brittle and lack the pliability necessary to conform to irregular forms.[107,110,111] Even with these structural restrictions, HA cements have been approved for clinical use in non-stress-bearing craniofacial, dental, and orthopedic defects[106,112] because they integrate into the bone and can be easily shaped to fit unique 3D structures.[113] Clinical experience with one of the HA bone cements in 100 patients over a minimum of two years demonstrated a success rate of 97% and a low rate of infection.[111] As an alternative, synthetic materials can be used because they are more readily available, capable of providing sufficient structural support, and chemically and physically customizable (e.g., degradation rates). The most common synthetic materials used in 3D scaffolds include PLA, PGA, poly-lactic-co-glycolic acid (PLGA), poly caprolactone, poly anhydrides, and poly carbonates.[103,105,106,114] Because most materials alone have shown some form of limitation, researchers are now fabricating composite materials that combine polymers and inorganic minerals in order to achieve optimal and controllable degradation and mechanical properties and enhance bone formation.[94,115] The composites that investigators have evaluated include calcium phosphate–chitosan, calcium phosphate–PLA, HA–collagen scaffolds,[116] PLGA–beta-tricalcium phosphate (β-TCP),[117] and PLGA–collagen–apatite.

Scaffolds are also often embedded within or coated with a variety of osteoinductive growth factors to promote formation of new bone and help promote vascularization.[94,118,119] BMP2 and BMP7 have been shown to be involved in production and maturation of bone and osteoblast and osteoclast differentiation. The benefit and efficacy of BMPs in improving bone healing for a variety of bone defects has been demonstrated in preclinical studies involving many different animal models (rats, rabbits, dogs, and sheep) and in at-risk patients with complex fractures such as spinal fusions, internal fixation of fractures,

treatment of bone defects, and reconstruction of maxillofacial conditions.[120–130] In human patients, studies report successful use of rhBMP2 as an effective adjunct for bone healing in foot and ankle surgery.[131,132] Aside from osteogenic growth factors, like BMP2 and BMP7, scaffold constructs also contain other growth factors that aid in osteoblast and osteoprogenitor cell proliferation, differentiation, and migration.[94,133]

Vascularization

Although there is significant potential for bone regeneration, current bone tissue engineering strategies are limited by the lack of vascularization, which leads to poor graft integration and failure of engineered substitutes.[102] Therefore, there are ongoing efforts to improve bone tissue regeneration by enhancing vascularization in engineered constructs.[94]

The two primary approaches used to vascularize a bone graft are: (1) to rely on angiogenesis of the donor, or (2) to form a vascular network within the graft prior to implantation. The majority of bone graft substitutes depend on vascularization through angiogenesis from the donor after implantation of the cell-seeded scaffold. In order to enhance and accelerate vascularization in engineering bone constructs, various strategies have been attempted, including (1) growth factor delivery, (2) using co-culturing systems, (3) applying mechanical stimulation, (4) using biomaterials/scaffolds with appropriate properties, and (5) incorporating microfabrication techniques.[94,102,134–136]

One method to improve vascularization is to stimulate angiogenesis on the graft. This may be accomplished by adding one or more endogenous, pro-angiogenic growth factors such as vascular endothelial growth factor (VEGF),[137,138] platelet-derived growth factor-BB (PDGF-BB),[139] transforming growth factor-β (TGF-β), or sonic hedgehog (Shh) in order to direct cellular behavior.[94,139–146] Cross-talk between osteoblasts and ECs is essential to successful vascular growth and osteoblast differentiation. Many studies have demonstrated that dual delivery of growth factors such as BMP2 and VEGF can enhance de novo bone formation.[94,147,148] Another alternative has been to utilize scaffolds with appropriate mechanical stiffness and pore characteristics to improve oxygen/nutrient perfusion and vascular cell alignment.[143] Cell-seeded scaffolds can also be subjected to mechanical stimulation (e.g., shear stress of fluid flow) during co-culture in order to enhance bone tissue formation and improve vascularization in a VEGF-mediated manner.[94]

Attempts have also been made to vascularize the graft before implantation by heterotopic bone induction to form a vascular network within the graft in vitro or in vivo.[149–151] Warnke and colleagues reported a successful extended mandible reconstruction by growth of a custom titanium mesh bone transplant that was initially implanted into the lattisimus dorsi muscle for seven weeks, and then transplanted as a free bone–muscle flap to repair the mandibular defect of an adult male patient.[149] Since the publication of this seminal work, there have been other attempts to use an intramuscular endocultivation technique using the latissimus dorsi muscle, porous HA, and tricalcium phosphate or demineralized bone scaffolds to vascularize bone grafts.[151,152] These studies made use of various bone and vascular cell types, platelet-rich plasma, and growth factors to enhance the process. Future heterotopic bone induction strategies could also utilize an in vitro co-culture system to form a vascular network using ECs in a matrix that is later seeded with marrow cells and subsequently implanted.

A viable strategy for vascular enhancement within engineered bone tissue replacements is to co-culture EC types and osteoblast cell types together within a scaffold in order to promote osteogenesis and vascularization simultaneously.[94,102] Numerous 3D co-culture studies have shown that ECs and osteoblasts have an important, synergistic relationship with one another during bone formation, remodeling, and repair and, thus, both cell types are needed to create vascularized engineered bone constructs in vitro.[153–156] For example, studies have shown that EC–osteoblast co-culture systems can be applied to generate vascularized bone tissue in both ectopic and orthotropic sites in vivo.[157–163] Certain groups have reported successful co-culture of bone marrow MSCs (bmMSCs) and HUVECs in vitro,[164] although orthotopic models in animals have met with mixed results and still need to demonstrate the potential of MSC and EC co-culture systems to regenerate bone.[159,162] Thus, co-culture systems can be used to study concurrent angio-/vasculogenesis and osteogenesis and aid in improvement of vascularized bone regeneration.

Cell source

In order to create vascularized bone tissue, the general approach is to combine a osteogenic cell type with an endothelial cell type.[102] Osteogenic cells for bone engineering include mature osteoblasts, periosteal cells, and marrow and adipose MSCs. Similarly, a range of EC types or their progenitors can be used.

Mature osteoblasts and periosteal cells can be isolated from a biopsy of the calvarium, periosteum, or trabecular bone and serve as autologous, primary cell sources for bone engineering.[165–168] Mesenchymal stem cells are harvested less invasively via a marrow or adipose aspiration procedure and utilized for bone regeneration due to their multipotent phenotype.[169,170] Because MSCs have a large proliferative potential, they can be differentiated down osteogenic lineages using exogenous factors including hormones, growth factors (e.g., TGFβ and BMPs), and ECM molecules.[102] Friedenstein and colleagues were the first to describe MSC differentiation to osteogenic cells (e.g., osteoblasts); however, subsequent work has shown that MSCs can be induced to differentiate into chondrocytes, adipocytes, and myoblasts.[171,172] Specifically, MSCs improve bone tissue's osteogenic potential directly by differentiating into osteoblasts, and indirectly by releasing bone growth factors that enhance migration and differentiation of endogenous osteogenic cells.[103,173] Additionally, cells are also being genetically engineered to release growth factors (osteogenic and/or vasculo-genic) in order to accelerate cell homing, vascularization, and bone regeneration of the defect site.[79] Mesenchymal stem cell differentiation can also be directed via matrix/substrate stiffness, mechanical stimulation, and nanotopographical cues.

The most common cell source for bone tissue engineering applications is currently MSCs, because they can be easily harvested from patients with a relatively simple surgical procedure, have robust proliferative capacity, and avoid issues of immune rejection.[102,119] Goshima et al. were the first to take advantage of the potential of MSCs by seeding the cells onto a porous calcium–phosphate ceramic.[174] In a subcutaneous in vivo rat model, they demonstrated osteogenesis with an early bone growth phase resulting from the implanted mesenchymal cells and a late phase resulting from the host cells. Since the time of this seminal work, there have been many studies on the use of MSCs for bone tissue engineering applications.[102,103,158,175,176] The use of MSCs on biomaterial scaffolds has accelerated bone formation and bone integration in vivo.

Endothelial cell types for bone tissue engineering can be extracted from numerous tissue sources and used to self-assemble under the guidance of pro-angiogenic factors into vascular tubes. Commonly used ECs include human umbilical vein (HUVEC) dermal, microvascular, and progenitor ECs.[102] HUVECs have been shown to form capillary-like structures when co-cultured in 3D matrices with bone marrow and adipose MSCs.[177,178] ECs can also be isolated from the bone marrow directly or derived from an original progenitor cell, such as EPCs or bmMSCs however, these cells types are less commonly used.[179,180]

Preclinical and clinical studies

The evaluation of therapies for bone tissue engineering is predominately in the preclinical studies stages, with only a limited number of human clinical trials and case reports available. There have been many different large-animal studies, many of which have produced encouraging results, that have made it possible to investigate putative bone tissue engineering strategies.[181] Many studies demonstrate that a MSC-seeded scaffold produces significantly greater bone formation than cell-free grafts, and in most of the studies the MSC-seeded scaffolds resulted in similar bone formation as bone grafts.[182,183] For example, work by Geuze and colleagues have achieved ectopic bone formation in a goat model, using EPCs and bmMSCs on biphasic calcium phosphate scaffolds.[184] In addition to the use of calcium phosphate as the scaffold, investigators have also used coral. The rationale for coral as a scaffold is the porous structure and more rapid degradation of coral in comparison to calcium–phosphate-based materials.[185] The more rapid degradation time of the coral may reduce the inflammatory response and allow for growth of new bone tissue more quickly.[186] Since the treatment of large bone defects poses a continuous challenge in orthopedic surgery, only a limited number of groups are studying the use of a biomaterial in combination with a cell source to repair large osseous defects in animal models; however, there are many studies involving smaller defects.[181,187–189] Although current data have provided complex information on bone-healing pathways, many questions remain.[190] The number of cells seeded may be an important variable for bone growth in the implanted graft. High cell density at the time of seeding may have a negative impact on the graft by not allowing the cells to spread out on the graft and proliferate. Another consequence of high cell density without adequate vascularization is the formation of a hypoxic environment in the center of the graft.[186]

Case reports have described bone tissue engineering in clinical practice. Vacanti et al. reconstructed a distal thumb avulsion with periosteal cells and a coral scaffold.[191] At three months, the patient was able to return to work, and at 28 months the thumb had normal length and strength. In a separate study, Sandor et al. documented in situ bone formation to treat large mandibular defects using adipose stem cells, β-TCP granules, and BMP2.[192] The patient fully recovered and had successful osseointegration. Thus, in appropriately selected patients, it appears that bone tissue engineering concepts can be applied to repair bone defects in humans. In addition to case reports, there have been a handful of human clinical trials relating to bone repair and regeneration worldwide.

Challenges still remain in the inability to reproduce an engineered bone replacement that accurately mimics natural bone with well-formed, stable blood vessels. In order to achieve clinical success for the regeneration of large bone defects, vascularization of engineered bone tissue must be achieved. Attempts to vascularize bone tissue have yet to be validated in preclinical large-animal models. Once it is possible to generate well-vascularized bone tissue in a large animal, then clinical translation of cell-based approaches to bone tissue engineering will be expedited.[102]

Conclusion

Bone tissue engineering has the potential to provide better treatment options for bone reconstruction in orthopedic, craniofacial, and plastic surgery, which will likely eliminate many of the complications associated with use of auto- and allografts. Engineering novel bone replacements may result in the development of materials that will integrate into native bone for a complete functional recovery, without the morbidity associated with autologous donor bone harvest. An optimized, biocompatible scaffold with integrated marrow MSCs, sufficient vascularization, and some combination of osteoinductive factors (e.g.: BMPs) will enhance the local environment for bone growth and remodeling by the native tissue. Although a key area of ongoing research, identification of the optimal and most efficient technique(s) to vascularize large bone grafts is critical to improved bone graft survival and overall quality of the engineered construct. The challenge remains to create products that address the wide spectrum of clinical needs, from pliable materials for facial reconstruction to the strength required for long bone reconstruction. In order to do so, bone tissue engineering must synergistically focus on bone development and defect repair processes in order to emulate aspects of normal bone tissue development and remodeling.

Cartilage Tissue Engineering

Osteoarthritis, the most common cause of arthritis, is the leading cause of disability in the United States.[193] Over 80% of people 75 and older suffer from osteoarthritis, and 50% of patients over 50 years of age show radiologic evidence of this disease.[194] As the "baby boomer generation" continues to age, the demand for suitable treatments permit patients to maintain an active lifestyle will increase. Alternative cartilage disorders such as cartilage injuries, herniated disc, chrondrosarcoma, chrondromalacia, polychrondritis, and costochrondritis are caused by disease, trauma, or congenital abnormalities. Currently, the primary surgical options are limited to arthroscopic surgery or joint replacement—although the efficacy of arthroscopy with debridement or joint irrigation of the knee has undergone scrutiny.[195] Joint replacement surgery is required when the patient no longer responds to nonpharmacologic and drug treatments. Creating replacements for muscoskeletal tissues has proven to be challenging. Over the past several years, however, engineered cartilage has become a viable treatment option for patients with cartilage degeneration.

Structure and function of cartilage

Cartilage is the connective tissue that covers the ends of bones in a joint. The primary function of cartilage is to reduce friction of articulating bones and to assist with load bearing.[196] Structurally, cartilage is composed of a dense ECM with embedded chondrocytes.[196] The ECM includes collagen type II fibers, elastin fibers, and proteoglycans that give cartilage viscoelastic and mechanical properties. Because cartilage is avascular, it relies on diffusion for nutrients, oxygenation, and removal of waste. There are three types of cartilage, including hyaline, elastic, and fibrocartilage. The most common form of cartilage, hyaline cartilage, is primarily composed of type II collagen and proteoglycans. During the embryonic state, hyaline cartilage forms the nascent skeleton and is later converted to bone as the embryo matures. In adults, hyaline cartilage is found in tracheal rings, nose, bronchus, load-bearing joints, and costal regions of ribs. Elastic cartilage is composed of collagen type II and elastin fibers; it is found in the pinna of the ear and forms the epiglottis. Elastic cartilage is more cellular than hyaline cartilage. Fibrocartilage contains more collagen (types I and II) than hyaline, and is found in areas that require great load-bearing capacity. Fibrocartilage is found in several regions of the body: at segments connecting tendons or ligaments to bone, and between invertebral discs or articulations of the hip.[196]

Cell-based therapies

One cell-based treatment for the repair of cartilaginous lesions is autologous chondrocyte implantations (ACIs); ACI has been used as a biological therapy for over two decades. To perform an ACI, cartilage from a non-load-bearing region of bone is initially harvested. Chondrocytes are subsequently isolated from the harvested tissue and expanded. The cartilaginous lesion is then surgically debrided, and the chondrocytes are implanted under a periosteal flap. Although chondrocyte-based therapy has the capacity to slow down the progression of OA and delay partial or total joint replacement surgery, currently used procedures are associated with the risk of serious adverse events. Complications of ACIs can include disturbed fusion, delamination, hypertrophy, and ultimately graft failure.[200,201] In 2005, reviews of available evidence by the National Institute of Clinical Excellence concluded that autologous chondrocyte implantation is not recommended over alternative treatments.[202] Fortunately, second-generation ACI procedures using chondrocytes embedded in collagen sheets dramatically reduce adverse events, hypertrophy, and delamination.[203] Furthermore, third-generation ACIs with resorbable scaffolds are also promising.[204] MSCs also show considerable promise for cartilaginous repair, but there are many complications including sourcing, a lack of established guidelines from governmental agencies, and a lack of consensus of their long-term therapeutic potential.[205]

Cell source

An ideal cell source for tissue-engineered cartilage would be easily isolated and expanded, capable of synthesizing abundant cartilage-specific ECM (e.g., aggrecan and type II collagen), and be readily available. Currently, cell sources are typically harvested primary chondrocytes or stem cells that are induced to differentiate into chondrocytes (Table 42.3). Primary chondrocytes can be harvested

Table 42.3 Selected cartilage engineering in vivo studies

Reference	Model	Cell Source	Scaffold	Outcome
Xu[197]	Nude Mice	Human derived chondrocytes	3D printed PGA/PLA	8 weeks post subcutaneous implant, cell morphologies remained normal
Batioglu-Karaalti[198]	Rabbit	Mesenchymal stem cells (MSCs)	Decellularized trachea	90 days post implant, ciliated epithelium present
Liu[199]	Rabbit	iPSC-derived chondrocytes	Electrospun PCL/gelatin scaffolds	Higher cartilage-specific gene expression, protein levels and subchondral bone regeneration than controls
Kafienah	Athymic mice	Human nasal and articular chondrocytes	PGA	Cartilage engineered from human nasal cells survived during implantation (6 weeks), whereas articular cartilage recellularized tissues did not.

from articular, septal, auricular, and costal cartilage.[206,207] With respect to cartilage sources, nasal cartilage may be a better cell source than articular cartilage for tissue engineering applications. Nasal chondrocytes proliferate more rapidly than articular chondrocytes and possess a higher chondrogenic potential.[208]

Unfortunately, only a small number of autologous chondrocytes are readily available, and chondrocyte expansion in monolayers causes dedifferentiation (characterized by aberrant ECM production).[209] Furthermore, chondrocytes from older human donors generally proliferate more slowly and are less metabolically active than younger sources, limiting autologous cell sourcing to younger patients.[210] There is evidence to show that primary chondrocytes can be stimulated to proliferate and differentiate by various factors: with the addition of growth factors, by forming pellets at a high cell density, and by growth in a 3D scaffold.[211,212]

In order to optimize bone marrow stem cells' (BMSCs) differentiation into chrondrocytes, many growth factors and combinations of growth factors have been investigated. Basic FGF (FGF-2) is a potent mitogen that can promote chondrogenesis and proliferation of MSCs.[213] The formation of cartilage from MSCs was superior with FGF-2 in comparison to other growth factors, such as insulin-like growth factor, epidermal growth factor, and platelet-derived growth factor.[214] Another growth factor, BMP2, is found in the mesenchyme of the developing limb and is known to stimulate cartilage formation in culture. Furthermore, the addition of BMP2 to mesenchymal pellet culture system appeared to produce cartilage with higher amounts of proteoglycans in comparison to BMP4 or BMP6.[215] Adipose-derived stem cells (ADSCs) have also been shown to differentiate into chondrocytes in the presence of ascorbate, dexamethasone and TGF-β.[216,217] Production of cartilage-specific matrix components and an increase in mechanical properties were observed. Although ADSCs can differentiate into chondrocytes, their chondrogenic potential remains lower than that of BMSCs—more research needs to be done to improve the chondrogenic potential of these cells.

Scaffold

Scaffold materials utilized in the production of engineered cartilage are primarily composed of collagen, hyaluronan, fibrin sealant, and synthetic polymers. Collagen (Type I and II) is often used in these applications as it is biocompatible, biodegradable, formable, and can sustain chondrocyte phenotype in culture.[218] One method to reduce the dedifferentiation of chondrocytes in collagen scaffolds is to include hyaluronic acid in the construction of the engineered tissue.[219] Hyaluronan, a proteoglycan that acts to lubricate joint surfaces and assist cartilage in withstanding compressive forces, must be modified by esterification or other means for ensure anchorage to the collagen scaffold and to optimize solubility, hydration, and degradation.[220]

A fibrin matrix can also support the growth of chondrocytes, and has been demonstrated in the regeneration of cartilage within articular cartilage defects in vivo.[221] In vitro cultures have shown to induce chondrocyte proliferation and glycosaminoglycans and collagen Type II production.[221] One limitation in working with fibrin gels are that they shrink in size and degrade in a very short time.[221] Synthetic polymers such as PLA and PGA were initially investigated as cartilage scaffolds early in the study of cartilage tissue engineering. In vitro studies demonstrated the biocompatibility of PGA with chondrocytes, and early rabbit model studies demonstrated a better healing response of PGA seeded with chondrocytes over PGA scaffold alone.[222] PGA-seeded scaffolds have resulted in

the greatest production of glycosaminoglycans by chondrocytes at 20 days in comparison to alginate, fibrin, and collagen.[223] A concern with the application of PLA–PGA polymers is an inflammatory reaction that develops after hydrolysis of the polymer. However, a laryngotracheal rabbit model with a PLA–PGA copolymer had appropriate clinical function of the implants at the time of harvest at 12 months. The scaffolds were completely resorbed without signs of a chronic inflammatory response.[224] Despite the success in animal models, no PLA–PGA-based materials have progressed to clinical trials.

Novel potential sources for the creation of acellular scaffolds are decellularized donor tissues;[225] after 90 days in vivo, implants in rabbits show MSC-seeded tissues reintegrated with native trachea.[198] The construction of these decellularized tissues involves the removal of donor cells and materials using detergents, with the general tissue architecture remaining intact. Another recent advancement in scaffold construction has been the rise of 3D printing. In one study, 3D scaffold was coated with MSCs seeded in fibroin. The engineered tracheas were covered in regenerated respiratory mucosa, and after eight weeks, there was no graft rejection.[226] Although few studies are currently available, recellularized tracheas from decellularized or 3D printed sources show great promise.

Bioreactor culture system with mechanical stimulation

In the design of a bioreactor culture system, the primary factors to consider are the cell seeding density, mass transfer as modulated by shear stress, and compressive forces imparted onto resident cells.[227] The choice of cell seeding density must consider the balance of ECM production and mass transfer of nutrients. Limited mass transfer can result in non-uniform cell distribution with higher cell numbers at the surface of the scaffold, or even cell death in regions deeper into the tissue. Methods to apply shear stress and enhance mass transfer include mechanically stirring the media, perfusion of medium through scaffolds, and/or a rotating-wall bioreactor that imparts low shears and stirring.[227] In addition to enhanced ECM production, stirred mechanical systems also induce an even distribution of cells over the scaffold. To enable direct perfusion, a flow system is necessary where media or a cell suspension can directly pass through the inlet or pores of the 3D scaffold. Compared to statically cultured controls, a direct perfusion system can increase cell proliferation and glycosaminoglycans content.

Compressive forces are required for chondrocyte health, stimulate differentiation of MSCs to chondrocytes, and also contribute to structural maintenance of articular cartilage in vivo. In vivo, hydrostatic pressure is imparted onto chondrocytes via the synovial fluid contained in the cartilage matrix.[227] Physiological levels of hydrostatic pressure range from 7 to 10 MPa, and as cartilage is incompressible in this range, only minimal tissue deformation occurs.[228,229] Variables included in compression-dependent cell behaviors are the duration of hydrostatic pressure, total time of application, and magnitude of compression. In literature, these loads range from 0.1 to 15 MPa, and the frequency of compression ranges from 0.05 to 1 Hz.[204,230] Chondrocytes embedded in an agarose scaffold, cycled to 3–10% strain (at a frequency of 1 Hz) for 4 to 6 weeks have an increase in the amount of proteoglycan and collagen in comparison to static cultures.[231,232] Waldman and colleagues embedded bovine chondrocytes into a calcium polyphosphate scaffold, loaded this system to 5% compression (400 cycles/day) at a frequency of 0.5 Hz.[233] The engineered tissues were stimulated intermittently (every other day) for 1 to 4 weeks under

5% shear. Tissues that underwent compression and shear increased collagen synthesis by 76% and proteoglycan synthesis by 73% over static controls.

Clinical applications

Although significant improvements have been made toward the production of functional engineered cartilage, the translation of these technologies to the clinic has been severely limited. Currently, there are no FDA-approved engineered cartilages available in the United States. In Korea, however, there is one readily available engineered cartilage. Cartistem (Medpost, Korea), an umbilical cord blood-derived MSC on polymer scaffold, in 2012 was approved to treat arthritis and cartilage injury in Korea.[234] Recently, Cartistem was approved to enter Phase I/IIa clinical trials in the United States.[234] The FDA approval of Cartistem will enable the progress of tissue-engineered products for the treatment of cartilage repair and regeneration.

Future challenges

The challenge of cartilage tissue engineering remains to develop a therapeutic treatment for cartilage disease or injury. Difficulties in tissue engineering cartilage include (1) sourcing sufficient autologously sourced chondrocytes; (2) establishing a scaffold that can support cells, have clinically significant dimensions, and be able to withstand large mechanical loads; and (3) establishing an optimal culture regimen for engineering neocartilage. Future success criteria should be based on native cartilage physiology and the associated regulatory pathways. These criteria will inform future development of stem cell–based tissue-engineering technologies.

Cardiac tissue engineering

Cardiovascular disease is the leading cause of mortality in the United States. The number of people in the United States with one or more types of cardiovascular disease exceeds 1 in 3, costing over $300 billion each year.[31] Heart disease causes approximately one in four deaths in the United States each year, and the readmission rates have increased for related complications following treatment.[235,236] Patients who survive a myocardial infarction experience myocardial damage that can eventually result in congestive heart failure. Other causes of heart failure include hypertension, cardiomyopathy, valvular disease, and cardiac arrhythmias. The pathophysiology of heart failure is the inability of the heart to maintain adequate cardiac output because of injury to the cardiac myocytes that causes an increase in wall stress and forward pumping failure.[237]

Traditional treatment options for severe heart failure include pharmacologic therapy, heart transplantation, and other interventions such as cardiac resynchronization, coronary revascularization, and left ventricular assist device implantation. The number of people requiring heart transplantation continues to increase, but immune rejection and morbidity remain major problems for elderly recipients of hearts.[238] The one-year survival for heart transplants is approximately 81%, and the five-year survival is approximately 69%.[238]

Design goals for cardiac tissue regeneration

The heart is a muscular organ that functions as a pump through rhythmic cycles of contraction and relaxation. It is composed of three layers: the epicardium, the myocardium, and endocardium.[36] To prevent friction during heartbeats, the epicardium provides a smooth surface with reduced friction. The endocardium functions to interact with the circulating blood and create an antithrombotic surface on the interior of the myocardial wall. Between these two layers lies the primary layer of the heart: the myocardium. Myocardial tissue is involuntary muscle and consists of striated cardiac muscle cells with many branching cells that are joined by unique intercalated disks. The intercalated disks are gap junctions that permit electrical communication of impulses to a large area of the heart wall, thereby stimulating contraction.

Originally, cardiac tissue engineers found most success in constructing patches of myocardium to replace specific areas of diseased heart tissue. In addition to replacing damaged cardiac tissue, cardiac tissue engineering can be used to reconstruct pediatric congenital defects. Pediatric heart valves and pulmonary arteries have been engineered with some success, and future advances might include treatment of malformations including single ventricles and septal defects in the ventricles or atria.[239,240] It is substantially more difficult to engineer an entire heart with the ability to contract appropriately with separate chambers, adapt appropriately to physiologic stimuli, and respond to further cardiac disease progression. However, decellularized porcine hearts repopulated with neonatal cardiac cells have shown promising results in vitro, inviting further studies to assess viability in vivo.[241] Microfabrication and 3D printing techniques also hold the promise of meeting these complex structural requirements.

The alternative, cell-based therapy to cardiac tissue engineering is injection of cardiomyocytes, marrow-derived cells, or cardiac stem cells directly into the myocardium. Transplantation of cardiomyocytes has been studied in animal models by directly injecting fetal or neonatal cardiomyocytes into the injured myocardium. Administering embryonic cardiomyocytes after infarction has yielded beneficial effects on the remodeling process and ventricular ejection fraction in animal studies.[242] However, transplantation of fully differentiated cardiomyocytes has not successfully replaced scar tissue and restored synchronously contractile muscle.[243,244] The infusion of skeletal myoblasts received some attention as a potential therapy, but clinical trials so far have not yielded conclusive evidence of this treatment's efficacy.[245,246] Furthermore, hESC-derived cardiomyocytes have yielded myocardial remuscularization with native electromechanical coupling on injection into damaged myocardium.[247] Injection of induced pluripotent stem cells (iPSCs) has yielded more promising results, with a significant reduction in apoptosis and increase in myocardial function following injection two weeks after myocardial infarction.[248] One potential drawback, however, is the perpetuation of undifferentiated pluripotent cells in vivo rather than assumption of cardiomyocyte fates.[249]

In cell-injection therapies, approximately 90% of infused cells are lost to systemic circulation, which limits the viability of these therapies even for optimal cell types.[250] Injecting the cells into the myocardium directly (rather than the vasculature) improves the specificity of localization, and in situ polymerizable hydrogels help further with this.[251]

Cell source

Cells from autologous sources are desirable to mitigate immunogenic responses. In some studies, bone marrow–derived stem cells have been shown to differentiate into cardiac myocytes.[252,253] However, increasing evidence suggests that a paracrine signaling mechanism is primarily responsible for the improved myocardial function and vascularization seen in clinical trials.[254,255] Rat marrow–derived cardiac cells expressed proteins consistent with cardiomyocytes in vitro; in a rat infarct model, the transplanted cells improved cardiac structure and function.[256] In addition, other rodent myocardial infarct animal models with cardiac cells derived from marrow have shown improved cardiac function and better ejection fraction with less remodeling of the left ventricle.[253,256] Other sources include cardiomyocytes derived from hESCs or iPSCs, both of which have demonstrated efficacy in large-animal studies.[248,251]

Primary cardiac cells do not appear to be a viable cell source for cardiac engineering in humans because they are difficult to harvest and do not readily expand. Cardiac progenitor cells derived from induced pluripotent stem cells, however, have seen success in animal models and may be tested in future clinical trials.[257] In preclinical trials, transplanted sheets of skeletal myoblasts appear to enhance myocardial recovery, but concerns about arrhythmia have created controversy over their use.[258,259]

Scaffold

Both synthetic polymers and natural materials have been used for cardiac tissue engineering scaffolds. In a study comparing cardiac patches of polyglycolide (PGA), gelatin, and polylactide copolymer with polycaprolactone (PCL) using rat aortic smooth muscle as the cell source, PCL material yielded better ingrowth of cells in vitro and improved cellular architecture as compared to PGA and gelatin.[260] The gelatin scaffold induced an inflammatory reaction, which was attributed to the xenogeneic (bovine) protein in the gelatin. As an alternative material, natural alginate-based scaffolds can form a 3D structure with a uniform distribution of cardiomyocytes.[261] When a graft composed of fetal cardiac cells in an alginate scaffold was implanted in a rat myocardial infarct model, it was found to undergo intensive neovascularization and prolong cell survival. The alginate scaffold was almost completely degraded after nine weeks, and it was well invested with differentiated cardiomyocytes.[262]

Collagen gels have been used to form 3D scaffolds that support cardiomyocytes. Using a 3D collagen matrix, neonatal rat cardiomyocytes can form myocardial tissue.[263] These constructs were prepared by adding a cell solution to preformed, commercially available collagen that was allowed to gel over four hours. The collagen matrix supported the attachment, proliferation, and synchronous contractions of the neonatal cardiomyocytes in 3D. Furthermore, the spontaneous and synchronous contractions were maintained for up to 13 weeks.

Other investigators have created engineered heart tissue by mixing a solution of neonatal rat cardiac cells with both collagen gel and Matrigel (Becton Dickinson, Franklin Lakes, NJ).[264] After a few days, the constructs were placed in a custom-made stretch device to provide mechanical stimulation. The in vitro tissue demonstrated histologic features of native differentiated myocardium and contractile characteristics of native myocardium. Stretch stimulation seems particularly important in myocardial development, as contractile force was greater than twofold in the stretch group compared to the statically grown tissue.[265]

As an alternative to scaffold-based techniques, some investigators have used temperature-responsive polymer called poly(N-iso-propylacrylamide) (PIPA Am) that covalently attaches to tissue culture polystyrene to support the growth of cells. When the temperature is lowered to 32 °C, the PIPA Am—with the cells—spontaneously detaches from the underlying polystyrene. The intercellular mechanical junctions of the sheet on the upper surface, however, remain intact.[266] PIPA Am has been applied to rat neonatal cardiac

cells to create sheets that can be layered together to form a 3D myocardial tissue structure. Preclinical trials suggest that the implantation of these sheets leads to improved cardiac function after myocardial infarction.[266,267] Furthermore, these sheets can be layered in 3D printing to produce grafts of increasing thickness. After implanting a thin graft onto the damaged tissue, neovascularization occurs.[251] Repeating this process, in turn, allows surgeons to build up healthy, vascularized tissue.

To avoid the need for multiple surgeries, other groups have attempted to vascularize thicker grafts by loading growth factors (often VEGF) into matrices or by electrospinning a polymer–cell mixture.[268–271] Microfabrication is another promising method for including the heterogeneous microscale structures needed for the formation of vasculature. Soft lithography, in particular, has greatly reduced the cost and complexity of creating scaffolds for microcapillaries, which are then populated during cell seeding.[272,273]

The requisite complexity of scaffolding has been a major obstacle in myocardial engineering. In addition to ensuring anisotropic, near-native mechanical properties, it is difficult to confer proteomic heterogeneity and to allow for vascularization. Using decellularized organs as scaffolds helps overcome these issues. The native ECM remains intact and is repopulated with endothelial cells and cardiomyocytes under conditions of electrical stimulation and mechanical strain. During in vitro tests, the resultant bioartificial hearts showed modest functionality, but seeding protocols must improve before the engineered hearts are suitable for in vivo studies.[274]

Bioreactors

The objective of bioreactor development in cardiac tissue engineering is to stimulate the growth of a 3D structure that is conditioned by mechanical or electrical stimulation. A bioreactor system with a spinner flask causes turbulent flow that results in improved mixing for nutrient and oxygen delivery in comparison to static cultures.[275] Stretching and compression results in improved proliferation, a more uniform and organized distribution of cardiomyocytes on the scaffold, and a more abundant ECM.[276] Electrical stimulation also has aided the development of structures similar to those of native myocardium and increased their contractile response in comparison to nonstimulated cultures.[277]

For whole-organ engineering, media is perfused through the decellularized vasculature in a pulsatile fashion, and electrical stimulation is provided at physiologically relevant locations in the epicardium.[274] The preload and afterload also can be adjusted to optimize repopulation. In 2015, Bursac et al. engineered human myobundles by encapsulating myogenic cells derived from biopsy in a fibrinogen and Matrigel composite. These myobundles, cultured in a dynamic bioreactor, exhibited native responses to applied drugs and generated contractile forces similar to those of human fetal muscle.[278]

Preclinical studies

Many cell-based therapies have advanced to large animal studies. In particular, injection of hES cell-derived cardiomyocytes into an ischemic region of monkey ventricle following myocardial infarction yielded excellent graft survival and electromechanical coupling.[247] Another promising study involved seeding marrow mesenchymal stem cells (MSCs) onto a scaffold of a composite collagen and polylactic acid (PLA) reinforced with polytetrafluoroethylene (PTFE).[279] Four weeks after implantation into a nonfunctioning rat left ventricle, the marrow cells integrated into the host and formed differentiated cardiac muscle as evidenced by cell morphology and cytoplasmic reactivity of anti-Troponin C. Although the authors noted that mice are relatively resistant to arrhythmias, they suggested a cardiac patch could be implanted for human use to replace myocardial scar after infarction concurrently with coronary revascularization. In another promising preclinical study in rats, injecting a hydrogel composed of hyaluronic acid led to a 200% increase in wall thickness following myocardial infarction.[280]

Another group engineered grafts with fetal cardiac cells using 3D alginate scaffolds for the regeneration of infarcted myocardium.[262] The porous alginate scaffold was seeded with fetal cardiac cells and incubated for four days before implantation. The graft was implanted seven days after myocardial infarction in a rat model. Nine weeks after transplantation, the rats with grafts demonstrated attenuation of left ventricular dilatation and no change in left ventricular contractility. In contrast, the control group developed significant left ventricular dilatation with progressive deterioration in left ventricular contraction. The cardiac grafts were found to have intensive neovascularization that contributed to the survival of the cells in the graft. However, the beneficial effects of the graft on cardiac contractility were not likely directly caused by contraction of the implant because only a small fraction of the implanted cardiac cells survived after nine weeks. Other investigators reported the potential viability of injecting an alginate material with insulin-like growth factor-1 and hepatocyte growth factor: compared to a control at four weeks, the treatment increased angiogenesis, reduced apoptosis, and limited the spread of the infarct.[281]

Zimmermann has reported the construction of an engineered heart tissue composed of a suspension of neonatal rat heart cells, liquid collagen, and Matrigel formed in circular molds and subjected to mechanical strain that can improve contractile function of an infarcted rat model.[282] The engineered heart tissue showed electrical coupling comparable to the native myocardium, without evidence of arrhythmia, at 28 days. Furthermore, the engineered heart tissue proved superior to control implants in preventing further dilation and inducing systolic wall thickening of infarcted myocardial segments.[282] Similar results were observed in a preliminary human trial: when mononuclear bone marrow cell-seeded collagen matrices were placed atop post-infarction scars, the ejection fraction increased, and cardiac wall stress was closer to physiological values.[283] However, this study was confounded by the addition of a coronary artery bypass graft. Randomized controlled trials ought to be conducted to further evaluate this treatment's clinical utility.

Sheets of cells also have demonstrated success in preclinical trials. After myocardial infarction in a mouse, investigators grafted a scaffold-free sheet of adipocytes onto the surface of the ventricle.[284] The ejection fraction and survival rate were superior compared to a control group at one month after infarction. Cardioprotective effects were lost for sheets of adiponectin-knockout adipocytes, suggesting a role for adiponectin in modulating the ventricular remodeling process.[284]

Future challenges

The main challenges for cardiac tissue engineering are securing a reliable autologous cell source, combating arrhythmias, and improving engineered whole hearts. However, it is difficult to procure viable cardiac cells from older patients with diabetes and other diseases with impaired proliferative and functional capacities.[285] Fetal or neonatal cardiac progenitor cells, hiPS- or hES-derived cardiomyocytes, and multipotent cardiac progenitor cells and bone marrow–derived mononuclear cells have emerged as promising cellular candidates.[286] Refining methods of isolating, differentiating, and proliferating marrow-derived cells and induced pluripotent stem cells will help alleviate this issue.

Arrhythmias are commonly observed in myocardial grafts, though their exact cause is not known. One hypothesis is that the conduction velocity of grafts is lower than that of the surrounding tissue.[247] However, the arrhythmias often resolve spontaneously by three weeks following implantation, and some implanted grafts do not yield observable arrhythmias.[282]

Engineered whole hearts from decellularized scaffolds—which overcome concerns about vascularization—have shown great promise in murine and rat models, but many obstacles remain before they are clinically useful.[287] Among the most significant challenges are insufficient contractile force and the potential for immunogenic response on implantation.[288,289] Modern techniques in cardiac engineering show the potential for concurrent augmentation of the scar tissue formed at coronary revascularization. With further developments in the repopulation of decellularized scaffolds, future clinical applications may include reconstruction of congenital cardiac defects and even whole-heart engineering.

Urology tissue engineering

The urinary system is exposed to a variety of insults that require reconstruction as a treatment, including congenital abnormalities, cancer, trauma, infection, and iatrogenic injuries. Tissue-engineering techniques have been explored for the urethra and phallus, and to restore testicular function; most attention, however, has been devoted to the repair of the urinary bladder.[290]

As it stands today, bladder and urethral reconstruction most commonly uses gastrointestinal tissue. One congenital anomaly that may require such a reconstruction is exstrophy of the bladder, a condition with a prevalence of 3.3 births per 100,000.[291] The initial treatment for this bladder defect is early primary closure. In some cases, however, the bladder is too small for closure or the bladder does not develop to maintain continence. In these cases, tissue harvested from the small bowel or colon is used to augment its size.[291]

Cancer of the urinary bladder is the sixth most common cause of cancer death in America.[291] Invasive bladder cancer is treated by radical cystectomy with urinary diversion. The use of selective bladder preservation or partial cystectomy is inferior to radical cystectomy for invasive cancer, meaning that total bladder replacement could significantly enhance quality of life for these patients. Blunt trauma is another cause of urinary tract injury, often associated with pelvic fractures or straddle injuries for the urethra. In the case of large defects that require diversion of the urinary system, the use of gastrointestinal tract tissue is the only option. Bowel segments that are mobilized for bladder reconstructions are associated with various complications, including mucus production, chronic bacteruria, stone formation, rupture, electrolyte imbalance, and metabolic acidosis with a range of incidence from 5% to 44%.[292–294]

Design goals for urinary tissue

The objective of urinary tissue engineering is to provide an alternative source of tissue that is more similar to native bladder or urethra. A successful tissue-engineered bladder must act as a reservoir for urine, contract until empty, integrate with sites of anastomosis to prevent leakage, have mechanical strength to prevent rupture, and must not cause excessive stone formation. Structurally, the bladder is a hollow muscular organ that functions as a reservoir to hold urine until time of excretion through the urethra. The bladder wall is comprised of a transitional epithelium, the lamina propria, a muscular layer, and an adventitia, with the transitional epithelium forming a layer of only four to five cells when the bladder is empty, and two to three cells when the bladder is distended.[295] The viscoelastic properties of the bladder are derived from the smooth muscle, layer, a collagen content of approximately 50%, and an elastin content of approximately 2%.[291] The bladder has a physiologic compliance that contains neural input to set the volume for micturition.[291]

Cell source

The most common cell source for bladder tissue engineering is a primary cell source from urothelial cells and visceral smooth muscle cells. Primary urothelial cells are autologous and have been demonstrated expanding from a surface area of 1 cm^2 to 4202 cm^2 over a period of eight weeks, though wall muscle growth is more challenging.[296] An important question in diseased organ regeneration, however, is whether the autologous cells will reproduce the original disease process: Will neuropathic bladder smooth muscle cells, for instance, grow neuropathic grafts? In early trials, harvested and cultured human visceral smooth muscle cells from normal, exstrophic, and neuropathic bladders showed no differences in phenotype or degree of contractility.[297] In more recent studies on pediatric neuropathic bladders, however, urothelial source cells—not even thought to be the target tissue of the disease process—demonstrated less growth and inferior barrier formation when compared to normal controls, leaving it an open question.[298]

Alternative potential cell sources are bone marrow stem cells, embryonic stem cells, and induced pluripotent stem cells that have not been exposed to fibrotic or malignant changes. A recent study showed successful bladder wall growth from the MSCs of spina bifida patients, albeit with thin and fragile urothelium. Adding CD34$^+$ HSCs to these MSCs induced robust urothelium, alongside markedly increased neurvasculogenesis, a relative weakness of many bladder-engineering approaches.[299]

Scaffold

The main scaffold types for urologic tissue engineering are synthetic polymers, natural materials like collagen and alginate, and acellular tissue matrices derived from bladder or intestinal submucosa. It has been demonstrated that the adherence and proliferation of bladder smooth muscle cells appears to be similar across synthetic polymers (e.g., poly[lactic-co-glycolic] acid [PLGA] and PCL).[300] Hybrid materials, such as a PLGA meshcollagen gel, have also been shown to support the growth of urothelial and smooth muscle cells. Hybrid scaffolds aim to take advantage of the mechanical strength of the synthetic polymers and the cell adhesion properties of the collagen gel.[301] Tissues that are used to create an acellular matrix for bladder scaffolds are small intestine submucosa, native bladder tissue, and bladder submucosa.[302,303] Bladder replacement grafts composed of small intestine submucosa have demonstrated regeneration of normal bladder with urothelium, smooth muscle, and serosal layers in canine and rat models, and have recently been modestly successful in improving bladder capacity in human trials.[302,304]

Preclinical and clinical trials

The tissue-engineered bladder is progressing from in vitro models to clinical trials of partial organ replacement. Trials have been performed in a wide variety of species, with pigs and dogs appearing to be more representative of bladder size changes in humans than rats or rabbits.[305] Early efforts by the Atala group successfully proliferated the bladder urothelial and smooth muscle cells from a small biopsy, and used a cell-free bladder construct as the scaffold. They demonstrated in a canine 50%-cystectomy model that the cell-seeded graft had a 99% increase in the capacity of the bladder.[303] Histologic analysis confirmed the presence of nerve fibers in the tissue-engineered bladders. In a study by Kropp in 2004, well-expanded bladders were generated with acellular porcine small intestine submucosa (SIS) in a canine cystectomy model using cell-free grafts.[302] In a later study of a canine 90% bladder-replacement cystectomy, cell-seeded and cell-free scaffolds produced similar results of poor bladder regeneration: the authors attributed the lack of bladder regeneration to a poor vascular network and increased inflammation produced by the large implants.[306] The viability of the implanted graft depends on vascular ingrowth from the surrounding tissues, and the vascular network may not have been able to develop at a rapid enough rate to support such a large tissue graft. More recently, nanoparticles have been used in a porcine model enhance angiogenesis.[307] Attempts have been also made to study diseased animal models, although results have varied in their demonstrated differences with healthy controls.[308,309]

Table 42.4 Human trials of tissue-engineered bladder grafts

Reference	Year	N	Pathology	Cell Source	Scaffold	Outcome
Atala et al.[310]	2006	7	Myelomeningocele	Autologous urothelial/ smooth muscle	De-cellularized BSM w/ and w/o omental wrap, composite BSM/ PGA matrix.	Encouraging improvement in bladder capacity and compliance in omental wrap groups.
Caione et al.[312]	2012	5	Exstrophy-epispadias	Unseeded	Small intestine submucosa	+30% improvement in compliance and capacity at 6 and 18 months; poor muscle histology, and no significant clinical benefit.
Shaefer et al.[313]	2013	6	Multiple	Unseeded	Small intestine submucosa	Poor muscle histology, and no significant clinical benefit.
Joseph et al.[311]	2014	10	Myelomeningocele	Autologous urothelial/ smooth muscle	PGA matrix	Marginally improved compliance in 5 patients at 36 months, no improvement in capacity; no significant clinical benefit. Numerous adverse events.
Zhang/Liao[304]	2014	8	Multiple	Unseeded	Small intestine submucosa	Limited bladder regeneration in cell-seeded and cell-free group

BSM, bladder submucosa.

Table 42.4 lists currently published clinical trials of cystoplasty using tissue-engineering techniques in human patients. In 2006, Atala *et al.* generated considerable excitement by translating bladder tissue engineering into human trials.[310] The study identified seven patients, ages ranging from 4 to 19, with primary diagnoses of myelomeningocele and poorly compliant bladders. Using decellularized bladder submucosa or collagen/PGA matrices, autologous cells from bladder biopsies were seeded and cultured: seven to eight weeks elapsed between bladder biopsy and implantation of the final product. Patients, followed for a median of 46 months, demonstrated similar urodynamic results to those with gastrointestinal segment augmentations but without the associated complications. This positive preliminary data led to a Phase II trial on 10 spina bifida patients, published in 2014.[311] Although five patients seemed to show improved bladder compliance at 36 months, the difference was not statistically or clinically significant, nor was there any change in bladder capacity. Ultimately, a majority of patients underwent traditional ileocystoplasties, in part due to an unexpectedly high number of adverse events.

Though seeded substrates show superior performance in some animal models,[291] separate trials have also examined the implantation of acellular small intestine submucosa scaffolds into five patients with extrophic bladders,[312] six patients with microbladder from a variety of causes,[313] and eight patients with myelomeningoceles or spinal cord injury.[304] Though small improvements in capacity and compliance were evident in some patients, smooth muscle developed poorly in the first two studies, and patients did not achieve long-term continence. Zhang and Liao report a better outcome despite using a larger graft size, with significant increases in bladder capacity and compliance.[304] Histological samples still noted small amounts of muscle fiber, and further study is likely needed to confirm clinical efficacy.[314]

Future challenges

The use of tissue-engineered bladders in a clinical application demonstrates the exciting opportunities in the field of urothelial tissue engineering. Disappointing clinical results, however, have called into question the suitability of healthy animals as models for diseased bladders,[305,315,316] and have renewed emphasis on the importance of neovascularization factors and the proper selection of cell source.[311] Another potential clinical application is bladder reconstruction after cancer resection, utilizing harvested cells from an area of bladder without any neoplastic changes. The application of bladder tissue engineering for large cystectomies may require a vascular network before implantation, as suggested by data from the canine model.[306] Neuronal integration of the graft is important to restore the natural voiding mechanism. Improvements in existing approaches may rise from the use of marrow stem cells as a smooth muscle cell source, using HSCs in co-culture, stimulation of neuronal integration into the graft, continued optimization of the scaffold, and possibly the use of angiogenic nanoparticles.[299,307] Although there is conflicting evidence to suggest that viable bladder cells can still be harvested from diseased tissue, bladder smooth muscle derived from marrow stem cells may be a more attractive alternative cell source. Optimization of the scaffold for improved mechanical characteristics and improved control over degradation in response to tissue remodeling are two key issues. As tissue-engineered products progress from case studies to commercial applications, process methods to reduce the potential of infection and to achieve high-quality standards will be important issues for these new medical devices.

Corneal tissue engineering

A bioengineered cornea has the potential to restore vision when the loss is caused by corneal opacification. The cornea is a crucial part of the eye's refractive apparatus and functions to protect the eye against infection and structural damage. Causes of opacification are varied, but include abnormal corneal shape, infections that lead to corneal scarring, congenital disorders of the cornea, vitamin A deficiencies, parasites, and—especially in children—trauma.[317] Corneas are the most commonly transplanted tissue in the world, by an impressive margin, and demand for donor corneas often far outstrips supply. This imbalance generates considerable demand for engineered alternatives.

Objectives of tissue-engineered cornea

The cornea is composed of an outer epithelial layer; a thick, collagen-based stroma; and an inner endothelial layer. Altogether, the cornea is approximately 500 μm thick at the pupil center, increasing to 700 μm near the limbus, where the cornea and sclera meet.[318]

The epithelium is a stratified squamous layer approximately four to six cells thick. The most superficial cells are flat, polygonal cells with microvilli that interact directly with the 7 μm tear film responsible for providing the eye's optically smooth surface. Tight junctions between these epithelial cells provide a barrier to bacteria and tears. Underneath these lie the wing cells, and adjacent to the stroma lies the basal cell layer: a single 20 μm sheet of columnar cells that divides to supply the layers above. This basal cell layer is itself supplied by a pool of inwardly migrating epithelial stem cells at the limbus. The epithelium turns over completely every 7–10 days, and surface defects in a healthy eye are rapidly repaired. Damage to the cellular substrate—potentially caused by herpetic infections, chemical burns, or dystrophies—can prevent the normally rapid healing of surface defects, as can damage to the limbal stem cell (LSC) population.[318]

The corneal stroma comprises roughly 85% of the corneal thickness, largely consisting of carefully aligned collagen fibrils and specialized proteoglycans. Keratocytes, predominately located in the anterior stroma, maintain the stroma's ECM and are responsible for injury repair.[318]

The corneal endothelium is a hexagonal monolayer responsible for maintaining a high stromal water content of around 78%, thus ensuring continued transparency. This monolayer rests on a 10 μm basement membrane—known as Descemet's membrane—and exhibits very little mitotic potential, making the endothelium extremely vulnerable to any destructive process. Corneal cell counts below 500 cells/m^2 risk the development of an opacifying corneal edema.[318]

Treatments for severe corneal disease initially utilized penetrating keratoplasty (PK), a full-thickness allograft transplantation that replaced all corneal layers. In the past decade, however, full-thickness transplant has increasingly been replaced by more selective therapies: anterior lamellar keratoplasty (ALK) replaces only the epithelial layer and a portion of the stroma, leaving Descemet's membrane and the endothelial layer intact; endothelial keratoplasty (EK) replaces only Descemet's membrane and the endothelium. Both procedures exhibit improved complication rates.[317] In traditional PK, rejection is a major cause of graft failure and reportedly affects around 20% of patients at five years.[319] EK procedures likely carry similar rejection risk, whereas, in epithelial or stromal disease, ALK greatly reduces the odds of rejection by preserving the patient's own endothelium.[317]

Synthetic corneal replacements, or keratoprostheses (KPros), provide an alternative treatment option for those patients who are not candidates for allograft corneal transplantation. Synthetic corneal prostheses use a flexible material with an optically clear core surrounded by a microporous skirt designed to encourage fibroblast ingrowth and collagen deposition.[320] Multiple synthetic keratoprostheses have been tested clinically, including the Puntucci and AlphaCor KPros, but only the Boston (or *Dolman-Doane*) keratoprosthesis has met with enduring success.[321]

Approved by the FDA 1992, the Boston keratoprosthesis consists of a "collar-button" design with a front plate, a central core of transparent polymethylmethacrylate (PMMA), and a titanium back plate.[322] Unfortunately, the design currently requires corneal donor tissue—although not of transplant quality—to form a rim of attachment to the patient.[323] The most favorable outcomes using the Boston device are for patients with multiple failed grafts, repeated immunologic rejection of corneal allografts, and neovascularization of a corneal graft. The postoperative course must be closely followed for retroprosthetic membrane formation, glaucoma, retinal detachment, and endophthalmitis, but many patients retain useful vision over a multiyear period.[324] As of 2013, approximately 7500 devices had been implanted.[325]

Cell source

Severe ocular surface diseases such as Stevens–Johnson syndrome, ocular cicatricial pemphigoid, and chemical or thermal burns often destroy existing limbal epithelial stem cells (LESCs) along with the corneal epithelium.[326] In unilateral conditions, the obvious cell source for epithelial regrowth is the autologous LESC of the unaffected eye. To minimize damage to the stem cell pool, ex vivo expansion can reduce required limbal biopsy size in a process known as cultured limbal epithelial transplantation (CLET).[327] This is generally accomplished with xenogeneic or allogeneic feeder cells, and subsequent seeding onto transplantable carriers for surgical insertion.

In the earliest report of autologous cultivated corneal epithelial cells by Pellegrini, a biopsy from the limbus of the uninjured eye was obtained.[328] The autologous cultured corneal epithelium was implanted onto the cornea of two patients, and was found to restore the corneal surface with a significant improvement in visual acuity. Clinical CLET studies using autologous LESCs have now seen follow-up across a decade or longer,[329] and a review of CLET studies published over a 13-year period indicated an approximate success rate of 76% in autologous transplants.[330]

In patients who have bilateral LSC deficiencies, either allogeneic cultured epithelial cells or cells from another tissue in the patient must be used. The risk of using allogeneic cultured epithelial cells is an increased incidence of rejection and poor clinical outcome, alongside the potential necessity of long-term immunosuppressive therapy. Interestingly, Baylis *et al.* report no obvious difference in outcome between autologous and allogeneic CLET studies in their meta-analysis, although this result may be confounded by varying study designs and different injury etiologies in patients with bilateral symptoms.[330] To obviate immunorejection associated with allogeneic cells in bilaterally affected patients, epithelial cells from the oral mucosa have also been used in multiple clinical studies for corneal applications.[331,332] Although sample sizes were small, and oral mucosal cells may be more prone to corneal neovascularization, initial results have been encouraging.[327] Similar attempts have proceeded with conjunctival epithelium,[333] epidermis,[334] and hair follicle cells.[335] Preclinical studies have further

demonstrated the growth of cells resembling corneal epithelium from sources as diverse as bone marrow–derived mesenchymal stem cells,[336] umbilical cord stem cells,[337] and induced pluripotent stem cells,[338] among others.

Human corneal endothelial cells (HCECs) have also attracted considerable interest in recent years. Although EK procedures have greatly improved surgical outcomes, they still require valuable donor corneas, and there is much to gain from bypassing this requirement. Multiple preclinical studies have reported culturing HCECs in vitro with a variety of scaffolds.[339-344] As with their epithelial counterparts, a diverse array of HCEC precursor cells have been demonstrated in the literature in an attempt to overcome the immunogenicity of allogeneic sources, the paucity of HCEC sources, and the relatively limited proliferation capacity of HCECs in vivo.[345] These include rat neural crest cells,[346] corneal stroma,[347] umbilical cord mesenchyme,[348] and, most recently, mesothelial cells.[345]

Scaffold

The scaffolds for epithelial tissue engineering often function more as carrier substances than as conventional structures. The most clinically validated material choices are human amniotic membrane and fibrin-based materials. Amniotic membrane is a single layer of epithelial cells and basement membrane that surrounds the embryo during gestation. It is readily available, and early trials indicated very limited immunogenicity alongside inherent antimicrobial properties.[349] Though successfully employed in multiple clinical trials, its variability among donors, costly screening requirements, lack of optical transparency, and potential ability to pass viruses from donors have prompted a search for alternatives.[350]

Fibrin and fibrin-based carriers have also demonstrated success for corneal epithelial systems: biodegradable, they will readily integrate with the surrounding tissue. Fibrin scaffolds are readily available, clinically approved, standardized, and have acceptable optical and mechanical properties.[327] Human studies have demonstrated success in transplanting cultured corneal limbal cells onto fibrin carrier from the healthy eye to the contralateral eye.[329,351] Collagen scaffolds are under study in an attempt to mimic stromal architecture, and techniques exist to improve mechanical and optical properties.[327,352] Other groups have explored keratin,[353] silk,[354] chitin,[355] and electrospun synthetics.[356] Some approaches do not involve scaffolds at all: one group treated 25 patients with oral mucosal epithelial cells grown on temperature-sensitive culture wells, which allowed release of intact cell sheets upon cooling.[357] Finally, natural substrates have also been pursued, including decellularized donor cornea successfully seeded with corneal epithelial cells.[358] Many of these same substrates have been employed in preclinical trials of endothelial engineering, including chitosan,[339] decellularized human[340] and porcine corneal stroma,[342] hydrogel,[341] and pericellular matrix prepared using mesenchymal cells as a non-xenogeneic substrate for subsequent implantation.[343]

Clinical applications

Corneal epithelial engineering has been in clinical trials for some time; a 2013 meta-analysis examined results from around 400 separate eyes, and demonstrated an overall success rate of 76% across a wide variety of groups and techniques.[330] Encouragingly, in the setting of bilateral ocular surface diseases, replacement cell sources comprising autologous oral mucosal epithelial cells and conjunctival epithelium cells both demonstrated feasibility in clinical trials. With continued interest and progress, important steps can be taken toward standardization of result reporting across the CLET community, better facilitating comparisons between one study and the next.[330] Furthermore, moves toward completely xenobiotic-free culture systems, improved understanding of the homeostasis of epithelial maintenance, and increased focus on biologically appropriate scaffolding material will likely speed the development of a reliable product for widespread implementation.[327]

Engineering of corneal endothelium has lagged far behind its endothelial counterpart, facing more troublesome obstacles to cell culture and more challenging surgical collection and implantation. Although results have been promising in primate models,[359] endothelial trials have not yet produced significant clinical results.[360] The popularization of the safer EK surgical technique, however, alongside continual improvement in HCEC culturing abilities and increasing demand for donor corneas have caused interest in endothelial engineering to persist. Indeed, a recent cost analysis has already indicated considerable potential economic advantage to the technique over the standard regimen of donor testing.[361]

All in all, these studies demonstrate that corneal engineering is a promising treatment for patients with severe ocular disease who fail transplantation, or for patients who are poor candidates for conventional corneal transplantation. Continued progress toward reliable and reproducible graft success can position corneal tissue engineering as an important alternative to conventional donor-based techniques.

Key References

A full reference list for this chapter is available at: http://www.wiley.com/go/simon/transfusion

74 Roh, J.D. *et al.* Tissue-engineered vascular grafts transform into mature blood vessels via an inflammation-mediated process of vascular remodeling. *Proceedings of the National Academy of Sciences of the United States of America* **107**, 4669–4674 (2010).

75 Dahl, S.L. *et al.* Readily available tissue-engineered vascular grafts. *Science translational medicine* **3**, 68–69 (2011).

164 Tsigkou, O. *et al.* Engineered vascularized bone grafts. *Proceedings of the National Academy of Sciences of the United States of America* **107**, 3311–3316 (2010).

169 Hoch, A.I.& Leach, J.K. Concise review: optimizing expansion of bone marrow mesenchymal stem/stromal cells for clinical applications. *Stem cells translational medicine* **3**, 643–652 (2014).

247 Chong, J.J.H.& Murry, C.E. Cardiac regeneration using pluripotent stem cells—Progression to large animal models. *Stem Cell Research* **13**, 654–665 (2014).

273 Berthiaume, F., Maguire, T.J.& Yarmush, M.L. Tissue engineering and regenerative medicine: history, progress, and challenges. *Annual review of chemical and biomolecular engineering* **2**, 403–430 (2011).

274 Ott, H.C. *et al.* Perfusion-decellularized matrix: using nature's platform to engineer a bioartificial heart. *Nat Med* **14**, 213–221 (2008).

278 Madden, L., Juhas, M., Kraus, W.E., Truskey, G.A.& Bursac, N. Bioengineered human myobundles mimic clinical responses of skeletal muscle to drugs. *eLife* (2015).

317 Tan, D.T.H., Dart, J.K.G., Holland, E.J.& Kinoshita, S. Ophthalmology 3 Corneal transplantation. *Lancet* **379**, 1749–1761 (2012).

356 Sharma, S. *et al.* Cellular response of limbal epithelial cells on electrospun poly-epsilon-caprolactone nanofibrous scaffolds for ocular surface bioengineering: a preliminary in vitro study. *Molecular vision* **17**, 2898–2910 (2011).

Specialized clinical practice

CHAPTER 43

Obstetric transfusion practice

Marieke B. Veenhof,[1] Jos J.M. van Roosmalen[1,2] & Anneke Brand[3]

[1]Department of Obstetrics, Leiden University Medical Center, Leiden, the Netherlands
[2]Section of Health Care and Culture, Athena Institute, VU University, Amsterdam, the Netherlands
[3]Sanquin Blood Bank & Department of ImmunoHematology and Blood Transfusion, Leiden University Medical Center, Leiden, the Netherlands

Due to physiological hypervolemia in a healthy pregnant woman, a certain amount of blood loss after the birth of a child is tolerated.[1] Postpartum hemorrhage (PPH) up to 1000 ml in a healthy mother therefore does not lead to disturbances in hemodynamics. PPH of more than 1000 ml in 24 hours occurs in circa 5% of the deliveries in well-resourced countries and in up to 20% in underresourced countries.[1] In women with anemia or poor increase in blood volume during pregnancy (e.g., in preeclampsia), PPH less than 1000 ml can be hazardous to the mother. From a global health perspective, it is wise to conform to the World Health Organization (WHO) definition of PPH of more than 500 ml. Blood loss in pregnancy, with consequences in oxygen carrying capacity, does lead to additional danger for the fetus.

A worldwide survey shows huge variation of the lifetime risk of maternal mortality from bleeding, from one in six in the poorest countries to one in 30,000 in Northern European countries.[2] It is associated with nearly one-quarter of all maternal deaths globally and is also the leading cause of maternal mortality in most low-income countries.[3]

Obstetric hemorrhage and preeclampsia together account for 50% of maternal deaths in poor as well as rich countries.[2,4] Women with preeclampsia in the Netherlands had an aOR 1.53 (95% confidence interval [CI], 1.46 to 1.60) of postpartum hemorrhage.[5] Pregnancy complications and management differ in various parts of the world because of differences in blood groups, genetic and environmentally acquired diseases, poverty, and logistic and cultural factors.

Blood loss in pregnancy

Obstetrical causes

Delivery poses the highest risk for blood loss during pregnancy. If administration of at least four units of red blood cell transfusion is used as a surrogate definition for major obstetric hemorrhage, major obstetric hemorrhage is found in 4.5 per 1000 births in a Dutch national survey on severe maternal morbidity.[6] Of a total of 358,874 maternities during the study period from August 2004 until August 2006, overall severe maternal morbidity occurred in 2552 women (7.1 per 1000 births), of whom 1606 women needed four or more units of transfusions, indicating that 70% of severe pregnancy complications are associated with severe hemorrhage. Data were available on 1590 of the 1606 women related to the cause of bleeding. Table 43.1 shows the most frequent etiologies.[6] In 1480 women (93%), blood loss occurred during the postpartum period. Antepartum hemorrhage occurred in 135 women (8.5%), and major bleeding in early pregnancy was registered in 51 women (3.2%). These percentages are above 100, because in 76 women both antepartum and postpartum diagnoses were made. Because only women in need of at least four units of blood were included, the most frequent causes of obstetric blood loss before birth (like miscarriage and unexplained minor antepartum hemorrhage) are relatively underrepresented in these figures.

Assuming that the 270 women who received nine or more units of blood would have died if they had not received these transfusions, the maternal mortality ratio (MMR) would stand at 87 instead of the actual 13 per 100,000 live births.[7] For comparison, the MMR for Jehovah's Witnesses is estimated to be 68 per 100,000 live births. This is almost similar to the likely MMR if blood had not been available for those women who received nine or more units of red cells. This underscores the impact of a functioning blood transfusion service on the reduction of maternal mortality. Lack of access to sufficient blood will lead to a higher frequency of hysterectomy to stop the bleeding. Although hysterectomy may be a life-saving procedure for some women, it adds to the risk of dying in others.

Women who are Jehova's Witnesses have a risk of 14 per 1000 births to experience serious maternal morbidity because of obstetric hemorrhage. They also have a six times increased risk for maternal death and a 3.1 times increased risk for serious maternal morbidity compared to the general Dutch population. There is a 130 times increased risk of maternal death from major obstetric hemorrhage.[8]

Hematological causes

Maternal diseases, such as diabetes, renal failure, hemoglobinopathies, systemic lupus, and antiphospholipid syndrome, are not associated with primary bleeding but rather with increased maternal and fetal morbidity and mortality due to thrombotic and vascular complications

Rossi's Principles of Transfusion Medicine, Fifth Edition. Edited by Toby L. Simon, Jeffrey McCullough, Edward L. Snyder, Bjarte G. Solheim, and Ronald G. Strauss.

Table 43.1 Primary diagnosis in major obstetric hemorrhage defined as the need for at least 4 units of blood

Timing	Diagnosis[†]	n	(%)
Early pregnancy (n = 51)	Ectopic pregnancy	29	(56.9%)
	Spontaneous abortion	10	(19.6%)
	Termination of pregnancy	10	(19.6%)
	Miscellaneous[‡]	2	(3.9%)
Antepartum (n = 135)*	Abruptio placentae	61	(45.5%)
	Placenta praevia	54	(40.3%)
	Miscellaneous[§]	7	(5.2%)
	Unknown diagnosis	12	(9.0%)
Postpartum (n = 1480)*	Retained placenta or placental rests	703	(47.8%)
	Uterine atonia	567	(38.5%)
	Hemorrhage following CS	183	(12.4%)
	Perineal tears/episiotomy	148	(10.1%)
	Clotting disorders	116	(7.9%)
	Placenta acreta/increta/percreta	109	(7.4%)
	Rupture of cervix	58	(3.9%)
	Uterine rupture	44	(3.0%)
	Uterine inversion	13	(0.9%)
	Miscellaneous	65	(4.4%)
	Unknown diagnosis	10	(0.7%)

Source: Zwart et al. (2008).[6] Reproduced with permission of Wiley.

* In 76 cases, both antepartum and postpartum diagnoses were coded.

[†] Up to three diagnoses could be coded postpartum.

[‡] Molar pregnancy and placenta percreta.

[§] Rupture of uterine/ovarian artery, rupture of ovarian cyst, placenta percreta, vasa praevia, retroplacental haematoma, and rupture of uterine vein.

leading to preeclampsia, thrombo-embolism, and placental insufficiency. A few maternal diseases associated with maternal thrombocytopenia and (iatrogenic) coagulopathies can pose primary bleeding problems during pregnancy and delivery, but in the absence of obstetric complications rarely lead to maternal mortality.

Maternal thrombocytopenia

Gestational thrombocytopenia, ITP and HELLP

A platelet count below 150×10^9/L is a rather frequent finding in pregnancy. Spurious thrombocytopenia due to laboratory errors or EDTA agglutination is excluded by examination of a blood film or platelet counting in citrated blood.

Thrombocytopenia of $80-150 \times 10^9$/L of unknown origin, often referred to as *gestational thrombocytopenia* (GT), occurs in approximately 6% in the third pregnancy trimester and accounts for the vast majority of maternal thrombocytopenias.[10,11] Its cause and significance are often unknown. GT has been considered as subclinical idiopathic thrombocytopenic purpura (ITP) or as a precursor of HELLP (hemolysis, elevated liver enzymes, and low platelets) syndrome.[12,13] GT is a diagnosis of exclusion. If, in uncomplicated pregnancy, the blood film is normal in an otherwise healthy female without a history of immune thrombocytopenia (ITP) or antiphospholipid antibodies, no diagnostic tests are needed. These women should be carefully monitored for aggravation of thrombocytopenia, and if the platelet count drops below $70-80 \times 10^9$/L other causes of thrombocytopenia must be reconsidered.[14] After delivery, they may be at higher risk for postpartum HELLP syndrome.[12]

ITP has an estimated incidence of 3–4/100,000 new cases per year, with female predominance and a median age at presentation of 37 years.[15,16] Consequently, a past or present history of ITP is frequently encountered in pregnancy (estimated to be 1–5 cases per 10,000 pregnancies).[17] Often, the mother has a history of ITP with or without a low platelet count, although first presentation of ITP or accidentally discovered ITP in pregnancy also occurs. During pregnancy, platelets decrease with a nadir in the third trimester.[18,19]

Antenatal treatment is given exclusively on maternal indication and aims to maintain the platelet count above 20×10^9/L or higher in case of bleeding symptoms, generally using corticosteroids as first-line treatment.[19,20] Intravenous immunoglobulin (IVIG) is often reserved as second-line treatment or used to prepare for delivery, and if necessary it is combined with platelet transfusions. A platelet count $>50 \times 10^9$/L is considered safe for delivery. Although British guidelines recommend a platelet count $>80 \times 10^9$/L for caesarian section (CS) and epidural anesthesia,[21] uncomplicated procedures have been reported with platelet counts of $50-75 \times 10^9$/L.[22,23] ITP is not associated with severe maternal bleeding during delivery and is not an indication for caesarean delivery.[24] Mode of delivery is based on obstetric indications, with avoidance of procedures associated with increased hemorrhagic risk to the fetus.[21] There is no demonstrated effect of maternal treatment with corticosteroids or IVIG on the fetal platelet count.[25–27] Perinatal mortality in ITP is estimated around 0.6%.[28] The risk for neonatal thrombocytopenia below 50×10^9/L ranges from 4.9% directly after birth to 38% in the first two weeks after birth.[28–30] Intracranial hemorrhage (ICH) or other severe bleeding is not increased in fetuses from a mother with ITP. In large series, ICH in the neonate is reported to be 0–1.5%.[19,20,31,32] Nevertheless, brain imaging after birth is recommended in case of platelet counts $<50 \times 10^9$/L (American Society of Hematology guidelines).[19] The nadir of the neonatal platelet count and the highest risk for bleeding is 4 (1–7) days after delivery.[17–19] Most studies reported only weak correlations between the fetal platelet count at birth and the maternal platelet counts, the presence of antibodies in the maternal serum, or a history of splenectomy.[19,20] Although in individual cases the risk for fetal thrombocytopenia below 50×10^9/L cannot be predicted from the maternal platelet count, women refractory to corticosteroids and splenectomy and who cannot maintain a platelet count above 30×10^9/L despite immunosuppressive treatment are at higher risk for bleeding and neonatal thrombocytopenia.[18,19,33] In asymptomatic women, severe fetal thrombocytopenia is rare and approaches the background rate of circa 1% in term newborns. In multigravidae, absence of thrombocytopenia in a previous child predicts in approximately 70% of the cases a similar good outcome in the next child.[29,34] Passive thrombocytopenia in the neonate can persist for months, without an obvious adverse effect of breastfeeding.[35]

HELLP syndrome belongs to the micro-angiopathic hemolytic anemias, also referred to as *thrombotic microangiopathic anemias* (TMAAs), which can complicate pregnancy and puerperium.[36,37] The peak incidence has a relationship with the weeks of gestation (Figure 43.1), but there is considerable overlap. HELLP occurs in 0.2–0.8% of pregnancies. In 70–80%, there is also preeclampsia.[38] Its peak incidence is at 36 weeks, although in one-third HELLP presents up to seven days after a normal delivery not complicated by preeclampsia and in 10% prior to the 27th week of gestation.[39] Typical symptoms are right-upper abdominal pain, nausea, and vomiting. HELLP is not associated with overt disseminated intravascular coagulation (DIC), although in 70% the antithrombin III (ATIII) level is found decreased, in contrast to thrombotic thrombocytopenic purpura (TTP) and hemolytic uremic syndrome (HUS).[40] Due to vasoconstriction in preeclampsia, severe bleeding rarely occurs. However, severe neglected HELLP, often due to delayed delivery, leads to DIC, pulmonary edema, acute renal failure, abruptio placentae, and liver hematoma. Maternal mortality is as high as 20%, and neonatal death ranges from 10% to 60% depending on intervention with elective preterm deliveries that reduce the risk of death to mother and fetus. Mild thrombocytopenia and schistocytes are found in 50% of the neonates and resolve

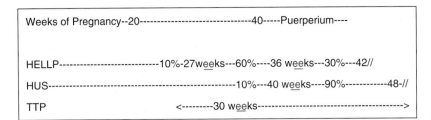

Figure 43.1 Pregnancy-associated microangiopathic thrombocytopenias.

without treatment or transfusions. Because termination of pregnancy is the definitive treatment, elective birth should be considered. Severe preeclampsia and HELLP will subsequently resolve 1–10 days after termination of pregnancy. The ranges of laboratory values that can be found in HELLP, collected by Sibai[36] in 442 cases, is shown in Table 43.2.

TTP and HUS

TTP and HUS share clinical features and may be difficult to distinguish from each other and other TMAAs. In many reports, the clinical difference described is the presence of acute renal failure, which is dominant in HUS and minimal or absent in TTP.

The time of onset of HUS is variable but affects mainly children and young adults.[21] Atypical HUS (aHUS), the most common form in pregnancy, typically presents from two days post delivery onward (mean 26 days), although in 5–10% antepartum HUS has been described. At presentation, 50% of females have thrombocytopenia below 100×10^9/L.[11] Atypical HUS is associated with complement dysregulation due to mutations in one or more complement genes;[21] in 6–10%, aHUS is due to acquired antibodies against complement factor H. Plasma exchange is often applied and can resolve anemia and thrombocytopenia, but almost half of the patients with aHUS experience persisting renal failure.

TTP results from an antibody-mediated reduction in the level of a von Willebrand factor (vWF) cleaving protease (ADAMTS13). TTP is most often seen in the second and third trimesters and requires treatment with plasma exchange similar as TTP in nonpregnant situations. TTP has no relationship with preeclampsia, and there is no need to terminate pregnancy. Patients with a history of TTP can have a relapse in pregnancy, but after stable remission pregnancy is not contraindicated, although close monitoring of the ADAMTS13 level is recommended.[41]

Early diagnosis of TTP and HUS is essential to start treatment, because most fatal events occur in the first few days. Plasma exchange is the most effective therapy for TTP and is also effective in patients with aHUS due to antibodies against factor H.[21,42] Based on laboratory results obtained afterward (ADAMTS13 <10% in TTP and low complement factors in aHUS), treatment can be adjusted. Eculizumab inhibiting the terminal complement pathway

may be useful in the treatment of aHUS.[43] Platelet transfusions for thrombocytopenia in TTP and HUS are only indicated in case of severe bleeding and not for prophylaxis in case of low platelet counts or intervention such as insertion of a central line. Delivery is—if possible—postponed until laboratory values are normalized.

DIC is seen in far advanced TMAA syndromes, but is predominantly caused by primary obstetric or septic pathology, such as abruptio placentae and severe intrauterine infection. 20–40% of obstetric patients with critical illness have symptoms of DIC. In pregnancy and puerperium, the use of a DIC score, based on decreased platelet count, increased D-dimers, decreased fibrinogen, and prolonged prothrombin time, is less reliable because D-dimers start to increase in first trimester and are always increased after the 35th week. Fibrin deposition in DIC not only contributes to multiple organ failure, but also, due to consumption coagulopathy with massive and ongoing activation of coagulation, results in depletion of platelets and coagulation factors with severe bleeding. Treatment aims to resolve the underlying condition. In cases of low platelet counts ($<50 \times 10^9$/L) and active bleeding, platelet transfusions are recommended, and plasma and fibrinogen (or cryoprecipitate) transfusions are indicated in case of persisting low fibrinogen and bleeding.[44]

Antiphospholipid antibody syndrome (APS) is an acquired condition of hypercoagulability, often associated with systemic lupus erythematosus (SLE). APS is characterized by arterial and venous thrombosis and gestational vascular complications leading to recurrent fetal loss, growth retardation, and prematurity. In patients with suspected clinical symptoms, antibodies against β2-GPI (Glycoprotein 1), anticardiolipin autoantibodies, and/or prolongation of plasma clotting time (lupus anticoagulant/LA) are present.[45] Based on randomized studies, women with recurrent abortion are treated with a combination of low dosages of aspirin and low-molecular-weight heparin.[31,45,46] There is no risk for fetal bleeding, but the mother has a slight increased risk for bleeding during delivery.

Inherited bleeding disorders

Pregnancy in women with hereditary thrombocytopenia carries a potential risk of bleeding for both mother and child. A retrospective survey conducted by a European Haematology Association (EHA) scientific working party identified that the prevalence (2–3/100,000 mainly Italian patients) of inherited thrombocytopenia is more common than hitherto assumed. They reported on 339 pregnancies with 13 different forms of inherited thrombocytopenia (50% with MYH9-related diseases). Surprisingly, there was no aggravation of thrombocytopenia or bleeding during pregnancy. The majority had a vaginal delivery, and 5% received platelets and/or red cells, which is higher than in the general population. A maternal history of bleeding events and severe thrombocytopenia was associated with delivery-related bleeding. None of the 156 children who inherited the disorder showed intrauterine bleeding, but the authors

Table 43.2 Laboratory values in 442 cases of HELLP

	Median	Range
Platelets 10^9/L	57	7–99
ALAT U/L	249	70–6193
LDH U/L	853	564–23.584
Bilirubin μmol/L//mg/dl	26//1.53	8.6–436//0.51–25.65
Creatinine μmol/L//mg/dl	97//1.10	53–1414//0.6–16.1
Urine acid μmol/L//mg/dl	462//7.7	174–900//2.9–15

Source: Sibai (1990).[36]

mentioned that such bleedings have been reported in the literature. Five newborns had petechiae, and two suffered a cerebral hemorrhage.[47] During pregnancy, required transfusions are thus limited; after delivery, blood transfusions may be unavoidable, and this can be problematic in cases where the patient is extensively immunized. Planned delivery and an individualized treatment plan are needed for these women. Such a policy also applies to woman with severe inherited platelet dysfunction such as Glanzmann thrombasthenia or Bernard Soulier syndrome, for which tranexamic acid with or without rVIIa is recommended.[48]

Woman with von Willebrand disease (vWD) are at increased risk for postpartum hemorrhage up to 6–20% and have an up to fivefold higher risk of needing transfusions.[49] As bleeding in vWD or more rare inherited coagulation factor deficiencies can persist or reappear up to two weeks or longer after delivery, substitution of postpartum replacement factors (desmopressin, vWF concentrates, or specific clotting factor concentrates) is recommended up to at least 3–5 days after delivery.[50]

Chronic maternal anemia

Physiological anemia is due to plasma volume expansion and is maximal around the 25th week of pregnancy. The WHO defines *anemia in pregnancy* as an Hb <6.8 mmol/L (11 g/dL), which is most often caused by nutritional deficiencies. Below an Hb of 5.5–6.2 mmol/L (9–10 g/dL), growth retardation and prematurity are reported, although it is not known whether this is related to the underlying disease or the lower Hb level itself.[51–53]

For chronic hemolytic diseases, such as thalassemia, hypertransfusion is applied to maintain Hb levels above 6.2 mmol/L (10 g/dl) in order to depress hemolysis of autologous red cells.[54] Patients with paroxysmal nocturnal hemoglobulinuria (PNH) not only are at increased risk for thrombosis requiring antithrombotic treatment but also can suffer a hemolytic crisis requiring transfusions in pregnancy. Randomized studies have only been performed in pregnant patients with sickle cell anemia disease (SCD) and showed that maintenance of a hematocrit above 33% with less than 35% sickle cells showed no better pregnancy outcome, although painful crises were significantly reduced.[55] Because patients with chronic hemolytic anemias are high antibody responders, they receive in well-resourced countries nowadays at least Rh- and Kel1-matched red blood cell transfusions. In poor-resourced countries, these patients receive less transfusions and the incidence of antibody formation is less well studied.

Assessment of amount of blood loss

Visual estimation is frequently used in routine practice to assess the amount of blood loss. This is, however, inaccurate, and health workers tend to underestimate blood loss considerably.

In a nicely researched experiment using pictorial guidelines to facilitate visual estimation (Figure 43.2), all professionals involved in obstetric care underestimated blood loss.[56] Compared to anesthetists, surgical nurses, and midwives, obstetricians tended to underestimate blood loss to a higher degree. The guidelines used in this study can be used as an effective tool to train health workers to improve their skills to estimate. The guidelines are available from http://www.bmfms.org.uk.

Other methods to estimate are the actual measurement of blood loss with a weighing scale or by measuring the peripartum Hb change. Measurement, however, has to be corrected because the amount of amniotic fluid is cumbersome. Peripartum Hb change has been shown to be unrelated to visually estimated blood loss.[57]

In other studies, the need for additional therapeutic uterotonic drugs or blood transfusion is taken as an indication of the amount of blood loss.[58] This is not relevant for clinical practice, but it is important for audit purposes.

Maternal transfusions

Prevention of postpartum hemorrhage can be achieved by active management of the third stage of labor.[58] Although active management consists of a package of the use of oxytocic drugs, early cord clamping, and active efforts to deliver the placenta, actual practices in different countries and even within countries use different packages, sometimes including selective radiological embolization of uterine vessels, and sometimes only consisting of prescribing oxytocic drugs.[59] Postpartum hemorrhage may occur in any laboring woman. Risk factors, however, will help the clinician anticipate the problem (Table 43.3). A recent study from Australia showed that the rates of obstetric blood product transfusion have increased from 1.2% in 2001 to 1.6% in 2010 across 891,914 pregnancies. Risk factors were women with bleeding or platelet disorders (relative risk [RR] in vaginal births, 7.8; 99% CI 6.9–8.7; RR after CS, 8.7; CI 7.7–9.7) and placenta previa (RR vaginally, 4.6; CI 3.4–6.3; and RR after CS, 5.7; CI 5.1–6.4). Operative vaginal deliveries had increased risk compared with nonoperative births (forceps RR, 2.8; CI 2.5–3.0; and vacuum RR, 1.9; CI 1.7–2.0). The increase was mainly true for red cells only, not for platelets or coagulation factors.[60]

Indications
Major obstetric bleeding

Preeclampsia, placental abruption, and amniotic fluid embolism are the most important obstetric disorders that may be accompanied by clotting problems. A woman with preeclampsia is already in a hypovolemic condition before hemorrhage starts, and this needs special attention. Urinary output is the best indicator of renal perfusion in a bleeding or preeclamptic woman and should be at least 30 ml/hour. Life-threatening massive bleedings after delivery result mostly from uterine atony, and, after conventional treatment with crystalloids, oxytocin, misoprostol, and prostaglandin, vascular embolization or surgical interventions and finally hysterectomy may follow to escape from death. Therefore, a standardized PPH management protocol must be in place for patients with active bleeding after more than 1–2 L blood loss aiming to reduce maternal morbidity and mortality.[61] This is in line with recent complex trauma protocols that advocate that when massive bleeding is anticipated, the patient should be transfused earlier without waiting for consumption and dilutional coagulopathies. Coagulation screens should be performed in case of active ongoing bleeding after 500 ml blood loss.[50] In case of uncontrollable excessive bleeding, prompt transfusions with an optimal ratio of RBC, plasma, platelets, tranexamic acid, and fibrinogen should be considered because it has been shown that hypofibrinogenemia develops early during major obstetric hemorrhage.[50,62–65] This has been shown to reduce total blood use and mortality in trauma.[66,67] Whether earlier administration of recombinant VIIa, currently mostly given as last ditch to prevent exsanguination, reduces hysterectomy is uncertain.[50,68] Control of bleeding and early transfusion and correction of coagulopathy must be carried out during the window of

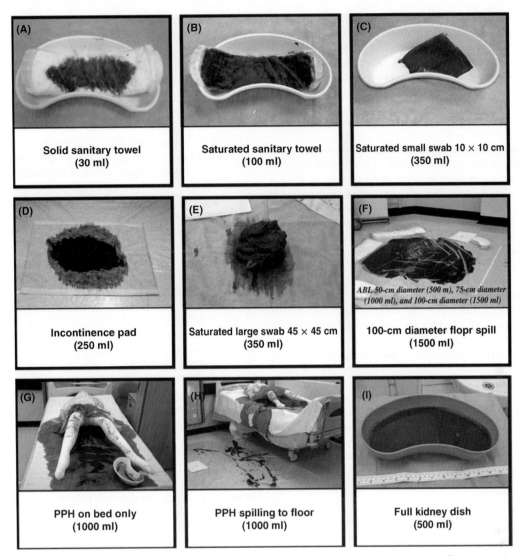

Figure 43.2 Pictorial guidelines to facilitate visual estimation of blood loss at obstetric hemorrhage. Source: Bose (2006).[56]

opportunity, which may be less than two hours, before the vicious circle initiated by hypothermia, acidosis, and irreversible coagulopathy leads to death.

Transfusion indications for postpartum anemia

As discussed, the blood loss is, however, difficult to estimate.[56] In a recent Swedish study, the incidence of PPH of more than 1000 ml was 4.6%, and in the Dutch study of Prick in the Netherlands it was 4.5%.[69,70]

Table 43.3 Risk factors for postpartum hemorrhage

- Overdistended uterus (multiple pregnancy, large fetus, and polyhydramnious)
- Prolonged labor
- Induction of augmentation of labor
- Postpartum hemorrhage in previous pregnancy
- Chorioamnionitis
- High parity
- Coagulation disorders (e.g., HELLP syndrome or placental abruption)

Although guidelines suggest a transfusion threshold at a hemoglobin concentration of 4–5 mmol/l (7.0–8.0 g/dL), lower concentrations above 3 mmol/L (5.0 g/dL) are usually well tolerated if isovolemia is maintained. In a study on healthy individuals, Weiskopf *et al.* found that acute isovolumetric reduction of hemoglobin concentration to 3.1 mmol/L (5.0 g/dl) does not appear to cause inadequate tissue oxygenation.[71] In healthy women with a postpartum median Hb level of 6.5 mmol/L(10.5 g/dl; range 7–15 g/dl), at three to six weeks after delivery no relationship between Hb level and the quality of life was observed.[72] A randomized study compared women 12–24 hours after PPH with a hemoglobin of 3–4.9 mmol/L (4.8–7.9 g/dL) who had not received ($n = 262$) or had received ($n = 259$) a median of two RBC units. Physical fatigue at three and seven days postpartum was only slightly better in the transfused group, but quality of life and physical complications up to six weeks after delivery showed no differences. In the non-intervention group, 33 women received RBC transfusions because of anemic symptoms.[73]

The results underscore that in case bleeding stopped, posthemorrhage transfusion is only required for symptomatic anemia.

There are limited data available on outcomes at Hb concentrations below 3.1 mmol/L (5.0 g/dL). Two retrospective studies on patients who declined blood transfusion, mostly Jehovah's Witnesses, found that morbidity and mortality rates were extremely high below this level,[74,75] but survival has in some cases been reported at Hb rates below 2.0 g/dl and even as low as 1.4 g/dl.[76,77]

Platelet transfusions during pregnancy and for delivery

During pregnancy, thrombocytopenias result from enhanced platelet phagocytosis in ITP or consumption in TMAAs, both disorders in which platelet transfusions are reserved for therapeutic and not for prevention of bleeding. Similarly, for patients with inherited thrombocytopenia, a restricted transfusion policy is in place to prevent alloimmunization. Whatever the cause of thrombocytopenia, most guidelines recommend a platelet count above 50×10^9/L for vaginal delivery. Below, a platelet count of 50×10^9/L a platelet transfusion can be considered, although in ITP also in case of lower platelet counts delivery is uneventful.[21,23] Local anesthesia is safe if the platelet count is above 100×10^9/L, but guidelines differ in their threshold for giving local anesthesia; most guidelines advise 50 or 80×10^9/L. Because of different pathophysiology and bleeding history, an individual treatment plan for every pregnant patient with thrombocytopenia is required.[78] Except in case of TTP posing a relative contraindication for platelet transfusions, platelet transfusions are not contraindicated in other TMAAs, nor in ITP or DIC. However, because platelet survival is shortened, other supportive treatments aimed to improve the cause of thrombocytopenia are required (see Chapter 21).

Blood products used and special precautions
Industrialized countries

Red cell transfusions

Pregnancy and transfusions both stimulate irregular red cell antibody formation. A survey of the transfused population in Western countries shows that women have 3–4 times more irregular antibodies than males and children.[79,80] In Western countries, females are routinely screened early in pregnancy to identify RhD negativity and irregular antibodies as a potential cause for hemolytic disease of the newborn (HDN) or for the availability of blood in case an indication for maternal transfusion should arise. In particular, antibodies against Rhc and Kel1 can cause hemolytic disease of the newborn (HDN) as severe as RhD HDN.[81] In cases of HDN due to Rhc/Kel1, in more than 40% of the cases the women had received prior transfusions.[82] Transfusions of Rhesus and Kel1-compatible donors to females prior or during fertile life can reduce non-RhD HDN. Most national guidelines have already implemented the use of Kel1-negative (often also Rhc-compatible) donors for woman up to the age of 45–50 years.

Platelet transfusions

Platelet transfusions can contain minimal contamination with erythrocytes, sufficient to immunize against the RhD antigen. If RhD$^+$ platelets are given to RhD^{neg} females before or during the fertile age, RhD prophylaxis with 375 IU anti-D is indicated.[83]

With increasing numbers of pregnancies, females produce leukocyte (HLA) antibodies against paternal antigens, which may impair recovery of platelet transfusions from random donors.[84,85] HLA antibodies must be excluded if it is expected that platelet transfusions are required for delivery. Because pregnancy stimulates immune anti-A and anti-B antibodies major ABO-incompatible platelet transfusions may also show reduced recovery.[86]

Immunoglobulin

High-dose intravenously administered immunoglobulin preparations are used during pregnancy for immunomodulatory purposes for increasing the maternal platelet count in ITP and to reduce severe fetal bleeding in fetal or neonatal thrombocytopenia (FNAIT). To prevent RhD HDN, RhD-negative woman are given intramuscular anti-D IgG between the 28th and 34th week of gestation, and preferentially within 72 hours after delivery of an RhD+ child.[87] This reduces RhD HDN to less than 1% of RhD-negative women. In recent years in several countries, noninvasive fetal D typing in maternal plasma determines the fetal blood type. Also, typing for C, c, E, and Kel1 (and even for HPA-1a) is possible. In case the fetus is D-negative, the pregnant woman will not receive the treatment unnecessarily.[88] Nevertheless, RhD HDN is still the most frequent and severe HDN. The residual immunization is due to medical, laboratory, and clerical errors, or anti-D is given in a too-low dose after larger fetomaternal hemorrhages during delivery or after trauma and obstetrical interventions.[89,90]

Special safety aspects of transfusion products

Besides enhanced induction of alloantibodies, blood products can transmit CMV and parvo-B19 V infections that may harm the fetus. During pregnancy for seronegative women, cellular blood products are selected to reduce cytomegalovirus (CMV) transmission. In some countries also, parvovirus B19 (parvo-B19V)-safe blood is administered. Leucocyte removal by filtration of cellular blood products virtually abolishes CMV transmission. Pooled plasma products (e.g., IVIG) must by regulation contain less than 10^4 parvo-B19 V copies, a load that is neutralized by antibodies present in the product, but this does not protect against parvo-B19 V in individual cellular products. In order to avoid graft-versus-host (GVH) reaction in the fetus, blood products must be irradiated with 25 Gy shortly prior to transfusion.

Low-income countries

In low-income countries, blood transfusion services are still deficient and generally not able to deliver the needed amount of units to save the life of women with massive obstetric blood loss. Bates *et al.* searched the literature for studies with a focus on "near misses" due to obstetric hemorrhage. They found that at least one-quarter of all maternal deaths could be prevented by rapid access to blood transfusion.[91] In many places, blood donation at the spot by relatives after the adverse event had taken place is the only available option. Transmission of hepatitis and HIV is a serious risk. Transfusion or injection of unsafe blood is responsible for 8–16 million hepatitis B, 2.3–4.7 million hepatitis C, and 80,000–160,000 HIV infections annually.[92] It is estimated that about 80% of the world's population has access to only 20% of the world's blood supply.[93]

In Tanzania, for instance, a National Blood Transfusion Service has been developed in response to a serious train crash in 2002 and the HIV epidemic. In 2006, voluntary nonremunerated donors have donated 67,000 units of blood. These have been proven to be safer donors than relatives.[94] However, these numbers are not sufficient, and patients will remain dependent on relatives as important sources for blood.[95] Improvement of a system of repeat replacement donors is feasible and is worth giving more attention to avoid first-time relatives who have high rates of hepatitis and HIV infections.[92]

Because anemia resulting from malaria, iron and folic acid deficiency, sickle cell disease, and infectious disease is rampant in low-income countries, a relatively small amount of blood loss is often disastrous. This is the reason why WHO defines *postpartum hemorrhage* as a bleed of >500 ml, whereas in many industrialized countries the threshold is >1000 ml.

Anemia should thus rigorously be treated during pregnancy in order to reduce the consequences of postpartum hemorrhage.[96] The use of bednets, nutritional supplements, antihelmintics, presumptive treatment of malaria, folic acid, and ferrous medication during antenatal care and active management of the third stage of labor will all help women to overcome the problems created by hemorrhage during childbirth. These strategies may reduce the need for blood transfusion. This is important as one should realize that unnecessary blood transfusion in a setting with limited resources is, firstly, a waste and, secondly, will increase exposure to transfusion-related risks and infections.[93]

A paper from Nigeria reports a blood transfusion rate of 25.2% during CS, a high rate that indicates the risk of surgery in low-resource settings.[97] A strategy that will safely reduce the number of caesarean sections will also reduce the need for blood transfusion.

Fetal transfusions

In this section, we will discuss aspects of fetal transfusion focusing on red cell immunization and the management of fetal and neonatal (alloimmune) thrombocytopenia.

Alloimmune hemolytic disease

The first fetal transfusion for hemolytic disease of the fetus was performed in 1963 by Liley.[98] After amniography and fetography, red cells were transfused under X-ray guidance in the intraperitoneal cavity of the fetus. This method of treatment of fetal anemia is based on the fact that red cells are absorbed from the peritoneal cavity and enter the circulation. Limitations of this technique include less uptake of the red cells in case of severe fetal hydrops. Reported survival rates at the time were approximately 50%.[99]

The advent of real-time ultrasound ushered a complete new era in the prenatal management of the fetus. Since the 1980s, all fetal transfusions are performed under real-time ultrasound-guided puncture, preferentially of the umbilical vein.[100] In recent decades, intravascular transfusions have been performed in thousands of pregnancies worldwide. Although randomized trials comparing intraperitoneal versus intravascular transfusions have not been performed, results of this latter technique, which is feasible from 16 weeks onward, are widely considered as superior.

Fetal blood sampling (FBS) is indicated when fetal anemia is suspected by Doppler velocity measurements of the fetal (medial cerebral artery) vessels[101] or in case of hydrops. The most frequent indication for fetal blood transfusion is anemia caused by red cell alloimmunization of the mother (see Chapter 45). Other indications for fetal blood transfusion include human parvovirus B19 infection,[102,103] severe fetomaternal hemorrhage,[104] placental chorioangiomas,[105] and homozygous α-thalassemia.[106]

FBS is also applied for the management of other conditions such as thrombocytopenia or severe tachyarrhythmia of the unborn.

The technique

The principle of fetal transfusion is to get access to the circulation with a 20–22 gauge needle, aspirate blood for diagnosis, and deliver red cells, platelets, or drugs in the fetal circulation. The most frequent used site of transfusion is the umbilical vein when the placenta is inserted anteriorly. The umbilical vein is preferred for several reasons. Firstly, the vein has a larger diameter than the arteries. Secondly, due to the eccentric location of the vein in the cord, an overshoot or slip of the needle does not in general lead to a hematoma in the Wharton's jelly but to a leakage in the amniotic cavity. A puncture in the artery may lead to leakage in the Wharton's jelly, inducing spasm of the artery and subsequent fetal bradycardia. Thirdly, fetal transfusion in the vein allows the operating team to monitor the flow of the transfused blood sonographically during the procedure. In some centers, an intravascular transfusion is combined with an intraperitoneal approach. When the umbilical vein at the placental insertion cannot be reached safely, the fetus is punctured in the intrahepatic vein.

Premedication to the mother is used for relief of maternal anxiety and sedation of the fetus. Routine intravenous or intramuscular administration of muscle relaxants such as atracurium or pancuronium is advocated to achieve fetal paralysis and thus prevent needle displacement due to fetal movements.[107]

Donor blood, volume, and rate of transfusion

The blood used is leukocyte reduced by filtration, irradiated, and mostly O RhD-negative and compatible with any maternal antibodies that are present. Because intrauterine transfusions easily stimulate new additional antibodies against fetal or donor red blood cell antigens, a cross-match with a freshly derived maternal blood sample should be carried out before every subsequent transfusion.[108]

The product should not carry the risk of transmitting CMV and preferentially not Parvo B19V, and it should not cause graft-versus-host disease. To have optimal survival profit, the red cells are stored as briefly as possible, and prior to transfusion supernatant solutions containing potassium, ABO antibodies, and red cell preservation solution are often removed and replaced by saline. An 80% packed red cell concentrate in 0.9% saline, irradiated with 25 Gy just prior to transfusion, can correct extreme low Hb values.

After access to the fetal circulation, 1–2 ml blood is aspirated and promptly examined for hemoglobin, hematocrit, and mean corpuscular volume. The volume of blood transfused is calculated by using a formula in which the pretransfusion fetal hematocrit, estimated fetal placental blood volume, and hematocrit of the donor blood are included.[109] The blood is transfused at a rate of 5 to 10 ml per minute.[109] During transfusion, the blood flow and the fetal heart rate are monitored by ultrasound and Doppler. The second transfusion is given 1–2 weeks after the first, and thereafter the fetal erythropoiesis is depressed and the fetus is completely dependent on transfusions every 3–4 weeks. However, at the end of treatment, more than 70% of women with HDN requiring intrauterine transfusions have multiple erythrocyte antibodies.[108] Selection of donors compatible with the mother for clinical relevant antigens could reduce this alloimmunization, although in more than half of the cases additional antibody formation cannot be circumvented as they are evoked by fetal red cells.[108]

Outcome of treatment

After birth, exchange transfusions or top-up transfusions may be required. Two randomized controlled trials showed no benefit of IVIG to the neonate in reducing the needs for exchange transfusion.[110,111]

At Leiden University Medical Centre, treatment of 593 ultrasound-guided intravascular transfusions, given between 17 and 35 gestational weeks, have been performed in 210 fetuses between 1988 and 1999, and they resulted in an overall survival rate of 86%.[81] In the period from 1999 to 2009, the survival rate improved to 98%.[112] Although there was a reduction of procedure-related complications, the main improvement in survival rate is due to a lower number of cases presenting with severe irreversible hydrops after implementation of routine screening for red cell antibodies early in pregnancy in 1997.[81]

A follow-up study of 291 infants treated with intrauterine transfusion at a median age of 8 years showed neurodevelopmental impairment in 4.8%, which is not statistically significant different from the general population. Hydrops, associated with the deepest intrauterine anemia, and prematurity were identified as risk factors.[113]

Fetal or neonatal alloimmune thrombocytopenia

In 0.3% of the newborns, thrombocytopenia with an immunological origin, such as fetal or neonatal alloimmune thrombocytopenia (FNAIT) or ITP, is encountered as a major cause of isolated severe thrombocytopenia with an incidence of circa 1:1000 live births.[114,115] Another cause of fetal thrombocytopenia is red blood cell alloimmunization, observed in 10–30% of severely hydropic fetuses.[116] Presumably, the mechanism causing thrombocytopenia is the increased erythropoiesis inhibiting myelo- and thrombopoiesis. Early after birth, almost 20% of (near-)term infants with perinatal asphyxia develop platelet levels below 50×10^9/L.[117]

Because except in NAITP severe in utero (intracerebral) bleeding is not documented in these conditions,[19,20,24,31] intrauterine platelet transfusions are not indicated as the risk of complications of the procedure exceeds the risk of bleeding during parturition.

In contrast, the risk for ICH in fetal/neonatal alloimmune thrombocytopenia (FNAIT) is estimated around 20% and can occur as early as in the 20th week of gestation.[118] In Caucasians, 2% of the pregnant women are negative for HPA-1a, and anti-HPA-1a antibodies are responsible for the majority (85%) of cases of FNAIT.[119] About 5–25% of FNAIT is caused by other anti-HPA antibodies, most frequently anti-HPA-5b, anti-HPA-3a, and anti-HPA-15.[120] In Asians, HPA-4b is more often implicated.[121] In 15–20% of FNAIT cases, no antibodies can be detected. Antibodies against private antigens and new antigens causing FNAIT are still discovered.[121] In platelet-alloimmunized pregnant women carrying a fetus positive for the offending antigen, the risk for thrombocytopenia can be as high as 85%. The incidence of ICH varies from 7% (in case of a sibling without ICH) to 80% (in pregnant women and a sibling with ICH).[122] It is assumed that the majority of ICH occurs antenatally between 30 and 35 weeks of gestation.

For antenatal management, it is important to know whether the father is homozygous or heterozygous for the offending antigen. In case of heterozygosity of the father, it is indicated to perform genotyping of the fetus. Although genotyping is possible by using polymerase chain reaction (PCR) on either chorionic villi or amniocytes (amniocentesis in the second trimester is preferable because of its lower risk of boosting antibodies), nowadays in several countries it is possible to assess the fetal HPA type on fetal DNA in maternal plasma. When the fetus is positive for the offending antigen, the pregnancy should be managed in or in collaboration with a specialized fetal center.

As HPA screening is not routine, FNAIT is mostly only recognized after an affected sibling. The antenatal management protocols in a subsequent pregnancy with FNAIT aim to prevent ICH. Unfortunately, monitoring anti-HPA antibodies by titration and quantification is still controversial, despite more recent studies

indicating that it is helpful in predicting the severity of fetal thrombocytopenia.[123–125] In order to diagnose fetal thrombocytopenia, FBS beginning as early as 20 weeks would be required.[126,127] Although FBS is a reliable tool for direct monitoring of the fetal thrombocytopenia, the cumulative procedure-related risk for fetal loss is high and approximates 6% per pregnancy.[128,129] The cumulative risk for emergency delivery due to FBS is 13–17%.[130,131] Currently, most centers have adopted noninvasive strategies and, in case of HPA antibodies or a previous sibling with FNAIT, blindly start weekly high-dose maternal IVIG. Some centers add corticosteroids as first-line treatment or toward delivery. Although the effect of IVIG is undoubted,[130,131] combinations with corticosteroids are more variable. Bussel et al. were the first who reported in 1988 that weekly maternal IVIG (1.0 g/kg maternal weight) was effective at elevating the fetal platelet count, since this is used as the standard dose.[132] Not all fetuses show a substantial increase in platelet count with this treatment, and the reported response rate in the literature varies between 30% and 85%. Even in nonresponders to IVIg with a sustained low platelet count, maternal IVIG reduced the risk of ICH,[131,133,134] possibly by downregulation of endothelial activation by platelet antibodies that cross-react with endothelial epithelial cells.[135]

There has been a gradual change in antenatal treatment of FNAIT pregnancies, from an invasive approach with repetitive FBS to a less invasive approach (FBS prior to IVIG and platelet transfusions before delivery) to a completely noninvasive approach (IVIG only). At Leiden University Medical Centre, treatment of 22 pregnancies (22 neonates; 2 with and 20 without a sibling with ICH) resulted in live births without ICH in all neonates, except in one case where an ICH was detected at 27 weeks just before starting the treatment.[134,136] Long-term follow-up of the infants, treated antenatally with IVIG, showed no adverse effects.[136,137]

The mechanism of action of IVIG in FNAIT is still unclear. There are several possible mechanisms that may synergize. Firstly, in the maternal circulation, the IVIG causes enhanced catabolism of the high level of IgG and will dilute the anti-HPA antibodies, resulting in a lower proportion of anti-HPA antibodies among the IgG transferred via the Fc-receptors (Fc-Rs) in the placenta. Secondly, in the placenta, IVIG may block the placenta receptor (Fc-R) and decrease the placental transmission of maternal antibodies, including anti-HPA-antibodies. Thirdly, in the fetus, IVIG may block the Fc-Rs on the macrophages and prohibit the destruction of antibody-covered platelets. At last, IVIG may downregulate maternal B cells producing anti-HPA. Ni et al. presented a murine model of FNAIT, measuring response to IVIG therapy. This model demonstrates that maternal IVIG administration has multiple effects on the amelioration of FNAIT, including decreased maternal antiplatelet antibody, decreased fetal platelet clearance, reduced bleeding, and increased fetal survival.[138]

Cost-effectiveness analysis performed by Thung et al., comparing noninvasive empiric intravenous immunoglobulin with FBS-guided treatment, concluded that noninvasive IVIG is a cost-effective strategy.[139]

In other developed countries, frequent ultrasounds in high-risk pregnancies and a preterm planned CS are performed to prevent ICH, and washed maternal platelets or HPA1a-negative platelets can be administered in case of neonatal thrombocytopenia.[140,141]

In low-income countries, very little information exists about fetal thrombocytopenia. This is because of either lack of tools of appropriate diagnosis or, presumably, less severe manifestation of the disease due to non-HPA1a antibodies.

Fetal transfusions for other indications

Parvovirus B19 infection during pregnancy may lead to an arrest in maturation of hematopoetic stem cells and thus anemia and thrombocytopenia. Parvo B19V is a frequent cause of nonimmune hydrops fetalis, and 46% of hydropic fetuses have thrombocytopenia below 50×10^9/L. The platelet count will further decrease after transfusion of red blood cells.[142] After confirmation of diagnosis of infection of the mother and elevated middle cerebral artery peak velocity at Doppler investigation, intrauterine transfusion is indicated. Usually, one intrauterine red blood cell transfusion is sufficient.[103]

Massive fetomaternal (transplacental) hemorrhage is a rare, unexpected, and serious complication in pregnancy resulting in severe fetal anemia, hydrops, and death. Reduced fetal movement is the only recognizable sign for the pregnant woman. The diagnosis can be confirmed when a sinusoidal pattern is observed at cardiotocogram registration and/or an increased flow in the middle cerebral artery is measured.[143] Fetal red cells in the maternal circulation can be confirmed with the Kleihauer–Betke test.[139] In the preterm period, fetal red cell transfusion is a realistic option.

After the introduction of laser coagulation of placental anastomosis as treatment for severe twin-to-twin transfusion syndrome (TTTS), TAPS (twin anemia–polycythemia sequence) is described as a new syndrome.[144] After laser coagulation, very small residual anastomosis may lead to chronic anemia and polycythemia in one of the twins.[145] Robyr *et al.* described 13 cases of TAPS (13% of their group of TTTS cases).[146] In 12 of the 13 cases, 1–5 fetal red cell transfusions was performed. Slaghekke described that, when the Solomon laser technique was used, the incidence of TAPS decreased from 16% to 3%.[147]

Because expectant management can also lead to a favorable outcome, further research in this field is needed. Very rare indications for fetal transfusions are placental chorioangioma and alpha-thalassemia.

Conclusion

Postpartum hemorrhage is a serious risk factor in obstetrics. Protocols for both prevention and management should be available in all labor and delivery wards. In industrialized countries, most maternal mortality can be prevented using oxytocics, embolization of uterine vessels, and blood transfusion. Unfortunately, both control of bleeding and early transfusion cannot be achieved in most low-income countries. In these countries, blood transfusion services are generally deficient to help women in need for red cells. Blood donation at the spot is often the only available option. This fact does bear a serious risk for transmission of infections such as hepatitis and HIV. The option of fetal transfusion, a widely used treatment of the unborn in the industrialized world, is not available for all in low-income countries.

Acknowledgement

We are grateful to Mrs. Ivanka Bekker for expert secretarial assistance in the preparation of this chapter.

Key References

A full reference list for this chapter is available at: http://www.wiley.com/go/simon/transfusion

1 Carrolli G, Cuesta C, Abalos E, Gulmezoglu AM. Epidemiology of postpartum haemorrhage: a systematic review. *Best Pract Res Clin Obstet Gynaecol* 2008;**22**:999–1012.

2 Ronsmans C, Graham WJ. Maternal mortality: who, when, where, and why. *Lancet* 2006;**368**:1189–200.

6 Zwart JJ, Richters JM, Ory F, Bloemenkamp KWM, De Vries JIP, Van Roosmalen J. Severe maternal morbidity during pregnancy, delivery and puerperium in the Netherlands: a nationwide population-based study of 371 000 pregnancies. *BJOG* 2008;**115**:842–50.

27 Rayment R, Brunskill SJ, Soothill PW, Roberts DJ, Bussel JB, Murphy MF. Antenatal interventions for fetomaternal alloimmune thrombocytopenia. *Cochrane Database Syst Rev* 2011;**5**:CD004226.

31 Neunert C, Lim W, Crowther M, Cohen A, Solberg Jr. L, Crowther MA, American Society of Hematology. The American Society of Hematology 2011 evidence-based practice guideline for immune thrombocytopenia. *Blood* 2011;**117**:4190–207.

38 Abildgaard U, Heimdal. Pathogenesis of the syndrome of hemolysis, elevated liver enzymes, and low platelet count (HELLP): a review. *Eur J Obstet Gynecol Reprod Biol* 2013 Feb;**166** (2):117–23.

47 Noris P, Schlegel N, Kiersy C, *et al.* Analysis of 339 pregnancies in 181 women with 13 different forms of inherited thrombocytopenia. *Haematologica* 2014;**99**: 1387–95.

61 Shields LE, Wiesner S, Fulton J, Pelletreau B. Comprehensive maternal hemorrhage protocols reduce the use of blood products and improve patient safety. *Am J Obstet Gynecol* 2015 Mar;**212** (3):272–80.

88 Daniels, G, Finning K, Martin P. Noninvasive fetal blood grouping: present and future. *Clin Lab Med* 2010 Jun;**30**:431–2.

91 Bates I, Chapotera GK, McKew S, van den Broek N. Maternal mortality in sub-Saharan Africa: the contribution of ineffective blood transfusion services. *BJOG* 2008;**115**:1331–9.

CHAPTER 44

Fetal and neonatal hematopoiesis

Robert D. Christensen[1] & Martha C. Sola-Visner[2,3]

[1]Division of Neonatology, University of Utah School of Medicine, Salt Lake City, UT, USA
[2]Division of Newborn Medicine, Children's Hospital Boston, Boston, MA, USA
[3]Harvard Medical School, Harvard University, Boston, MA, USA

Hematopoiesis is the process of creating the cellular elements of blood. In adults, the primary purpose of the hematopoietic system is to produce sufficient hemic cells to balance hemic cellular losses. In the fetus, three unique hematopoietic needs are also present: (1) The marked and constant somatic growth rate of the fetus generates a need to constantly increase the blood volume, (2) the relatively low oxygen tensions but high metabolic rates of fetal tissues require a system of oxygen delivery fundamentally different from that in adults, and (3) the typically sterile intra-amniotic environment results in less need, compared with adults, for antimicrobial systems, yet the fetal hematopoietic system must generate a fully operational antimicrobial phagocytic system for immediate use following birth (Table 44.1).

The CBC (complete blood cell count) is one of the most commonly performed laboratory tests in ill neonates. Efforts to better understand developmental hematopoiesis can inform clinical neonatology by enhancing appreciation of the capacities and inherent limitations of the granulocytopoietic, erythropoietic, and thrombopoietic systems of prematurely delivered and term neonates. Cytopenias are common in neonatal intensive care units (NICUs). Depending on the definitions used for each cytopenia, neutropenia typically occurs in 5% to 8% of patients in NICUs, regardless of gestational age;[1] thrombocytopenia in 25% to 30%;[2] and anemia in perhaps as many as 50%.[3] The prevalence of each cytopenia is higher among those delivered at the earliest gestational ages. Transfusion is the principal means of managing severe cytopenias among neonates, but alternatives are emerging.

Developmental hematopoiesis can be viewed as occurring in three anatomic stages—mesoblastic, hepatic, and myeloid. Mesoblastic hematopoiesis occurs in extraembryonic structures, principally the yolk sac, and begins between the 16th and 19th days of gestation. By about six weeks of gestation, the extraembryonic sites of hematopoiesis begin to ablate and hepatic hematopoiesis is initiated. By the 10th to 12th weeks, mesoblastic hematopoiesis ceases, and a small amount of hematopoiesis is evident in the bone marrow. In humans, it seems that the clavicle is the first bone to develop a marrow cavity.[4] The first cells present in the developing marrow space have macrophage surface markers and phenotypes. These are followed by myeloperoxidase-positive cells with the characteristics of neutrophils. However, the liver remains the predominant hematopoietic organ until the last trimester of pregnancy.

The anatomic site of hematopoiesis does not simply transfer from yolk sac to the liver to the bone marrow.[5] Rather, each organ subsequently houses distinct hematopoietic populations. For example, at 18 to 20 weeks of gestation, more than 85% of the cells in the fetal liver are erythroid, and few neutrophils are present. At the same time, fewer than 40% of the cells within the bone marrow are erythroid, and most are neutrophils. The mechanisms responsible for the changing anatomic sites of hematopoiesis and for the differences in hemic cells produced in the mesoblastic, hepatic, and myeloid sites have not been determined. Regardless of gestational age or anatomic location, production of all hematopoietic tissues begins with pluripotent cells capable of self-renewal and clonal maturation into all blood cell lineages. Progenitor cells differentiate under the influence of hematopoietic growth factors, which include those listed in Table 44.2.

Granulocytopoiesis

Sites of neutrophil production in the fetus

The human yolk sac contains no neutrophils. Its hematopoietic activity is limited to erythropoiesis and production of a small number of macrophages.[5] Similarly, the human fetal liver produces few, if any, neutrophils. The few neutrophils found in photomicrographic sections of human fetal liver are not arranged in clusters of hematopoietic nests but are widely separated and found surrounding the blood vessels, as if they were carried in by the circulation, not produced in the organ. Moreover, the spleen is not a granulocytopoietic organ in human fetuses like it is in fetal rodents.[6] No granulocytopoietic nests are found in human fetal spleen, and the neutrophils within it are mostly mature and evenly dispersed. This finding suggests they were carried there in the blood, not produced locally.

Where, then, do neutrophils originate in the human fetus? The first neutrophils are present approximately five weeks after conception and are clustered in the periaortic tissue. These first fetal neutrophils contain myeloperoxidase, and they mature into cells with band and segmented nuclei, but beyond these features, any differences or similarities between them and the neutrophils of adults have not been reported.[7] The function of these cells in the fetus and the explanation for this location of origin are unclear. The fetal bone marrow space begins to develop approximately eight

Rossi's Principles of Transfusion Medicine, Fifth Edition. Edited by Toby L. Simon, Jeffrey McCullough, Edward L. Snyder, Bjarte G. Solheim, and Ronald G. Strauss.

Table 44.1 Inherent differences in hematopoietic systems of the fetus, neonate, and adult

Fetus

Exists in a sterile environment. Until near term, does not generally need an antibacterial defense system.

Must produce a functional neutrophil reserve in preparation for extrauterine life.

Fetal hematocrit and blood platelet concentration increase from 20 weeks to term, whereas blood volume increases approximately 10-fold. Thus, erythrocyte and platelet production must be extremely rapid during this period to keep pace with the rapid expansion of blood volume. In the case of platelets, this process is aided by a longer survival of fetal/neonatal compared to adult platelets.

Neonate

At birth, the fetus moves from a sterile into a nonsterile environment and must have a fully operational neutrophil system to survive in this environment.

At birth, oxygen delivery to tissues markedly increases, as PaO_2 increases from 27 to >90 mm Hg. This effectively shuts off erythropoietin production. Consequently, erythropoiesis temporarily ceases, resulting in the physiologic anemia of infancy.

Rapid growth and blood volume expansion continue. However, platelet concentration does not change, and platelet lifespan is longer in neonates compared to adults.

Adult

The rapid somatic growth and blood volume expansion of infancy and childhood cease. Thus, the previous need to accelerate hematopoiesis to keep pace with somatic growth ends.

The neutrophil system must continue to be responsive to rapid increases in demand for cells.

Blood platelet concentration and hematocrit remain relatively constant throughout healthy life.

---

weeks after conception (Figures 44.1 and 44.2). The space is lined by osteoclast-like cells with cell-surface characteristics of macrophages. These cells appear to core out the space from the primitive cartilage. Eight to ten weeks after conception, the bone marrow space progressively enlarges, but no neutrophils are present within the space until 10.5 to 11 weeks[4] (Figure 44.3). The first neutrophils in the marrow do not have band or segmented nuclei, but they contain myeloperoxidase and express the cell surface characteristics of myeloblasts and promyelocytes. From 14 weeks to term, the most common cell type in the fetal bone marrow space is the neutrophil, although the marrow space is not nearly so densely packed with cells as it becomes in older children and adults.[4,7]

Macrophages are crucial to fetal morphogenesis because they aid in shaping organs and scavenging debris and apoptotic cells. Although neutrophils and macrophages have a common progenitor cell, the discordant temporal appearance of neutrophils and macrophages in the fetus and the divergence of their anatomic locations are striking.[8] Recent observations have cast doubt on long-held theories about the origins of macrophages in the human fetus. For example, it was believed that macrophages originate from precursor cells in the bone marrow and mature through a progression of cell types from monoblast to promonocyte to monocyte, which then migrate to various tissues and differentiate into macrophages. Observations of human fetuses do not support this origin of macrophages. Firstly, macrophages appear in the yolk sac, liver, lung, and brain long before the bone marrow cavity has been formed. Secondly, promonocytes and monocytes are absent in the yolk sac and liver, but macrophages are present there nevertheless. Thus, the macrophages in the yolk sac may develop directly from stem cells without passing through a monocyte stage. It is not clear whether these primitive macrophages migrate from the yolk sac to populate the lungs, liver, brain, and other organs.[9]

Regulation of neutrophil production

The mechanisms that regulate neutrophil production during human fetal development are not clear. Granulocyte colony-

Table 44.2 Hematopoietic growth factors

Growth Factors	Molecular Mass (kd)	Chromosomal Location	Principal Target Cell
Erythropoietin	30.4	7q11–22	CFU-E, fetal BFU-E
Colony-stimulating factors			
G-CSF	18.8	17q11.2–21	CFU-G
GM-CSF	14.4	5q23–31	All CFC
M-CSF	26 (dimer)	1p13–21	CFU-M
SCF	15–20 (dimer)	12q2–24	Primitive CFC
Interleukins			
IL1α	17	2q13	Primitive CFC, hepatocyte, macrophage
IL1β	17	2q13	Primitive CFC, hepatocyte, macrophage
IL2	15–20	4q26–27	T cell
IL3	14–15	5q23–31	All CFC
IL4	16–20	5q23–31	T cell, B cell
IL5	13.2 (dimer)	5q23–31	CFO-EOS
IL6	20.8	7p21–24	Primitive CFC
IL7	25	8q12–13	B cell
IL8	8–10	4	Neutrophil, endothelial cell
IL9	16	5q31–32	BFU-E, primitive CFC
IL10	23	1	Macrophage, lymphocyte
IL11	22	19q13	Primitive CFC, BFU-MK, CFU-MK
IL12	70–75		T cell, NK cell, macrophage
Thrombopoietin	35	3q26–28	BFU-MK, CFU-MK

BFU-E, primitive erythroid progenitor; BFU-MK, primitive megakaryocyte progenitor; CFC, colony-forming cells; CFO-EOS, eosinophil colony-forming unit; CFU-G, granulocyte colony forming unit; CFU-MK, mature megakaryocyte progenitor; G-CSF, granulocyte colony-stimulating factor; GM-CSF, granulocyte-macrophage colony-stimulating factor; IL, interleukin; M-CSF, macrophage colony-stimulating factor; NK, natural killer; SCF, stem cell factor.

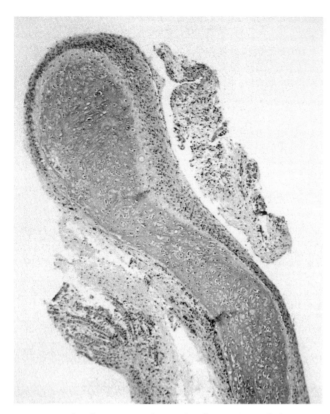

Figure 44.1 Clavicle approximately 7 weeks after conception, before any marrow space is present. In the human fetus, the first bone to contain a developing marrow space is the clavicle, followed closely by the other long bones. (Hematoxylin and eosin stain; original magnification, ×100.)

stimulating factor (G-CSF) and macrophage colony-stimulating factor (M-CSF) are present in the developing fetal bone as early as six weeks after conception and in the fetal liver as early as eight weeks.[10] Cells that generate granulocyte macrophage colony-stimulating factor (GM-CSF) are widely distributed in fetal tissues, including pulmonary epithelium. Stem cell factor messenger RNA (mRNA) is present in the yolk sac, liver, and bone marrow at the earliest stages of their respective development.[5] The specific signal (s) inducing neutrophil production in the fetus are not known. Similarly, the precise signals that initiate the production of macrophages in the embryo and fetus are not known.

It is curious that the actions of G-CSF, M-CSF, GM-CSF, erythropoietin, thrombopoietin (TPO), and stem cell factor are not limited to hematopoiesis in the fetus and neonate. Receptors for all of these factors are located in distinct areas of the fetal central nervous system and gastrointestinal tract, where their patterns of expression change with development. Important undefined developmental roles clearly exist for these factors that are beyond those known for hematopoiesis. Although not fully characterized, these roles appear to predominantly be anti-apoptotic, perhaps providing some degree of protection during adverse conditions such as hypoxemia or acidosis. Better definition of the physiological non-hematopoietic roles of these factors during human development is needed, to inform investigators, as well as clinicians testing the administration of these factors in the NICU, about potential unwanted and unplanned effects.

Although neutrophil production in the bone marrow space clearly is present by 14 weeks of gestation, the blood of the fetus,

even through 20 weeks, contains few neutrophils. Forestier *et al.* reported that fetuses at 20 weeks of gestation had a mean absolute blood neutrophil concentration of only 190/μl, a range of 0 to 490/μl, and a mode concentration of zero.[11] Despite the near absence of circulating neutrophils in the first trimester, and the relative scarcity (by adult standards) of neutrophils in the second trimester, progenitor cells with the capacity to generate neutrophils in vitro (CFU-GM) are abundant in the early human fetal liver, bone marrow, and blood.[12–17] In rodents, the number of CFU-GM per gram of body weight is far fewer in animals delivered prematurely than in those delivered at term and is lower in term animals than in adults. The quantity of neutrophilic progenitor cells per gram of body weight in the developing human fetus has not been reported.[18] Thus it is not clear whether, as in experimental animals, preterm human infants have a relatively small supply of granulocytic progenitors. The venous blood of adults contains approximately 20 to 300 CFU-GM per milliliter. In contrast, the blood of term infants contains approximately 2000 CFU-GM per milliliter. Even higher concentrations are present in the blood of infants delivered prematurely. The high concentrations of CFU-GM in fetal blood, however, do not necessarily indicate a large total body quantity of CFU-GM. It is likely that a significant percentage of fetal CFU-GM are in the circulation.[16]

When fetal CFU-GM are cultured in vitro in the presence of recombinant G-CSF, they undergo maturation into colonies of neutrophils. Fetal CFU-GM often clonally mature into larger colonies and contain more cells than do CFU-GM obtained from the bone marrow of adults.[19] The physiologic role of G-CSF includes upregulation of neutrophil production. This appears to be the case for the fetus and neonate as well as for the adult. Thus, the low quantities of circulating and storage neutrophils in the midtrimester human fetus may be due in part to low production of G-CSF. Supporting this hypothesis are observations of poor production of G-CSF by cells of human fetal origin.[19,20] Monocytes isolated from the blood of adults produce G-CSF when stimulated with a variety of inflammatory mediators, such as bacterial lipopolysaccharide or interleukin-1. In contrast, monocytes isolated from the umbilical cord blood of preterm infants and from the liver and bone marrow of aborted fetuses up to 24 weeks of gestation generate only small quantities (10 to 100 times less per cell) of G-CSF protein and mRNA after lipopolysaccharide or interleukin-1 stimulation.[19,20] Despite the poor capacity to generate G-CSF, it appears that G-CSF receptors on the surface of neutrophils of newborn infants are equal in number and affinity to those on adult neutrophils.

Neonatal neutropenia

Relatively few neutrophils are present in the human embryo and early fetus, and neutrophil production is a relatively minor component of hematopoiesis in the midtrimester fetus. On this basis, one might anticipate that neonates delivered extremely prematurely would be at high risk of serious bacterial infection. Indeed, of all the risk factors for neonatal infection analyzed in the national collaborative study on neonatal infections, premature birth had the strongest correlation. One might also anticipate that premature neonates delivered at the limits of viability (22 to 25 weeks gestation) would have a high likelihood of developing neutropenia. This propensity is indeed seen. For instance, if neutropenia is defined as a blood neutrophil concentration <1000/μL, 40% of neonates weighing <1000 g at birth develop neutropenia at some time during their hospital stay.[21] Most such cases are detected on the first day after

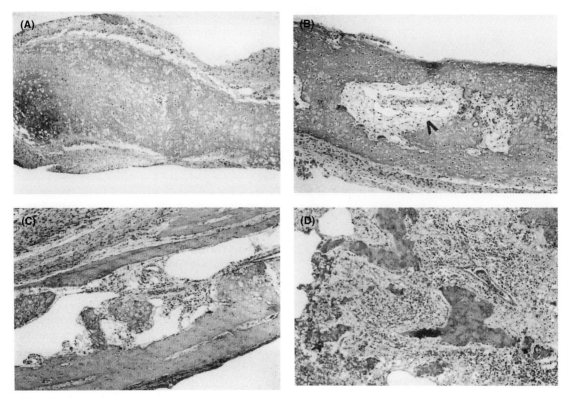

Figure 44.2 Photomicrographs of clavicles 6 to 14 weeks after conception (hematoxylin and eosin stain; original magnification, ×100). (A) Six weeks after conception. Clavicles at this stage consist of primitive cartilage and contain no marrow cavity and no myeloperoxidase positive cells. (B) Nine weeks after conception. Clavicles at this stage have the beginning of a marrow cavity (*arrowhead*) but no myeloperoxidase-positive cells. (C) Eleven weeks after conception. Clavicles at this stage have an elongated marrow cavity and small hematopoietic islands of myeloperoxidase-positive cell in the marrow space. (D) Fourteen weeks after conception. Spiculation has begun, and the volume of hematopoietic marrow has begun to increase. Source: Slayton *et al.* (1998).[4] Reproduced with permission of Elsevier.

birth. Most are associated with maternal hypertension, or with a birth weight less than the 10th percentile for gestation, and most are relatively transient, with counts exceeding 1000/μL within a few days. When neutropenia first appears after the third day of life, the underlying cause is usually obscure.[21] Neutropenia among extremely low-birth-weight neonates, although common, is only viewed as problematic in one of two situations: (1) neutropenia during an infectious illness among these patients is a very poor prognostic sign (see Chapter 30 for more information), and (2) neutropenia that is severe and prolonged is important to

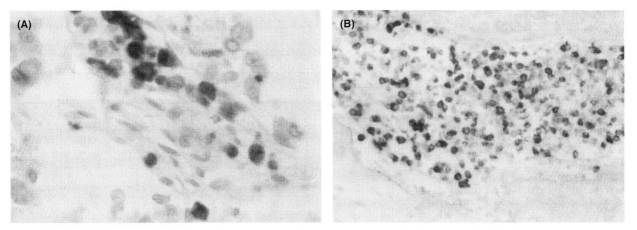

Figure 44.3 Appearance and subsequent expansion of neutrophils within the clavicular marrow cavity 12 to 15 weeks after conception. (A) At 12 weeks of gestation, a small number of myeloperoxidase-positive cells are present in the developing marrow cavity. Many of these cells have the morphologic appearance of neutrophils with segmented or band nuclei, and they appear in discrete clusters within the marrow cavity. (Myeloperoxidase stain; original magnification, ×400.) (B) At 15 weeks, clavicles have a marrow cavity that contains numerous myeloperoxidase-positive cells. (Original magnification, ×200.) Source: Slayton *et al.* (1998).[4] Reproduced with permission of Elsevier.

recognize, because it might be one of the syndromes of genetic abnormalities involving severe chronic neutropenia.

Erythropoiesis

Erythropoietin in the fetus and neonate

A constant supply of amino acids, lipids, iron, specific vitamins, and trace nutrients is needed to support fetal erythropoiesis, and limitations in any of these can thwart red blood cell production.[22] However, the rate of erythrocyte production is not physiologically regulated by any of these factors, but primarily by the concentration of erythropoietin. Erythropoietin is an 18.4-kd glycoprotein that binds to specific receptors on the surface of erythroid precursors and various other cells and supports their clonal maturation by inhibiting apoptosis.[23] In addition, erythropoiesis can occur from embryonic stem cells using mechanisms that are erythropoietin independent.[24]

In the human fetus, erythropoietin is produced by a variety of cells: hepatocytes and cells of monocyte–macrophage origin in the liver, kidney interstitial cells and proximal tubules, and adrenal cortex.[25,26] The absence of erythropoietin or its receptor, as has been produced in murine knockout models, leads to profound anemia and fetal death on approximately embryonic day 13.[27,28] Postnatally, erythropoietin is produced almost exclusively by peritubular cells of the kidney, with a small fraction produced by liver and neuronal and glial cells in the central nervous system. Although some erythropoietin production occurs in the fetal kidney, it is minimal. Anephric fetuses have normal serum erythropoietin concentrations and hematocrits, indicating that the majority of fetal erythropoietin production is nonrenal.[29]

The factors that regulate the switch of erythropoietin production from the liver to the kidney are not known. Some investigators have suggested that, among preterm neonates, this switch does not occur until at or near term gestation; thus, this physiological delay is responsible for the relatively low concentrations of circulating erythropoietin in the common hyporegenerative anemia known as *anemia of prematurity*.[30]

The actions of erythropoietin in the human fetus are not limited to erythropoiesis. Functional erythropoietin receptors are expressed on the surface of cells within a wide variety of fetal tissues, including intestinal villi, endothelium, mesangium, smooth muscle, placenta, and neurons.[25,26,31,32] Erythropoietin has an anti-apoptotic effect on several of these cell types. Erythropoietin occurs in relatively high concentration in human amniotic fluid, colostrum, and milk—fluids that are swallowed in large amounts by the fetus and neonate.[33] A healthy midtrimester human fetus may swallow 200 to 300 ml of amniotic fluid per kilogram of body weight per day. With an amniotic fluid erythropoietin concentration of 200 mU/ml, the fetus would swallow approximately 60,000 mU/kg a day—an amount that, if given systemically to a neonate, would have a marked erythropoietic effect. Erythropoietin receptors are present along the villous border of the fetal and neonatal intestine.[25,33] Erythropoietin in amniotic fluid, colostrum, and human milk is not absorbed into the circulation and has no systemic effect but acts locally in the intestine as a trophic and antiapoptotic factor. Erythropoietin in amniotic fluid, colostrum, and milk tends to resist digestive conditions present in the fetal and neonatal gastrointestinal tract.[33,34]

Erythropoietin is present in concentrations of 20 to 50 mU/ml in the spinal fluid of neonates. Markedly greater spinal fluid concentrations of erythropoietin are seen after perinatal asphyxia, and this erythropoietin appears to be derived within the brain as opposed to crossing the blood–brain barrier.[35] Erythropoietin crosses the blood–brain barrier poorly, and modifications of the epo molecule permit better central nervous system penetration after IV dosing, for neuroprotection.[35,36]

The biologic roles of erythropoietin and erythropoietin receptors in the fetal and neonatal intestinal tract and central nervous system are not known. One potential function for erythropoietin in the fetal brain is as a neuroprotectant.[37] This postulate is supported by the observations that erythropoietin production increases in the brain during fetal hypoxia, and that recombinant erythropoietin protects neurons in tissue culture from hypoxemic damage and does so by diminishing apoptosis, which is analogous to the function it has in erythropoiesis.

Fetal erythroid progenitors

Culture of bone marrow cells in tissue culture has added to the understanding of erythropoietic regulation. When bone marrow cells are placed in semisolid media culture systems for 5 to 7 days, the erythropoietin-sensitive precursors (CFU-Es) clonally mature into clusters containing 30 to 100 normoblasts.[38] Erythroid-specific progenitors that are less well differentiated than CFU-Es, and hence more primitive cells, are called *burst-forming units-erythroid* (BFU-Es). Twelve to 14 days after bone marrow cells are placed in semisolid culture systems, BFU-Es have developed into large clusters of normoblasts, each containing 200 to more than 10,000 normoblasts. BFU-Es from human fetuses respond in a slightly different manner than do BFU-Es isolated from adults. Specifically, BFU-Es of fetal origin generally develop into erythroid clones more rapidly and generally develop substantially more normoblasts than do BFU-Es of adult origin.[39,40] Also, BFU-Es from adult bone marrow require a combination of erythropoietin plus another factor, such as interleukin-3 or GM-CSF, to clonally mature, whereas many fetal BFU-Es mature in the presence of erythropoietin alone.[39,40]

Physiological hemolysis after birth

Mild to moderate jaundice is so common during the first few days after birth as to warrant the name *physiological jaundice of the newborn*. The source of the bilirubin giving rise to this transient condition is heme catabolism,[41] a process that stoichiometrically generates carbon monoxide and bilirubin. The carbon monoxide generated by heme catabolism can be quantified in exhaled breath, serving as a measure of the hemolytic rate.[42] A unique aspect of the fetal-to-neonatal transition involves a period of accelerated hemolysis, persisting for a few days after birth, and providing a bilirubin load that contributes to *physiological jaundice of the newborn*, as shown in Figure 44.4. Mechanisms underlying this transient physiological hemolysis are the topic of current investigation.

Embryonic, fetal, and adult hemoglobins

Tissues must receive a constant supply of oxygen. The development of oxygen-carrying proteins increases the ability of blood to transport oxygen. The binding of oxygen and its dissociation from hemoglobin are accomplished without expenditure of metabolic energy.[43] Hemoglobin consists of iron-containing heme groups and globin, a protein moiety. An interaction between heme, globin, and 2,3-diphosphoglycerate (also called 2,3-bisphosphoglycerate) gives hemoglobin its unique properties in the reversible transport of oxygen. Hemoglobin is a tetrameric molecule composed of two

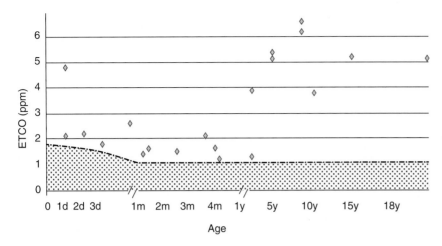

Figure 44.4 Physiological hemolysis during the first days after birth. The reference range (shaded zone) for end-tidal carbon monoxide is shown for healthy neonates and children. During the first day after birth, values are twice that of neonates after 1 to 2 weeks. Values from neonates and children with known hemolytic disorders (shown as diamonds) are all above the reference. Source: Christensen *et al.* (2014)[42] Reproduced with permission of Elsevier.

pairs of polypeptide chains, each encoded by a different family of genes; the α-like globin genes on chromosome 16 and the β-like globin genes on chromosome 11. The main hemoglobin of normal adults (HbA) is made up of one pair each of α and β chains ($\alpha_2\beta_2$). Six distinct hemoglobins can be detected within the erythrocytes of the human embryo, fetus, child, and adult—Gower-1, Gower-2, Portland, fetal hemoglobin (HbF), and the adult hemoglobins HbA and HbA_2. The time of appearance and quantitative relations among the hemoglobins are determined by complex developmental processes that are not well defined.

Human embryos have the slowly migrating hemoglobins Gower-1, Gower-2, and Portland. The ζ chains of Hb Portland and Gower-1 are structurally similar to α chains. Both Gower hemoglobins contain a unique polypeptide chain, the ε chain. Gower-1 Hb has the structure $\zeta_2\varepsilon_2$, and Gower-2 has $\alpha_2\varepsilon_2$; Portland Hb has the structure $\zeta_2\gamma_2$. Four to eight weeks after conception, the Gower hemoglobins predominate, but by 12 to 14 weeks, they are no longer detected.

Fetal hemoglobin contains γ chains in place of the β chains of HbA and is represented as $\alpha_2\gamma_2$. The resistance of HbF to denaturation by strong alkali usually is used in its quantitation. After the eighth postconceptional week, HbF is the predominant hemoglobin. At 24 weeks of gestation, it constitutes 90% of total hemoglobin. Thereafter a gradual decline in HbF occurs, so that at birth the average is 70% of the total. Synthesis of HbF decreases rapidly postnatally, and by 6 to 12 months of age only a trace is present. Fetal hemoglobin is heterogeneous because of two types of γ chain synthesis directed by two sets of genes. The chains differ at position 136 in the presence of either a glycine (Gγ) or an alanine (Aγ) residue. In the neonate, the relative proportion of Gγ to Aγ chain is 3:1.

Trace quantities of HbA can be detected in embryos. Thus, it is possible to make an early prenatal diagnosis of major β-chain hemoglobinopathy. Prenatal diagnosis is based on techniques used to examine the rates of synthesis of β chains or the structure of newly synthesized β chains or on molecular techniques from sampling the chorionic villus tissue or amniotic fluid. Gene deletion disorders, such as α-thalassemia, can be detected with the same methods.

At 24 weeks of gestation, approximately 5% to 10% of hemoglobin in a fetus is HbA. Thereafter a steady increase follows, so that at term, the proportion of HbA averages 30%. By one year of age, the normal adult hemoglobin pattern appears. The minor adult hemoglobin component (HbA_2) contains δ chains and has the structure $\alpha_2\delta_2$. It is seen only when significant amounts of HbA are present.

At birth, less than 1% of HbA_2 is present, but by 12 months, the normal level of 2% to 4% is attained. Throughout life, the normal ratio of HbA to HbA_2 is approximately 30:1.

In the fetus and neonate, the rates of synthesis of γ and β chains and the amounts of HbA and HbF are inversely related. This has been attributed to a switch mechanism, but the developmental processes that direct the switch from predominantly γ-chain synthesis in utero to predominantly β-chain synthesis after birth are unclear. Primitive erythrocyte progenitors undergoing clonal maturation in culture (BFU-Es) predominantly generate HbF. This may be the basis for the increased levels of HbF that occur in anemia with severe erythropoietic stress. Alternative explanations involve more basic genetic regulators in the DNA sequences that flank the hemoglobin gene complexes.

Because hemoglobins containing ε chains are normally present only very early in intrauterine life, they are largely of theoretic interest. Small amounts of the Gower hemoglobins have been detectable in a few neonates with trisomy 13. Increased levels of Hb Portland have been found in cord blood of stillborn infants with homozygous α-thalassemia.

The normal adult level of HbA_2 (2.4% to 3.4%) is seldom altered. Levels of HbA_2 exceeding 3.4% are found in most persons with the β-thalassemia trait and in those with megaloblastic anemia secondary to vitamin B_{12} and folic acid deficiency. Decreased HbA_2 levels are found in those with iron deficiency anemia and thalassemia major.[44]

Erythrocytes of the midtrimester fetus and preterm infant are large (Figure 44.5). At 22 to 23 weeks gestation, the mean corpuscular volume (MCV) can be 135 fL or more, compared with a value of 88 ± 8 fL in adults. Similarly, at 22 to 23 weeks gestation, the mean cell hemoglobin (MCH) can be over 45 pg, compared with 29 ± 2 pg in adults.[45] Even at term, the MCV and MCH are strikingly higher than the upper limit of normal among healthy adults. However, throughout gestation, the mean corpuscular hemoglobin concentration is essentially the same as in adults.[45] Presumably, these very large and hemoglobin-laden erythrocytes are advantageous to the early fetus, although it is not clear what those advantages are. Perhaps the very high content of hemoglobin carried by these large cells somehow constitutes a fetal advantage. Whether large erythrocytes are also advantageous for prematurely delivered neonates *ex utero* is not known. Many preterm neonates have large phlebotomy losses in the first week of NICU care and are transfused with much smaller erythrocytes from adult donors. The consequences of this change in erythrocyte size are not known.

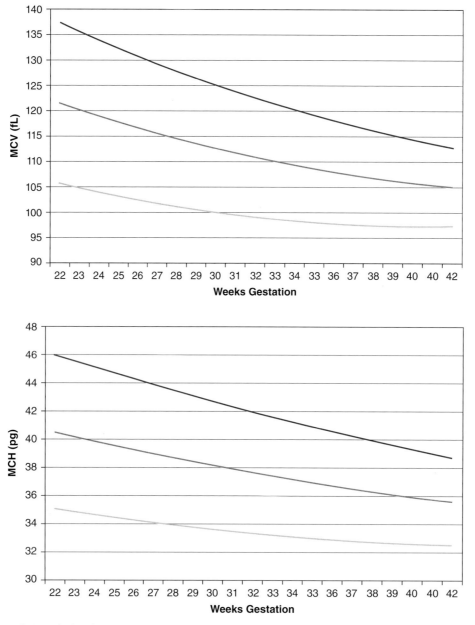

Figure 44.5 The expected range of values for mean corpuscular volume (MCV; part a) and for mean corpuscular hemoglobin (MCH; part b) for neonates of 22 weeks through 42 weeks gestation, as measured on the first day after birth. The upper and lower boundaries incorporate 95% of the measured values. Source: Christensen *et al.* (2008). Reproduced with permission of Nature Publishing.

Thrombopoiesis

Platelets were described in the early part of the nineteenth century, but it was not until 1882 that their role in hemostasis was recognized. The origin of platelets from megakaryocytes was reported in 1906,[46] and since then the study of mechanisms responsible for platelet production has focused on megakaryocytes. The megakaryocyte compartment in the bone marrow consists of two pools of cells.[47] One is composed of cells that are morphologically unrecognizable but are committed to the megakaryocyte lineage. These cells, the megakaryocyte progenitors, retain a high proliferative capacity and ultimately determine the number of megakaryocytes in the bone marrow. The other pool consists of nondividing cells that are morphologically recognizable as megakaryocytes and undergo endoreduplication or endomitosis, a process in which the

ploidy of the cell increases without cellular division. There is some degree of overlap between these two pools.

Fetal and neonatal megakaryocyte progenitors

Progenitor cells committed to the megakaryocyte lineage can be identified by two methods: a culture system, in which they are identified by their ability to form megakaryocyte colonies, and immunologic staining, which allows characterization according to the specific antigens expressed on their membranes. With these methods, two different megakaryocyte progenitor cells have been identified: the burst-forming unit megakaryocyte (BFU-MK), which is a more primitive megakaryocyte progenitor,[48,49] and a later progenitor known as the colony-forming unit megakaryocyte (CFU-MK).[47,50] In culture, CFU-MK–derived colonies are smaller

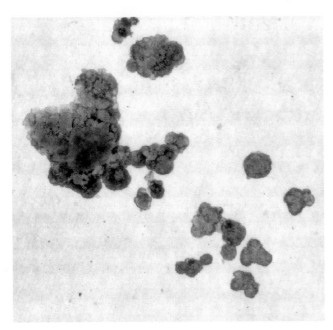

Figure 44.6 Photomicrograph showing a megakaryocyte colony derived from a megakaryocyte progenitor (CFU-MK) from the bone marrow of a thrombocytopenic preterm neonate. (Original magnification, ×400.) Light-density mononuclear cells isolated from the bone marrow were cultured in collagen-based serum-free media with 50 ng/ml of recombinant human thrombopoietin. After fixation, the colonies were stained with a monoclonal antibody against glycoprotein IIb/IIIa to allow accurate identification of megakaryocytes.

(3 to 50 cells per colony) and primarily unifocal (Figure 44.6), whereas BFU-MK–derived colonies are larger (>50 cells per colony) and have multiple foci of development. When immunologically phenotyped, CFU-MKs express CD34 and HLA-DR, whereas BFU-MKs express CD34 but not HLA-DR. Recent studies in mice have also identified a subtype of hematopoietic stem cell that resides at the apex of the hematopoietic stem cell hierarchy and has enhanced propensity for short- and long-term platelet reconstitution. This platelet-biased stem cell is characterized by surface expression of von Willebrand factor (vWF).[50]

There are no differences between fetal and adult megakaryocyte progenitors in regard to the expression profile of CD34 and HLA-DR.[51] However, fetal BFU-MK–derived colonies are significantly larger than adult BFU-MK–derived colonies and are usually composed of only one or two foci of development. Adult BFU-MK–derived colonies are typically multifocal.[52] In addition, a unique megakaryocyte progenitor present in fetal bone marrow has an unusually high proliferative potential and gives rise to very large unifocal colonies (>300 cells).[53] This cell, not found in adult bone marrow cultures, may represent a more primitive megakaryocyte progenitor. The development of miniaturized assay systems to study megakaryocyte progenitors has made it possible to study these cells in the peripheral blood of neonates. Using these techniques, it has been shown that preterm neonates (24 to 36 weeks) have higher circulating concentrations of all megakaryocyte progenitors than do term neonates.[54,55]

Fetal and neonatal megakaryocytes

Unlike their progenitors, megakaryocytes have no proliferative abilities but undergo a complex maturational process. Through this process, they evolve from small, mononuclear cells to very large, polyploid cells easily recognized in the bone marrow as mature

megakaryocytes.[56,57] The modal ploidy is 16N in normal adult bone marrow.[58]

In the human fetus, megakaryocytes are first detected in the circulatory system at eight weeks of gestation, and the first platelets appear at five weeks.[59] Compared with the megakaryocytes of adults, fetal megakaryocytes are significantly smaller at all stages of maturation. Their ploidy distribution is also shifted to the left, with a higher proportion of low ploidy megakaryocytes.[60–62] The modal ploidy in the bone marrow of near-term fetuses is 8N.[63] Against prior paradigms, it is now understood that the small size and low ploidy of neonatal megakaryocytes are not a reflection of their immaturity. In fact, 2N and 4N cord blood–derived megakaryocytes are more cytoplasmically mature than adult peripheral blood–derived megakaryocytes of similarly low ploidy, based on the surface expression or maturation markers (CD42b), the presence of alpha granules, the development of a well-formed demarcation membrane system, and the ability to form proplatelets.[64] Thus, the phenotype of fetal and neonatal megakaryocytes is the result of a developmentally unique maturational pattern, characterized by rapid proliferation followed by full cytoplasmic maturation, without polyploidization (Figure 44.7).

Umbilical cord blood has higher concentrations of circulating megakaryocytes than adult blood. As in the fetus, cord blood megakaryocytes from term infants are considerably smaller than adult circulating megakaryocytes,[65] although they are otherwise phenotypically mature megakaryocytes. A recent study evaluating the timing of the transition from neonatal to adult megakaryocytes in human bone marrow samples found that neonates have megakaryocytes of uniform small sizes, which diverge into separate clusters of smaller and larger cells beginning at two years, and finally transition to larger (adult-like) megakaryocytes by four years.[66] Because cord blood–derived megakaryocytes have been shown to generate less platelets than adult-derived megakaryocytes,[67] it has been postulated that the normal platelet counts of fetuses and neonates are maintained by the increased proliferative potential of the fetal and neonatal megakaryocyte progenitors (Table 44.3).

The process of platelet production and release is one of the less well-understood steps of thrombopoiesis. However, recent work has substantially enhanced our understanding of this process, and has painted a graphic picture of how megakaryocytes—in their final hours—convert their cytoplasm into branched proplatelet extensions that elongate based on a process of microtubule sliding and polymerization.[68] Organelles and platelet-specific granules are delivered to the nascent platelets (at the tips of each proplatelet extension) by a mechanism involving both traveling of the organelles along the microtubules and movement of the linked microtubules relative to each other.[69] The role of blood flow–induced shear stress on platelet release has also been evidenced by a recent study using intravital microscopy to observe in vivo platelet release in intact murine bone marrow,[70] or recent studies using fluidic microreactor devices that attempt to reproduce the effects of shear stress in the bone marrow or blood vessel environment on platelet production.[71] In these studies, megakaryocytes were observed to extend dynamic proplatelet-like protrusions into microvessels (or their in vitro equivalent). These intravascular extensions were then sheared from their transendothelial stems by flowing blood, resulting in the appearance of preplatelets in peripheral blood. The signals regulating the direction of proplatelet extensions into the blood vessels and the separation of preplatelets from their parent megakaryocytes are just beginning to be understood, but recent work has identified sphingosine-1-phosphate as a critical mediator of these processes.[72]

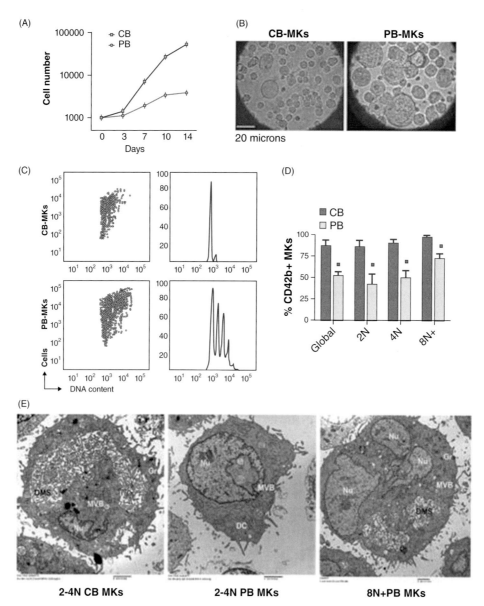

Figure 44.7 Comparison of neonatal and adult megakaryopoiesis. (A) Number of cells derived from CD34+ cells obtained from cord blood (CB) and adult peripheral blood (PB) during culture in a serum-free liquid system with TPO as the only growth factor. The figure indicates the mean number of cells (per 1,000 CD34+ cells plated) at each time point ± SEM. (B) Photomicrograph of CB- and PB-derived MKs at the end of the 14-day culture period. Both pictures were taken at a magnification of 600x. (C) Ploidy levels of CB- and PB-derived megakaryocytes (MKs) were measured by flow cytometry following propidium iodide staining. (D) Percentage of MKs expressing CD42b at each ploidy level. Compared to PB-MKs, CB-MKs exhibited significantly higher percentages of CD42b+ (mature) cells at each ploidy level. The bars represent the mean and SEM of three independent experiments (* p<0.05). (E) Human MKs of different ploidy levels were flow-sorted following anti-human CD41-FITC and Hoechst 33342 staining and then examined by transmission electron microscopy. *Left*: Representative flow-sorted 2N/4N CB-MK. The majority of these MKs were mature, and exhibited abundant platelet granules (Gr) and well developed demarcation membrane systems (DMS). Center: In contrast, 77% of flow-sorted 2N/4N PB-MKs were immature, as evidenced by the absence of demarcation membranes and a paucity of granules. *Right*: 54% of all flow-sorted 8N PB MKs were ultrastructurally similar to the mature neonatal 2N/4N MKs, although they were of larger size. Source: Liu and Sola-Visner (2011) (Curr Opin Hematol 18:330–337.) Reproduced with permission of Lippincott, Williams & Wilkins.

Thrombopoietin and thrombopoietin mimetics

TPO, the main physiologic regulator of platelet production, was first isolated in 1994.[73] The gene that encodes TPO has been localized to the long arm of human chromosome 3.[74] TPO mRNA is expressed primarily in the liver, and to a lesser extent in other tissues, including kidney and bone marrow stromal cells.[75] In vitro, TPO acts as a potent stimulator of all stages of megakaryocyte growth and development, except platelet release.[76] It also plays roles in platelet activation, mostly by

priming the platelets to the effects of other agonists.[77] TPO and TPO receptor knockout mice models have been generated.[78,79] These mice have megakaryocyte and blood platelet concentrations of only 10% to 15% those of control mice. These studies confirmed that TPO is the primary regulator of platelet production, but also proved that alternative pathways exist for megakaryocytopoiesis.

Much attention has also been directed to the effects of TPO on other hematologic cell types. In vitro, TPO alone stimulates the

Table 44.3 Differences in megakaryocytopoiesis between neonates and adults

	Adults	Neonates
TPO concentrations	Very high in hyporegenerative thrombocytopenia	Not as high in thrombocytopenic neonates (mostly SGA) as in thrombocytopenic adults
Megakaryocyte progenitors	Sparse in the blood	Abundant in the blood
	Give rise to small colonies	Give rise to large colonies
	Less sensitive to TPO	More sensitive to TPO
Megakaryocytes	Large	Small
	High ploidy levels	Low ploidy levels
	Mature only at ≥8N	Mature at 2N and 4N
Effects of rTPO	Stimulates megakaryocyte proliferation	Stimulates megakaryocyte proliferation

SGA, Small for gestational age; TPO, thrombopoietin; rTPO, recombinant thrombopoietin.

Source: Sola-Visner (2006) (Haematologica Reports 2006;2:65–69).

proliferation and survival of erythroid, myeloid, and multipotential progenitors.[80] TPO also enhances erythropoietin-induced erythroid burst formation, an effect mediated by its ability to inhibit apoptosis of erythroid progenitors.[81] Further studies have shown that TPO acts on early hematopoietic progenitors (including hematopoietic stem cells), thus disclosing an important role for this cytokine in hematopoiesis in general, in addition to its megakaryopoietic functions.[82,83] These findings have significant clinical implications for patients with mutations in the TPO receptor that render it unresponsive to TPO, such as in congenital amegakaryocytic thrombocytopenia, who frequently progress to aplastic anemia.

Results of several animal studies have confirmed the role of TPO as a potent stimulator of platelet production. The recombinant human full-length TPO molecule (rTPO) and a recombinant human polypeptide that contains the receptor-binding N-terminal domain of TPO (rHuMGDF) were the subject of several studies. When injected into normal animals, rTPO and rHuMGDF induced marked thrombocytosis.[84,85] Administered to animals exposed to myelosuppressive chemotherapy, rHuMGDF not only was able to ameliorate the associated thrombocytopenia but also accelerated red blood cell and neutrophil recovery.[86,87]

Several phase I and II trials in human subjects also demonstrated the efficacy of rTPO and rHuMGDF as stimulators of platelet production in adults without thrombocytopenia[88] and in patients with chemotherapy-induced thrombocytopenia.[89,90] However, the appearance of thrombocytopenia and ultimately aplastic anemia secondary to the generation of cross-reactive anti-TPO antibodies in a small number of patients receiving rHuMGDF[91] led to the discontinuation of all clinical trials involving any of the forms of

recombinant TPO. As an alternative, much interest has been recently directed to the development of TPO-mimetic molecules. These are small molecules that have no sequence homology to TPO, but bind to the TPO receptor and have biologically comparable effects. The lack of homology represents a significant advantage over recombinant forms of TPO, because it should preclude the development of cross-reactive neutralizing antibodies against endogenous TPO. At least five different TPO receptor agonists have been described, and two are currently approved by the US Food and Drug Administration (FDA) for the treatment of patients with chronic ITP not responsive to other therapies: romiplostim (AMG 531), an engineered peptibody composed of a recombinant protein carrier FC domain linked to multiple c-mpl-binding domains,[92,93] and eltrombopag (SB-497115), an oral, nonpeptide TPO receptor agonist.[94] Both compounds have been effective in patients with refractory ITP, and have a favorable safety profile in children and adults. Eltrombopag is also approved for the treatment of severe aplastic anemia and of chronic hepatitis C infection–associated thrombocytopenia, to allow the initiation and maintenance of interferon-based therapy.

TPO in the fetus and neonate

Little is known about the role of TPO or the theoretical benefits of administration of rTPO or TPO-mimetic compounds to neonates. Recombinant TPO certainly supports the growth of megakaryocyte colonies from the blood or bone marrow of neonates. In fact, bone marrow progenitors from neonates are more sensitive to rTPO than progenitors from adults in vitro (Figure 44.8).[95] Similarly, newborn rhesus monkeys are highly sensitive to rTPO in vivo (Figure 44.9)

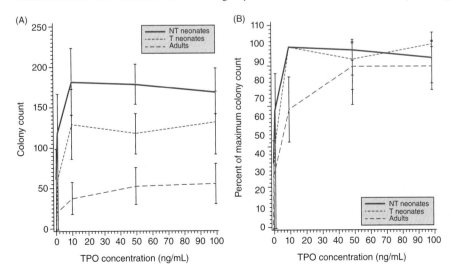

Figure 44.8 (A) Dose response to recombinant thrombopoietin of megakaryocyte progenitors obtained from the bone marrow of neonates with thrombocytopenia (*T*), neonates without thrombocytopenia (*NT*), and healthy adults. The marrow obtained from neonates generated approximately three times more colonies (per 10^5 low density cells) than the marrow obtained from adults. (B) In a percentage of maximal colony count versus recombinant thrombopoietin concentration curve, the curves for the neonates with thrombocytopenia and those without thrombocytopenia reached a plateau at 10 ng/ml, compared with 50 ng/ml for the adults. This indicates that megakaryocyte progenitors from neonates are more sensitive to recombinant thrombopoietin in vitro than are their adult counterparts. Source: Sola *et al.* (2000). Reproduced with permission of Wiley.

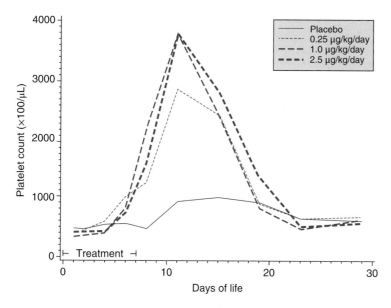

Figure 44.9 Dose–response to polyethylene glycol (PEG)–rHuMGDF (a truncated form of recombinant human full-length TPO molecule, or rTPO) of the blood platelet concentration in newborn rhesus monkeys, demonstrating the sensitivity of megakaryocyte progenitors of neonates to rTPO in vivo. The monkeys received daily subcutaneous injections of placebo or PEG–rHuMGDF at doses of 0.25, 1.00, or 2.50 µg/kg a day for seven days. Each line represents the average platelet counts of the two monkeys in each treatment group sampled on study days 2, 4, and 6, and then twice weekly until day 28. The peripheral platelet count increased on day 6 of treatment, peaked on day 11, and returned to baseline by day 23. The two higher doses generated similar increases in platelet count. Source: Pastos *et al.* (2006). Reproduced with permission of American Society of Hematology.

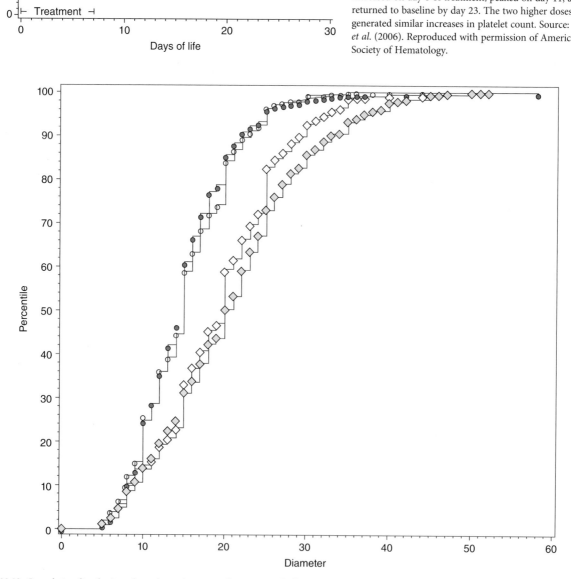

Figure 44.10 Cumulative distribution plots of megakaryocyte diameters in the bone marrow of thrombocytopenic neonates (dark circles), non-thrombocytopenic neonates (clear circles), thrombocytopenic adults (dark diamonds), and non-thrombocytopenic adults (clear diamonds). The megakaryocyte diameters are displayed on the *x*-axis, and their cumulative distribution on the *y*-axis. Both adult curves are shifted to the right compared to the neonatal curves, indicating the predominance of larger megakaryocytes in these samples. Furthermore, the curve for the thrombocytopenic adults is also shifted to the right compared to that for the non-thrombocytopenic adults, indicating a higher percentage of large megakaryocytes. In contrast, the curves of thrombocytopenic and non-thrombocytopenic neonates are overlapping, indicating no change in the megakaryocyte size distribution in this cohort of thrombocytopenic neonates compared to controls. Source: Sola-Visner *et al.* (2007). Reproduced with permission of Nature Publishing.

and respond to lower doses (per kilogram body weight) than those required in adult rhesus monkeys to achieve a similar effect.[96] Megakaryocyte progenitors from preterm neonates with or without thrombocytopenia also seem to be more sensitive to rTPO than progenitors from term neonates.[97] However, there are substantial qualitative differences in the response of neonatal and adult megakaryocytes to TPO, as demonstrated by a recent study evaluating the maturation of megakaryocytes cultured either in TPO alone or in adult bone marrow stromal conditioned media.[98] In that study, adult megakaryocytes reached the highest ploidy levels when cultured in serum-free medium with maximal concentrations of rTPO, whereas neonatal megakaryocytes reached their highest ploidy when cultured in marrow stromal cell–conditioned media *in the absence* of rTPO. In fact, the addition of supraphysiologic concentrations of this cytokine (≥ 1 ng/mL) inhibited the polyploidization of neonatal megakaryocytes. Whether rTPO or any of the TPO-mimetic peptides will be clinically useful as an alternative to platelet transfusions in the care of neonates with thrombocytopenia remains to be determined. However, it is clear that there are substantial developmental differences in megakaryocyte regulation, which will have to be taken into account when considering both the possible efficacy and the potential toxicity of thrombopoietic growth factors in this population.

Neonatal thrombocytopenia

When a fetus is delivered prematurely, the thrombopoietic system can be taxed by new demands. For instance, endothelial damage from infection or from the presence of intravascular catheters can accelerate platelet usage well beyond that normally experienced by the fetus. Moreover, disorders that tend to shorten gestation, such as pregnancy-induced hypertension and placental insufficiency, appear to have suppressive effects on fetal platelet production.[99] Because of these and other issues, thrombocytopenia is a very common problem in the NICU, manifested in 20–30% of all NICU patients, and in 75% or more of the extremely low-birth-weight population.[100] Recent work has suggested that when a fetus or preterm neonate requires an increase in platelet production as a compensation for accelerated platelet usage or destruction, they might face developmental limitations in their ability to upregulate thrombopoiesis. Specifically, TPO concentrations in small-for-gestational-age neonates with hyporegenerative thrombocytopenia are less elevated than those reported in adults with hyporegenerative thrombocytopenia, suggesting that—at least in this group of neonates—lower than expected TPO concentrations might contribute to the thrombocytopenia.[101] Furthermore, thrombocytopenic neonates in general do not seem to increase the size of their megakaryocytes as compared to their non-thrombocytopenic counterparts, thus blunting one of the mechanisms by which adults increase platelet production in response to platelet demand[102] (Figure 44.10). Similar results were obtained in a murine model of immune-mediated fetal thrombocytopenia, in which fetuses failed to increase their megakaryocyte size in response to platelet consumption.[103] The mechanisms underlying the small size of neonatal megakaryocytes are not clearly understood, but recent studies suggest that they involve a combination of cell-intrinsic factors and factors in the fetal/neonatal microenvironment. Indeed, as demonstrated by stem cell transplant experiments, the adult environment is more conducive to megakaryocyte maturation than the fetal environment, but cell-intrinsic factors (such as the response to TPO) nevertheless limit the ultimate size and ploidy that neonatal megakaryocytes can achieve.[104,105]

Key References

A full reference list for this chapter is available at: http://www.wiley.com/go/simon/transfusion

4 Slayton WB, Li Y, Calhoun DA, *et al.* The first appearance of neutrophils in the human fetal bone marrow cavity. *Early Hum Dev* 1998;**53**:129–44.

7 Charboard P, Tavian M, Humeau L, *et al.* Early ontogeny of the human marrow from long bones: an immunohistochemical study of hematopoiesis and its microenvironment. *Blood* 1996;**78**:4109–19.

19 Schibler KR, Liechty KW, White WL, *et al.* Production of granulocyte colony-stimulating factor in vitro from monocytes from preterm and term neonates. *Blood* 1993;**82**:2269–89.

37 Rangarajan V, Juul SE. Erythropoietin: emerging role of erythropoietin in neonatal neuroprotection. *Pediatr Neurol* 2014;**51**:481–8.

45 Christensen RD, Jopling J, Henry E, Wiedmeier SE. The erythrocyte indices of neonates, defined using data from over 12,000 patients in a multihospital healthcare system. *J Perinatol* 2008;**28**:24–8.

52 Zauli G, Valvassori L, Capitani S. Presence and characteristics of circulating megakaryocyte progenitor cells in human fetal blood. *Blood* 1993;**81**:385–90.

61 Hegyi E, Nakazawa M, Debili N, *et al.* Developmental changes in human megakaryocyte ploidy. *Exp Hematol* 1991;**19**:87–94.

64 Liu ZJ, Italiano J, Ferrer-Marin F, Gutti R, *et al.* Developmental differences in megakaryocytopoiesis are associated with up-regulated TPO signaling through mTOR and elevated full length GATA-1 levels in neonatal megakaryocytes. *Blood* 2011;**117**:4106–17.

66 Fuchs DA, McGinn SG, Cantu CL, *et al.* Developmental differences in megakaryocyte size in infants and children. *Am J Clin Pathol* 2012;**138**:140–5.

102 Sola-Visner MC, Christensen RD, Hutson AD, Rimsza LM. Megakaryocyte size and concentration in the bone marrow of thrombocytopenic and nonthrombocytopenic neonates. *Pediatr Res* 2007;**61**:479–84.

CHAPTER 45

Hemolytic disease of the fetus and newborn

Bjarte G. Solheim,[1] Morten Grönn,[2] & Thor Willy Ruud Hansen[3,4]

[1]Institute of Immunology, Oslo University Hospital-Rikshospitalet and University of Oslo, Oslo, Norway
[2]Department of Child and Adolescent Medicine, Akershus University Hospital, Nordbyhagen, Norway
[3]Neonatal Intensive Care, Women and Children's Division, Oslo University Hospital, Oslo, Norway
[4]Institute for Clinical Medicine, Faculty of Medicine, University of Oslo, Oslo, Norway

The changing spectrum of hemolytic disease of the fetus and newborn (HDFN)

Status in developed countries

During the past 30 to 40 years, the spectrum of HDFN has changed profoundly. In the late 1960s and early 1970s, HDFN was a common neonatal problem dominated by Rh(D) alloimmunization. Overt fetal or neonatal hemolysis, with marked anemia and hyperbilirubinemia in the neonate, were commonly observed symptoms. The neonates were often severely affected and unstable at birth, and required multiple exchange transfusions. HDFN was associated with considerable neonatal morbidity and mortality.

Introduction in the 1970s of routine postpartum prophylactic Rh immune globulin (RhIG or anti-D) to D-negative women (with D-positive infants), and after pregnancy termination or abortion, has changed the picture dramatically and reduced D alloimmunization by about 90%.[1] After introduction of additional antepartum prophylactic RhIG, the frequency of D alloimmunization is now well below 0.2%.[2] The introduction of prophylactic RhIG ranks as one of the great success stories of modern perinatal care and immunology.

Programs for antibody screening and ABO/Rh typing of pregnant women allow focus on fetuses and neonates at risk, and have paved the way for the vastly improved antepartum surveillance and therapy outlined in Chapter 43.

Finally, postpartum therapy has improved considerably.[3] Exchange transfusion, although first described in the 1920s, was simplified and became common in the late 1940s with the use of umbilical catheters. Phototherapy was first discovered in England in the late 1950s and was initially met with considerable skepticism in both Northern Europe and North America, in contrast with immediate acceptance and enthusiasm in Latin America. Today modern phototherapy, in many centers combined with high-dose intravenous immunoglobulin (HDIVIG), has reduced the need for exchange transfusion to single figures even in large centers, although disagreement as to the efficacy of HDIVIG continues. The practical execution of exchange transfusion is rapidly becoming a "lost art," as most current graduates of pediatric training programs consider themselves lucky if they even get the chance to observe an exchange transfusion, and are highly unlikely to ever get to perform one. This raises serious challenges in order to keep the necessary competence in the practical execution of exchange transfusion.[3]

Alloantibody frequencies in populations of mostly European ancestry before and after introduction of postpartum prophylactic RhIG treatment are indicated in Table 45.1.

Status in countries with low human development index

Programs for antibody screening and ABO/Rh typing of pregnant women and introduction of postpartum routine prophylactic RhIG treatment have posed both organizational and economic challenges in countries with a low human development index (HDI). Improved neonatal surveillance and therapy have been introduced only to a limited degree, and antepartum treatment is often nonexistent. HDFN is, therefore, still a major cause of morbidity and mortality in these countries.[4]

Serologic and clinical features

Development of immune HDFN requires maternal immunoglobulin G (IgG) antibodies directed against paternal antigens on fetal red cells. Immunization can occur when fetal red cells pass through the placenta to the mother's circulation or the antigens were present in previous transfusions of the mother. Only maternal IgG antibodies can cross the placenta. The transport is an active process dependent upon interaction between maternal IgG and syncytiotrophoblast Fc receptors, and is most active in the third trimester.[7] IgG antibodies can be elicited by most blood group antigens (Tables 45.1 and 45.2, and Chapter 16). The immune response to peptide antigens (e.g., D) typically requires T-cell help and is dominated by IgG antibodies. Because the D antigen is extraordinarily immunogenic and induces high-affinity anti-D IgG, it has been a major cause for HDFN in Caucasian and African populations, where 10–15% of people lack the D antigen. This is not the case in East Asia (particularly China), where >99% of the population is D-positive (see Chapter 14). In addition, IgG autoantibodies causing maternal hemolytic anemia can result in HDFN. The common occurrence of antibodies reacting with carbohydrate antigens of the ABO, Hh, Ii, Lewis, and P systems without prior exposure to allogeneic red cells is a result of the wide distribution of these antigens in nature. IgM is generally the dominating antibody, but IgG anti-A, anti-B, and more rarely anti-H, are also present. Because the I antigen and antigens of the Lewis and P systems are

Rossi's Principles of Transfusion Medicine, Fifth Edition. Edited by Toby L. Simon, Jeffrey McCullough, Edward L. Snyder, Bjarte G. Solheim, and Ronald G. Strauss.

Table 45.1 Red cell antibodies in 1967 and 1995[5,6]

Antibody	1967 (Minnesota, 7 years)	1995 (Sweden, 12 years)
D	1864 (63.1%)	159 (19.0%)
E	80 (2.7%)	5 (6.1%)
C	448 (15.2%)	36 (4.3%)
C[w]	4 (0.14%)	10 (1.2%)
c	68 (2.3%)	38 (4.5%)
e	2 (0.07%)	1 (0.1%)
K1	93 (3.1%)	48 (5.7%)
Duffy	17 (0.6%)	26 (3.1%)
MNSs	45 (1.5%)	35 (4.2%)
Kidd	7 (0.2%)	10 (1.2%)
Lutheran	—	13 (1.6%)
P1	27 (0.9%)	48 (5.7%)
Lewis	94 (3.2%)	241 (28.8%)
I	13 (0.4%)	—
Others	194 (6.6%)	120 (14.4%)
Total	2,956	836
Blood samples	43,000	110,765

almost lacking on fetal cells, they are not associated with HDFN.[8] Table 45.2 summarizes antibody frequencies and severity of HDFN caused by relevant blood group antigens in populations of European and African ancestry.[9]

The direct antiglobulin test (DAT) (see Chapter 16) is one of the cornerstones for the diagnosis of HDFN. It detects IgG antibodies on the surface of red cells, and the number of IgG molecules bound to the erythrocyte surface determines the strength of the reaction. Using the spin antiglobulin test, the detection limit is 100 to 150 IgG molecules per red cell; when over 1000 are bound, the DAT is strongly positive (all cells are agglutinated).[10] Transplacental passage of maternal IgG results in antibody coating of the fetal red cells. High alloantibody concentrations lead to a strong DAT, whereas low concentrations or binding affinity result in a weak or, by traditional methods, often negative DAT. A strong positive DAT is observed, particularly with anti-D; however, the reaction is more variable with alloantibodies against other Rh antigens and antigens

Table 45.2 Blood group antigens and hemolytic disease in the neonate[9] in populations of European and African ancestry

Antigen	Antibody frequency (per 1000 pregnant women)	Severity of HDFN in infants with the antigen		
		None/Mild	Moderate	Severe
A, B, AB	Not relevant	Not HDFN, but antibody in 90%	<10%	<1%
D	2.6	51%	30%	19%
c, cE	0.9	70%	23%	7%
E	2.0	Almost all	—	Rare
C, Ce, C[w], e	0.7	86%	14%	Rare
Le[a], Le[b]	3.0	Not HDFN		
Kell (K1)	3.2	30–50%	30–37%	13–38%
Fy[a]	0.8	67–94%	16%	6–16%
Fy[b]	Rare	Rare cause of mild HDFN		
Kidd (Jk[a])	0.2			Rare
M	0.5			Rare
N	0.1			Rare
U	Rare			Rare
N	0.03	Not HDFN		
P (P1)	0.03	Not HDFN		

such as Kell, Duffy, Kidd, and MNSs, which are well expressed on fetal red cells.[7] Because ABO antigens are not fully developed on fetal red cells and A and B substances are expressed by most tissues, the DAT in ABO incompatibility is often negative. However, with very sensitive techniques (e.g., automated analyzer with low-ionic-strength medium with enhancing agents), IgG can almost always be demonstrated on the red cells in ABO incompatibility.[11] As a basic test, the DAT has poor predictive value in identifying neonates requiring treatment. Only 23% of newborns found to be DAT positive on neonatal screening have been reported to develop hyperbilirubinemia requiring treatment, but when the DAT was strongly positive (generally because of anti-D), all required treatment.[12] It should also be borne in mind that after antepartum treatment of D-negative women with prophylactic RhIG, neonates may demonstrate a positive DAT without signs of hemolysis.[13] Thus, although obtaining a DAT test in cord blood has been considered compulsory in infants of RhD-negative mothers, The British Committee for Standards in Haematology recently suggested that this should no longer be a routine.[14]

In the affected fetus, anemia is the most important pathological component of HDFN, whereas in the newborn, both anemia and hyperbilirubinemia may cause physiological perturbations. Bilirubin, by virtue of being lipophilic, crosses the placenta during pregnancy and is removed by the mother's liver. However, because of the immaturity of the neonate's liver, plasma levels of unconjugated bilirubin after birth can quickly become high enough to cause serious central nervous system damage in the newborn. The anemia causes increased fetal erythropoiesis, which in severe cases leads to erythroblastosis with widespread extramedullary hematopoiesis and many nucleated red cells (erythroblasts) in the circulation. If untreated, the most severe stage of erythroblastosis, hydrops fetalis, can lead to stillbirth and is characterized by severe anemia, massive edema, and hypoproteinemia.

In severe erythroblastosis, examination of a blood film will show massive presence of nucleated red cells, but only a few spherocytes due to the rapid destruction of the red cells (e.g., serious Rh HDFN). In less severe HDFN, spherocytes will dominate the blood film, and only a few nucleated red cells are observed (e.g., ABO HDFN). This explains why examination of a blood film can be of diagnostic importance in neonates with pronounced jaundice.[3]

Persistent or prolonged jaundice in neonates is a common feature of HDFN, not infrequently has a cholestatic component, and can be observed in virtually all conditions mentioned in this chapter. Achieving the correct diagnosis is important for the neonate and can have implications for other family members as well.

Hemolytic disease predicted by antepartum maternal antibody screening

Although the majority of cases of acute neonatal hyperbilirubinemia caused by hemolysis currently occur without antepartum warning in high-HDI countries, there remain a number of neonates for whom HDFN is predicted by antepartum screening. Almost all blood group antibodies of IgG type can cause HDFN. However, the severity and frequency of HDFN vary, and anti-D still remains the most common cause of severe HDFN.[3] The most frequent alloantibodies are directed against Rh antigens (anti-D, anti-E, anti-c, and anti-C), Kell antigens (anti-K1), Duffy antigens (anti-Fy[a]), Kidd antigens (anti-Jk[a]), and MNSs antigens (Table 45.2). Anti-D, anti-c, anti-E, and anti-K are found in about 1 per 1000 pregnant women. Anti-K is mostly caused by transfusion, and the frequency of HDFN due to anti-K is much lower than that due to anti-D.[7] However, anti-Kell can cause severe fetal anemia because the antibody also inhibits fetal erythropoiesis.[15] The frequency and severity of HDFN caused by the other antibodies mentioned here are low (Table 45.2). A positive antepartum maternal antibody screening should be followed by frequent antepartum monitoring and makes treatment with intrauterine transfusions possible (see Chapter 43).

Antepartum diagnosis and postpartum management of neonates affected by HDFN require close collaboration among obstetric, neonatal, and transfusion medical teams. Delivery is generally induced around 36 weeks of gestation. All neonates at risk should have cord blood taken for measurement of hemoglobin, DAT, and bilirubin (see Chapter 43), although the utility of the DAT in this context has recently been questioned.[14] Because of the use of intrauterine transfusions, many neonates have normal hemoglobin at birth and develop only modest hyperbilirubinemia. In these neonates, the DAT demonstrates few antibody-covered red cells, and typing barely reveals the neonate's original blood type. However, all potentially affected neonates should remain in the hospital until hyperbilirubinemia and/or anemia is under control and appropriate follow-up is organized, even if phototherapy, high-dose IVIG, and exchange transfusions may not be required. Red cell transfusions can be indicated when anemia develops during the first weeks after birth. Severe anemia (hemoglobin <10 g/dL) at birth or rapidly increasing hyperbilirubinemia should be treated as discussed later in this chapter.

Early-onset/rapidly progressive hemolytic disease not predicted by maternal antibody screening

Today, neonatal pediatricians in countries with high HDI most often observe HDFN in relatively full-term infants whose mothers' antepartum screening was negative. Within the first 48 hours of life, such newborns develop early-onset jaundice with a total bilirubin already exceeding 20 mg/dL (342 μmol/L).[3] Because the problem in such cases was not predicted by antepartum screening for maternal antibodies, therapy would not have been started. The most common causes of HDFN presenting in this way are as follows:

- ABO incompatibility;
- Hemoglobinopathies;
- Erythrocyte enzyme defects; and
- Disorders of the red cell membrane.

The reader is referred to Chapter 11 for detailed information on the three latter conditions.

ABO incompatibility

ABO incompatibility is now the leading cause of HDFN in high-HDI countries.[12] HDFN resulting from ABO incompatibility generally occurs only in offspring of women of blood group O because IgG anti-A and anti-B are far more common in group O than in group A or B mothers, and are confined to the 1% with high antepartum titers of IgG antibodies.[16] Unlike in non-ABO HDFN, even the first ABO-incompatible infant of a mother is at risk for significant hemolysis, because ABO antibodies are present before pregnancy. If a mother has born an infant with significant ABO incompatibility, subsequent siblings are at greater risk of having the same problem. Minor degrees of red cell destruction are common, as shown by the increased incidence of neonatal jaundice, albeit the

hemoglobin values may be normal or slightly lower in ABO-incompatible infants compared to ABO-compatible infants.[7] With respect to ethnic groups, the prevalence of maternal-newborn ABO incompatibility ranges from 31% in those of European ancestry to 50% in Asians. For the most part, ABO HDFN causes only mild to moderate neonatal jaundice, which is detected 24 hours after delivery. In very rare cases, however, hemolysis is severe enough to cause hydrops.[17] The frequency of HDFN caused by anti-A is only about 1 in 150 births, and even lower for anti-B.[3] The higher frequencies that have been reported from Africa and Saudi Arabia are probably related to more potent anti-A and anti-B (caused by environmental factors) and a relatively strong expression of A and B antigens.[7]

Antepartum and postpartum serologic tests are poor predictors of ABO hemolytic disease. The results of the DAT in HDFN caused by ABO incompatibility are very different from those observed with HDFN caused by anti-D (not treated antepartum). In the latter, a positive DAT can be observed even in cases showing minor clinical symptoms. However, in ABO incompatibility only 20% to 40% of incompatible pairs demonstrate a positive reaction, and significant hemolysis can be observed with a negative or only weakly positive DAT. In infants with a positive DAT result, the test differentiates poorly between newborns with clinical hemolysis and unaffected newborns. Only about 10% of the DAT-positive, ABO-incompatible maternal-fetal pairs develop clinically significant HDFN. However, in infants with clinically significant hemolysis, >80% have a positive DAT.[12,18] Also, the clinical symptoms differ in that anti-A and anti-B HDFN result mainly in hyperbilirubinemia detected within 24 hours after delivery, but do not evince the significant fetal or neonatal anemia observed in anti-D HDFN. This is explained by the few and unbranched A and B antigen sites on fetal red cells, allowing antibody-coated cells to remain in the circulation longer than in anti-D HDFN. Another important factor is that ABO antigens are expressed on virtually all cells in the body, whereas D antigen is restricted to red cells. Thus, anti-D is "focused" to red cells, whereas anti-A and anti-B are absorbed by tissues and neutralized by soluble A and B substances in plasma. As a reflection of this, the blood film in anti-A or anti-B HDFN shows a large number of spherocytes, with little or no increase in nucleated red cells. In anti-D HDFN, there are few spherocytes but large numbers of nucleated red cells. However, in ethnic groups that express strong (many and branched) A and B antigen sites, severe anemia, nucleated red cells, and significant antepartum morbidity (even with hydrops fetalis) can be observed.[3]

Management of ABO HDFN is usually successful with modern phototherapy alone. Close monitoring of affected neonates is important, as HDIVIG adjuvant therapy and occasionally even exchange transfusion may be required. The latter is particularly relevant in individuals from certain ethnic groups who express strong A and B sites.[3] However, it should be noted that there is no consensus on the use of HDIVIG for ABO incompatibility. Thus, although some report a very salutary effect, others find no effect and remain critical.[19,20]

Hemoglobinopathies

Except for α-thalassemia major, hemoglobinopathies generally do not cause antepartum or neonatal problems. Some occasional structural mutations in α and γ genes that give no symptoms in adults can, however, result in transient hemolytic anemia in neonates. Mutations in the β genes (e.g., sickle cell disease or β-thalassemia) give no symptoms at birth because of the predominance of fetal hemoglobin.

α-thalassemia major occurs when all four α-globin genes on the homologous chromosome 16 are deleted (α°), and it is predominantly seen in some Mediterranean island populations and in Southeast Asia. The lack of α-globin production leads to the dominating production of fetal γ_4 hemoglobin (hemoglobin Bart's), which has a very high oxygen affinity and is physiologically useless. Infants are usually stillborn between 28 and 40 weeks, demonstrating the typical picture of hydrops fetalis with pallor, generalized edema, and massive hepatosplenomegaly. The few that are live-born expire within the first hours after birth. Postpartum management has no impact on survival unless combined with carefully planned antepartum therapy, and it has to be followed up with lifelong red cell transfusions or hematopoietic stem cell transplantation. Checking blood samples from the parents will show whether they are carriers of the α° gene (hypochromic, microcytic red cells). The diagnosis is confirmed by hemoglobin electrophoresis.

α- and γ-globin chain structural abnormalities are generally clinically silent, but can result in occasional neonatal hemolytic anemia due to formation of unstable αγ-hemoglobin. When the fetal γ-globin is replaced by adult β-globin, the hemolytic anemia resolves. Diagnosis is confirmed by hemoglobin high-performance liquid chromatography. For further details and information, see Chapter 11.

Red cell enzyme defects

The important enzyme defects in the neonatal period are glucose-6-phosphate dehydrogenase (G6PD) deficiency and pyruvate kinase (PK) deficiency, but pyrimidine 5′ nucleotidase deficiency should also be remembered. They may present with early-onset, often severe hyperbilirubinemia. The blood smear is normal in G6PD and PK, and anemia is rare. Family medical history and measurement of the relevant pretransfusion enzyme activities are of diagnostic importance.

G6PD deficiency is transmitted in an X-linked recessive form, and seen in all ethnic groups; however, its highest prevalence is in central Africa (20%) and the Mediterranean region (10%). It has been shown that the genes for three important enzymes in bilirubin metabolism can interact to produce significant hyperbilirubinemia. These are, in addition to the G6PD gene, the genes for uridine diphosphate glucuronosyl transferase 1A1 (UGT1A1) and solute carrier organic anion transporter polypeptide (SLCO1B1).[21] Variants in the gene for UGT1A1, known as Gilbert syndrome, have also been shown to interact with the gene for hereditary spherocytosis to augment neonatal jaundice.[22,23] Thus, because patients with known or suspected heredity for one or more of these genes can develop severe hyperbilirubinemia, close monitoring is important.[24] Interaction with other risk factors for hyperbilirubinemia in the newborn, as well as a number of medicines (e.g., sulphonamides and primaquine), infections, chemicals, and foods (fava beans are particularly infamous for their role in precipitating severe hemolysis in G6PD deficiency), can severely aggravate the clinical picture.

Pyruvate kinase deficiency is autosomal recessive, and it is the second most common red cell enzyme defect in neonates. The severity varies from hydrops fetalis to severe early-onset neonatal hyperbilirubinemia, and mild hyperbilirubinemia mimicking physiologic jaundice. For further details and information, see Chapter 11.

Pyrimidine 5′ nucleotidase deficiency is the third most common red cell enzyme defect, and has on occasion presented with neonatal jaundice that was sufficiently severe to require multiple exchange transfusions.[25] The blood film is notable for marked basophilic stippling of the red cells. Inheritance is autosomal recessive, the gene is localized on 7p15-p14, and the complementary DNA (cDNA) has been cloned and sequenced.[26]

Red cell membrane defects

The main clues that a neonate has a red cell membrane disorder are a family history, DAT-negative hemolysis (with a sensitive method), and an abnormal blood film. Red cell membrane electrophoresis from pretransfusion samples is diagnostic.

Hereditary spherocytosis is the most common red cell membrane defect. It occurs in 1 in 5000 live births in couples of North European ethnicity, but is less frequent in other population groups. It is inherited as an autosomal dominant trait.[3] Blood films have a similar appearance to those in ABO HDFN; the DAT is negative. Some neonates require one or two red cell transfusions during the first months of life.

Hereditary elliptocytosis is a more complex autosomal dominant disorder. In heterozygotes, the only findings are elliptocytes in the blood smear. Neonates who have more than one mutation in a red cell membrane protein (homozygotes or compound homozygotes) have severe, transfusion-dependent, hemolytic anemia. The blood film is characteristic, showing a high proportion of bizarre fragmented red cells and microcytes (mean corpuscular volume <60 fL). Red cell transfusion is often necessary until splenectomy can be carried out. For further details and information, see Chapters 11 and 46.

Management of immune-mediated hemolytic disease of the fetus and newborn

Surveillance and tests

Antepartum surveillance and treatment are detailed in Chapter 43. After adequate intrauterine transfusion treatment, fetal erythropoiesis is suppressed, and the red cell mass maintained by compatible transfused cells. As a result, most of these neonates present neither neonatal jaundice nor anemia of clinical importance after birth, and very few require exchange transfusion postpartum. In contrast, late anemia is common in the newborn because of suppression of erythropoiesis caused by intrauterine transfusions and the continued presence of hemolyzing maternal antibodies. Therefore, the neonates need follow-up with monitoring of hemoglobin, blood film, reticulocyte count, and bilirubin in order to determine when hemolysis has stopped and endogenous red cell production takes over.[3] In any consideration of red cell transfusions, the neonate's general condition, growth, and development are of major importance in determining the appropriate hemoglobin level for intervention (see Chapter 46).

In countries with low HDI, antepartum treatment is mostly unavailable, and even antibody screening and ABO/Rh typing are often not performed in the pregnant mother. In such areas, the clinical picture can be more like that seen in high-HDI countries in the 1960s, with serious anti-D HDFN (erythroblastosis, hyperbilirubinemia with grave anemia on the first postpartum day, and, in serious cases, hydrops fetalis or even stillbirth).

Phototherapy

Improved delivery and understanding of phototherapy since its introduction in the late 1950s have had major effects on the clinical treatment of HDFN. The efficacy of phototherapy depends on the following factors:[27]

- Spectral qualities of the delivered light (wavelength range 400–520 nm, with peak emissions of 460 nm);

Norwegian guidelines for management of neonatal jaundice†

Date and time (h/min) of birth........../.........-......... h.......min.........

Birthweight.............. g   Maternal blood group...................   Infant's blood group.................

DAT (Coombs).............. Gestational age (weeks) ....

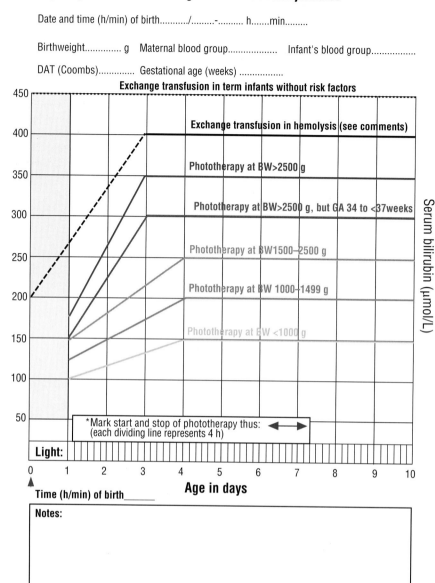

Figure 45.1 Guidelines for treatment of neonatal jaundice as currently practiced in Norway. Birth weights are used in lieu of gestational ages to reflect the impact of varying maturation. When considerable hyperbilirubinemia persist, other diagnosis should be considered. This graph is presented for illustration purposes only. Local and national variations in epidemiology and healthcare delivery systems may suggest other approaches. Source: Norwegian Pediatric Association. Reproduced with permission.

†By consensus at the fall meeting of the Norwegian Pediatric Society, 2006.

- Intensity of light (irradiance) delivered to the skin surface;*
- Skin surface area receiving phototherapy;*
- Distance from infant's skin to light source;
- Total serum bilirubin concentration at the start of phototherapy;
- The cause of jaundice; and
- Duration of exposure.

Modern phototherapy devices with high-intensity gallium nitride light-emitting diodes (LEDs) are small, efficient, and easy to use.[27] The total radiation applied to a neonate has vastly increased and made *intensive phototherapy* an important alternative to exchange transfusion, even in the treatment of severe HDFN. *Intensive*

phototherapy implies radiation in the blue-green spectrum (wavelengths ~430–490 nm) of at least $30\,\mu W/cm^2/nm$ (measured at the infant's skin) and delivered to as much as possible of the infant's body surface area.[28] Figure 45.1 shows the Norwegian Pediatric Association guidelines for phototherapy in neonates with hyperbilirubinemia. The levels shown are approximations adapted to the infant's age. Note that birthweight strata are used in lieu of gestational ages to (approximately) represent the impact of varying maturation.

Please note that in showing these guidelines, the authors do not mean to suggest that these could or should be applied uncritically in other countries with different healthcare delivery systems. Specific factors as regards how birthing and neonatal care and follow-up are organized must be taken into consideration. Such factors, and not merely where intervention lines are drawn on a chart, can

---

* *Spectral power* is a key concept in phototherapy, and is the product of the irradiance and the size of the irradiated area. Practically speaking, high irradiance is of limited benefit if the size of the irradiated area is small.

contribute to the ability of a country to avoid kernicterus, the devastating neurological sequelae of severe jaundice.[29] In addition, we recommend a close study of the American Academy of Pediatrics (AAP) guidelines.[28] These are carefully researched and well argued, and contain a wealth of information, which is very important to the understanding of the mechanisms and practical execution of jaundice treatment. Thus, they merit careful study by anyone planning to formulate or adapt local or national guidelines for jaundice management.

Today, the "typical" neonate with HDFN presents in countries of high HDI as a well, term neonate with ABO incompatibility and a total serum bilirubin often in excess of 20 mg/dL (342 μmol/L) but without significant anemia. Intensive phototherapy, during the 2 to 6 hours it often takes to organize an exchange transfusion, may result in a significant decrease in total serum bilirubin, thus frequently removing the indication for exchange transfusion.[3] In addition, conversion of a significant amount (25% or more) of circulating bilirubin to more water-soluble isomers could theoretically lessen the transfer of bilirubin across the blood–brain barrier and into the brain.[30] When HDIVIG is given as adjuvant to phototherapy, the need for exchange transfusion may be even further reduced.

High-dose intravenous immunoglobulin

Since the beginning of the 1990s, several studies have reported the effect of HDIVIG as an adjuvant to standard therapy for HDFN. Two systematic reviews have performed a meta-analysis of the impact of HDIVIG on the use of exchange transfusion, comparing IVIG plus phototherapy with phototherapy alone.[31,32] The conclusion of both reviews was that IVIG significantly reduced the risk for exchange transfusion. However, the authors of the two systematic reviews differ with respect to their recommendation as to the use of HDIVIG. The Cochrane review[31] concludes that the number and quality of studies, and the number of infants included, is too small to recommend the use of adjuvant IVIG in HDFN, and suggests further well-designed studies. However, the other review[32] supports the use of high-dose IVIG, and also shows that when IVIG is used in addition to phototherapy in HDFN, both duration of phototherapy and hospital stay are reduced to a point that equals the cost of the IVIG in the United Kingdom. Recently the IVIG Hematology and Neurology Expert Panels have recommended that HDIVIG be offered to neonates with HDFN as treatment for severe hyperbilirubinemia[33] and endorsed the recommendations outlined in the AAP guidelines on the treatment of hyperbilirubinemia. The AAP guidelines state:

> In isoimmune hemolytic disease, administration of IVIG (0.5–1.0 g/kg over 2 hours) is recommended if the total serum bilirubin (TSB) is rising despite intensive phototherapy or the TSB level is within 2 to 3 mg/dl (34–51 μmol/L) of exchange level. If necessary, this dose can be repeated in 12 hours.

It has been argued that the results of several HDIVIG studies were confounded by the concurrent introduction of newer phototherapy devices with much higher irradiance.[20] Although this cannot be ruled out completely, Huizing et al., in a study with a historical control cohort, found no effect of change of phototherapy devices, while confirming the salutary effect of HDIVIG in both Rh- and ABO-HDFN.[19] Two recent prospective studies failed to find a significant effect of HDIVIG as far as reducing the need for exchange transfusion.[34,35] None of these studies are, due to design and patient selection, comparable to the cited study by Huizing

et al.[19] Thus, of the Rh-disease patients in the Dutch study,[34] 66% had been treated with intrauterine transfusions, signifying very aggressive immunization. It is not surprising that with such a high load of circulating Rh antibodies, a relatively moderate dose of IVIG should not be sufficient to block or reduce the effect. In the Brazilian study,[35] HDIVIG or placebo was given prophylactically, and thus was not targeted toward infants most likely to need exchange transfusion. In comparison, in the retrospective study by Huizing et al.,[19] HDIVIG was only given to infants who had crossed, or were just about to cross, the intervention line for exchange transfusion. Thus, this strategy targeted infants who would have been exchanged using the historical algorithm. A similar strategy was employed by Elalfy et al.[36] with findings also supporting the utility of IVIG.

Exchange transfusions are associated with a mortality of 2% and serious complications in 12% of the patients, and with decreasing opportunities to attain and maintain the necessary procedural skills, these numbers are unlikely to improve. Conversely, phototherapy, when properly performed, is largely considered to be an innocuous procedure, although some concern has recently been raised about increased lethality in tiny, immature infants of <750 g birthweight.[37] It must be remembered that IVIG is a pooled plasma product, which before the introduction of adequate pathogen inactivation was involved in several cases of viral transmission. However, since 1994, there has been no transmission of blood-borne infections with pathogen-inactivated IVIG prepared from selected donors[33] (see also Chapter 31). Of some concern is a recent report that HDIVIG increased the risk of necrotizing enterocolitis in term and near-term infants with hemolytic disease.[38] Of note, this study was retrospective, whereas in another retrospective study no such side effects were described.[19] Thus, whether further randomized studies, as suggested by the authors of the Cochrane meta-analysis,[31] are called for or appropriate may be a matter for discussion and careful evaluation.

Exchange transfusions

The criteria used to assess the need for exchange transfusion include total bilirubin level, hemoglobin level, and clinical symptoms. Traditional guidelines suggest exchange transfusion in the following circumstances:

Within 12 hours of birth if:

- Cord blood bilirubin concentration exceeds 3 to 5 mg/dL (50–85 μmol/L) for preterm infants, and 5 to 7 mg/dL (85–120 μmol/L) for term infants, or the rate of increase is >0.5 mg/dL/hour (8.5 μmol/L/h); and
- Severe anemia: hemoglobin <10 g/dL combined with hyperbilirubinemia.

After 24 hours of birth if:

- Total bilirubin concentration >20 mg/dL (342 μmol/L) or a bilirubin increase of >0.5 mg/dL/hour (8.5 μmol/L/h), or hemoglobin <10 g/dL combined with hyperbilirubinemia.

Today, the effect of intensive phototherapy and reduction of hemolysis by HDIVIG treatment almost always results in a considerable decrease in bilirubin levels during the 2 to 6 hours needed to set up an exchange transfusion. Thus, the clinical indication for exchange transfusion may be removed, but the need for simple transfusion increases.[3] Exchange transfusions are considered indicated when intensive phototherapy, with or without IVIG, fails to adequately reduce bilirubin concentration or when the initial serum bilirubin places the infant at risk for kernicterus. Also, depending on the medico-legal situation in the area of practice, some would argue that regardless of the effect of high-intensity phototherapy and

HDIVIG on total serum bilirubin levels, an exchange transfusion should be carried out if the infant has shown signs of acute intermediate-to-advanced bilirubin encephalopathy (discussed further here). Factors potentiating bilirubin toxicity include immune-mediated hemolysis, acid–base disturbances, asphyxia, free heme groups, and other byproducts of hemolysis or drugs that displace bilirubin from albumin and other plasma-binding proteins.[9]

Figure 45.1 shows current Norwegian guidelines for exchange transfusion as well as phototherapy in neonates with hyperbilirubinemia.[29] As stated in this chapter regarding the phototherapy part of the guidelines, the authors do not mean to suggest that these guidelines for exchange transfusion in neonates could or should be applied uncritically in other countries with different healthcare delivery systems.. Treatment decisions after the first 24 hours are dependent upon degree of maturity versus immaturity (here approximately represented by birthweights), bilirubin concentration, the rate of its increase and risk factors that have a potentially negative effect on bilirubin–albumin binding, the permeability of the blood–brain barrier, and the susceptibility of brain cells to damage by bilirubin. Such factors may include hemolysis, acidosis, septicemia, low serum albumin concentration, or an infant appearing generally sick. In the presence of one or more such risk factors, clinical judgment may suggest performing an exchange transfusion at TSB levels 50–100 μmol/L lower than those indicated by graph lines. Immediate exchange transfusion is recommended if the infant shows signs of acute bilirubin encephalopathy.

Exchange transfusions supply the neonate with compatible red cells and fresh plasma, while incompatible red cells, bilirubin, and maternal antibodies in plasma are removed. A standard exchange transfusion of twice the infant's blood volume reduces incompatible fetal red cells by about 85%; bilirubin and maternal antibody concentrations are reduced by 25% to 45%.[8] The amount of blood needed for an exchange transfusion is 170 mL/kg (200 mL/kg in preterm infants), with 25–50 mL added to compensate for dead-space in tubing and blood warmer. An exchange transfusion consists of hemoglobin S-negative red cells that are compatible with maternal serum and/or plasma and are reconstituted with fresh frozen group AB plasma to obtain a hematocrit of 45% to 60%, depending on the desired end result as far as hematocrit. The blood should be leukocyte-reduced (to prevent transmission of cytomegalovirus), irradiated, and preferably <5 days old. Platelet addition needs only be considered if an infant's platelet count is seriously compromised, or after multiple exchange transfusions.

In view of the declining number of exchange transfusions and the risks involved with the procedure, it is important that maternity and neonatal services develop, maintain, and teach appropriate written guidelines for the use of exchange transfusion in HDFN and the performance of the procedure itself.

Conclusion

In immune-mediated HDFN, maternal IgG antibodies—usually related to the ABO, Rh, or Kell blood groups—cross the placental barrier, causing hemolysis of fetal red cells. HDFN caused by hereditary red cell disorders is less frequent, but in some geographic areas the possibility of co-occurrence of genetic variants relevant to bilirubin metabolism needs to be kept in mind. Although HDFN can be fatal, advances in diagnosis, treatment, and prevention have made immune-mediated HDFN increasingly controllable in countries with high HDI. Diagnostic modalities include maternal assays, antepartum treatment, and routine prophylactic RhIG given to D-negative women at risk. Postpartum management includes treatment of hyperbilirubinemia and anemia. Hyperbilirubinemia is usually treated by means of *intensive phototherapy*, and adjuvant HDIVIG may be given to reduce hemolysis. In addition, anemia is corrected by simple transfusion of red cells. These approaches have reduced the indications for exchange transfusion to very severe HDFN or when intensive phototherapy combined with IVIG fail to reduce hyperbilirubinemia to levels that are considered safe. With further improvement of phototherapy equipment and practice, IVIG treatment could reduce the need of exchange transfusions and change the spectrum of HDFN treatment even more. Administration of D-penicillamine and/or metalloporphyrins to reduce bilirubin formation are therapies that may turn out to be useful in the future,[39] but none of these drugs have thus far received regulatory approval for use in jaundiced neonates.

Although mortality and morbidity of HDFN have been greatly reduced in countries with high HDI, HDFN still poses a serious challenge in many countries with low HDI. In these countries, introduction of maternal assays, routine prophylactic RhIG treatment, and affordable phototherapy should be encouraged. Currently, studies are underway in low-resource settings to filter sunlight, using sheets of films that remove most ultraviolet and significant levels of infrared light, while transmitting effective levels of therapeutic blue light.[40] Because high-dose IVIG often will be beyond economic reach, phototherapy combined with drugs to reduce the postpartum formation of bilirubin could be of interest.[39]

Disclaimer

The authors have disclosed no conflicts of interest.

Key References

A full reference list for this chapter is available at: http://www.wiley.com/go/simon/transfusion

1 Crowther CA, Middleton P, McBain RD. Anti-D administration in pregnancy for preventing Rhesus alloimmunsation. *Cochrane Database Syst Rev* 2013;**2**: CD000020. doi: 10.1002/14651858.CD000020.pub2

2 Fung Kee Fung K, Eason E, *et al*. Prevention of Rh alloimmunization. *J Obstet Gynecol Can* 2003;**25**:765–73.

3 Murray NA, Roberts IAG. Hemolytic disease of the newborn. *Arch Dis Child Fetal Neonatal Ed* 2007;**92**:F83–8.

7 Haemolytic disease of the fetus and newborn. In: Klein HG, Anstee DJ. *Mollison's blood transfusion in clinical medicine*. 12th ed. Oxford: Wiley-Blackwell, 2014:499–548.

10 Blood grouping techniques. In: Klein HG, Anstee DJ. *Mollison's blood transfusion in clinical medicine*. 12th ed. Oxford: Wiley-Blackwell, 2014:303–55.

13 Cortey A, Brossard Y. Prevention of fetomaternal rhesus-D alloimmunization. Practical aspects. *J Gynecol Obstet Biol Reprod (Paris)* 2006;**35** (1 Suppl.):1S123–30.

21 Watchko J, Lin Z. Exploring the genetic architecture of neonatal hyperbilirubinemia. *Semin Fetal Neonat Med* 2010;**15**:169–75.

28 American Academy of Pediatrics Subcommittee on Hyperbilirubinemia. Management of hyperbilirubinemia in the newborn infant 35 or more weeks of gestation. *Pediatrics* 2004;**114**:297–316.

32 Gottstein R, Cooke RWI. Systematic review of intravenous immunoglobulin in haemolytic disease of the newborn. *Arch Dis Child Fetal Neonatal Ed* 2003;**88**: F6–10.

33 Anderson D, Ali K, Blanchette V, *et al*. Guidelines on the use of intravenous immune globulin for hematologic conditions. *Transfus Med Rev* 2007;**21**:S9–56.

CHAPTER 46

Red blood cell transfusions for neonates and infants

Ronald G. Strauss

LifeSource/Institute for Transfusion Medicine, Chicago, IL, USA

The majority of preterm neonates and/or infants, particularly those with birthweight below 1.0 kg, receive transfusions. Because of the frequency of transfusions to these tiny patients and the many controversial aspects of neonatal and infant transfusion management, this chapter will focus on neonates and infants. For the most part, older children are transfused following guidelines similar to those for adults, and they will not be discussed further in this chapter.

Many aspects of hematopoiesis are either incompletely developed in preterm infants or adapted to serve the fetus (i.e., the intrauterine counterpart to a live-born preterm neonate that may possess characteristics of extremely low-birthweight infants). This lack of complete development and/or adaptation to extrauterine life diminishes the capacity of the neonate to produce red blood cells (RBCs), platelets, and neutrophils—particularly during the stress of life-threatening illnesses encountered after preterm birth such as sepsis, severe pulmonary dysfunction, necrotizing enterocolitis, and immune cytopenias. Similarly, hepatic function is immature, and the result is low levels of both plasma clotting and anticoagulant proteins. The serious medical and surgical problems of preterm birth can be further complicated by phlebotomy blood losses, bleeding, hemolysis, and consumptive coagulopathy. Thus, preterm infants begin life with quantities of blood cells and hemostatic proteins that are barely adequate. Furthermore, these infants have a diminished ability to further increase production adequately to compensate for the hematologic problems they experience. These circumstances lead to the need for blood component transfusions—of which RBC transfusions are the most numerous and will be discussed in this chapter (see Chapter 47 for platelet and plasma transfusions).

Preterm infants, especially those with a birthweight less than 1.0 kg and with respiratory distress, are given numerous RBC transfusions early in life because of several interacting factors. Neonates delivered before 28 weeks of gestation (birthweight <1.0 kg) are born before the bulk of iron transport has occurred from mother to fetus via the placenta and before the onset of marked erythropoietic activity of fetal marrow during the third trimester. Hence, preterm infants of very low birthweight enter extrauterine life with low iron stores and a small circulating volume mass of RBCs. Soon after preterm birth, severe respiratory disease can lead to repeated blood sampling for laboratory studies and, consequently, to replacement RBC transfusions. As a final factor, preterm infants are unable to mount an effective erythropoietin (EPO) response to decreasing numbers of RBCs; this factor contributes to the diminished ability to compensate for anemia and enhances the need for transfusions.

The physiology of hematopoiesis in the fetus and newborn is discussed in detail in Chapter 44, hemolytic disease of the fetus and newborn in Chapter 45, and congenital hemolytic anemias in Chapter 11. Accordingly, only the aspects of physiology and pathophysiology that pertain to neonatal transfusion medicine, in general, are included here. The emphasis is on transfusion management during the first several weeks after birth.

Red cell transfusion

Pathophysiology of anemia of prematurity

During the first weeks of life, all infants experience a decline in the number of circulating RBCs caused by physiologic factors. In sick preterm infants, phlebotomy blood losses also contribute to the decline. In healthy term infants, the nadir blood hemoglobin value rarely decreases to less than 9 g/dL (mean = 11 to 12 g/dL) at an age of approximately 10 to 12 weeks.[1] Because this postnatal decrease in hemoglobin level is universal and is well tolerated by term infants, it is commonly called the *physiologic anemia of infancy*. Among preterm infants, this decline occurs at an earlier age and is more pronounced in severity. Mean hemoglobin concentration decreases to approximately 8 g/dL in infants of 1.0 to 1.5 kg birthweight and to 7 g/dL in infants weighing less than 1.0 kg.[2] In preterm infants, this marked decline in hemoglobin frequently is exacerbated by phlebotomy blood losses and may be associated with symptomatic anemia that necessitates RBC transfusions, making the *anemia of prematurity* unacceptable as a "purely physiologic" event.

Physiologic factors that influence erythropoiesis and the biologic characteristics of EPO are critical in the pathogenesis of the anemia of prematurity. Growth is extremely rapid during the first weeks of life, and RBC production by neonatal marrow must increase commensurately to avoid a decreasing hematocrit caused by an insufficient number of circulating RBCs being diluted within the expanding blood volume. It is widely accepted that the circulating life span of neonatal RBCs in the bloodstream is shorter than that of adult RBCs. This shorter survival of neonatal RBCs, quite possibly, is an artifact in part because studies of transfused autologous RBCs

Rossi's Principles of Transfusion Medicine, Fifth Edition. Edited by Toby L. Simon, Jeffrey McCullough, Edward L. Snyder, Bjarte G. Solheim, and Ronald G. Strauss.
© 2016 John Wiley & Sons, Ltd. Published 2016 by John Wiley & Sons, Ltd.

labeled with biotin or radioactive chromium may underestimate RBC survival in the infant's bloodstream for technical reasons. In healthy adults—when body size is stable so that blood and RBC volumes are constant (i.e., not increasing with growing body size and commensurate increase in erythropoiesis), when no transfusions are given, and when large volumes of blood are not being taken for laboratory studies—the gradual disappearance of transfused labeled RBCs, caused by dilution with RBCs produced endogenously by the marrow, accurately reflects RBC survival in the bloodstream. In contrast, one or more confounding factors (i.e., growth, RBC transfusions, and phlebotomy) exists in infants—particularly, sick preterms—thus introducing error into the calculations performed when RBC survival is determined, based on disappearance of labeled RBCs.

In addition, a key clinical factor is the need for repeated blood sampling to monitor the condition of critically ill neonates. Small preterm infants are the most critically ill, require the most frequent blood sampling, and suffer the greatest proportional loss of RBCs because their circulating cell volumes are smallest. In the past, the mean volume of blood removed for sampling has been reported to range from 0.8 to 3.1 mL/kg/day during the first few weeks of life for preterm infants requiring intensive care. Promising "in-line" devices that withdraw blood, measure multiple analytes, and then reinfuse the sampled blood have been reported.[3,4] They have decreased the need for RBC transfusions. However, until these devices are proven more extensively to be practical, effective, and safe, replacement of blood losses from phlebotomy will remain a critical factor responsible for transfusions given to critically ill neonates—particularly, transfusions given during the first four weeks of life.

A key reason that the nadir hemoglobin values of preterm infants are lower than those of term infants is that preterm infants have a relatively diminished EPO plasma level in response to anemia.[5] Although anemia provokes EPO production in premature infants, the plasma levels achieved in anemic infants, at any given hematocrit, are lower than those observed in comparably anemic older persons.[6] Erythroid progenitor cells of preterm infants are quite responsive to EPO in vitro—a finding suggesting that inadequate production of EPO (not marrow unresponsiveness) is the major cause of physiologic anemia.[7]

The mechanisms responsible for the diminished EPO output by preterm neonates are only partially defined and likely are multiple. One mechanism is that the primary site of EPO production in preterm infants is in the liver, rather than kidneys.[8] This dependency on hepatic EPO is important because the liver is less sensitive to anemia and tissue hypoxia—resulting in a relatively sluggish EPO response to the decreasing hematocrit. The timing of the switch from the liver to kidneys is set at conception and is not accelerated by preterm birth. Viewed from a teleologic perspective, decreased hepatic production of EPO under in utero conditions of tissue hypoxia may be an advantage for the fetus. If this were not the case, normal levels of fetal hypoxia in utero could trigger high levels of EPO and produce erythrocytosis and consequent hyperviscosity. Following birth, however, diminished EPO responsiveness to tissue hypoxia is disadvantageous and leads to anemia because it impairs compensation for low hematocrit levels caused by rapid growth and RBC losses caused by phlebotomy, clinical bleeding, hemolysis, and so on.

Diminished EPO production cannot entirely explain low plasma EPO levels in preterm infants, because extraordinarily high plasma levels of EPO have been reported in some fetuses and infants.[9,10]

Moreover, macrophages from human cord blood produce normal quantities of EPO messenger RNA and protein.[11] Thus, additional mechanisms contribute to diminished EPO plasma levels. For example, plasma levels of EPO are influenced by metabolism (clearance) as well as by production. Data in human infants[12] have demonstrated low plasma EPO levels resulting from increased plasma clearance, increased volume of distribution, more rapid fractional elimination, and shorter mean plasma residence times than comparative values in adults. Thus, accelerated catabolism accentuates the problem of diminished EPO production, so that the low plasma EPO levels are a combined effect of decreased synthesis plus increased metabolism.

Red cell transfusion practices

RBC transfusions are given to maintain the hematocrit at a level judged best for the clinical condition of the infant.[13] General guidelines acceptable to most neonatologists are listed in Table 46.1. However, many aspects of neonatal RBC transfusion therapy are controversial and vary from center to center. This lack of consistency stems from incomplete knowledge of the cellular and molecular biology of erythropoiesis during the perinatal period, of the pathophysiologic effects of neonatal anemia, and of the infant's physiological response to RBC transfusions. In some instances the value of RBC transfusions is clear (e.g., to manage anemia that has caused congestive heart failure), but in others it is not (e.g., to correct irregular patterns of heart or respiratory rates), and practices are based largely on logical assumptions. Although well-designed clinical trials are being reported,[14,15] they are not completely mutually supportive and questions remain. Therefore, it is important that pediatricians critically evaluate the guidelines in Table 46.1 and apply them in light of neonatal practice at their respective institutions.

An important controversy that is still unresolved is the wisdom—or lack thereof—of prescribing RBC transfusions for neonates using restrictive guidelines (i.e., low pretransfusion hematocrit values) versus liberal guidelines (i.e., conventional, relatively high pretransfusion hematocrit values). Two of the three randomized controlled trials will be discussed.[14,15] Although many of their initial results agreed, they disagreed in one extremely important way—specifically, whether preterm infants were at increased risk of brain injury when given RBCs per restrictive guidelines (i.e., due to undertransfusion). In both trials, preterm infants were randomly assigned to receive small-volume RBC transfusions per either restrictive or liberal guidelines—with guidelines based on a combination of the pretransfusion hematocrit or hemoglobin level, age of the neonate, and clinical condition at the time each transfusion was given.

Both studies found that neonates in the restrictive transfusion group received fewer transfusions without an increase in mortality or morbidity based on several clinical outcomes. However, one critical discrepancy was present. Bell et al.[14] found increases in apnea, intraventricular bleeding, and brain leukomalacia in infants transfused per restrictive guidelines, whereas Kirpalani et al.[15] found no differences between infants in the restrictive versus liberal groups. Moreover, rates of serious outcomes were fairly high in both groups of the Kirpalani study—perhaps a result of the extreme prematurity of the infants. However, because neonates in the liberal transfusion group of Bell et al. likely had substantially higher hematocrit and hemoglobin levels than neonates in the liberal group of Kirpalani et al. (an average hematocrit of 6% or a hemoglobin level of 2 g/dL higher), it was speculated that the higher

Table 46.1 Guidelines for small-volume red cell transfusions

- Maintain >35% to 40% hematocrit for *severe* cardiopulmonary disease.
- Maintain >30% to 35% hematocrit for *moderate* cardiopulmonary disease.
- Maintain >30% to 35% hematocrit for *major* surgery.
- Maintain >20% to 25% hematocrit for infants with *stable* anemia, especially with:
  Unexplained breathing disorders
  Unexplained tachycardia
  Unexplained poor growth.

Words in italics must be defined locally. For example, *severe* pulmonary disease may be defined as requiring mechanical ventilation with >0.35 FiO_2 and *moderate* as less intensive assisted ventilation.

hematocrit levels, in some way, protected liberally transfused infants in the Bell study.[14,15]

However, long-term neurologic follow-up studies for the US trial—performed years later when the subjects were approximately 11 years old—surprisingly revealed that intracranial volumes were substantially smaller in the transfused infants in the liberal arm than in those in the restrictive arm. In addition, the children in the liberal arm also were found to perform more poorly than those in the restrictive arm on measures of fluency, visual memory, and reading.[16,17] In the multicenter Canadian study, long-term follow-up at age approximately 18 months revealed no statistically significant difference in combined death or severe adverse neurodevelopmental outcomes—supporting their initial conclusions. However, to add to the confusion, in a post hoc analysis there was a significant difference favoring the liberal transfusion strategy. Thus, it is unclear whether a relatively high pretransfusion hemoglobin value is *neuroprotective* or *neurodamaging*. To this end, a definitive randomized clinical trial, Transfusion of Prematures (TOP), commenced in 2013 and will randomly assign 1824 very-low-birth-weight (VLBW, <1000 g) infants to a liberal or restrictive RBC transfusion protocol. The pretransfusion hemoglobin thresholds will be based on the presence of respiratory support and postnatal age, with the primary outcome of death or significant neurodevelopmental impairment in survivors at a corrected age of 22–26 years. Hopefully, this trial will definitively answer the question of whether liberal or restrictive RBC transfusion guidelines are best for premature infants.

Until more definitive data are available, the rationale underlying the recommendations for RBC transfusions in Table 46.1 are as follows.

Maintain hematocrit >35% to 40% for severe cardiopulmonary disease

In neonates with severe respiratory disease, such as those requiring high volumes of oxygen with ventilator support, it is customary to maintain the hematocrit at approximately 40% (hemoglobin concentration at 13–14 g/dL)—particularly when blood is being drawn frequently for testing. This practice is based on the belief that transfused donor RBCs, containing adult hemoglobin with its superior interaction with 2,3-diphosphoglycerate (2.3-DPG), will provide optimal oxygen delivery throughout the period of diminished pulmonary function. Consistent with this rationale for ensuring optimal oxygen delivery in neonates with pulmonary failure, it seems logical to maintain the hematocrit around 40% in infants with congenital heart disease that is severe enough to cause either cyanosis or congestive heart failure.

Maintain hematocrit >30% to 35% for moderate cardiopulmonary disease

Following similar logic, it seems reasonable to maintain the hematocrit above 30% to 35% for moderate cardiopulmonary disease (Table 46.1).

Maintain hematocrit >30% for major surgery

Definitive studies are not available to establish the optimal hematocrit for neonates facing major surgery. However, it seems reasonable to maintain the hematocrit >30% because of the limited ability of the neonate's heart, lungs, and vasculature to compensate for anemia. Additional factors include the inferior off-loading of oxygen to tissues by the infant's own red cells because of the diminished interaction between fetal hemoglobin and 2,3-DPG plus the developmental impairment of neonatal pulmonary, renal, hepatic, and neurologic function. Because this transfusion guideline is simply a recommendation—not a firm indication—it should be applied with flexibility to individual infants facing surgical procedures of varying complexity (i.e., minor surgery may be judged not to require a hematocrit >30%). The amount of anticipated blood loss must be strongly considered in preoperative transfusion decisions—with a likelihood of large blood loss, some physicians might like the preoperative hematocrit to be relatively high.

Maintain hematocrit >20% to 25% for stable infants with symptomatic anemia

The clinical recommendations for RBC transfusions in preterm infants who are not critically ill but, nonetheless, develop moderate anemia (hematocrit <25% or hemoglobin level <8 g/dL) are extremely variable. In general, infants who are clinically stable with modest anemia do not require RBC transfusions, unless they exhibit significant clinical problems that are ascribed to the presence of anemia or are predicted to be corrected by donor RBCs.[19,20] As an example, proponents of RBC transfusions to treat disturbances of cardiopulmonary rhythms believe that a low blood level of RBCs contributes to tachypnea, dyspnea, apnea, and tachycardia or bradycardia because of decreased oxygen delivery to the respiratory center of the brain. If true, it follows that RBC transfusions might decrease the number of apneic spells by improving oxygen delivery to the central nervous system. However, results of clinical studies have been contradictory.[14,18,19]

Another controversial clinical indication for RBC transfusions is to maintain a reasonable hematocrit level as treatment for unexplained growth failure. Some neonatologists consider poor weight gain to be an indication for transfusion, particularly if the hematocrit is <25% and if other signs of distress are evident (e.g., tachycardia, respiratory difficulty, weak suck and cry, and diminished activity).[20] In this setting, growth failure has been ascribed to the increase in metabolic expenditure required to support the work of labored breathing. In the past, a hematocrit below 30% was of concern and often led to transfusion. However, results of clinical studies have not supported this practice,[18,19] and no apparent rationale exists to justify maintaining any predetermined hematocrit level by prophylactic, small-volume RBC transfusions in stable, growing infants who seem to be otherwise healthy.

In practice, the decision of whether to transfuse is based on the desire to maintain the hematocrit concentration at a level judged to be most beneficial for the infant's clinical condition. Investigators who believe this "clinical" approach is too imprecise have suggested the use of "physiologic" criteria such as red cell mass,[21] available oxygen,[22] mixed venous oxygen saturation, and measurements of oxygen delivery and utilization[23] to develop guidelines for transfusion decisions. In one study of 10 human infants with severe (oxygen-dependent) bronchopulmonary dysplasia, improvement of physiologic endpoints was shown (increased systemic oxygen transport and decreased oxygen use) as a consequence of small-volume RBC transfusions.[23] However, these promising but technically demanding methods are, at present, difficult to apply in the day-to-day practice of neonatology. The application, in infants, of data obtained from studies of animals and adult humans that correlate tissue oxygenation with the clinical effects of anemia and the need for RBC transfusions is confounded by the differences between infants and adults in hemoglobin oxygen affinity, ability to increase cardiac output, and regional patterns of blood flow.

Another physiologic factor considered in transfusion decisions is use of the circulating red cell volume/mass rather than the hematocrit or hemoglobin level. Although circulating red cell volume/mass is a potentially useful index of the blood's oxygen-carrying capacity, it cannot be predicted accurately from hematocrit or hemoglobin concentration levels; hence, it must be measured directly.[24] Unfortunately, circulating red cell volume/mass measurements and other "physiologic" criteria for transfusions are not widely available for clinical use.

Red blood cell products to transfuse

RBCs from fresh versus stored units

Most transfusions are given to preterm infants as small-volume transfusions (10 to 20 mL/kg body weight) of RBCs in extended-storage media (additive solution AS-1, AS-3, AS-5) at a hematocrit of approximately 55% to 60% (Table 46.2). Alternatively, some neonatologists prefer RBCs stored in citrate-phosphate-dextrose-adenine (CPDA) solution at a hematocrit of approximately 70%—in my view, an unfortunate practice because the superiority of CPDA solution over extended-storage media has not been shown by clinical trials, and the insistence to transfuse CPDA RBC units creates inventory management problems for blood suppliers. As shown later in this chapter, AS-1 and AS-3 have been shown in

randomized clinical trials to have similar efficacy and safety to CPDA in small-volume RBC transfusions.

Some centers prefer to centrifuge RBC aliquots before transfusion to prepare a uniformly packed RBC concentrate (hematocrit >80%).[25] Most RBC transfusions are infused slowly over 2 to 4 hours. Because of the small quantity of extracellular fluid (storage media) infused very slowly with small-volume transfusions, the type of anticoagulant–preservative solution used poses no risk for most premature infants.[26,27] Accordingly, the traditional use of relatively fresh RBCs (<7 days of storage) has been replaced in many centers by the practice of transfusing aliquots of RBCs from a dedicated unit (or part of a unit) of RBCs stored up to 42 days in efforts to diminish the high donor exposure rates among infants who undergo numerous transfusions.[27–29] Neonatologists who object to prescribing stored RBCs and insist on transfusing fresh RBCs generally express the following four concerns: (1) the increase in the level of potassium in the plasma (i.e., supernatant fluid); (2) the decrease in the level of 2,3-DPG; (3) the possible risks of additives such as mannitol and the relatively large amounts of glucose (dextrose) and phosphate present in extended-storage preservative solutions; and (4) the changes in red cell shape and deformability that may lead to poor flow through the microvasculature. Although these concerns often are legitimate for large-volume (≥ 25 mL/kg) transfusions, particularly when infusion is rapid, they do not apply to small-volume transfusions for the following reasons.

After 42 days of storage in extended-storage media (AS-1, AS-3, and AS-5) at a hematocrit of approximately 60%, extracellular ("plasma") potassium levels in RBC units approximate 50 mEq/L (0.05 mEq/mL), a value that at first glance seems alarmingly high. Simple calculations, however, show that the actual dose of ionic potassium transfused in the extracellular "plasma" fluid is small. An infant weighing 1 kg given a 15-mL/kg transfusion of RBCs stored 42 days in extended-storage media at a hematocrit of 55% to 60% receives only 0.3 mEq. The potassium concentration of RBCs stored in CPDA solution at a hematocrit of 70% increases to 70 to 80 mEq/L after the 35 days of permitted storage, and the dose of potassium infused with a 15-mL/kg transfusion to a 1-kg infant is 0.3 to 0.4 mEq. These doses are quite small when compared to the usual daily potassium requirement of 2 to 3 mEq/kg and have been shown in several clinical studies not to cause hyperkalemia.[27]

By 21 days of storage, 2,3-DPG is totally depleted from RBCs as reflected by a P_{50} value that decreases from approximately 27 mm Hg in fresh blood to 18 mm Hg in stored RBCs at the time of outdate. Because of the effects of high fetal hemoglobin levels in neonatal RBCs, the 18 mm Hg value of RBCs transfused after maximum storage corresponds to the expectedly low P_{50} value obtained from studies of RBCs produced by many healthy preterm infants at birth. Thus, both older stored RBCs and endogenous RBCs from neonates have a similarly reduced ability to off-load oxygen compared with fresh adult RBCs. However, older adult RBCs in banked RBC units provide an advantage over the infant's own cells because 2,3-DPG and the P_{50} of transfused adult cells (but not endogenous infant RBCs) increase rapidly after transfusion. When studied by a randomized clinical trial, in the setting of small-volume (15 mL/kg) transfusions, 2,3-DPG levels were maintained in infants given stored AS-1 RBCs.[28]

The quantity of additives present in RBCs in extended storage media is unlikely to be dangerous for neonates given small-volume transfusions (15 mL/kg).[26,27] Regardless of the type of suspending solution, the quantity of additives is quite small in the clinical setting in which a neonate would receive a single, small-volume

Table 46.2 Formulation of red cell anticoagulant–preservative solutions

Constituent	CPDA	AS-1	AS-3	AS-5
Volume (mL)	63*	100†	100†	100†
Sodium chloride (mg)	None	900	410	877
Dextrose (mg)	2010	2200	1100	900
Adenine (mg)	17.3	27	30	30
Mannitol (mg)	None	750	None	525
Trisodium citrate (mg)	1660	None	588	None
Citric acid (mg)	206	None	42	None
Sodium phosphate (monobasic) (mg)	140	None	276	None

* Approximately 450 mL of donor blood is drawn into 63 mL of CPDA solution. One red blood cell unit (hematocrit, ~70%) is prepared by means of centrifugation and removal of most plasma. Results of calculations will be slightly different if 500 mL of donor blood is drawn.
† When additive solution AS-1 or AS-5 is used, 450 mL of donor blood is first drawn into 63 mL of CPD, which is identical to CPDA except it contains 1610 mg dextrose per 63 mL and has no adenine. When AS-3 is used, donor blood is drawn into CP2D, which is identical to CPD except it contains double the amount of dextrose. After centrifugation and removal of nearly all plasma, the cells are resuspended in 100 mL of the additive solution (AS-1, AS-3, or AS-5) at a hematocrit of approximately 55% to 60%.
CPD, citrate–phosphate–dextrose; CPDA, citrate–phosphate–dextrose–adenine.

Table 46.3 Quantity (Total mg/kg) of additives infused during a transfusion of 15 mL/kg AS-1, AS-3, or AS-5 RBCs at hematocrit 60%

Additive	AS-1	AS-3	AS-5	Toxic Dose*
Sodium chloride	54.0	24.6	52.6	137 mg/kg/day
Dextrose	132.0	66.0	54.0	240 mg/kg/hour
Adenine	1.6	1.8	1.8	15 mg/kg/dose
Citrate	Trace	37.8	Trace	180 mg/kg/hour
Phosphate	Trace	16.6	Trace	>60 mg/kg/day
Mannitol	45.0	None	31.5	360 mg/kg/day

* The accuracy of a toxic dose is difficult to predict because infusion rates are slow, allowing metabolism and distribution of additives from blood into extravascular sites. In addition, dextrose, adenine, and phosphate enter red cells and are somewhat sequestered and not immediately "available" in the extracellular solution. Data on potential toxic doses from Luban et al.[26]
Calculations for quantity of additives infused assumed the following: (1) total volume of RBC unit = 300 mL, consisting of 100 mL additive solution + 180 mL completely packed red cells + 20 mL of primary anticoagulant trapped between the red cells; (2) 15 mL/kg transfusion = 9 mL red cells + 6 mL additive solution; (3) quantity of additive solution infused per single RBC transfusion = quantity in 100 mL/(100 × 6); and (4) trace amounts of trisodium citrate, citric acid, and phosphate were carried over by primary anticoagulant trapped between red cells.

transfusion over 2 to 4 hours. With AS-1, AS-3, and AS-5 as examples (Table 46.3), the dose of extended-storage media additives transfused during a typical small-volume transfusion is estimated to be far less than levels believed to be toxic.[26] This assumption was proved correct in clinical studies in which infants received one or more transfusions.[27] The safety and efficacy of transfusing stored RBCs are documented by the results of several laboratory tests performed before and after small-volume RBC transfusions in preterm infants (Table 46.4).

During storage in conventional preservative solutions, red cells sustain decreases in 2,3-DPG and adenosine triphosphate, and they undergo membrane and cytoskeletal changes that lead to the formation of echinocytes and microvesicles and to decreased deformability. The last changes may lead to diminished perfusion of the microvasculature and, consequently, to tissue and organ dysfunction. For the past few years, an argument has raged over whether critically ill adult patients are harmed by receiving "old" RBC units (usually defined as stored ≥15 or ≥21 days), and whether mortality, multi-organ failure, infections, need for mechanical ventilation, length of stay in intensive care units and in the hospital,

Table 46.4 Mean change in blood chemistry levels during RBC transfusions[28,29]

Value	Change*	
	1 to 21 Days of Storage (n = 78)	22 to 42 Days of Storage (n = 42)
Hematocrit (%)	+12 ± 5	+12 ± 4
Glucose (mg/dL)	−12 ± 24	−16 ± 28
Lactate (mmol/L)	−0.6 ± 1.1	−0.2 ± 0.3
pH	0.00 ± 0.08	0.00 ± 0.06
Calcium (mg/dL)	−0.1 ± 0.5	0.0 ± 0.8
Sodium (mEq/L)	+0.3 ± 4.6	−0.4 ± 4.7
Potassium (mEq/L)	+0.2 ± 0.8	+0.2 ± 0.6

* Change (±SD) is posttransfusion value minus pretransfusion value. Statistical tests used were t test for pH, sodium, potassium, and glucose (normal distribution) and Wilcoxon rank sum test for hematocrit, calcium, and lactate (abnormal distribution). No statistically significant differences were found (p values all >0.05) when comparing 1 to 21 days versus 22 to 42 days of storage.

and so on could be diminished by transfusing only fresh RBC units. Older, largely observational studies generally support the idea that "old" RBC units put critically ill patients at risk, particularly if they receive multiple transfusions. Several studies challenged this concept and cautioned against insisting on transfusions of fresh RBCs.[31,32]

The controversy over transfusion of fresh versus stored RBCs is similar for neonatal RBC transfusions (i.e., neonates are often critically ill, and questions about morbidity caused by transfusing stored RBCs have been raised). However, well-designed randomized clinical trials have addressed their short-term efficacy and safety, and, within the limits of the number of infants studied, fresh and stored cells have been documented to be equivalent.[14,27–29] Similarly, the relatively long-term outcomes of transfusing fresh versus stored RBCs to VLBW premature infants have been assessed in a double-blind, randomized clinical trial involving 377 infants with birthweights <1250 g.[33] The age of the fresh RBCs, by definition, was no more than seven days (mean = 5.1 days). In contrast, the age of the stored RBCs ranged from two to 41 days (mean = 14.6 days). The primary outcome was a composite measure of necrotizing enterocolitis, retinopathy of prematurity, bronchopulmonary dysplasia, intraventricular hemorrhage, and death—measured up to 90 days after randomization. The occurrence of the outcome was nearly identical in both groups—52.7% of infants transfused with fresh RBCs versus 52.9% of infants transfused with stored RBCs.

In addition to the results of randomized clinical trials, described above, that establish the short-term and relatively long-term efficacy and safety of stored RBCs for small-volume transfusions given to neonates and infants, the posttransfusion circulating kinetics of transfused "stored/aged" donor RBCs has been reported to be nearly identical to that of "fresh" donor RBCs. The intravascular recovery 24 hours after transfusion (short storage = 98.6% vs. long storage = 96.9%) and long-term survival (short storage = 81.2% vs. long storage = 87.5%) of donor red cells was normal, when measured in human infants using biotinylated red cells.[34] In conclusion, because the risks of multiple donor exposure can be nearly eliminated by giving infants cells taken from dedicated, stored RBC units and because the increased risks of transfusing stored versus fresh cells have not been demonstrated, it seems prudent to transfuse stored RBCs for small-volume transfusions.

Cytomegalovirus (CMV)-"safe" RBC units

The combined "belt-and-suspenders" approach (i.e., transfusing units that are known to be both leukocyte-reduced *and* sero-negative for antibody to CMV) has been shown in a recent non-randomized observational study to completely prevent transfusion-transmitted CMV in VLBW preterm infants.[35] However, this approach will delay transfusions when sero- and antibody-negative units are not readily available, and it significantly increases the costs compared to using leukocyte reduction alone. Thus, it is important to be mindful of three other nonrandomized observational studies that found leukocyte reduction alone to strikingly reduce[36] or completely prevent[37,38] transfusion-transmitted CMV in hematopoietic progenitor cell (HPC) transplant recipients—patients known to be profoundly immunosuppressed. Based on their findings, authors of all three of the HPC reports recommended against the use of blood from CMV sero- and antibody-negative donors and favored leukocyte-reduced blood alone for HPC transplant patients.[36–38] Because randomized controlled trials comparing the efficacy to prevent transfusion-transmitted CMV of transfusing blood from sero- and antibody-negative donors versus leukocyte-reduced units alone versus combined sero- and antibody negative units that have been leukocyte-reduced are highly unlikely to ever be performed, practice decisions must be made on a logical assessment of all available data.

Accordingly, because there is no documented benefit of using the combined belt-and-suspenders approach of transfusing sero- and antibody negative units that have also been leukocyte-reduced versus transfusing units leukocyte-reduced without regard for CMV antibody status, and because of the adverse effects of delaying necessary transfusions plus the additional costs of CMV antibody testing, the best approach to preventing transfusion-transmitted CMV is to transfuse blood that has been leukocyte-reduced using strict quality control by the blood supplier. The usual recommended practice is to give leukocyte-reduced blood components to both CMV sero- and antibody-negative *and* sero- and antibody-positive infants. This is because sero- and antibody-positive infants will catabolize maternal CMV antibodies during their first months of postnatal life, at poorly predictable rates, and will lose their protective effects. Moreover, infants with passive maternal antibody have not been truly infected with CMV and, accordingly, will neither produce their own antibodies nor develop cellular immunity against CMV. Thus, all newborns are at potential risk for transfusion-transmitted CMV, whether or not they test positive for CMV antibody.

Irradiated RBC units

Neonates, particularly those who are extremely preterm, are believed by many to be at risk for transfusion-associated graft-versus-host disease (TA-GVHD).[27] However, the extent to which they are at risk and the consequent justification to mandate transfusion of irradiated cellular blood components are controversial. Although the immune system of neonates and infants unquestionably exhibits diminished function when compared to the immunity of older children and adults, TA-GVHD has been reported almost exclusively in infants from recognized high-risk groups—infants who already must receive irradiated cellular blood components for reasons independent of prematurity.[27,39] In most hospitals caring for preterm neonates and infants, a blanket policy exists to transfuse irradiated cellular blood components to all infants to a specified age, and it is justified because not all neonates and infants with severe immunodeficiency disorders are recognized as such when they are first transfused (i.e., irradiated blood, which is indicated, may not be ordered). Accordingly, many hospitals irradiate cellular blood components transfused to all pediatric patients until the age at which their physicians believe severe immunodeficiency disorders become clinically evident—usually until the age of 4 or 6 months, or even 12 months, with some physicians justifying intervals to several years of age, depending on the likelihood that immunodeficient infants will be admitted to their hospitals.

Practical blood banking aspects of RBC transfusions

For most blood banks serving neonatal intensive care units, a key principle is to limit allogeneic donor exposures by transfusing RBCs from dedicated RBC units stored as long as permitted by local policies or regulations (e.g., 42 days for RBCs preserved in extended-storage anticoagulant–preservative solutions). To illustrate, at the University of Iowa DeGowin Blood Center, preterm infants who need small-volume (15 mL/kg) transfusions are assigned to dedicated RBC units that have been prestorage leukocyte-reduced and suspended in extended-storage (42-day) solutions. At the time the first transfusion is ordered, a freshly collected unit (stored ≥ 7 days) is dedicated to the preterm infant, and the volume ordered is withdrawn. When subsequent transfusions are ordered, aliquots are removed sterilely and issued.[25] Although dedicated units are used throughout 42 days of storage, if an unassigned RBC unit has been stored 14 days without being dedicated to an infant, it has become relatively old (i.e., 14 of its 42 storage days have lapsed), and it enters the general inventory to be used for other patients. This plan has been demonstrated to be cost-effective.[40] Aliquots of RBCs are irradiated at the time of issue. Aliquots must be filtered through a standard blood filter (approximately 180 microns) either when drawn into the syringe for transfusion or at the time of infusion. Generally, small-volume transfusions are infused via a pump over a 2–4-hour period.

Larger volume (>25 ml/kg) RBC transfusions, as might be needed for surgery, are issued as entire or one-half RBC units—depending on anticipated transfusion needs. They are selected and processed (i.e., leukocyte-reduced and irradiated) similarly to small-volume transfusion aliquots and are infused at rates indicated by the clinical situation—with attention to possible potassium toxicity. Data from randomized clinical trials are not available to guide clinical practices, but in terms of potassium safety, it is customary to infuse RBCs as rapidly as needed if they have been stored no longer than seven days or if they have been freshly washed. For urgent transfusions, when units with <7 days storage or freshly washed units are not available, RBC units can be infused safely at a rate of 0.5 ml/kg/min—based on the assumption of an average potassium concentration of 30 mEq/L in older stored RBC units and a maximum safe infusion rate for potassium of 0.016 mEq/kg/min.

Acknowledgments

This work was supported by US National Institutes of Health grants P01 HL46925 and RR00059.

Disclaimer
The author has disclosed no conflicts of interest.

Key References

A full reference list for this chapter is available at: http://www.wiley.com/go/simon/transfusion

3 Widness JA, Madan A, Grindeanu LA, *et al.* Reduction in red blood cell transfusions among preterm infants: results of a randomized trial with an in-line blood gas and chemistry monitor. *Pediatrics* 2005;**115**:1299–306.

12 Widness JA, Veng-Pedersen P, Peters C, *et al.* Erythropoietin pharmacokinetics in premature infants: developmental, nonlinearity, and treatment effects. *J Appl Physiol* 1996;**80**:140–8.

14 Bell EF, Strauss RG, Widness JA, *et al.* Randomized trial of liberal versus restrictive guidelines for red blood cell transfusions in preterm infants. *Pediatrics* 2005;**115**:1685–91.

15 Kirpalani H, Whyte RK, Andersen C, *et al.* The Premature Infants in Need of Transfusion (PINT) study: a randomized, controlled trial of a restrictive (low) versus liberal (high) transfusion threshold for extremely low birth weight infants. *J Pediatr* 2006;**149**:301–7.

17 Nopoulos PC, Conrad AL, Bell EF, *et al.* Long-term outcome of brain structure in premature infants: effects of liberal vs restricted red blood cell transfusions. *Arch Pediatr Adolesc Med* 2011;**165**:443–50.

27 Strauss RG. Data-driven blood banking practices for neonatal RBC transfusions. *Transfusion* 2000;**40**:1528–40.

33 Fergusson DA, Hebert P, Hogan DI, *et al.* Effect of fresh red blood cell transfusions on clinical outcomes in premature, very-low-birth-weight infants: the ARIPI randomized trial. *JAMA* 2012;**308**:1443–51.

36 Kekre N, Tokessy M, Mallick R, *et al.* Is cytomegalovirus testing of blood products still needed for hematopoietic stem cell transplant recipients in the era of universal leukoreduction? *Biol Blood Marrow Transplant* 2013;**19**:1719–24.

39 New HV, Stanworth SJ, Engelfriet CP, *et al.* International forum: neonatal transfusions. *Vox Sang* 2009;**96**:62–85.

CHAPTER 47

Platelet and plasma transfusions for infants and children

Jeanne E. Hendrickson[1] & Cassandra D. Josephson[2,3]

[1]Departments of Laboratory Medicine and of Pediatrics, Yale School of Medicine, Yale University, New Haven, CT, USA
[2]Department of Pathology and Laboratory Medicine, Emory University School of Medicine, Atlanta, GA, USA
[3]Children's Healthcare of Atlanta, Blood Tissue & Apheresis Services, Atlanta, GA, USA

Physiologically speaking, infants and children are not simply small adults when considering causes and treatments of thrombocytopenia and coagulopathy. Gestational age, congenital diseases, immature liver, maternal factors, and transplacental antibody transfer must all be considered when evaluating and treating neonates with thrombocytopenia, bleeding, or coagulopathy. Bleeding tendencies and diseases prevalent in childhood must be understood for optimal transfusion support. Special consideration must be given to the product(s) transfused to infants and children with thrombocytopenia or coagulopathy, those undergoing surgery and exchange transfusion, and those supported by extracorporeal membrane oxygenation. These considerations include ABO compatibility, total blood volume, immunosuppression, immunodeficiencies, and blood donor exposure. This chapter will briefly review the etiology of thrombocytopenia and coagulopathy in infants and children, with a general overview of platelet, plasma, and cryoprecipitate transfusion support.

Platelet transfusion

Pathophysiology of thrombocytopenia in infants

Platelet counts in developing fetuses are typically higher than 150,000/µL by the end of the first trimester,[1,2] with most healthy term newborns typically having counts above this level.[3] The prevalence of neonatal thrombocytopenia varies by study, with 1–5% of all neonates affected by platelet counts lower than 150,000/µL.[4–6] Preterm infants and those born small for gestational age are more likely to be affected by thrombocytopenia than term infants,[5] with up to 25% of all neonates admitted to neonatal intensive care units (NICUs) having mild, moderate, or severe thrombocytopenia at some point during their hospital stay. Babies in the NICU with extremely low birth weights are quite likely to have low platelet counts, with 73% of infants weighing under 1000 grams reported to have platelet counts lower than 150,000/µL in one study.[5]

Neonatal thrombocytopenia can be caused by decreased platelet production, increased platelet destruction, or a combination of these. The pathophysiology of neonatal thrombocytopenia noted at or soon after birth may be due in part to maternal hypertension, placental insufficiency, and/or perinatal hypoxemia;[7] such conditions are more likely to be present in preterm than term infants. Perinatal infections such as Group B *Streptococcus* or *E. coli* may also be associated with early neonatal thrombocytopenia, as may congenital infections such as toxoplasmosis, rubella, cytomegalovirus (CMV), or herpes simplex virus (HSV).[7] Thrombocytopenia that develops after the first few days of life may be due to postnatally acquired sepsis, disseminated intravascular coagulopathy (DIC), or necrotizing enterocolitis (NEC).[6]

Unique to neonates, transplacental transfer of maternal alloantibodies may contribute to thrombocytopenia in otherwise "well-appearing" infants.[8] Maternal antibodies against human leukocyte antigens (HLAs) as well as human platelet-specific glycoprotein antigens (HPAs) are capable of crossing the placenta, binding to the platelets of fetuses, and leading to neonatal alloimmune thrombocytopenic purpura (NAITP).[9,10] Antibodies against HPA-1a are the most well-known causes of NAITP in Caucasians, with women lacking the HPA-1a antigen and expressing the HLA DBR3∗0101 being at particularly high risk of developing these antibodies during pregnancy with HPA-1a expressing fetuses.[10] Antibodies against HPA-5b, HPA-15a, or other HPA antigens may also lead to NAITP.[11] Rarely, maternal autoantibodies such as those found in mothers with ITP or other autoimmune diseases like systemic lupus erythematosus may lead to neonatal thrombocytopenia.[12] Thus, it is prudent to check the maternal history and the maternal platelet count in instances of unexpected neonatal thrombocytopenia.

Although NAITP and sepsis are at the top of the differential of a term neonate with thrombocytopenia, conditions such as proprionic academia or methylmalonic academia, Wiscott Aldrich syndrome, X-linked thrombocytopenia, or congenital amegakaryocytic thrombocytopenia may also lead to persistent thrombocytopenia in neonates and children.[13] Chromosomal abnormalities such as trisomy 13, 18, or 21 may be associated with persistent neonatal thrombocytopenia, with transient abnormal myelopoiesis (TAM) being present in some neonates with trisomy 21.[14] Thrombocytopenia absent radius (TAR), although rare, should be in the differential diagnosis of unexplained neonatal thrombocytopenia,[15] as should Kasabach–Merritt syndrome.

Platelet dysfunction may also contribute to bleeding in infants and children, be the etiology congenital (such as in Glanzmann's thrombasthenia or Bernard Soulier) or medication induced.

Rossi's Principles of Transfusion Medicine, Fifth Edition. Edited by Toby L. Simon, Jeffrey McCullough, Edward L. Snyder, Bjarte G. Solheim, and Ronald G. Strauss.
© 2016 John Wiley & Sons, Ltd. Published 2016 by John Wiley & Sons, Ltd.

Table 47.1A Neonatal platelet transfusion thresholds

Situation	Platelet Transfusion Threshold
Clinically stable term neonate	20,000–25,000/μL
Clinically stable preterm neonate	25,000–50,000/μl*
Clinically unstable neonate or bleeding neonate	50,000–100,000/μL
Need for invasive procedure	50,000/μL
NAITP	30,000–50,000/μl#
ECMO	50,000–100,000/μl#

* Platelets for Neonatal Transfusion – 2 Study ongoing.
# Transfusion threshold dependent on past and present bleeding.

Medications given to mothers prior to delivery (including Ketorolac)[16] may potentially impact neonatal platelet function. Medications used in NICUs, including indomethacin and nitric oxide, may also impact platelet function. The transfusion threshold in these instances is not well established, but may be higher than described for other infants.

Platelet transfusion in infants

Ongoing debate exists regarding ideal platelet transfusion thresholds for neonates, with a paucity of data in existence to guide clinical decision making. Most neonatal platelet transfusion guidelines are thus based on consensus rather than on evidence.[17,18] Some institutions prophylactically transfuse stable term and preterm infants at platelet counts of 25,000/μL and 30,000/μL, respectively,[19] whereas others transfuse stable infants at platelet counts of 50,000/μL. A recent study showed no relationship between platelet count and major intracranial hemorrhage, with more that 91% of neonates with platelet counts under 20,000/μL demonstrating no bleeding.[20] Table 47.1A lists potential guidelines for neonatal platelet transfusions.

A single randomized trial of premature infants in their first week of life, completed more than two decades ago, demonstrated that a pretransfusion threshold above 150,000/μL was not associated with fewer bleeding episodes, including intraventricular hemorrhage, than a transfusion threshold above 50,000/μL.[21] A retrospective study of newborns <32 weeks of gestational age born in two different cities showed no difference in intracranial hemorrhage rates between neonates transfused with restrictive (transfusion for platelet count less than 50,000/μL in bleeding or sick infants) compared to liberal (transfusion according to institutional guidelines) criteria.[22] Another recent study of preterm, low-birth-weight infants (<1500 g) demonstrated that more restrictive transfusion thresholds (transfusion for platelet count less than 50,000/μL in sick infants or less than 25,000/μL in stable infants) were associated with no greater bleeding than more liberal thresholds.[23] Intracranial bleeding is likely associated with a number of variables, with platelet count being just one such variable. Platelets for Neonatal Transfusion—Study 2 (PlaNeT-2) is an ongoing, two-stage, randomized trial comparing outcomes of preterm neonates receiving prophylactic platelet transfusions to maintain counts above 25,000/μL or above 50,000/μL.[24]

Two neonatal populations worthy of mention include those on extracorporeal membrane oxygenation (ECMO) and those with NAITP. Babies on ECMO are at high risk of bleeding, due in part to thrombocytopenia, platelet dysfunction, and heparinization of the circuit. Thus, platelet transfusion thresholds between 50,000/μL and 100,000/μL are typically utilized in these babies, dependent on bleeding status.[25,26] Neonates with NAITP are also at high risk

of bleeding. Babies with NAITP and a documented intracranial bleed should be maintained at platelet counts above 50,000/μL for at least the first week of life. Neonates with NAITP and no bleeding are typically maintained at platelet counts above 30,000/μL and often higher for the first week of life. Random donor (banked) platelets may be transfused for babies with NAITP, and will typically increase the neonate's platelet count at least transiently.[8,27,28] Platelets lacking the HPA-1a, HPA-5b, or other offending antigen may be requested from blood donor centers for neonates thought to have NAITP mediated by these respective antibodies, although emergent transfusions should never be withheld while antigen negative platelets are being located. Maternal platelets are another therapeutic option, yet they may be difficult to obtain and they *must* be washed to remove offending antibodies prior to transfusion.[9] IVIG is often given to affected neonates in an attempt to increase the platelet circulatory half-life; it is also administered during pregnancy to women carrying fetuses at risk for NAITP, with dose and schedule determined by risk stratification.[28–30]

Pathophysiology of thrombocytopenia in children

Thrombocytopenia in children is typically caused by decreased production, increased destruction, or sequestration of platelets.

Hypoproliferative thrombocytopenia occurs in children treated with chemotherapy or radiation, with the majority of platelet transfusions in childhood given in these patient populations. A subset of anti-epileptic drugs, along with drugs in other categories, may decrease platelet production in children. Myelodysplasia, marrow infiltrative processes, and aplastic anemia also lead to decreased platelet production. Lastly, a number of hereditary bone marrow failure syndromes and other congenital disorders such as Wiscott Aldrich syndrome lead to impaired platelet production.

Although platelet transfusions are rarely indicated, the most common cause of destructive thrombocytopenia in children is idiopathic thrombocytopenic purpura (ITP). The majority of children who present for medical care with acute ITP have isolated thrombocytopenia with platelet counts lower than 20,000/μL, and may have the abrupt onset of bruising and bleeding. Platelet count alone has not been shown to predict bleeding severity in ITP.[31] Intracranial hemorrhage is a rare but life-threatening complication of acute ITP,[32] occurring in less than 1% of cases. A 2009 study of 40 children with ITP and intracranial hemorrhage showed that 90% had a platelet lower than 20,000/μL, 33% had head trauma, and 22% had hematuria.[33]

Other destructive thrombocytopenias in children include chronic ITP, autoimmune diseases, heparin-induced thrombocytopenia, HIV, posttransplant thrombocytopenia, posttransfusion purpura, and neoplasm-associated immune thrombocytopenias. Nonimmune causes of destructive thrombocytopenias in children include hemophagocytic syndromes, Kasabach–Merritt syndrome, DIC, infectious etiologies, congenital heart disease, type 2B von Willebrand disease (vWD), and platelet-type vWD. Thrombotic microangiopathies, including hemolytic uremic syndrome (HUS), thrombotic thrombocytopenia purpura (TTP), and drug or bone marrow transplant associated microangiopathy, also occur in children.

Mild thrombocytopenia may occur in children with hypersplenism or splenic sequestration, with platelet counts rarely dropping below 50,000/μL. Thrombocytopenia may also be associated with liver disease. Laboratory artifact may rarely lead to "spurious" thrombocytopenia (e.g., platelet counts reported to be low by automated counters, but not truly low), with EDTA-dependent

Table 47.1B Pediatric platelet transfusion thresholds

Situation	Platelet Transfusion Threshold
Bleeding patient	Situation dependent
Bleeding on ECMO or during surgery	50,000–100,000/µL
Prophylaxis for hypoproliferative thrombocytopenia	10,000/µL[*]
Prophylaxis for line placement	20,000/µL
Prophylaxis for lumbar puncture	50,000/µL[#]
Prophylaxis for CNS bleeding in children with sickle cell disease undergoing transplantation	30,000–50,000/µL
Prophylaxis for major surgery	50,000/µL[%]
Platelet dysfunction with bleeding or in need of invasive procedure	Not applicable

[*] stem cell transplant thresholds may be 15,000–20,000/µL.
[#] with consideration of 100,000/µL when circulating blasts are present.
[%] prophylaxis for CNS surgery may be higher.

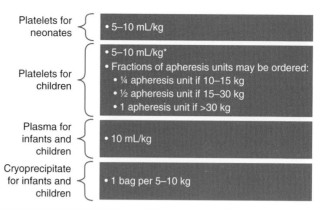

Platelets for neonates
- 5–10 mL/kg

Platelets for children
- 5–10 mL/kg*
- Fractions of apheresis units may be ordered:
  - ¼ apheresis unit if 10–15 kg
  - ½ apheresis unit if 15–30 kg
  - 1 apheresis unit if >30 kg

Plasma for infants and children
- 10 mL/kg

Cryoprecipitate for infants and children
- 1 bag per 5–10 kg

*Higher platelet doses increase the length of time between transfusion episodes in patients with hypoproliferative thrombocytopenia, but have not been shown to decrease bleeding rates.

Figure 47.1 Platelet, plasma, and cryoprecipitate dosing for infants and children.

antibodies, cold agglutinins, and drugs being known to cause pseudothrombocytopenia

Platelet transfusion in children

As with transfusions in neonates or adults, platelet transfusions in children may be given (1) in the setting of an acute hemorrhage, or (2) as prophylaxis to decrease bleeding in at-risk patients. The first category is relatively straightforward, and thresholds for the latter continue to be debated. Young children with treatment-associated hypoproliferative thrombocytopenia may be at higher risk for bleeding than adults,[34,35] with factors beyond platelet count likely contributing to this risk. These factors may include chemotherapy intensity as well as functional differences in interactions between the vascular endothelium and platelets.[34]

Platelet transfusion in children with active bleeding

Platelet transfusion should be considered in any pediatric patient with thrombocytopenia and active bleeding, with transfusion thresholds being situation dependent (Table 47.1B). Patients with congenital platelet disorders and active bleeding may also benefit from platelet transfusions in addition to adjunctive therapies, regardless of platelet count.

Children with hypoproliferative thrombocytopenia from chemotherapy or radiation, those undergoing bone marrow transplantation, those on ECMO, or those undergoing surgery who are bleeding may benefit from platelet transfusions. Children with ITP and acute, life-threatening bleeding should receive 1–2 doses of platelets (with a dose defined as 5–10 mL/kg; Figure 47.1), in addition to 0.8–1 g/kg of IVIG and 30 mg/kg of methylprednisolone.[36,37] Repeat platelet dosing may be needed due to rapid antibody-mediated removal post transfusion. Rarely, emergent splenectomy is also needed in children with ITP and life-threatening bleeding. Although platelet transfusion thresholds are not applicable and alloimmunization may result, platelet may be effective at controlling bleeding in children with Glanzmann's thrombasthenia, Bernard Soulier, and other congenital causes of severe platelet dysfunction.[38,39] However, other treatments, including topical therapies, antifibrinolytics, desmopressin, or recombinant factor VIIa, may also be used in some of these disorders.

Prophylactic platelet transfusion in children

Thresholds for prophylactic platelet transfusions in children are not well established. Pending additional pediatric specific studies and guidelines, prophylactic platelet transfusion guidelines in adults may be considered.

The 2014 AABB guidelines recommend that adult patients with hypoproliferative thrombocytopenia be transfused at a platelet count of 10,000/µL to prevent spontaneous bleeding.[40] However, equipoise currently exists among pediatric hematology/oncology clinicians regarding platelet transfusion thresholds for children with hypoproliferative thrombocytopenia.[41,42] A recent single-institution study evaluating transfusion practice over 10 years showed the median platelet count for which pediatric oncology patients with hypoproliferative thrombocytopenia were transfused was 16,000/µL.[43] A 2013 survey of Children's Oncology Group Stem Cell Transplant Directors described that 69% of institutions transfused non-transplant oncology patients for platelet counts below 10,000/µL, with 27% of institutions transfusing these patients for platelet counts below 15,000/µL.[42] This study found transfusion thresholds for stem cell transplant patients to be higher: 47% of institutions prophylactically transfused their transplant patients for platelet counts below 10,000/µL, and 44% of institutions prophylactically transfused for platelet counts below 20,000/µL.[42]

Of the multiple large transfusion studies performed to date on patients with hypoproliferative thrombocytopenia, only one (Optimal Platelet Dose Strategy to Prevent Bleeding in Thrombocytopenia Patients [PLADO]) has included a separate pediatric analysis.[44] PLADO enrolled 200 pediatric patients from 0 to 18 years of age,[34] and was designed to evaluate the relationship between platelet transfusion dose and bleeding. The transfusion threshold for the study was a platelet count less than 10,000/µL, with a low (1.1×10^{11}/m^2), a medium (2.2×10^{11}/m^2), and a high (4.4×10^{11}/m^2) platelet dose randomly assigned. Platelet dose was not found to predict bleeding. Of note, the children in the study had a higher risk of World Health Organization grade 2 or higher bleeding than the adults (86% of children 0–5 years of age, 88% of children 6–12 years of age, and 77% of children 13–18 years of age, compared to 67% of adults). In addition, the children in this study had more days of grade 2 or higher bleeding than adults, with a median of three days (compared to one day in adults). Bleeding was most pronounced in the pediatric patients undergoing stem cell transplantation. Taken in combination, these results suggest that factors beyond platelet counts alone impact bleeding risk in pediatric patients and demonstrate the need for additional studies.

Children with sickle cell disease undergoing stem cell transplantation are at especially high risk of central nervous system (CNS) bleeding[45,46] given vascular issues, prior cerebrovascular accidents

(CVAs, or strokes), and transplant-associated hypertension. The prophylactic platelet transfusion threshold for this patient population has thus been set higher than that of other pediatric transplant patients, with 50,000/μL historically being utilized;[45,47] some centers have recently dropped their transfusion threshold to 30,000/μL.[48]

Adult guidelines that are reasonable to translate to pediatric patients include transfusion for platelet counts less than 20,000/μL prior to central line placement and for platelet counts less than 50,000/μL prior to non-CNS surgeries.[40] The 2014 AABB guidelines recommend transfusing platelets for adult patients with platelet counts less than 50,000/μL prior to lumbar puncture (LP); extrapolating these guidelines to LPs in children *without circulating blasts* is reasonable. It must be noted, however, that traumatic LPs in children with circulating blasts have been shown to decrease event-free survival.[49–51] Two studies have identified a platelet count under 100,000/μL as a risk factor for a traumatic LP in pediatric leukemia patients.[52,53] Thus, transfusing children with new-onset leukemia to platelet counts above 100,000/μL prior to their initial LP may be considered, although national pediatric guidelines currently suggest a count of 50,000/μL.[54]

Prophylactic transfusions of functional platelets in the perisurgery or peripartum period may be indicated in patients with congenital or acquired platelet function defects; adjunctive therapies are often necessary as well. Careful care coordination and treatment planning between multiple specialties are necessary in these cases, to minimize the likelihood of operative or delayed postoperative bleeding.

Conditions in which platelet transfusions should generally be avoided include those associated with consumptive coagulopathies such as TTP and HUS. At least one pediatric case report documents a cerebral infarct in a three-year-old child with TTP following a platelet transfusion.[55] Although the risks associated with platelet transfusion in TTP patients prior to line placement for plasmapheresis may be lower than historically thought,[56] the general recommendation is to avoid transfusions in these circumstances[57] due to the known role of platelets in microvascular thrombus formation.

Platelet product selection for infants and children

Platelets chosen for transfusion to neonates and children in the United States may be from apheresis or whole blood donors, with many centers preferentially utilizing apheresis platelets. ABO-compatible platelets or identical platelets are ideally selected for transfusion into pediatric patients, in an attempt to (1) minimize the passive transfer of incompatible plasma,[58,59] and (2) to minimize the destruction of platelets expressing incompatible antigens.[60] An additional consideration in neonates is the need for any chosen platelets also to be compatible with maternally derived isohemagglutinins that may be transiently present in the neonate's circulation. Transfusion of Rh(D)-positive platelet products into Rh(D)-negative children should be avoided if possible, given the presence of a small number of contaminating red blood cells (RBCs) expressing the Rh(D) antigen. Although the likelihood of an Rh(D)-negative patient forming an anti-D after exposure to an Rh(D)-positive platelet unit is extremely low,[61–64] prophylaxis with Rh immune globulin (RhIg) (although not without controversy) may be considered in children. A 300 μg dose of RhIg can suppress immunization to 15 mL of packed RBCs.[65]

Irradiation prevents transfusion-associated graft-versus-host disease. Given that neonates may have undiagnosed immunodeficiencies,[66]

some institutions irradiate all cellular products transfused to neonates.[67] Other institutions selectively irradiate products transfused to neonates weighing less than 1200 g. Neonates or children with known or suspected cellular immunodeficiencies, receiving intensive chemotherapy, undergoing bone marrow transplantation, receiving HLA-matched products, or receiving directed donor products also require irradiated cellular blood products.[67,68] Leukoreduction decreases HLA alloimmunization, febrile transfusion reactions, and transmission of viruses harbored in white blood cells (WBCs);[69] thus, leukoreduced platelets are typically recommended for transfusion to neonates and children. Leukoreduced platelets are generally considered to be "CMV safe," with an ongoing debate in very-low-birthweight infants (≤1500 g) and extremely low-birthweight infants (≤1000 g) regarding whether leukoreduced platelets from CMV-seronegative donors lead to lower rates of CMV transfusion transmission than leukoreduced platelets from CMV untested or seropositive donors.[70–75]

5–10 mL/kg of platelets are typically infused as a single "dose," with a maximum dose regardless of weight typically being one apheresis unit or one "pool" of whole blood–derived platelets (4–8 donors). Some centers provide fractions of apheresis platelet units in a weight-based fashion (e.g., 5–10 mL/kg to neonates, ¼ apheresis unit to children <15 kg, ½ apheresis unit to children between 15 and 30 kg, and a whole apheresis unit to children >30 kg), and others provide platelets derived from a single whole blood unit for every 10 kg of body weight. Small volumes of platelets are often transferred prior to transfusion from parent units into syringes, with these aliquots retaining acceptable in vitro characteristics for up to six hours after transfer.[76–78] Volume reduction is not typically recommended, given the loss and activation of product that occurs during this modification.[79] Transfusion rates vary based on recipient condition, but each dose must be infused within four hours. Post-transfusion platelet increases are dependent in part on the platelet count of the transfused unit, the recipient's condition, and the degree of donor–recipient ABO matching. With a transfusion threshold of 10,000/μL, the pediatric subanalysis of the PLADO study showed no differences in bleeding rates in children transfused with low, middle, or high doses of platelets.[34] However, patients transfused with low doses of platelets ultimately received a larger median number of platelet transfusions than did patients on the middle- or high-dosage arms.[80,81]

Transfusion reactions in the pediatric population

In addition to infectious complications of transfusion, other noninfectious hazards of transfusion should also be considered.[69] A 2014 study at a single institution found that 6.2/1000 pediatric transfusions were associated with a reported transfusion reaction compared to 2.4/1000 adult transfusions, with platelets being the most likely blood product to result in a transfusion reaction. 2.7/1000 pediatric transfusions (vs. 1.1/1000 adult transfusions) were associated with an allergic transfusion reaction. 1.9/1000 pediatric transfusions (vs. 0.47/1000 adult transfusions) were associated with a febrile nonhemolytic transfusion reaction. 0.29/1000 pediatric transfusions (vs. 0.078/1000 adult transfusions) were associated with hypotension.[82] Another 2014 study reviewed the charts of pediatric patients at a single institution being transfused with platelets and found 116/805 platelet transfusions to be associated with a potential acute transfusion reaction; only four of these 116 potential reactions were reported to the hospital transfusion service.[83] In combination, these studies suggest that transfusion reaction rates in pediatric patients may be higher than previously appreciated, with additional studies being warranted.

One complication of platelet transfusion, particularly of concern in patients lacking a portion of the platelet glycoprotein, is the development of platelet glycoprotein alloantibodies. The largest study to date, published in 2004, found 16/54 Glanzmann's patients developed platelet glycoprotein alloantibodies after transfusion, 8/54 developed HLA alloantibodies, and 5/54 developed both platelet glycoprotein and HLA alloantibodies.[84] HPA and HLA alloantibodies increase the risk of platelet refractoriness, and HPA alloantibodies may lead to neonatal alloimmune thrombocytopenia.[85,86] These antibodies may also be relevant to donor selection, should subsequent stem cell transplantation be considered.

Plasma transfusion

Development of the coagulation system

Quantitative and qualitative differences in coagulation factors, coagulation inhibitors, and fibrinolytic proteins exist in neonates compared to older children and adults. Plasma levels of the vitamin K–dependent coagulation factors (II, VII, IX, and X) and the contact factors (XII, XI, high-molecular-weight kininogen, and pre-kallikrein) at one day of age are 70% lower than values seen in adults.[87,88] By six months of age, levels of all of these coagulation factors in both premature and full-term infants are within normal adult ranges. On the other hand, levels of fibrinogen, FV, FVIII, and FXIII, and von Willebrand factor (vWF) are all greater than 70% of adult values on the first day of life in both premature and full-term infants. Fibrinogen levels are lower in premature infants than in full-term infants. Inhibitors of coagulation (AT, protein C, and protein S) are also lower in infants than adults. In the fibrinolytic system, plasminogen levels are lower in infants than adults and significantly lower in preterm than term infants.[89]

Activated partial thromboplastin time (aPTT) has been shown to be the most prolonged coagulation test in both premature and full-term infants on day one of life compared to adults, being 1.2 to 1.5 times longer in term infants and 1.4 to 2.4 times longer in preterm infants.[89] This prolongation has been attributed to the quantitative and qualitative deficiencies of contact factors. In full-term infants, aPTT values are similar to adult values by three months of age, and in premature infants aPTT normalization occurs by six months of age. Values of prothrombin time (PT) are less prolonged in neonates than aPTT values, with reported values ranging from being not significantly different from adult values to being 1.15 to 1.3 times longer.[89] All diagnoses and treatment decisions must be made within the context of these age-dependent ranges.[90]

Plasma transfusion in infants and children

Plasma is one of the most inappropriately utilized blood products. Many infants and children receive plasma transfusions, with a 2012 study analyzing more than 3 million admissions of infants and children showing that 2.85% received plasma.[91] A 2014 study of multiple NICUs in Italy reported that 60% of 609 plasma transfusions given to neonates were noncompliant with published recommendations.[92] Other studies and surveys have also shown relatively high rates of plasma transfusion to nonbleeding infants and children, despite limited evidence of efficacy.[92–95]

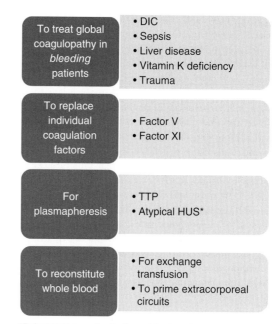

*Refer to text regarding Eculizumab treatment.

Figure 47.2 Plasma transfusion indications in infants and children.

Drawing on experience, past publications,[68,96] and adult guidelines,[97] Figure 47.2 lists plasma transfusion indications in infants and children. Plasma may be used in infants and children to (1) treat global coagulopathy, (2) replace individual coagulation factors, (3) treat diseases such as TTP requiring plasmapheresis, and (4) reconstitute whole blood, for exchange transfusions or extracorporeal circuit priming.

Plasma to treat global coagulopathy

Causes of coagulopathy in infants and children include sepsis, DIC, liver disease, trauma, and dilutional effects. With the realization that treatment of the underlying cause of DIC is essential, plasma may be transfused for DIC-associated bleeding. Plasma is also indicated for liver failure with active bleeding and prior to invasive procedures, although the hemostasis observed after FFP infusion is typically quite transient. Empiric infusion of plasma is not recommended for an elevated INR in the absence of bleeding.[98,99] Although Vitamin K is the first-line therapy for neonates with congenital or acquired vitamin K deficiency, plasma or prothrombin complex concentrates are also indicated in cases of life-threatening bleeding.[89,100,101] Trauma-associated coagulopathy has been demonstrated in children independent of dilutional effect, with adverse outcomes.[102] Pediatric massive transfusion protocols typically treat trauma and dilutional coagulopathy by providing RBCs in addition to plasma, cryoprecipitate, and platelets for resuscitation. Ongoing studies are investigating whether this practice of balanced transfusion resuscitation will improve outcomes in pediatric patients,[103–106] as has been shown in adult patients.

Plasma to replace individual coagulation factors

Plasma is indicated for replacement of coagulation factors, in situations where specific factor concentrates are not available.[98] If a child has a suspected congenital bleeding deficiency but the etiology is not apparent, initial therapy with 10 mL/kg of plasma is reasonable while awaiting definitive factor testing.[89] Plasma remains the treatment of choice in the United States for replacement of factors

V and XI,[99,107,108] although two factor XI concentrates are available outside the United States.[109,110] Reviewed in more detail in Chapters 30 and 31, recombinant or virally inactivated plasma-derived factors VII, VIII, IX, XIII, vWF, and fibrinogen have replaced the need for plasma or cryoprecipitate in patients congenitally deficient in these factors.

Plasma for plasmapheresis

Plasma or cryo-poor plasma is used for plasmapheresis procedures in children with acquired TTP.[111,112] Plasmapheresis removes IgG autoantibodies against ADAMTS13, and replenishes the ADAMTS13 cleaving enzyme. Atypical hemolytic uremic syndrome (aHUS), due to congenital or acquired abnormalities of complement regulatory proteins, may also initially be treated with emergent plasmapheresis utilizing plasma.[111] Complement regulatory and complement-activating proteins should be measured in children suspected of having aHUS, with eculizumab (a humanized anti-C5 monoclonal antibody) recently demonstrating treatment efficacy in children and adults.[113–115]

With the exception of TTP and aHUS, most plasmapheresis procedures completed in children utilize albumin as a replacement fluid. In some instances, patients undergoing frequent plasmapheresis procedures with albumin may become depleted of fibrinogen and other coagulation factors. In these instances, plasma may need to be substituted for albumin in some future procedures (e.g., half albumin and half plasma could be utilized for one procedure to replace such factors, with the following procedure reverting back to albumin as a replacement fluid).

Congenital TTP is due to a deficiency of ADAMTS13. Unlike acquired TTP, plasmapheresis is not necessary because inhibitors are not present. Potential treatments include periodic infusions of plasma or cryoprecipitate; vWF products containing ADAMTS13 recently have been shown to have treatment efficacy.[116,117]

Plasma to reconstitute whole blood (for extracorporeal circuit priming or exchange transfusion)

Transfusion support of pediatric cardiothoracic surgery patients is complex, with dual risks of thrombosis and bleeding. RBCs, fresh whole blood, plasma in combination with RBCs, or nonblood products are used to prime cardiothoracic surgery circuits.[118] Studies show conflicting data with regard to which components in a prime result in less bleeding, fewer transfusion requirements, and better outcomes.[119–122]

ECMO is increasingly being utilized to treat a number of pediatric conditions nonresponsive to traditional ventilatory support.[25] Circuit and coagulopathy maintenance is complicated, with some institutions combining albumin, RBCs, and other additives to prime ECMO circuits.[67] Plasma is transfused in children on ECMO for bleeding in some instances and for elevated INRs (ranging from 1.5 to 2) in other instances.[26,123] A protocol that includes factor Xa monitoring, thromboelastography, and antithrombin monitoring, in addition to traditional coagulation testing, has recently been shown to decrease bleeding, to decrease transfusion requirements, and to increase circuit life in pediatric ECMO patients.[123]

Neonatal exchange transfusions are typically completed using group O RBCs (lacking offending cognate minor antigens) reconstituted with AB plasma, to an Hct of 50–55%; fresh whole blood is utilized instead of reconstituted whole blood in a few regions of the United States. The primary indication for exchange transfusion in neonates, reviewed in detail elsewhere, is hemolytic disease of the newborn with hyperbilirubinemia.[124]

Plasma product selection for infants and children

FFP is frozen to −18 °C within 6–8 hours of phlebotomy; FP24 is frozen within 24 hours of phlebotomy. These products are used interchangeably, unless single factor V or VIII replacement is needed.[125,126] Thawed plasma is FFP or FP24 stored at 1–6 °C for up to five days, with degradation of coagulation factors over time. This product may be useful in situations such as traumas, in which plasma is rapidly needed;[127] however, few pediatric studies have been completed involving thawed plasma. Plasma cryoprecipitate-reduced (also known as cryo-poor plasma) is utilized in some centers as a second-line product and in some centers as a product equivalent to FFP or FP24 for TTP plasmapheresis.

Plasma chosen for transfusion should ideally be ABO compatible, although Rh(D) matching is not required. Plasma is considered an acellular product, and thus irradiation is not necessary. 10–15 mL/kg of plasma typically raises coagulation factors by approximately 30%.

Cryoprecipitate transfusion

Cryoprecipitate is made from the cold, insoluble, high-molecular-weight proteins removed from thawed plasma, including fibrinogen, factor VIII, factor XIII, vWF, and fibronectin. Each individual bag of cryoprecipitate must include 80 IU of factor VIII and 150 mg of fibrinogen, typically in 5–20 mL of plasma.[125] Many blood manufacturers pre-pool 2–10 individual bags of cryoprecipitate for transfusion convenience.

Cryoprecipitate may be used to increase fibrinogen levels in infants and children with hypofibrinogenemia and hemorrhage due to liver disease or DIC[128] (Figure 47.3). Cryoprecipitate may be used to increase fibrinogen levels in older adolescents and young women with postpartum hemorrhage.[129] Cryoprecipitate may be used to replenish fibrinogen levels in pediatric trauma patients, a subset of whom have been reported to have trauma-associated

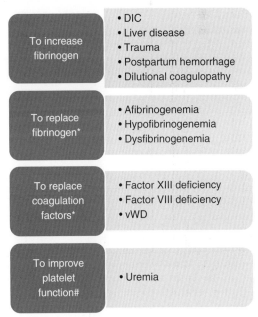

*If recombinant or human derived concentrates are not available or indicated.
#Mechanism of action of cryoprecipitate in uremia is unclear.

Figure 47.3 Cryoprecipitate transfusion indications in infants and children.

hypofibrinogenemia independent of dilutional coagulopathy.[102] In addition, cryoprecipitate can be used in combination with FFP to replace fibrinogen plus coagulation factors in instances of dilutional coagulopathy. Cryoprecipitate may also be used as a second-line therapy to treat uremia-associated bleeding.[130]

Historically, cryoprecipitate has been used for bleeding or prophylaxis in hemophilia, vWD, factor XIII deficiency, congenital afibrinogenemia, or hypofibrinogenemia. These diseases are increasingly being treated with recombinant or human-derived concentrates,[131] although cryoprecipitate remains a second-line therapy should such concentrates be unavailable.

Transfusion thresholds for fibrinogen have not been extensively studied in children, although extrapolation of adult guidelines would suggest that fibrinogen levels should be maintained above 80–100 mg/dL.[98,132] Recent adult studies suggest that fibrinogen levels above 150 mg/dL may be more ideal.[129,133]

In children, one unit of cryoprecipitate per 5–10 kg of body weight is estimated to raise the fibrinogen level by 60–100 mg/dL (Figure 47.1);[95,128] this equates to approximately 2–5 mL of cryoprecipitate per kilogram.[98,134] The half-life of fibrinogen (3–5 days), along with the indication for transfusion, will determine the recommended frequency of cryoprecipitate transfusion. Cryoprecipitate chosen for transfusion should ideally be ABO compatible in children; it is considered an acellular product and thus does not require irradiation for recipients at risk for transfusion-associated graft-versus-host disease. Potential adverse effects of cryoprecipitate transfusion, including the risk of thrombosis, are discussed in more detail elsewhere.

Disclaimer

The authors have disclosed no conflicts of interest.

Key references

A full reference list for this chapter is available at: http://www.wiley.com/go/simon/transfusion

7 Chakravorty S, Roberts I. How I manage neonatal thrombocytopenia. *Br J Haematol* 2012;**156** (2):155–62.

21 Andrew M, Vegh P, Caco C, *et al.* A randomized, controlled trial of platelet transfusions in thrombocytopenic premature infants. *J Pediatr* 1993;**123** (2):285–91.

23 Borges JP, dos Santos AM, da Cunha DH, Mimica AF, Guinsburg R, Kopelman BI. Restrictive guideline reduces platelet count thresholds for transfusions in very low birth weight preterm infants. *Vox Sang* 2013;**104** (3):207–13.

28 Peterson JA, McFarland JG, Curtis BR, Aster RH. Neonatal alloimmune thrombocytopenia: pathogenesis, diagnosis and management. *Br J Haematol* 2013;**161** (1):3–14.

34 Josephson CD, Granger S, Assmann SF, *et al.* Bleeding risks are higher in children versus adults given prophylactic platelet transfusions for treatment-induced hypoproliferative thrombocytopenia. *Blood* 2012;**120** (4):748–60.

40 Kaufman RM, Djulbegovic B, Gernsheimer T, *et al.* Platelet transfusion: a clinical practice guideline from the AABB. *Ann Intern Med* 2015 Feb 3;**162** (3):205–13.

54 C17 Guidelines Committee. Guideline for platelet transfusion for pediatric hematology/oncology patients. Edmonton, AB: C17 Council, 2011.

60 Julmy F, Ammann RA, Taleghani BM, Fontana S, Hirt A, Leibundgut K. Transfusion efficacy of ABO major-mismatched platelets (PLTs) in children is inferior to that of ABO-identical PLTs. *Transfusion* 2009;**49** (1):21–33.

95 Poterjoy BS, Josephson CD. Platelets, frozen plasma, and cryoprecipitate: what is the clinical evidence for their use in the neonatal intensive care unit? *Semin Perinatol* 2009;**33** (1):66–74.

132 Gibson BE, Todd A, Roberts I, *et al.* Transfusion guidelines for neonates and older children. *Br J Haematol* 2004;**124** (4):433–53.

CHAPTER 48

Perioperative transfusion needs

Leanne Clifford,[1] Daryl J. Kor,[1] & James R. Stubbs[2]

[1]Department of Anesthesiology, Mayo Clinic, Rochester, MN, USA
[2]Division of Transfusion Medicine, Department of Laboratory Medicine and Pathology, Mayo Clinic, Rochester, MN, USA

Background

Anemia, thrombocytopenia, and derangements in coagulation parameters are common in the perioperative setting.[1–4] Historically, concerns for surgical hemorrhage associated with adverse patient outcomes have driven liberal transfusion practices in these surgical populations. Indeed, recent estimates suggest that approximately 50% of the 24,000,000 annual transfusions in the United States continue to take place in the perioperative environment.[5,6] However, a growing body of evidence supports more conservative transfusion practices.[7,8] These sentiments are largely based upon accumulating evidence suggesting a lack of efficacy with liberal transfusion practices,[8,9] increased awareness regarding the risks of transfusion therapies,[10–12] and an increased appreciation of blood components as a valuable health care resource—in terms of both supply limitations and associated costs.[13,14] In light of these findings, dedicated patient blood management (PBM) programs have been implemented, aiming to cultivate more evidence-based transfusion practices.[15] Despite these advances, the literature continues to describe the liberal and highly variable utilization of transfusion therapies in surgical populations.[16,17] Examples include red blood cell (RBC) administration for the correction of stable asymptomatic anemia, and plasma administration for correction of abnormal coagulation parameters in the absence of bleeding.[18–21]

Although the risk for hemorrhage must be considered in all patients undergoing invasive procedures, it is important to recognize that our ability to accurately predict bleeding risk remains disappointingly limited.[17,21,22] Likewise, the determinants of when to transfuse RBCs to a bleeding surgical patient remain poorly defined. Moreover, it must also be acknowledged that the prophylactic administration of either plasma products or platelet components with the intention of modifying bleeding risk is largely devoid of evidence and may be potentially harmful.[23–25] This leaves us with challenging questions: What is the best way to assess my patients' risk of perioperative bleeding? What is the best approach to mitigating this bleeding risk? How much bleeding is acceptable before we should decide to transfuse? To what extent should derangement in laboratory tests be tolerated before transfusion? In this chapter, we discuss the preoperative evaluation of potential transfusion needs, indications for and goals and risks of perioperative blood product transfusion, interpretation of coagulation tests, and special perioperative transfusion situations.

Anemia and surgery

Many decades ago, the World Health Organization (WHO) defined *anemia* as hemoglobin (Hb) levels <11.0 g/dL for children 0.50 to 4.99 years, <11.5 g/dL for children 5.0 to 11.99 years, <12.0 g/dL for children 12.0 to 14.99 years and nonpregnant women ≥15.0 years, <11.0 g/dL for pregnant women, and <13.0 g/dL for men ≥15.0 years.[26] Anemia, as defined here, is a widespread condition, affecting approximately 25% of the world's population.[27] Not surprisingly, anemia is the most common preoperative hematologic abnormality encountered in the surgical patient population. Estimates of the prevalence of preoperative anemia range from 30% to more than 50% for cardiac surgery patients[1,28–32] to 76% for patients with advanced colon cancer.[33] Anemia is often a sign of underlying diseases or conditions that could negatively impact surgical outcomes. Such negative consequences are not restricted to severe anemia. Adverse outcomes such as renal injury, stroke, and even death have been shown to be associated with surgical patients categorized as having mild or moderate anemia.[28,29,34,35] Perioperative anemia, therefore, imparts significant added risk for surgical patients. To address the problems associated with anemia, RBC transfusions are frequently administered perioperatively.

Impact of anemia on surgical outcomes

Musallam and colleagues recently evaluated the effects of preoperative anemia on patients undergoing major noncardiac surgery. Data from 2008 were obtained from the American College of Surgeons' National Surgical Quality Improvement Program database derived from 211 hospitals worldwide.[28] Of the 227,425 patients from whom data were obtained, 69,229 (30.44%) had preoperative anemia. Anemia was defined as *mild* (hematocrit [Hct] >29% but <39% in men and >29% but <36% in women) or *moderate-to-severe* (≤29% in men and women). Multivariate logistic regression analysis was used to evaluate the impact of anemia on 30-day mortality and composite morbidity (cardiac, central nervous system, respiratory, sepsis, urinary tract, venous

Rossi's Principles of Transfusion Medicine, Fifth Edition. Edited by Toby L. Simon, Jeffrey McCullough, Edward L. Snyder, Bjarte G. Solheim, and Ronald G. Strauss.

thromboembolism, and wound). The odds of 30-day postoperative mortality were higher in patients with anemia (odds ratio [OR] 1.42, 95% confidence interval [CI] 1.31–1.54). When mild and moderate-to-severe anemia were evaluated separately, the increased odds of mortality persisted (OR 1.41, 95% CI 1.30–1.53 for mild anemia; and OR 1.44, 95% CI 1.29–1.60 for moderate-to-severe anemia). Similar findings were obtained for 30-day postoperative composite morbidity (OR 1.35, 95% CI 1.30–1.40 for anemia; OR 1.31, 95% CI 1.26–1.36 for mild anemia; and OR 1.56, 95% CI 1.47–1.66 for moderate-to-severe anemia).

Wu and colleagues retrospectively analyzed data from 310,311 elderly veterans (>65 years old) who underwent noncardiac surgery to determine if preoperative anemia was associated with cardiac events or mortality.[36] Preoperative Hct was found to be inversely correlated with cardiac events and mortality with such events steadily increasing with decreasing Hct levels. A 10% increase in such events was seen when associated with mild anemia (Hct 36.0–38.9), and this rose to a 53% increase in association with more severe anemia (Hct 18.0–20.9).

In a single-center cohort study of noncardiac surgical patients, Beattie and colleagues assessed the relationship between preoperative anemia and postoperative mortality.[37] Data were collected on 7759 consecutive noncardiac surgical patients between the years 2003 and 2006. The WHO definitions of anemia for adult men and nonpregnant adult women were used in the study. Preoperative anemia was found in 39.5% of men and 39.9% of women. Logistic regression analysis demonstrated an association of preoperative anemia with increased mortality (OR 2.36, 95% CI 1.57–3.41). When a propensity-matched cohort of patients was used for analysis, preoperative anemia continued to be associated with increased mortality (OR 2.29, 95% CI 1.45–3.63).

Micelli et al. evaluated the effect of preoperative anemia on outcomes in patients undergoing cardiac surgery.[38] Data were obtained on a cohort of 7738 consecutive heart surgery patients between April 2003 and February 2009. The WHO definitions of anemia for adult men and nonpregnant adult women were utilized for the study. Preoperative anemia was present in 1856 patients. Overall mortality for the total cohort was 2.1%. The incidence of mortality for patients with preoperative anemia was significantly higher than for nonanemic patients (4.6% vs. 1.5%, p < 0.0001). Propensity-adjusted multivariable logistic regression analysis demonstrated preoperative anemia as an independent predictor of mortality (OR 1.44, 95% CI 1.02–2.03), postoperative renal dysfunction (OR 1.73, 95% CI 1.43–2.1), and a >7-day hospital length of stay (OR 1.3, 95% CI 1.15–1.47).

In a study evaluating the effects of anemia and cardiovascular disease on surgery-associated morbidity and mortality, Carson et al. studied 1958 patients who refused blood transfusion for religious reasons.[39] Overall, increased 30-day risk of mortality was associated with decreasing preoperative Hb levels, especially for patients with an Hb of 6 g/dL or lower. The risk of mortality was particularly high in patients with cardiovascular disease who had a preoperative Hb of 10 g/dL or less.

To assess the impact of postoperative anemia on surgical outcomes, Carson and colleagues published a retrospective cohort analysis (1981–1984) of patients 18 years of age or older who declined to receive RBC transfusions on religious grounds, underwent surgery, and had a postoperative Hb of 8 g/dL or lower.[40] The primary outcome measure was in-hospital mortality in the 30 days following surgery. The combination of 30-day mortality or 30-day in-hospital morbidity (arrhythmia, congestive heart failure,

infection, or myocardial infarction [MI]) was the secondary outcome measure. Postoperative Hbs of 8 g/dL or lower were present in 300 of 2083 patients reviewed. The majority (70.3%) of the study subjects were female, and the mean age was 57 years (standard deviation [SD] ±17.7 years). There were 0 deaths (upper 95% CI 3.7%) in 99 patients with a postoperative Hb of 7.1–8.0 g/dL, whereas morbidity occurred in 9 (9.4%, 95% CI 4.4%–17.0%) of 96 patients evaluated in the 7.1–8.0 g/dL Hb range. In contrast, when the postoperative Hb was 4.1–5.0, 11 (34.4%, 95% CI 18.6–53.2%) of 32 patients died and 15 (57.7%, 95% CI 36.9–76.6%) of 26 evaluated patients died or experienced 30-day morbidity. Following adjustments for age, Acute Physiology and Chronic Health Evaluation II score, and cardiovascular disease, the odds of death increased 2.5 times (95% CI 1.9–3.2) for every successive 1 g decrease in postoperative Hb, with 54.2% (13 of 24) and 100% (7 of 7) 30-day mortality in patients with post-operative Hbs of 2.1–3.0 g/dL and 1.1–2.0 g/dL, respectively. This study demonstrated that the risks of mortality and morbidity in surgical patients became very high when the postoperative Hb fell below 5.1 g/dL (e.g., the mortality rate for postoperative Hb 5.1–7.0 g/dl = 9.0% [10 of 110], whereas the mortality rate for postoperative Hb 3.1–5.0 g/dl = 30.0% [18 of 60]).

A similar study was published 12 years later by Shander et al.[41] This retrospective study included patients 18 years of age or older who underwent surgery between 2003 and 2012, could not be transfused, and had at least one postoperative Hb of 8.0 g/dL or less. The primary outcome was mortality in the 30 days following surgery. Postoperative morbidity (arrhythmia, congestive heart failure, deep wound infection, and myocardial infarction pneumonia) in the 30 days following surgery or until discharge (whichever time frame was shorter) was also measured. Two-hundred ninety-three patients were included in the study. The mean age of the study subjects was 61.5 years (SD ± 16.9 years), and 74.1% of the subjects were female. Overall, 24 study subjects died (overall mortality rate 8.2%, 95% CI 5%–11.3%). There were two deaths (1.5%) in 133 patients with a postoperative Hb of 7.1–8.0 g/dL, while composite morbidity/mortality occurred in 31 (23.3%) of patients. When the postoperative Hb was 4.1–5.0, 6 (19.4%) of 31 patients died, and composite morbidity/mortality occurred in 13 (41.9%) of patients. Three (50%) of 6 patients with a postoperative Hb 2.1–3.0 g/dL died. Following adjustments for age, American Society of Anesthesiology score, and age, the odds of death increased 1.82 times (95% CI, 1.27–2.59) for every successive 1 g decrease in postoperative Hb. The authors concluded that their study confirmed the previously documented low risk of mortality for a nadir Hb in the 7.1–8.0 g/dL range. They also observed similar progressively higher mortality risks in association with the lower range postoperative Hbs.

Additional publications also demonstrate anemia as an independent risk factor for postoperative morbidity and mortality in association with noncardiac and cardiac surgery.[42–44]

Impact of RBC transfusions on surgical patient outcomes

As previously noted, RBC transfusions are widely utilized in the perioperative setting. Studies show that 40–70% of all RBC transfusions are given in association with surgical procedures.[45–47] The report from the 2011 AABB National Blood Collection and Utilization Survey (NBCUS) documented that surgical departments used 19.8% of all RBCs distributed.[48]

A common rationale for RBC transfusions is to enhance oxygen delivery (DO_2) in patients with a decreased red cell mass, often inferred by the presence of a low Hb, who are considered to have a low tolerance for such a state due to impaired compensatory mechanisms, such as when there is coexisting cardiovascular disease. As previously outlined, numerous studies have shown an association between anemia and morbidity and mortality in surgical patients. What is not known conclusively are the specific thresholds when RBCs should be administered to resolve anemia and improve outcomes.

The influence of RBC transfusions on outcomes in surgical patients has been assessed in multiple studies. A recent study evaluated postoperative morbidity, in-hospital mortality, and long-term survival of Jehovah's Witness patients who underwent cardiac surgery compared to a similarly matched group of cardiac surgery patients who received RBC transfusions.[49] Between January 1, 1983, and January 1, 2011, 322 Jehovah's Witness and 87,453 non–Jehovah's Witness patients underwent cardiac surgery. Transfusions were given to 48,986 of the non–Jehovah's Witness patients. When compared to matched patients who received transfusions, Jehovah's Witnesses had better outcomes for the following:

- Myocardial infarction, 0.31% versus 2.8% ($p = 0.01$)
- Additional operation for bleeding, 3.7% versus 7.1% ($p = 0.03$)
- Prolonged ventilation, 6% versus 16% ($p < 0.001$)
- Intensive care unit length of stay (15th, 50th, and 85th percentiles), 24, 25, and 72 versus 24, 48, and 162 hours ($p < 0.001$)
- Hospital length of stay (15th, 50th, and 85th percentiles), 5, 7, and 11 versus 6, 8, and 16 days ($p < 0.001$).

The 95% one-year survival in Jehovah's Witness patients was significantly higher than the 89% one-year survival of transfused patients ($p = 0.007$). In contrast, 20-year survival was similar (34% vs. 32%; $p = 0.90$). The results of this study suggest that nontransfused cardiac surgery patients are not at increased risk for morbidity or mortality compared to similar patients who receive perioperative transfusions.

Carson and colleagues studied the impact of RBC transfusions on 30-day and 90-day postoperative mortality in a retrospective cohort study of 8787 consecutive patients, 60 years of age or older, who underwent surgery for the repair of hip fractures at 20 hospitals between 1983 and 1993.[50] The "trigger" Hb for transfused patients was defined as lowest value prior to the first transfusion, and this was compared to the lowest Hb in nontransfused patients. The overall mortality rates were 4.6% ($n = 402$) at 30 days and 9.0% ($n = 788$) at 90 days. Postoperative transfusions were given to 3,699 (42%) patients. Transfusions were given to 55.6% of patients with an Hb between 8.0 g/dL and 10 g/dL and to 90.5% of patients with an Hb less than 8.0 g/dL. After adjustment for trigger Hb, cardiovascular disease, and other risk factors for death, the odds ratios for 30-day (0.96; 95% CI, 0.74–1.26) and 90-day mortality (1.08; 95% CI, 0.90–1.29) showed no influence of postoperative RBC transfusions on mortality. There was also no difference in 30-day postoperative mortality when patients who received preoperative RBC transfusions were compared to those who did not (adjusted OR, 1.23; 95% CI, 0.81–1.89). It was concluded that perioperative RBC transfusions at an Hb transfusion trigger of 8.0 g/dL or higher in this elderly patient population did not influence 30-day or 90-day mortality. Assessment of the influence of RBC transfusions on mortality at an Hb transfusion trigger of less than 8.0 g/dL in this population could not be made because 90.5% of patients received RBC transfusions.

The Transfusion Requirements in Critical Care (TRICC) trial is an important randomized clinical trial designed to assess RBC transfusion-related outcomes in critically ill patients.[51] In this trial, 838 critically ill, normovolemic patients with an Hb of less than 9 g/dL within 72 hours of admission to an intensive care unit were randomized to either restrictive or liberal RBC transfusion strategies. There were 408 patients in the restrictive group and 420 patients in the liberal group. RBC transfusions were administered to restrictive-group patients for an Hb less than 7 g/dL in order to maintain the Hb between 7 g/dL and 9 g/dL. RBCs were administered to liberal-group patients for an Hb less than 10 g/dL in order to maintain the Hb between 10 g/dL and 12 g/dL. Thirty-day mortality was not statistically different between the restrictive and liberal RBC transfusion groups, although the raw mortality rate was lower in the restrictive group (18.7% vs. 23.3 %, $p = 0.11$). The mortality rates were lower in the restrictive transfusion group (8.7% in the restrictive group vs. 16.1% in the liberal group, $p = 0.03$) when less acutely ill patients (Acute Physiology and Chronic Health Evaluation II score of ≤20) as well as when patients younger than 55 years of age (5.7% in the restrictive group vs. 13.0% in the liberal group, $p = 0.02$) were compared. The restrictive-strategy group also had lower rates of myocardial infarction (0.07% vs. 2.9%, $p = 0.02$), pulmonary edema (5.3% vs. 10.7%, $p < 0.01$), and mortality during hospitalization (22.3% vs. 28.1%, $p = 0.05$). The restrictive and liberal groups had similar mortality rates for patients with a primary or secondary diagnosis of cardiac disease (20.5% vs. 22.9%, $p = 0.69$). The average Hb and the number of RBC units transfused were significantly lower in the restrictive group. It was concluded that the restrictive RBC transfusion strategy with a transfusion trigger of 7 g/dL was at least as effective, and possibly superior to, a trigger of 10.0 g/dL in critically ill patients, with the possible exception of patients with acute MI and unstable angina.

In a large study designed to determine the optimal perioperative RBC transfusion threshold, the Transfusion Trigger Trial for Functional Outcomes in Cardiovascular Patients Undergoing Surgical Hip Fracture Repair (FOCUS) studied 2016 patients with known cardiovascular disease or cardiovascular risk factors who were randomized to restrictive or liberal postoperative RBC transfusion groups following surgical repair of hip fractures.[9] All study patients were at least 50 years of age (mean age, 82 years), and all had a postoperative Hb less than 10 g/dL. Patients in the liberal RBC transfusion group received one RBC transfusion immediately after enrollment and additional RBC transfusions to maintain the Hb higher than 10 g/dL. Patients in the restrictive RBC transfusion group received RBCs if they developed symptoms warranting RBC transfusions or when the postoperative Hb dropped below 8 g/dL (even in the absence of symptoms). Symptoms triggering RBC transfusions were chest pain felt to be cardiac in nature, orthostatic hypotension or tachycardia unresponsive to fluid challenge, or congestive heart failure. The primary study outcome was mortality or the inability to walk 10 feet across a room without assistance at the 60-day evaluation point. Also evaluated was a combined outcome of death, in-hospital MI, or unstable angina. Another secondary outcome was death beyond the 60-day evaluation point for any reason. For the primary study outcome, similar rates were observed for the liberal and restrictive RBC transfusion groups (35.2% vs. 34.7%, OR 1.01, 95% CI 0.84–1.22). Similar rates for the liberal and restrictive groups were found for the composite endpoint of death, in-hospital MI, or unstable angina (4.3% vs. 5.2%, OR 0.82, 99% CI 0.48–1.42). When evaluated individually, the rate of MI was higher (although not statistically significant) in the restrictive group (3.8% vs. 2.3%, relative risk [RR] 1.65, 95% CI 0.99–2.75). The death rates for the liberal and restrictive groups at 60 days were similar (7.6% vs. 6.6%, OR 1.17, 99% CI 0.75–1.83). The FOCUS trial demonstrated that, when compared to a liberal postoperative RBC transfusion strategy at a threshold of 10 g/dL, a restrictive RBC transfusion strategy (threshold of 8 g/dL or for symptoms) was not associated with worse outcomes in hip fracture repair patients with cardiovascular disease or cardiovascular risk factors. The only exception to this conclusion might be related to the risk for MI where there was a marginally increased rate in the restrictive RBC transfusion group. The results of this trial, therefore, support the concept that, for patients with a postoperative Hb of 8.0 g/dL or higher, RBC transfusion decisions can be guided by symptoms rather than a higher Hb threshold.

Two studies in cardiac surgery patients provide support for the concept that an Hb of 8 g/dL is a safe RBC transfusion trigger.[52,53] In the first study, 428 consecutive coronary artery bypass graft (CABG) patients were assigned to one of two postoperative RBC transfusion groups.[52] One group was transfused with RBCs for an Hb <8 g/dL, whereas the other group was transfused for an Hb <9.0 g/dL. No between-group differences in mortality or morbidity were seen. The restrictive group, however, received fewer RBC transfusions (0.9 vs. 1.4 RBC units/patient), which resulted in a reduction of 500 RBC transfusions per 1000 CABG procedures.

In the second cardiac surgery trial, 502 consecutive patients were randomized to liberal or restrictive RBC transfusion strategies.[53] Patients in the liberal strategy were transfused to maintain the Hct at or above 30% throughout surgery and the postoperative period. Patients in the restrictive strategy were transfused to maintain the Hct at or above 24% throughout surgery and postoperative period. The combination of 30-day all-cause mortality, acute renal injury requiring dialysis or hemofiltration, acute respiratory distress syndrome (ARDS), and cardiogenic shock were chosen as the composite primary outcome. No difference in the rates of the composite endpoints was observed (liberal group 10% vs. restrictive group 11%). Overall, regardless of restrictive or liberal RBC transfusion strategy, the number of RBC transfusions were correlated with death and other clinical complications (HR 1.2 per transfused RBC unit). These two trials support a restrictive RBC transfusion approach (i.e., Hb or Hct transfusion triggers of 8 g/dL or 24%) in cardiac surgery patients.

A recent Cochrane review evaluated strategies for guiding allogeneic RBC transfusion decisions.[54] Nineteen randomized trials comparing lower (restrictive) versus higher (liberal) RBC transfusion thresholds involving a total of 6264 medical and surgical patients were identified. Most of the studies assessed outcomes in patients transfused at Hb thresholds between 7 g/dL and 10 g/dL, although specific thresholds differed between trials. The analysis showed that, when compared to liberal RBC transfusion strategies, restrictive transfusion strategies resulted in:

- A lower rate of receiving RBC transfusions (46% vs. 84%, RR 0.61, 95% CI 0.52–0.72);
- 1.19 fewer RBC units transfused per patient;
- Trends suggesting lower 30-day mortality (RR 0.85, 95% CI 0.70–1.03) and overall infection rates (RR 0.81, 95% CI 0.66–1.00) (no differences seen in pneumonia rates, however);
- No differences in functional recovery, hospital length of stay, or intensive care length of stay; and
- No differences in MI risk when all trials were evaluated (RR 0.88, 95% CI 0.38–2.04).

The two largest studies included in the Cochrane analysis, the TRICC trial and the FOCUS trial, however, showed different results

pertaining to the risk of MI associated with a restrictive RBC transfusion strategy.[9,51] The TRICC trial documented a lower risk of MI in the restrictive group (0.7% vs. 2.9%, RR 0.25, 95% CI 0.07–0.88), and the FOCUS trial showed a higher (although not statistically significant) risk in the restrictive group (3.8% vs. 2.3%, RR 1.65, 95% CI 0.99–2.75).

With regard to RBC transfusion decisions in patients with active bleeding, in a single center trial, 921 patients with acute upper GI bleeding were randomized to a restrictive (threshold Hb 7 g/dL) or a liberal (threshold Hb 9 g/dL) RBC transfusion strategy.[8] Excluded from the study were patients with acute coronary syndrome, massive bleeding, a history of peripheral vascular disease, a history of stroke, or an Hb more than 12 g/dL. Emergent upper endoscopy was performed on all patients, and endoscopic therapy was provided as necessary. The patients in the restrictive RBC transfusion group, as compared to the liberal group had:

- Lower percent of patients receiving RBC transfusions (49% vs. 86%);
- Fewer number of RBC units transfused (mean 1.5 units vs. 3.7 units);
- Fewer complications (40% vs. 48%);
- Lower percent of patients having subsequent bleeding (10% vs. 16%, hazard ratio [HR] 0.62, 95% CI 0.43–0.91);
- Lower mortality due to uncontrolled bleeding (0.7% vs. 3.1%); and
- Lower all-cause mortality (5% vs. 9%, HR 0.55, 95% CI 0.33–0.92).

The results of this study suggest that a restrictive RBC transfusion strategy might be safe and associated with improved outcomes in actively bleeding, hemodynamically stable patients when there are no additional comorbidities that impart risk such as unstable coronary artery disease, and when surgical intervention is promptly available.

Predictive value of coagulation tests

The international normalized ratio (INR) and activated partial thromboplastin times (aPTTs) are frequently used to guide hemostatic interventions, particularly in the perioperative setting where the risk for hemorrhagic events is increased. Indeed, several societal guidelines make reference to the degree of derangement in the INR that may warrant treatment, typically citing the somewhat arbitrary threshold of >1.5 times the upper limit of normal.[24,55,56] Importantly, however, the interpretation of coagulation test results is fraught with challenges. In part, this is the result of long-standing misconceptions regarding the relationship between INR or aPTT values with in vivo coagulation factor concentrations and clinical coagulation or hemostasis.[22,25] Indeed, this misinformation almost certainly contributes to the well-documented inappropriate use of plasma products.[57,58] To this point, it has now been demonstrated in a variety of clinical settings that the INR and aPTT are poorly predictive of clinical coagulopathy or periprocedural bleeding.[59] Furthermore, the subsequent administration of plasma often fails to produce an effective and sustained correction in coagulation factor content. In fact, for mild to moderate prolongations in INR (1.1–1.85), plasma administration frequently fails to "normalize" the coagulation test.[17,19]

The poor correlation between coagulation screening tests, in vivo coagulation factor levels, and clinical coagulopathy is perhaps best explained by the nonlinear relationship between the INR and serum coagulation factor levels[60] (Figure 48.1). In a healthy subject, coagulation factor levels exceed those required to achieve

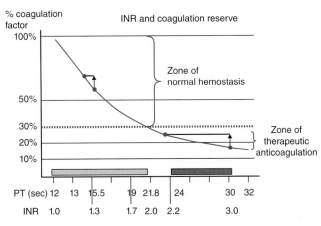

Figure 48.1 The nonlinear relationship between the concentration of coagulation factors and coagulation test results. The concentration of factors (y-axis) is shown as a function of the international normalized ratio (INR) or prothrombin time (PT, in seconds). In general, a concentration of 30% is adequate for biologic hemostasis. Note that when starting at an elevated INR, a small increase in the concentration of factors will have a large impact on the measured INR. In contrast, an equivalent rise in the concentration of factors will have a negligible effect on mildly elevated INR values. The curve is a generalized view and will vary for individual patients.

hemostasis as approximately 30% of normal factor levels can still produce normal coagulation.[61] At this level of coagulation factor activity, the INR may be expected to rise to a level as high as 1.6.[25,62,63] Thus, the INR will be outside of the normal range well before clinical coagulopathy is encountered. In addition, it should be recognized that the INR assay itself is predominantly driven by concentrations of factor VII. Therefore, patients with isolated mild deficiencies of factor VII can have abnormal INRs despite normal levels of other coagulation factors and an absence of clinical coagulopathy. This is a commonly encountered phenomenon in hospitalized patients whose acute illness may render them vitamin K deplete, with impaired hepatic synthetic function. Furthermore, administration of antibiotics, catabolic states, and subclinical impairment of the enterohepatic circulation may all effect factor VII levels.[64]

Beyond isolated Factor VII deficiency, when multiple mild factor deficiencies exist, such as in liver disease or with vitamin K depletion, the INR and the aPTT have been shown to further overestimate abnormalities in coagulation.[65] This point was highlighted by Burns and colleagues, who observed that an in vitro plasma mixture containing a single coagulation factor at 75% activity and all the remaining factors at 100% activity produced normal INR and aPTT results.[66] In contrast, an in vitro plasma mixture containing two coagulation factors at 75% activity and all the remaining factors at 100% activity resulted in prolonged INR and aPTT values.[66]

With growing concern regarding the ability of INR and aPTT to predict bleeding events, in addition to the their frequently unacceptable turnaround times for results, recent focus has shifted toward the use of modern viscoelastic assays such as thromboelastography (TEG) and rotational thromboelastometry (ROTEM).[67–70] These tests appear able to provide a more accurate and timely point-of-care assessment of thrombus formation in whole blood.[71] Although used most extensively in cardiac surgery and liver

transplantation, early data suggests that these tools may better guide individual transfusion decisions and reduce overall blood product exposure.[72,73] Indeed in 2011, Görlinger and colleagues found the use of ROTEM in cardiac surgical patients resulted in increased utilization of specific factor concentrates, whereas also resulting in an overall reduction in blood product transfusions, without any associated increase in morbidity or mortality.[74]

Management of perioperative anticoagulation and antiplatelet therapies

Management of anticoagulation in the perioperative period can be challenging. Clinicians must weigh the risk of thromboembolic complications versus procedural bleeding and determine the best overall strategy for optimizing outcomes (e.g., active reversal with vitamin K or coagulation factor replacement versus bridging with heparin therapy). Currently, there is little strong evidence in the literature from randomized clinical trials to provide definitive recommendations and many of the existing guidelines are based upon expert opinion. In clinical practice, thromboembolic and bleeding risks depend upon both patient and procedural characteristics. Therefore determining the optimal management strategies will depend upon specific individual risk factors and procedural details. For patients with mechanical heart valves, the risk of thromboembolism is highest in the first three months after valve surgery, particularly when considering the mitral valve.[75] In this instance, simple measures such as avoiding elective surgery during this time frame can help to avoid unnecessary interruptions in anticoagulation that would place the patient at greatest risk of thromboembolic complications. In 2012, the American College of Chest Physicians (ACCP) recommended careful planning of elective procedures with cessation of warfarin seven days before surgery thus allowing INR to gradually normalize and avoiding the need for vitamin K administration that may prolong the achievement of an effective antithrombotic state with warfarin postoperatively.[76] This guideline also stressed the importance of regular INR checks during this time to allow for initiation of bridging anticoagulation (either with heparin or low-molecular-weight heparin) until the time of surgery.[76] An INR check is specifically endorsed on the day prior to surgery to allow for low-dose oral vitamin K supplementation if clinically indicated.[76]

For patients with atrial fibrillation (AF), the risk of thromboembolism may be best characterized using existing risk stratification scores such as the CHADS2 or CHADS2-VASc.[77] However, it must be recognized that these scores have not been specifically validated for predicting risk of thromboembolism in the postoperative period.[77] Of note, the **R**andomized **E**valuation of **L**ong-Term Anticoagulant Therap**y** (RELY) trial recently evaluated thromboembolic risk in patients with nonvalvular AF.[78] This investigation found a rate of thromboembolic complications (including stroke, pulmonary embolus or cardiovascular death) of 1.2%, with the greatest risk seen in patients undergoing urgent surgery.[78]

Finally, for patients whose indication for anticoagulation is thromboembolic disease, risk of subsequent thromboembolism with anticoagulant interruption is believed dependent on the time from the initial thromboembolic event. Where feasible, deferring surgery and anticoagulation interruption may be of benefit.[79,80] In the event that emergency surgery is required, bridging with heparin is often endorsed.[81] However, further randomized trials are warranted in this area in order to determine the optimal perioperative management of anticoagulation in this setting.

For patients taking newer oral anticoagulants (NOACs) including factor Xa inhibitors such as rivaroxaban and apixaban, or direct thrombin inhibitors such as dabigatran, evidence guiding perioperative interruption is more limited. Based on their elimination half-lives (7–11 hours for factor Xa inhibitors and 12–14 hours for thrombin inhibitors in patients with normal renal function),[82] these agents are typically interrupted for 2–3 days ahead of elective surgery to minimize surgical bleeding.[83,84] This interval may be extended in particularly high-risk operations or shortened in particularly low-risk procedures. Importantly, coagulation studies are not routinely indicated in NOAC-treated patients, indeed INR and aPTT have not been validated for the assessment of coagulation status in these patients.[85] However, for emergent operations or in those presenting with a bleeding episode, assessment of coagulation status may be desired. Factor Xa levels may help to guide management of factor Xa inhibitors.[86] The prothrombin time will also typically be prolonged in patients taking factor Xa inhibitors, however significant interassay variability exists and so its measurement is not considered a first-line measure if factor Xa assays are available.[85] In addition, factor Xa inhibitors will also produce a dose-dependent prolongation of R and K time on ROTEM with no change in maximal amplitude[86] If rapid correction of anticoagulation with rivaroxaban is required, prothrombin complex concentrates (PCCs) may be effective.[87,88] At present, specific antidotes remain under investigation.[89]

For patients treated with direct thrombin inhibitors, aPTT levels have been advocated to assess coagulation status;[90] however, this method lacks sufficient evidence to make strong recommendations for its use. At present, dabigatran anticoagulation may be best measured using the thrombin time or dilute thrombin time.[91] Importantly, in the setting of acute bleeding, dabigatran may be successfully filtered by hemodialysis,[92] offering a unique method for reversing anticoagulation. Ongoing randomized clinical trials are needed to determine the best way to reverse NOACs.[89] As with warfarin, decision making regarding interruption of anticoagulation should weigh the risk of thrombosis versus the risk of bleeding for each individual patient and procedure. Due to the rapid onset of action of these agents relative to warfarin, bridging with heparin is often not required when reinitiating therapy postoperatively.

With an aging population, use of antiplatelet agents, such as aspirin and clopidogrel, is widespread in order to manage the risk of major cardiac and vascular thromboembolic events. As with anticoagulants, similar risk to benefit assessments must be made ahead of elective surgery.[93] Both aspirin's and clopidogrel's antiplatelet properties last for the lifespan of the platelet due to their irreversible inhibition of cyclooxygenase 1/2 and the platelet adenosine diphosphate (ADP) P2Y12 receptor, respectively.[94] Due to concern for increased perioperative bleeding,[95–97] historically antiplatelet agents have been withheld for 7–10 days preoperatively. Most recently, this notion was supported by findings from the Perioperative Ischemic Evaluation (POISE-2) randomized controlled trial in which aspirin administration was not associated in any significant decrease in risk of death or nonfatal myocardial infarctions, however major perioperative bleeding was increased.[98] Of note, patients with recent coronary stents and those taking thienopyridines or Ticagrelor were excluded from this study, raising concern about the generalizability of these findings. Moreover, prior observational studies have suggested that early perioperative aspirin use may reduce both death and ischemic complications in patients undergoing cardiac surgery.[99,100] Similarly, Biondi-Zoccai and colleagues

noted a threefold increase in thrombotic complications in moderate- to high-risk patients in whom aspirin was withheld perioperatively.[93] This controversy has led to a re-exploration of the risks and benefits of antiplatelet therapies in the perioperative setting. Indeed the 2012 ACP Guidelines suggest continuing aspirin around noncardiac surgery in those deemed to be at moderate to high risk of cardiovascular events (with aspirin cessation for 7–10 days in those at low risk).[76] Of note, these guidelines were published ahead of the POISE-2 trial findings becoming publically available.

In light of the ongoing equipoise, an individual assessment of risk-to-benefit ratios are required for each patient. In general, currently accepted evidence is in favor of withholding antiplatelet agents when prescribed only for primary prevention (low thrombotic risk) and/or when bleeding risk may be life-threatening, for example with intracranial or ophthalmic surgery. Conversely, patients with bare metal stent placement within six weeks or drug eluting stent within six months should not routinely discontinue antiplatelet therapy for elective surgery. For these patients requiring urgent surgery with an intermediate or high risk of bleeding, options include discontinuation of clopidogrel with continuation of aspirin, or discontinuation of both agents with bridging therapy around the time of surgery.

Conservative versus liberal transfusion

Historically, blood products have been transfused liberally to treat mild derangements in laboratory parameters under the assumption that the normalization of these laboratory abnormalities would improve patient outcomes. Indeed, in the middle of the last century, it was recommended that RBCs be transfused to maintain an Hb concentration >10 g/dL based upon the assumption that increasing the patient's Hb would improve tissue oxygenation.[101] This became a longstanding, accepted standard of practice for surgical patients for many years. Even now, plasma continues to be administered to correct modest abnormalities in INR in the absence of active bleeding.[19,23,62,102] Importantly, a significant proportion (approximately 50%) of these "liberal" transfusions take place in the perioperative setting,[5] which makes it a prime setting to achieve more appropriate blood product utilization moving forward.

A growing body of literature has begun to specifically focus on which clinical situations truly warrant transfusion and at what threshold. As outlined above, multiple RBC transfusion studies have demonstrated the safety and effectiveness of restrictive practices.[8,9,51–53] Similar results have been obtained in liver resection patients[103] as well as in patients with sepsis,[104] and traumatic brain injury.[105] Additionally, Yu et al. identified a positive dose response relationship between the number of blood products transfused and risk of adverse outcomes in patients undergoing cardiac surgery.[106] In aggregate, the prevailing conclusion of available literature suggests that liberal RBC transfusion practices do not offer a morbidity or mortality advantage.[107,108] To the contrary, the growing body of observational research suggest that restrictive transfusion practices may be associated with a higher probability of survival and fewer complications such as infection, acute respiratory distress syndrome, cardiogenic shock, acute kidney injury and multi-organ dysfunction.[109–111]

Despite the growing evidence for restrictive RBC transfusion strategies, widespread implementation of conservative transfusion practices in the operating room environment has not been without challenges. Although many societal guidelines and patient blood management programs now advocate conservative transfusion strategies,[112–115] transfusions continue to be frequently administered outside of published guidelines. In an effort to improve the intraoperative transfusion practice, the American Society of Anesthesiologists' (ASA) practice guidelines recommend: (1) periodic visual assessment of the surgical field and communication with the surgical team, (2) continuous monitoring for evidence of inadequate perfusion and oxygenation of vital organs, and (3) RBC administration when the Hb falls below 6 g/dL, in quantities necessary to achieve adequate organ perfusion, also noting that RBC transfusion is generally unnecessary when the Hb is >10 g/dL.[24] Furthermore, these guidelines endorse the use of blood recovery techniques and permissive hypotension to decrease blood loss, when appropriate. Outside of massive transfusion protocols, it is also recommended that RBC transfusions occur one unit at a time, with subsequent evaluation of the clinical response before determining the need for additional RBC transfusions.[24] Similar conservative approaches to transfusion therapies have been echoed by the STS/SCA and the AABB clinical practice guidelines.[113]

Blood avoidance techniques

In light of the potential for transfusion-related adverse events as well as the limited supply of blood component therapies and the occasional religious objection to blood transfusion, avoidance of transfusion—in some situations—may be a safer and more cost-effective and morally acceptable option. Although blood transfusion is not always avoidable, several interventions may be employed to facilitate the avoidance of blood component therapies. Prior to elective surgery, phlebotomy should be limited to only tests essential for clinical decision making.[116] The rationale for limiting phlebotomy is based on a growing body of data outlining the prevalence, severity, and implications that hospital-acquired anemia (HAA) has on patient outcomes. A large observational study by Koch and colleagues describes an incidence of HAA of 74%.[117] Although felt to be multifactorial, phlebotomy has been highly correlated with HAA. Data suggest a decrease in Hb of 0.08 g/dL for every 1 ml of blood drawn,[118] or an 18% increased risk of developing moderate-to-severe HAA with every 50 ml of blood drawn.[119] Equally, if not more important, HAA has been associated with increased hospital length of stay, hospitalization costs, and in-hospital mortality.[117] Minimizing phlebotomy volumes has been previously demonstrated to reduce transfusion requirements in critically ill patients, and should be a standard measure employed as part of blood avoidance.[120] In certain populations, particularly patients with preexisting anemia, and in those who refuse transfusion, erythropoietin and iron supplementation should be considered, especially if preoperative autologous blood donation will take place.[121] If safe to do so, cessation or avoidance of blood thinning drugs—including nonsteroidal anti-inflammatory drugs, antiplatelet agents, and anticoagulants—is prudent.[122]

Intraoperatively, there should be meticulous attention to hemostasis and rapid control of hemorrhage.[116] Permissive hypotension may be considered as a method to minimize precipitous blood loss.[123,124] To this end, a recent randomized trial evaluating resuscitation of trauma patients demonstrated that patients resuscitated to a mean arterial pressure (MAP) of 50 mmHg required significantly fewer blood products and reduced crystalloid resuscitation volumes compared with those resuscitated to a MAP goal of 65 mmHg.[123] These patients also had a lower early postoperative mortality and experienced coagulopathy less frequently and with a lesser severity.[123] Other measures to minimized intraoperative

blood loss include the avoidance of hypothermia,[125,126] and when possible, cell salvage mechanisms should be utilized to facilitate rapid autologous transfusion. Modern cell salvage technologies are unique in their ability to provide rapid, large volumes of blood to patients without the need for preoperative donation or hemodilution that may be limited by patient tolerance and hemodynamic reserve. These methods have been most extensively used in hepatic,[127,128] cardiac,[129–131] and orthopedic[132] surgeries and have been shown to be cost-effective and safe. Research is ongoing regarding use of these methods in patients with active malignancy and bacteremia.[133,134]

Although infrequently employed, acute normovolemic hemodilution remains a viable option.[135–137] Although aprotinin is no longer approved for use by the US Food and Drug Administration, lysine analogs such as ε-aminocaproic acid and tranexamic acid are advocated by some, including the Society of Thoracic Surgeons and Society of Cardiovascular Anesthesiologists (STS/SCA), to minimize total blood loss.[138] Efficacy for these agents is most robust in the settings of cardiac surgery, orthopedic surgery, and trauma resuscitation. In addition, topical hemostatic agents may be utilized. Postoperatively, iatrogenic anemia can again be minimized through the judicious use of phlebotomy.

Topical hemostatic therapies

Topical therapies for localized bleeding offer a variety of effective hemostatic options that may avoid the need for transfusion. While suture ligation of a damaged vessel remains the single most effective method for hemostasis, this is not always technically feasible. In this situation, use of electrocautery, sclerosing agents, argon laser beam coagulation, and direct packing and compression have been common practice.[139] More recently various topical sealants, thrombins, and antifibrinolytic agents have become available for treatment of topical oozing.[140,141] Of note, none of these agents are effective in the management of occult hemorrhage. Fibrin sealants consist of the simultaneous application of topical fibrinogen with either topical thrombin or aprotinin.[142] They are applied in the form of a liquid, spray, or dressing and are typically helpful in aiding hemostasis along vascular anastomosis suture lines.[143–145]

Topical thrombin is also available in isolation. Currently, bovine, human, and recombinant thrombins are available. The use of bovine-derived thrombin has been associated in a minority of patients with the development of antibodies directed against bovine coagulation proteins in the preparation.[146] These antibodies include Factor V antibodies and thrombin antibodies. In some patients, these antibodies can cross-react with human coagulation proteins, resulting in the development of a coagulation inhibitor. In some of these patients, the inhibitor can be clinically significant and represents a serious adverse effect of bovine thrombin. However, clinically significant inhibitors are very infrequent and this risk of inhibitor formation should be further reduced with the advent of human and recombinant thrombin.[147] These agents may be applied as a powder or reconstituted and applied as a liquid spray for topical hemostasis. In patients without an identified source of bleeding—such as the trauma patient with disseminated intravascular coagulation—packing with antifibrinolytic-soaked gauzes (e.g., Amicar) may be used to achieve temporary hemostasis until definitive control of bleeding can be achieved.

In addition to the above agents, sterile topical collagen, cellulose, and gelatin agents—such as Floseal, Surgicel, and Gelfoam—may be applied and left inside the body to help produce a mechanical hemostatic effect until they dissolve.[143] Very little is known about the toxicity of these agents.

Perioperative transfusion guidelines

Red blood cells: indications, threshold, and dose

Evidence-based indications for RBC transfusion in nonbleeding, hemodynamically stable patients have been revised and subsequently reaffirmed many times in recent decades.[112,113,148] Unfortunately, few of these investigations provide meaningful guidance for surgical populations, particularly when clinically significant active bleeding is encountered.[24,138] In this specific clinical circumstance, the unwavering take home message is that appropriate RBC transfusion practices require more than an arbitrary hemoglobin-based transfusion trigger. Rather, the decision to transfuse RBCs in this context should be based upon patient-specific symptoms (e.g., hemodynamic instability or evidence of tissue hypoxia) and details relating to the surgical course (e.g., expected ongoing blood loss).[24,138] To this point, the most compelling indication for intraoperative RBC transfusion remains acute hemorrhage with associated hemodynamic instability or evidence of inadequate oxygen delivery. In contrast, generalized mucosal oozing, gradual blood loss over a prolonged period of time, and asymptomatic anemia related to chronic disease or hemodilution are perhaps more frequent clinical scenarios that prompt decisions regarding the appropriateness of intraoperative RBC administration. In 2006, the ASA's taskforce on perioperative blood transfusion were among the first to encourage more conservative transfusion practices for surgical populations.[24] The authors appropriately noted that the literature was insufficient to define a transfusion trigger in surgical patients with substantial blood loss. They concluded that the decision to transfuse should be based upon regular assessment of the surgical field, communication with the surgical team, estimated blood loss, Hb concentration, and an assessment of organ perfusion. Assessment of organ perfusion includes heart rate, blood pressure, urine output, evidence of ischemia, and, where appropriate, mixed venous oxygen saturations and echocardiography. All members of the panel agreed that RBCs should be administered when the Hb is <6 g/dl and that transfusion is rarely necessary when the Hb >10 g/dl.[24]

Beyond the setting of acute hemorrhage, available guidelines generally support conservative transfusion practices, considering individual patients' need for RBC transfusion only when the Hb falls below 7 g/dL. This recommendation is endorsed by the Society of Critical Care Medicine and the Eastern Association of Surgery for Trauma's 2009 joint clinical practice guidelines.[112] Specifically, this guideline intended to address indications for RBC transfusion in the critically ill, those presenting with trauma, requiring mechanical ventilation or with known stable coronary disease. However, ongoing equipoise exists regarding optimal transfusion thresholds in patients with coronary artery disease. Although similar recommendations were repeated in the AABB 2012 clinical practice guidelines, a more modest Hb threshold of 8 g/dL was suggested for patients with stable coronary disease and postoperative surgical patients in the presence of symptoms such as chest pain, orthostatic hypotension, tachycardia unresponsive to fluid resuscitation, or congestive heart failure.[113] Of note, this slightly higher threshold of 8 g/dL was predominantly chosen based upon findings of the FOCUS trial in which liberal (Hb <10 g/dL) transfusion strategies were compared to a more restrictive approach (Hb <8 g/dL or

symptomatic) in surgical patients with known stable cardiovascular disease.[114] For patients with acute coronary syndromes, an Hb threshold of 8–10 g/dL is typically desired. In 2011, the STS/SCA again echoed the appropriateness of a more restrictive transfusion practice. Specifically they emphasized that RBC transfusion is *most often* necessary when Hb falls <6 g/dL, *may* be required <7 g/dL, and is *never* required when Hb >10 g/dL.[149]

The primary goals of perioperative blood product transfusion are to maintain tissue oxygenation and ensure hemostasis. Although improved oxygen carrying capacity is certainly achieved with RBC transfusion, the association between RBC transfusion and improved tissue oxygenation remains much more controversial.[150–152] Multiple studies have attempted to address this very question; even though oxygen delivery was consistently found to be increased following RBC transfusion, very few studies were able to demonstrate a reciprocal increase in tissue oxygen consumption.[112,152] Although the underlying mechanisms remain under investigation, it is hypothesized that this observation may be secondary to a diminished capillary diameter in critically ill or injured patients, or as a function of the many biochemical changes that occur in stored RBCs.[153]

In the absence of acute blood loss, the desired endpoints following perioperative RBC transfusion are less well defined. Available literature suggests that an individualized assessment for evidence of ischemia or hemodynamic stability with signs or symptoms suggestive of inadequate end-organ perfusion and oxygenation should guide decisions on RBC administration.[24] Where none of the above criteria are satisfied, further transfusion is unlikely to result in meaningful clinical benefit. However, respecting well-thought-out guidelines supporting RBC transfusion when the Hb falls below 7 g/dL, it would not be unreasonable to transfuse patients to a target above this threshold.

In summary, modern perioperative RBC transfusion practice has seen a move toward more conservative transfusion strategies. This substantial reevaluation of our RBC transfusion practice has been largely driven by evolving evidence showing an association between liberal transfusion practices and adverse patient outcomes, including infection, acute respiratory distress syndrome, multi-organ dysfunction, and mortality. Although the association between liberal RBC transfusion practices and these adverse patient outcomes remains a matter of much debate, the absence of evidence suggesting the potential for harm with restrictive transfusion therapies would appear to support recommendations to avoid RBC transfusion in nonbleeding, hemodynamically stable patients when the Hb is >7 g/dL.

Plasma: indications, threshold, and dose

It has been estimated that approximately one-third of plasma products are transfused for non-evidence-based indications.[19–21] In the United States, the most frequently cited rationale for deviation from published guidelines is to correct abnormal preprocedural coagulation screening tests in nonbleeding patients.[60] The rationale for transfusing plasma in this context is based on three basic assumptions: (1) an elevated INR reliably predicts bleeding complications, (2) administration of plasma will normalize the INR, and (3) administration of plasma will prevent bleeding complications. Importantly, all three assumptions rest on minimal evidentiary support and when considering the growing body of evidence suggesting a poor correlation between coagulation screening test abnormalities[22,60] and periprocedural bleeding complications alongside the increasingly appreciated risks of transfusion, such practice is strongly discouraged.

In the absence of massive transfusion or hemorrhagic shock, anticoagulant therapy, or consumptive disorders, such as disseminated intravascular coagulation, de novo coagulation factor depletion as an underlying etiology for clinically significant bleeding is rare. Indeed, it is understood that adequate coagulation persists with approximately one-third of normal clotting factor concentrations and fibrinogen levels ≥75 mg/dL.[62,154] Although these abnormalities will result in derangements of laboratory coagulation parameters, clinical coagulopathy does not typically correlate. With improved understanding of in vivo coagulation, as well as the risks of transfusion therapies, there have been notable changes in the clinical indications for perioperative plasma transfusion. Indeed, the historic use of plasma as a volume expander is now obsolete. At present, the strongest indication for plasma transfusion is for the treatment of active hemorrhage that is believed related to multiple coagulation factor deficiencies.[62,102,148,155] Recent military data have also strongly supported the use of liberal plasma transfusion strategies (e.g., 1:1 RBC–plasma) in the setting of massive hemorrhage in attempt to avoid trauma-induced coagulopathy.[156–158] The rationale for this more aggressive plasma resuscitation practice is that it may circumvent the need for more persistent and unrelenting transfusion requirements that may otherwise result from delayed and/or inadequately dosed plasma transfusion with resultant coagulopathy. The absence of accurate and timely point-of-care laboratory tests reflecting the current coagulation status during active resuscitation has further supported this simplified approach to coagulation factor management in the setting of massive transfusion.[159]

Although such liberal approaches to plasma transfusion have been investigated in civilian trauma populations,[160] equipoise remains. Recent literature has suggested that fixed-ratio plasma resuscitation strategies may reduce early transfusion requirements, and potentially improve survival in civilian populations.[161–163] However, additional literature raises concern that such liberal approaches to plasma resuscitation may not translate well to civilian populations in whom there is often far greater prevalence of comorbid disease. Indeed, such populations may be at risk for adverse outcomes with more liberal plasma transfusion strategies.[164–166] Additionally, the issue of survival bias in the observational studies investigating hemostatic resuscitation strategies has also raised concern as to the true impact of these liberal transfusion practices on patient important outcomes.[167–171] Of note, the modern viscoelastic assays, TEG and ROTEM (discussed in the "Predictive value of coagulation tests" section), may enable physicians to make point-of-care decisions regarding a patient's ability to form thrombus and thereby afford a more individualized and evidence-based approach to plasma transfusion in the setting of trauma or massive hemorrhage. Indeed, a better understanding of the translatability of fixed-ratio plasma resuscitation strategies to civilian populations as well as a robust comparison of fixed-ratio plasma resuscitation strategies to strategies incorporating viscoelastic testing are highly anticipated areas of future research.

Beyond massive bleeding, indications for plasma transfusion are notably sparse. Specific examples of evidence-based indications for plasma transfusion include:

1 Replacement of inherited single coagulation factor deficiencies for which no virus-safe fractionated product exists;[102]

2 Replacement of specific protein deficiencies;[172]

3 Replacement of multiple coagulation factor deficiencies with associated severe bleeding, massive transfusion, and/or disseminated intravascular coagulation;[102,173]

4 As a component of plasma exchange in patients with thrombotic thrombocytopenic purpura;[102] and

5 Urgent reversal of warfarin anticoagulation when severe bleeding is present and PCCs are not available.[102]

Notably, the frequently cited indication of ≥1.5-fold prolongation of aPTT/PT is particularly controversial based on the knowledge that elevated INR/aPTT does not necessarily correlate well with clinical coagulopathy.[60] Haas and colleagues recently conducted a comprehensive review of the literature pertaining to the value of INR/aPTT in perioperative coagulopathy. Their study found that 6 of the 11 published guidelines for management of perioperative bleeding continued to endorse the ≥1.5-fold prolongation threshold; however, referenced evidence supporting this recommendation was from generally small, poor-quality studies and expert panel recommendations.[59] Use of plasma for correction of abnormal coagulation tests prior to specific invasive procedures and in patients with liver disease is discussed in this chapter.

Specific contraindications to plasma transfusion include the presence of an isolated coagulation factor deficit when specific factor concentrates are available, reversal of oral anticoagulation therapy in the absence of bleeding, and treatment of hypovolemia. For patients who are anticoagulated with vitamin K antagonist therapies (e.g., warfarin), discontinuation of the oral anticoagulant therapy and supplementation with vitamin K are the primary therapeutic modalities when reversal is needed and there is no evidence for active bleeding or requirements for emergent high-risk surgery. In the presence of clinically significant active bleeding, PCCs should be considered ahead of plasma transfusion due to their potential for more rapid reversal of the oral anticoagulant effect.[174,175] In addition, these agents are felt to carry a lower risk of transfusion-associated pulmonary and infectious complications.

In the absence of massive bleeding, plasma is typically dosed at 10–15 ml/kg predicted body weight[155] with an expected increase in clotting factor levels of 25–30%. This equates to approximately 1 L of plasma in a typical 70 kg patient. Importantly, however, recent studies have suggested that this dosing regimen may often result in an inadequate repletion of clotting factors. Indeed, recent evidence suggests that upward of 30 ml/kg of plasma may be needed to reliably achieve desired coagulation factor levels, thereby ensuring adequate hemostasis.[176] However, a primary concern with this plasma dosing regimen is the potential for volume overload, particularly in those with baseline predisposing factors (e.g., congestive heart failure and advanced renal disease).

The efficacy, or lack thereof, of plasma transfusion outside of massive hemorrhage is discussed in detail above (predictive value of hemostatic tests). Importantly, much of these data does not relate to patients with liver disease, casting yet more uncertainty over interpretation of INR values with regard to bleeding risk. A recent in-depth evaluation of in vivo coagulation status in patients with liver disease by Lisman et al. provides a comprehensive contemporary summary of "rebalanced hemostasis."[177] In this review, they summarize the evidence for the simultaneously enhanced procoagulant state (due to elevated von Willebrand factor and factor VIII, along with decreased ADAMTS-13, proteins C and S, antithrombin, and plasminogen) as well as an anticoagulant state (due to thrombocytopenia and platelet dysfunction; depletion of factors II, V, VII, IX, X, XI and XIII; vitamin K deficiency; dysfibrinogenemia; along with elevated tissue plasminogen activator, nitric oxide, and prostacyclins).[177] To this end, Spector and colleagues articulated the important fact that transfusion of additional plasma in an attempt to correct these patients' INRs typically only resulted in a temporary correction.[178] Although a number of observational studies have attempted to examine the efficacy of plasma transfusion, no randomized trials have evaluated liberal versus conservative plasma transfusion strategies as has been seen with RBCs. This will be an important future step in refining current transfusion practice.

Platelets: indications, threshold, and dose

As with other blood component therapies, platelet transfusion is generally considered appropriate in the presence of thrombocytopenia or abnormal platelet function with clinically significant active bleeding.[179–183] Recommendations for nonneuraxial surgery advocate single unit platelet transfusion with a target platelet count of $\geq 50 \times 10^9$/L[182]. In patients undergoing invasive neurologic or ophthalmologic procedures, a slightly higher threshold of 100×10^9/L has been recommended.[184] As with plasma transfusion, early military data suggest a potential role for early transfusion of platelets in order to avoid persistent bleeding following massive transfusion. Specifically, when the application of a 1:1:1 ratio of RBCs, plasma, and platelets was applied in military populations, improved survival was noted.[156,158] However, the data supporting this strategy are far less robust when compared to liberal plasma transfusion. Moreover, the translatability of the military experience to civilian populations remains incompletely defined. This again is an area in critical need of additional scientific study.

Current evidence suggests that the risk of bleeding due to thrombocytopenia is minimal when the platelet count is $\geq 50 \times 10^9$/L.[185] Importantly, however, this assumes that platelet function is normal. Frequently, there are clinical scenarios that may result in platelet dysfunction despite normal platelet counts (e.g., cardiopulmonary bypass, antiplatelet therapies, and congenital disorders). In these specific circumstances, the role of platelet transfusion is often unclear.[182] Indeed, recent recommendations from the AABB have highlighted these uncertainties.[182] Increasingly, thromboelastography, platelet aggregometry and platelet mapping assays have been advocated to help inform clinical decisions in these specific settings.[186] As an example, a maximal amplitude <54 mm on TEG has been noted to represent abnormal platelet count and/or function with impaired whole blood clot formation.[187] Platelet aggregometry with an ADP-induced aggregation <31 units has been shown to be independently associated with bleeding events and transfusion in cardiac surgery.[188] Similarly, platelet mapping provides an estimate of the degree of platelet inhibition due to aspirin or ADP–receptor antagonists and has been shown to correlate well with light transmission aggregometry.[189] Nonetheless, no well-validated guidelines currently exist with regard to platelet transfusion thresholds using these more advanced laboratory testing strategies.

Aside from active bleeding, evidence-based guidelines suggest the administration of platelet components for platelet counts $<10 \times 10^9$/L to prevent spontaneous hemorrhage ($<20 \times 10^9$/L when fever, sepsis, heparin therapy, DIC, or other conditions leading to increased platelet consumption coexist). These indications are mostly supported by a number of studies evaluating transfusion strategies in patients with leukemia and bone marrow failure and do not focus specifically on the needs of nonbleeding surgical populations.[190–192] Therefore, the optimal platelet count triggering platelet transfusion in the nonbleeding postoperative patient remains poorly defined and specific recommendations are largely lacking.

In terms of the expected response to platelet transfusion, the expected increment in platelet counts are typically around $5–10 \times 10^9$/L per unit transfused in a typical 70 kg adult.[193] These expected increments should be used to guide dosing with the aforementioned transfusion goals in mind. Platelet transfusion is generally efficacious with a predictable rise in platelet count. Occasionally platelet refractoriness may be seen in patients with hematological malignancies.[193] Questions related to dosing and efficacy of platelet transfusion have been further examined by the platelet dose (PLADO)[194] and prospective randomized optimal platelet and plasma ratios (PROPPR)[160] trials.

The role of plasma transfusion in special circumstances

Central venous catheter (CVC) insertion

Serious complications of CVC placement are rare and include pneumothorax, air embolus, and hemothorax. In fact, significant bleeding following subclavian vein catheterization occurs in patients with perfectly normal hemostasis and results from inadvertent laceration of the subclavian artery.[195] Among patients with advanced liver disease, the insertion of a central venous catheter for transvenous hepatic biopsy provides an excellent model to demonstrate the failure of abnormal coagulation tests to predict bleeding complications at the time of central line placement. Goldfarb and Lebrec[196] reported results of 1000 consecutive CVC placements in patients with liver disease, all of whom had abnormalities of laboratory coagulation tests. Only one patient experienced a significant hematoma. Similarly, Foster et al.[197] performed central line insertions on 259 patients with advanced liver disease awaiting transplantation, all of whom had serious coagulation derangements. Importantly, no preprocedure products were given and no important bleeding complications were observed.

Comparable results have been replicated in multiple subsequent studies. Petersen et al.[198] compared bleeding complications in anticoagulated (aPTT of 1.5 times control) versus nonanticoagulated patients undergoing CVC placements. Of the 22 hematomas observed, 13 were found in anticoagulated patients and nine were in nonanticoagulated patients. None of the patients with hematomas required treatment beyond topical care. Of note, among 22 episodes of inadvertent puncture of the carotid artery, the incidence of subcutaneous hematoma formation was the same in both the anticoagulated patients (4/12) and the nonanticoagulated patients (3/10).

Fisher et al.[199] reported results of 658 cannulations in patients with advanced liver disease (median INR 2.4, median platelet count 81×10^9/L) in which no preprocedural plasma or platelets were given. INR values >5.0 and platelet counts $<50 \times 10^9$/L were associated with a higher incidence of superficial hematomas or site oozing; however, the strongest predictor (OR 8.0) of a procedure-related hematoma was a failed guide wire attempt. This paper underscored the fact that technical mishaps remain the dominant cause of hematoma formation, and that bleeding complications other than skin hematoma or oozing are rare regardless of the coagulation test results.

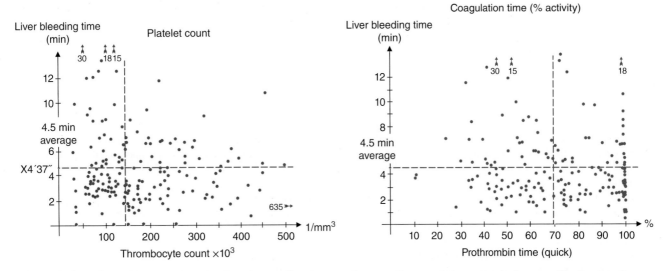

Figure 48.2 Lack of correlation between bleeding from the site of liver biopsy and preprocedure coagulation test or platelet count. The duration of bleeding from the site of puncture of the liver (*y*-axis) is plotted as a function of the preprocedure platelet count (left-hand panel) or the preprocedure coagulation test (expressed as % activity, right-hand panel). There is no correlation between preprocedure laboratory test results and the duration of bleeding. Source: Ewe (1981).[201] Reproduced with permission of Springer.

Liver biopsy

Closed liver biopsy has generally been considered one of the higher risk bedside invasive procedures due to the fact that patients with liver disease often have multiple derangements of coagulation test and biopsies are performed without the aid of direct pressure on the wound sites. For these reasons, there is a strong desire to identify which patients are at increased risk for bleeding. In some instances, abnormalities in hemostasis screening tests sway providers to preferentially perform open surgical or laparoscopic biopsy over closed biopsies or a biopsy followed by Gelfoam plugging.[200]

One of the earliest studies evaluating hemostasis in patients with liver disease found that among 200 patients with nonmalignant liver disorders undergoing laparoscopic liver biopsy, most patients had at least one abnormal coagulation test but none were treated with blood components preprocedurally.[201] These investigators found no correlation between the length of time the liver bled after puncture and the preprocedure laboratory values (Figure 48.2). Similar findings have been duplicated by others, including Terjung et al.[202] In this study, patients undergoing percutaneous liver biopsies with at least one abnormality in preprocedural coagulation tests were evaluated for bleeding outcomes. The authors found no correlation between bleeding risk and mild to moderate abnormalities in the preprocedure INR, aPTT, platelet count, or bleeding time.

Given the strong (albeit unfounded) reliance on the INR as a key measure of hemostasis in liver disease, and the dependence of the INR test on factor VII, it is not surprising that investigators might explore the role of recombinant factor VIIa given before liver biopsy. Jeffers et al.[203] studied 71 patients who received recombinant Factor VIIa in doses ranging from 5 to 120 µg/kg 10 minutes before laparoscopic liver biopsy. Although prothrombin time correction was fairly uniform, especially with the 20, 80, and 120 µg/kg doses, hemostasis at 10 minutes failed in 26% of patients, and an 80 µg/kg "rescue" dose of recombinant factor VIIa was administered. No toxicity was observed. This study unfortunately lacked a control group, and no follow-up testing for hematoma formation was performed. Although the ability of recombinant factor VIIa to improve the INR in patients with liver disease readily occurs, the

fundamental question is whether preprocedure treatment with it is superior to treatment with FFP or to no treatment at all. This would be best answered in a prospective, randomized controlled clinical trial.

Thoracentesis and paracentesis

Given the lack of evidence in favor of preprocedure transfusions for CVC placement or for closed liver biopsy, it is not surprising that published evidence also fails to support the use of preprocedure prophylaxis for less invasive procedures such as thoracentesis or paracentesis. McVay and Toy[204] reported a retrospective review of outcomes in 608 consecutive procedures. Patients were not transfused before the procedure, and no patient had serious bleeding. The proportion of procedures that were accompanied by a decline in Hb was comparable in the group with normal INR/aPTT/platelet values versus abnormal INR/aPTT/platelet values.

Bleeding following paracentesis was also examined by Webster et al.,[205] who reported a retrospective analysis of 179 outpatients. Four patients developed intra-abdominal or abdominal wall bleeding that required a transfusion of RBCs. The INR values of these four were indistinguishable from those of the 175 patients who did not bleed.

Procedures on the upper airway, bronchoscopy, and transbronchial lung biopsy

Special care to provide good hemostasis is prudent when procedures are being performed on the oropharynx, trachea, or bronchi, given that excessive bleeding can be rapidly fatal. Tonsillectomy was an early subject for studies assessing preoperative hemostatic screening. As with other surgical procedures, the predictive value of an isolated abnormal coagulation screening test for bleeding at tonsillectomy or adenoidectomy is very poor. The majority of patients who bleed during these procedures have normal presurgical tests.[206]

Tracheotomy is commonly performed in very ill patients in intensive care, many of whom may have abnormal laboratory tests for coagulation. Auzinger et al.[207] studied patients with severe liver disease undergoing percutaneous tracheotomy. In this study, all but two patients had derangements of laboratory coagulation tests or platelet count. Only one patient had excessive bleeding (defined as >150 mL), which was external (extratracheal). Similar findings have been confirmed in multiple small observational studies.[208,209] In aggregate, these publications appear to refute the notion that mild to moderate prolongation of the INR or aPTT or mild to moderate thrombocytopenia represent absolute contraindications to safe tracheotomy.

In 1994 Kozak and Brath[210] reviewed 274 patients undergoing fiberoptic bronchoscopy and biopsy procedures. Abnormal coagulation screening tests were found in 10% ($n = 28$) of patients. Overall, 35 patients bled, 32 of whom had normal preprocedure laboratory values. Three patients had severe bleeding, and each of them had normal preprocedure test results. A larger retrospective review of bronchoscopies by Diette et al.[211] found that bleeding did not correlate with coagulation parameters or platelet count, and that performing a transbronchial biopsy did not independently increase the risk of bleeding. Such findings have now been replicated several times over in both human and animal models.[212,213]

Epidural anesthesia, diagnostic lumbar puncture, and neurosurgical procedures

Because bleeding in the closed space of the subarachnoid or epidural region can produce paraparesis or paraplegia following lumbar puncture (LP), avoiding preventable bleeding is more important for lumbar punctures and epidural anesthesia than for most invasive procedures. Nevertheless, several studies provide evidence that thrombocytopenia is not a major contraindication to diagnostic LP. Howard et al. reported an extensive experience with >5000 LP procedures performed in 958 children with leukemia.[214,215] Despite the fact that platelets in these children may have been dysfunctional due to leukemia or antibiotics in addition to the varying degrees of thrombocytopenia observed (10 to 100×10^9/L), no patient developed spinal hematoma or a clinical bleeding complication. The authors noted that the likelihood of finding >500 red cells/μL in the spinal fluid was slightly higher in patients with platelet counts $<100 \times 10^9$/L compared to those with counts $>100 \times 10^9$/L. However, among patients with counts $<100 \times 10^9$/L, the likelihood of an LP with >500 red cells/μL did not increase as the platelet count declined to levels as low as 10×10^9/L, thus the authors concluded that a platelet count of 10×10^9/L was adequate to perform a routine LP for administration of intrathecal chemotherapy. Similar findings have subsequently been confirmed in adult populations,[216,217] although the authors recommended prophylactic transfusions be given if the platelet count were $<20 \times 10^9$/L.[216] These studies provide evidence that an LP, if of diagnostic importance, should not be delayed or withheld because of thrombocytopenia.

In contrast to thrombocytopenia, the chance of peridural hematoma appears to be increased among patients with full-dose anticoagulation who undergo placement or removal of an epidural catheter for spinal anesthesia. Ruff and Dougherty[218] reported five cases of paraplegia among 342 patients who received a diagnostic LP followed by administration of full-dose heparin. In addition, the introduction of low-molecular-weight heparin treatment in the United States was accompanied by an observed increase in reported spinal hematomas among patients with epidural catheters, estimated to occur at a rate of 1 in 10,000 patients.[219] In patients with low-dose anticoagulation undergoing vascular surgery, Rao and El-Etr[220] did not find evidence of epidural/peridural hematomas following placement of either an epidural catheter or a subarachnoid catheter. In a similar manner, low-dose heparin was

not associated with spinal hematoma in over 5000 patients undergoing spinal or epidural anesthesia.[221]

Interestingly, in 2001 Schramm et al.[222] reviewed outcomes among 1211 patients undergoing craniotomy, spinal surgery, or other neurosurgical procedures at the Royal Melbourne Hospital in Australia. The authors found that 17% of preoperative laboratory tests were abnormal, but neither prolongation of the INR nor depression of the platelet count predicted excessive surgical bleeding. Of note, procedure-related bleeding was associated with patients who gave a history of bleeding and those who demonstrated a prolonged aPTT. These authors concluded that these patients may have had von Willebrand disease.

Angiography

The increasing use of interventional radiology and cardiology has created a new cohort of patients at risk for arterial bleeding following angiography. Not surprisingly, there is little evidence that preprocedure blood components are indicated for angiographic procedures. Darcy et al.[223] prospectively studied 1000 consecutive patients undergoing femoral arterial puncture for diagnostic or therapeutic vascular procedures. Analysis was restricted to patients with INR values <1.5. The incidence of hematoma formation was the same in patients without any abnormality in preprocedural INR (9.7%) as those with abnormal results (8.1%). Neither the INR nor the aPTT was predictive of hematoma formation; however, hematoma formation was more common among patients with platelet counts $<100 \times 10^9$/L, with the use of catheters larger than 5 Fr, and among patients with a documented history of bleeding disorders.

Key references

A full reference list for this chapter is available at: http://www.wiley.com/go/simon/transfusion

8 Villanueva C, Colomo A, Bosch A, et al. Transfusion strategies for acute upper gastrointestinal bleeding. *N Engl J Med* 2013;**368**:11–21.

9 Carson JL, Terrin ML, Noveck H, et al. Liberal or restrictive transfusion in high-risk patients after hip surgery. *N Engl J Med* 2011;**365**:2453–62.

23 Roback JD, Caldwell S, Carson J, et al. Evidence-based practice guidelines for plasma transfusion. *Transfusion* 2010;**50**:1227–39.

24 American Society of Anesthesiologists Task Force on Perioperative Blood Transfusion and Adjuvant Therapies. Practice guidelines for perioperative blood transfusion and adjuvant therapies. *Anesthesiology* 2006;**105**:198–208.

50 Carson JL, Duff A, Berlin JA, Lawrence VA, et al. Perioperative blood transfusion and postoperative mortality. *JAMA* 1998;**279**:199–205.

53 Hajjar LA, Vincent JL, Galas FR, et al. Transfusion requirements after cardiac surgery: the TRACS randomized controlled trial. *JAMA* 2010;**304**:1559–67.

54 Carson JL, Carless PA, Hébert PC. Transfusion thresholds and other strategies for guiding allogeneic red blood cell transfusion. *Cochrane Database Syst Rev* 2012: CD002042.

76 Douketis JD, Spyropoulos AC, Spencer FA, et al. Perioperative management of antithrombotic therapy: antithrombotic therapy and prevention of thrombosis. *Chest* 2012;**141** (2 Suppl.):e326S–50S.

102 O'Shaughnessy DF, Atterbury C, Bolton Maggs P, et al. Guidelines for the use of fresh-frozen plasma, cryoprecipitate and cryosupernatant. *Br J Haematol* 2004;**126**:11–28.

112 Napolitano LM, Kurek S, Luchette FA, et al. Clinical practice guideline: red blood cell transfusion in adult trauma and critical care. *Crit Care Med* 2009;**37**:3124–57.

113 Carson JL, Grossman BJ, Kleinman S, et al. Red blood cell transfusion: a clinical practice guideline from the AABB. *Ann Int Med* 2012;**157**:49–58.

116 Goodnough LT, Shander A. Blood management. *Arch Pathol Lab Med* 2007;**131**:695–701.

122 Goodnough LT, Shander A, Spence R. Bloodless medicine: clinical care without allogeneic blood transfusion. *Transfusion* 2003;**43**:668–76.

125 Tieu BH, Holcomb JB, Schreiber MA. Coagulopathy: its pathophysiology and treatment in the injured patient. *World J Surg* 2007;**31**:1055–64.

138 Ferraris VA, Ferraris SP, Saha SP, *et al.* Perioperative blood transfusion and blood conservation in cardiac surgery: the Society of Thoracic Surgeons and The Society of Cardiovascular Anesthesiologists clinical practice guideline. *Ann Thorac Surg* 2007;**83** (5 Suppl.):S27–86.

148 Szczepiorkowski ZM, Dunbar NM. Transfusion guidelines: when to transfuse. *Hematology Am Soc Hematol Educ Program* 2013;**2013**:638–44.

149 Ferraris VA, Brown JR, Despotis GJ, *et al.* 2011 update to the Society of Thoracic Surgeons and the Society of Cardiovascular Anesthesiologists blood conservation clinical practice guidelines. *Ann Thorac Surg* 2011;**91**:944–82.

157 Sihler KC, Napolitano LM. Massive transfusion: new insights. *Chest* 2009;**136**:1654–67.

159 Pham HP, Shaz BH. Update on massive transfusion. *Br J Anaesth* 2013;**111** (Suppl.):i71–82.

160 Holcomb JB, Tilley BC, Baraniuk S, Fox EE, *et al.* Transfusion of plasma, platelets, and red blood cells in a 1:1:1 vs. a 1:1:2 ratio and mortality in patients with severe trauma: the PROPPR randomized clinical trial. *JAMA* 2015;**313**:471–82.

170 Murad MH, Stubbs JR, Gandhi MJ, *et al.* The effect of plasma transfusion on morbidity and mortality: a systematic review and meta-analysis. *Transfusion* 2010;**50**:1370–83.

182 Kaufman RM, Djulbegovic B, Gernsheimer T, *et al.* Platelet transfusion: a clinical practice guideline from the AABB. *Ann Intern Med* 2015;**162**:205–13.

219 Horlocker TT. Thromboprophylaxis and neuraxial anesthesia. *Orthopedics* 2003;**26** (2 Suppl.):s243–9.

CHAPTER 49

Transfusion therapy in the care of trauma and burn patients

John R. Hess,[1] John B. Holcomb,[2] Steven E. Wolf,[3] & Michael W. Cripps[3]

[1]Department of Laboratory Medicine and Hematology, University of Washington School of Medicine; and Transfusion Service, Harborview Medical Center, Seattle, WA, USA
[2]Center for Translational Injury Research, University of Texas Health Science Center, Houston, TX, USA
[3]Department of Surgery, Division of Burn/Trauma/Critical Care, University of Texas Southwestern Medical Center, Dallas, TX, USA

The oldest reports of successful blood transfusions for trauma come from the American Civil War. However, it was more than 50 years later, at the end of World War I, that recognizably modern blood banking was developed.[1] Useful blood storage was possible only after three critical discoveries. First was the discovery that bacteria caused infections, which allowed the development of sterile fluid-handling techniques. Second was the discovery of ABO blood groups, which allowed donors and recipients to be crossmatched and universal donor blood types identified. Third, the discovery that citrate was a safe anticoagulant for human blood at low doses allowed blood donors and recipients to be separated in time and space, which in turn allowed the building of blood inventory and the institution of blood product quality control.[2] Taking advantage of these discoveries and a transfusion bottle of his own design, Oswald H. Robertson then developed a system for delivering typed and syphilus-tested whole blood in bottles in ice chests to casualty clearing stations and base hospitals, and demonstrated the lifesaving value of stored blood transfusion for combat casualties.[3] The approximately 30,000 Robertson bottle transfusions performed in 1918 were a model of how a blood transfusion service could function. After the war, organized blood banks disappeared because of their high overhead requirements, although direct transfusions continued, until individuals and institutions started to rebuild blood services. Lundy at the Mayo Clinic in 1935,[4] Bethune and Duran-Jorda in the Spanish Civil War in 1936,[5,6] Fantus at Cook County in 1937,[7] and DeGowin at Iowa in 1938[8] all contributed to the rebirth of blood banking, but the largest impetus came from the London Blood Transfusion Service, the British Army, and the joint US Army, Navy, and American Red Cross programs in World War II. The London Blood Transfusion Service was able to provide half a million units of whole blood during the London Blitz of 1940,[9] the British Army developed acid–citrate–dextrose (ACD) solution for the safe three-week storage of whole blood and showed that it could be delivered around the world,[10] and the American war effort ultimately collected and processed 13 million whole blood collections.[11] These efforts became the basis for national blood systems.

During the Korean War (1950–1953), the US Army's Surgical Research Team studied blood loss, the evolution of shock, and the effects of fluid resuscitation with the tracer deuterium heavy water.[12] Furthermore, they reported on the safety of massive transfusion with stored universal donor blood and on the use of plastic bags for fluid and blood administration. A decade later in the Vietnam War, these concepts and products were integrated into systems for early resuscitation, rapid transportation, massive transfusion, and early surgical intervention, which reduced the death rate from wounds in field hospitals to 3%.[13,14] Altogether, the US armed forces transfused 600,000 units of whole blood or red cells in Vietnam.[15] They further demonstrated the relative safety of the 100,000 units of group O universal donor red cells given, in that all seven fatal hemolytic transfusion reactions in Vietnam occurred in patients receiving crossmatched but mistransfused blood. By the end of the 1960s, ambulances in US cities were taking injured civilians to regional trauma centers.[16]

The Coconut Grove nightclub fire in Boston, Massachusetts, on November 28, 1942, was the critical event in the history of burn care. It led to the first burn resuscitation formula, the first systematic evaluation of the use of blood plasma in burn resuscitation, and the first burn unit in the United States.[17,18] The first two concepts remain controversial, but the ready availability of blood and blood components has improved survival among elderly burned patients and patients with associated medical problems who otherwise would not have tolerated a low hemoglobin level.[19] Interoperative transfusion allowed wider more complete debridement procedures, rapidly reducing the inflammatory burden of irrevocably damaged tissue, and thereby decreasing the number of surgical procedures and the length of hospital care needed by a burned patient.[20]

The development of trauma centers and burn units in the late 1960s coincided with the development of blood bags and blood component therapy and with a general increasing demand for blood components in hospitals to support more advanced surgery and the war on cancer.[21] In an expanding blood supply system,[21] blood products were frequently in short supply, especially universal donor group O-negative red cells and group AB plasma. Managing a limited inventory of AB plasma meant keeping it frozen in the blood bank until the patient had a blood type and an indication in the form of a prothrombin time (PT) or activated partial thromboplastin time (aPPT) greater than 1.5 times normal.[22] By the time the American College of Surgeons' Acute Trauma Life Support (ATLS) guidelines were written, the system of delaying plasma was so ingrained that many thought there was science behind it.[23,24]

Rossi's Principles of Transfusion Medicine, Fifth Edition. Edited by Toby L. Simon, Jeffrey McCullough, Edward L. Snyder, Bjarte G. Solheim, and Ronald G. Strauss.
© 2016 John Wiley & Sons, Ltd. Published 2016 by John Wiley & Sons, Ltd.

A mistaken prejudice about injury and the physicians who cared for injured patients also shaped the development of trauma transfusion.[25] In war, the banked blood was going to "our nation's finest," but in peacetime, injury was viewed as a problem to be prevented with engineering and social controls like collapsible steering columns and divided highways or seatbelt and helmet laws. The injured were assumed to be the poor and the drunk. The civilian health research establishment was slow to recognize the need for trauma research. In the 1960s, the National Academy of Sciences and the National Institutes of Health debated building a National Institute of Trauma to address the nation's leading cause of early death and ultimately decided not to do so.[26] The problems of trauma treatment were viewed as local and organizational, not national and scientific. Care of the injured was felt to revolve around prevention, rapid transport, and better surgical care, with little requirement for basic or translational research. The perceived needs did not blend with the molecular biology agenda of the time. As a result, injury research has been relatively underfunded compared to its impact for decades.[27]

The local and organizational issues surrounding trauma and burn care became the major focus of building in the 1970s and 1980s. Ultimately, 1082 trauma centers in the United States and Canada were accredited by the Committee on Trauma of the American College of Surgeons at various levels of service based on resources and programs, and 164 burn centers were built as well.[28] The Committee on Trauma trained and accredited a generation of physicians and surgeons in the principles of ATLS, teaching basic injury epidemiology and a clinical approach focused on simple clinical skills such as managing the airway, checking for tension pneumothorax and hemopericardium, controlling accessible hemorrhage, rapidly moving patients to the operating room, and the resuscitation of hemorrhagic shock. Nationally, the program was viewed as a success as the number of moderately injured patients who died of surgically preventable causes decreased markedly.

The resuscitation of hemorrhagic shock became a focus of research.[29] In animals, poor tissue perfusion secondary to hypovolemic hypotension became life threatening after approximately 30% blood loss, but perfusion could be restored by volume replacement with crystalloid fluids.[30] With continued blood loss and volume replacement, red cell mass became critically low next after 60% of total blood volume blood loss. Red cell transfusion corrected this problem. Decreasing colloid osmotic activity led to blood flow–limiting edema after 120% blood volume removal. With concomitant albumin, volume, and red cell replacement, hemorrhagic complications occurred spontaneously after 180% volume, red cell, and albumin replacement that were related primarily to plasma coagulation factor deficiency, and platelets became limiting only after 220% removal and replacement of the other blood components. These isovolemic models of controlled hemorrhage and blood component replacement suggested that volume and oxygen transport were the critical early issues in the treatment of hemorrhagic shock and that coagulopathy was largely dilutional and a late complication. This logic was codified as the ATLS resuscitation algorithm, in which injured patients were given crystalloid fluids to maintain volume and red cells to maintain oxygen transport if more than 2 L of crystalloid fluid were required to maintain blood pressure.[31] Plasma was to be given based on laboratory measures of a prolonged PT or aPTT greater than 1.5 times normal, platelets when the platelet count was less than 50,000/μL, and cryoprecipitate when the fibrinogen was less than 100 mg/dL. Again, the system worked well for moderately injured patients and led to reduced overall mortality, especially from renal failure.

However, in severely injured patients with initially uncontrolled hemorrhage, the use of large volumes of crystalloid fluid led to massive tissue edema and severe coagulopathy. Tissue edema made closing wounds difficult. Attempting to close the abdomen over swollen bowel led to compression of the inferior vena cava, trapping blood in the legs, decreasing venous return to the heart, and worsening shock. Leaving the abdomen open led to prolonged hospitalizations, many complications, and secondary mortality. Cold crystalloid resuscitation caused hemodilution and hypothermia, which in turn caused coagulopathy and more bleeding, a phenomenon that came to be known as the *bloody vicious cycle*. The combination of acidosis, hypothermia, and coagulopathy was the *triad of death*. In the face of difficult-to-control bleeding, surgeons performed *damage control laparotomies* where normal anatomy was sacrificed in favor of stabilizing critical vascular integrity and limiting fecal, urinary, and biliary contamination in the hopes of getting the procedure performed in less than 40 minutes.[32] Nevertheless, for patients who needed 10 units of red blood cells (RBCs), mortality was typically 40%, and for those who needed 20 units, it was 50%.[33]

In the past two decades, three areas of clinical investigation led to the use of more plasma and less crystalloid in the resuscitation of severely and profoundly injured patients. The first line involved reducing the amount of crystalloid fluid given for volume expansion because there were situations in which it was not necessary and certain patients appeared to do better without the extra volume. The second line involved experiences, almost entirely military, in which dramatically better hemostasis was achieved with the use of fresh whole blood. The third involved the purposeful administration of plasma early in resuscitation to prevent coagulopathy, because once coagulopathy had developed it proved difficult to treat with conventional blood components.

A dramatic demonstration that crystalloid resuscitation could be deadly was conducted by Bickell and colleagues in a model of aortic tear in swine.[34] In the model, a loop of stainless-steel suture was placed in the aorta and brought out through the skin. A week later, with the animal awake, the suture was torn out to create an 0.45 cm aortic tear. Pigs sustaining this injury typically lay down, dropped their blood pressure to 30 Torr systolic for an hour while the injury bleeding clotted firmly, and then the blood pressure slowly returned to normal with 85% of the animals surviving. Attempting to resuscitate the swine with crystalloid raised their blood pressure, causing further bleeding and hemodilution that preventing the bleeding from ever clotting and resulted in 100% fatality. On the basis of this demonstration, a large study was performed in patients in Houston sustaining penetrating trucal trauma.[35] Moderately hypotensive patients were randomized to be either resuscitated or not prior to exploratory surgery. Mortality was higher (69 vs. 60%, $p = 0.04$) in the resuscitated group. A second smaller randomized study conducted by Dutton and colleagues also showed no benefit to early resuscitation in the short time between admission and exploratory surgery in moderately hypotensive injured patients in a level 1 trauma center.[36]

US military experience with the use of fresh whole blood to treat battlefield casualties in situations where platelets were not available also led to a widening appreciation of the ability of whole blood to rapidly achieve hemostasis in badly injured soldiers. In the first Iraq war, Somalia, Bosnia, Kosovo, and then Afghanistan and the second Iraq war, situations repeatedly occurred where casualties with uncontrolled coagulopathic bleeding after resuscitation with red cells and crystalloid were able to achieve hemostasis after the administration of fresh whole blood.[37] In one early and informative case from Mogadishu in 1993, a soldier was bitten by a great white shark, losing the back of a thigh. By the time he arrived at the American combat support hospital, he was in profound shock. His surgeons proceeded to give him all 50 units of RBCs in additive solution that were available in the country, leading to more free bleeding with each unit he was given until they ran out. At that time, they switched his resuscitation to fresh whole blood collected from the arms of group O soldiers in his unit, and with the administration of each successive unit, his coagulopathy improved until he stopped bleeding altogether after 16 units of fresh whole blood. Stories like this one spread rapidly among surgeons, and the dramatic photographs of the extent of the injury and success of the hemorrhage control further emphasized the take-home messages that red cells alone can lead to a profound dilutional coagulopathy and that fresh whole blood can correct it.

The recognition that crystalloid fluids and red cells did not prevent coagulopathy led to many attempts at more balanced resuscitation. Hiipala wrote about the importance of early administration of plasma in the massively bleeding trauma patient in the 1990s, but groups like the British Committee for Standards in Haematology continued to advocate for limiting plasma use and strict transfusion triggers.[38,39] However, with the descriptions of the acute coagulopathy of trauma in 2003 and reports of ever more devastating injuries from improvised explosive devices in the second Iraq war at the same time, the need to prevent and reverse coagulopathy early in resuscitation came to the fore.[40] The US military published its first theater guideline recommending early initiation of balanced hemostatic resuscitation in 2004; held a small international expert panel in San Antonio, Texas, in May 2005; and published a national recommendation in 2007 stating red cells, plasma, and platelets be given in 1:1:1 ratios to the most seriously injured.[41] Since that time, Holcomb has led a series of consecutively more rigorous studies of the resuscitation of massive hemorrhage—the Trauma Outcomes Group study (2009), the Prospective Observational Multicenter Massive Transfusion Trial (PROMMTT, 2012), and the Pragmatic Randomized Optimal Plasma and Platelet Ratios trial (PROPPR, 2015)—that constitute the best evidence for resuscitation of massive hemorrhage using balanced ratios of conventional blood products. The American College of Surgeons has followed with educational projects such as the Educational Initiative on Critical Bleeding in Trauma and the Trauma Quality Improvement Project for 2012, and with requirements that hospitals and trauma centers have massive transfusion protocols and that they utilize hemostatic ratios of blood products.[42,43] In Northern Europe, a similar process has been led by Johansson through his work at the University of Copenhagen and in the Scandinavian Conferences on Critical Bleeding.[44]

The epidemiology of physical injury

Injury is common, and over the last decade mortality has increased.[45,46] In the United States, approximately one individual in 10 receives a significant physical injury requiring medical attention every year, and one in 100 is hospitalized because of such an injury annually. Approximately one in 1000 individuals receives a blood transfusion for injury each year, and just over 180,000 people die of physical injury annually. Costs are greater than $400 billion each year. About 95,000 of these deaths are the result of unintentional injury, with the remainder divided between suicides using physical methods and deaths from injuries purposely inflicted by others. Injury is the third leading cause of death overall, and because it occurs so frequently in children and young adults, it is the leading cause of loss of years of productive life through age 75. As noted, to deal with these injuries, the United States and Canada have built more than a thousand trauma centers and more than a hundred burn centers.

Motor vehicle–related injuries, interpersonal violence, and falls are the most common causes of fatal injuries. Work and recreational accidents also contribute to the toll. All of the common causes of injury are subjects of ongoing efforts at primary prevention through engineering and social controls, but faster cars, higher caliber handguns, and a rising elderly population limit the decline in the overall incidence of both injuries and deaths.

Half of all injury-related deaths in civilians occur outside the hospital, either because of rapid death from massive injury or because they occur in remote or unobserved locations so that movement to advanced care is too late. In the Vietnam War, 85% of battlefield deaths occurred in the field with 40% occurring essentially instantaneously, 65% being dead within five minutes, 80% within 30 minutes, and 90% within two hours of injury.[47] For civilian casualties that arrive at the hospital alive and subsequently die a hemorrhagic death, a similar compression of early deaths occurs with 50% of such patients dead in two hours and 80% dead in six hours (Figure 49.1). Later deaths are caused largely by central nervous system injury or multiple organ failure.[48] Autopsy series of those who die in the field suggest that 15 to 20% have a potentially correctable hemorrhagic cause of death.

Blood use in the injured is strongly related to injury severity. In an examination of blood usage rates in a trauma center, only 8% of all admissions received RBCs, and only 3% of all admissions received 10 or more units.[49] Increased anatomic injury severity was strongly associated with increased RBC use and mortality. Nevertheless, there does not appear to be an upper limit to the number of RBC units that can be successfully transfused, and survivorship after massive transfusion was 60%, after 20 units of RBC was about 50%, and after hypermassive transfusion for trauma is reported in the 15–20% range. This means that massive transfusion is not a marker of therapeutic futility.

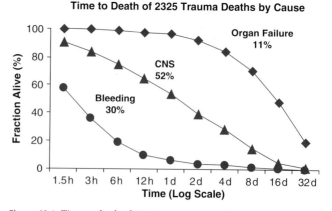

Figure 49.1 Time to death of 2325 trauma patients directly admitted to Maryland Shock-Trauma who survived at least 15 minutes and died in care. Median time to death for patients with uncontrolled hemorrhage as their major cause of death was two hours. Only 4% of all admissions died during their primary hospital admission. Source: Data from Dutton *et al.* (2010).[48]

Because of the spatial distribution of the population in the United States and Canada, only about half of seriously injured patients are treated initially in level 1 trauma centers. Blood products for the immediate care of the severely injured are often limited in smaller facilities to liquid red cells and frozen plasma, and plasma administration is often delayed. The consequences of this delay creates a need for alternative blood products for austere environments such as freeze-dried plasma and frozen platelets.[50] These products and their potential uses will be discussed in greater detail in this section.

Trauma-associated coagulopathy

The human coagulation system is slow and weak. Sustain a small laceration, and it typically takes at least five minutes for bleeding to stop. Brush the clot, and it bleeds again. The clotting system is also limited in capacity. The effectors of blood coagulation, fibrinogen and platelets, exist in limited amounts in the whole body. For fibrinogen, that amount is about 300 mg/dL in 3 L of plasma or about 9 g of fibrinogen altogether in the blood of healthy individuals. Platelets are present in similarly small amounts. The normal 250,000 platelets/μL fill only 0.2% of the blood volume or 10 mL of the normal 5 L of blood. Laid out side-by-side as $3 \times 3\,\mu$m discs, all the platelets in the circulation will cover only 10 m^2. However, the body has 100 m^2 of capillaries in the lung and 3000 m^2 of capillaries altogether. Thus, the body starts with 2 teaspoons of fibrinogen and 2 teaspoons of platelets, and initial blood losses after severe injury can mean that 40% of that is already lost before care ever begins. Only blood product transfusion can provide more of these critical materials rapidly.

Furthermore, the physiology of massive injury leads to rapid degradation of the body's already limited coagulation capacity. Dilution, acidosis, hypothermia, consumption, and fibrinolysis all contribute to an inability to take full advantage of the limited blood-clotting resources that the body starts out with.[51] In combination, they insure that many severely and most profoundly injured patients are coagulopathic when they arrive at medical care.

Loss of coagulation factors and platelets starts with the acute blood loss of injury, which can be in excess of 40% in patients arriving in deep shock. Attempts to raise blood pressure with asanguinous fluid to sustain tissue perfusion will lead to further blood loss through uncontrolled defects in vascular integrity. Dilution of platelet counts and coagulation factor concentrations occurs naturally as remaining intravascular blood is watered down by physiologic vascular refill. Normally, blood pressure pushes water into the tissues, which returns through the lymphatic circulation. As blood pressure falls in hemodynamic shock, water moves back into the vascular space down a concentration gradient to dilute the colloid osmotic activity of plasma proteins.

Acidosis, which develops rapidly with tissue hypoprofusion, has profound effects on plasma coagulation. Normally, activated plasma coagulation factors assemble into complexes on negatively charged phospholipid rafts on the surfaces of exposed subendothelial cells, platelets, and endothelium in ways that increase the clotting activity of the enzymes in these complexes by 10,000 to a millionfold. The increased concentration of protons that are low pH destabilizes these coagulation factor complexes and reduces their activities. The reduction is 50% at pH 7.2, 70% at pH 7.0, and 80% at pH 6.8.[52] All these levels are commonly seen in patients suffering severe hemorrhagic shock.

Hypothermia also affects the plasma coagulation enzymes, reducing their activities by about 10% per degree Celsius, but it has a much greater effect on platelet activation. Normally, platelets activate when they adhere to exposed subendothelium through bridging von Willebrand factor. The von Willebrand factor binds to the platelet glycoprotein receptor Ib with one end and to type III collagen on the other, creating traction and torsion of the receptor leading to platelet activation. However, this receptor torsion–platelet activation coupling is lost with mild cooling and is essentially gone at 30 °C.[53] In the past, the combination of a low core temperature and severe injury with uncontrolled bleeding was viewed as fatal, but now the combination of extracorporeal blood warming, avoidance of blood dilution, and an array of hemorrhage control strategies allows many trauma patients who present with severe hypothermia to survive.

Consumption of platelets and coagulation factors can occur both within wounds and diffusely with the embolization of tissue factor–bearing tissue fragments and phospholipids and with the diffusion of thrombin. In high-energy blunt or penetrating trauma, the extent of endothelial disruption may extend to billions of endothelial microtears, each associated with the exposure of tissue factor–bearing cells and subendothelial basement membrane collagen. Under these circumstances, factors VII, VIII, and V and platelets can be depleted. Factor VII is present normally in only nanomolar amounts, so the exposure of a few hundred grams of mesothelial cells presents enough tissue factor to bind all of the factor VII available. Factors VIII and V are classically consumable factors, activated by thrombin and inactivated by protein C. The blood can be exposed to multiple cycles of activation and inactivation in its course through injured tissue with resultant comsumptive loss of much procoagulant activity. Finally, platelet activity can be consumed with either reduction in platelet number or depletion of platelet granule contents, membrane, and energy. Severely injured patients typically present with normal numbers of platelets that then decline over the first hour in the hospital, and their remaining platelets appear to have reduced activity, a phenomenon called *platelet fatigue*.[54]

Fibrinolysis, in the context of trauma-associated coagulopathy, is the early and inappropriate breakdown of fibrin clot, resulting in the loss of hemostasis and the substrate for further coagulation and vascular healing. Pathologic fibrinolysis following trauma is typically caused by plasmin or neutrophil elastase. Plasmin is activated by tissue plasminogen activator released in response to low blood flow, and its breakdown is delayed by early destruction of plasminogen activator inhibitor by protein C. Neutrophil elastase is released in large amounts in injured tissue, and its signature fibrin fragments are found in large amounts following severe injury.

In severely injured patients, all of these activities limiting stable clot formation can be going on at once. In a review of the risks for uncontrolled coagulopathy following injury, Cosgrove and colleagues found that the risks were additive.[55] Patients with severe injury but without shock, acidosis, or hypothermia were rarely coagulopathic. With profound injury, about 10% were coagulopathic at presentation; and with shock requiring diluting resuscitation, the rate increased to 40%. With profound injury and hypothermia coagulopathy was present in 50%, and with acidosis in 60%, of all patients. However, when three or more of these factors were present simultaneously, the incidence of coagulopathy increased to 85–98%. Thus, the most severely injured patients will develop coagulopathy.

What was not widely recognized until a decade ago is that about one in four of severely and profoundly injured patients arrive at the hospital with coagulopathy already established. In 2003, Brohi and his colleagues described a thousand patients arriving at the Royal

London Hospital by helicopter from motor vehicle collisions on the London ring-road; they had received only 400 mL of crystalloid fluids on average before arrival, and yet one-quarter had their prothrombin time (PT) prolonged beyond 1.5 times normal.[56] Moreover, the quarter with the prolonged PT had a fourfold excess in-hospital mortality. Brohi called the finding the *acute coagulopathy of trauma*. A month later, MacLeod and her colleagues from the Ryder Trauma Center in Miami reported a similar finding in 20,000 patients seen over a five-year period.[57] In their series, 28% of all seriously injured patients had a prolonged PT that was associated with a 35% excess in-hospital mortality, and 8% had a prolonged partial thromboplastin time (PTT) that was associated with a 426% excess in-hospital mortality. In 2009, Hess and his colleagues described the prevalence of abnormal coagulation, which was measured at admission in 35,000 direct admissions to the Cowley Shock-Trauma Center in Baltimore over a seven-year period; this coagulation showed greater prevalence of abnormalities of the PT, PTT, fibrinogen, and platelet count with increasing injury severity, and the increasing severity of each of the abnormalities was associated with increasing in-hospital mortality.[58] At the highest levels of injury severity observed, the prevalence of abnormal admission coagulation tests was 45%, and in-hospital mortality was 80%. In a search for clinical and mechanistic drivers of the acute trauma of coagulopathy, Cohen and his colleagues from the Prospective Observational Multicenter Massive Transfusion Trial (PROMMTT) found that the fraction of 1198 severely injured patients with an INR ≥1.3 was 42% and that they generally had depressed concentrations of factors I, II, V, and VIII, and evidence of increased concentrations of activated protein C.[59] Decreased concentrations of platelets on admission are much less frequent. As noted, most patients with severe injury present with normal platelet counts, but when the admission counts are low, they are associated with very high in-hospital mortality.

There has been an argument in the literature about whether the acute coagulopathy of trauma is a separate pathophysiologic entity or is just the early and hypocoagulable form of disseminated intravascular coagulation (DIC).[60] The International Society of Thrombosis and Hemostasis used trauma as their example of the early and hypocoagulable form of the condition. On the other hand, calling a condition *DIC* that is not disseminated, intravascular, or coagulation-related but is the product of multiply local injuries, extravascular or at least extra-endothelial, and hemorrhagic is confusing and imprecise, whereas the term *acute coagulopathy of trauma* is concise and descriptive. This argument is purely semantic.

Damage control resuscitation

Several large autopsy series suggest that the majority of potentially savable lives that are currently lost to injury are in the group of seriously injured patients with uncontrolled hemorrhage who die in the early hours after presentation.[61,62] The autopsy series suggest that such patients may represent 8–19% of all injury deaths, and the deaths represent a combination of missed diagnostic and therapeutic opportunities that in turn result in delayed hemorrhage control. As these deaths clearly overlap with the excess mortality associated with the acute coagulopathy of trauma, designing resuscitation systems to limit coagulopathy is a priority.

In an instructive case, a young soldier seen in the combat support hospital in Baghdad with massive injuries from an improvised explosive device received 18 units of RBCs in the approximately 50 minutes of his hospital care and died before type-specific plasma was thawed. In reviewing the case among the hospital staff in Baghdad, the surgeons pointed to the need to get plasma into the patient sooner, whereas the supporting transfusion service pointed to the limited supplies of universal donor group AB fresh frozen plasma (FFP) and the potentially massive waste of plasma products associated with the legal requirement to use thawed FFP within six hours of thawing. The transfusion service had adopted the protocol of first obtaining the patient's ABO type and only then thawing type-specific plasma to provide the best matched product, limit frozen plasma wastage, and balance usage by ABO type. However, the end result was dead patients. An outside consultant suggested that the problem could be partially ameliorated by the simple expedient of relabeling thawed FFP as thawed plasma, which can be kept for five days; that keeping four units of AB plasma thawed at all times would provide a buffer of plasma for immediate use; and that patients might benefit as well from prompt initial treatment of the acute coagulopathy of trauma. After confirming the legal definitions of thawed plasma and assuring a continuing supply of AB FFP, this plan was adopted. It was further agreed that units of red cells and plasma would be given alternately to the profoundly injured to keep the combined hematocrit of the administered products close to 30% and provide an easy protocol for administration in the chaotic situation of a massive injury resuscitation (Figure 49.2).

The clinical results were dramatic. All involved in the immediate care of the subsequent wounded casualties thought that they did better. More patients appeared to survive initial resuscitation, their tissues handled better in the operating room with less spontaneous bleeding and edema, and the required duration of ventilator support

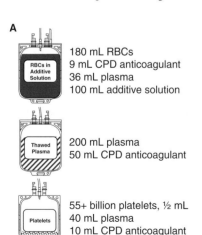

A

180 mL RBCs
9 mL CPD anticoagulant
36 mL plasma
100 mL additive solution

200 mL plasma
50 mL CPD anticoagulant

55+ billion platelets, ½ mL
40 mL plasma
10 mL CPD anticoagulant

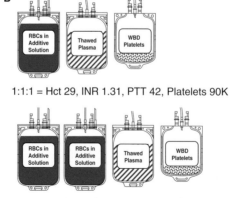

B

1:1:1 = Hct 29, INR 1.31, PTT 42, Platelets 90K

2:1:1 = Hct 39, INR 1.55, PTT 50, Platelets 60K

Figure 49.2 (A) Whole blood–derived blood components processed by the platelet-rich plasma method have the average contents shown above. (B) Giving RBC, plasma, and platelets in a 1:1:1 unit ratio results in a hematocrit (Hct) of 29%, a plasma concentration of 65%, and a platelet concentration of about 90 K/mcL. An additional unit of RBC dilutes the plasma to 52% and the platelet count to 60 K/mcL while raising the Hct unnecessarily. Source: Data from Arman and Hess, 2003 (Transfus Med Rev 2003 Jul;17[3]:223–31) and Kornblith *et al.*, 2014 (J Trauma Acute Care Surg 2014 Dec; 77[6]:818–27).

was shorter because patients appeared to get less blood and fluids altogether. Other surgical groups in theater, both US and allied and in Iraq and Afghanistan, adopted the procedures, and by the end of 2004 the use of 1:1 unit ratios of red cells and plasma for resuscitation had become a theater guideline. A retrospective review of cases performed at the Baghdad hospital showed a strong correlation between the ratio of plasma units to red cells given and survival.[63]

Because the 1:1:1 resuscitation strategy was at variance both with conventional surgical dogma as outlined in the ATLS manual and with evolving transfusion medicine doctrine as exemplified by the drive to reduce plasma usage generally, the authors felt it necessary to gather a panel of experts and review the findings. Expert review panels were recruited and asked to develop data and position papers on critical issues surrounding early massive transfusion for trauma. The meeting took place at the US Army Institute of Surgical Research in San Antonio on May 25–27, 2005, and the results were published as a supplement to the *Journal of Trauma* in September 2006.[64] There were several major findings. First, there was essential agreement on the epidemiologic association of injury severity, number of units of RBCs transfused, and admission coagulation measures with time to death and in-hospital mortality between the German Trauma Registry and the US Miami and Baltimore Trauma Registries.[65] Second, in contacting 80 academic trauma centers, formal massive transfusion protocols were rare.[66] Third, a number of high-volume trauma centers, including those in Sydney, Baltimore, and Helsinki, had learned to switch their resuscitation blood orders from emergency uncrossmatched to type-compatible 1:1:1 as soon as a blood type was available. Fourth, concerns about the safety of red cell and plasma transfusion were widespread, especially among groups writing standards, but the size of the associated risks and the effects of risk reduction strategies such as leukoreduction were not known. Fifth, for the group of severely injured patients with ongoing massive uncontrolled hemorrhage, resuscitation with a 1:1:1 unit ratio of red cells–plasma–platelets was recommended as long as resuscitation was running ahead of available laboratory data. Finally, it was widely admitted that there was a general lack of useful data to allow the identification of injured patients at risk for massive transfusion, and also regarding what the best clinical and laboratory tests were to guide subsequent transfusion and what safety and efficacy trade-offs were involved in blood product–based resuscitation. Early balanced resuscitation appeared to reduce morbidity and mortality, no group was performing such resuscitation in an ideal way, and the trauma community was poorly positioned to gather the data that would be needed to justify the costs and risks of such a commitment of resources. The meeting was a watershed event.

In the five years following the conference, a number of retrospective studies of massive bleeding were published that described differences in outcome associated with differences in resuscitation on large, essentially consecutive series of patients. Borgman and his colleagues published the results of the Baghdad series showing a 50% reduction in mortality with high-plasma versus low-plasma resuscitation of combat injuries. Johansson and colleagues reported a 33% drop in massive transfusion mortality at the University of Copenhagen Hospital after instituting hemorrhage control resuscitation.[67] Cotton and colleagues reported a 40% improvement in 30-day survival after damage control laparotomy when damage control resuscitation was used.[68] Holcomb and the Trauma Outcomes Group gathered 466 cases of massive transfusion from the records of 16 trauma centers, which showed a strong relationship of the plasma-to–red cell transfusion ratio with outcome.[69] Also noted

was a strong relationship of platelet count on admission and platelet transfusion to outcome. However, all of these important studies were subject to the criticism that it was impossible to separate out the effects of receiving blood products from the effects of surviving long enough to receive the products, or *survival bias*.[70] In a review of 10 published series, Stansbury and her epidemiologic colleagues pointed out a number of reasons for believing that the reported effect of a high plasma-to-RBC ratio was real, most importantly the declining overall mortality, but ultimately concluded that randomized and prospective data would be necessary to overcome the biases introduced by patient selection and time to treatment differences.[71]

Obstacles to conducting randomized trials in trauma patients are multiple. They include problems with study design, informed consent, study team building, and support. The trials of recombinant human blood-clotting factor VIIa (rFVIIa) conducted by its manufacturer and of hypertonic saline by the Resuscitations Outcomes Consortium provided experience and object lessons. In the rFVIIa hemorrhage trials, informed consent turned out to be a particular problem as half of all hemorrhage deaths occurred in the first two hours after arrival in the trauma center and the mean time to obtaining consent from next of kin or another legally authorized representative was three hours. This meant that a $40 million trial with a planned mortality of 40% had only 11% mortality and a statistically negative outcome in the patients who could be consented.[72] The hypertonic saline trials provided experience with conducting large publically funded resuscitation research under the exception from informed consent (EFIC) rules of the US government. They were successfully conducted and showed no benefit for this low-volume resuscitation technique.[73]

The first large prospective trial of hemostatic trauma resuscitation, PROMMTT, was observational only.[74] Designed to gather data in preparation for a randomized trial, in 15 months it screened 12,560 patients with highest level trauma team activations at 10 level 1 trauma centers and enrolled 1245 patients with apparent uncontrolled hemorrhage who survived at least 30 minutes and received at least one unit of red cells within six hours of admission. A subset of 905 of these patients who went on to receive at least three blood products in the next six hours became the analysis cohort. In the first six hours of observation, 95 patients died, including 77 of uncontrolled hemorrhage, whereas in the period between six hours after admission and 30 days only 18 of 125 further deaths were associated with uncontrolled bleeding. A Cox proportional hazards analysis showed that deaths in the first six hours were strongly associated with the ratio of plasma to red cell units given, with hazard ratios for death four times greater in the patients receiving plasma-to–red cell ratios less than 0.5. However, even with the strong association with outcome, the centers had trouble delivering plasma in a timely manner, with 65% of patients receiving no plasma in the first hour, 40% receiving no plasma in the first two hours, and 20% receiving none in the first three hours. Infusion times for platelets were even slower. Median time to hemorrhagic death was 2.6 hours. Ultimately, 25% of patients in the evaluation cohort died, of whom only a third died of hemorrhage, and most of them during the first six hours when active resuscitation was occurring. The study showed that it was possible to gather accurate time of transfusion data on large numbers of trauma patients in a short time period, but that the process was labor intensive, required screening large numbers of patients to enroll the few patients likely to benefit, and even in the best centers was still subject to risks of survival bias because of long delays in delivering plasma and platelets to the bedside. However, the size of the possible therapeutic benefit of timely administration of balanced resuscitation appeared to be as large as a 75% reduction in hemorrhage-related mortality.

The PROMMTT study suggested that a prospective randomized test of 1:1:1 transfusion in severely injured and massively bleeding trauma patients was possible. However, such a trial would require access to more than 10,000 trauma patients and the ability to screen patients and enroll those at high risk for active ongoing hemorrhage while simultaneously excluding those with severe head injury unlikely to benefit from resuscitation. It would need to submit them to randomized treatment quickly with EFIC, and to treat them promptly with blood products available within minutes after arrival so that there was no delay between the time of randomization and treatment to create survival bias.

The PROPPR study was conducted between August 2012 and January 2014.[75] It screened 14,000 patients and enrolled 680 who had an Assessment of Blood Consumption score of 2 or more and no evidence of unsurvivable head injury. The 12 participating trauma centers had to prove that their transfusion service could make six units of universal donor RBCs and plasma available within 10 minutes of notification and have six more available within 20 minutes of patient arrival. The patients were randomized to receive plasma–platelets–red cells in either 1:1:1 or 1:1:2 unit ratios and followed to 24-hour and 30-day mortality endpoints. The trial was completed with better than 97% protocol compliance and 100% follow-up for the primary endpoint.

The results are complicated only in the sense that the US Food and Drug Administration (FDA) required that the primary endpoints be 24-hour and 30-day survival as a condition of granting the permission to conduct the study under EFIC rules. The study results were not significant at these primary endpoints. However, over the course of resuscitation from 10 minutes to three hours, a significantly greater proportion of patients treated with the 1:1:1 ratio survived, and the absolute difference in mortality was significant at the end of resuscitation and persisted from three hours to the end of the study (Figure 49.3). The number of hemorrhage deaths occurring during resuscitation was reduced by almost 50%, and the

relative reduction in total deaths over 30 days was 18%. Overall mortality in the treated arm was 18%, down from 40% to 70% in series reported a decade ago.

What the PROPPR study did not tell was whether the benefit of balanced hemostatic resuscitation was the result of the extra plasma, the platelets, or both. It addresses only the difference between resuscitation with a 1:1:1 ratio of blood components and a 2:1:1 ratio. Planned blood sampling at admission and two hours after admission will miss most of the intermediate differences that led to excess early deaths in the 2:1:1 arm.

Rapid delivery of balanced hemostatic resuscitation is the new standard of care. It has been adopted by the American College of Surgeons in their Trauma Quality Improvement Guidelines for Massive Transfusion Protocols required for trauma center accreditation.[76] It is required for Patient Blood Management program accreditation through the AABB.[77] It saves lives, and it saves blood.

Clinical approach to the trauma patient

There are general phases of trauma care: prehospital, emergency room, operative care, and postoperative care. The phases of care are more blurred now as hemostatic resuscitation has been pushed further forward even into the prehospital phase of care with the provision of red cell and plasma products to some helicopter emergency patient transport systems, and associated with improved outcomes and minimal wastage.

Half of all civilian trauma deaths occur in the prehospital environment. Rapid movement of patients from the area where injury occurred to a trauma center provides the greatest benefit because most rapidly fatal injuries are truncal and require surgical or radiographically guided access for care. Nevertheless, opportunities exist and should not be lost to limit extremity bleeding through the use of tourniquets. Neck, scalp, and truncal soft tissue bleeding can be reduced by the application of direct pressure and hemostatic bandages. Keeping patients warm and limiting blood dilution are also important goals. The administration of crystalloid

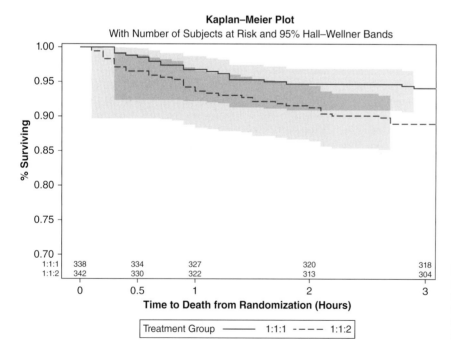

Figure 49.3 Mortality in the resuscitation phase of the PROPPR trial comparing resuscitation with a 1:1:1 unit ratio of RBC–plasma–platelets with a 2:1:1 ratio as a Kaplan–Meier plot with 95% Hall–Wellner confidence intervals. Data from Holcomb *et al.* (2015).[75]

fluids in the field to prevent acute renal failure does not appear to be necessary with modern casualty evacuation times, and raising blood pressure is associated with the loss of more of the patient's blood through vascular defects. In situations where red cells and plasma are available in the field or in transport, they can be given, but only about 15% of patients undergoing helicopter transport to trauma centers appear to be candidates for transfusion even when blood products are available.[78]

In the emergency room, there is an emphasis on rapid and systematic evaluation. The primary survey (ABCDEs) of *a*irway, *b*reathing, *c*irculation, neurologic *d*isability, and full *e*xposure is followed by a more systematic evaluation and the mobilization of teams to deal with specifically identified problems. Hypotension and penetrating injury suggest major internal bleeding and urgent need to move to the operating room (OR), as do significant tachycardia and the presence of fluid in body cavities assessed in a focused ultrasonographic survey for trauma (FAST). A combination of these two pairs of signs as the Assessment of Blood Consumption score has close to 80% power to predict massive transfusion and served as a major inclusion criterion in the PROPPR study.[79] For patients with less urgent needs to go directly to the OR, staged further studies leading to a complete secondary survey of the patient are the next goal. Hemorrhage remains a concern. There are multiple body cavities where it is possible to lose enough blood to cause shock from hypovolemia: pleural spaces and the mediastinum in the chest; peritoneal and retroperitoneal spaces in the abdomen, pelvis, and thighs; as well as subcutaneous spaces. Whole-body imaging is important for patients stable enough to tolerate it, and computerized tomographic (CT) scanning identifies additional sites of injury such as intracranial bleeding, pericardial hemorrhage, major vascular disruption, major organ fracture or laceration, and bowel, biliary, and urinary tract disruption that need prompt attention. Moreover, musculoskeletal injuries are frequent and need at least initial stabilization to make patients movable for nursing care. Simply placing a pelvic binder to hold the pelvic ring together can often limit venous bleeding and prevent further arterial injury in the early phases of patient assessment.

In the OR, time remains of the essence. The historic problem that 40 minutes of wide-open abdominal exposure in a hemorrhaging trauma patient led to the loss of a degree centigrade in core temperature through evaporative cooling from the exposed wet tissue surfaces is not true anymore as balanced resuscitation prevents gut swelling with evisceration and has the result that fluid and body warmers can now keep up. However, the requirement to obtain hemorrhage control can supersede the demands of normal operative patient setup, so that vascular access for resuscitation may be limited and resources for patient warming altogether missing in the early phases of emergently opening a body cavity for hemorrhage control. As a result, a decision on the goals of the exploratory surgical procedure needs to be made early. Massive organ disruption or soft tissue injury may lead to a decision to pack wounds for hemorrhage control with the concomitant need to change or remove packing a day (or at most two days) later and therefore a need to leave the wound open. The decision to pursue only hemorrhage control, restoration of critical organ perfusion, and limitation of wound contamination with bowel tie-off and bile and urinary drainage is classic damage control. However, damage control surgery rates are plummeting as iatrogenic resuscitation injury is avoided.[80] More frequently, surgical exposure allows the identification of correctable sources of bleeding that can be dealt with by vascular repair or ligation, repair or removal of injured organs, and closure.

Increasingly, close collaboration between surgeons and interventional radiologists (IRs) has led to procedures that are partially performed by one specialty and partially by the other. These procedures occur with the patient being moved in the middle of the procedure from the OR to the IR suite or can occur in modern hybrid ORs where the interventional radiology cameras can be brought to the patient and the two groups can work together simultaneously.[81] Transfusion support for such highly complex and high-blood-loss situations is similar to other massive transfusion situations and involves ongoing balanced resuscitation shaped to the clinical situation and the available laboratory data.

At the end of such procedures, patients are moved to recovery rooms or directly to intensive care units (ICUs) for continued resuscitation. Bleeding is often slowed but not stopped, and provision for continuing blood product support and planning for potential return of frank hemorrhage if packing fails or is reinitiated with unpacking is prudent. In the recovery room or ICU, bleeding is usually slow enough that its replacement can be guided by laboratory measures. It is still important to remember that the limitations of resuscitation imposed by multiple different blood components diluting each other make it prudent to avoid components such as platelets in additive solution that do not maximize plasma dose.

Clinical approach to the mass casualty trauma situation

Mass casualty trauma situations are uncommon, and those requiring large amounts of blood are rare. In the United States between the years 1975 and 2000, there were only four such events that required more than 100 units of RBCs to treat all of the resulting casualties in their first 24 hours of care.[82] The largest domestic use of RBCs for a mass casualty event was 224 units given for injuries from falling glass from the World Trade Towers into crowds of pedestrians below. The London and Madrid train bombings used even more RBCs (338 and 696, respectively) on the first day, but each involved the care of hundreds of casualties spread across multiple hospitals in a large urban area. Blood use in the Boston Marathon 2013 bombings has been described.[83]

The rarity of massive blood use in multicasuality events is to be contrasted with the frequency of massive blood use in a single individual when polytrauma or transplant more commonly creates situations where one individual uses more than 100 units of RBCs in 24 hours. A critical difference between these situations is the need to have well-practiced protocols to maintain the unique identity of each patient in multicasualty settings. The use of universal donor products in disaster situations where casualties may be unidentified or, more importantly, misidentified is an important precaution. It should be remembered that more than 100,000 universal-donor whole blood and red cell units were given in the Vietnam War and that all seven fatal acute hemolytic reactions there were associated with the misidentification of recipients of crossmatched red cells.

Mass casualty trauma situations are major media events, and the media frequently encourage the population to donate blood as a response to disaster. During the Clapham Junction railway disaster in London in 1988, the number of volunteer donors responding effectively shut down the Richmond blood center. The 600,000 extra units of blood collected nationwide after the September 11, 2001, terrorists attacks were unnecessary and largely had to be destroyed.

Initial resuscitation of the burn patient

The resuscitation of patients with severe burns is different than that of patients with penetrating and/or blunt force trauma. Trauma patients in hemorrhagic shock with ongoing acute blood loss are generally resuscitated with blood products. Burn patients typically have a higher initial hemoglobin concentration associated with redistribution of plasma water into the interstitium and intracellular space. Therefore, their initial resuscitation utilizes crystalloid and occasionally colloid solutions, and blood product transfusion is rare during burn resuscitation. However, later during the treatment course, cumulative blood loss associated with eschar excision and grafting, anemia of critical illness, and laboratory testing increases. It is during this latter period in the hospital course that attention should be given to the type and quantity of blood transfusions given to patients with severe burns.

In the initial period (24–48 hours after injury), resuscitation is conducted according to standard burn resuscitation formulas; however, no single formula replaces the role of the physician, who must continually assess the adequacy of resuscitation. Utilizing the Parkland formula, most patients receive 2 to 4 mL/kg of fluid per percentage of total body surface area (BSA) burned in the first 24 hours after injury. This fluid is generally lactated Ringers' solution. The first half of the calculated volume is given over the first eight hours from injury, not from the beginning of resuscitation; the rest is given over the next 16 hours.[84,85] Children also should receive maintenance fluids containing dextrose in addition to the resuscitative fluid. The presence of inhalation injury can increase the volume of fluid to achieve adequate resuscitation. Whether colloid is used in the first 24 hours is determined on a case-by-case basis; administration of colloid should not be routine, but is utilized in the severely burned patient who is not hemodynamically responsive to crystalloid resuscitation. Urinary output of 0.5–1 mL/kg/hour is the most commonly used measure of resuscitation adequacy.

Release of vasoactive mediators from injured tissue results in a diffuse capillary leak starting soon after injury. This loss of microvascular integrity results in extravasation of crystalloid and colloid solutions for the first 18 to 24 hours after injury. This pathophysiologic process explains the enormous fluid volumes given to burned patients for the first 24 hours, which can be up to 40 L. This is the reason that most burn resuscitation formulas incorporate the use of colloid after 24 hours; microvascular integrity is restored at that time, and colloid remains largely intravascular. Colloid, generally 5% albumin, is infused at a dose based on burn size (generally, 0.3 to 0.5 mL/kg per percentage of total BSA burned over 24 hours). During this period, crystalloid utilization decreases markedly.

Transfusion therapy in the care of the severely burned

Patients with less than 10% total BSA burns rarely receive transfusions.[86] Those with increasing burn size, age, and presence of anticoagulants significantly increase the use of blood transfusions, but deciding when to transfuse can be difficult.[87] The hypermetabolic response to severe burn significantly alters normal physiologic parameters that are commonly relied upon to determine transfusion indications. When considering transfusions in burn patients, several factors are evaluated, including the acuity of the anemia, the risk-benefit of transfusions, blood loss mitigation techniques, and potential physiologic benefit.

During the initial resuscitative period, burned patients will have an acute blood loss anemia that is not associated with large-volume blood loss, but rather from destruction of erythrocytes within the cutaneous circulation and by hemorrhage into the burn wound. This initial anemia is typically not significant enough to require transfusion, as evident by data showing an average of 5.3 +/− 0.3 days from admission to the first transfusion.[88] The critical point of highest blood loss, and subsequently the use of large-volume transfusions, occurs during burn wound excision and grafting. Further blood loss can occur from postoperative dressing changes. During burn wound excisions, most estimates suggest that 1 mL of reconstituted whole blood will be used for each square centimeter of excised wound. Therefore, if 1000 cm^2 will be excised, approximately two units of packed RBCs and two units of FFP should be available. Platelets are rarely transfused unless the platelet count is less than 10,000/mm^3 in the absence of other coagulopathies.

Efforts made to mitigate the use of transfusions during eschar excision include the use of hemostatic techniques such as topical thrombin, epinephrine-soaked gauze, tourniquets, and fibrin sealants.[89,90] It is well known that intraoperative blood loss is the limiting factor of the extent of excision and grafting performed. Initial steps to control hemorrhage use electrocautery devices or pressure. Thrombin spray and laparotomy pads saturated with thrombin and epinephrine can be applied directly to the wound bed to limit intraoperative blood loss. The use of tourniquets for excision and grafting of extremities can further decrease blood loss, but should be tempered by the risk of ischemia resulting in graft loss.[91] Recently, the use of activated thrombin mixed with fibrin that is sprayed onto the wound has become popular and may prove effective. Results of preliminary studies of the use of intraoperative blood recovery techniques show recovery and reinfusion of approximately 40% of shed blood without adverse inflammatory or infectious complications.[92] As in the care of trauma patients, the importance of normothermia in preventing coagulopathy is recognized, and patients are actively warmed or more importantly not allowed to get cold at the time of surgery.

Data from a multicenter study evaluating the effects of blood transfusion in severe burns revealed that 70% of blood transfusions for burn victims occur outside of the operating room.[5] These transfusions are done to treat the persistent anemia of chronic illness that affects most critically ill patients, including burn patients. This anemia is multifactorial in origin and due in part to mild ongoing blood loss from dressing changes and phlebotomy, impaired RBC production from erythropoietin insensitivity, malnutrition, and metabolic demands. As with operative excisions, some efforts can be undertaken to mitigate this anemia as well. Minimizing blood draws and using pediatric blood collection tubes can decrease blood volumes wasted. Maintaining adequate nutrition is important for all patients, and some studies have identified up to 13% of critically ill patients as deficient in nutrients necessary for erythrogenesis.[93] Administration of exogenous erythropoietin has been extensively studied in multiple critically ill populations but has yet to show any efficacy in patients with burns.

Transfusing patients with thermal injuries must be tempered with the known risks and benefits of blood and blood products. Increasing hemoglobin concentrations is the only method to increase oxygen carrying capacity, but the known transfusion-associated morbidity documented in multiple specialties is also seen in burn patients. The safety of a restrictive transfusion strategy demonstrated in the Transfusion Requirements in Critical Care (TRICC) trial has been investigated in patients with thermal injuries.[94] Mann *et al.* retrospectively found a fivefold decrease in the volume of blood transfused per percentage total BSA without adverse cardiac complications or increased morbidity.[95] Sittig and Deitch found a greater than threefold decrease in transfusion requirements when a more selective transfusion policy was implemented whereby 86% of blood transfused was given at the time of an operative procedure.[6] In another retrospective analysis, Kwan *et al.* implemented a restrictive transfusion protocol to maintain hemoglobin of 7 g/dl and found a significant decrease in both 30-day mortality (38% for liberal vs. 19% for restrictive) and overall hospital mortality (46 liberal vs. 22% restrictive).[96] In a large, multicenter retrospective analysis of 666 patients, the number of infections per patient increased with each unit of blood transfused. This translated to a 13% increase in developing an infection per unit of blood transfused.[5] These studies should be confirmed with a randomized prospective analysis (which is underway). Despite the laudable push for a generally more restrictive RBC transfusion threshold, burn patients with underlying cardiovascular disease probably will benefit from more liberal red cell use.

The appropriate use of plasma during intraoperative blood loss from burn wound excision is not well defined. Increasing the volume of plasma in relation to packed RBCs has shown definitive benefit in trauma patients with hemorrhagic shock. In one study comparing higher FFP usage in burn patients (1:1 vs a 4:1 (RBC:FFP)), there was a decrease in overall blood product usage and a trend toward shorter duration of hospital stay, fewer infectious complications, and less organ dysfunction in the 1:1 group.[97] However, in military patients with severe thermal injuries, the use of plasma was associated with the development of acute respiratory distress.[98] There is a recent trend to use viscoelastic analysis in guiding transfusion resuscitation, and early use during burn wound excision shows promise in minimizing the amount of plasma transfused, but further investigation is warranted.[99]

Adjuncts in transfusion therapy for trauma and burn patients

Tranexamic acid

Tranexamic acid (TXA) and ε-aminocaproic acid are lysine analogs used as antifibrinolytics.[100] Newly formed fibrin polymer has exposed lysine residues that serve as binding sites for plasmin and facilitate the plasmin-dependent breakdown of fibrin polymer. During normal coagulation, a strong thrombin burst activates the thrombin-activated fibrinolysis inhibitor (TAFI), which removes these lysine residues to prevent fibrin breakdown.[101] However, after trauma and especially with the acute coagulopathy of trauma, the intensity of thrombin activation is reduced and as a result TAFI is not activated. However, activation of plasmin by tissue plasminogen activator secreted in response to hypotension and inactivation of plasminogen activator inhibitor by activated protein C lead to high plasmin activity. The combination of high plasmin activity and widely available plasmin binding sites on fibrin leads to rapid degradation of fibrin polymer. Using TXA to inhibit fibrinolysis stabilizes newly formed clot and reduces blood loss.

TXA has been demonstrated to reduce blood loss in several nontrauma settings such as in knee and hip joint replacement, in craniosynostosis surgery, and after tooth removal in patients with hemophilia. Knee and hip joint replacement trials have shown reduced blood drainage after surgical site irrigation with a suspension of the drug.[102] In infants undergoing craniosynostosis surgery,

a randomized trial demonstrated an almost 50% reduction in blood loss and red cell replacement requirements with intravenous administration.[103] In hemophilia patients undergoing dental extraction, oral wash with a suspension of the drug reduced duration of bleeding.[104]

For trauma patients, the international CRASH II trial and the MATTERs study are the basis for recommendations for wide use of the drug. The CRASH II trial was a large simple randomized trial of TXA use or nothing in 20,211 trauma patients in 274 hospital in 40 countries.[105] Use of the drug led to a 1.5% reduction in overall mortality with a reduction in the odds of hemorrhagic mortality by 15%. However, in patients treated more than three hours after injury, mortality was increased. The Military Application of Tranexamic Acid in Trauma Emergency Resuscitation study (MATTERs) is a retrospective review of 896 consecutive admissions to a British Army medical facility in Afghanistan that demonstrated better survival in patients treated with TXA.[106] The mortality benefit observed in patients receiving TXA was almost 50% in those receiving more than 10 units of RBCs.

Despite occasional reports of thrombotic complications after TXA administration, a large meta-analysis of randomized trials of the drug did not reveal excess thrombosis or mortality after its use. This suggestion of broad safety has led to recommendations that TXA be given in prehospital situations. A large Australian study of the use of TXA in the prehospital setting and in facilitating the movement of patients from remote locations to trauma surgical centers is underway, and in the United States, the Resuscitation Outcomes Consortium is starting a trial of TXA in head-injured patients. The drug is rapidly becoming a standard of care.

Plasma-derived coagulation factors

In Central Europe, especially in Austria, recent work has focused on using plasma-derived coagulation factor concentrates to rapidly restore activity in the coagulation system in severely injured patients. The two products that have received the most attention are four-factor prothrombin complex concentrates (PCCs) and fibrinogen concentrates.[107] Chapter 27 describes these products.

Four-factor PCCs provide enough factors VII, X, and II to reconstitute the extrinsic pathway coagulation enzymes, and fibrinogen concentrate provides both fibrinogen and factor XIII. Given early in the course of trauma, they appear effective in multiple uncontrolled case studies, but the exact effects of the lack of factors V, VIII, and XI are unknown. Moreover, the factor concentrates are expensive.

The potential advantages of using these pharmaceutical plasma-derived products are several. Their excellent storage properties and ease of reconstitution mean that they can be kept on the anesthesiologist's cart or even used in the field, ambulance, or helicopter. Their high concentrations of extrinsic pathway factors allow rapid restoration of extrinsic pathway function, the most common coagulation defect seen in severely injured patients with the acute coagulopathy of trauma. They are blood-type independent, are immunologically well tolerated, contain low concentrations of other proteins, have low volume, and are virologically safe because of pathogen reduction steps integrated into their manufacture.

Disadvantages include the need for reconstitution, which can take 20 minutes and requires another set of hands; the lack of other plasma proteins; and the lack of the full complement of coagulation factors. Although reconstitution is relatively easy, the anesthesiologist is busy in managing other aspects of the care of these most severely injured trauma patients, and time to reconstitution delays the onset of therapy. Also, severely injured patients need volume, so PCCs have frequently been given with other colloids such as starches, which interfere with platelet coagulation. Finally, the PCCs lack factors I, V, VIII, XI, and XIII, and the most seriously injured patients often have deficits of factors I, V, and VIII, with those that do having very high mortality.

As noted, factors I and XIII are present in fibrinogen concentrate, so fibrinogen concentrate is typically given with PCCs, but fibrinogen concentrates have also been given alone. Healthy individuals have relatively low fibrinogen concentrations, which become markedly higher in the days following injury. Providing fibrinogen early to severely injured patients who are still capable of generating a normal thrombin burst takes advantage of the normal extra thrombin capacity to lay down the added extra fibrinogen as fibrin to make stronger clots. For this reason, fibrinogen has been viewed as an attractive field medical agent to be given early to reduce blood loss in patient transport. These concepts have been demonstrated in animal studies and small human trials where they are clearly better than classic ATLS resuscitation. However, how the advantages of rapid restoration of extrinsic pathway function and increased fibrinogen balance with the problems created by missing factors and the modest time delay involved in mixing is not known. Direct comparisons with 1:1:1 blood product resuscitation are needed.

Recombinant activated human factor VII

Recombinant activated human coagulation factor VII (rVIIa) was developed as a factor VIII bypass activity for use in the treatment of hemophilia patients with inhibitors. It saw use in trauma first in Israel, then more widely, and finally was tested in randomized trials. The failure of the drug to alter mortality in the randomized trials was discussed in this chapter in relation to time to death in trauma patients with uncontrolled hemorrhage and the trial requirements for informed consent.

rVIIa is grown in mammalian cell culture, isolated and activated by chromatography, and freeze dried. Milligram doses reproduce the normal nanomolar concentrations of the active factor in plasma, but the half-life is only two hours. A quarter of severely injured trauma patients had an abnormal PT in the early reports of the acute coagulopathy of trauma and appeared likely to benefit from treatment, but an isolated elevated PT was associated with only a modest increase in mortality. Early trials showed that the drug reduced blood use in situations such as prostate surgery, but as a vitamin K–dependent coagulation factor, rVIIa's activity is highly pH dependent and is reduced in acidic patients and environments.

The combination of inappropriate claims that the drug was a *universal hemostat*, failure to demonstrate a mortality benefit in the randomized trauma trials, an alleged association with increased posttrauma thrombosis, and perceived high cost have reduced usage.[108] If the drug has a use, it is probably early after injury rather than late, and in combination with products such as fibrinogen concentrates to reduce bleeding in transport. Avoiding crystalloid use and more balanced forms of resuscitation have largely replaced the need for rVIIa in trauma center care.

Hemorrhage control bandages

It is possible to make excellent hemorrhage control bandages that provide for rapid control of even arterial bleeding when applied to accessible sites with appropriate pressure. Dry fibrin sealant dressings (DFSDs) containing fibrinogen and thrombin freeze-dried on an absorbable mesh backing have been approved for use, and even better prototypes have been demonstrated.[109] Many of the same hemostatic effects can be achieved with hydrophobically modified chitosan and other synthetic hemostatic agents, which can be made into wound-adhering bandages and are inexpensive as well.[110]

Animal experiments with the Army/American Red Cross DFSD prototype showed reduced blood loss and improved survival in experimental models of grade V liver injury and groin injury. In its one human use in a groin injury with femoral artery rupture above a level compatible with tourniquet, it proved lifesaving. Nevertheless, its relatively high cost and use of plasma-derived products created manufacturing problems. The currently available licensed versions use lower concentrations of thrombin and fibrinogen that are less effective against arterial hemorrhage, but can still be used in liver surgery. Making low-cost synthetic hemorrhage-control bandages with appropriate short-term stability and midterm biodegradation will be a major advance in the care of large superficial wounds, accessible but not-tourniquet-compatible hemorrhage, and wound stabilization and hemorrhage control during trauma and other forms of surgery.

Artificial oxygen carriers

Hemoglobin and perflurocarbon-based oxygen carriers have a long and complex history. Cell-free hemoglobin can support life for a few hours in patients with profound hemolysis from clostridial sepsis, in animals following exchange transfusion to lethally low hematocrits, and occasionally in patients given hemoglobin-based blood substitutes. However, most patients do not tolerate the materials, and 11 randomized trials using four different commercial products all had excess mortality in the treated groups.[111] For this reason, it is hard to imagine a public health agency such as the FDA approving a material that consistently kills more people than it helps.

Tetrameric cell-free hemoglobin will stay in the circulation for several hours and functions in oxygen delivery during that time, but all the while it disassociates into dimers that are cleared by haptoglobin binding and glomerular filtration and oxidizes to met-hemoglobin and hemichromes, heme, iron, and globin precipitates. Free hemoglobin leads to renal proximal tubular injury as its classic toxicity. It also binds endothelium-derived nitric oxide, causing vasospasm with hypertension and increased vascular resistance; serves as a primary nutrient for bacterial pathogens such as *Streptococcus aureus* and *Escherichia coli*; and presents bacterial endotoxin to the immune system in a more active form. Hemoglobin breakdown products cause oxidative injury, including monocyte and endothelial activation, excitatory neurotoxicity, and the production of lysophospholipids and cyclic endoperoxides with secondary immune consequences.[112]

Modified hemoglobins, whether internally cross-linked tetramers, polymerized tetramers, or conjugates, can be made to reduce one or more of these extracellular toxic mechanisms, but usually at the expense of exacerbating another. The polymerized bovine and human hemoglobins could not eliminate vasoactivity, but lost cooperativity and some oxygen carrying capacity as a result and had inflammatory side effects as well. Polyethylene glycol–conjugated hemoglobin is highly osmotically active, meaning that it has both limited bulk oxygen carriage and significant colligative interference with plasma coagulation proteins. Even though these oxygen carriers carry oxygen, they do not improve the outcome of injured patients.

Oxygen can be dissolved in perfluorocarbon oils, and the oils can be emulsified to be miscible in water, but a safe and effective combination of these properties has not been achieved. The original product, a mixture of perfluorodecalin and perfluorotriprolyl amine emulsified with a polar detergent (Fluosol, Green Cross Corp., Tokyo, Japan), failed a human trial in patients refusing red cell transfusion for religious reasons.[113] The product had the side effect that the perfluorocarbon lipids could not be metabolized or excreted, and so they accumulated in liver, spleen, and marrow macrophages at a rate of a pound per dose, and a dose functioned for only a few hours. Subsequent development of the volatile perfluorocarbon oils perfluoroctyl bromine and perfluorodichloro octane, which had high oxygen solubility and low vapor pressures compatible with both air breathing and simultaneous excretion of the fluorocarbon through the lung, failed because the high dose of emulsion necessary to carry useful amounts of oxygen led to complement activation, fever, and hypotension.

Despite the well-understood physicochemical limitations of all available alternative oxygen carriers and the well-characterized toxicities of the second-generation products that have undergone human trials, there continues to be interest in these blood substitute materials. Approximately 100 articles are published each year on their possible roles in trauma resuscitation. This literature largely ignores the toxicities and colligative activities of all such alternative oxygen carriers that make them largely incompatible with the restoration of blood coagulation function at the heart of modern trauma care.

Summary

The reduction in blood transfusion in the care of burned patients has been dramatic (three- to fivefold), as burn surgeons have learned to manage blood loss and accept lower transfusion triggers. This is an example of patient blood management evolving in a surgical field largely independent of transfusion medicine.

In the last decade, improvements in trauma resuscitation and trauma care have led to an almost 50% reduction in the incidence of hemorrhagic deaths in trauma centers carrying out damage control resuscitation. These improvements center on the early administration of balanced hemostatic resuscitation with plasma and platelets aimed at early correction of the acute coagulopathy of trauma. These improved outcomes have been validated in the PROPPR study, a large randomized clinical trial.

The challenges of extending these improvements in care to injured patients arriving in smaller centers and to soldiers and civilians in the field will center on developing ways to deliver current blood products earlier in care and the wider use of hemostatic adjuncts such as tranexamic acid, hemostatic bandages, and fibrinogen concentrates. It will require a national commitment to collecting the amounts of universal donor blood products needed to make the system work. This will be facilitated by developing a new generation of blood products such as freeze-dried plasma, more effective plasma derivatives, and frozen platelets.

Key references

A full reference list for this chapter is available at: http://www.wiley.com/go/simon/transfusion

40 Brohi K, Singh J, Heron M, Coats T. Acute traumatic coagulopathy. *J Trauma* 2003 Jun;**54**(6):1127–30.

44 Johansson PI, Stensballe J, Oliveri R, Wade CE, Ostrowski SR, Holcomb JB. How I treat patients with massive hemorrhage. *Blood* 2014 Nov 13;**124**(20):3052–8.

48 Dutton RP, Stansbury LG, Leone S, Kramer B, Hess JR, Scalea TM. Trauma mortality in mature trauma systems: are we doing better? An analysis of trauma mortality patterns, 1997–2008. *J Trauma* 2010;**69**:620–6.

58 Hess JR, Lindell AL, Stansbury LG, Dutton RP, Scalea TM. The prevalence of abnormal results of conventional coagulation tests on admission to a trauma center. *Transfusion* 2009 Jan;**49**(1):34–9.

75 Holcomb JB, Tilley BC, Baraniuk S, *et al.*, on behalf of the PROPPR Study Group. Transfusion of plasma, platelets, and red blood cells in a 1:1:1 vs a 1:1:2 ratio and mortality in patients with severe trauma: the PROPPR Clinical Trial. *JAMA* 2015 Feb 3;**313**(5):471–82.

77 *AABB, PBM Standards Unit. Standards for patient blood management.* Bethesda, MD: AABB, 2014.

82 Schmidt PJ. Blood and disaster—supply and demand. *N Engl J Med* 2002;**346**:617–20.

105 CRASH-2 trial collaborators, Shakur H, Roberts I, Bautista R, *et al.* Effects of tranexamic acid on death, vascular occlusive events, and blood transfusion in trauma patients with significant haemorrhage (CRASH-2): a randomised, placebo-controlled trial. *Lancet* 2010 Jul 3;**376**(9734):23–32.

CHAPTER 50

Transfusion support for the oncology patient

Wade L. Schulz & Edward L. Snyder

Department of Laboratory Medicine, Yale School of Medicine, Yale University; and Blood Bank, Yale-New Haven Hospital, New Haven, CT, USA

Transfusion support for patients with cancer is a complex, multi-faceted medical therapy meant to assist in the management of complications related to chemotherapy, radiation, transplantation, or widespread metastatic disease. Oncology patients often require chronic transfusion support and present several unique challenges to the provider. For these patients, greater attention must be paid to the selection, preparation, modification, and response to blood components to help ensure better outcomes. This chapter highlights the most challenging aspects of transfusion therapy for oncology patients encountered by clinicians and transfusion services on a routine basis.

Red cell transfusion

Indications

The goal of red blood cell (RBC) transfusion in oncology patients is the same as in other populations—to increase the oxygen carrying capacity of whole blood for patients with anemia. Unfortunately, there are no evidence-based laboratory criteria upon which to determine when transfusion is appropriate for oncology patients. Studies in other critically ill patient populations have shown that hemoglobin levels of 7 to 10 g/dL can be tolerated without the need for allogeneic transfusion.[1] There is no evidence to suggest that higher hemoglobin levels provide any therapeutic benefit. Indeed, there is evidence to suggest that "hypertransfusion" may actually be detrimental to patient outcomes.[2] Therefore, oncology patients should be transfused for symptomatic anemia or at predetermined hemoglobin or hematocrit levels defined by a hospital's oncology service.

Selection of ABO group for RBC transfusion

For most oncology patients, no special consideration is needed for the appropriate selection of ABO group for RBC units. However, for patients who have received an allogeneic hematopoietic stem cell transplant (HSCT), the choice of appropriate ABO group can be more difficult. This is particularly true in the case of ABO mismatch between the hematopoietic progenitor cell (HPC) donor and recipient. Although a blood group mismatch between donor and recipient ABO type does not seem to have any long-term drawbacks,

providing appropriate transfusion support in the period after transplantation can be complex.[3,4] These patients are known to require more transfusions due to delayed cellular engraftment and red cell aplasia. They are also at risk for acute and delayed red cell hemolysis from ABO incompatibility while engraftment takes place.[4,5] Although some controversy exists, ABO-mismatched HSCT does not appear to adversely impact outcome or long-term survival in either pediatric or adult populations.[3,4,6]

An ABO mismatch can lead to concerns during HSC infusion as well as post transplantation. In the setting of allogeneic transplantation, there are several possibilities for ABO antibody mismatch. When the donor possesses antibodies against recipient red cells, patients are deemed to have a minor mismatch. An example of a minor mismatch is when a patient (recipient) with group A red cells receives HPCs from a group O donor. A major mismatch is when the recipient has antibodies targeted to donor red cells. This would occur when a group O patient (recipient) receives HPCs from a group A donor. Finally, there is "two-way" incompatibility, where both major and minor mismatches occur, for example when a group A patient (recipient) receives HPCs from a group B donor. Table 50.1 summarizes both major and minor incompatibility by blood group. The key to successful transfusion for any of these mismatches is to reduce hemolysis during HPC infusion. For patients with a minor mismatch, this can be achieved by plasma reduction of the HPCs to significantly lower the amount of offending antibody. For patients with major mismatch, red cell depletion of the HSC product can be used to prevent acute hemolysis during infusion.[7]

Antibodies can persist for weeks to months after transplantation, which can lead to ongoing issues in the selection of proper blood components.[8,9] Patients can also present as chimeras after HSCT, with two distinct blood groups seen by routine blood typing.[8] Fortunately, standardized strategies have been developed to provide the most compatible ABO components for these patients. For patients with major incompatibility from recipient anti-A or anti-B directed to donor red cells, recipient-type RBC units are necessary until ABO antibodies are no longer detected.[10–12] For patients with minor incompatibility, recipient-type plasma and platelets should be used until the recipient's red cells are no longer detected. Donor-type RBC units can be used immediately after HSCT for patients with minor incompatibility.[10–12] Patients with two-way

---

Table 50.1 Compatibility by ABO Group in hematopoietic stem cell transplantation

Recipient ABO Blood Group	Donor ABO Group			
	O	A	B	AB
O	C	M	M	M
A	m	C	Mm	M
B	m	mM	C	M
AB	m	m	m	C

C = compatible; M = major incompatibility; m = minor incompatibility; mM = both major and minor incompatibility ("two-way" incompatibility).

Table 50.2 Transfusion protocol for HSCT patients

Recipient	Donor O			Donor A			Donor B			Donor AB		
	RBC type	FFP/PLT type	2nd choice PLT	RBC type	FFP/PLT type	2nd choice PLT	RBC type	FFP/PLT type	2nd choice PLT	RBC type	FFP/PLT type	2nd choice PLT
O	O	O	A or B	O	A	O	O	B	O	O	AB	A
A	O	A	O	A	A	O	O	AB	A	A	AB	A
B	O	B	O	O	AB	A	B	B	O	B	AB	B
AB	O	AB	A	A	AB	A	B	AB	B	AB	AB	A or B

NOTE: Rh positive recipients with Rh negative donors receive Rh negative products. Rh negative recipients with Rh positive donors receive Rh positive products.

incompatibility require group O RBC units and group AB plasma and platelets until offending antibodies and cells are no longer detectable. Table 50.2 provides a transfusion protocol that can be followed for ABO-mismatched HSCT.[10–12]

Alloimmunization to red cell antigens

Despite significant immunosuppression, patients with malignancy can still mount immune responses to foreign red cell antigens, which can complicate transfusion and increase the risk for hemolysis.[13,14] Rates for red cell alloimmunization in oncology patients have been most studied in patients with hematologic malignancies undergoing HSCT. These studies have shown that alloimmunization occurs in 2% to 8% of patients in these populations.[15,16] Additional studies are needed to better assess the rate of red cell alloimmunization in patients with solid tumors or other oncologic conditions.

Component modification: leukocyte reduction and irradiation

A major advance in blood component modification has been the implementation of prestorage leukocyte reduction techniques. Decreased numbers of white blood cells within transfusion components have been shown to reduce the risk of alloimmunization to human leukocyte antigens (HLA).[17] In addition, leukocyte reduction can lower the rate of blood-borne transmission for pathogens that are carried within white cells, such as cytomegalovirus (CMV).[18] According to the 2011 National Blood Collection Utilization Survey, approximately 85% of all red cell units in the United States were leukocyte reduced, most before storage.[19]

Despite the use of leukocyte-reduced units, many oncology patients are still at risk for transfusion-associated graft-versus-host disease (TA-GVHD) because of their immunocompromised state. In cases of TA-GVHD, donor lymphocytes generate a profound immune response against the recipient's cells.[20] The underlying causes and manifestations of TA-GVHD are discussed in Chapter 60. Prevention of TA-GVHD can be accomplished by gamma irradiation of cellular blood components.[21] Some within the field of transfusion medicine have argued for a policy of universal

blood component irradiation, as the process has few side effects and may prevent cases of TA-GVHD in patients whose high-risk status is not known.[22] However, the practicality and cost-effectiveness of such a policy have not been determined.[22] The main disadvantage of irradiation is the induction of a potassium leak within the red cell membrane, thereby shortening the shelf of an RBC unit to no more than 28 days from the date of irradiation or the original expiration date, whichever comes first. There are no such concerns regarding the irradiation of platelets or plasma products, the latter of which does not require irradiation.

Alternatives to allogeneic red cell transfusion

For oncology patients undergoing a surgical intervention, intra-operative blood recovery—a process where shed whole blood is centrifuged, washed of contaminants, and then reinfused—may be of benefit to reduce allogeneic blood usage.[23] Although concern has been raised about the promotion of tumor cell metastasis with the use of such blood recovery in some cancer patients, several trials conducted in patients with hepatobiliary and genitourinary cancers have shown no evidence of decreased patient survival.[24–26] Additional techniques including acute normovolemic hemodilution (ANH) and the use of preoperatively donated autologous whole blood can also be considered. However, these techniques are often not feasible in oncology patients who are too anemic and who can require surgery at unpredictable times. The lack of cost-effectiveness for preoperative autologous donation also limits its utility to oncology patients undergoing major surgery.[27]

Another alternative to allogeneic red cell transfusion is the administration of erythropoietin-stimulating agents (ESAs). However, the chronic use of ESAs in patients with cancer and other critical illnesses has been found to have potential serious adverse effects. Several studies have found that ESA administration can lead to an increased risk for thrombosis.[28] In addition, it has been postulated that erythropoietin may accelerate tumor growth and lead to decreased survival. Finally, studies have also shown that use of ESAs does not significantly decrease the need for allogeneic transfusion in critically ill patients.[29,30] These findings led to a black box warning for the use of ESAs in the setting of cancer-related anemia.[31]

Platelet transfusion

Indications

Platelet transfusion is intended to stop or prevent bleeding in thrombocytopenic patients. The use of platelet transfusion is a first-line therapy for acute hemorrhage in patients with thrombocytopenia or those receiving antiplatelet medication. However, some controversy exists over the use of platelet transfusion for bleeding prophylaxis. Initial studies that supported the use of platelets for bleeding prophylaxis arose from trials in leukemic patients who were noted to have decreased bleeding episodes after platelet transfusion.[32] Later studies also demonstrated that prophylactic transfusion resulted in better outcomes and lower mortality compared to the use of therapeutic transfusion in patients with hematologic malignancy.[33] In the early 1990s, the goal for routine bleeding prophylaxis was to keep platelet counts greater than $20,000/\mu L$.[34] However, more recent trials have shown that spontaneous hemorrhage is unlikely, even with platelet counts as low as $5,000$ to $10,000/\mu L$. In addition, patients transfused under more stringent criteria appear to have no change in morbidity and use significantly fewer blood products, thereby reducing the risks of chronic transfusion exposure.[35–40]

Multiple clinical trials have shown that there is no increase in bleeding complications associated with the use of stringent platelet transfusion criteria. However, one retrospective study of patients after HSCT showed increased mortality in severely thrombocytopenic patients (platelet counts $<10,000/\mu L$), even though there was no increased risk of bleeding.[41] Although difficult to completely interpret given the retrospective nature of the study, these data may imply a protective benefit from platelet transfusion other than bleeding prophylaxis in transplant patients. Prospective studies on survival and outcome that compare stringent and conservative approaches to platelet transfusion are still needed to determine the best course of treatment for thrombocytopenic oncology patients.

Selection of ABO group and Rh type for platelet transfusion

Platelets express ABO antigens, although interactions between these antigens and host antibodies do not usually mediate clinically significant transfusion reactions.[42] Although type-specific platelets are preferred, most blood banks will transfuse ABO-mismatched platelets to adults without significant concern for incompatibility. However, the use of ABO-mismatched platelets in oncology patients can result in decreased therapeutic benefit or adverse reactions. For instance, a form of platelet refractoriness is mediated by ABO antibodies, with mismatched platelets cleared from circulation minutes to hours after infusion.[42] Furthermore, there is some evidence to suggest that ABO incompatibility can promote the development of HLA alloimmunization in multitransfused patients.[42] Another concern is the possibility that high-titer ABO antibodies in the plasma of donor platelets units may lead to hemolytic transfusion reactions in ABO-incompatible recipients.[43–45] Children in particular may demonstrate clinically significant hemolysis to ABO-incompatible platelet transfusions owing to their small blood volume. Therefore, it is recommended that oncology patients with low platelet counts receive ABO-compatible

platelet products when feasible. For populations undergoing HSCT, other considerations regarding major and minor mismatches are also relevant. Table 50.2 summarizes guidelines for platelet transfusion therapy in the peritransplant period.

Even though platelets lack Rh antigens, there remains a small concern for Rh alloimmunization during platelet transfusion due to the potential exposure to small numbers of residual red cells in the products collected from Rh-positive donors. Because of the immunogenicity of the D-antigen, even a few milliliters of red cells can lead to alloimmunization in Rh-negative recipients, yet the overall rate of alloimmunization is quite low.[46] There is evidence to suggest that, in part due to immunosuppression, both adult and pediatric patients with hematologic malignancies are unlikely to form anti-D responses to Rh-incompatible platelet transfusions.[47,48] Thus, the provision of Rh-incompatible platelet products is unlikely to cause D alloimmunization in oncology populations. This risk may be further reduced through the use of apheresis platelets, as these units have been shown to have fewer residual red cells.[46] Nonetheless, it is still advisable to prevent Rh alloimmunization in children and females of childbearing potential because of the consequences of anti-D development in these populations. Alloimmunization can be prevented with a dose of $50\,\mu g$ to $300\,\mu g$ of Rh immunoglobulin (RhIg) provided within 72 hours of D antigen exposure.[49] Care must be used to ensure that the intramuscular-only formulation of RhIg is never given intravenously.

Selection of platelet products

Historically, the majority of platelet products were derived from whole blood by centrifugation. These individual units were then pooled into groups of four to five to yield a product intended to raise platelet counts by approximately $50,000/\mu L$.[50] With advances in apheresis technology in the 1970s, an increasing number of platelet units were obtained from single donors that provided a platelet dose equivalent to the pooled product.[50,51] The decision to use platelet pools versus platelets from individual donors relates to concerns about exposure to multiple donors, risk of alloimmunization, risk of adverse reactions, and platelet quality rather than increases in baseline platelet count as both products have similar viability and recovery.[52] The risk for many of these issues are not specific to oncology and are discussed in greater detail in Chapters 18 and 20.

One particular concern for oncology patients is a possible increase in risk for platelet alloimmunization due to the large number of transfusions administered to these patients. This was a significant concern prior to the era of leukocyte reduction, especially for pooled platelet products. However, several studies, including the Trial to Reduce Alloimmunization to Platelets (TRAP), have demonstrated that the risk of alloimmunization is identical between leukoreduced pooled platelets and apheresis units.[17] Once a patient has become alloimmunized, the use of platelet pools may be advantageous until crossmatch-compatible or HLA-matched units are available. In this scenario, an alloimmunized patient may be more likely to respond by chance to one of the four or five donors whose units constitute a platelet pool. Therefore, in alloimmunized patients, apheresis platelets should be used only if the unit is crossmatch-compatible or HLA-matched.[50]

Platelet refractoriness and alloimmunization

Chronically transfused oncology patients often experience lower than expected platelet increments after transfusion, which is known as platelet refractoriness. This can be due to either immune or nonimmune causes. Platelet alloimmunization and refractoriness are discussed in detail in Chapter 18. In oncology patients, over 70% of cases of platelet refractoriness are due to nonimmunologic factors.[50] Unfortunately, few clinical management options exist for patients with nonimmunologic platelet refractoriness. When possible, correcting the underlying cause (e.g., splenectomy for hypersplenism, removal of offending medications) can alleviate refractoriness. For the acutely bleeding patient or for hemorrhage prophylaxis, strategies of continuous platelet infusion (*platelet drip*) have been attempted with moderate success.[53] The *platelet drip*, wherein a dose of platelet concentrate is infused slowly over a four-hour period, is intended to provide an ongoing source of platelets to maintain vascular integrity, while addressing the practical concern of blood bank platelet inventory management.

Although they constitute a minority of cases, the underlying cause of refractoriness in the remaining 20–30% of oncology patients is likely due to an antibody to a platelet antigen. Platelets express class I HLA and numerous other platelet-specific antigens. Human leukocyte antigens are the most common mediator of immunologic platelet refractoriness, although studies have shown that alloantibodies can develop to any platelet antigen.[50,54] The treatment strategy for immune-mediated refractoriness is to provide antigen-negative components. Although often not a cause of true refractoriness, the first approach is to provide ABO-compatible units, which may lead to a more sustained increase in platelet count. The next option is to provide crossmatch-compatible platelets from the hospital blood bank or donor center. This involves crossmatching the patient's serum with a variety of donor platelets and selecting units that do not cause agglutination.[55] Crossmatch-compatible platelets have been proven to be as effective as HLA-matched platelets in raising platelet counts in alloimmunized patients.[50,54,55] Thus, the decision to provide HLA-matched platelets should depend upon factors such as quality of the HLA match, severity of alloimmunization, and availability of crossmatched products. If a majority of tested donors are incompatible and HLA-matched products are needed, the recipient can be HLA typed to provide antigen-matched products.[50,54] Polymorphisms of HLA class I antigens can complicate compatibility testing and make the process of finding fully matched donors difficult.

Unfortunately, once alloimmunization has occurred, immune modulation with corticosteroids, plasmapheresis, and intravenous immunoglobulin (IVIG) is of little benefit.[56] Therefore, the overall best strategy to reduce immune-mediated platelet refractoriness is prevention of HLA and platelet antigen exposure. Leukocyte reduction has helped reduce the incidence of alloimmune platelet refractoriness by limiting exposure to HLA.[17] Conservative transfusion strategies have also helped prevent exposure to HLA and platelet-specific antigens, and may play a role in reducing the frequency of alloimmunization.

Component modification: irradiation, leukocyte reduction, and volume reduction

As is the case with RBC units, platelets can be modified to maximize safety for oncology patients. Despite leukocyte reduction, platelet units contain small amounts of white cells. Thus, patients at risk for TA-GVHD should receive irradiated platelets.[20] As mentioned previously, leukocyte reduction of platelet products helps reduce the rate of alloimmunization.[17] According to the 2011 National Blood Collection and Utilization Survey, approximately 70% of all whole blood–derived platelet units were reported as leukocyte reduced.[19] In addition, nearly all apheresis platelets are leukocyte reduced as part of the collection process.

Volume reduction of platelet products via centrifugation and resuspension in saline should be considered for oncology patients who have experienced severe allergic or anaphylactic reactions to platelet products.[57] Volume reduction is also efficient at removing the plasma fraction of platelet products to reduce the risk of hemolysis associated with ABO-incompatible transfusion as well as the risk of volume overload.[57]

Alternatives to platelet transfusion

For patients unwilling to undergo platelet transfusion, or for severe platelet refractoriness, several medical therapies may be beneficial during bleeding episodes. A commonly prescribed drug, 1-deamino-8-D-arginine vasopressin (DDAVP or desmopressin), acts to stimulate the release of von Willebrand factor from endothelial cells, which can enhance platelet activity even at very low platelet counts.[58] DDAVP is also of proven benefit for platelet dysfunction and bleeding associated with uremia.[59] Antifibrinolytic therapies have also been employed as an adjunct to platelet transfusions for the bleeding patient. Medications such as aminocaproic acid, tranexamic acid, and aprotinin have all been successfully used to reduce hemorrhage and allogeneic transfusion requirements in the bleeding patient.[60,61]

Chemical and cytokine-based stimulation of the marrow to endogenously increase platelet production has also been attempted. Agents such as thrombopoietin (TPO) and megakaryocyte growth factors have been synthesized, but clinical trials with some of these drugs led to the development of neutralizing antibodies and thrombocytopenia in some recipients.[62,63] TPO and TPO-like growth factors are now used for some conditions such as immune thrombocytopenic purpura (ITP), and studies in oncology populations have been promising.[64] Several agents, such as romiplostim and eltrombopag, have been licensed by the US Food and Drug Administration. Interleukin-11 (IL11), a cytokine that drives megakaryocyte production and division, has also been approved for use in thrombocytopenia.[62,63]

Plasma and plasma-derived product transfusion

Indications for plasma transfusion and product selection

The indications for transfusion of plasma and plasma-derived products, such as cryoprecipitated antihemophilic factor (AHF), is similar between oncology and other patient populations. For the majority of oncology patients, no additional consideration is given to the selection of ABO group for plasma or cryoprecipitate so long as the unit is ABO compatible with the recipient. Donor and recipient Rh types are not a consideration for infusion of plasma or cryoprecipitate. As mentioned in this chapter, for patients who have undergone allogeneic HSCT, the choice of ABO group can be complex and should be based upon consideration of major and minor mismatches. Table 50.2 summarizes guidelines for plasma transfusion therapy in the peritransplant period. The guidelines for cryoprecipitated AHF are identical to those for plasma. Because these products are acellular, there is no need for gamma irradiation, even in transplant and immunosuppressed oncology patients.

Alternatives to plasma transfusion

For some oncology patients, plasma transfusion may be contraindicated, may be ineffective, or may not provide rapid enough reversal of coagulopathic states. For these conditions, there are several alternatives to plasma products, consisting of concentrated or recombinant coagulation factors. Among the most commonly used agents for acute moderate to severe bleeding is recombinant activated factor VII, a potent activator of the coagulation cascade.[65] Successful use of factor VIIa has been reported to help control massive bleeding in a variety of oncology patients.[66–68] There is also a role for use of factor VIIa as a bypass agent for those oncology patients who acquire inhibitors to circulating coagulation factors, mainly factor VIII.[69] However, factor VIIa failures in bleeding oncology patients have been reported for gastrointestinal bleeding and alveolar hemorrhage.[70,71]

The instances of factor VIIa usage cited above highlight the difficulty of recommending broad application of this therapy to the bleeding oncology patient. The most significant problem with making an evidence-based recommendation is that the vast majority of uses of factor VIIa in the literature are in the form of case reports. Few adequate clinical trials have been conducted to determine the safety and efficacy of this drug in oncology populations. Furthermore, appropriate dosing regimens are imprecise and mostly based on data gathered in trials performed in other critically ill patient populations. Factor VIIa also carries a number of risks, chief of which is the possibility for development of severe or even fatal arterial and venous thromboembolism.[72] Thus, Factor VIIa may be considered as an alternative to plasma infusion, but should be used only after other interventions have failed.

Intravenous immunoglobulin

IVIG is used to provide passive immunity in highly immunosuppressed individuals and has also been used as an immunomodulatory therapy for patients with conditions such as immune thrombocytopenic purpura (ITP).[73,74] For recipients of HPC products, IVIG has been associated with improved immune defense against pathogens such as CMV and has helped to decrease the complications of acute GVHD.[75,76] The benefit of IVIG administration for chronic GVHD and infection prophylaxis in marrow transplantation is not clear and warrants further study.[76]

IVIG infusion is usually tolerated without significant adverse events in oncology patients. The common side effects include myalgia, headache, fever, and fatigue.[77] A rare but serious complication of IVIG administration is acute renal failure seen with particular formulations that use sucrose as a globulin stabilizer.[77] Thus, oncology patients with chronic renal insufficiency should be closely monitored during IVIG administration. Current IVIG products have not transmitted hepatitis B, hepatitis C, or human immunodeficiency virus, but there are rare case reports of transmission of parvovirus B19, a serious pathogen for oncology patients.[78] Plasma is now screened for this virus before being pooled for fractionation.

Granulocyte transfusion

Indications

Historically, granulocyte infusions have been used in oncology patients with severe neutropenia to treat life-threatening, antibiotic refractory infections. The decision to initiate granulocyte transfusion usually represents failure of other forms of therapy. Only patients with a reasonable chance at sustainable marrow recovery after resolution of the underlying infection are candidates for granulocyte products.[79] It has been shown that humans should produce approximately $2–3 \times 10^{11}$ polymorphonuclear cells daily to clear significant bacterial or fungal infections. For oncology patients

whose marrow cannot support this level of production, doses of 1×10^{11} granulocytes per square meter of body area can be used to support the immunologic response.[80]

Granulocyte donation and donor preparation

A number of trials have been performed to evaluate the safety and efficacy of granulocyte transfusion using G-CSF stimulation in healthy donors. Several studies have suggested that granulocyte infusions from these donors are modestly effective for the treatment of bacterial and fungal infections.[81] However, it has been hypothesized that improved outcomes may be seen with higher granulocyte doses. To obtain a larger number of granulocytes, the recently completed Safety and Effectiveness of Granulocyte Transfusion in Resolving Infection in People with Neutropenia (RING) study used G-CSF and dexamethasone to stimulate donors. Although this multicenter trial found that there was no difference in success rates between antibiotic and granulocyte therapies, only a small number of patients were enrolled.[82]

Healthy donors who qualify for granulocyte transfusion should be ABO-compatible with the intended recipient, and products must be crossmatched before infusion as granulocyte products may contain 6–12% red cells. A popular granulocyte mobilization regimen used in donors consists of the administration of 5 to 10 μg/kg G-CSF subcutaneously administered approximately 12 hours before leukapheresis.[83] Historically, dexamethasone was also administered for granulocyte mobilization, but it is no longer routinely given. Granulocyte collections can be performed serially over 4–5 days to yield multiple doses for neutropenic patients. The side effects of granulocyte donation are usually mild and include bone pain, headache, fatigue, and fluid retention caused by G-CSF administration and apheresis.[79,84,83]

Alloimmunization

Alloimmunization is of significant concern given the large number of white cells, red cells, and platelets contained within a granulocyte product.[85] In addition, patients previously alloimmunized to HLA often demonstrate a reduced response to granulocyte infusion.[86] Thus, the expectation for successful response to granulocyte therapy should be tempered in an individual who has previously demonstrated HLA alloimmunization. If granulocyte transfusion is necessary for these patients, antigen matching for HLA may be required for an appropriate response to granulocyte transfusion.

Granulocyte storage, component modification, and infusion

Granulocytes must be stored at 20 to 24 °C without agitation for a maximum of 24 hours from the time of collection.[87] Because of the limited lifespan of neutrophils, it is preferred that granulocyte products be transfused within 6 to 8 hours of collection. Before issuance, the granulocyte products should be irradiated to prevent recipient TA-GVHD. Granulocytes should be infused through a 150–260-μm filter, but leukocyte reduction filters must never be used.[88]

Adverse reactions to blood transfusion

Oncology patients undergoing transfusion therapy are subject to the same set of adverse reactions as any patient receiving blood components. However, oncology patients are at increased risk for many types of adverse reactions. In addition, discerning between an adverse transfusion event and exacerbation of an underlying condition can be difficult.

Because they are often immunosuppressed, oncology patients are at increased risk for TA-GVHD (discussed in Chapter 60) and many transfusion-transmitted infections. In particular, CMV is one of the most problematic transfusion-transmitted infections for oncology patients. The virus is highly prevalent with a seroprevalance of 50–70% and has been found in the mononuclear cells of both seropositive and seronegative blood donors.[89,90] Although CMV infections are rarely significant in immunocompetent hosts, infection can lead to severe pathology in immunosuppressed patients. These latter patients can develop CMV-related pneumonia, gastrointestinal inflammation, and delayed HSCT engraftment. Although CMV-seronegative blood can be obtained, availability is often limited due to the high seroprevalence in the general population. In addition, as noted above, even seronegative individuals can harbor infectious viral particles. Because CMV is present within mononuclear cells, the use of leukocyte reduction to prevent CMV transmission has also been employed. Several studies have found that leukocyte reduction is as effective as the use of seronegative units, but it does not completely eliminate the risk of CMV transmission.[91,92] Thus, while the use of donor screening and leukocyte reduction is beneficial, oncology patients are still at some degree of risk for CMV exposure from blood transfusion.

Adverse effects of hematopoietic progenitor cell infusion

The majority of adverse events associated with HPC infusion are associated with the dimethyl sulfoxide (DMSO) content of the progenitor product. DMSO is a chemical modifier used in a majority of cryopreservatives that allows for the controlled freezing and thawing of mononuclear cells without development of membrane lysis.[93] However, *in vivo*, DMSO is a toxic substance and has been linked to fever, nausea, vomiting, and chills during and immediately after HPC infusion. DMSO has also been linked to pulmonary and cardiovascular problems during HPC infusion, including dyspnea, hypotension, bradycardia, and arrhythmia.[93,94] Due to the amount of DMSO infused, small children and those patients receiving multiple HPC units are more susceptible to DMSO-related problems.[93] If the total infusion volume exceeds 10 mL/kg of recipient body weight, infusions are usually divided to reduce the risk of adverse reactions.

Researchers have also begun to evaluate whether HPC components other than DMSO can lead to infusion toxicity. Several recent studies have correlated adverse events to the numbers of granulocytes present in HPC products.[95,96] These studies found that even after DMSO depletion, over half of patients undergoing HPC infusion experienced an adverse event such as fever, rigors, or dyspnea. It is therefore possible that the dyspnea associated with HPC infusion is not entirely caused by DMSO, but that granulocytes may contribute through transfusion-related acute lung injury (TRALI)-like mechanisms. These studies argue that a reduction in granulocyte content of the final HPC product would lead to fewer reactions. However, this is technologically challenging to achieve as removal of granulocytes would also remove the HPCs.

Bacterial contamination of HPC products can occur during collection or processing of the cells.[97] Adequate field sterilization practices during stem collection and the processing of HPC products in sterile areas with air-controlled biosafety cabinets can reduce the risk of bacterial contamination.[98] However, due to the significant handling of HPC products, contamination can be a frequent issue, particularly for marrow specimens.[99] Because of this risk, units are routinely cultured and, if bacterially contaminated, provided to patients in conjunction with prophylactic, broad-spectrum antibiotics. Interestingly, one study has demonstrated that, of 33 patients who received bacterially contaminated HPCs, only six developed evidence of bacteremia and none had any long-term complications.[100] Thus, bacterial contamination of an HPC product need not be an absolute barrier to infusion.

Summary

Transfusion support is a major therapy for many patients with hematologic and oncologic disorders. However, given their frequent exposure and often immunosuppressed state, they are often at more risk for adverse events due to transfusion. Compared to other patient populations, oncology patients are at increased risk for TA-GVHD, certain transfusion-transmitted diseases, alloimmunization to cellular antigens, and immunomodulation. In addition, HPC transplant patients present unique challenges to transfusion services, as they require specific assessment for potential ABO incompatibility. Careful selection of blood components and component modification is therefore necessary to provide appropriate therapy to these patients. Significant advances have been made in transfusion therapy, including more sensitive donor testing and blood component alternatives, which will continue to improve the safety of transfusion for oncology patients.

Acknowledgments

The authors acknowledge the outstanding work of Christopher Tormey, MD, and the late Margot S. Kruskall, MD, whose text for the third and fourth editions of *Rossi's Principles of Transfusion Medicine* formed the template for this chapter in the fifth edition.

Key References

A full reference list for this chapter is available at: http://www.wiley.com/go/simon/transfusion

1 Corwin HL. Anemia and red blood cell transfusion in the critically ill. *Semin Dial* 2006; **19**: 513–16.

4 Stussi G, Halter J, Schanz U, Seebach JD. ABO-histo blood group incompatibility in hematopoietic stem cell and solid organ transplantation. *Transfus Apher Sci* 2006; **35**: 59–69.

12 Lapierre V, Kuentz M, Tiberghien P. Allogeneic peripheral blood hematopoietic stem cell transplantation: guidelines for red blood cell immuno-hematological assessment and transfusion practice. *Bone Marrow Transplant* 2000; **25**: 507–12.

19 Department of Health and Human Services. The 2011 National Blood Collection and Utilization Survey Report. Washington, DC: DHHS, 2012.

20 Higgins MJ, Blackall DP. Transfusion-associated graft-versus-host disease: a serious residual risk of blood transfusion. *Curr Hematol Rep* 2005; **4**: 470–6.

34 Consensus conference. Platelet transfusion therapy. *JAMA* 1987; **257**: 1777–80. PMID: 3820494. http://jama.jamanetwork.com/article.aspx?articleid=365357

42 Cooling L. ABO and platelet transfusion therapy. *Immunohematology* 2007; **23**: 20–33.

51 Burgstaler EA. Blood component collection by apheresis. *J Clin Apher* 2006; **21**: 142–51.

53 Slichter SJ. Platelet transfusion therapy. *Hematol Oncol Clin North Am* 2007; **21**: 697–729.

54 Rebulla P. A mini-review on platelet refractoriness. *Haematologica* 2005; **90**: 247–53.

73 Sandler SG, Tutuncuoglu SO. Immune thrombocytopenic purpura—current management practices. *Expert Opin Pharmacother* 2004; **5**: 2515–27.

SECTION V

Hazards of transfusion

CHAPTER 51

Transfusion-transmitted virus infections (TTVIs)

Erhard Seifried & Michael Schmidt

Institute of Transfusion Medicine and Immunohematology, German Red Cross, Frankfurt/M, Germany

Introduction

Ever since the advent of the global human immunodeficiency virus (HIV) epidemic, transfusion medicine has maintained a heightened awareness of the potential risk of transmitting infection through blood transfusions. This has paradoxically increased despite the actual infectious risks of blood transfusion being lower than ever in developed countries. The enhanced level of safety has resulted from a series of stepwise interventions and policies in blood services throughout the world. Microbial risks were once mainly related to persistent infections such as HIV, hepatitis B virus (HBV), and hepatitis C virus (HCV), where viral carriage and latency were the key factors predisposing an agent to transmission by transfusion. More recently, several acute infections have posed a threat to blood safety when they have occurred at high incidence in certain populations. West Nile virus (WNV) in North America is a good example of this, but other infections such as Chikungunya virus and the specter of respiratory viruses such as pandemic influenza have made transfusion microbiologists widen their areas of vigilance. These issues are reflected in this chapter.

Hepatitis virus infections (A, B, C, D, and E)

Hepatitis A virus infections

Hepatitis A (formerly known as infectious hepatitis) is an acute infectious disease of the liver caused by the hepatitis A virus (HAV).[1] Many cases have little or no symptoms, especially in youth. The time between infection and symptom development is between two to six weeks.[2] Clinical symptoms are nausea, vomiting, diarrhea, jaundice, fever, and abdominal pain.[3,4] Acute liver failure occurs rarely, mostly in elderly people. It is usually spread by contaminated food or drinking water with infected feces. It can also be spread through close contact with or blood products from an infectious person. Children are often asymptomatic and can infect others.[5,6] After an infection, people develop an immune response for the rest of their lives. The diagnosis requires blood tests for antibodies or nucleic acid amplification (NAT).[7–10] Vaccinations are effective prevention.[11,12] Other preventive measures include handwashing and cooking food properly. A specific antiviral treatment is currently not possible. Patients are treated for nausea or

diarrhea. The human body is usually able to eradicate the virus without severe liver disease. The treatment of acute liver failure is a liver transplantation.

Worldwide, approximately 1.5 million symptomatic cases occur each year with probably millions of asymptomatic infections. HAV infections are more common in regions of the world with poor sanitary conditions and limited resources of clean water. In developing countries, about 90% of children have already been infected at age 10.[13]

The risk of symptomatic infections is directly related to age, with more than 80% of adults with symptoms of acute viral hepatitis.

After ingestion, HAV will be transported into the bloodstream through the epithelium of the oropharynx or intestines. The blood carries the virus to its target, the liver, where it multiplies within hepatocytes and Kupffer cells (liver macrophages). Virions are excreted into the bile and bloodstream. HAV is secreted in large amounts from about 11 days before the onset of symptoms or appearance of anti-HAV IgM antibodies in the blood (Figure 51.1). Therefore, donors could be asymptomatic but still viremic. The incubation period is 15–50 days and mortality of less than 0.5%.[14,15] Within the liver hepatocytes, the RNA genome is released from the protein coat and converted by its own ribosome in the cell.

The HAV is a non-enveloped picornavirus and contains a single-stranded RNA in a protein shell packed. There is only one serotype of the virus, but multiple genotypes exist.

A serotype and seven different genetic groups (four human and three monkeys) have been described. The human genotypes are numbered I–III. Six subspecies have been described (IA, IB, IIA, IIB, IIIA, and IIIB). The monkeys' genotypes were numbered IV–VI.[16] A single isolate of genotype VII isolated in man was also described. Genotype III has been isolated from human and monkey.[17] Most human isolates are from genotype I.

The virus spreads by the fecal-oral route and infections often occur in areas poor hygiene and overcrowding.[18] HAV can also pass through the parenteral route through blood and blood products. About 40% of all acute viral hepatitis is caused by HAV. It is resistant to detergent, acid (pH 1), solvents (such as ether and chloroform), drying and temperatures up to 60 °C. It can survive for months in fresh and salt water.

In developed countries, on the other hand, the infection primarily strikes susceptible young adults, most of whom get it when traveling

Rossi's Principles of Transfusion Medicine, Fifth Edition. Edited by Toby L. Simon, Jeffrey McCullough, Edward L. Snyder, Bjarte G. Solheim, and Ronald G. Strauss.

© 2016 John Wiley & Sons, Ltd. Published 2016 by John Wiley & Sons, Ltd.

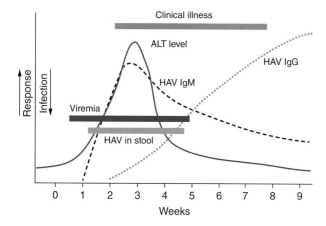

Figure 51.1 Scheme of HAV infections and immune response.

to countries with a high incidence of the disease or by contact with infectious people.

During the acute phase of infection, the liver enzyme alanine transferase (ALT) is in the blood at concentrations much higher than normal. The enzyme is derived from the liver cells destroyed by the virus.

There is no specific treatment for hepatitis A. Patients are advised to rest, avoid fatty foods and alcohol, eat a balanced diet, and stay hydrated.

In the United States in 1991, there was a low mortality rate for hepatitis A of four deaths per 1000 cases for the general population, but a higher rate of 17.5 per 1000 in those aged 50 years and older. The risk of death from acute liver failure by HAV infection increases with age and underlying chronic liver disease.[19]

Keynotes: hepatitis A virus

Virus	Region	Transmission	Screening	Inactivation	Vaccination
Picornaviridae, RNA, 7 genotypes	South America, Africa, Asia	Fecal-oral, blood components	NAT, antibody screening	Reduced efficiency	Yes

Hepatitis B virus infections

The hepatitis B virus (HBV) has a complex coiled genomic structure.[20,21] An envelope embeds the core of the virus. The virus belongs to the virus family Hepadnaviridae. Based on the replication cycles the DNA virus is close to the retroviridae. Therefore they are named DNA retroviruses. The surface antigen of HBV was first described in 1963 by B.S. Blumberg as a new serum protein in Australian Aboriginals.[22–24] He named the new antigen the Australia antigen. In 1968 a correlation was made between the Australia antigen and the transmission of hepatitis B. Therefore the antigen was renamed HBsAg for *hepatitis B surface antigen*. HBsAg is embedded by lipid envelopes and approximately 25 μm round or filamentous subviral particles can be present in huge numbers of up to 10^{13} particles/ml or 10^6 ng/ml in serum. The complete HBV particle diameter is from 45 to 52 μm. Inside the HBsAg envelope the hepatitis B core antigen (HBcAg) is located.[25,26] Inside of that is the HBV genome, with a length of 3200 base pairs. The HBV genome is a complex virus particle with round structure and characteristic properties (Figure 51.2).

Characteristics of DNA molecules of hepatitis B genomes

Open circular open-coiled structure with overlapping ends of the double-strand DNA (dsDNA) genome

- Single-string gap, place for the endogenous DNA-polymerase
- Covalent lineage of the virus protein coding DNA minus strand
- (5′-position) with the virus DNA–polymerase
- Lineages of the DNA plus strand with a RNA primer

HBV infection pathomechanism

The virus infects liver cells by the bloodstream.[27,28] Via currently unknown receptors, the virus genome is transported into the liver cells. Cellular repair enzymes build a covalently closed circular DNA (ccc-DNA) that activates the cellular gene expression, producing messenger RNA (mRNA). The mRNA represents the complete genome and works as a matrix for the core protein and the viral DNA-polymerase. Those proteins assemble together to the core particle and embed the mRNA (self-assembly).[29,30] In the next step, the viral DNA-polymerase transcribes the core particles of the RNA into DNA. The RNA is cleaved after producing the viral DNA plus strand. The residual 18 5′ terminal bases of the RNA pre-genome represent the primer for the plus strand. In parallel to the genome maturation, subgenomic mRNA molecules are expressed. They are named as 3-DO-carboxy-terminal HBs proteins, S (small), M (middle), and L (large), with preS1, preS2, and S protein structures.[31] The HBs proteins are released into the endoplasmic reticulum. Within the endoplasmic reticulum, the HBs particle embeds the circlet core particle and builds the final HB-virus. The HBsAg as well as the HB virus are released via Golgi apparatus into the bloodstream.

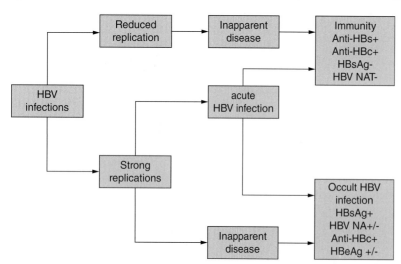

Figure 51.2 Different HBV forms.

In addition, HBV is coding for two nonstructure proteins, named HBeAg and HBx.[32-34] HBeAg is a nonessential form of HBcAg and has an immune modulating function. HBx has several effects on viral and cellular gene expression. Based on this transcription-regulating mechanism, including a reversed transcription enzyme, HBV is at risk of new genomic variants based on mutation of viral enzymes. The reason is caused by the missing proofreading function of the reversed transcriptase enzymes. Nevertheless, due to a longtime adaptation between the host and virus without selection pressure, HBV viruses are characterized by eight stable wild-type viruses. Currently, their genotypes are known as HBV genotype A to H. The most predominant genotypes in Asia are B and C, whereas the most predominant genotypes in Europe are A and D.[35] With an immune selection pressure, HBeAg negative mutants named *escape mutants*, with mutation within the HBs proteins can develop.[36-38]

HBV pathogenesis between virus and host

HBVs are strictly species specific and hepato-autotrophic.[39] Other cells like leukocytes are rarely infected. The reason for the species specificity is currently unknown. HBV and all genome products are usually under nonpathogenic conditions; therefore, HBV-infected persons produce virus copies in a high concentration without showing clinical symptoms or damage of liver cells. HBV is not directly cytopathic and liver cells are usually a privileged region of the human body, where immune cells can be unable to attack the infection for months or years or indefinitely. Newborns, children, or immunodeficient patients usually cannot produce efficient immune reactions. Therefore, an asymptomatic infection with a high viral concentration can persist.[40] Chronic HBV infections are defined with the detection of HBsAg or HBV-DNA over a period of six months.[41,42] About 10% of all HBV infections become chronic. Seroconversion from HBeAg to anti-HBe antibodies reduces HBV replication and concentration. Nevertheless, patients with anti-HBe antibodies and HBsAg have sometimes still had a high viral concentration were observed. Patients with a chronic HBV infection are at high risk for liver cirrhosis and liver cancer, approximately 10% for each.[43-46]

After an HBV infection, a liver disease of three different unapparent conditions can be possible:

1 immunotolerance and high infectivity;
2 partial immune control with HBsAg positivity and low-level infectivity; and
3 natural acquired immunity.

The humoral and cellular immune response can depress virus replication in most cases, but the ccc-DNA form of HBV is rarely completely eliminated in the hepatocytes. Therefore, patients infected with HBV can re-amplify the virus, especially when their immune situation is changed, such as after immunosuppression. Stopping immunosuppression puts patients at high risk of a severe immune reaction including a fulminant hepatitis B reaction. Liver cell carcinoma develops most frequently in HBV-infected middle-aged patients from Asia and Africa after longtime virus persistence. The probability of liver cell cancer is increased with exposition of aflatoxin or by a coinfection with hepatitis C virus.[47-52]

HBV transmissions

Infected patients contain HBV virus in blood, saliva, semen, breast milk, vaginal, and sore secretions, which all can cause infection by percutaneous or transmucosal route. In high epidemic regions transmissions from mother to child are important, especially because most child infections have no clinical symptoms.[53-56] The vertical infection from mother to child accrued usually in utero, at the end of pregnancy, or during nativity. Transmissions by heterosexual or homosexual contact are reported. Contaminated, inefficiently sterilized medical devices like endoscopes are possible infection sources, as are personal devises such as toothbrushes, razors, and so on. Also, thorns and branches accidentally contaminated with blood have transmitted HBV during sport activities such as orienteering races.

To prevent transfusion of infections by blood components,[57-60] all blood components are screened in most countries for HBsAg and approximately 30–40% of all blood donations in developed countries are in addition screened by HBV nucleic amplification technique (NAT).[10,61,62] In countries with low epidemic prevalence, anti-HBc screening is often also implemented for the detection of chronic infected HBV donors (occult hepatitis infections [OBI]).[36,63,64]

Approximately 50% of the world population has been exposed to HBV. World Health Organization (WHO) estimates that approximately 350 million HBsAg-positive people exist. Major epidemic regions are Africa north of the Sahara, Southeast Asia, and major regions of Russia. Middle risk accrued in Southeast Europe, South America, India, North America, Australia and Northern, Central, and Western Europe. The prevalence of HBV infection is age-dependent, approximately 15% of the world population older than 60 is affected.[65] Although exact data regarding the prevalence of HBV exist, data regarding Hepatitis B incidents are still limited or missing. Most patients die due to long-term clinical diseases of liver cirrhosis and liver failure.[66,67]

The clinical symptoms of HBV infection depend on the immunopathogenesis and demonstrate a broad range:

1 Light liver damage only detectable by a small increase of transaminases and spontaneous healing. Chronic hepatitis decompensated liver cirrhosis and hepatitis cellular carcinoma are possible if virus replication continue;
2 Liver disease with extrahepatic manifestation like arthritis, exanthema, glomeruli nephritis, and polyarteritis nodosa caused by immune complex with high concentration of HBV;
3 Acute hepatitis with high levels of liver enzyme (ALT values much increased); and
4 Fulminant hepatitis with complications of liver cirrhosis and liver carcinoma (less than 1%).

Most cases achieve immunity against HBV within three to six months, but virus replication can continue at a low level over many years. Only highly sensitive NAT assays could detect these low-level carriers (NAT sensitivity should be less than 10 IU/ml). A chronic HBV infection with only mild symptoms should also be treated, to prevent severe clinical complication like liver cirrhosis and carcinoma, which can develop after more than 10 years, or to protect others from HBV infections.

Diagnostic opportunities

Important for HBV diagnostics are HBV antigens (HBsAg, HBeAg), HBV antibodies (Anti-HBc, Anti-HBs, and Anti-HBe) in patient serum and plasma,[64] and HBV detection by NAT,[59,61,68-70] as shown in Figure 51.3.

Finally, histopathological investigations can amend diagnostics of serum/plasma. There is no correlation between the detection of virus parameters (antigens or antibodies) and inflammation activity. Antibodies against HBV, especially anti-HBc, can be detected lifelong in most cases.[25,26,71] The antibody titer against HBsAg (anti-HBs) represents one's immunity status. Vaccinated people

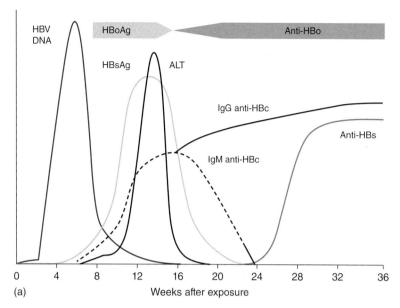

(a)

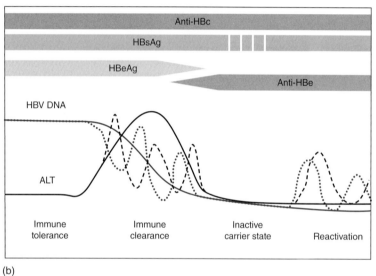

(b)

Figure 51.3 Clinical, serologic, and virologic course of acute and chronic HBV infection. (A) Schematic profile of serologic and virologic markers of a typical acute resolving hepatitis with the average timing of detection of serum HBV DNA, HBsAg, and HBeAg and their corresponding antibodies, with respect to the ALT elevation reflecting immune-mediated liver cell destruction after HBV replication (as reflected by serum HBV DNA levels) has been mostly controlled by noncytolytic mechanisms. (B) Course of chronic hepatitis B after perinatal or early-childhood-acquired infection. The four distinct phases shown are: immune tolerance (high-level HBV replication with normal ALT levels), immune clearance (high ALT level, lower HBV DNA levels and frequent hepatitis flares, depicted with dashed lines for both HBV DNA and ALT, which may lead to loss of HBsAg and anti-HBe seroconversion), inactive carrier state (normal ALT, presence of anti-HBe and low or even undetectable HBV DNA), and reactivation phase after many years of inactive carrier state (lower and fluctuating HBV DNA and ALT levels in the presence of anti-HBe), commonly associated with selection of core or precore HBV variant. (Reproduced from Figure 46.2 in Alter & Esteban-Mur, Chapter 46, Rossi's Principles of Transfusion Medicine, 4th Edition)

should have an anti-HBs titer higher than 100 U/L to have a sufficient response against HBV. Breakthrough infections were reported in the United States with people with a reduced anti-HBs titer of less than 100 U/L.[72,73] The most important parameter is the analysis of HBsAg in serum/plasma. Commercial enzyme immunoassays (EIA) for HBsAg are very sensitive (detection limit less than 0.1 ng/ml) and very specific (higher 99.9%). The diagnostic window for HBsAg is approximately 32–38 days.[70,73–75] HBsAg can be detected after vaccination for up to one week in the serum. False negative results due to escape mutants are rare. In some cases, HBsAg will be negative in the acute infection period. Therefore, detection of hepatitis B should be supplemented by anti-HBc IgM and HBV NAT.[61] Patients more than six months positive for HBsAg develop a chronic occult hepatitis B infection (OBI).[36] NAT can be positive or negative in OBI patients. The last decade saw improvement in NAT systems, which now have an analytical sensitivity of app. 2 IU/ml which represent a diagnostic window of approximately 20 days for HBV infection. Most NAT systems detect HBV, HCV and HIV-1 simultaneously in a multiplex assay.

Therefore, blood donor screening by NAT follows these three parameters, although in many countries, HBV NAT screening is voluntary. As shown by Roth et al.,[76] screening of more than 114 million blood donations for HBV by NAT, detected 1728 NAT only positive blood donors (negative for HbsAg, Anti-Hbc, anti-HBs and anti-Hbe). Highly sensitive HBV screening by NAT can prevent more infections than for hepatitis C or HIV-1. HBV concentration can increase, especially in immunosuppressed patients, up to 10^{10} genome equivalents per ml (geq/ml). In OBIs, the HBV-DNA concentration is reduced to low levels, 1 to 10 geq/ml, or under the detection limit of the NAT system. The doubling time of HBV in a mouse model is very long, approximately 2.56 days. Therefore, the diagnostic window is much longer compared to Hepatitis C (app. 11 h) or to HIV-1 (app. 18 h).[77]

HBV therapy

In principle, the eradication of HBV might be possible because the virus infects only the human population and a sufficient vaccine is available. If more than 95% of the human population can be vaccinated, the virus will not be able to survive in order to find nonvaccinated humans. Unfortunately, only monoclonal agents are used for vaccines. They induce an efficient immune protection against genotype A. Therefore, high anti-HBs titers are necessary to protect against other HBV genotypes.

At the end of the 1970s, interferon-α (IFNα) was detected as efficient against HBV. Treatment with IFNα reduced the viral load within a few days.[78] Unfortunately, it increased again after IFNα therapy was ended. Interferon has nasty flulike side effects, justifying a continuation of therapy when its antiviral effect is proven by follow-up of HBV DNA. A permanent cure can be assumed if an initially positive HBeAg and HBV NAT is negative six months after the end of therapy. Considerably more tolerable than interferon is the nucleoside analog lamivudine therapy known from the HIV therapy.[79,80] Lamivudine inhibits reverse transcriptase of HBV DNA, causing chain termination. Of special significance is lamivudine for prophylaxis of re-infections after liver transplantation and in case immunosuppression causes HBV reactivation. Nucleoside analogs effective against herpes viruses, such as famciclovir and ganciclovir, have only a small effect on HBV. If the treatment is not perfect or widely applied, the HBV infection can cause liver failure or hepatocellular carcinoma formation. In these cases, a liver transplant might be the only valid therapy, and even then, one must prevent a HBV re-infection of the transplanted organ.

within the transaminase peak of an acute infection which will be in a range of 50–70 days.

The antibodies are stable over 10–15 years after the hepatitis C infection. Screening by NAT and HCV antibodies can differentiate between an acute HCV infection (NAT positive, HCV AB negative) and a chronic HCV disease (NAT pos. and HCV AB positive). The quantitative HCV RNA determination is suitable for the control of the antiviral treatment.[88,89]

The efficiency of the HCV antiviral therapy depends on the HCV genotype.[90] Genotype knowledge is essential for recognition of epidemiological correlations and detection of HCV infection chains. The diagnostic window for HCV is long for antibody development: still about 55 days.[91,92] That window could be cut, however, by the introduction of NAT in the blood donor screening. Depending on different NAT methods, the current diagnostic window is between 6–8 days if the virus is in the replication process (ramp-up period). Roth et al. found in a worldwide donor screening of more than 300 million investigations[76] 680 HCV infected donors with only NAT positive screening.

Hemovigilance data from Germany showed clearly the efficiency of blood donor screening by NAT for HCV (Figure 51.5). Before 1999, approximately 6–8 transfusion-transmitted HCV infections were reported annually in Germany. In 1999, all blood donations began being screened by minipool NAT. Since then, only one additional HCV transmission has occurred, in 2005. The virus

Keynotes: hepatitis B virus

Virus	Region	Transmission	Screening	Inactivation	Vaccination
Hepadnaviridae, DNA, retrovirus, 8 genotypes (A–H)	Worldwide	Blood components, sexual activities, blood infected utensils	NAT, antigen (HBsAg, HbeAg), and AB (Anti-HBc, Anti-HBe, Anti-HBs)	Possible up to 6 log	Yes, titer should be >100 IU/l

Hepatitis C virus

The 1989 genetic methods were able to identify hepatitis C virus (HCV), which was shown to be responsible for most blood-borne cases of nonAnonB (NANB) hepatitis (Figure 51.4). HCV has a genome of approximately 9600 base pairs,[81,82] which is a single-strand RNA (ssRNA) with a plus strand polarity. From the viral RNA, a continuous open reading frame of 3010–3033 amino acids long poly-protein is synthesized. Resulting from a post-translational cellular signal peptidase and two viral proteases, 10 different structural or nonstructural proteins are produced. By sequencing of HCV genome, so far six different genotypes with numerous subtypes can be identified.[83] Due to taxonomic characteristics, the HCV genome belongs to the Flaviviridae family. Worldwide, approximately 170 million people are currently infected with HCV.[84–86] Epidemiological data indicate a high HCV prevalence in certain risk groups, such as hemophiliacs (60–90%) dialysis patients (30–40%), and intravenous drug users (>80%). Compared to HBV, the risk of HCV transmission through sexual or close family contact is considered low. In approximately 40% of all HCV infections, the transmission pathway cannot be detected. The diagnosis of HCV infection is essentially based on the detection of antibodies against the core protein and the nonstructural proteins NS3 to NS5.[87] However, the presence of antibodies does not provide information about whether a self-limiting or chronic HCV infection occurred. Also, the determination of IgM antibodies cannot differentiate between acute or chronic infection. HCV antibodies occur usually

concentration in the infective donor was only 10 IU/ml, and below the detection limit of the minipool screening method.[93]

Even a reduction from minipool to individual donation NAT might not have prevented this HCV transmission. Due to the high doubling time in the ramp-up phase of about 11 hours, diagnostic window for HCV differs only about one to two days between blood donor screening in minipools of 96 samples or testing on an individual NAT basis.

The long-disputed question of whether early treatment of acute HCV infections can prevent chronicity of the disease was solved in 2001 when Nakamuta et al. reported the kinetics of the HCV during interferon therapy.[94] They showed that high concentrations of interferon alpha could prevent a chronic disease.[95] The coupling of interferon with a branched-chain polyethylene glycol molecule (Peg-interferon) leads to a compound with prolonged action compared to unmodified interferon through a longer absorption, a slower clearance and a correspondingly higher half-life. Peg-interferon therefore only needs to be injected once a week to treat chronic HCV infections.[96–98] New Daclatasvir (Daklinza) is an inhibitor of the NS5A complex,[99–102] and may be used in combination with other drugs to treat infections of chronic hepatitis C. Another possible new drug is cyclophilin B.[103–106] This treatment inhibits virus protein and cell protein interactions. Immuno-suppressant agents like cyclosporine can also inhibit protein interactions. The group of Zeuzem et al. showed that a combination therapy that includes sofosbuvir over a period of 12 weeks leads to a healing rate of over 90%.[107] Thus, a healing of HCV infections can be the usual prognosis of HCV treatment.

Keynotes: hepatitis C virus

Virus	Region	Transmission	Screening	Inactivation	Vaccination
Flaviviridae, RNA, 6 genotypes, 30 subtypes, residual risk TTID: <1:1 million	Worldwide	IVD drug user, medical instruments, blood components, sexual activities	NAT, antigen (NS3, NS5), AB (Anti-HCV)	Possible up to 6 log	Not available

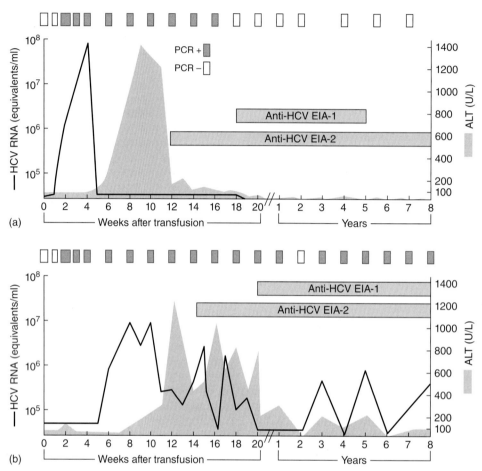

Figure 51.4 Biochemical, serologic, and molecular biologic profile of acute and chronic transfusion-associated hepatitis C virus (HCV) infection. Acute, resolving hepatitis C is shown in (A) and chronic hepatitis C in (B). Resolving disease cannot be differentiated from progressive disease by the time of onset of detectable HCV RNA by means of polymerase chain reaction (PCR), the magnitude of HCV RNA elevation as measured by means of branched DNA assay, the interval to the first elevation in the level of alanine aminotransferase (ALT), the magnitude of ALT elevation in the acute phase, or the interval between exposure and the first appearance of antibody. Progression to chronic disease cannot be predicted in the acute phase, and the only distinguishing features in these patterns are the persistence of ALT elevation and the persistence of HCV RNA in persons with chronic hepatitis C. The acute, resolving pattern (A) occurs in 10% to 15% of patients with transfusion-associated hepatitis C and the chronic pattern (B) in 85% to 90%. Note: (1) HCV RNA is detectable soon after exposure. Here, the PCR results was positive two weeks after exposure, but it can become positive even sooner. (2) HCV RNA may be detected by means of branched DNA assay coincident with PCR reactivity, but the reaction may be delayed, as shown here. (3) The major peak of viral replication (assessed with HCV RNA level) occurs before the first increase in ALT level and before any clinical or biochemical evidence of hepatitis; it is presumed that persons might be most infectious in this interval before the acute phase. (4) In acute resolving infection, HCV RNA levels increase rapidly before the decline in serum ALT level. (5) In chronic infection, HCV RNA level diminishes and can remain low, fluctuate, or become undetectable; HCV RNA levels sometimes show a periodicity that parallels the fluctuations in ALT level; in (B), the level of HCV RNA increases a short time before ALT level does and decreases before the decline in ALT. (6) Second-generation anti-HCV assays shorten the seronegative window in HCV infection much more than do first-generation assays; nonetheless, anti-HCV was not detectable for 12 to 15 weeks after exposure and for six to seven weeks after the first significant rise in ALT level. Antibody to HCV (detected with second-generation assays) almost always persists in chronic cases and generally persists in acute resolving cases. Antibodies detected with the first-generation assay (anti-C100, anti-5-1-1) generally disappear in resolving cases. (Reproduced from Figure 46.4 in Alter & Esteban-Mur, Chapter 46, Rossi's Principles of Transfusion Medicine, 4th Edition)

Hepatitis D virus infections

Hepatitis D virus was discovered by M. Rizetto 1975 in liver biopsies from patients with chronic hepatitis B infection.[108] By immunofluorescence analysis, he found a new antigen of HBV. At that time, only three were known: HBsAg, HBeAg, and HBcAg. The new antigen was named HBV-D antigen. Later, it was shown that the D-antigen referred to a new hepatitis virus, hepatitis D virus (HDV).[109,110] The D-antigen is embedded in HDV with proteins of HBV. HDV genome

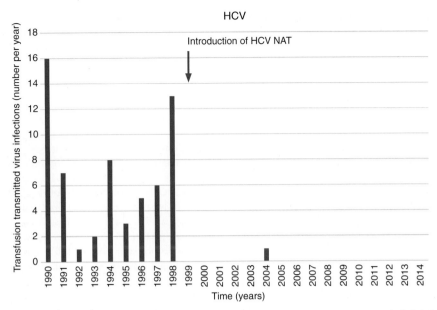

Figure 51.5 HCV transfusion transmitted infections in Germany. Source: Funk *et al.* Hemovigilance report 2011, Paul-Ehrlich-Institute, Germany, Frankfurt. Reproduced with permission.

contains a small (approximately 1700 bases long), covalently closed, circular, single-stranded RNA that is complementary to itself over a wide range and therefore looks like a partial double-stranded virus.[111–115] Such genomic structure had then been found only in viroids. In addition to this viroid-like behavior, HDV genome segment had a gene that encoded HDAg. HDV are approximately 38 nm large round particles with an HBsAg envelope. HDAg exists in a short form (SHDAg) with 195 amino acids and a longer form (LHDAg) with 214 amino acids. SHDAg is necessary for the regulation of the HDV genome replication, whereas LHDAg inhibits the replication process. LHDAg is required for the translation of the envelope of HDV ribonucleoprotein. The HDV ribozyme has become an important tool in molecular biology, because it can cut RNA molecules precisely. The helper virus HBV essentially determines the host and cell tropism of HDV. HDV can replicate intracellularly without HBV and spread from cell to cell, but cannot develop a complete infection.

Superinfections of HDV in chronic HBV carriers (HDV infection after HBV infection) often lead to persistent chronic HDV infection.[116–118] In co-infected patients (who have HBV and HDV at the same time) the HDV infection is often mild.[116,119–121] The pathogenicity of HDV is controversial because some studies show a high cytotoxicity of SHDAg, but SHDAg-producing cell cultures are viable. In patients with severe HDV/HBV infection, a microvesicular steatosis is found in liver tissue. Coinfection with HDV and HBV sometimes leads to a biphasic course. Often both viruses multiply in parallel. The HB viremia is reduced by HDV in general. However, the course of acute hepatitis is not necessarily more difficult than for HBV mono-infection. The persistence rate in HBV/HDV co-infections is not increased. HDV superinfection of HBsAg carriers is unfavorable. The HDV genotype is also important for the course of the infection. HDV seems to be dominant in this constellation to HBV. Patients with chronic HDV/HBV infection are three times more likely (60–70%) to develop liver cirrhosis and liver than cancer patients with HBV mono-infection. The overall mortality is about three times higher in superinfected HDV/HBV patients.

HDV virus concentration reaches high levels in the acute infection period: 10^{11} geq/ml (genomic equivalents/ml). In this period, patients are

very infectious. In the next phase the virus titer usually decreases to concentrations of 10^6 geq/ml. Prenatal infections are possible if HBV is transmitted. Typical transmission pathways are unsanitary injections (intravenous drug use) and contact with open wounds in tropical regions. Worldwide, approximately 350 million people have HBV, and approximately 15 million are co-infected or superinfected with HDV (relation is 1:23).[122–125] Epidemic areas are the Mediterranean, Southeast and Eastern Europe, Central and East Asia, and local areas in tropical South America and Africa. With intravenous drug users often co-infections by HDV with HCV and HIV are reported. In many countries, the incidence rate of HDV has decreased in the last 10 years. Since blood donations are tested for HBV infections in general, a special screening for HDV for blood products is not required because HDV infections are observed only in conjunction with HBV. The most sensitive and reliable detection of HDV is done by NAT.[126] No anti-viremic therapies for HDV yet exist. Its treatment with interferon and/or lamivudine has little effect on its chronicity.[127–130] For fulminant hepatitis D cases with terminal liver failure, a liver transplantation is the final therapeutic approach.[131–133] After transplantation, a graft re-infection with HBV is lower than with HBV mono-infections compared to HDV/HBV infections. When HBV re-infection is suppressed by lamivudine and/or hyperimmune globulin, the overall prognosis is favorable. Otherwise, re-infections of HDV are also possible.

Keynotes: hepatitis D virus

Virus	Region	Transmission	Screening	Inactivation	Vaccination
Deltasvirus, RNA	Worldwide	Blood components, sexual activities	NAT in development, antibody screening	Possible up to 6 log	Not available

Hepatitis E virus infections

In 1980, hepatitis E virus (HEV) infections were first reported in studies of oral-fecal transmitted hepatitis in India.[134] The experimental transmission in nonhuman primates and the virus visualization and characterization became possible in 1983. The early 1990s saw the HEV genome sequenced and serological and molecular screening tests developed.[135–139] HEV is an ssRNA with a diameter of 32–34 nm. It is a non-enveloped spherical particle with a genetic heterogeneity. The importance of these genetic variants of clinical courses is currently not clear. Type 1 genotype was found in Asia and North Africa, Type 2 was isolated in the United States, Type 3 was found in Europe, and Type 4 was detected in isolates from China and Taiwan. To date, the taxonomic classification of HEV is not entirely clear. Similarities exist to the caliciviruses.[140–142]

HEV is generally transmitted via the fecal-oral route, and mainly through contaminated drinking water. According to WHO the incubation period ranges from three to eight weeks, with a mean of 40 days. The period of communicability is unknown. HEV causes acute sporadic and epidemic hepatitis, which usually is self-limiting. Symptomatic infection is most common in adults between 15 and 40 years. It is frequent in children, but then mostly asymptomatic. In rare cases fulminant hepatitis with liver failure and death can occur. Severe clinical courses with mortality between 0.5% and 4% mainly occur during pregnancy.[143–146]

WHO estimates annually worldwide 20 million HEV inbfections, 3 million acute cases of HEV and 56,000 HEV-related deaths. Highest seroprevalence rates are observed in regions with low development index. WHO estimates indicate that over 60% of all HEV infections and 65% of all HEV related deaths occur in East and South Asia, where seroprevalence rates of 25% are common in some age groups; in Egypt, half of the population aged over five years is serologically positive for HEV. Investigations by Baylis *et al.* show high incidence rates in Japan, the United Kingdom, Germany, and Sweden, between 1:4500 and 1:8500.[147–149] HEV antibodies are usually developed in infected patients after 3–4 months (Figure 51.6). Because neutralizing antibodies' concentration can wane over time, re-infection with HEV might be possible.

In addition to the nutritional infection pathway, HEV transmission by blood products is clearly confirmed in several publications.[3,150–154] However, general blood donor screening for HEV is not recommended at the moment, but some countries like Japan started in 2014 with a 100% blood donor screening for HEV by NAT. Pathogen inactivation of HEV is limited, because the virus is not protein-embedded or lipid coated. A licensed vaccine has recently been developed in China.

Keynotes: hepatitis E virus

Virus	Region	Transmission	Screening	Inactivation	Vaccination
Caliciviridae, RNA, 4 genotypes in humans	Worldwide	Fecal-oral, blood components	NAT, antibody screening	Reduced efficiency	Vaccine recently licensed in China

Hepatitis F virus

Indian scientists found virus particles that could not associate with the known hepatitis A through E. Therefore, it could be a new standalone virus (hepatitis F) or a mutation and new genotype of the hepatitis B virus. It is believed that hepatitis F can cause liver inflammation. Since the existence of the hepatitis F virus is currently not clearly understood, it is only assumed that the main transmission pathway could equal that of a hepatitis A or hepatitis E infection via the fecal-oral route through contaminated drinking water or food. (Note to reader: Keynotes for hepatitis F are currently not available.)

Hepatitis G virus/GBV-C

Hepatitis G virus or GBV-C is an enveloped RNA virus and a member of the Flaviviridae family (which also includes HCV).[155–157] The viral genome is similar to HCV in structure, but has only 25% homology with it. Several genotypes are reported, mainly restricted to the various continents. GBV-C was discovered in patients with sporadic "non-A, non-B" hepatitis. This led to the conclusion GBV-C was the cause of viral hepatitis, but further study found it was not, nor did it have any other hepatotropic or pathological role. It was just a "passenger" virus isolated at random. Although parenteral transmission is highly efficient for GBV-C/HGV (58% of recipients of GBV-C/HGV RNA-positive blood products and 32% of aplastic anemia patients), it appears that sexual and vertical transmission are the most common transmission routes.[158]

The prevalence of GBV-C RNA in blood donors ranges from 1% to 5% depending on geographic location. Antibodies, such as anti-E2, are usually three to four times more likely than viral RNA.[159–162] Blood screening is not recommended.

Keynotes: hepatitis G virus

Virus	Region	Transmission	Screening	Inactivation	Vaccination
Flaviviridae, RNA	Worldwide	Fecal-oral, blood components	NAT in principle possible, antibody screening	Possible	Not available

Retroviruses

Retroviruses are lipid coated and widely distributed in nature, with examples in insects, reptiles, and almost all mammals. There are four main pathogenic human retroviruses—namely, HIV-1 and HIV-2, belonging to the lentivirus group of the retrovirus family, and human T-cell lymphotropic viruses (HTLV-I and HTLV-II) belonging to the oncona group. It is generally accepted that HTLV-I and HTLV-II evolved from simian T-lymphotropic retroviruses that were transmitted to humans centuries ago. HIV-1 is also thought to have derived from a simian ancestor, as simian immunodeficiency viruses are endemic in chimpanzees in Central Africa. HIV-2 originated from sooty mangabey monkeys in West Africa. It is thought that transmission to African natives occurred only over the last century.

Retroviruses are membrane-coated, ssRNA viruses that require the essential enzyme, reverse transcriptase, to transcribe their RNA to complementary double-stranded DNA that will be integrated into the host cell chromosome. The host cell enzymes aid the virus to complete its life cycle by synthesizing virions that bud from the plasma membrane to infect other cells or organisms.

Lentivirus diseases

Lentiviruses constitute the basis of their genetic features of a subset of the family of retroviruses and are responsible for a variety of neurological and immunological disorders. Typical representatives

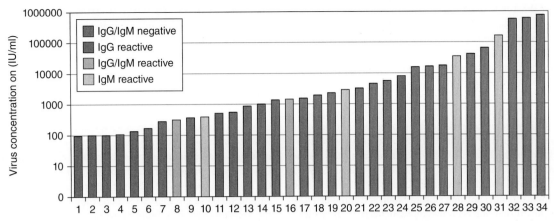

Figure 51.6 HEV NAT and HEV antibody status in 34 donor samples. Virus concentration was in range between 100 and 10^6 IU/ml. In 25/34 (73.5%) cases no HEV specific antibodies were detected. Source: Prof. M. Schmidt, German Red Cross, Frankfurt. Reproduced with permission.

are visna-maedi virus of sheep (VMV), infectious anemia virus of horses (EIAV), and arthritis-encephalitis virus of goats (CAEV) and the immunodeficiency viruses of monkeys (SIV), bovine (BIV), and cats (FIV).

Human immune deficiency virus-1

Human pathogenic lentiviruses are the human immunodeficiency viruses type 1 and 2 (HIV-1, HIV-2). Due to a distinct genetic entity in the variable Env gene (V3 loop) and the Gag protein (p17), they are subdivided into groups and subtypes. Currently, HIV-1 is classified into four groups with a total of 12 known subtypes (Figure 51.7):
- Group M (major): subtype A-K
- Group O (outlier): subtype 1, 2
- Group N (new)
- Group P (pending the identification of further human cases)

In 1983, an unusual accumulation of rare skin tumors (Kaposi's sarcoma), and atypical pneumonia (pneumocystis pneumonia carnii, PCP) was observed in homosexual men in the United States.[163–165] It turned out that the cause of these diseases was a reduced cellular immune defense, probably caused by a viral infection. This hypothesis was confirmed in 1983 by Luc Montangnier[166,167] and 1984 by Robert C. Gallo,[168,169] who isolated a novel human retrovirus from affected patients. In addition to the genetic information for the structural proteins, Gag, Pol, and Env genes encoded a number of proteins with regulatory and accessory functions.[170] In HIV-1, the following proteins are included:
- Tat
- Rev
- Nef
- Vif
- Vpr
- Vpu

After activation of the integrated proviral DNA by cellular transcription factors that bind to the 5′ LTR, a de novo synthesis of viral mRNAs starts. These transcripts are spliced twice in the nucleus, and transported into the cytoplasm for translation to the regulatory proteins Tat, Rev, and Nef.[171,172] After the splicing process, Tat is transported again into the nucleus and increases the viral RNA synthesis rate by a factor of 100–1000.

The Nef protein can interact with different kinases to bind to the lambda chain of the T-cell receptor and cause a downregulation of the CD4 receptor on the surface of the host cell. Thus, the Nef protein has multiple interactions in signal transduction and in the metabolism of the host cell. Experiments show that HIV-1 can infect a variety of cells: other B lymphocytes, natural killer cells, endothelial cells, megakaryocytes, astrocytes, and glial cells. Nevertheless, CD4 T-lymphocytes, macrophages, and dendritic cells (DCs) are its primary targets. Besides the CD4+ surface marker, which acts as the primary HIV-1 receptor, other co-receptors are necessary for a successful infection. In recent years, it has been found that these are chemokine receptors. The CCR5 molecule was identified as an HIV-1 co-receptor on CD4+ positive macrophages and dendritic cells.[173,174]

Acquired immune deficiency syndrome (AIDS) was first described in 1981 in the United States and later in Western Europe as striking at-risk male homosexuals and drug addicts. These groups were early excluded from blood donation due to indications for transmission of AIDS by blood transfusions. Even after introduction of highly sensitive blood testing for HIV, most countries still practice lifelong exclusion from blood donation for the risk groups.

Infections with HIV-1 since developed into a pandemic, with a major infection pathway by heterosexual transmissions. According to estimates by UNAIDS and the WHO at the end of 2013, about 35 million people were living with HIV-1 and 2.1 million were infected anew each year.[175–177] 90% of all infected residents live in third world countries. The sub-Saharan region has a high number of them, about 30 million.

HIV strongly challenged transfusion medicine and the safety of blood products. In addition to blood component recipients, patients with coagulation disorders (hemophilia A and B) were

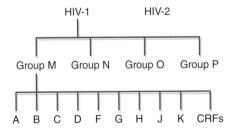

Figure 51.7 Taxonomic of HIV-1 and HIV-2. Source: Prof. M. Schmidt, German Red Cross, Frankfurt. Reproduced with permission.

infected in the 1980s (and 1990s) by contaminated factor concentrates.[178–180] This led nations like Germany to classify blood products as medical products, subject to the regulatory requirements of the Medical Act.

Blood products can be screened for antibodies to HIV-1/-2, the p24 antigen and in addition to HIV NAT. Roth et al.[158] reported more than 270 million investigations in which 244 samples turned up only NAT positive, preventing HIV-1 transmission by blood components. The diagnostic window depends on the analytical sensitivity of the detection method and is calculated for NAT systems between 6–8 days. Despite the high level of blood safety a calculated residual transfusion HIV-1 infection risk of 1:1,000,000 remains in the literature. Schmidt et al.[181] described an HIV-1 transmission by blood components after introduction of blood screening of HIV-1 by NAT. The cause of the transmission was a false negative HIV-1 NAT test result based on mutations in the primer/probe region of the detection method. The mutations reduced amplification efficiency. In 2012, Chudy et al.[182,183] reported further cases with false negative NAT screening results. One case was a HIV-1 transmission by a red blood cell concentrate. The reason for these negative HIV NAT results is that the reverse transcriptase from RNA into cDNA does not have a proofreading function. Errors in transcription are therefore neither registered nor corrected.

Based on these reports, a new requirement to screening systems will be mandated in many countries in 2015. Blood donor screening for HIV-1 by NAT should be done on a dual target basis, with amplification in at least two independent genome regions, to reduce the risk of mutations in one of the primer/probe areas.

HIV-1 therapy

The current applied antiretroviral therapy (ART) focuses on the inhibition of viral protein reverse transcriptase (RT) and protease (PR).[184–186] Furthermore, various drugs are in clinical trials that pursue the inhibition of various viral and cellular functions. ART should begin as early as possible after an infection, with three or more antiretroviral drugs. With the use of a combination therapy (highly active antiretroviral therapy [HAART]), the rate of severe illness has decreased remarkably. The following reverse transcriptase inhibitor (RTI) drugs are available:

- Nucleoside analogs (zidovudine/Retrovir, didanosine/Videx, zalcitabine/Hivid; stavudine/Zerit; lamivudine/Epivir, abacavir/Ziagen);
- Nonnucleoside RTIs (NNRTIs; Nevirapine/Viramune, efavirenz/Sustiva, delavirdine/Rescriptor); and
- Inhibitor of viral protease (PI) (saquinavir/Fortovase, nelfinavir/Viracept, amprenavir/Agenerase; Lopinarvir/Kaletra).

Patient discipline is necessary because drug side effects are frequent. Incomplete medication leads viruses to build up resistance; this leads in time to treatment failure. In addition, in some patients, a lack of bioavailability of individual drugs exists. Therefore, drug level monitoring is very important.

Human immune deficiency virus-2

Most HIV-2 infected people are living in Central and West Africa. The first case in the United States was reported in 1987.[187] There are currently eight different subtypes known for HIV-2 (A to H). Subtypes A and B are epidemic. Subtype A is particularly common in West Africa, but also in Angola, Mozambique, Brazil, India, and very limited in Europe or the United States. Subtype B is mainly restricted to West Africa.[188]

HIV-2 is closely related with the simian immunodeficiency virus in sooty mangabeys (Cercocebus Atys Atys) (SIVsmm), a species of monkeys that inhabit the forests of the coast of West Africa. Phylogenetic analyzes show that the SIVsmm is most related to the two strains of HIV-2, which are connected to spread in humans (A and B HIV-2 groups). SIVsmm is found in sooty mangabeys of the Tai Forest, west of Ivory Coast.

The multi-spot HIV-1/HIV-2 Rapid Test is the only FDA-approved method to differentiate between HIV-1 and HIV-2. Modern enzyme immunoassays (ELISA) can detect HIV-1 and HIV-2 in parallel. Confirmation of an HIV-2 infection can be made by HIV-2 specific immunoblot pattern (Western blots) or by HIV-2 NAT. The National Institute of Health (NIH) in the United States recommends a differential diagnosis of HIV-2 when a person had sexual contacts with persons from West Africa or shared syringes with persons from that region. People from West Africa are at the highest risk of HIV-2 infections, as West Africa is the origin of the virus.[189,190] In most countries, blood donor screening is only implemented for HIV-2 by serological methods. The next generation NAT systems have already integrated a simultaneous detection of HIV-1 and HIV-2.

HIV-2 was found to be less pathogenic than HIV-1. The pathomechanism of HIV-2 is not clearly understood, but its transfer rate is much lower than HIV-1's. Both infections can lead to AIDS in individual patients, and both viruses can mutate to resist drugs. Treatment of patients with HIV-2 infections includes clinical evaluation and CD4+ cell counts during ART with nucleoside RTIs (NRTIs), protease inhibitors (PIs), and NNRTIs with the addition of CCR5 co-receptor antagonists and fusion inhibitors. Selections for the first and/or second-line treatment for HIV-2 are currently not defined. HIV-2 appears intrinsically resistant to NNRTIs, but sensitive to NRTIs, thought the mechanism is poorly understood. PIs have shown variable effect, while integrase inhibitors are also evaluated. Combinations of the above therapies are being reviewed and show variable effects depending on their types. Although the mechanisms are not clearly understood for HIV-1 and HIV-2, they are known to use different therapeutic combinations. HIV-2 infections had lower mortality than HIV-1 infections, but co-infection is also possible. The progress of co-infections depends on which virus was first. Co-infection seems to be a growing problem globally as time progresses, with most cases identified in West African countries, but some in the United States.[191,192]

Keynotes: HIV-1

Virus	Region	Transmission	Screening	Inactivation	Vaccination
Lentiviridae, RNA, 4 groups (M, O, N, P), 12 subtypes, residual risk TTID: <1:1 million	Worldwide, Africa	Blood components, sexual activities	NAT, antigen (p24), antibody screening	Possible, 4–6 log	Not available

Keynotes: HIV-2

Virus	Region	Transmission	Screening	Inactivation	Vaccination
Lentiviridae, RNA, 8 genotypes (A–H)	Worldwide, West Africa	Blood components, sexual activities	NAT, antigen, antibody screening	Possible, 4–6 log	Not available

Human T-cell lymphotropic virus

Human T-cell lymphotropic virus (HTLV-I) was identified and isolated in a Japanese patient in 1978.[193] The virus was found that causes adult T-cell leukemia and lymphoma (ATL) and tropical spastic paraparesis (TSP), which can also be found as HTLV-I-associated myelopathy. The virus is now known worldwide, but endemic in Japan, the Caribbean, South America and West and Central Africa, where infection rates are often more than 1%. HTLV-II was originally identified in 1982 in a patient with hairy cell leukemia.[194,195] HTLV-I and HTLV-II show 65% homology. HTLV-II is found in Native American populations and in some populations of injecting drug users.

The overall prevalence in blood donors in the United States is about 9.6/100,000 person years and the incidence is 0.239/100,000. HTLV-II is more common than HTLV-I in blood donors.[196] Current HTLV donor screening tests offered only on antibody detection by ELISA or chemiluminescent (ChLIA). The more sensitive assays use recombinant HTLV proteins in a sandwich assay format. Assays test both HTLV-I and HTLV-II in parallel.

Confirmatory testing of reactive HTLV donation is more complex than a confirmatory test for HIV, in part because of the relatively poor Western blots, which are commercially available. NAT could be an alternative to confirm reactive HTLV-1/-2 antibody screening results, but no commercial test is currently available.[74,197]

Most British HTLV-positive blood donors have been shown to be of Afro-Caribbean origin or sexual partners of someone Afro-Caribbean origin. Therefore, it is important that sexual partners and other family members are also tested for HTLV in a clinical follow-up.

The diagnostic window for HTLV antibodies is about 51 days. A study by the US transfusion recipients estimated a residual risk of HTLV infections at 1:128,000.[198] In general transfusion transmitted infectious risk for HTLV is transmitted by cellular components (leukocytes). Therefore, leukocyte depletion is able to improve blood safety.[199]

Although most HTLV-positive donors show no clinical signs of disease, a small percentage (2% to 4%) can develop an acute T-cell leukemia (ATL) up to 40 years after infection.[200,201] HTLV-I is also associated with uveitis.

An asymptomatic HTLV infection should usually not be treated with drugs, because of the small chance of development of clinical disease. Chemotherapy for the treatment of ATL is often less effective than other forms of leukemia or lymphoma. Therefore, there is a high mortality associated with this disease.

Keynotes: HTLV-1 and HTLV-2

Virus	Region	Transmission	Screening	Inactivation	Vaccination
Retroviridae, RNA	Japan, Caribbean, South America	Blood components, sexual activities	Antibody screening	Possible, 4–6 log	Not available

Flaviviruses

Dengue virus infections

Dengue virus infections pose a major international public health concern. According to WHO, approximately 2.5 billion people in more than 100 countries are at risk of infection, 50 to 100 million dengue virus infections occur every year, and approximately 1.25 million people may die due to dengue fever, dengue hemorrhagic fever (DHF), or dengue shock syndrome (DSS).[139,202–204] A very recent study suggests that dengue infections are underreported and that annual infection rates may be even three- to fourfold higher than estimated by the WHO. Dengue fever can therefore be considered to be the most important mosquito-borne viral disease.[205–207] As an arthropod-borne infection, the major transmission pathway occurs by mosquitoes from the *Aedes* genus;[208] however, transmission by blood components or organ transplants has also been documented.[209–211]

Dengue virus is a ssRNA virus belonging to the Flaviviridae family. The mature virion has three structures (core, membrane, and envelope) and seven nonstructural (NS1, NS2a, NS2b, NS3, NS4a, NS4b, and NS5) proteins. There are four serotypes classified according to their immunological properties: DEN-1, DEN-2, DEN-3, and DEN-4.[212–215] The primary vector is *Aedes aegypti*, but other vectors, like *Aedes albopictus* or *Aedes polynesiensis*, are also possible. Female mosquitoes acquire the virus by biting infected humans during the viremic period and become infective after an incubation period of 7–14 days. Subsequently, infected mosquitoes can transmit the virus during every feeding.

Laboratory diagnosis can be done using NAT, antibody screening, or dengue antigen tests. The diagnostic window is 3–5 days for IgM antibodies and 2–3 days for NAT.[216,217] The diagnostic window for the NS1 antigen test may also be very short. IgG antibodies are detectable after approximately 9–10 days. Cross-reactivity with other flavivirus infections is possible and can be explained by sharing common antigenic epitopes. Commercial NAT systems for blood donor screening are available with a 95% level of detection of 14.9 geq/ml.

Fever is the predominant symptom in adults, whereas people younger than 15 often have asymptomatic infections or an undifferentiated febrile illness with maculopapular rash. Dengue fever (DF) and dengue hemorrhagic fever (DHF) are characterized by severe headaches, sudden onset of high fever, hemorrhagic manifestations, thrombocytopenia, and evidence of plasma leakage. Dengue shock syndrome has a high mortality rate and often acts as a pathway to disseminated intravascular coagulation (DIC). There are no specific antivirals currently available for dengue; therefore, its management is symptomatic and supportive.

In Germany, 594 total imported cases of dengue fever were reported in 2010; 75% were imported from Asia, and 21% came from South and Central America.[218] The last dengue epidemic in Continental Europe occurred from 1927 to 1928 in Greece. Since then, Europe has been the only populated continent without autochthonous dengue virus infections until in 2010, when cases of autochthonous dengue virus infections were reported from southern France and Croatia.[219,220]

In both countries, *Aedes albopictus* mosquitoes have become domestic and were the implicated vectors in the transmission cases. *Aedes albopictus* has become increasingly established in the European Union. It is assumed that the import of mosquito larvae during the transport of car tires, in combination with rising average temperatures in Europe due to climate change, are important factors of this process.

Today, *Aedes albopictus*, the so-called Asian tiger mosquito, is established in many European countries, such as Greece, Albania, Italy, Croatia, Montenegro, and Spain, and it is spreading further. During mosquito monitoring activities in 2011, *Aedes* species were also detected in the Upper Rhine Valley in Baden-Württemberg.

Aedes albopictus is not only a very efficient vector for dengue virus, but also for numerous other arboviruses, such as the Chikungunya virus. Consequently, if travelers with arboviral infections acquired abroad return home, where *Aedes albopictus* has become domestic, there is the risk of causing a local outbreak. Likewise, infected tourists could import infections, as happened during the Chikungunya outbreak in northern Italy in 2007, which was probably caused by a tourist from India.

Although the primary pathway for dengue virus is through the mosquito vector, vertical transmission through intrapartum transmission, nosocomial transmission through needlestick injury, transmissions by organ and bone marrow transplantation, and transfusion of blood components have all been reported. Even though the diagnostic window is assumed to be very short, asymptomatic donors could be the source of such transmissions. In some cases, however, the differentiation between non-mosquito transmission and mosquito-borne infection is difficult in endemic areas where the vector is widespread.

Transfusion-transmitted dengue virus infection has been confirmed in two cases from Hong Kong and Singapore.[221–225] As a first step to improve blood safety, with regard to dengue virus, many countries have implemented a temporary donor deferral program for travelers returning from highly endemic areas. These deferral strategies might be helpful if only a few donors will be affected (e.g., less than 1%). If more than 5% of the donor population will be involved, there is a high risk of unnecessary donor deferral because donors might not come back, even if the deferral is temporary.

Testing for dengue virus is also an option. In the most recent outbreak of dengue fever on Madeira, in the Atlantic Ocean, Portuguese authorities implemented blood donor screening by NAT for dengue virus RNA. Additionally, an ELISA test for the NS1-antigen of dengue virus is available that allows early detection of an infection. Another approach is the implementation of pathogen-reduction methods.

For Germany, however, the main strategy should be the implementation of strict vector control measures, such as insecticiding and reducing potential breeding sites, in order to avoid the spread of *Aedes* species throughout the country.

Keynotes: Dengue virus infections

Virus	Region	Transmission	Screening	Inactivation	Vaccination
Flaviviridae, RNA, Genotypes 1–4	Japan, Caribbean, South America	Vector transmitted (Arbovirus) blood components	NAT, antibody screening	Possible, 4–6 log	Not available

West Nile virus infections

The WNV is known since 1937. It has a structure similar to dengue fever virus, and both belong to the genus *Flavivirus* within the family *Flaviviridae*. WNV is an enveloped RNA virus with a positive-sense, single strand of RNA, which is between 11,000 and 12,000 nucleotides long.[226,227] The virus occurs in tropical as well as temperate areas. It infects mainly birds, but can spread to humans, horses, and other mammals.[228,229] The vector of the virus is through mosquitoes of different genera, such as *Culex*, *Aedes*, or *Ochlerotatus*. The European/Asian tiger mosquito, *Aedes albopictus*, can transfer it to human and birds.

From 1999 to 2003, there was a large spread of a new strain (strain New York, lineage 1) of West Nile virus in the United States from the East Coast to the West Coast.[230,231] A huge number of infections, some fatal, led the FDA to mandate blood donor screening for West Nile Virus by NAT in 2003. The virus concentration in humans was in a range between 10^1 geq/ml and 10^5 geq/ml. Thus, a blood donor screening in small pool sizes (1–8 donations per mini pool) was required to reduce the diagnostic window to a minimum of three days.[223,224,232–237] After about 11–12 days, infected patients developed IgM antibodies and got a natural protection against the virus infection. In recent years, the incidence of WNV disease in Europe increased from year to year (data by ECDC), particularly in Greece, Russia, Hungary, and northern Italy.[238–240] All donors who visited a country with WMV infections have to be deferred from blood donations for 28 days. As an alternative, blood donors can be screened for WNV by NAT with a sensitive method or antibody assays. But the diagnostic window for antibody assays is 11–15 days. Therefore, they are not feasible to detect infected blood donors in the early infection period and the specificity of the commercial antibody tests is limited. Cross-reactivities with other flaviviruses cannot be ruled out.

Keynotes: West Nile virus infections

Virus	Region	Transmission	Screening	Inactivation	Vaccination
Flaviviridae, RNA, 5 lineages	USA, Greece, Russia, Hungary	Vector transmitted (Arbovirus) blood components	NAT, antibody screening	Possible, 4–6 log	Not available

Alphavirus infection

Chikungunya virus infections

Chikungunya virus (CHIKV) is an enveloped ss (+) RNA virus and belongs to the genus Alphavirus in the family Togaviridae, a group of arboviruses. Infection is mostly transmitted by the bite of arthropods. The pathogen was discovered in 1953.[241] In humans, the virus causes chikungunya fever.[242,243] The virion has a diameter of about 60 nm, making it one of the smaller viruses. It has a length of about 11,700 base pairs that code for 2474 amino acids. The protein NSP4 takes presumably over the function of an RNA polymerase.

Chikungunya occurs in Africa, Asia, and the Indian subcontinent. In 2005/2006, there was a CHIKV epidemic on the island La Réunion, with a total of 270,000 infections (about 35% of the population) and a total of 254 documented, related deaths.[244,245] A year later (2007), an epidemic occurred in northern Italy in Ravenna.[246,247] Here, 197 suspected cases of chikungunya fever were registered. Currently, there is a local epidemic of CHIKV in the Caribbean, Latin America, and the northern part of South America. WHO reports indicate that by October 2014, over 776,000 suspected cases of Chikungunya have been recorded in the Caribbean islands, Latin American countries and some south American countries. 152 deaths have also been attributed to this disease during the same period. In El Salvador, the Food and Drug Administration reported more than 30,000 suspected cases this year, and about 1700 have been registered in Venezuela.[248–250] Most infections are in the

Dominican Republic. According to the reports of the Pan-American Health Organization OPS, CHIKV has spread to at least two dozen countries and territories in the Western Hemisphere since the first case was detected on the Caribbean island of St. Martin at the end of 2013.[251]

Survivors develop usual neutralizing IgG antibodies that protect them from a second infection for their lives. In the early infection period, an asymptomatic viremic phase may occur; therefore, CHIKV epidemics represent a challenge for blood donor services in endemic countries. Blood donor screening can be made by NAT, but currently no commercial NAT systems are available. These are eagerly awaited.

Keynotes: chikungunya virus infections

Virus	Region	Transmission	Screening	Inactivation	Vaccination
Chikungunya virus, RNA	Africa, Asia and the Indian subcontinent, Caribbean Island, northern part of South America	Mosquitos, blood components	Commercial NAT in development	Yes	Not available

Herpesvirus infections

Herpesviruses are spread all over the world and can infect all creatures. Humans are known as the host for various herpesviruses. All human herpesviruses (HHVs) have the ability to rest in tissues after acute infection. Depending on the immune system and stress factors replication of herpesviruses can start again and cause a re-infection.

Human cytomegalovirus (CMV or HHV-5) is the most transfusion-relevant herpesvirus infection for humans.[252–254] Herpes simplex (HHV-1 and HHV-2) and herpes varicella zoster (HHV-3) have limited target cells, but CMV can manifest itself in many different organs. CMV represents a major challenge in immunosuppressed patients exposed to transfusion therapy. Special patient groups at risk are the following:

- Transplant recipients;
- Patients with severe immune deficiency;
- Fetuses (intrauterine transfusion);
- CMV-negative pregnant women;
- Low-birth-weight premature infants and neonates; and
- Multitransfused patients.

It is important to distinguish between CMV infection by serological tests or viral isolation and CMV disease by laboratory evidence of infection in connection with specific symptoms that identify the virus. Most CMV infections are asymptomatic, but high fever, sore throat, and symptoms similar to flu and glandular fever occur. Reactivation of CMV can occur when the immune system is weakened.

The target cells of CMV are monocytes and macrophages. Therefore, leucocyte depletion is effective at reducing residual infection risk. The main infection risk is during childhood or the early adult years via sexual activities. At the age of 40, about 60–70% of all donors in Western Europe have anti-CMV IgG antibodies as a sign of a past CMV infection.

Most blood transfusion services are using ELISA-based assays to test blood for the presence of anti-CMV.[255–260] Hemagglutination assays can detect both classes of antibodies, and some commercial tests can now be performed on automated blood group analyzers (PK7300 systems).

CMV transmission by transfusion is now relatively rare in developed countries, particularly those in which all blood components are leukocyte reduced. It is believed that only 12% to 62% of CMV-seropositive blood units infect CMV-seronegative recipients depending on the interval to the last seronegative donation.[261] The incubation time of the primary CMV infection varies between four and eight weeks. The residual risk of transfusion-associated CMV infection of anti-CMV negative blood components (not reduced leukocytes) is 1.2% to 1.6% per donation, whereas the risk for leukocyte-reduced blood components is of 2.3% to 3.0%.[262] The residual risk for both procedures has currently not been investigated.

In marrow transplantation, CMV is one of the most important infections, and responsible for about 15% of mortality before the introduction of good antivirals.[263–265]

Antiviral drugs, active against CMV, include ganciclovir, foscarnet, cidofovir, and valacyclovir.[266–269] Drugs may be prescribed for prevention, suppression, or treatment.

Epstein–Barr virus (EBV or HHV-4) is responsible for infectious mononucleosis, Burkitt's lymphoma, and nasopharyngeal cancer, and may also be transmitted by transfusion.[270]

Human herpesvirus 6 effects (HHV-6) is *roseola infantum* or *sixth disease*—a childhood rash. Primary infection in adults is rare.

Human herpesvirus 8 (HHV-8) is the causative agent for Kaposi's sarcoma and other tumors such as Castleman disease. Infections with HHV-8 are also associated with polyneuropathy, organomegaly, and endocrinopathy. As with CMV and EBV, HHV-8 appears to cause a persistent infection within the host immune cells.[271–273]

EBV and HHV-6 have a very high prevalence in the general population (>80%). HHV-8 has a seroprevalence in blood donors, between 0 and 20%. African populations have been reported to have a prevalence of 35% to 75% to 50%, which shows evidence of HHV-8 DNA, 10%. In the United Kingdom, HHV-8 was more common among MSM-reported STD clinics, and that was a factor in the decision to exclude this population as blood donors.

Transfusion-transmitted EBV infections are usually asymptomatic, but some present as infectious mononucleosis with a slight fever, loss of appetite, and nausea. Most HHV-4 infection is benign with a low frequency of disease development.[274–276]

Keynotes: herpes virus infections

Virus	Region	Transmission	Screening	Inactivation	Vaccination
Herpesviridae, DNA, 8 genotypes (HHV 1–8)	Worldwide	Human to human contacts, blood components	NAT, antibody screening	Possible, 4–6 log	Not available

Parvovirus B19 infections

The parvoviruses still form the only family of viruses whose genome consists of single-strand, linear DNA, and the only known human pathogen is parvovirus B19. It was isolated in 1975 by Yvonne Cossart and employees from blood associated with the clinical picture of erythema infectiosum, also known under the names of *fifth disease* or *slap-cheeked syndrome* in young children.[277–279]

Parvoviruses, as the name indicates, are among the smallest known viruses. The virus capsids have a diameter of only 18–26 nm and are not surrounded by a membrane or an envelope. They have an iso-octahedral structure and consist of 60 capsomeres, which are 95% the structural protein VP2, and 5% VP1 protein. VP2 is identical to the carboxy-terminal region of VP1 sequence. The capsids mediate the absorption of the parvovirus B19 to its target cells. The linear DNA single strands of parvovirus B19 is 5600 bases long. The genome has two large open reading frames: The first location is for the nonstructured protein NS1 (MW 71,000). The protein activates the promoter and has important functions in the replication of virus DNA. Furthermore, after the replication, the protein induces apoptosis of the infected cells. The second reading frame is located in the 5′ half of the genome and is coding for the structural proteins VP1 and VP2.

Parvovirus B19 infects erythropoietic precursors[280,281] (red blood cells in different stages of differentiation in the BFU-E [erythrocyte-forming unit], CFU-E [erythrocyte colony-forming unit], and the erythroblasts in the bone marrow, as well as pronormoblasts in the fetal liver) by binding to the P antigen, a glycosphingolipid, which is the membrane receptor on the target cells.[282] Various other cell types also contain this receptor explaining the widespread manifestations of parvovirus B19 infection. Individuals lacking the P blood group antigen are naturally immune to parvovirus B19 infection.

Parvovirus B19 is usually transmitted by droplet infection. In the bloodstream of infected persons, the virus concentration can increase to very high concentrations of 10^{11}–10^{13} geq/ml.[283–286]

Infections by parvovirus B19 occurred mainly in the early childhood. Therefore, 40–50% of adolescents aged 15 years already have virus-specific antibodies. The percentage grows up to 80% at the age of 40, which could explain why few transfusion-transmitted cases are reported.

After parvovirus B19 infection, the body forms IgM and IgG antibodies directed against the capsid proteins VP1 and VP2. The first IgM antibodies appear approximately 6–10 days after infection with B19. From the 12th day, IgG antibodies are detectable. The virus concentration will be diminished under the NAT detection limit within 3–4 weeks after infection in about 80% of all cases. Low B19 virus concentration can be detectable up to 12 months. CD4-positive T lymphocytes are in addition involved in the elimination of B19 virus.

The clinical symptoms of B19 infections are manifold. The course of the infection and severity of the disease depend on the patient's hematological and immunological status. Possible clinical manifestations include acute anemia, arthritis, transient aplastic crisis, chronic arthritis, thrombocytopenia, neutropenia, pure red cell aplasia, hydrops fetalis, pancytopenia, chronic anemia, myocarditis, pericarditis, hepatitis, acute liver failure, meningitis, acute liver failure, uveitis, vasculitis, and pneumonia. About 33% of children have no symptoms.[287–290] Generally, clinical symptoms are mild also. In adults, however, complications can occur, especially in women. In 50% of adults, pains in the small joints of both hands and feet can occur. In immunosuppressed patients, such as those with congenital immunodeficiency, transplant and cancer patients, and HIV-infected persons, parvovirus B19 can cause a long, life-threatening infection persistent over months or years. B19-associated mortality in transplant patients is estimated to be about 7%. Before parvovirus B19–specific antibodies are formed, large amounts of B19 virus (up to 10^{13} geq/ml) can be detected in the blood.

Despite the high virus concentration, many infections are asymptomatic, so that infected people can come to a blood donation and be accepted as donors. The virus may also be present in the final blood components products such as factor VIII and IX in relevant concentrations because chemical or physical pathogen inactivation methods are less efficient since B19 virus has no lipid or protein

membranes. Commercial NAT systems are available and should detect all three genotypes of B19 viruses. Many blood transfusion services have introduced screening for plasma products by NAT.[149,291–294] Pools of source plasma for fractionation are only acceptable with less than 10 000 geq/ml of parvovirus B19. This level of activity is ascertained by considering the level of parvovirus antibodies that also are present in the pool and their ability to neutralize small concentrations of the virus.

At present, there is no effective vaccine against parvovirus B19 or antiviral chemotherapeutic agents for the treatment of the infection.

Keynotes: parvovirus B19 infections

Virus	Region	Transmission	Screening	Inactivation	Vaccination
Parvovirus B19, DNA, small virus, 3 genotypes	Worldwide	Droplets, blood components	NAT antibody screening	Yes, but less efficient	Not available

Filoviridae

Ebola virus infections

Marburg virus (MBG) and Ebola virus (EBOLA) are nonsegmented negative-stranded RNA viruses and belonged to the family of Filoviridae within the order Mononegavirales.[295–297] The species Ebola virus can subdivide into subspecies from Reston, Sudan and Zaire. The virions are filamentous and extremely polymorphic. The total length is up to 14 μm compared to the uniform diameter of about 80 nm. The lipid envelope surrounding the nucleocapsid consists of genomic RNA and four structural proteins.

- Nucleoprotein;
- Viral structural protein (VP) 30;
- Viral structural protein (VP) 35; and
- Viral polymerase.

The viral polymerase controls the transcription and replication in the cytoplasm of the cell. VP 35 appears to be a cofactor of the viral polymerase.[298] The nucleoprotein envelopes the RNA and interacts with VP30, which in the case of Ebola acts as a transcription factor.

Filovirus-related hemorrhagic fever was first diagnosed in 1967 in Europe (Marburg, Frankfurt, and Belgrade). The first patient was a lab worker who had contact with monkeys imported from Uganda (*Cercopithecus aethiops*). A total of 26 primary and six secondary infections were registered, with seven death cases. The Ebola virus hemorrhagic fever was first described in 1976 during two outbreaks in Sudan and the Democratic Republic of Congo (Yambuku).[299,300] A total of 602 cases were registered, and the mortality rate was 88%. The natural hosts are humans and other primates. Experimental hosts, including guinea pigs, hamsters, and mice, are often the primary infection. The initial transmission pathway (zoonosis) is currently unclear. The transmission from humans to humans occurs through close contact with infected people and their excretions (often nosocomial). Sexual, neonatal, and airborne transmissions are possible, but epidemiologically of minor importance. The incubation period is usually between one and 21 days.[301,302] Animal studies indicate Ebola viruses are very infectious, so small viral concentrations might be sufficient to infect new people. The disease progresses with severe clinical symptoms like high hemorrhagic fever and loss of fluid (up to 10 L/day). Therefore, patients will have numerous medical complications, including renal insufficiency. Secondary bacterial infections can be added. In the acute period, patients need intensive medical care. Since clinical symptoms begin immediately at the time of viremia, Ebola infection has only a low relevance for transfusion medicine. Asymptomatic infectious patients have not been observed. Of particular importance to medical transfusion is the care of these patients, since cross-matching must be carried out under high security and safety conditions. A challenge for blood transfusion service is to produce convalescent plasma from patients with neutralizing antibodies against Ebola virus infections.

Keynotes: Ebolavirus infections

Virus	Region	Transmission	Screening	Inactivation	Vaccination
Filoviridae, Ebola virus, RNA	West Africa	Human-to-human contacts, droplets, blood products	Commercial NAT available	Probably yes, no data available	Not available

Pandemic influenza

Influenza viruses are lipid enveloped negative-stranded RNA viruses of the orthomyxoviridae family. There are three types of influenza virus, A, B, and C, which give rise to each their type of influenza. Influenza C gives few clinical symptoms, and infects only humans. Influenza B generally only infects humans, whereas influenza A can infect a number of species. Influenza A and B can cause serious disease, and are the two virus types that cause epidemics each winter.

Influenza pandemics are a persistent threat due to frequent mutations in the genetic code of the virus. Therefore, a persistent efficient immune response is not possible. The lethal influenza viruses that have infected humans have so far been managed by the existing public health measures. This was helped by the relative inability of the "bird flu" virus (H5N1) to infect people.[303-305] However, there is concern that eventually a mutation or mixed infection of these deadly viruses will spread into the public. Since there have been a series of bird flu cases in humans involving H5N1, it is assumed that any new influenza threat will probably be closely related. Vaccines have been prepared, but like normal human flu vaccines, they have good efficacy in immunocompetent individuals, but are of limited use to those at highest risk from such a pandemic (the old and the very young). It is believed that transfusion-transmitted influenza is relatively rare but theoretically possible. But the timeframe of an asymptomatic viremia is very limited, probably only a few hours. At the height of each epidemic, the use of blood is probably severely limited, because of the cancellation of planned operations, but also because of the shortage of health workers and blood donors. Commercial NAT detection systems are available, but a routine blood donor screening is not recommended. Only in case of a global pandemic should this question be raised again to improve blood safety.

Keynotes: influenza infections

Virus	Region	Transmission	Screening	Inactivation	Vaccination
Orthomyxo-viridae, influenza virus, RNA	Worldwide	Human-to-human contacts, human contacts with birds, pigs and other animal	Antibody screening, commercial NAT available	Possible	Yes, but vaccination has to be updated annually

Other viruses

Lymphatic choriomeningitis (LCMV)

LCMV was first described in 1931 as one of the main causes of meningitis.[306,307] LCMV is a lipid enveloped ssRNA virus, and one of the Arenaviruses. Its main reservoir is mice, but it can infect other animals or humans. Eight solid organ transplantations have been infected with LCMV from two organ donors, raising the concern that LCMV can also be a transfusion-transmitted virus.[308,309] A French study found a low prevalence in the blood donor population, suggesting a low risk of transmission. However, the researchers suggest that the history of the last rodent contact should lead to a temporary deferral of potential donors. This could have an important impact on donor deferrals. Based on the low prevalence rate, a general blood donor screening is currently not recommended.

Keynotes: lymphatic choriomeningitis virus

Virus	Region	Transmission	Screening	Inactivation	Vaccination
Arenavirus, LCMV, RNA	Worldwide	Contacts with rodents and mice, blood components not proven	In development	No data available	Not available

TT virus (TTV)

TTV was discovered in the search for the elusive reason for the smaller (non-C) component of the "non-A to E" post-transfusion hepatitis. The virus was discovered in a post-transfusion hepatitis patient with the initials TT and first reported by T. Nishizawa in 1997.[310,311] TTV is a small (18–50 nm), non-enveloped DNA virus and belongs to the family Anelloviridae. Isolates have been classified into five main clades numbered 1 to 5. TTV genogroup 3 also includes the eight virus strains known as SENV-A to H.[312] TTV can be transmitted by transfusion and has a prevalence of TTV RNA between 5% and 80%; there are again significant geographical differences in infection rates with higher prevalence in Africa (up to 80%). It is assumed that 50% of African children of one year have been infected with TTV. Sensitive NAT assays demonstrate a high percentage of viral infections in blood donors. The relevance of TTV in transfusion is limited due to the absence of clinical symptoms.

Keynotes: TT virus

Virus	Region	Transmission	Screening	Inactivation	Vaccination
Anelloviridae, TTV, RNA	Worldwide	Blood components possible	In development	No data available	Not available

Summary

Blood safety is an important topic in transfusion medicine with subtopics like prevention of the incorrect blood transfusion,[313] prevention of transfusion-related acute lung injury (TRALI),[314] and of course prevention of transfusion-transmitted virus infections.[315] After the AIDS scandal, blood safety was improved regarding transfusion-relevant viruses like HIV-1, HBV, and HCV. The introduction of NAT and serological screening assays comprised big milestones in hemovigilance and reduced the residual infectious risk to less than 1:1,000,000 for HIV-1 and HCV.[316]

But viruses are not stable. They change their genetic information and sequence due to mutation pressure. RNA viruses have no proofreading function for reverse transcriptase. Therefore, risks of mutation within the primer and probe binding region exist and were the cause for several cases of transfusion-transmitted HIV-1 with NAT-negative blood. Therefore, manufacturers of diagnostic assays must be on alert to adapt their system to new genotypes.

Secondly, people travel the world. A new virus can be spread around the world within 48 hours. Therefore, new pathogens can become relevant for all countries or for some regions like West Nile virus for the United States and probably for Europe within the next years.

Nevertheless, blood safety is a global challenge for all transfusion services. The scientific exchange within international societies is inspiring, and cooperation within WHO a necessity. Safe blood products should be available on the same safety level to all patients in the world.

Disclaimer

The authors have no conflicts of interest.

Key references

A full reference list for this chapter is available at: http://www.wiley.com/go/simon/transfusion

3   Stramer SL. Current perspectives in transfusion-transmitted infectious diseases: emerging and re-emerging infections. *ISBT Sci Ser* 2014;**9**:30–6.

22   Blumberg BS, Alter HJ, Visnich S. A "new" antigen in leukemia sera. *JAMA* 1965;**191**:541–6.

58   Guertler L. Virus safety of human blood, plasma, and derived products. *Thromb Res* 2002;**107** (Suppl. 1):S39–45.

74   Dodd R, Kurt Roth W, Ashford P, Dax EM, Vyas G. Transfusion medicine and safety. *Biologicals* 2009;**37**:62–70.

76   Roth WK, Busch MP, Schuller A, *et al.* International survey on NAT testing of blood donations: expanding implementation and yield from 1999 to 2009. *Vox Sang* 2012;**102**:82–90.

152   Hewitt PE, Ijaz S, Brailsford SR, *et al.* Hepatitis E virus in blood components: a prevalence and transmission study in southeast England. *Lancet* 2014;**384**:1766–73.

159   Allain JP. Emerging viruses in blood transfusion. *Vox Sang* 2000;**78** (Suppl. 2):243–8.

167   Montagnier L. Origin and evolution of HIVs and their role in AIDS pathogenesis. *J Acquir Immune Defic Syndr* 1988;**1**:517–20.

183   Chudy M, Weber-Schehl M, Pichl L, *et al.* Blood screening nucleic acid amplification tests for human immunodeficiency virus Type 1 may require two different amplification targets. *Transfusion* 2012;**52**:431–9.

236   Leiby DA. Emerging infectious agents. *Dev Biol (Basel)* 2005;**120**:11–5.

CHAPTER 52

Transfusion transmission of parasites

Bryan R. Spencer

American Red Cross, Dedham, MA, USA

Summary

Blood recipients in the United States (US) generally face a low risk of being transfused with a component contaminated with parasites. Quantifying the risk often depends on parameters that are unknown or poorly characterized, but estimates have remained stable in recent years at one transmission of parasitic infection per million transfusions.[1-2] This round figure obscures divergent trends for some of the agents of highest visibility as well as considerable differences in local risks across the country.

A comprehensive review of 68 pathogens by the AABB's Transfusion Transmitted Diseases (TTD) Committee[3] identified four protozoan parasites among the agents of greatest concern, based on empirically established transfusion risk and regulatory/public perception. Human mobility patterns continue to be important factors associated with risk, due to high rates of international travel by US residents, the movement of military personnel, and large migration flows. Increased awareness, more refined risk assessments, and ongoing development of molecular tools and improved diagnostics are helping clarify the risks. For *Babesia microti* and other *Babesia* species, recent research suggests that transfusion transmission has been historically undercounted, given that transfusion transmission can easily go undetected, especially when transfused to immunocompetent patients. Implementation of screening for *Trypanosoma cruzi*, the etiological agent of Chagas disease, has significantly curbed the risk of transmission associated with immigrants from endemic countries in Latin America, while raising questions about the frequency of autochtonous transmission within the US. Transfusion of malaria parasites continues to be a rare occurrence in the US, with prevention strategies that rely wholly on deferral of at-risk donors. This chapter will discuss the parasitic agents most likely to be found in blood donors, the risks from each, and the strategies for eliminating or diminishing these risks.

Babesiosis

Concern about the risk for transfusion-transmitted babesiosis has grown more acute in the US over the last several years. Increased medical awareness, enhanced public surveillance, and greater scrutiny by regulators and blood centers have documented an expanding range of transmission in nature and more precise estimates of transfusion risk in endemic areas. *B. microti* is responsible for the large majority of clinical cases and transfusion transmission events

in the US, but is one of at least four distinct genotypes documented within the country. In Europe, *Babesia divergens* causes most human illness from babesial infection, with increasingly more countries reporting human cases. Multiple *Babesia* species have been documented in Asia, which together with isolated reports from Africa, Australia, and South America indicate the emergence of human babesiosis as a global phenomenon.

Transmitted primarily by ixodid ticks, over 100 species of these intra-erythrocytic protozoan parasites infect a large number of vertebrate species worldwide.[4] *Babesia* infection is often clinically silent, with symptomatic infections more common with advancing age.[5] Clinical infections begin 1–6 weeks following tick bite and are frequently nonspecific, presenting with flulike symptoms including fever, headache, and myalgias. Risk for severe disease is higher in the elderly, the immunocompromised, and the asplenic; complications can include thrombocytopenia, hemolytic anemia, and renal, heart, or respiratory failure.[6] The case fatality rate can range from 5% to 10% for *B. microti*[6] to 42% for *B. divergens*.[7] That nearly all reported cases of *B. divergens* have occurred in asplenic hosts[7] almost certainly contributes to this disparity.

Human babesiosis is an emerging disease both within the US and globally. Since the first case of human babesiosis was recorded in the US in 1966,[8] fewer than 2000 cases were reported in the country over the next four decades.[9] During that time, the seven states considered "endemic"—Massachusetts, Connecticut, New York, Rhode Island, and New Jersey in the Northeast, and Minnesota and Wisconsin in the Upper Midwest—established their own reporting and surveillance systems. Isolated cases were sporadically identified in other states, sometimes in connection with a transfusion case. In 2009, the Council of State and Territorial Epidemiologists voted to make human babesiosis a nationally notifiable disease, with standardized laboratory, clinical, and epidemiologic criteria developed for diagnosis of tick-borne or transfusion-associated cases. Following implementation in 2011, the number of states adopting the reporting criteria has grown considerably and the number of cases reported has more than doubled the totals from the prior 45 years (see Table 52.1). The seven "endemic" states consistently account for 95% or more of all reported cases, but the number and distribution of locations finding cases outside these states (see Figure 52.1) suggest that the enhanced surveillance capacity may lead to higher numbers in future.

The primary agent responsible for human babesiosis in the US is *B. microti*. It is transmitted by the black-legged deer tick (*Ixodes*

Rossi's Principles of Transfusion Medicine, Fifth Edition. Edited by Toby L. Simon, Jeffrey McCullough, Edward L. Snyder, Bjarte G. Solheim, and Ronald G. Strauss.
© 2016 John Wiley & Sons, Ltd. Published 2016 by John Wiley & Sons, Ltd.

Table 52.1 History of reporting of babesiosis in US before and after it was made a nationally notifiable disease (2011)*

	1966—2010	2011	2012	2013	2014
Number of states reporting	≈7	18	22	27	31
Number of states with cases	Varies	15	14	22	20
Number of cases reported	<2000	1124	911	1762	1571
Number transfusion cases	159**	10	7	14	Unknown

* Data from Spencer (2009)[9] and CDC (2011, 2012, 2015).[10–13]
** Reported in Herwaldt et al. for 1979–2009.[14]

scapularis, previously known as I. dammini), the vector of Lyme disease. Heightened awareness and scrutiny, together with increased molecular characterization of patient isolates of Babesia parasites, present a complex picture of Babesia transmission in nature. B. microti is now considered a species complex composed of three distinct clades with identical morphology but partly distinct vertebrate hosts and potentially differing levels of pathogenicity for humans.[15] Babesia duncani, first recognized in the early 1990s, is morphologically identical to B. microti but antigenically and genetically distinct, and has been found in humans, dogs, and wildlife in the Western US.[16] Babesia sp. MO1 was originally thought to be the primary European parasite B. divergens, but it has been shown to be distinct on the basis of genetic sequence difference and in vitro characteristics. All three human cases (in Missouri, Kentucky, and Washington) were in splenectomized patients, and this genotype has also been found in rabbits in Massachusetts and Texas.[17–19] Additional genotypes designated Babesia sp. CA-type (CA1–CA4) are morphologically indistinct and serologically cross-reactive with B. duncani but are genetically distinct, and have caused severe illness in four patients all of whom lacked their spleen.[16] Finally, the first human case in Tennessee, found in an immunocompromised hunter with heavy tick exposure, has been characterized as "genetically distinct" from previously identified zoonotic agents.[20] Investigation of the patient's rural property found Babesia sp. MO1 in Eastern cottontail rabbits, but detailed characterization of the patient's isolate remains unpublished to date.[19–21] Outside of B. microti, very little is known about the geographic distribution, vertebrate reservoirs, tick vectors, or virulence in humans of other Babesia species. That nearly all patients are asplenic suggests that most transmission goes undetected. In sum, at least four distinct genotypes of Babesia protozoa are known to cause human illness in the US, with very little still known about the risk posed to human health and the blood supply by the newly described species and isolates.

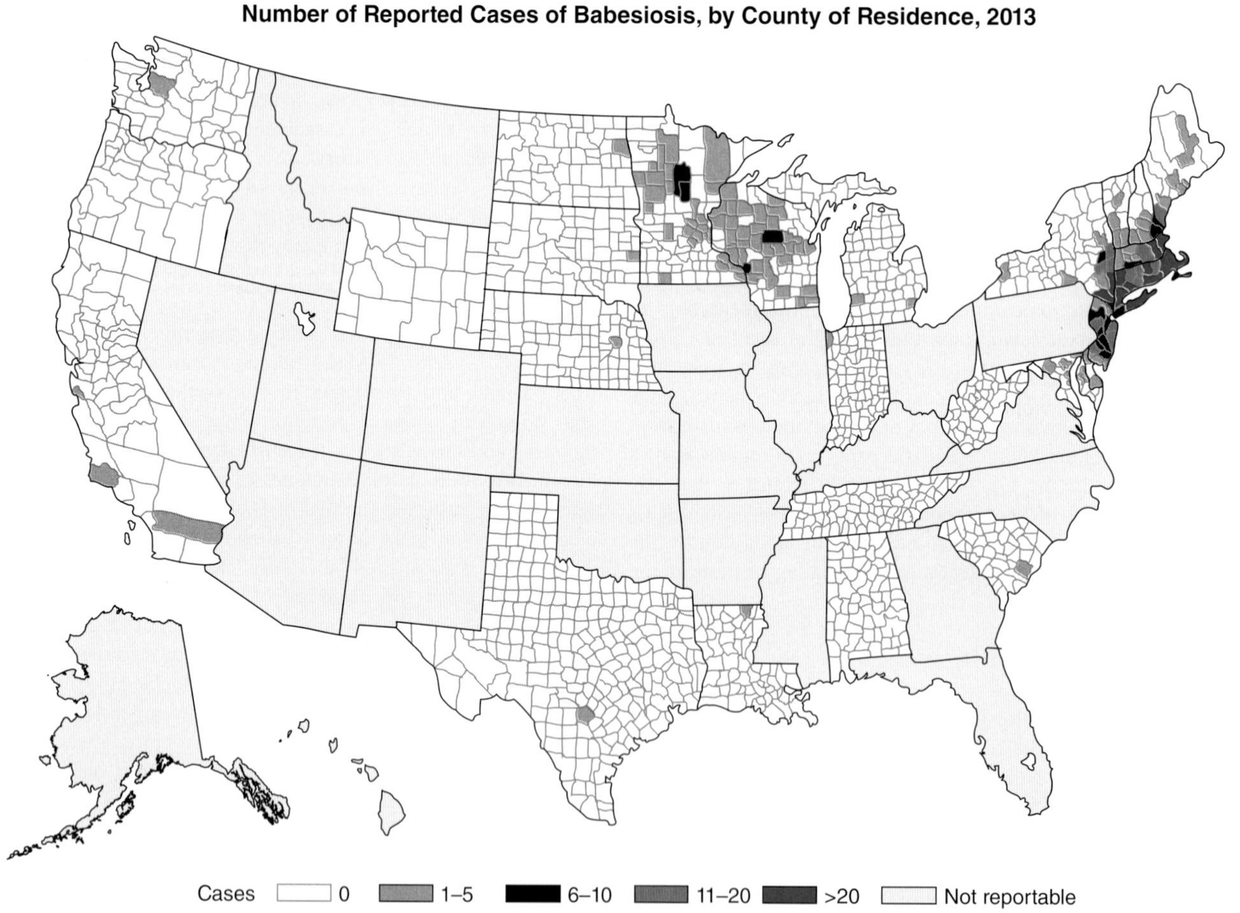

Number of Reported Cases of Babesiosis, by County of Residence, 2013

Cases: 0 · 1–5 · 6–10 · 11–20 · >20 · Not reportable

Figure 52.1 Distribution of reported cases of babesiosis in the US in 2013. Image courtesy of US Centers for Disease Control and Prevention. N = 1750; county of residence was unknown for 12 of the 1762 patients. Cases are mapped to the patients' county of residence, which was not necessarily where they became infected. One or more cases were reported by 22 of 27 states that conducted surveillance. Source: US Centers for Disease Control and Prevention (http://www.cdc.gov).

A similar picture of increasing complexity is also emerging in Europe. Reports of human babesiosis are rare, with fewer than 50 human cases reported since the first report in 1957, a fatal case in a splenectomized Yugoslav farmer.[7] Most European cases are attributed to *B. divergens*, a bovine pathogen, with cases reported from several countries in Western Europe, the former Yugoslavia, and the former USSR.[22] Risk for human infection correlates geographically with the presence of infected cattle populations and areas infested by the tick vector, *Ixodes ricinus*; little is understood about the role that spleen-intact human populations and silent carriage of *B. divergens* might play in terms of risk to the blood supply.[22] A new variant isolated from asplenic patients in Italy, Austria, and Germany has been designated *B. venatorum*.[7] Also, a single case of autochtonous *B. microti* has been identified in Europe due to this agent, likely by blood transfusion,[7] although entomologic[23] and serologic[24] evidence suggests transmission is much more common than recognized.

Finally, in East Asia, the first case of autochtonous human babesiosis in Japan has been confirmed, due to transfusion-acquired *B. microti*–like infection;[25] asymptomatic *B. microti*–like infection has been documented in Taiwan;[26] and the first case of human babesiosis has been reported from Korea, with the isolated parasite designated KO1 and appearing to be related to *Babesia* species that infect sheep.[27] Dozens of cases have been newly reported from China, in both healthy and immunocompromised populations.[28–29] Isolated reports from Africa, Australia, and South America reflect the ubiquity of the parasite in vertebrates worldwide.[19]

The two most important characteristics of *B. microti* infection driving transfusion risk are the probability that most infections are clinically silent[30] and the ability of immunocompetent persons to carry infection for lengthy periods.[31] There is little direct evidence for the proportion of infections that are asymptomatic, but one recent review suggests that one-half of children and one-fourth of immunocompetent adults have no symptoms with *B. microti* infection.[5] This figure may overstate the clinical attack rate in children, who do not seem to face lower risk of acquiring *Babesia* infection than adults[32] but whose case counts[11–12] and population-adjusted incidence rates[33] are much lower than those of persons aged 60 and older. Moreover, a comparison of seropositivity rates of blood donors with symptomatic cases reported to public health departments also supports a high ratio of clinically silent to apparent infections. For example, New London County in southeastern Connecticut reported an average annual case rate of 14 cases per 100,000 population from 2011 to 2013,[34] but serological testing in 8000 blood donors across eight years showed 1.8% with *B. microti* antibodies, a 130-fold difference.[35] A similar comparison of testing performed on islands off the coast of Massachusetts yields 1.4% seropositivity in donors compared to 24 cases per 100,000 population,[33] a 57-fold difference. The ratio of inapparent to apparent infections is not estimable from these numbers without also considering the duration of detectable antibody, but available evidence suggests elevated antibody titers lasting 6–12 months, especially in the presence of extended parasitemia.[31] This latter characteristic, of course, is the primary driver of transfusion risk, and early research confirmed the ability of the parasite to persist for several months in untreated individuals.[31] In vitro studies indicate that while cold storage reduces viability, some parasites do survive storage at 4 °C and can remain infective for 21 to 31 days.[36,37] The implications of long-term carriage of *B. microti* are amply demonstrated in a case in Minnesota, where an asymptomatic donor infected recipients from each of four donations over a six-month period.[38]

A recent review published by the CDC summarizes 162 transfusion cases in the US from 1979 to 2009.[14] Of these, 159 were due to *B. microti*, most of which occurred in the seven "endemic" states, but another 13% occurred in 21 different states due to interstate movement of blood donors or blood components. The overall mortality rate was 18%, consistent with the advanced age (median age 65) and also the compromised immune status of many recipients, due to asplenia or other morbidity. The median range from transfusion to diagnosis was six weeks, although in some cases it extended over seven months. The overwhelming majority of implicated components were red cells, with a median storage age at time of transfusion of 16 days and four cases where red cells were between 35 and 40 days old. Another three cases were caused by *B. duncani* and occurred in California and Washington. Outside the US, transfusion transmission of *B. microti* has been documented once each in Canada, Germany, and Japan, the only countries besides the US to report transfusion cases of *Babesia*.[39] Only Germany and Japan's cases reflect autochthonous transmission, however, whereas in Canada the donor acquired infection while on holiday in the United States.

Few studies have directly measured the risk for transfusion transmission of *Babesia* parasites. Given the absence of symptoms in healthy individuals, studying paired donor–recipient specimens is the most secure way of estimating the risk in endemic areas. One study estimated that 1/617 units (0.17) of PRBCs might be at risk for transmitting *B. microti* in the state of Connecticut, and that the risk from platelets was estimated as zero.[40] In another Connecticut study, analysis of paired donor–recipient specimens involving chronically transfused patients indicated one possible *B. microti* seroconversion out of nearly 2000 evaluable transfusions.[41] Infectivity of different blood components is not easy to determine given that the likelihood both of establishing infection in the recipient and of that infection becoming clinically detected are likely to depend on the dose of parasites, the length of storage, and the recipient's immune status. In the aforementioned case in Minnesota, one of three recipients of platelets became infected with *B. microti*, whereas three of three surviving recipients of red cells became infected.[38] In another case, out of six individuals transfused with RBCs from an asymptomatic donor, two neonates and one elderly adult became infected, whereas two other neonates and a child remained aparasitemic.[42] Lookback studies in Connecticut found that 13% of seropositive or parasitemic donors transmitted infection, but 50% of recipients of red cells from an index donation became infected, compared to only 10% of those receiving red cells from the donor's prior donation.[43] Investigational testing performed under research protocols in endemic New England states suggests a residual risk of 1 per 20,000–30,000 transfused units[44] Published numbers at present suggest a frequency of transmission of 1 per million, but the authors note that the 162 recorded cases "undoubtedly represent a fraction of those that occurred."[14]

Traditional diagnosis of *Babesia* infection relies on microscopic exam of Giemsa-stained blood films. This method, however, requires an experienced microscopist, and a high enough index of clinical suspicion to perform the exam. In US transfusion cases, diagnosis is often made incidentally and not due to clinical suspicion.[14] Immunofluorescent assay (IFA) diagnosis is both sensitive and specific for measuring exposure, but it is too time consuming for mass screening and involves subjectivity on the reader's part. Automated IFA assays have been employed under investigational protocols with high throughput and strong performance characteristics.[45] Inoculation of blood from suspected human cases into laboratory animals offers both high sensitivity and specificity, but its utility is limited to research investigation. Real-time polymerase chain reaction (PCR) appears to be highly sensitive and a valuable complement to serological methods.[44–48]

Human babesiosis has historically been treated with clindamycin and quinine (CQ), but atovaquone with azithromycin has emerged as the first-line recommendation in the US given the fewer collateral effects.[5] Treatment with CQ continues to be recommended for severe cases. In severe cases, partial or whole blood exchange transfusion might be indicated, especially for severe infections of *B. divergens*.[5]

In the absence of a licensed screening assay, prevention of transfusion-transmitted babesiosis currently relies exclusively on a question asking the donor if they have ever had babesiosis. This strategy is insufficient in that only donors whose *Babesia* infection was symptomatic and properly diagnosed will self-report a risk. Because the majority of *B. microti* infections are silent or remain undiagnosed,[5] parasitemic donors can escape detection. In the American Red Cross, only about 1 in 20,000 donors in Massachusetts or Connecticut reports a history of babesiosis during health history, showing the low sensitivity of the question.[49] Seasonal deferral in endemic areas would adversely impact the blood supply, and would not address the issues of nonresidents who travel to endemic areas and the transfer of blood products from endemic to non-endemic areas.[39] The predictive value of self-reported exposure to ticks in relation to serological status has proven low in Wisconsin and Connecticut donors.[39] Available evidence indicates that neither serology nor nucleic acid detection alone will be sufficient to effectively mitigate risk.[45–47] Cost-effectiveness modeling suggests that screening for *Babesia* will be costly even if limited to the most highly endemic parts of the US, estimated at $5 to 6 million per quality-adjusted life-year.[50]

As with other protozoan infections, pathogen inactivation methods hold promise in reducing the risk from transfusion-transmitted babesiosis. Photochemical treatments currently under development indicate parasite reductions of 5 logs in whole blood.[51] Equivalent efficacy has been shown in platelets and plasma.[52] Market interest in *Babesia*-screened red cell products is not well defined in the United States given the recent, and limited, availability to transfusion services.

Chagas disease

Risk for transfusion transmission of *Trypanosoma cruzi* infection has declined considerably in the United States with the widespread implementation of donor screening in 2007. Prior to that, concern had grown from the late 1980s forward with documentation of a small number of transfusion transmissions along with recognition of the potentially large human reservoir population due to the growing Hispanic population in the United States. Endemic in Central and South America and in Mexico, this protozoan hemoflagellate is transmitted in nature by reduviid bugs, or triatomines. These bugs have a tendency to bite on the face (and hence are called *kissing bugs*), but do not directly inject the parasite in their bite. Rather, the insect vector deposits the infective metacyclic forms of the trypanosomes in its feces during or soon after the blood meal, which is rubbed into the wound or transferred to susceptible membranes in the eye or mouth by the sleeping host. Triatomids competent for transmitting *T. cruzi* are widespread in the Americas, including in the United States, where autochthonous transmission occurs.[53] The agent is readily transmitted by blood transfusion, solid organ transplantation, and congenital transmission.[54] Rare outbreaks from contaminated food or drinks have also been reported.[55] Symptoms during the acute phase last four to six weeks

and are characterized by mild symptoms, including fever, malaise, and edema of the face, as well as lymphadenopathy and hepatosplenomegaly.[56] The fatality rate in the acute phase is usually less than 5%, and many cases go unrecognized. During this period, parasites are readily detectable in peripheral blood.[54] The ensuing chronic phase is lifelong, with infections that remain asymptomatic and parasitemia that is low grade and intermittent.[56] Ten to 30 years later, 30–40% of carriers will develop serious sequelae involving the cardiac and/or digestive features (megacolon and mega-esophagus). Chagas is estimated to kill about 12,000 people annually, mostly due to cardiac complications.[57] Acute stage treatment with benznidazole or nifurtimox leads to cure in 50–80% of cases, but treatment during the chronic phase is less effective at eliminating infection, and therapies for slowing disease progression once symptomatic are mostly experimental but are under active investigation.[56]

Public health authorities have achieved considerable success in reducing risk and morbidity from Chagas disease in the last three decades. Whereas in the early 1980s an estimated 17 million residents of Latin America were infected and 100 million lived in areas at risk for transmission, current estimates are roughly eight million infected and 65 million at risk for insect transmission.[56] Annual incidence of cases has dropped more sharply, from 700,000 new cases annually to 28,000 or so currently, a 96% decline.[56–57] This success began with the Southern Cone Initiative, inaugurated in six South American countries in 1991, which sought to eliminate domestic infection by *Triatoma infestans* (the primary vector in several countries) and to interrupt transfusion transmission through universal donor screening.[58] Subsequent efforts were adopted in the remaining regions of Latin America, tailored to the different species of vectors and the ecologic conditions found throughout.

The adoption of universal blood screening in Latin American countries has dramatically lowered the risk for transfusion transmission in endemic countries. Whereas in the early to mid-1990s only four of 17 Latin American countries for which data were compiled had achieved universal donor screening, now 20 of 21 have implemented universal testing.[57] Estimates within the last 20 years were that nearly 2000 transfusion transmission events might occur annually across the region[59] or even within Mexico alone,[60] but the adoption of universal screening based on assays of high sensitivity[61] suggests a sharply lower risk today.

Clearly, the risk in the United States and other receiving countries of Latin American immigrants depends on their immigrants' risk for acquisition of infection extending decades into the past. Recent US census figures estimate that 54 million Hispanics live in the United States, of whom two-thirds are of Mexican origin,[62] 4.8 million are Central American, and 3.1 million are of South American origin. Roughly one-third of these residents are foreign-born, and 40% of them arrived to the US prior to 1990,[62] before the intensification of control programs in endemic countries. This suggests that a very large number of Hispanic immigrants might have been exposed long before entering the US. Current estimates project that 300,000 Hispanic immigrants in the US may be infected with *T. cruzi*.[54] Canada and Australia are estimated to have more than 1000 *T. cruzi*–infected immigrants each,[63] and Europe between 68,000 and 123,000, nearly entirely undiagnosed.[58] Within the US, 55% of Hispanic residents are found in California, Florida, and Texas, and eight states have a Hispanic population of 1 million or greater. Hence, the Hispanic population in the US is concentrated in few states, but risk for transfusion transmission of *T. cruzi* can be found countrywide.[62]

Until the licensure of a screening test in December 2006, there were seven reported cases of *T. cruzi* transfusion transmission in the

United States and Canada,[64] and five cases of transmission associated with solid organ transplantation.[65,66] The actual number of transfusion cases was undoubtedly higher, in that all seven cases were detected in immunocompromised patients.[64] Although platelet products were implicated in six of these seven events, robust estimates for infectivity of different blood components were not available until recently. Prior estimates of ≈20% risk of transmission from a *T. cruzi*–infected donor were based on studies conducted in endemic countries where transfusion of fresh whole blood is common.[59] Lookback studies based on large numbers suggest that risk of transmission by blood is less than 2% overall, ranging from 0% in PRBCs or plasma to 13% in platelets.[67] A higher inoculum of parasites in platelet concentrates compared to plasma and whole blood might partially explain this difference.[68]

The approach for screening blood donors for *T. cruzi* is different in countries that are endemic for active transmission than for those where risk derives entirely or nearly so from immigrants from Latin America. As noted above, all but one of 21 endemic countries in the Americas have adopted universal screening. Given that infection is lifelong, seroprevalence and potential risk in blood donors remain elevated for decades longer than achievement of full or partial control of natural transmission. Available data on numbers at risk and prevalence in donors support the current practice of testing all donors at each donation in Latin America.[56,59] Elsewhere, however, selective testing has become the norm. Canada, France, England, and Japan have all implemented testing, but it is limited to presenting donors with identifiable risk factors relating to own or maternal birth in Latin America or exposure through travel or residence in the region.[69–72] Donor loss is mitigated, costs are reduced, and the residual risk following testing is vanishingly small.

In the United States, the widespread screening for *T. cruzi* that followed licensure of the first serological screening test by the US Food and Drug Administration (FDA) provided an abundance of data on the prevalence and distribution of Chagas in the US. Data from the first two years of testing yielded seroprevalence of 1:7000 donors,[73] with 25% of repeat reactive donations confirmed by RIPA (radioimmunoprecipitation assay), a non-FDA-licensed confirmatory assay. On the basis of very strong performance characteristics of the commercial enzyme-linked immunosorbent assay (ELISA) used for screening, together with the very low risk for incident infection in donors with a negatively screened donation, the FDA's Blood Products Advisory Committee endorsed selective testing for US donors where one negative donation would qualify them going forward, formalized in guidance issued by the FDA in 2010.[74] More recent seroprevalence studies reflect lower prevalence of 1 per 40,000 donors, possibly due to culling of prevalent infections from the donor pool in the earliest years of testing.[75] In areas with high numbers of Hispanic donors, such as Texas, rates may be several-fold higher, such as the 1:6500 confirmed antibody-positive rate in Texas.[76] As of February 14, 2015, the AABB Chagas Biovigilance website indicates 2032 confirmed positive donations in the United States from January 2007 forward, with cases widely distributed but concentrated in California, Florida, Texas, and other states with large Hispanic populations.[77]

An interesting finding triggered by the investigations of seropositive donors in the US and their risk profiles is documentation of a number of presumed autochthonous cases. At least nine of the 11 triatomines species found in the US are competent vectors of *T. cruzi*, and two dozen or more vertebrate species serve as natural wildlife hosts of the parasite.[54] Although domestically transmitted cases had previously been documented,[53] they were very rare, and

the number of cases has now increased from 7 to 23.[78] Hence, unlike in other countries that have embraced selective testing strategies, risk in the US includes that from local transmission in addition to that from migrants. Current estimates suggest a seroprevalence of 1:354,000 donors due to local transmission, but prevalent risk would be mitigated by the testing of all donors at their first donation. The risk for incident infections in humans in the US is unknown, but new evidence suggests that triatomine feeding on humans may be more common than previously thought[79] and that domestic dogs might be the bridge between sylvatic cycles and peridomestic transmission.[80] Developing estimates of risk for autochtonous transmission in the US will help in the management of risk by blood transfusion as well as that from mother to child.

Aside from testing, additional options for risk reduction include donor exclusion, pathogen removal, and pathogen inactivation. Until Canada adopted selective testing of donors with identifiable risk factors, it simply excluded donors on the basis of residence and travel history in endemic areas. Such an approach is not specific and is likely feasible only where such donors constitute a small portion of the donor pool. Leukoreduction filters have been shown to lower the concentration of trypanosomes in blood,[81] but at least one case of transfusion transmission in platelets was from a leukoreduced, and irradiated, product.[64] A variety of photochemical treatment methods in platelets,[82] plasma,[83] and red cell components[84–85] all show promise in reducing the parasite load by several logs.

Malaria

Human malaria is caused by one of five species of protozoan parasites: *Plasmodium falciparum*, *Plasmodium vivax*, *Plasmodium malariae*, *Plasmodium ovale*, and *Plasmodium knowlesi*, the last of which has only recently been described.[86–87] Malaria is a significant cause of global morbidity and mortality, responsible for an estimated 200 million clinical cases annually and over half a million deaths, and it is especially severe among young children in sub-Saharan Africa.[86] Natural infection with malaria typically occurs through the bite of an infective female *Anopheles* mosquito. Less frequently, parasites might be transmitted through blood transfusion, organ transplant, parenteral exposure, or mother-to-child transmission.[88] The US recorded an average of three cases of transfusion-associated malaria per year between 1963 and 1989.[89] More recently, there were 13 cases recorded during the 1990s and seven from 2000 to 2012, dropping from about an average of one case per year to one every other year, equivalent to less than 0.05 per million donations.[90–97] This compares favorably to the historical estimate of 0 to 2 cases per million donations in non-endemic areas, as contrasted with an incidence of 50 cases per million donations in endemic countries.[98]

In malaria-endemic settings, where frequent boosting by infective mosquito bites helps induce and maintain protective immune responses, severe infection is rare for those who survive beyond early childhood.[99] In a non-immune population, such as that in the United States, clinical malaria presents as a febrile illness with paroxysms, possibly at regular intervals, with accompanying flulike symptoms. Complications can include severe anemia, hepatic involvement, cerebral alterations, renal failure, and shock.[100] The case fatality rate for malaria is generally low (less than 1% in developed countries)[101,102] but can surpass 10% in recipients of blood products.[89]

Once endemic throughout large parts of the country, malaria in the United States is now due almost exclusively to imported infections.[91–97] In a typical year, ≈1500 malaria infections are diagnosed in the US, more than 95% of which are found in US civilians who have visited endemic areas and in foreign civilians from endemic countries. A comprehensive review of transfusion-transmitted malaria in the US indicates that many of these infections were preventable, with >60% having occurred due to deviations from the prevailing deferral guidelines.[89] Of the cases in which donor exclusion guidelines were followed, *P. malariae* has a disproportionate effect, accounting for 65% of transfusion cases compared to representing only 4% of cases diagnosed in US travelers. This fact reflects the ability of *P. malariae* to remain at subpatent levels for lengthy periods, even up to 40 years.[103] Indeed, because malaria parasites from the four primary *Plasmodia* remain viable in blood stored at 4 °C for at least one week, there exists risk from these four species,[88] and presumably from *P. knowlesi* as well. *P. falciparum* malaria has been transmitted in blood stored for 19 days, as well as in units of platelets.[104] Interval to onset in transfusion cases is likely to vary by species, with *P. falciparum* being the quickest to develop at about 10 days, *P. vivax* taking 16 days, and *P. malariae* taking 40 days or more.[88] Where a donor has been implicated, recent history in the US implicates presumably semi-immune visitors from endemic areas. Over a 20-year period, only one US civilian without previous residence in malaria-endemic countries has been implicated in transfusion transmission, in contrast to 28 former residents of endemic countries.[89]

In the absence of an FDA-approved blood-screening assay, prevention of transfusion-transmitted malaria in the United States has long relied on exclusion of presenting donors with elevated risk for malaria infection. The criteria are oriented to determining risk on the basis of prior infection with malaria, prior residence in a malarial country, or recent travel to a malaria risk area. In 2013, the FDA issued new guidance[105] that provided significant changes to draft guidance issued in 2000 and a 1994 memo that were the basis of previous policy. Continuity of policy exists in many important respects, including deferral for:

1 History of malaria within three years;
2 Residence in a malaria-endemic country within three years; and
3 Travel to a malaria-endemic area within one year.

Important clarifications or definitions were added, however, that represented meaningful change from the prior policy:

1 A *malaria-endemic* area was now defined as any area with malaria where CDC recommends antimalarial chemoprophylaxis in travelers in *The Yellow Book*, whereas previously any nonzero risk was considered *endemic*.
2 *Travel to a malaria-endemic area* was now defined as travel of duration between 24 hours and five years, whereas previously even the briefest exposure –including land travel through a risk area—could trigger deferral.
3 *Residence in a malaria-endemic country* was now defined as a continuous stay of longer than five years in a country or countries having any malaria-endemic areas.
4 Donors who meet the definition of a *resident in a malaria-endemic country* will be deferred for three years following travel to a malaria-endemic country unless they have lived for three continuous years in a non-endemic country.

These first two changes followed published evidence[106–107] and discussion at Blood Products Advisory Committee meetings that showed a vanishingly small risk for infection with the large majority of donors receiving the one-year travel deferral, but a significant impact on availability equivalent to ≈1% of presenting donors. The third change acknowledges the lengthy exposure typically required

to acquire partial immunity that allows for asymptomatic carriage, whereas the final change reflects caution against the possibility that partial immunity may be boosted and sustained by return to endemic areas.[99]

Advances in diagnostics have created opportunities for non-endemic countries to implement strategies that lessen the impact of malaria deferrals while minimizing risk of transfusion transmission. In Europe, regulations published by the Council of Europe in 2006 and subsequently updated[108] endorse the use of validated immunological tests to shorten the deferral period of donors with potential malaria risk who test negative: Those donors who have lived for six months or more in a malaria-endemic area are acceptable as blood donors if they test antibody-negative at least four months after their last visit to a malaria area, as opposed to being permanently deferred. Likewise, donors who report a travel history of less than six months in duration to an endemic area may be accepted as blood donors if they test antibody-negative at least four months after their last visit to a malaria area, in contrast to a one-year (no malaria symptoms reported) or three-year deferral (malaria-like symptoms within six months of return from endemic area).[108] Since 2001, England has used an enzyme immunoassay (EIA) based on three recombinant *P. falciparum* antigens and one *P. vivax* antigen (all to the erythrocytic merozoite stage) to shorten the deferral period for at-risk donors to six months for those testing negative.[109] Australia also seeks to reinstate deferred donors on the basis of this same test,[110] and a few other countries employ malaria donor-screening tests on a routine basis.[111] Although not all five *Plasmodia* are screened for in the assay adopted by England, it accounts for the two species causing most cases of transfusion transmission and does appear to have some cross-reactivity with other species.[112] Immunofluorescent antibody tests (IFATs) for malaria antibody detection tend to be sensitive, but have the limitations of being time-consuming and subjective. Direct methods for detection of malaria infection are also available. Most widely used for malaria diagnosis worldwide is Giemsa- or Wright-stained blood films, although their use is not practical for mass screening in non-endemic areas, where labor costs are prohibitive and the expertise is lacking. Assays detecting circulating parasite antigens such as histidine-rich protein 2 (HRP) and lactate dehydrogenase (LDH) offer sensitivity equivalent to microscopy for *P. falciparum* but are less sensitive for *P. vivax* below a parasite density of 200 parasites per microliter,[100] still insufficient to prevent transfusion transmission.

A variety of nucleic amplification assays allow for detection of one or more malaria species. Conventional[113] and seminested PCR[114] screening of blood bank samples have detection thresholds on the order of 10^{-3} parasites/μl. Similar to *Babesia* infection, malaria transfusion risk cannot fully be mitigated by serologic or nucleic acid detection alone. Although biological outliers, a small proportion of individuals retain low-level infection that lasts for several years, including beyond the exclusion period for prior residents of endemic countries.[115–117] With an infectious dose theoretically as low as 1–10 parasites per unit of blood, however, even the most sensitive nucleic acid detection methods cannot reduce the risk to zero. Malaria antibody duration is proportional to length of exposure, however,[118] and is hence an informative complement to direct parasite detection methods for reducing transfusion risk.

Leishmaniasis

Leishmania species are a large group of protozoan parasites with broad distribution worldwide.[119] *Leishmania* are transmitted in nature by the bite of a female phlebotomine sandfly, but can be transmitted in blood components and, rarely, congenitally or sexually.[120] Clinical manifestations can vary widely, ranging from asymptomatic infection to severe illness with visceral, cutaneous, or mucosal involvement. The visceral form (kala-azar) is characterized by fever, wasting, hepatosplenomegaly, and pancytopenia, and if untreated is usually lethal.[120] Cutaneous forms involve progressive skin lesions that become ulcerative, sometimes with mucosal involvement. Although endemic in about 88 countries, the public health burden is hardly uniform. More than 90% of visceral cases appear in Bangladesh, Brazil, India, Nepal, and Sudan, and about 90% of cutaneous leishmaniasis occurs in Afghanistan, Brazil, Peru, Iran, Saudi Arabia, and Syria.[120] The World Health Organization estimates that two million new infections occur annually, about 1.5 million due to cutaneous leishmaniasis (CL) and half a million due to visceral leishmaniasis (VL), and that as many as 12 million people worldwide are infected.[120] The distribution is expanding due to myriad factors that include ecological disturbances, growing urbanization in developing countries, and the growing numbers of people immunocompromised by HIV infection or other reasons.[120] The United States is home to both phlebotomine sandflies and *Leishmania* parasites, but autochtonous transmission is limited to infrequent and isolated outbreaks,[121–122] with fewer than 50 human cases documented.

The infective form of *Leishmania* parasites in the sandfly is the flagellated promastigote; in humans and other vertebrate hosts, the parasite takes the form of an oval amastigote that is typically found in phagocytic vacuoles of macrophages and other mononuclear phagocytes.[120] Diagnostic methods include microscopic visualization of amastigotes in the tissue aspirates or biopsies from spleen, bone marrow, or lymph nodes, or in the peripheral blood buffy coat. The duration of parasite circulation in the blood can vary across the >20 *Leishmania* species, but in any case rarely lasts more than one year.[123] The immunological response differs according to the clinical syndrome, with VL leading to a stronger and more enduring antibody production than CL.[124] The conventional treatment of leishmaniasis has been pentavalent antimony, but new strategies include lipid formulations of amphotericin B, injectable paromomycin, and miltefosine.[124]

The risk for transfusion transmission of *Leishmania* may be underappreciated and its occurrence underreported, with about a dozen probable or confirmed cases having been reported in the literature[125] over the past 60 years. Interestingly, half of these cases were in infants, and nine of 10 were in children six years old or younger.[119] The average incubation period was over seven months, with fever and hepatosplenomegaly being the most common symptoms.[119] Studies from endemic areas, as well as studies of US military personnel returning from operations in southwest Asia, highlight the potential risk. Viscerotropic *L. donovani* and *L. tropica* isolated from US servicemen have been shown to survive at least 25 days in whole blood or PRBCs stored at 4 °C, at least five days in platelet concentrates at 24 °C, and at least 35 days in glycerolized RBCs frozen at −70 °C. Further, *L. tropica*–spiked whole blood stored at 4 °C for 30 days retained infectivity to healthy mice. Fresh frozen plasma did not support parasite survival.[126]

Because transfusion transmission would likely be mistaken for sandfly transmission in endemic areas, and because infection may be subclinical and intermittent in immunocompetent individuals, assessing the risk for transmission in blood is a challenge. A number of studies performed on blood donors across Southern Europe and Brazil indicate rates of detectable parasitemia reaching 10% or more

in some areas,[127] whereas a recent review compiles several reports documenting the widespread nature of asymptomatic infection in healthy populations.[128] Numbers of this magnitude suggest that the actual transfusion risk might be quite a bit higher than indicated by published reports, which represent cases detected in largely immunosuppressed individuals.

The options to blood banks to prevent distribution of *Leishmania*-contaminated blood are limited. Targeted donor exclusion is practiced selectively in the United States, specifically relating to the risk of armed services personnel and other travelers to theaters of war in Iraq harboring *Leishmania* species upon return. To prevent this, AABB established a 12-month deferral during Operation Desert Storm in Iraq in the early 1990s, and again in 2003.[125] Given the broad distribution of *Leishmania* across 88 countries, travel-based deferrals might prejudice blood availability if strictly applied, but the existing malaria deferral no doubt lowers the risk associated with travel to the 68 countries also endemic for malaria transmission.[3] Because serological status correlates poorly with asymptomatic infection,[123] antibody tests hold little promise for donor screening. Photochemical inactivation of different *Leishmania* species has shown 4-log reduction of amastigote and promastigote forms in pheresis platelets,[129] and another study demonstrated 5 to 6-log reductions in both platelets and plasma.[130] Another study utilizing riboflavin and ultraviolet light was only partially effective in whole blood, with a 2.3-log reduction in parasite load.[131] Furthermore, filtration of leukocytes at both the point of collection and the bedside has been shown to dramatically lower free and intracellular *Leishmania* parasites.[132]

Toxoplasmosis

Toxoplasma gondii is an obligate, intracellular protozoan that has felines as a definitive host but can grow in any mammalian or avian organs or tissues.[133] Felines become infected in nature by consuming intermediate rodent hosts with infective *Toxoplasma* cysts in the brain or skeletal muscle. The parasite is ubiquitous in nature and can infect a wide variety of animals, including sheep, cattle, and pigs, developing into cysts that remain infective for years. Human infection can occur through many modes of transmission. Most commonly, they include consumption of raw or undercooked meat containing *Toxoplasma* cysts, and accidental ingestion of *T. gondii* oocysts from soil or cat litter contaminated with excreted oocysts. Increasingly, water is implicated as a vehicle for transmission.[133] There are rare reports of infection acquired via solid organ transplantation and blood transfusion.[133] Finally, congenital transmission can occur when the mother acquires primary infection during pregnancy, but the probability of transmission to the fetus (and clinical outcome) depends on the timing of infection.[133]

Up to one-third of the world's population is estimated to be infected with *T. gondii*. About 90% of primary infections are subclinical, and they appear to be lifelong. Illness in those with symptomatic infections is usually nonspecific and self-limiting, typically involving fever and isolated swollen lymph nodes. More rarely, infection might lead to myocarditis, pneumonitis, hepatitis, or encephalitis.[133] Toxoplasmosis is usually severe in immunocompromised hosts, and it has emerged as a common opportunistic infection of persons with AIDS. Estimates of seroprevalence across countries vary from less than 10% to greater than 90%, and the acquisition of infection depends on an array of local and household factors that include hygiene and sanitation, source and preparation of food, exposure to felines, and climatic factors influencing the survivability of oocysts in nature.[133] In the United States, the National Health and Nutrition Examination Survey (NHANES) from 1999 to 2004 indicated an age-adjusted seroprevalence <10%, with foreign-born residents three times as likely as US-born residents to be antibody-positive, 24.8% to 8.2%.[134]

Transfusion transmission of toxoplasmosis was reported nearly 40 years ago, in a case where patients with acute leukemia were transfused with leukocytes from donors with chronic myelogenous leukemia.[135] Despite the scarcity of reports of transfusion transmission, the risk has been well documented in cardiac transplant patients as well as liver and kidney recipients.[133] Seroprevalence studies in healthy blood donors indicate a broad range of antibody prevalence from 7.4% in Durango, Mexico,[136] to 75% in northeastern Brazil.[137] Antibody presence is long-lived and does not necessarily denote infectivity. Unfortunately, little information is available on the long-term kinetics of antibody development and patent parasitemia over long periods of time, and parasite isolation or detection by PCR is rarely useful in immunocompetent patients, except in diagnosis of ocular toxoplasmosis.[138] Otherwise, parasitemia in healthy individuals seems to be low-grade and intermittent, with low probability of detection. The ability of the parasite to survive 50 days at 4 °C[135] and the isolated reports of transfusion transmission in the literature both establish an element of risk.

Prevention of transfusion-transmitted toxoplasmosis is not feasible with either donor exclusion or serologic screening. In most places, discarding units from seropositive donors would heavily prejudice blood availability, with unclear indications that positive antibody status of the donor implies risk for parasitemia. In high-prevalence countries, many blood recipients are likely to have been previously exposed. In an immunocompetent recipient, transfusion transmission is likely to go undetected. Given the parasite's ability to readily invade and replicate in leukocytes,[139] leukocyte filtration might diminish the risk in similar fashion as with cytomegalovirus. Whether inactivation treatments being evaluated for other protozoa might be of use for *Toxoplasma* remains unexplored.

Microfilariasis

Filarial worms are arthropod-borne macroparasites that can be caused by a number of different organisms. *Wuchereria bancrofti* and *Brugia* spp. cause lymphatic filariasis; *Loa loa*, *Onchocerca volvulus*, and *Mansonella streptocerca* cause nonlymphatic, subcutaneous filariasis; and *Mansonella ozzardi* and *Mansonella perstans* cause nonlymphatic infections of different body cavities and are typically asymptomatic or mild.[3] The filariases occur in more than 80 countries, and the health and socioeconomic burdens from lymphatic filariasis and *O. volvulus* are particularly severe, with an estimated prevalence of 120 million and 37 million infections, respectively.[140] These organisms share similar life cycles and are all transmitted by hematophagous arthropods. In each, adult female worms produce larvae called *microfilaria*, which for most species circulate in the bloodstream, sometimes with periodicity timed to their primary vector's feeding habits. The microfilaria are the infective form for insects, but when transmitted by transfusion they are incapable of propagating further.[141]

The lymphatic forms of filariasis, which cause elephantiasis, have been targeted by the World Health Organization as potentially eradicable, primarily by eliminating the human reservoir of microfilaria that infect the mosquito vectors through repeated mass administration of curative drugs.[140] Results from low- to moderate-prevalence areas in Egypt[142] and from moderate- to high-

prevalence parts of Papua New Guinea[143] indicate dramatic success in lowering human infections and even, surprisingly, reversing the pathology associated with infection.

There is little published information on the risk for transfusion transmission of filariasis. In most endemic areas, the risk for vector-acquired infection would be orders of magnitude greater than that from transmission for the average individual, given the relative degree of exposure to infective insect vectors and the limited rate of blood transfusion. However, limited studies from Nigeria have shown prevalence of microfilaria of 3.5% with *Loa loa*;[144] 15.6% with *M. perstans* and 1.3% with *L. loa*;[145] and 1.3% with unspecified microfilaria.[146] There has been at least one report of an American blood donor being found with microfilaria.[141] Isolated case reports of transfusion transmission exist from Italy[147] and India,[148] in both cases indicating that the outcome in blood recipients might often be no more severe than mild allergic reaction response to microfilarial antigens.

The microfilaria of both *W. bancrofti*[149] and *L. loa*[150] survive routine storage conditions for blood. Those from *M. ozzardi*[151] and from *B. malayi* and *W. bancrofti*[152] have been successfully recovered following cryopreservation in research laboratories. Given the modest clinical consequences even with direct transfusion, most countries appear to consider the risk to blood recipients too small to merit donor or component screening.

Summary

The current risk for transfusion transmission of parasites in the United States is not high, but it is likely greater than the prevailing estimate of one per million units. Until the recent licensure of a screening assay, it appears probable that hundreds of individuals donated annually while infected with *T. cruzi*, the result of demographic changes in the United States and its donor population. Although that implies potentially several cases of transfusion transmission annually, the adoption of testing for all donors at least once has brought the incident risk to near-zero.

Silent infection in semi-immune donors constitutes at least some risk for malaria transmission in blood products in the absence of serological and nucleic acid screening, but recent years have seen an average of one case every other year. Meanwhile, most presenting donors hold very small risk from travel exposure, and the three-year deferral for prior residency has high (even if imperfect) efficacy. Both serological and direct detection assays can contribute to enhanced safety against these and other parasitic agents. Broadly effective methods such as pathogen removal or inactivation also appear promising.

Perceived risk for *Babesia* species in blood is growing and represents the most commonly transmitted parasite in the United States. A recent review indicates growing recognition of transfusion-associated cases, and surveillance data following its publication document a frequency of roughly one per million transfusions. Undoubtedly, though, many cases remain undetected. The combination of asymptomatic infection in healthy donors, the lack of a licensed screening assay, and the mobility of both people and blood products altogether imply risks that are higher and geographically less circumscribed than appreciated.

Other parasites with wide global distribution are rarely documented as transfusion transmitted. *Leishmania* parasites frequently produce asymptomatic infection, but malaria travel exclusion policies interrupt risk from some donors while the adoption of universal leukoreduction in many countries further reduces the risk.

Toxoplasma gondii is a common infection worldwide, but parasitemia is not commonly found except in immunocompromised patients, who are not part of the donor population. Microfilaria of different species can be transmitted in blood products, but as a self-limiting infection producing allergic reaction is considered of modest clinical consequence. In sum, the potential for transfusion transmission exists from other parasites that cause human illness, but they are generally not considered significant enough to merit specific interventions.

Key references

A full reference list for this chapter is available at: http://www.wiley.com/go/simon/transfusion

3 Stramer SL, Hollinger FB, Katz LM, *et al.* Emerging infectious disease agents and their potential threat to transfusion safety. *Transfusion* 2009;**49**:1S–29S.

5 Vannier E, Krause PJ. Human babesiosis. *N Engl J Med* 2012;**366**:2397–407.

14 Herwaldt BL, Linden JV, Bosserman E, *et al.* Transfusion-associated babesiosis in the United States: a description of cases. *Ann Intern Med* 2011;**155**:509–19.

30 Ruebush II TK, Juranek DD, Chisholm ES, *et al.* Human babesiosis on Nantucket Island: evidence for self-limited and subclinical infections. *N Engl J Med* 1977;**297**:825–7.

54 Bern C, Kjos S, Yabsley MJ, Montgomery SP. *Trypanosoma cruzi* and Chagas' disease in the United States. *Clin Microbiol Rev* 2011;**24**:655–81.

57 Pan American Health Organization. Chagas fact sheet 2014. http://www.paho.org/hq/index.php?option=com_topics&view=readall&cid=5831&Itemid=40743&lang=en

89 Mungai M, Tegtmeier G, Chamberland M, Parise M. Transfusion-transmitted malaria in the United States from 1963 through 1999. *N Engl J Med* 2001;**344**:1973–8.

CHAPTER 53

Bacterial contamination of blood components

Richard J. Benjamin

Cerus Corporation, Concord, CA, USA

Bacterial contamination of blood components is a persistent but often overlooked problem in transfusion medicine. Although public attention has focused on transfusion-transmitted viral infection, improved methods of screening through donor questioning and testing have greatly reduced the transmission of hepatitis viruses and retroviruses. Given the reduction of viral transmission via allogeneic blood, the risk of bacterial contamination has emerged as the greatest residual threat of transfusion-transmitted disease. Before recent developments in skin preparation, diversion, and testing for bacterial contamination, the incidence of platelet bacterial contamination was approximately 1 in 1000 components and septic reactions were reported with 1 in 15–100,000 transfusions.[1] This chapter provides a brief overview of risks associated with blood components. The main focus is on approaches to minimize or eliminate the risk of bacterial contamination.

Transfusion-transmitted bacterial infection by red blood cells (RBCs)

Sepsis associated with the transfusion of bacterially contaminated RBC components is generally regarded as a very rare event, and appears to be declining in incidence. Prospective bacterial cultures of whole blood or RBC units show that 1–3000 units may be culture positive, mostly with skin commensals such as *Staphylococcus* spp. or *Propionibacterium* spp., but these proliferate poorly during storage at 1 to 6 °C. Organisms that grow well in the cold are more likely to be involved in septic reactions and then only after weeks of storage due to slow growth at those temperatures. An example of such a cryophilic organism is *Yersinia enterocolitica* where most cases of contamination occur after storage for 25 days.[2] Historical reports from New Zealand indicated a *Y. enterocolitica* transfusion-transmitted incidence rate of 1 in 65,000, with a fatality rate of 1 in 104,000 RBC units transfused.[3] Sepsis associated with the transfusion of Gram-negative bacterially contaminated RBCs is typically severe and rapid in onset. Patients frequently develop high fevers (temperatures as high as 109°F [42–43 °C] have been observed) and chills during or immediately following transfusion. From 1987 to 1996, 20 cases of *Yersinia*-infected RBC units in 14 states were reported to the US Centers for Disease Control and Prevention (CDC).[4] Twelve of the 20 recipients died in 37 days or less following transfusion. The median time from transfusion to death was 25 hours. Of the seven who developed disseminated intravascular coagulation, six died. Since that time, passive reporting studies from the United States,[5] France,[3] and the United Kingdom[6] of contaminated RBCs that caused symptoms of infection show a relative paucity of *Yersinia* spp. cases (Table 53.1).

From 1995 to 2004, 25 fatalities thought to be secondary to contamination of whole blood or RBC units were reported to the US Food and Drug Administration (FDA; Table 53.1). 20 of 25 (80%) were caused by Gram-negative organisms.[10] The risk of death from a bacterially contaminated RBC transfusion in the United States was estimated to be 0.13 per million in 1998–2000 in one independent study and can be estimated at 1:4,800,000 (0.21 per million) from the above FDA data over the longer time period of 1995–2004.[5] More recently, FDA reports document only four fatalities caused by contaminated RBC between 2005 and 2013, all caused by Gram-negative bacteria, including a single case of *Y. enterocolitica*. This translates to an estimated incidence of 1:32,500,000 (0.031 per million).[9] Similarly, French investigators reported 25 septic reactions associated with 4.1 million RBC transfusions (~1:141,000 transfusions), including four fatalities (1:1,025,000 transfusions) during a two-year period in 1996–1998. All fatalities were due to Gram-negative organisms; however, Gram-positive organisms comprised 13 of 29 (45%) isolated species, with a single case of *Y. enterocolitica* found in an autologous unit.[8] In contrast, between 2000 and 2008, 18 million RBC transfusions were transfused and only seven septic reactions were reported (1:2,571,000 transfusions), including two deaths (1:9,000,000 transfusions), and none were linked to Gram-positive units. A single fatality was caused by *Y. enterocolitica*. The dramatic decline in incidence of sepsis associated with RBC transfusion in the United States and France is unexplained, but may be linked to the widespread introduction of prestorage leukoreduction in both countries during the latter time periods.[7] Asymptomatic donors with transient bacteremia are presumed to be the source of most Gram-negative bacterial contamination. Leukoreduction during manufacture may decrease the risk of such contamination, as bacteria are ingested by leukocytes in the collected product and removed during processing.[11]

For *Y. enterocolitica*, implicated donors are typically found to have elevated immunoglobulin M (IgM) antibody titers, implying blood collection during an asymptomatic bacteremia following a recent infection.[4,12,13] In one case, an outbreak of *Serratia marcescens* sepsis was linked to contamination of RBCs in Denmark and Sweden.[14] The contamination was thought to involve the manufacturing process, because the sterile bag sets were autoclaved and put in a clean but not sterile outer plastic package. It was thought

Rossi's Principles of Transfusion Medicine, Fifth Edition. Edited by Toby L. Simon, Jeffrey McCullough, Edward L. Snyder, Bjarte G. Solheim, and Ronald G. Strauss.
© 2016 John Wiley & Sons, Ltd. Published 2016 by John Wiley & Sons, Ltd.

Table 53.1 Bacterial species involved in septic transfusion reactions and fatalities after RBC transfusions as reported to the french national hemovigilance program and the US FDA[7–9]

	France Sepsis (Fatalities)		United States Fatalities	
	1996–1998	2000–2008	1995–2004	2005–2013
Total Transfusions (Millions)	4.1	18	~120[#]	~126[#]
Gram-positive bacteria				
Staphylococcus aureus	2[%]	0	1	0
Coagulase-negative staphylococci	3	0	4	0
Enterococcus faecalis	1[&]	0	0	0
Streptococcus spp.	4[*]	0	0	0
Bacillus cereus	2	0	0	0
Propionibacterium acnes	1	0	0	0
Total Gram-positive bacteria	**13**	**0**	**5**	**0**
Gram-negative bacteria				
Enterobacter spp.	1 (1)	1	1	0
Escherichia coli	3[&]	1	3	1
Klebsiella spp.	1	3	3	0
Serratia spp.	2 (1)	0	5	1
Yersinia enterocolitica	1	1 (1)	2	1
Acinetobacter spp.	5 (1)[%]	1 (1)	0	0
Pseudomonas spp.	2 (1)	0	4	1
Proteus mirabilis	1	0	0	0
Pantoea agglomerans	0	0	1	0
Gram-negative bacilli	0	0	1	0
Total Gram-negative bacteria	**16 (4)**	**7 (2)**	**20**	**4**
TOTAL	**29 (4)**	**7 (2)**	**25**	**4**
Rate of sepsis	1:141,379	1:2,571,429	-	-
Rate of fatality	1:1,025,000	1:9,000,000	1:4,800,000	1:32,500,000

[*] in two cases two isolates of *Streptococcus spp.* were isolated from the implicate bag.
[%] In one case *S. aureus* and Acinetobacter spp. were both isolated from the implicated bag.
[&] In one case *Enterococcus spp.* and *E. coli* were both isolated from the implicated bag.
[#] estimated from the National Blood Collection and Utilization Surveys.[47]

that *S. marcescens* present in the dust in the factory contaminated the outside of the containers, and in the presence of moisture and a nutrient (the plasticizer diethylhexylphthalate), the bacteria proliferated and gained entry into the bag.[15]

Although autologous blood is generally considered a "safer" blood component than allogeneic blood, there have been at least six reported cases of bacterial contamination of autologous RBC units, five from Y. enterocolitica[16–20] and one from *Serratia liquefaciens*.[16] Fortunately, all reactions were nonfatal, presumably assisted by preformed immunity. Upon retrospective questioning, all patients infected by *Yersinia* spp. recalled gastrointestinal symptoms in the days before donation. In the case of *Serratia* spp. contamination, the patient's infected toe ulcer was presumed to be the source.

Transfusion-transmitted bacterial infection of plasma, cryoprecipitate, and derivatives

Cell-free products such as plasma and cryoprecipitate are stored in the frozen state and thus are rarely associated with significant contamination, as documented by the lack of any reported cases to the French National Hemovigilance Program between 2000 and 2008. However, *Pseudomonas cepacia* and *Pseudomonas aeruginosa* have been cultured from cryoprecipitate and plasma thawed in contaminated waterbaths.[21,22] The increasing use of thawed plasma and the advocacy for the use of liquid, never-frozen plasma[23] that may be stored at 1–6 °C for up to five days and 26 days, respectively, before transfusion imply that physicians need to be increasingly vigilant for septic reactions with these components.[24]

Products derived from blood components may also be contaminated with bacteria. Human serum albumin is a good culture medium and preserves the viability of contaminants. The heating step (60 °C for 10 hours) in the manufacturing of albumin is performed to inactivate certain viruses, not to ensure bacterial sterility.[25] This would require autoclaving (superheated under pressure), which would cause albumin to denature. On occasion, specific lots of albumin product have been found to be contaminated with bacteria, typically *Pseudomonas* spp.[26] These lots have produced endotoxic shock, transient bacteremias, and febrile reactions in recipients. Two patients in different hospitals developed *Enterobacter cloacae* septicemia after receiving albumin.[26,27] Cultures of unopened product grew *Stenotrophomonas multophilia* and *Enterococcus gallinarum* in addition to *E. cloacae*. This resulted in a worldwide recall of certain lots of 5% and 25% albumin. It is suspected that cracks in the glass bottles were responsible for the contamination. Manufacturing problems, therefore, are a source of bacterial risk from these derivatives.

Transfusion-transmitted syphilis

Treponema pallidum is a thin-walled, motile, spiral, Gram-negative rod or spirochete that cannot be visualized with Gram's stain and does not grow on bacteriologic media or cell culture. Although it is a bacterium, it is often treated as a distinct entity, different from other transfusion-transmitted bacterial organisms, and thus is addressed separately. Only 25% of patients with primary syphilis have a reactive serologic test for syphilis, and the test does not become routinely positive until the fourth week after the onset of symptoms; therefore, donors infected with *T. pallidum* may be asymptomatic with negative serology during periods of spirochetemia.[28,29] Although the organism does not survive prolonged storage at

4 °C, it may live for 1 to 5 days at these cold temperatures.[30,31] Therefore, a rare infection may be associated with transfusion of a fresh RBC unit from a donor who was in the seronegative phase at the time of donation. Platelets stored at 20 to 24 °C provide a more hospitable temperature for *T. pallidum*; however, this organism does not thrive with the high-oxygen tension in modern platelet storage bags. Since 1969, only three cases of transfusion-transmitted syphilis have been reported in the literature.[32–34] The extremely low rate of transfusion-transmitted syphilis infection likely results from the following: (1) donor questioning targeting high-risk behavior; (2) the cardiolipin-based assay, which, although an insensitive test in the acute post-infectious setting, does pick up a number of infected donors; (3) refrigerator storage, which results in the death of spirochetes; (4) antibiotics given to many patients at the time of platelet transfusion, which would be bactericidal for any viable organisms; and (5) donors excluded for a positive test for HIV, HCV, or HBV because of the high correlation between infection with *T. pallidum* and viruses such as these, even though the donors may have been in the seronegative phase of syphilis at the time of donation.[35] Because syphilis testing plays only a minor role in protecting the blood supply and is associated with a high degree of false-positive reactions, elimination of syphilis testing has been advocated. The counterargument is that such testing provides a surrogate marker for individuals at risk of other sexually transmitted diseases and, therefore, should be retained.

Transfusion-transmitted bacterial infection of platelets

Source of contamination

Platelets are stored at room temperature (20–24 °C) in oxygen-permeable bags with agitation for 5–7 days, which are excellent growth conditions for many aerobic and microaerophilic bacterial species. Bacteria most commonly enter the container at the time of phlebotomy through contamination of the needle during veni-puncture with skin commensals and contaminants, or more rarely through asymptomatic donor bacteremia with oral or enteric commensals. Investigation of the donors involved in the donation of contaminated components rarely identifies a focus of infection or source of contamination.[36] Skin commensal organisms such as *Staphylococcus epidermidis* and the anaerobic organism *Propioni-bacterium acnes* are the organisms most often detected as contaminants by culture methods.[37–38] Prior to the introduction of routine culture-screening processes, septic fatalities caused by platelet contamination were predominantly caused by enteric Gram-nega-tive organisms[10] (Table 53.2). Very rarely, contamination of the collection bag, tubing, or anticoagulant with improper sterilization during manufacturing, or contamination of products after collection due to failure of the closed storage system (e.g., defects in the bags or tubing), has been documented, and these may involve environmental contaminants such as *Serratia* spp., *Bacillus* spp., and *Pseudomonas* spp.

Table 53.2 Bacterial species involved in platelet septic transfusion reactions and fatalities as reported to the french national hemovigilance program, US FDA and american red cross hemovigilance program[7–9,39]

	France Sepsis (Fatalities)		United States FDA Fatalities Only		American Red Cross Sepsis (Fatalities)
	1996–1998	2000–2008	1995–2004	2005–2013	2006–2011
Total Transfusions (Millions)	0.47	1.94	~15[#]	~18[#]	4.1
Gram-positive bacteria					
Staphylococcus aureus	0	13 (4)	4	9	8 (3)
Coagulase-negative Staphylococci	5	11	11	5	22 (1)
Enterococcus faecalis	0	2 (1)	1		
Streptococcus spp.	0	3	4	3	4
Bacillus cereus	2	3	1		
Propionibacterium acnes	3	0			
Clostridium perfringens			1		1
Other Gram-positive bacilli			1		
Total Gram-positive bacteria	**10**	**32 (4)**	**23**	**17**	**35**
Gram-negative bacteria					
Enterobacter spp.	1	1	5		1
Escherichia coli	1	5 (2)	9	3	
Klebsiella spp.	2 (1)	3 (3)	11	2	1
Serratia spp.	1 (1)	3	5	2	
Yersinia enterocolitica	0	0			
Acinetobacter spp.	1	2		1	1
Pseudomonas spp.	0	2	2		
Proteus mirabilis	0	0			
Salmonella spp.			2		
Other Gram negative bacilli			1		
Morganella spp.			1	2	
Pasturella spp.			1		
Eubacterium limosum			1		
Total Gram-negative bacteria	**6 (2)**	**16 (5)**	**37**	**11**	**3**
TOTAL	**16 (2)**	**48 (9)**	**60**	**28**	**38**
Rate of sepsis	1:29,375	1:40,417	-	-	1:106,921
Rate of fatality	1:235,000	1:216,000	1:250,000	1:642,857	1:1,015,750

[#]estimated from the National Blood Collection and Utilization Surveys.[47]
American Red Cross data reflect apheresis platelets only, whereas French and US FDA data include both pooled WBD and apheresis platelets.

Clinical presentation

The clinical sequelae resulting from transfusion of bacterially contaminated platelets range from asymptomatic to mild fever (which may be indistinguishable from a nonhemolytic transfusion reaction) to acute sepsis, hypotension, and death. The clinical picture is much more varied and often less severe than that of patients infected by transfusion of bacterially contaminated RBCs.[40] Sepsis caused by transfusion of contaminated platelets is vastly underrecognized and underreported. Indeed, Jacobs et al. found that, during periods at their institution where active culture screening was in place, contaminated platelet components and sepsis were 32.0- and 10.6-fold more likely to be documented, than during a period when detection relied solely on clinician recognition and reporting.[41] Reaction severity was greater with components containing $\geq 10^5$ colony-forming units/ml and with higher bacterial virulence. At lower concentrations and with less virulent organisms, patients frequently displayed no immediate symptoms. Likewise, patients on antibiotic therapy or are neutropenic; they may not display classical signs of fever and sepsis, and, when they do, these are often ascribed to other infectious causes.

Patients may not react immediately after transfusion of contaminated platelets: In one well-documented outbreak of *Salmonella choleraseus*, seven patients were linked to one repeat donor with an occult chronic osteomyelitis. The time to the onset of illness ranged from 5 to 12 days (mean 8.6 days). In all cases, the platelet units were stored for less than one day.[42] In a similar situation, the CDC reported in 2006 a multistate outbreak of *Pseudomonas fluorescens* bloodstream infections. All cases could be traced to contaminated heparin flushes.[43] A total of 28 patients had delayed onset of *P. fluorescens* infections, ranging from 84 to 421 days after their last potential exposure.

Recognizing the potential harm of misdiagnosis of septic reactions, the AABB (formerly known as the American Association of Blood Banks) recommends active steps for all patients who, within 24 hours of a platelet transfusion, display a fever $\geq 38\,°C$ ($<100.4°F$) with a rise of $>1\,°C$ ($1.8°F$) plus rigors, hypotension, shock, tachycardia, dyspnea, or nausea/vomiting. Furthermore, any change in clinical condition leading to a suspicion of sepsis even in the absence of fever should lead to actions that include halting the transfusion, patient support, and investigation for possible transfusion of a contaminated component.[44] Indeed, broad-spectrum antibiotics should be considered for any patient who develops fever within six hours of platelet transfusion.[45-46]

Incidence

Sepsis resulting from transfusion of bacterially contaminated platelets is the most common transfusion-transmitted disease. Platelets are stored at room temperature ($20-24\,°C$), making them an excellent growth medium. Multiple aerobic culture surveillance studies have demonstrated that 1 in 1000 to 3000 platelet units are bacterially contaminated.[1] Based on the fact that approximately 10 million platelet units (apheresis plus whole blood derived) were transfused every year in the United States,[47] it was estimated that 2000 to 4000 bacterially contaminated platelets units were transfused every year before the advent of culture screening. Despite the estimates of contamination, the actual septic transfusion reaction rates were much lower at approximately 1 in 25,000 platelet units (range 1 in 13,000 to 100,000).[1] The French National Hemovigilance Program, utilizing active surveillance in the period 2000–2008, reports rates of ~1:40,000 (24.7 per million) and ~1:216,000 (5.14 per million) for sepsis and fatality, respectively.[8]

Following the introduction of methods to limit and detect contamination in 2004 in the United States, the American Red Cross described a ~70% decline in sepsis reported to their passive surveillance program, with current rates of 1:107,000 for sepsis and 1:1,016,000 for fatalities.[39] Likewise, the FDA described 60 fatalities caused by platelet transfusion in the 10-year period 1995–2004[10] (average 6.0/year; 62% caused by Gram-negative bacteria; ~1:250,000 transfusions) and only 28 in the nine-year period 2005–2013 (average 3.1/year; 36.1% caused by Gram-negative organisms)[9] (Table 53.2). Even with culture screening in place, Jacobs et al. estimate that at least 550 contaminated units are still transfused in the United States, as detected by a bacterial screening test performed at the time of transfusion.[48]

Prevention measures introduced in the United States

The College of American Pathologists (CAP) and AABB instituted steps to require the detection of bacteria in platelet products, beginning in 2002. CAP added an item to the Laboratory Accreditation Checklist[49] regarding the detection of bacteria that was modified in December 2004 to read, "Does the laboratory have a validated system to detect the presence of bacteria in platelet components?" In March 2004, AABB instituted a new standard that required blood banks or transfusion services to have steps in place to "limit and detect bacterial contamination" in all platelet products.[50] Subsequently, this was modified to include "limit, detect or inactivate bacteria" in recognition of the advent of approved pathogen inactivation technologies in many countries. Since that time, blood centers and transfusion services have implemented a variety of interventions to accomplish this goal.

The majority of US blood collectors implemented bacterial culture screening of all apheresis platelets using one of two FDA-approved tests, the BacT/ALERT™ system (BioMerieux inc, Durham, NC) or, less commonly, the Pall eBDS™ test (Haemonetics, Braintree, MA).[51] These tests are not suitable for screening individual random donor platelets derived from whole blood collections (WBD), and the AABB standards allowed the use of surrogate tests validated by individual users, including pH and glucose measurements at the time of poststorage pooling and release to patients. These assays were subsequently shown to be insensitive and nonspecific, providing suboptimal protection against bacterial contamination.[52] Two subsequent innovations were the introduction of the Pall Acrodose™ (Haemonetics) prestorage pooling system that allows the pooling of WBD before storage, facilitating the use of culture testing after manufacture, and FDA-approved point-of-issue tests, including the Platelet Pan Genera Detection assay (Platelet PGD™, Verax Biomedical, Worcester, MA) and the BacTx™ (Immunetics, Boston, MA) test.[48,53] These technologies allow bacterial testing at the time of issue. In 2010, the AABB published an interim standard effectively requiring the use of FDA-approved tests, or technologies shown to be equivalent, thereby preventing the use of surrogate tests. A survey performed by the AABB in 2011 revealed that the vast majority of platelets were derived from apheresis collections, and 89.5% of these were screened using the BacT/ALERT culture system.[54]

The American Red Cross began routine aerobic cultures using the BacT/ALERT system in March 2004, and in their first 10 months of testing, 226 of 350,658 platelet collections initially tested positive.[55] Sixty-eight of these were confirmed positives for a rate of bacterial contamination of one in 5157 distributed components. Despite universal testing of all platelet products, in the two-year period from

March 2004 through May 2006, the ARC reported 20 septic transfusion reactions caused by transfusion of bacterially screened units. Of the 20 septic reactions, three were fatal and involved *Staphylococcus* species.[37] All of the units involved with septic fatalities, and 13 of the units implicated in septic reactions, were associated with platelets transfused on the fifth day after collection. Of note, with BacT/ALERT culture screening, products are released for transfusion 12–24 hours after cultures are initiated; however, blood centers continue to hold the culture until the end of the components' shelf life. Therefore, an efficient communication system was put in place to recall platelet products from the hospital should a culture indicate reactivity after distribution from the blood center. Experience showed that slow-growing organisms that trigger late reactive cultures after transfusion has occurred are seldom associated with transfusion reactions.[36]

Since 2006, the Red Cross further refined its approach to bacterial safety by adopting inlet-line diversion of the initial 30–40 ml of blood post phlebotomy (which decreases the collection contamination rate), increased the volume screened from a 4 ml to 8 ml sample under aerobic conditions (which increases BacT/ALERT culture sensitivity), and converted from a two-step povidone–iodine skin preparation technique to the use of a single step with 2% chlorohexidine–isopropyl (Chloraprep, Cardinal Health, Leawood, KS) alcohol swabs.[38,56,57] The Red Cross also instituted the Acrodose prestorage pooling system with BacT/ALERT screening for WBD platelets, although these comprise only 5% of the platelet components distributed.[57]

With these changes in place, the Red Cross screened 2.2 M apheresis collections between 2006 and 2011 and detected 417 confirmed positive (188 per million: 1:5320) cultures, including ~22% highly pathogenic Gram-negative bacteria.[39] The majority of cultured organisms were Gram-positive (Figure 53.1), and transfusion was prevented in most cases. Nevertheless, 38 septic transfusion reactions were reported to the Red Cross hemovigilance program (Table 53.2), including four fatalities, for an overall rate

of sepsis of 1:107,000 distributed platelet components and 1:1,016,000 fatalities.[39] The fatalities were caused by *Staphylococcus aureus* (three cases) and coagulase-negative *Staphylococci* (one case). Most cases of sepsis were caused by Gram-positive organisms; however, three involved Gram-negative organisms and one implicated an anaerobe, *Clostridium perfringens*.[58] This represents a ~70% decline in the rate of sepsis and fatalities reported to the Red Cross Hemovigilance Program compared to the 10-month period in 2003–2004, immediately before bacterial culture was instituted.[55] During that period, 12 high-probability septic reactions, including two fatalities, were reported by passive surveillance, whereas ~500,000 platelet components were distributed.

A similar trend is seen in the fatality data reported to the FDA: From 1995 to 2004, 60 deaths caused by bacterially contaminated platelets were reported, averaging six deaths per year (Table 53.2) before the initiation of the AABB standard.[10] These were predominantly caused by Gram-negative organisms (37 of 60 = 62%). In the nine-year period since the Standard, 28 deaths were reported for an average of 3.1 deaths per year, with 39% (11/38) caused by Gram-negative bacteria.[9] Bacterial culture screening is therefore most effective at preventing the transfusion of platelets contaminated with rapidly growing Gram-negative bacteria.

Causes of false-negative bacterial culture screening tests

It is clear that there has been a significant improvement in platelet safety over the prior decade, but a substantial risk remains. All septic reactions reported to the Red Cross have been associated with negative bacterial cultures, suggesting that the sample inoculated into the culture bottles was sterile.[39] When performing bacterial culture screening, a sample is taken from the product 18–24 hours after collection in order to allow bacteria at very low concentrations (e.g., as low as 1 cfu/collection) to proliferate and reach concentrations of >1–10 cfu/ml, the demonstrated average lower sensitivity limit of the BacT/ALERT system when using an 8 ml sample.[11,59,60]

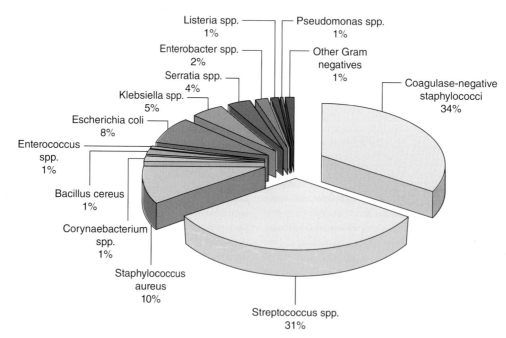

Figure 53.1 Distribution of bacterial species detected as confirmed positive by the BacT/ALERT culture screen in the American Red Cross between 2006 and 2011. Source: Benjamin *et al.* (2014).[39] Reproduced with permission.

Table 53.3 Results of bacterial screening assays performed late during storage or on outdate, on platelet components screened and found negative for bacterial contamination during manufacture

	#Tested	Confirmed Positives	Rate per Million	Sensitivity of Day 1 Test	Reference
PASSPORT Study	6,039	4	662 (1:1,509)	25.9%	[64]
Irish Blood Service Day 8	8,282	18	2,200 (1:460)	29.2%	[63]
Irish Blood Service Day 4	3,310	4	1,200 (1:828)		[63]
Welsh Blood Service	6,438	6	931 (1:1,073)	40.0%	[62]

It is thought that bacteria with a prolonged lag growth phase or slow doubling rate may avoid detection simply by virtue of low concentrations at the time of sampling (e.g., sampling error).[61] Some of these bacteria may enter a rapid-growth phase later in storage and reach clinically relevant concentrations by the time of transfusion. Further evidence in support of this hypothesis is provided by cultures performed later during storage or at outdate on components screened and found negative by culture assay at the time of manufacture. Three groups (Table 53.3) now report that reculture of platelets later during storage or at outdate using the BacT/ALERT system frequently reveals residual bacterial contamination, suggesting that early cultures may only detect 25–40% of contaminated units.[62–64] Similarly, Jacobs et al. showed that platelets previously screened and found negative by either the BacT/ALERT or eBDS system revealed bacterial contamination in 9 of 27,620 (~1:3000) tests using the Platelet PGD assay, suggesting that less than one-half of the contaminated units were detected by early culture.[48] Overall, there is a need to further improve the safety of platelets.

Strategies to reduce the risk of posttransfusion sepsis

Approaches to reduce the risk of posttransfusion sepsis can be grouped into four major categories: sepsis avoidance by appropriate platelet transfusion, reducing bacterial contamination, improving bacterial detection, and eliminating contaminating bacteria.

Sepsis avoidance by appropriate platelet transfusion

Platelets that are transfused when not indicated can be of no benefit and only harm patients. Recently, the AABB published an extensive evidence-based analysis of the indications for platelet transfusion.[65,66] The recommendations reemphasize the 10,000/uL trigger for prophylaxis in stable nonbleeding patients and provide guidance for surgery and other situations. Strict adherence to appropriate transfusion remains the most important safety measure for prevention of bacterial sepsis and other complications of transfusion.

Reduction of bacterial contamination
Donor screening

Donors are routinely asked whether they feel well on the day of donation and screened for a fever. Should the donor report a history of a recent infection, all antibiotic therapy must be complete before donation is permitted. The phlebotomy site is inspected to ensure a clean site without signs of inflammation or infection. Surgical wounds must be healed and dry. Unfortunately, asking donors about symptoms suggestive of infections is problematic. For example, 13% of donors have had gastrointestinal symptoms in the 30 days before donation yet are not indicative of risk.[67] Retrospective questioning of donors implicated in red cell sepsis associated with *Yersinia* spp. showed that only half had any gastrointestinal symptoms in the preceding 30 days.[4,13] Therefore, donor questioning

about gastrointestinal symptoms does not appear to be a specific predictor of *Yersinia* bacteremia. Likewise, most donors implicated in septic transfusion reactions or found to have positive bacterial screening cultures have no history, symptoms, or signs of infection. Although it is known that procedures such as brushing one's teeth and straining at stool may be associated with bacteremia, this is generally asymptomatic and screening is not effective. Rarely, an investigation may reveal pathology in the donor: Bacterial culture screening that reveals *Streptococcus bovis* should always lead to appropriate investigation for colonic pathology, as a number of cases of colonic polyps or carcinoma have been discovered in this fashion.[36,68] Likewise, a series of *Salmonella* spp. infections in one institution revealed a donor with chronic osteomyelitis.[42]

Skin preparation

Despite excellent technique, one cannot ensure a sterile venipuncture because organisms harbored in sebaceous glands and hair follicles cannot be completely removed or killed, and skin fragments drawn up into the collection bag during the initial phase of donation can provide a source of infectious organisms.[69–70] Scarring or dimpling of the venipuncture site from prior donation has also been recognized as a risk factor for bacterial contamination, because these areas frequently are difficult to disinfect.[71] In one case, phlebotomy at a dimpled venipuncture site of an apheresis donor resulted in three episodes of platelet contamination with Gram-positive organisms; sepsis occurred in four recipients of those platelets.

The effectiveness of skin preparation may depend on the disinfectant solution utilized, the number of applications (generally one or two), the dwell time during which the skin is exposed to the disinfectant, and the skill of the operator.[72] Blood centers have standard procedures that enforce optimal skin disinfection procedures. The FDA recognizes three principal disinfections solutions for blood donation—tincture of iodine (TI), chlorhexidine, and povidone–iodine—each usually suspended in isopropyl alcohol. Investigations of the residual contamination after disinfection show that *iodine solutions and 2% chlorhexidine are effective in reducing the donor skin bacterial burden* (Table 53.4), *whereas green soap and isopropyl alcohol are not.* Skin of donors who are allergic to iodine is often cleansed with a chlorhexidine solution.[73] In the United States, most blood centers now use a single-step 2% chlorhexidine swab process with 30-second dwell time, and that has been shown to be as effective as TI without the risk of staining clothes and allergy.[56]

Diversion

Diversion of the first milliliters of whole blood from the primary container has been shown to reduce the amount of bacterial contamination from the skin, presumably by capturing skin fragments or a shower of bacteria released at the time of phlebotomy. Bruneau et al.[74] collected the first and second 15 ml aliquots of 3385 whole blood collections and cultured these under aerobic and anaerobic conditions. Seventy-three were positive in the first

Table 53.4 Proportion of donors with bacterial growth after skin disinfection

Bacterial Colonies per Plate	Povidone Iodine	Isopropyl Alcohol + Tincture of Iodine	Chlorhexidine Gluconate	Green Soap and Isopropyl Alcohol
0	34–49%	63%	60%	0%
1–10	35–43%	34%	25%	17%
11–100	10–14%	2%	12%	47%
>100	0–13%	1%	3%	36%
p value compared to povidone iodine		<0.001	>0.3	<0.001

Source: Goldman *et al.* (1997).[72] Reproduced with permission of Wiley.

15 ml and 21 in the second, including four species not detected in the initial 15 ml. Overall contamination rate was 2.2%, mainly with Gram-positive *Staphylococcus* spp. and *Bacillus* spp. The residual risk of contamination in the collection was 0.6%, showing that diversion could significantly reduce the overall risk. A study from the Netherlands compared the bacterial contamination rates of whole blood collections with and without the removal of the first 10 mL. The diversion of the first 10 mL showed a significant decrease in bacterial contamination (18,263 collections with 0.39% contamination without diversion compared with 7115 collections with 0.21% contamination with diversion, $p < 0.05$).[75] Diversion is most effective at decreasing contamination with skin flora. A majority of bacteria-related fatalities involve Gram-negative organisms, which are likely not interdicted by diversion.

Similarly, the ARC data reported data between 2004 and 2006 where it is possible to compare the confirmed-positive bacterial culture rates with and without diversion (Table 53.5).[38] The authors report on the contamination rate of one-arm collections (which incorporated inlet-line diversion) and two-arm collections (which did not) on the same apheresis equipment. There was a 2.2-fold higher rate of skin contaminants with the two-arm procedure compared with the one-arm procedure, and this difference was apparent only for skin contaminants.

Apheresis versus whole blood–derived platelet concentrates

Therapeutic doses of platelets can be obtained from a single donor through an apheresis procedure, or from whole blood donations. Four to six platelets concentrates from whole blood donations are pooled to make a therapeutic dose; therefore, it would be expected that pooled platelets obtained from multiple donors would be at higher risk of bacterial contamination.

From 1986 to 1998, Johns Hopkins Hospital increased the use of apheresis platelets from 51.7% to 99.4% and saw a threefold reduction in septic transfusion reaction involving platelets, from one in 4818 transfusions to 1 in 15,098 transfusions.[76] With the introduction of AABB Standard 5.1.5.1 in 2004, most apheresis platelets were screened using culture methods, whereas WBD were screened by the transfusion service after pooling using surrogate markers (e.g., pH or glucose), as many institutions felt that culturing of individual WBD platelets was impractical. The Acrodose PL system is now available for prestorage pooling of WBD platelets, which allows institutions to pool WBD platelets and then store them for up to five days after collection.[57] By using prestorage pooling, the volume of the product is acceptable for culturing with either the BacT/ALERT or eBDS. The Red Cross reported that BacT/ALERT cultures performed on pools of five WBD were fivefold more likely to be contaminated than apheresis platelets, using identical screening processes, in keeping with the concept that pooled platelets are more likely to be contaminated than single-donor apheresis platelets.[57]

Table 53.5 Comparison of one- and two-arm apheresis platelet collections

Rate per 10^5 Cultures	Two-Arm Procedures	One-Arm Procedures*	OR (95% CI)
Skin contaminants	17.2	7.8	2.2 (1.5-3.3)
Nonskin organisms	5.5	4.1	1.3 (0.7-2.4)
Total confirmed positives	22.7	11.9	1.9 (1.4-2.7)

*An inlet-line diversion pouch was in place on the one-arm procedures only.

Source: Eder et al., 2008 [57]. Reproduced with permission of Wiley.

Prepooled WBD platelets prepared by the buffy coat method have been available in Europe since the early 1990s. Recently, Canada transitioned from the platelet-rich plasma method to the buffy coat method. The conventional wisdom in Europe is that the confirmed positive culture and sepsis rate of prepooled buffy coat platelets is equivalent to those of apheresis platelets,[77] perhaps due to the overnight incubation of whole blood in the presence of white cells before preparation of buffy coats and leukoreduction of the pooled product. Bacterial culture screening results, however, show wide variability, with some investigators showing a 2–5-fold increased confirmed positive culture rate with pooled products[62,75,78–80] and others showing no difference (Figure 53.2).[81]

In the United States, there has been a gradual move away from pooled platelets to apheresis platelets. A survey of AABB-accredited blood centers, hospital blood banks, and transfusion services in late

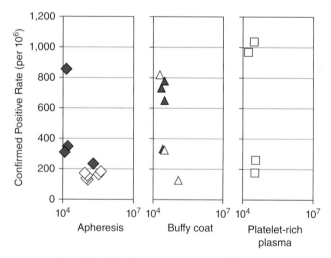

Figure 53.2 Rate of confirmed positive BacT/ALERT™ screening cultures broken out by platelet type, with data derived from 16 international studies. The *x*-axis in each panel represents the number of products tested varying from 1×10^3–1×10^7 on a logarithmic scale. Solid symbols represent the use of both aerobic anaerobic cultures conditions. Used with permission. Source: Benjamin and McDonald (2014).[78] Reproduced with permission of Elsevier.

2004 examined platelet usage, supply, and testing methods.[51] Between 2003 and 2004, there was an 11.3% reduction in the use of WBD platelets, and 77.2% of platelets transfused by the institutions surveyed were apheresis platelets. By 2011, the National Blood Collection and Utilization survey revealed that 91.1% of platelets were from apheresis collections.[82]

Reducing storage duration

Longer platelet storage time is associated with an increased probability of clinically significant contamination, as low initial concentrations of bacteria may proliferate over time. In 1983, in the United States, platelet storage for WBD platelets was transiently approved for seven days based on acceptable in vitro function, in vivo recovery, and survival data. However, because of anecdotal reports of bacterial proliferation over the extended storage time, the shelf life was returned in 1986 to five days. With the introduction of prestorage bacterial culture screening, the FDA again allowed the investigation of seven-day storage under the Post Approval Surveillance Study of Platelet Outcomes, Release Tested (PASSPORT) protocol, where each apheresis collection was screened under aerobic and anaerobic culture conditions.[64,83] This protocol successfully demonstrated improved platelet logistics and decreased wastage; however, poststorage culture revealed a substantial rate of residual contamination, and the protocol was closed. Even with five days of storage, reports of septic transfusion reactions and fatalities persist, especially on days 4 and 5 of storage (Table 53.2).

Only by severely reducing the storage time of platelets would one significantly impact the risk of bacterial overgrowth. However, operational changes affect the storage age of available platelets. With increased complexity of disease-marker testing, the availability of one-day-old platelets has decreased. For example, in the United States in 1982 the mean age of distributed platelets was 1.6 days, in 1983 (after extension of the dating period to five days) it was 2.0 days, and in 1992 (after addition of increased laboratory testing) it was 2.5 days. In 1983, only 5% of issued platelets were greater than three days old. In 1992, just 10% were older than three days. But with the introduction of centralized testing and bacterial screening, the mean age of issued platelets increased to 2.7 days, with 20% older than three days. With the addition of nucleic acid testing for HIV and hepatitis C virus (HCV), additional delays occurred. Not only can this decrease available shelf life of an already precariously limited supply of platelets, but also it can decrease the availability of fresh platelets, which are the most hemostatic and the least likely to be bacterially contaminated.

One US center that collects its own whole blood and apheresis platelets has focused on early transfusion as a means of ensuring bacterial safety:[84] All products are sampled and cultured for bacteria, but the components are transfused as soon as possible after sampling. Apheresis platelets are transfused within 48 hours, and pooled WBD platelets within 72 hours of collection. The authors report that after 23,199 transfusions, 71 products were shown to be contaminated, all with Gram-positive *Staphylococci* spp. or *Streptococci* spp., except for a single Gram-negative *Enterobacter cloacae* isolate. Only a single mild septic reaction was reported to a product contaminated by a coagulase-negative *Staphylococcus* spp. isolate. The authors argue for the safety of fresh products despite contamination by bacteria, especially in patient groups that are usually on prophylactic antibiotic therapy for other clinical indications.

Other countries limit the shelf life of platelets in order to improve safety: Japan limits platelets to a <3.5-day shelf life, and in 2009 the German Paul Erlich Institute limited storage to four days following a series of fatal sepsis cases.[85] Neither country employs bacterial culture screening. Germany allows transfusion on day 5 after collection if the product is screened using a culture system or point-of-release screen on day 4 or 5 (see below). In December 2012, the FDA Blood Products Advisory Committee suggested that the US centers similarly reduce shelf life to four days unless rescreened for bacterial contamination on day 4 or 5. At the time of writing, the FDA had not converted this recommendation into guidance, and US blood centers continue to label platelets for five days of storage.

Bacteria detection

Bacterial contamination of platelet products is thought to initially involve minimal numbers of bacteria, some of which may proliferate to high levels during storage. In vitro inoculation experiments confirm that the growth dynamics differ by bacterial species. In one study, bacterial growth characteristics were reported for 165 platelet units, each inoculated on the day of collection with 1–5 CFU/ml of one of the following organisms: *Bacillus cereus*, *P. aeruginosa*, *Klebsiella pneumoniae*, *S. marcescens*, *S. aureus*, and *S. epidermidis*.[86] All examples of *B. cereus*, *P. aeruginosa*, *K. pneumoniae*, *S. marcescens*, and *S. aureus* had concentrations $>10^2$ CFU/mL by Day 3 following inoculation. By Day 4, all units with these organisms contained $>10^5$ CFU/mL. Units contaminated with *S. epidermidis* showed slower and more varied growth. This study concluded that an assay capable of detecting 10^2 CFU/mL on Day 3 of storage would detect a vast majority of bacterially contaminated platelet units.

Based on these and similar observations, sensitive culture techniques that can detect 1–10 CFU/ml are used soon after manufacture, and rapid, less sensitive detection methods are used closer to the time of transfusion. Examples of screening systems with high sensitivity that may be used soon after manufacture are two culture-based systems that are FDA approved in the United States, the BacT/ALERT and eBDS systems mentioned in this chapter. These can theoretically detect as few as a single viable bacterium in a 4–10 ml sample. In practice, they are validated to detect 1–10 CFU/ml of a range of transfusion-relevant bacterial strains. In contrast, there are a number of detection systems that detect bacteria directly, such as the FDA-approved PGD assay (Verax Biomedical, Worcester, MA), BacTx (Immunetics, Boston, MA) assay, and other tests in development especially in Europe, including NAT assays and flow cytometry–based assays (BactiFlow™ ALS, BioMerieux, Durham, NC). These assays typically have a lower analytical sensitivity than culture methods ($\sim 10^2$-10^5 cfu/ml), but may be performed rapidly (1–4 hours) and so are suitable for use close to the time of issue when bacterial concentrations are likely to be higher.

Bacterial culture

The BacT/ALERT system uses an automated liquid culture system that includes culture broth under aerobic or anaerobic conditions. Each bottle contains a sensor that changes color as a consequence of increasing CO_2 produced by bacterial proliferation. The system monitors both the absolute color change and rate of change of the colorimetric sensor. The bottles are inoculated with a needle through a rubber stopper, rendering the system incompletely closed and susceptible to contamination by introducing bacteria into the bottle. The method reliably detects contamination of platelets inoculated to 10 CFU/mL and in many cases <5 CFU/mL (e.g., *B. cereus*, *S. marcescens*, *C. perfringens*, *S. epidermidis*, *S. pyogenes*, *E. coli*, *K. pneumoniae*, *S. aureus*, and viridans streptococci) in 12–26 hours.[60]

The BacT/ALERT system is widely implemented in the United States and around the world. There are several variables that may affect culture sensitivity, including the delay between collection and sampling; the volume of product inoculated into the culture bottle; and the use of both aerobic and anaerobic culture conditions.[78] Wagner and Robinette[88] used a model system of platelets contaminated in vitro with *S. epidermidis* or *E. coli* at 10, 1 or 0.1 cfu/ml and then sampled 0, 6, 24, or 48 hours later. 0.5, 1, or 2 ml were inoculated and incubated in 12 BacT/ALERT aerobic bottles for each data point. Their results clearly showed that higher initial concentrations, larger sample volumes, and longer delay before sampling were associated with a larger proportion of inoculated bottles signaling positive at any given time point. This work was subsequently replicated for a wider range of organisms.[60] Various laboratories around the world have implemented the test in different ways, as can be seen in Table 53.6. No definitive data yet support the superiority of any given conformation.

Assuming that the initial number of bacteria contaminating a clinical collection is very low, an increased time delay before sampling would make it more likely that a higher concentration of bacteria are available in any given sample. In the United States and Canada, most blood centers therefore wait >24 hours after collection before taking the sample; however, many European countries, including Ireland, Wales, and Holland, use shorter periods in order to facilitate workflow in the center.[54,78] Conversely, the English National Blood Service delays sampling until 36–48 hours after collection to maximize the probability of detecting contamination.[80] The shelf life of platelets is extended to seven days to increase the time available for transfusion in the hospitals. In a similar fashion, increasing the volume of sample inoculated might be expected to increase culture sensitivity. Theoretical calculations suggest that doubling the sample volume may increase the proportion of contaminated products detected by as much as 25%, and Eder *et al.* found that BacT/ALERT culture was 1.54 (1.05–2.27) fold more likely to detect bacteria using an 8 ml sample versus a 4 ml sample.[38,89] Further theoretical calculations have been provided by Tomasulo and Wagner, who advocate the use of a sample size that is a constant proportion of the product volume, in order to standardize the sensitivity of the assay for single, double, and triple collections.[90] Despite the theoretical consideration that larger volume products may be less safe if all collections are sampled at the same volume, Eder *et al.* report no difference in the septic transfusion

reaction rates between single, double, and triple collections.[91] The downside of increased volume inoculation is the loss of product volume for transfusion and decreased splits rates for multiple component collections.

Many centers inoculate both aerobic and anaerobic culture bottles in order to maximize culture sensitivity. Most clinically relevant bacteria found contaminating platelets grow under both conditions, although specific strains may grow faster in one condition than the other. This was best demonstrated for a single strain of *Streptococcus lugdenensis* implicated in a fatal transfusion reaction.[92] A small number of species are obligate aerobes (e. g., *Pseudomonas fluorescens*) or obligate anaerobes (e.g., *P. acnes* and *Clostridium* spp.). Utilizing both aerobic and anaerobic conditions allows the detection of a complete range of species, speeds up detection of some strains, and doubles the volume of product cultured, thereby increasing the sensitivity of the overall detection system. Nevertheless, most US blood centers use only aerobic culture conditions, as anaerobic conditions mostly detect *P. acnes*, a species that does not grow well under the aerobic conditions of platelet storage; are rarely implicated in transfusion reactions; and are detected after a median of ~120 hours of incubation, when most products are already transfused. Anaerobic conditions are necessary for the detection of *Clostridium* spp., a rare but potentially lethal contaminant of platelets.[58,93]

Even under optimized culture conditions that include both aerobic and anaerobic culture conditions, false-negative screening cultures continue to be detected. As outlined in Table 53.3, outdate cultures suggest that only 25–40% of contaminated products are intercepted and septic reactions continue to be reported.[62–64] Under the most sensitive conditions used by the English National Blood Service, no septic reactions have been reported despite >500,000 platelet transfusions; however, this finding is difficult to interpret as zero septic reactions were reported to the UK SHOT hemovigilance system for the two years prior to the introduction of culture screening.[80] The consensus view is that although culture screening has significantly reduced the risk of bacterial sepsis, especially for Gram-negative organisms, no iteration can ensure the absolute safety of platelets from contamination. Bacterial screening creates substantial logistic burdens due to delay of product release into inventory; product loss due to sampling, especially when large volumes are used; and the need for product recalls when culture screenings turn reactive after components are distributed to

Table 53.6 International approaches to assuring bacterial safety of platelet products utilizing bacterial culture (BacT/ALERT™), flow cytometry (BactiFlow™), or pathogen inactivation (Intercept™) technologies

| Country | Storage Duration (d) | Flow Cytometry | Pathogen Inactivation | Bacterial Culture | | | Ref. |
				Aerobic (A)/Anaerobic (An)	Volume (ml)	Delay (Hours)	
US	5	—	—	A	8–10	18–24	54
Canada	5	—	—	A	8–10	24	81
England	7	—	—	A/An	16–48	36–48	80
Ireland	5	—	—	A/An	15–20	>12	63
Wales	5	—	—	A/An	16–20	>16	62
Australia	5	—	—	A/An	16	—	93
Holland	7	—	—	A/An	15	16–22	94
Hong Kong	5	—	—	A	10		95
Switzerland	5	—	X	—	—	—	96
Germany	4	X*	—	—	—	—	85
France	5	—	—$	—	—	—	7
Japan	<3.5	—	—	—	—	—	95

* Allows extension to five-day storage.
$ One regional blood center and all overseas departments use pathogen inactivation routinely.

hospitals. Individual users have optimized the conditions of the culture assay to maximize analytical sensitivity while minimizing impact on logistics and blood availability, leading to the many different conformations shown in Table 53.6.

The second culture system is the enhanced Pall Bacterial Detection System (eBDS), which is utilized in a small number of US blood centers and hospitals. The system measures oxygen consumption in the headspace gas of a 4 ml sample pouch at a fixed time point (18 or 24 hours) and cannot detect obligate anaerobes. One study reported on the use of the eBDS system with 118,067 apheresis and WBD units from 23 US blood centers.[97,98] Investigators found 118 initially reactive (1 in 992) and 23 confirmed positive (1 in 5133) units. All true-positive units contained *Staphylococcus* spp. and *Streptococcus* spp. Ninety-five false-positive units were identified (1 in 1243). Of the false positives, 18 were caused by contamination and 56 had no bacteria present. There was one report of a missed detection with *S. epidermidis*. In a study by Fournier-Wirth *et al.*, 5 to 50 CFU/mL bacteria was inoculated into apheresis platelet units and tested in the eBDS.[99] No false-positive results were seen. After 18 hours of incubation, 61 of 63 units tested positive; and after 24 hours, all 63 tested positive. In the earlier incubation, two cases of *B. cereus* were not detected. The eBDS system uses a standard format and cannot be manipulated to increase sensitivity other than to elect to measure reactivity at 24 hours rather than 18 hours.

Rapid immunoassay for cell wall determinants

In September 2007, the FDA approved a rapid immunoassay for the detection of aerobic and anaerobic bacteria in leukocyte-reduced apheresis platelets as an adjunct quality control device. The Platelet PGD Test is a qualitative immunoassay that differentiates between Gram-negative and Gram-positive bacteria through the detection of lipopolysaccharides (LPS) and lipotechoic acid (LTA), respectively.[48] As approved, it is intended to be an adjunct safety test for leukocyte-reduced apheresis platelets within 24 hours of transfusion, after the use of an FDA-cleared bacterial culture method at the time of manufacture. The system is also approved as a quality control test for pooled WBD platelets within four hours of transfusion. In this case, the platelets are not required to be prescreened using a culture method. The Platelet PGD Test can detect *B. cereus*, *C. perfringens*, *E. aerogenes*, *E. coli*, *K. pneumoniae*, *P. aeruginosa*, *S. aureus*, *S. epidermidis*, and *S. agalactiae* at a level >10^5 CFU/mL and *S. marcescens* at a level of 8.6×10^5 CFU/mL. The test takes approximately 20–60 minutes to perform and is optimally performed after at least 72 hours of platelet storage. In a clinical study, the Platelet PGD test detected nine confirmed-positive components of 27,620 apheresis platelets (1:3069) previously screened and found negative for bacteria using the BacT/ALERT or eBDS culture systems. These were all Gram-positive organisms that were detected on days 3 (four occurrences), 4 (two occurrences), and 5 (three occurrences) after collection. In the same study, two false-negative tests of 10,424 tests (1:5212) were confirmed, and the false-positive rate was 0.51%.

Subsequently, the FDA approved the Immunetics BacTx test, a qualitative colorimetric assay that detects peptidoglycan, a ubiquitous component of bacterial cell walls.[53] Indications include utility as a quality control test in leukoreduced apheresis or pooled WBD platelets, with identical restrictions on use as the Platelet PGD test described above. The limit of detection for *Bacillus cereus*, *S. aureus*, *S. epidermidis*, *Clostridium perfringens*, and *P. acnes* is <10^4 CFU/ml and for *E. coli*, *Pseudomonas aeruginosa*, *Klebsiella oxytoca*, *Serratia marcescens*, and *Streptococcus agalactiae* is <10^5 CFU/ml in both apheresis and WBD platelets.

A US survey performed under the auspices of the AABB in 2012 suggests that rapid detection assays are not in widespread use, and are limited to a small number of transfusion services that pool WBD platelets at the time of transfusion, or as a confirmatory test when platelet components are implicated in transfusion reactions.[54]

NAT detection techniques

Several amplification methods have been described for the detection of bacterial contamination utilizing broad-range NAT assays targeting genes with multiple copies, such as 16S ribosomal DNA or 23S ribosomal RNA based on real-time technology, but none are available commercially.[100] Theoretically, PCR should be able to detect 1 CFU/ml of bacteria; however, the presence of bacterial DNA contaminating PCR reagents, and even in platelet products themselves, reduces the theoretical sensitivity of the assay to 20–1000 CFU/ml. Schmidt *et al.*[101] reported on the use of polymerase chain reaction (PCR) to detect 16S ribosomal RNA from *S. aureus*, *E. coli*, *B. cereus*, and *K. pneumoniae* in pooled platelet concentrates. At an inoculum of 10 CFU/mL, the PCR testing detected all four bacteria at 12, 16, 20, and 24 hours after spiking. With a lower inoculum of 10 CFU/bag, the PCR testing detected 60% of *E. coli*, 80% of *B. cereus*, 90% of *K. pneumoniae*, and 100% of *S. aureus* 12 hours after spiking. Another study compared 16S ribosomal DNA PCR with the automated culture system BacT/ALERT.[102] A total of 2146 platelet concentrates was tested with both methods. When comparing to the culture method, the PCR had a sensitivity and specificity of 100%. To date, because of the complexities associated with such tests and the 2–6-hour delay to obtain results, nucleotide-based amplification has not been routinely applied to bacterial screening of platelets.

Flow cytometry–based detection

A flow cytometry–based system has been developed for bacterial detection in platelets and other biological and food products.[103] Using the BactiFlow technology (bioMerieux, AES Chemunex, France), a nonfluorescent compound is taken up by viable cells and is cleaved by cellular esterases to produce a fluorescent product that is trapped within the bacteria.[104] Fluorescent viable bacterial cells are then detected by a commercial flow cytometry system that is both rapid (0.75–1 hour for 12 samples) and sensitive, being able to detect 150–500 CFU/ml.[105] BactiFlow is in routine use in Germany to extend shelf life from four to five days when performed on day 3 or 4 after collection. BactiFlow was shown to have an initial reactive rate of 3.6% in a pilot clinical study involving 472 products, of which 1.7% failed to confirm on retesting. The confirmed positive rate was 0.21%, and confirmed false-positive rate was 1.7%.[85] Results of a larger clinical study of this product are awaited.

Pathogen elimination

The ability to eliminate bacterial contaminants nonspecifically soon after collection offers a promising scenario for completely preventing septic reactions. In this light, AABB standard 5.1.5.1 recognizes that approved pathogen inactivation (PI) systems meet the intent of the standard as a method to prevent septic transfusion reactions. Three PI systems are described that are designed to substantially reduce the risk of transmission of a variety of infectious diseases by platelet transfusion. The Intercept™ (Cerus Corp., Concord, CA) system uses a psoralen-based compound amotosalen plus ultraviolet-A (UVA) light to crosslink nucleic acids to prevent pathogen replication, whereas the Mirasol™ system utilizes the vitamin riboflavin and ultraviolet B plus visible light to achieve a similar effect by damaging nucleic acids and forming mono-adducts.[106–107] These two technologies are CE marked in Europe and are in various stages of implementation in European blood centers. The Intercept system was approved by the FDA in December, 2014. A third technology, Theraflex™ UVC Platelets, is in development, and uses UV-C light alone to damage nucleic acids and prevent replication.[108] Efficacy in reducing the risk of bacterial contamination and sepsis is predicted by in vitro experiments: Each system has been evaluated by measuring the ability to reduce the titer of bacteria in artificially contaminated platelet products. In brief, components are inoculated with high concentrations of known bacterial species, and then the titer is assessed before and directly after pathogen inactivation treatment. If the bacteria are not detectable after treatment, the outcome is designated as "greater than" ($>$) the difference between the initial titer and the minimal detectable titer in the test assay. Table 53.7 shows published results for each technology.[106,109–111] It can be seen that the technologies differ widely in their ability to inactivate various species of bacteria, but all three are less able to inactivate spore-forming *Bacillus* strains. PI is performed soon after platelet collection, a time when bacterial concentrations are low; however, concentrations tend to increase with time as viable bacteria proliferate. In order to be effective, PI treatments must render platelet components "functionally sterile" (defined as negative bacterial cultures at outdate) in order to be effective. Because the components are stored for many days after treatment, even single viable bacteria may proliferate to sufficient concentrations to cause severe transfusion reactions. Furthermore, if PI is to replace bacterial culture screening, the technology must be effective against rapidly growing Gram-negative bacteria (e.g., *Klebsiella* spp., *E. coli*, etc.) that were known to be frequently associated with fatal transfusion reactions before the implementation of bacterial screening in the United States.[10] The robustness of PI shown in Table 53.7 may be viewed as an indication of how soon after collection the PI process should be performed.

For example, Goodrich *et al.* inoculated multiple platelet samples with each of 20 different bacterial strains, and performed PI two hours later.[110] They found that for components contaminated with <20 CFU/ml, PI was 98% effective at inducing functional sterility and substantially more effective than bacterial culture screening, whereas for components contaminated with 20–103 CFU/ml, PI was 91% effective and as effective as culture screening. These data suggest that Mirasol treatment performed within two hours of collection is likely to be as effective as BacT/ALERT culture screening at preventing transfusion reactions. If Mirasol were performed greater than two hours after collection, the effectiveness would likely be less than that of BacT/ALERT culture screening. In a similar experiment, Nussbaumer *et al.* inoculated double-dose apheresis platelet components with three different concentrations (1–10, 10–100, and 100–1000 CFU/ml) of each of seven different species of bacteria, performed Intercept PI on one split product 18–20 hours (W. Nussbaumer, personal communication) later, and compared the outcome to BacT/ALERT culture screening on days 1, 2, and 5 after inoculation.[112] Intercept was 100 percent effective at inactivating all species and more effective than BacT/ALERT culture screening. These data support the use of Intercept PI at late as 18 hours after collection. Recently, Schmidt *et al.* confirmed these findings with apheresis platelets contaminated with eight different bacterial species and Intercept-treated 12 hours after contamination. In the same experiment performed with whole blood collections contaminated with 100 cfu of bacteria, platelets manufactured 24 hours, and then Intercept treated 35.5 hours after collection were 100% sterile.[113]

Taken together, these data suggest that while pathogen inactivation systems are promising technologies for preventing septic transfusion reactions, clinical data will be needed to fully define their utility. The available technologies differ in their ability to inactivate clinically relevant strains, and blood collectors need to validate each technology and how it is implemented. Technologies with less robust inactivation should be performed close to the time of collection in order to be as effective as available culture screening techniques.[114] Clinical data with the Intercept system in routine use have begun to be published, and it is reported to be effective at preventing bacterial septic reactions.[95]

International comparison

There is wide variation in the way different countries approach the problem of bacterial contamination of platelets. An international survey published in 2007 of 12 countries revealed many approaches, with routine culture screening performed in a minority.[98] A similar survey in 2014 revealed that all but a few countries had implemented BacT/ALERT culture screening in some form. Almost all countries recognize the danger of contaminated platelets and have instituted routine screening of donors for risk factors, standardized skin preparation techniques, and diversion for the initial blood drawn during phlebotomy. With only these interventions, France reports a continued high risk of sepsis (1:40,000 transfusions) and fatality (1:216,000 transfusions) (Table 53.2). Pathogen inactivation utilizing the Intercept system was implemented in the EFS-Alsace Region in 2006 (and in the overseas French departments of Ile de La Reunion, Guadalupe, and Guyana).[95] Likewise, Switzerland implemented PI in 2011 (Table 53.7). The French and SwissMedic National Hemovigilance Programs document no cases of sepsis since implementation of PI with a total of >180,000 PI-treated transfusions reported.[95,96,111] In Germany, a pilot study where 52,243 platelet components were screened with both BacT/ALERT™ and eBDS™ cultures before release, documented a false negative result for one collection that lead to a fatality and severe reaction in the recipients of split units.[77] Culture screening was not implemented and subsequently in 2009 the Blood Working Party (Arbeitskreis Blut: National Advisory Board of the Federal Ministry of Health) mandated a shortened shelf-life of four days.[95,116]

Table 53.7 Log reduction of bacteria titer following pathogen inactivation with amotosalen/ultraviolet a (Intercept™, Cerus Corp. Concord, CA), riboflavin/ultraviolet (Mirasol™, Terumo, Lakewood, CO), and Ultraviolet-C Light (Theraflex™ UV platelets, macopharma, France)[106–107,109,111,115]

Bacterial Strain	Riboflavin/ UV	UVC Light	Amotosalen/ UVA
Staphylococcus coag. neg.	>4.6	4.8	>6.6
S. aureus	4.8	>4.8	6.6
Streptococcus spp.	2.6-3.7	—	>6.8
P. acnes	—	4.5	6.7
Bacillus spp.	2.6	4.3	3.6
E. coli	>4.4	>4.0	>6.4
Klebsiella spp.	2.8	4.8	>5.4
Pseudomonas spp.	>4.5	>4.9	4.5
S. marscescens	4.0	>5.0	>6.7
E. cloacae	—	>4.3	—
A. baumanii	1.8	—	—
Y. enterocolitica	3.3	—	—
L. monocytogenes	—	—	>6.3

Permission to extend shelf-life to five days has been granted based on bacterial screening with the BactiFlow system and with a CE-marked 16s RNA PCR system on day 3 or 4 after collection. Japan likewise restricts the shelf life of platelets and does not perform bacterial screening. Recently shelf life was extended from 72 hours to midnight on the third day effectively allowing up to 3.5 days shelf-life, in order to facilitate logistics of supplying hospitals. Seven septic reactions have been reported over the last six years with platelets two and three days old, including one fatality caused by *S. aureus*.

A recent systematic survey of reports of routine BacT/ALERT screening involving >10,000 components documented 16 reports, including countries where universal screening is performed. These included the United States, Canada, United Kingdom, Ireland, Wales, Australia, Hong Kong, and Holland (Table 53.6). Data from these studies are difficult to compare due to different definitions used to define the outcome of screening, incomplete reporting of the variables that might affect outcome and the results in terms of septic transfusion reactions, and the differences in details of how the screening system is implemented (Table 53.6). As outlined above, BacT/ALERT screening has clearly reduced the incidence of septic transfusion reactions reported to various hemovigilance programs, but reports of false negative tests and septic reactions persist. Although the sensitivity of the test is increased by delay between collection and sampling, increasing sample volume and the use of both aerobic and anaerobic conditions, blood centers have to balance the incremental sensitivity against the logistical impact of loss of product volume for testing, delay before release into inventory and increased product wastage due to more false positive results. We must await definitive publication of the outcomes of screening in terms of reported septic transfusion reactions before we can fully evaluate the effectiveness of culture screening as implemented in each country.

Conclusion

Bacterial contamination of blood components is the most common cause of transfusion-transmitted infectious disease. Septic transfusion reactions related to RBC transfusions have declined rapidly in the last decade, possibly related to the more universal application of leukoreduced blood products. Most cases of posttransfusion sepsis involve platelets that must be stored at room temperature under conditions conducive to bacterial proliferation. With the introduction of improved skin disinfection, diversion techniques and bacteria detection of platelets, the rate of clinically significant septic reaction has decreased however a substantial risk of septic transfusion reactions remains. Clinicians must be vigilant for these reactions and respond rapidly to support patients when they occur. There is a growing consensus that further interventions are necessary to further enhance platelet safety with respect to bacteria, including the use of point of transfusion bacterial assays or pathogen inactivation techniques.

Disclaimer

Richard Benjamin has disclosed relationships with Fresenius Kabi AG, Immucor, Inc., and Cerus Corporation.

Key references

A full reference list for this chapter is available at: http://www.wiley.com/go/simon/transfusion

1   Hillyer CD, Josephson CD, Blajchman MA, Vostal JG, Epstein JS, Goodman JL. Bacterial contamination of blood components: risks, strategies, and regulation: joint ASH and AABB educational session in transfusion medicine. *Hematology Am Soc Hematol Educ Program* **2003**:575–89.

11 Brecher ME, Jacobs MR, Katz LM, *et al.* Survey of methods used to detect bacterial contamination of platelet products in the United States in 2011. *Transfusion* 2013;**53**:911–8.

95 Pietersz RN, Reesink HW, Panzer S, *et al.* Bacterial contamination in platelet concentrates. *Vox Sang* 2014;**106**:256–83.

78 Benjamin RJ, McDonald CP. The international experience of bacterial screen testing of platelet components with an automated microbial detection system: a need for consensus testing and reporting guidelines. *Transfus Med Rev* 2014;**28**:61–71.

114 Benjamin RJ. Pathogen inactivation—defining "adequate" bacterial protection. *ISBT Science Series* 2014;**9**:124–30.

CHAPTER 54

Prion diseases

Marc L. Turner

Department of Cellular Therapy, University of Edinburgh; and Scottish National Blood Transfusion Service, Edinburgh, Scotland, UK

Prion diseases, or transmissible spongiform encephalopathies (TSEs), comprise a spectrum of diseases in animals and humans. In animals, these diseases include scrapie in sheep and goats, chronic wasting disease in deer and elk, and transmissible mink encephalopathy. Bovine spongiform encephalopathy (BSE) was first described in cattle in the United Kingdom (UK) in the early 1980s and developed into an epidemic of more than 180,000 bovine cases, spreading also to a range of other animals including domestic and exotic cats and exotic ungulates.

Sporadic or classical Creutzfeldt–Jakob disease (CJD), first described in the early 1920s,[1] occurs at an incidence of around one in one million per year. It presents at a mean age of 68 years with a rapidly progressive dementia, leading to death after about six months. Kuru, described in the Fore people of Papua New Guinea,[2] comprised an endemic disease presenting with cerebellar ataxia and a more prolonged clinical course. The disease is thought to have been spread through cannibalistic funeral rites. Although these cultural practices died out toward the end of the 1950s, there are still occasional people who develop new clinical disease, pointing to the potentially very prolonged incubation periods of these diseases. Iatrogenic transmission of sporadic CJD has occurred via neurosurgical instrumentation and electroencephalogram (EEG) electrodes, corneal and dura mater grafts, and cadaveric pituitary-derived growth and follicular stimulating hormones.[3] Those patients infected through direct central nervous system inoculation tend to manifest an incubation period of around two years and a rapidly progressive dementia reminiscent of sporadic CJD. Those infected through peripheral inoculation demonstrate a more prolonged and variable incubation period (mean 13–15 years) and a clinical syndrome similar to that of Kuru, suggesting that the route of infection has a significant impact on the incubation period and clinical manifestation of disease.

Finally, there are a group of rare inherited human prion diseases—including familial CJD, Gerstmann–Sträussler–Scheinker (GSS) disease, and fatal familial insomnia—related to polymorphisms within the gene for prion protein.[4] The pathology of these disorders is characterized by the accumulation of abnormal prion protein (PrP^{TSE}) within the central nervous system associated with neuronal degeneration and reactive gliosis, giving rise to the characteristic spongiform appearance from which these diseases took their original name.[5] There is patchy evidence of peripheral accumulation of PrP^{TSE} in patients with sporadic and familial forms of CJD, but little substantive evidence of infectivity in peripheral blood and tissues or of transmission by blood components, plasma derivatives, or cellular, tissue, or organ transplants.[6]

Variant CJD was first described in 1996.[7] The disease is characterized by a relatively early onset compared to sporadic disease (median 28 years, range 12–74 years); a clinical presentation consisting of behavioral disturbance,[8] dysesthesia, and ataxia followed by progressive neurologic deterioration;[9] and a prolonged clinical phase (median 14 months, range 6 to 48 months).[10] The pathologic features are also characteristic, with the presence of PrP^{TSE} not only within the central nervous system, but also in the follicular dendritic cells of peripheral lymphoid tissues, including tonsils, spleen, lymph nodes, and gut-associated lymphoid tissue. PrP^{TSE} has been demonstrated in two appendix samples removed eight months and two years before the onset of clinical disease.[11] The epidemiologic, pathologic, and experimental data are consistent with variant CJD having arisen from the oral transmission of BSE from infected cattle.

To date, 177 cases have been described in the UK, 27 in France; 5 in Spain; 4 each in Ireland and the United States (US); 3 in the Netherlands; 2 each in Italy, Canada, and Portugal; and 1 each in Japan, Saudi Arabia, and Taiwan.[12] Two of the Irish patients, two of those in the US, and those in Canada and Japan are thought to have been infected during travel in the UK. The overall incidence of clinical cases appears to be diminishing, with current mathematical models projecting a maximum likelihood of 70 (95% confidence interval [CI], 10–190) further clinical cases in the UK.[13] However, the possibility of a cohort of subclinically infected individuals[14] and four cases of transmission of variant CJD prions by blood components described in 2004 and 2006[15–17] raise concern that secondary and higher order transmissions by blood components, plasma derivatives, and cellular, tissue, or organ transplantation could extend the outbreak, particularly if compounded by other potential routes of transmission such as surgery and interventional medical procedures. Although blood service organizations have taken several precautionary measures,[18,19] the persisting uncertainties surrounding the nature, level, and distribution of infectivity; the prevalence of subclinical disease; and the overall transmissibility of the disease continue to undermine our ability to accurately judge the magnitude of this risk and evaluate the impact of current and proposed risk management strategies.

The molecular basis of prion diseases

Prion diseases are associated with a change in the secondary and tertiary conformation of a widely expressed glycoprotein termed prion protein (PrP^C). PrP^C is a 30- to 35-kD protein with two N-linked glycosylation sites and a glycosylphosphatidylinositol anchor. The secondary structure consists of around 40% alpha helix and 3% to 4% beta-pleated sheet. Prion infection is associated with a conformational transformation, resulting in an increase in the proportion of beta-pleated sheet. This, in turn, engenders a change in the physicochemical and biological properties of the molecule (PrP^{TSE}), including an increased resistance to degradation of biological and physical agents (PrP^{RES}).[20] The precise etiology of the conformational change remains unclear, with some authorities favoring a process of homodimerization and others preferring one of nuclear polymerization. The prion hypothesis[21,22] proposes that PrP^{TSE} is the direct cause of infectivity, although it is acknowledged that the relationship between PrP^{TSE}, PrP^{RES}, infectivity, and tissue damage is not straightforward. Some authorities suggest that a small nucleic acid–based agent may be the causative agent.[23,24]

The nature, concentration, and distribution of infectivity

Our current understanding of the pathogenesis of CJD is largely predicated on animal studies. Biochemical and biological assays point to the accumulation of high concentrations of PrP^{TSE} and infectivity in the central nervous system in all forms of prion disease.

Animal models of peripherally transmitted prion diseases[25,26] point to follicular dendritic cells (FDCs)[27,28] in the germinal centers of lymphoid tissue as the key cell in the establishment of infection, and not B lymphocytes as previously suggested.[29,30] The presence of abnormal prion accumulation in the FDCs in tonsil, spleen, and lymph nodes of all patients with variant CJD thus far examined postmortem suggests a similar pathophysiology for CJD in humans following primary (e.g., cattle BSE to humans) or secondary and higher order (human-to-human) transmission.[31]

The exact nature of infectivity in peripheral blood and tissues is uncertain. Recent work suggests that in brain homogenates, the maximum specific infectivity is associated with proteinase-resistant particles of 300 to 600 kD (i.e., oligomers of 14 to 28 PrP molecules).[32] There are also data suggesting that proteinase-sensitive forms of PrP^{TSE} could be infectious. Further work in this area, particularly relating to the physicochemical characteristics of the infectious prion in plasma, is a priority.

The World Health Organization (WHO) conducted a review of the data on the distribution of infectivity and PrP^{TSE} in peripheral tissues and organs in human prion diseases and in naturally and experimentally infected animal prion diseases.[6] Although the highest levels of infectivity are confined to neurologic tissues, lower levels of infectivity and/or PrP^{TSE} have been demonstrated in a wide range of other tissues.

Two sets of rodent studies are informative with regard to the likely concentration and distribution of infectivity in peripheral blood. The first studies were carried out in mice infected with the Fukuoka-1 strain of GSS disease[33,34] and provided the data on which the original risk assessments were based.[35] The second set of studies was carried out in hamsters infected with the 263 K strain of scrapie and has led to a review of blood infectivity assumptions.[36,37] The transmission of prion infection by blood components drawn from donor sheep during both the incubation period and clinical phase of disease has been demonstrated in two different model systems using mice and sheep recipients.[38–41]

In humans, the data on peripheral blood infectivity in sporadic and familial CJD are open to interpretation,[42] although recent data suggest that infectivity can be detected in the peripheral blood of patients with variant CJD using transgenic mice overexpressing bovine PrP.[43]

The spatial distribution of infectivity also varies between models. Brown et al.[33,34] mimicked to a certain extent clinical blood separation processes and demonstrated a four-to fivefold higher concentration of infectivity in the buffy coat (per unit volume) compared to plasma. Gregori et al. studied purified blood components and concluded that red cells and platelets have very little infectivity, and that approximately 40% of infectivity is associated with leukocytes, with most of the remainder residing within the plasma.[36,44] In contrast, the studies in sheep[38–41] and in humans[43] described above suggest that infection can be transmitted by all blood components.

The temporal development of infectivity in peripheral tissues during the incubation period is similarly uncertain. In rodent models, a variety of patterns of change in infectivity and PrP^{TSE} concentration have been observed.[45,46] In humans, the pattern of development of infectivity in peripheral blood and tissues during CJD infection is unknown, although, as noted, abnormal PrP has been detected in an appendix sample removed two years before development of clinical variant CJD.

Overall, the current working assumption is that level of infectivity in the peripheral blood of donors during the subclinical phase of variant CJD infection is likely to be in the order of 1 ID per unit of infected red cells prior to leukodepletion.[47,48]

Clinical transmissibility of CJD by blood and tissues

Although there are a handful of reports of patients who have developed sporadic CJD following exposure to blood components,[49] plasma derivatives,[50–53] or organ transplantation,[50] these reports have not established a convincing link with sporadic CJD in the donors. To the contrary, a large number of epidemiologic case control,[54–64] lookback,[65,66] and surveillance[67–70] studies over the past 30 years have demonstrated no clear evidence of transmission of sporadic CJD by blood transfusion or plasma derivatives. It should be borne in mind, however, that CJD is a rare disease and occasional cases of transmission by blood components could have been missed.

The Transfusion Medicine Epidemiology Review was established in the UK in 1996 in order to monitor potential linkage between CJD in donors and recipients.[71,72] Individuals who develop variant CJD are reported to the UK Blood Services by the National CJD Research and Surveillance Unit (NCJD-RSU) to establish whether they have previously been blood donors. If they have been donors, the recipients are traced and notified. In the reverse arm, NCJD-RSU determines whether individuals who have developed variant CJD have themselves received blood. If they have been transfusion recipients, the UK Blood Services trace and notify the donors. Individuals identified in this way are considered to be "at risk for public health purposes."[73] There are clear ethical and social tensions in adopting a notification strategy when the level of risk is uncertain, psychologic and social detriment may ensue, and no practical benefit accrues to the notified individuals.[74,75] No linkage has been identified between donors and recipients with sporadic or familial CJD in this study. However, 18 UK blood donors have gone on to develop variant CJD, and of their 66 traceable recipients (26 of whom are informative in the sense of having survived more than five years after transfusion), three have developed variant CJD and one showed evidence of subclinical infection at postmortem examination (having died of an unrelated condition).[15–17] In France, three blood donors have developed variant CJD, although of their 18 traceable recipients, none have developed variant CJD at the time of this writing.

Eleven of the above-noted UK blood donors also contributed 25 plasma donations to pools from which a total of 178 plasma batches were manufactured before the UK began importing plasma in 1999. No recipients of implicated products have thus far developed clinical variant CJD—although one patient with hemophilia showed evidence of subclinical infection at postmortem, having died of other causes. Again, following risk assessment, many of these people are now regarded as "potentially at risk for public health purposes."[73,76]

Cells, tissues, and organs are much less frequently transplanted, and many are derived from brain-stem-dead or non-heart-beating donors. In the absence of routine cadaveric testing, it is, therefore, not possible to know whether such individuals may have been incubating CJD at the time of their deaths.[77] There are no clearly substantiated reports of individuals having developed CJD as a result of cellular, tissue, or organ transplantation. However, both prion diseases and these transplant procedures are relatively uncommon events, and given that a significant tissue mass is transplanted, the concentration of infectivity that would be required to transmit infection is well below the level of sensitivity of current assay methods. Therefore, a precautionary assumption is that these tissues may be capable of transmitting disease should the donor be infected.

The prevalence and distribution of subclinical infection

It is the prevalence and epidemiologic distribution of pre- or subclinical disease that drive the risk of secondary transmission, rather than the incidence of clinical disease. Although the incidence of sporadic CJD is known, the incubation period is uncertain and the prevalence of pre- or subclinical disease is unknown. Iatrogenic and familial forms of CJD are fortunately rare; however, it appears likely that preclinical cases will occur in these forms of disease. Those individuals in at-risk groups can often be identified by family or medical history and excluded as donors.

The prevalence and distribution of subclinical variant CJD are also unknown; however, the available data provide some important hints.

Firstly, the median age of onset of disease has not altered over the past decade in the way one would expect where a cohort of individuals has been exposed to the risk of infection over a discrete period.[7,12,78] These data suggest the existence of age-related susceptibility and/or exposure between the ages of 10 and 20 years,[13,79,80] a cohort who would now be between 25 and 45 years old. The patients who have developed variant CJD in France have an older age profile (median age 37 years) than in those in the UK: the reason for this difference is unknown.

Mathematical modeling suggests a maximum likelihood of 3000 infected people (95% CI, 520–6810) in the UK, mainly in the 10- to 30-year age group.[13] The data generated by study of tonsil and appendectomy samples have also been revealing.[14,81,82] The first of the studies revealed three out of 12,674 samples positive for

abnormal prion protein on Western blot,[83] where the specificity is thought to be high but the sensitivity uncertain.[84] A more recent study demonstrated 16 out of 32,441 appendectomy samples positive for abnormal prion protein with similar prevalence across the 1941–1960 and 1961–1985 birth cohorts, gender, and geographic distribution.[85] This is at variance with the number of individuals projected to develop clinical disease and suggests a probability of subclinical infection of 0.93 (95% CI, 0.70–0.97).[13,86] The potential existence of a cohort of individuals in the population with long-term subclinical infection[87,88] is consistent with experimental animal data[89,90] suggesting that methionine–valine heterozygosity or valine homozygosity at codon 129 of the *PRNP* gene predisposes to a prolonged period of subclinical infection. Although all clinical cases of variant CJD thus far have been methionine homozygous at codon 129,[91] the second reported case of transfusion-transmitted variant CJD prions was shown to be methionine–valine heterozygous at codon 129.[16] Two of the three patients who tested positive in the retrospective study of tonsils and appendices have also recently been shown to be valine homozygous at this locus,[92] suggesting that codon 129 genotype (among other things) may influence the propensity of an infected individual to develop clinical disease. Long-term studies on patients who developed Kuru or iatrogenic CJD support this possibility. Individuals who were homozygous for methionine at codon 129 developed clinical disease sooner than those of other codon 129 genotypes, who have developed disease more sporadically and with longer incubation periods (in some cases, over 40 years from their likely infection).

Taken together, these data suggest that the underlying prevalence of subclinical disease in the UK could be around 1 in 2000 (95% CI, 1 in 1250 to 1 in 3500)[93] and that there could be further cases of clinical disease in individuals with other codon 129 genotypes. There are no specific data on which to estimate the prevalence in other countries. However, from the relative incidence of clinical disease, one might expect prevalence in Ireland to be approximately 20% of that in the UK, that in France to be approximately 10%, and that in the Netherlands to be around 5%.

Approaches to risk management

In the face of the uncertainties and extrapolated estimates, a precautionary set of assumptions is that it is likely that there exists a proportion of healthy people with subclinical variant CJD in the UK and other Western European countries, that infectivity is present in the peripheral blood of these individuals, and that transmission of disease is possible through blood and tissue products, but the exact magnitude of these risks is unclear. The best risk management approaches are those that are likely to have some beneficial impact over the widest range of plausible scenarios. However, the effectiveness of such precautionary strategies may be partial or unknown, and the potential for risk substitution and ethical dilemmas needs to be considered.

Donor selection

Residence in the UK (and, to a lesser extent, Ireland and France) is clearly a risk factor for variant CJD, and many countries exclude prospective donors who have lived in such countries.[94] The stipulated period of residence varies widely, depending on the negative impact on the blood donor base and the perceived differential risk.[95]

It has proved more difficult to delineate subpopulations who may be considered to be at higher risk of subclinical vCJD than the general population. Individuals considered to be "presumed infected" or "at risk for public health purposes" are deferred from blood transfusion and tissue transplantation.[73] Although blood transfusion by itself is thought unlikely to give rise to a self-sustaining outbreak, it is possible that transfusion in combination with other potential routes of transmission such as surgical or invasive medical procedures could result in such an event. Confirmation of clinical transmission of variant CJD via blood transfusion led to the introduction of deferral of donors in the UK who themselves have definitely or probably received blood components in order to reduce the risk of tertiary and higher order transmissions, at the cost of a 5% to 10% loss in blood donations. However, surveys have documented considerable inconsistency in donor recall of blood transfusion, undermining confidence in the effectiveness of such measures. Donor exclusion criteria are blunt risk management tools that have the potential for significant negative impact on individual donors and on the blood and tissue supply.

Donor screening assays

The development of peripheral blood assays aimed at the detection of subclinical CJD in donor populations is hampered by the absence of an antibody response or of detectable DNA associated with transmission of the infectious agent.

PrP^{TSE} detection remains the most promising route to development of a preclinical screening assay,[96,97] despite caveats about the precise relationship with infectivity. Achieving the required levels of sensitivity and specificity has, however, proved to be a major challenge. It has been estimated that the threshold of detection may need to be as low as 10^6 molecules of PrP^{TSE}/mL in peripheral blood.[98] Immunoblotting with proteinase K digestion and gel electrophoresis has been enhanced using phosphotungstic acid precipitation and chemiluminescence,[99] but is insufficiently sensitive to detect PrP^{TSE} in blood. Capillary immunoelectrophoresis following proteinase K digestion and competitive antibody binding was the first method to describe detection of PrP^{TSE} in blood,[100] but it has proved complex and difficult to reproduce in other laboratories.[101] A number of attempts have now been made to move away from the use of proteinase K resistance as the defining principle.[102]

Several assays use denaturation of PrP^{TSE} aggregates, the best characterized of which is the conformation dependent immunoassay.[103] A number of PrP^{TSE}-specific monoclonal antibodies have now been described, of which 15B3 is the best characterized.[104] Several groups have developed assays predicated on differential binding of other ligands, including polyanionic compounds,[105] synthetic polypeptides,[6] streptomycin/calyx-6-arene,[6] and palindromic peptides.[106] Some of these approaches have shown sufficient sensitivity to detect infectivity in the peripheral blood of prion-infected animals.

The MRC Prion Unit in London have developed a solid-state binding matrix to capture and concentrate PrP^{TSE} and have coupled this to direct immunodetection of surface-bound material. The resultant assay has proved to be highly sensitive and capable of detecting PrP^{TSE} in the peripheral blood of just over 70% of patients with clinical variant CJD[107] with acceptable specificity in normal controls.[108] Whether the failure to detect PrP^{TSE} in 30% of patients with clinical disease reflects insufficient sensitivity or an absence of abnormal prion in the blood and lymphoreticular tissue of some individuals is currently unclear.[109]

Finally, three approaches appear to amplify PrP^{TSE} and/or infectivity. Protein folding cyclic amplification (PMCA) uses repeated cycles of incubation and sonication to amplify PrP^{TSE} up to 10^7-fold,[44] whereas real-time quaking-induced conversion (RT-QuIC) measures the rate of formation of amyloid fibrils.[110] In vitro cell culture has also proved capable of amplifying murine scrapie.[111] Such amplification approaches might prove a valuable adjunct to other detection methods.

There are three key concerns relating to the introduction of donor screening assays.

1 The specificity of an assay is dependent not only on its technical properties, but also on the population in which it is deployed. An assay with a satisfactory positive predictive value in the context of patients with suspect disease may have a very poor positive predictive value in the context of general population screening. The potential impact of an assay with a low specificity on the false-positive rate of a healthy donor population is illustrated in Figure 54.1. Overall, there is a clear need for assays employing different analytical principles, one or more of which can be used for primary screening and others as supplementary or confirmatory assays to help control the false-positive rate.

2 The validation of such assays is problematic.[112–114] The standard approach to validation of microbiological screening assays uses large numbers of samples from patients known to have the disease in question. Patients with variant CJD in particular are fortunately now very rare, there being nobody alive with the disease at the time of writing. It is likely, therefore, that it will be necessary to carry out the development and validation of peripheral blood screening assays on spiked brain homogenates and endogenously infected animal models, raising concerns about the relevance of these models to the human peripheral blood setting.

3 Consideration will need to be given to the impact of introduction of a screening assay on donors. There are likely to be difficulties in the discrimination of false from true positives and, indeed, in understanding the "meaning" of a true-positive result in terms of the implications for the donor. Donors will have to be informed that they will be screened and notified of any positive result. The psychological and social impact on the individual is likely to be high, and the negative impact on the blood supply could be profound. Further, detailed consideration needs to be given

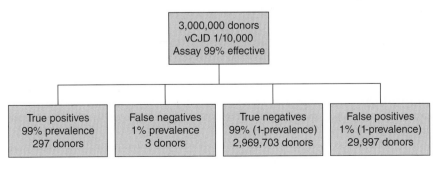

Figure 54.1 The impact of sensitivity and specificity of an assay for variant CJD on test results from a donor population.

to the practical and ethical implications of introducing an assay and the provision of adequate supporting resources.[115–117]

Blood component processing

Whole blood is now rarely transfused, the majority of components being collected via apheresis or derived from whole blood donation and processed into red cell concentrate (in additive solution), platelet concentrate, and fresh frozen plasma. In addition, in the UK, Ireland, France, and some other countries, all clinical blood components are subject to universal leukocyte reduction, which removes 3–4 $\log_{10}$ leukocytes.[118–120] The rodent studies of Brown *et al.*[33,34] and Gregori *et al.*[36] and the sheep studies of Houston *et al.*[40] and Andreoletti *et al.*[41] suggest that it is likely that component processing brings about some reduction in overall infectivity because of reduction in the amount of residual leukocytes and plasma, but it seems unlikely that this will completely remove infectivity in all donations.

Several companies have worked on the development of prion reduction filters for red cell components that offer the possibility of a further reduction in infectivity.[121,122] There are concerns about the evaluation of the efficacy of these technologies given that they have developed using spiked brain homogenates and endogenous infectivity animal models. Potential detrimental effects include additional blood loss in the dead volume of the filter and the possibility of alterations to red cell antigenicity or membrane properties.

Plasma derivative manufacture

It is unlikely that the virus inactivation steps used in the manufacture of plasma derivatives will have a significant impact on prion infectivity.[123] However, work based on consideration of the likely physicochemical characteristics of the prion agent and the partitioning effects of plasma fractionation suggests that a significant reduction in infectivity may occur during the fractionation process, resulting in a relatively low risk of transmission by plasma derivatives.[124] Studies of spiked brain homogenates support this prediction, but are unlikely to accurately reflect the physicochemical nature of the infectious agent in plasma.[125–128] A smaller number of endogenous infectivity studies have been carried out in animal models that again support the general premise, but are unable to demonstrate more than a 1- to 2-log reduction because of low concentrations of infectivity in the starting material.[34] Several manufacturers are using nanofiltration as a second virus reduction step, and these filters have, at least experimentally, demonstrated prion removal, mainly using brain homogenate spikes. One manufacturer has introduced a prion-binding affinity chromatography system as a risk reduction measure in solvent–detergent-treated plasma. There has been no documented case of transmission of sporadic CJD by plasma derivatives. Surveillance of patients exposed to large volumes of plasma products has shown one patient with hemophilia who showed evidence of abnormal prion accumulation in the spleen on postmortem, having died of unrelated causes. Most individuals exposed to large volumes of plasma products are considered to be "potentially at risk for public health purposes."[129]

Cellular, tissue, and organ transplantation

Many types of cells, tissues, and organs are transplanted.[130] As noted previously, the concentration of infectivity in such tissues is uncertain, although broadly speaking, a very low concentration would suffice to cause transmission of disease if the donor were infected. Deferral of transfused donors has proved to be complex because of the nature of the donor population(s), the shortage of some tissues, and the lifesaving nature of the procedure—particularly of organ transplantation. A feasibility study has been initiated to look at the possibility of testing tonsil from cadaveric donors for PrP^{TSE} accumulation. Broadly speaking, any processing that reduces the amount of cellular material and also avoids pooling is likely to be of benefit. There are ongoing studies of the applicability of, for example, washing method for bone processing. Agents that proved effective in the decontamination of surgical instrumentation are largely inapplicable to cells or organs, although some might be applicable to acellular tissues such as heart valves, bone, or tendons. Finally, it is possible that some of the compounds found to mitigate TSE infectivity in vitro and/or in vivo could be applicable to these products.[131,132] Substantial further research and development work will need to be carried out before results of these investigations can be translated to the clinical setting.

Ethical, legal, and societal considerations

Many of the issues raised in this chapter pose not only scientific and medical challenges, but also wider ethical, legal, and societal questions. Early uncertainty over the possibility of secondary transmission of CJD by blood transfusion or plasma derivatives led to the implementation of risk management strategies based on the precautionary principle, perhaps best articulated by the Krever Commission in Canada:[133,134]

> Preventive action should be taken when there is evidence that a potentially disease-causing agent is or may be blood borne, even when there is no evidence that recipients have been affected. If harm can occur, it should be assumed that it will occur. If there are no measures that will entirely prevent the harm, measures that may only partially prevent transmission should be taken.

The accumulating evidence of the existence of a cohort of individuals subclinically infected with variant CJD prions in the UK, along with recent reports of clinical transmission by blood transfusion, speak to the prudence of these measures. However, important uncertainties persist, and the effectiveness of current risk reduction measures including donor selection procedures, component processing, and plasma fractionation remains unclear. New technologies such as prion reduction filters and prion screening assays are under development, and the precautionary principle would speak to the need to implement these where possible. However, such measures are not without potential countervailing risks and ethical problems.[135] Donor deferral criteria can be considered discriminatory, and the introduction of a donor screening assay could have a serious impact on the psychological health of individuals who test positive, leading to difficulties in balancing nonmaleficence with regard to the patient against nonmaleficence with regard to the donor. Donor deferral and screening measures could have a serious negative impact on the sufficiency of blood and tissue supply, leading to a failure of beneficence.[136] Component-processing technologies such as universal leukocyte reduction[137] and prion reduction filters[138] offer the opportunity to circumvent these problems, but at significant financial cost, raising issues of equity of access to healthcare resources. Finally, compulsory notification of people at potentially increased risk of exposure to CJD infection through blood components or plasma derivatives raises the issue of respect for autonomy.[139]

In this context, continued efforts should be made to improve the evidence base regarding clinical blood transfusion and tissue transplantation;[140] to promote a conservative approach to the use of human blood and tissue products;[141] to ensure that patients are appropriately informed;[142,143] and to facilitate public understanding of, and engagement with, the uncertainties and ethical dilemmas inherent in managing this risk.[144]

Disclaimer

The author is Medical Director of the Scottish National Blood Transfusion Service and was a member of the UK Advisory Committee on the Safety of Blood, Tissues and Organs until December 2014.

Key references

A full reference list for this chapter is available at: http://www.wiley.com/go/simon/transfusion

12 The National CJD Research & Surveillance Unit. Current data on variant CJD cases worldwide. http://www.cjd.ed.ac.uk/documents/worldfigs.pdf

36 Gregori L, McCombie N, Palmer D, *et al.* Effectiveness of leucoreduction for removal of infectivity of transmissible spongiform encephalopathies from blood. *Lancet* 2004;**364**:529–31.

40 Houston F, McCutcheon S, Goldman W, *et al.* Prion diseases are efficiently transmitted by sheep. *Blood* 2008;**112**(12): 4739–45.

47 Gregori L, Yang H, Anderson S. Estimation of variant Creutzfeldt–Jakob disease infectivity titres in human blood. *Transfusion* 2011 Jan 3. doi: 10.1111/j.1537-2995.2011.03199x

48 Bennett P, Daraktchiev M. *vCJD and transfusion of blood components: an updated risk assessment*. Department of Health, February 14, 2013.

72 National Blood Service, Scottish National Blood Transfusion Service, Welsh Blood Service, Northern Ireland Blood Transfusion Service, National CJD Surveillance Unit. Transfusion medicine epidemiology review. http://www.cjd.ed.ac.uk/TMER/TMER.htm

93 Advisory Committee on Dangerous Pathogens (ACDP) TSE Risk Assessment Subgroup. Position statement on occurrence of vCJD and prevalence of infection in the UK population. 2012. http://media.dh.gov.uk/network/261/files/2012/08/ACDP-statement-vCJD-occurrence-and-prevalence-Jul-2012.pdf

107 Edgeworth JA, Farmer M, Sicilia A, *et al.* Detection of prion infection in variant Cruetfeldt-Jakob disease: a blood based assay. *Lancet* 2011 Feb 5; **377**:487–93.

122 Gregori L, Gurgel PV, Lathrop JT, *et al.* Reduction in infectivity of endogenous transmissible spongiform encephalopathies present in blood by adsorption to selective affinity resins. *Lancet* 2006;**368**:2226–30.

130 Galea G, Turner ML. Cell, tissue, and organ transplantation. In: Turner ML, Ed. *Creutzfeldt–Jakob disease: managing the risk of transmission by blood, plasma, and tissues*. Bethesda, MD: AABB Press, 2006: 215–43.

CHAPTER 55

Testing for pathogens in donors

Tho D. Pham[1] & Susan A. Galel[2]

[1]Stanford Blood Center and Department of Pathology, Stanford University School of Medicine, Palo Alto, CA, USA
[2]Blood Screening, Roche Molecular Systems, Pleasanton, CA, USA

Introduction

Without safe blood components and transfusions, much of modern medical intervention would be impossible. Because their use is so ubiquitous, the safety of blood components for recipients must be guaranteed to the furthest extent possible. To achieve this goal, two primary strategies are employed: donor questioning and testing.

One of the main strategies employed and required in ensuring blood safety is donor testing for various pathogens,[1] and this will be the focus of this chapter. The various modalities of testing and the tests themselves will be described. The factors underlying the effectiveness of testing in preventing transfusion-transmitted infection (TTI) are as follows: (1) the infectious agents are known to us and we test for them, and (2) the infectious agents or antibodies against them are present at detectable levels. Even with modern testing technologies being as sensitive as they are, transmission can occur in the absence of detection.

Donor screening tests

The efficacy of testing is dependent on the ability to detect certain markers of infection: either the presence of the infectious agent's genomic material (nucleic acid) or protein, or antibodies formed against the infectious agent. There are two general testing modalities: the first is nucleic acid testing (NAT), assaying for nucleic acid sequences (RNA or DNA) specific to the infectious agent's genome, and the second is assaying for viral protein or antibodies produced by the host specific to the infectious agent. Antibody testing can detect current infection, but in some cases it detects past or resolved infection. NAT testing is generally more sensitive and can detect evidence of infection earlier than can serologic methods. However, it does not provide information about past infection. For both methodologies, the time between donor acquisition of infection and a positive test is called the *window period*. Although it varies depending on the infection and test employed, this window period is generally shorter for NAT testing than it is for serologic/protein assays.

Serologic/protein assays

The body's first immunological response to an infection is guided by the innate immune system, involving neutrophils, monocytes/macrophages, and antigen presenting cells. This rapid response with its incumbent pro-inflammatory cytokines gives rise to the acute symptomatology exhibited in illness. As this acute response is being manifest, the adaptive immune system is being activated and makes antibodies against the offending pathogen. The first antibody made is immunoglobulin M (IgM), a pentameric immunoglobulin that, as a first-line antibody, lacks high affinity against the pathogen. As the B lymphocytes mature, they undergo somatic hypermutation, selection, and class switching to produce higher affinity IgG specific to the pathogen. The IgG-producing memory B cells can last in the circulation for years to decades, even if the infection is cleared. Therefore, in general, the first immunoglobulin to be detected by serologic methods is IgM and represents an acute or recent infection, whereas IgG detected may indicate either ongoing or past infection.[2–8]

Serologic tests can be divided into two categories based on testing platform technology: enzyme immunoassays (EIAs) and chemiluminescent immunoassays (ChLIAs). A brief description follows.

Using ChLIAs, microparticles are coated with proteins specific to the pathogen. Depending on the pathogen in question, a variety of purified or recombinant proteins are used. These antigen-coated microparticles are incubated with the donor's plasma (or serum). During the incubation step, any pathogen-specific antibodies stably bind to the antigen-coated microparticles. After the incubation period, the microparticles are enriched and incubated with either antihuman-immunoglobulin or antigens of the pathogen, conjugated to a chemiluminescent molecule that can be easily detected. The amount of light generated is directly proportional to the amount of antibodies in the donor plasma that are specific against the purified or recombinant proteins of the pathogen. Cutoff values that define a reactive result are established by the manufacturer. Tests used for screening of donations must be both highly sensitive (to detect most infections) and highly specific (to minimize *false-positive* results).

In an EIA testing platform, generally a two-step enzyme-linked immunosorbent assay (ELISA) scheme is used. The bottom of a well is coated with reagent infectious antigens, either purified or recombinant peptides. The donor plasma (or serum) is then added and incubated in the well. Pathogen-specific antibodies in the donor plasma (if present) bind to the immobilized reagent antigen. An enzyme-conjugated secondary antibody (antihuman-IgG and/or antihuman-IgM, depending on the test) is then added. A colorimetric substrate is subsequently added, which in the presence of the enzyme conjugated to the secondary antibody will produce a color

Rossi's Principles of Transfusion Medicine, Fifth Edition. Edited by Toby L. Simon, Jeffrey McCullough, Edward L. Snyder, Bjarte G. Solheim, and Ronald G. Strauss.

Table 55.1 FDA-approved serology/protein tests most commonly used in the united states

Target Protein Detected	Test Name	Test Method	Capture Target(s)
IgM and IgG against HBV core antigen	Abbott PRISM HBcore	ChLIA	Recombinant HBV core antigen
	ORTHO HBc ELISA Test System	EIA	Recombinant HBV core antigen
HBsAg	ABBOTT PRISM HBsAg	ChLIA	Mouse monoclonal anti-HBsAg IgM
	Genetic Systems HBsAg EIA 3.0	EIA	Mouse monoclonal anti-HBsAg IgM
IgG against HCV antigens	ABBOTT PRISM HCV	ChLIA	Recombinant peptides from HCV core, NS3, NS4, and NS5
	Ortho HCV Version 3.0 ELISA Test System	EIA	Recombinant peptides from HCV core, NS3, NS4, and NS5
IgG and IgM against HIV-1 (group M and O) and HIV-2	ABBOTT PRISM HIV O Plus	ChLIA	Recombinant HIV-1 Group M envelope and HIV-1 Group O envelope; recombinant and synthetic HIV-2 envelope
	Genetic Systems HIV-1/HIV-2 Plus O EIA	EIA	Recombinant HIV-1 gp160 and p24; HIV-2 gp36; synthetic HIV-1 group O polypeptide
Immunoglobulin against HTLV-I and HTLV-II	ABBOTT PRISM HTLV-1/HTLV-II	ChLIA	Purified HTLV-I and HTLV-II antigens
	Avioq HTLV-I/II Microelisa System	EIA	Purified HTLV-I viral lysate, a purified HTLV-II viral lysate, and a recombinant HTLV-I p21E antigen
Immunoglobulin (or IgG) against *T. cruzi* antigens	ABBOTT PRISM Chagas	ChLIA	Recombinant *T. cruzi* proteins FP3, FP6, FP10, and TcF
	ORTHO *T. cruzi* ELISA Test System	EIA	*T. cruzi* lysate

change. The color change generated is directly proportional to the levels of pathogen-specific antibodies in donor plasma.

A slight variation on the testing schemes mentioned above is employed in the tests used to detect hepatitis B surface antigen (HBsAg). In these tests, a monoclonal antibody specific for HBsAg is immobilized (on either the microparticles in ChLIA or well bottoms in EIA) and incubated with donor plasma, and HBsAg, if present in donor plasma, is subsequently immobilized. To this is added a second reagent, monoclonal anti-HBsAg antibody, that is appropriately conjugated to enable detection by simple spectrophotometric methods.

In the event that a donor screening serology/protein test is reactive to either ChLIA or EIA, the test is repeated in duplicate. If one or both of the repeat tests is reactive, the result for the donation is labeled "repeat reactive" (RR). At this point, regardless of the pathogen for which the test is RR, the unit will typically be discarded.[9]

The pathogens for which there are current US Food and Drug Administration (FDA)-approved serologic screening tests are shown in Table 55.1.[10]

Nucleic acid testing (NAT)

NAT decreases the window period of an infectious pathogen when compared to serologic/protein tests. Of the pathogens currently detected by NAT, only HBV is a DNA virus; the others are RNA. In general, a nucleic acid sequence specific to the pathogen in question is amplified and detected. There are two main strategies available for nucleic acid amplification and detection: polymerase chain reaction (PCR) with real-time fluorescence detection and transcription-mediated amplification with end-point chemiluminescence detection.

PCR has been used for decades, and many modifications and improvements have been made on the general process. The method is based on using a primer pair that flanks the nucleic acid region of interest. Within the sample is also the template DNA/RNA (in this case, it would be the donor's sample) and Taq DNA polymerase. Through a repeating series of temperatures in the thermocycler to produce melting, annealing, and amplification of the genetic region of interest, the target is exponentially amplified by the power of 2 (i.e., at the end of every cycle, there will be twice as many amplicons as compared to the beginning of the cycle). Therefore, if one were to successfully perform 35 PCR cycles on a sample with only initially four copies of pathogen, at the end of 35 cycles there would be a total of $4 \times 2^{35} =$ greater than 34 billion molecules. If the pathogen nucleic

acid material is RNA, the first round of amplification occurs with reverse transcriptase, creating cDNA that can then proceed with PCR as described. In real-time PCR, at each annealing step, a sequence-specific oligonucleotide probe with both a reporter and quencher dye in proximity to one another is allowed to anneal with the template, separate from the primers. As long as the reporter and quencher dye molecules are in close proximity, no signal is generated. Once primer-specific polymerase-mediated extension occurs, the exonuclease activity of the polymerase liberates the reporter from the quencher dye and consequently produces fluorescence. Because fluorescence is produced at every round of amplification, its rise is proportional to the amount of starting nucleic acid template (i.e., pathogen genome). Therefore, a higher concentration of pathogen genome at the start will produce a positive signal at an earlier round. This method of detection is called *real-time detection*.

The transcription-mediated amplification method rests upon amplification of the targeted area by RNA polymerase. Similar to PCR, primers targeting the sequence of interest are used. Once annealed, if the region of interest is RNA, it is reverse-transcribed to make cDNA, followed by a round of DNA amplification to produce a double-stranded DNA molecule. At this point, a highly efficient T7 RNA polymerase acts on its promoter (which is designed into the targeting primers above) to produce multiple RNA transcripts from the region of interest. These steps are then repeated, starting with reverse transcriptase. A key difference from PCR is that transcription-mediated amplification reactions are isothermal and do not require a thermocycler. At the end of amplification, a chemiluminescently labeled single-stranded oligonucleotide probe specific to the region of interest is added. It will hybridize with the amplified products, creating a double-stranded molecule. Nonhybridized single-stranded oligonucleotide probes are inactivated, and the remaining chemiluminescently labeled double-stranded molecules are measured. This is known as an end-point detection method.

In a multiplex assay, all the pathogen-specific primers for HIV, hepatitis C virus (HCV), and hepatitis B virus (HBV) are used in one reaction. The currently available NAT platforms allow testing multiple donors (a *minipool* [MP] of typically 6–16 donors) in a multiplex scheme to detect the presence of HIV RNA, HBV DNA, or HCV RNA. Therefore, if an MP-NAT result is positive, it means that one or more of the individual donors tested in the MP could be positive for any one or more of the viruses tested. The next step is to

Table 55.2 FDA-approved donor NAT tests most commonly used in the United States

Test Name	Assay Use	Targets Detected	Manufacturer	Amplification Method	Detection Method
cobas TaqScreen MPX Test	Multiplex screen	HIV-1 Group M RNA, HIV-1 Group O RNA, HIV-2 RNA, HCV RNA, HBV DNA	Roche Molecular Systems, Inc.	PCR	Real-time fluorescence
cobas AmpliScreen Tests	Single-virus screen or viral target discrimination	Single-virus tests for: HIV-1 RNA, HCV RNA, or HBV DNA	Roche Molecular Systems, Inc.	PCR	End point colorimetric
cobas TaqScreen MPX Test, v2.0	Multiplex screen and simultaneous viral target discrimination	HIV-1 Group M RNA HIV-1 Group O RNA HIV-2 RNA HCV RNA HBV DNA	Roche Molecular Systems, Inc.	PCR	Real-time fluorescence
cobas TaqScreen WNV	Single-virus screen	WNV RNA	Roche Molecular Systems, Inc.	PCR	Real-time fluorescence
Procleix Ultrio Plus Assay	Multiplex screen	HIV-1 RNA HCV RNA HBV DNA	Hologic, Inc.	TMA	End point chemiluminescence
Procleix Ultrio Plus discriminatory assays	Viral target discrimination	Single virus tests for: HIV-1 RNA, or HCV RNA, or HBV DNA	Hologic, Inc.	TMA	End point chemiluminescence
Procleix WNV	Single-virus screen	WNV RNA	Hologic, Inc.	TMA	End point chemiluminescence

FDA, US Food and Drug Administration; HBV, hepatitis B virus; HCV, hepatitis C virus; HIV, human immunodeficiency virus; NAT, nucleic acid testing; TMA, transcription-mediated amplification; WNV, West Nile virus.

do individual testing (IDT) of the donors in that initially reactive MP. In addition to identifying which donor sample is responsible for the positive signal, the specific viral target must also be identified (i.e., discriminatory testing). Some multiplex screening assays both detect and discriminate the viral target in one step. Other assays require secondary viral discriminatory tests to distinguish which viral target is present in the donor sample.

NAT screening may be performed as IDT rather than MP. This is more costly, but improves the sensitivity of the assay,[11] as individual donor samples containing very low levels of viral nucleic acid may not be detected if pooled with other samples for MP screening. IDT screening is primarily of benefit for detection of infections associated with very low levels of viremia, such as West Nile virus (WNV) infection and possibly occult hepatitis B infection (OBI), as discussed further in this chapter. For detection of very early HIV, HCV, or HBV infections, there is only a brief period of time where IDT would be of benefit over MP screening; this is because the concentrations of these viruses increase rapidly during early infection due to short virus doubling times. However, regions that have a high frequency of new HIV, HCV, or HBV infections among their blood donors may find value in IDT screening.[12,13]

The current most widely used FDA-approved NAT screens are shown in Table 55.2.[10]

Consequences of a reactive screening test

If a screening NAT result is reactive at the individual donor level, or if any serologic/protein test is RR, the unit in question is typically discarded according to FDA requirements. What happens thereafter and what additional tests are performed differ according to the pathogen for which the test is reactive. Additional testing may be required to guide decisions regarding donor management and counseling, retrieval and quarantine of previously donated components, and notification of prior recipients.

Confirmatory and supplemental testing

The serology/protein tests discussed above are FDA-licensed as blood or plasma donor screening tests, which are separate from approval as a diagnostic test. An RR result on a serology/protein screening test does not necessarily signify infection in the blood donor. Additional more specific supplemental testing is needed to distinguish whether the RR result represents a true or false-positive result. According to FDA regulation Title 21, CFR 610.40, supplemental testing is required for RR screening tests for HIV, HCV, HBV, and human T-cell lymphotropic virus (HTLV) when such tests are approved by the FDA for that purpose. Some virus-specific NAT tests, if positive, are approved by FDA as confirming RR serology/protein results. The serology/protein screening tests included in this category are HBsAg, anti-HCV, and anti-HIV-1/2. However, if the NAT is negative for the respective virus, additional serologic supplemental testing is required. HBsAg neutralization, HCV RIBA, HIV-1 IFA or Western blot, and HIV-2 EIA are the FDA-approved confirmatory tests for the respective serology/protein tests (however, HCV RIBA is no longer available). FDA has also approved HTLV and *Trypanosoma cruzi* antibody confirmatory tests.

Not all serology/protein tests have an FDA-approved confirmatory test, but performing additional unlicensed supplemental tests, or repeating the test on a second manufacturer's screening assay, may provide information useful for donor counseling.

Donor management and reentry testing

Donor management (eligibility for future donations) and counseling vary depending on which screening test is reactive and what the confirmatory testing shows, if one is available. If the donor is ineligible for future donations, the donor must be informed of the deferral. The specifics of donor management and reentry testing for different testing scenarios are outlined by the FDA and/or AABB in various documents that have been released over time.[9,14–24]

Reentry testing algorithms to qualify donors for future donations are only available for certain screening tests, and even then only in very specific scenarios, usually in conjunction with confirmatory testing and a waiting/deferral period. Reentry testing is available for tests relating to HCV, HBV, and HIV. As a general rule, reentry testing is available when the original reactive screening test is thought to represent a false-positive for infection. The general reentry testing procedures for each test are shown in Tables 55.3 and 55.4.[17,21–23]

Table 55.3 Criteria for reentry eligibility

Virus	FDA Guidance	Initial NAT	Initial Serology	Initial Confirmatory	Eligible for Reentry?	Waiting Period
HCV	Guidance for Industry; May 2010[23]	Neg/ND	RR	Neg/Ind/ND	Y	6 months
		Neg/ND	RR	Pos	N	NA
		Pos	NR	N.A	Y	6 months
		Pos	RR	Neg/Ind/ND	N	NA
		Pos	RR	Pos	N	NA
HIV	Guidance for Industry; May 2010[23]	Neg/ND	RR	Neg/Ind/ND*	Y	8 weeks
		Neg/ND	RR	Pos	N	NA
		Pos	NR	N.A	Y	8 weeks
		Pos	RR	Neg/Ind/ND	N	NA
		Pos	RR	Pos	N	NA

Virus	FDA Guidance	Initial NAT	Initial HBsAg	Initial anti-HBc	Eligible for Re-entry?	Waiting Period
HBV	Guidance for Industry May 2010[17]	Neg/ND	NR	RR	Y	8 weeks
	Guidance for Industry November 2011[21]	Neg/ND	RR/confirmed	NR	Y**	56 days***
		Neg/ND	RR/confirmed	NR	Y****	12 months
	Guidance for Industry October 2012[22]	Pos	NR	NR	Y	6 months
		Pos	NR	RR	Y	6 months
		Pos	RR/confirmed	NR	N	NA
		Pos	RR/confirmed	RR	N	NA
		Pos	RR/non confirmed	NR	Y	6 months
		Pos	RR/non confirmed	RR	N	NA

* HIV-1 WB or IFA indeterminate, unreadable, negative, or not done; HIV-1 p24 EIA2 negative; second, different HIV-2 test negative, or, if RR, investigational HIV-2 supplemental test (if performed) was not positive.

** If HBV vaccination given for possible future exposure, and vaccination given within 28 days prior to positive HBsAg test result.

*** No need to retest; donor eligible for reentry into donor pool after 56-day waiting period.

**** If HBV vaccination given as prophylaxis following exposure, and vaccination given within 28 days prior to positive HBsAg test result.

Confirmed, confirmed by HBsAg neutralization; Ind, indeterminate; NA, not applicable; ND, not done; Neg, negative; NR, nonreactive; Pos, positive; RR, repeat reactive.

Retrieval of prior donations and notification of prior recipients

Upon demonstration of a reactive NAT or RR serologic test, FDA requires not only quarantine of the current donation, but also quarantine and retrieval of components from prior donations made when the donor could have been harboring infection.[9,14,16,19,20,23,25–28] If supplemental testing confirms donor infection, in some cases the FDA and/or AABB recommend notification of prior recipients of their potential exposure to infection. Notification of potentially exposed recipients is required or recommended for donors with HIV, HCV, WNV, *T. cruzi*, and HTLV infections[9,14,16,19,23,25,27,28]

Residual risk for TTI

Despite our best efforts, blood products still carry an inherent risk (albeit small at this time) of TTI.[29–33] Even when the donor screening questionnaire and all the screening tests are negative, there is a residual risk that exists in every blood component. The sources for this residual risk can come from known and unknown pathogens.

Table 55.4 Reentry testing for HIV, HCV, and HBV

Follow-Up NAT*	Follow-Up Serology	Action
Neg	NR	Reinstate
Neg	NR	Further evaluation
Pos	RR	Defer permanently
Pos	NR	Defer permanently

* HBV follow-up NAT must have a sensitivity of ≤2 IU/mL.

HBV, hepatitis B virus; HCV, hepatitis C virus; HIV, human immunodeficiency virus; NAT, nucleic acid testing; Neg, negative; NR, nonreactive; Pos, positive; RR, repeat reactive.

Although the tests currently employed have high sensitivity, whatever testing method used will have a window period during which infection is not detectable. Therefore, in a modern blood bank where electronic control systems are in place to prevent release of untested or test-positive units, the most significant source of residual risk is an infected donor who donates during the window period. Although the window period for NAT is much shorter than for the respective serology/protein tests (about 9 days for HIV and 7.4 days for HCV with minipool NAT),[11,31] a window period nonetheless exists. Where epidemiologic risk factors are known, donor questioning to exclude individuals who may have been recently exposed to infection plays a critical role in protecting the blood supply from window-period donations.

The window period is just one aspect contributing to residual risk. The other contributing factors are unknown pathogens or pathogens for which there are no current tests. The risk for transmitting an as-yet-unidentified pathogen through blood is impossible to calculate. For known pathogens without available testing, one main defense is the donor questionnaire. Additionally, public health and infectious disease organizations play an important role in raising alert and scrutiny. The AABB Transfusion-Transmitted Diseases Committee maintains a website containing fact sheets about potential pathogens and potential mitigation strategies.[34–36]

A notable example of alertness to potential hazards, and recommendation of a mitigation strategy thereto, is the recent Ebola virus epidemic in West Africa in 2014. Although most potentially exposed individuals would be deferred from donating by the malaria questions, the secondary transmissions to healthcare workers in the United States who came in contact with infected individuals from West Africa prompted AABB to release a bulletin recommending a 28-day self-deferral for those who have had contact with infected persons.[37] As the time of this writing, there have been no reports of transfusion-transmitted Ebola either within or without the United States.

Variations in practice

International

It should be underscored that the infectious disease screening tests performed by blood centers of a certain country/region reflect a variety of factors that are unique to that country/region, particularly the prevalence of the infectious disease. For example, testing of donors for WNV is performed primarily in countries such as the United States and Canada, where there have been recurrent epidemics; some non-endemic countries perform WNV testing on donors who have recently traveled to regions where WNV is active. Testing for hepatitis E virus (HEV) RNA has been implemented in Japan and is being considered in other regions with an increased prevalence of this infection. In the United States and other places, donor screening for antibodies to the hepatitis B core antigen (anti-HBc) excludes donors who may have OBI.[38,39] However, in HBV hyperendemic countries such as China, excluding donors with anti-HBc is not practical. In these countries, sensitive NAT testing may be used to detect the low levels of circulating HBV DNA that are associated with OBI.

The pathway to access blood donor screening tests also differs by region. In some countries, such as the United States and China, clinical trials of donor screening tests are required for regulatory approval. In other countries, the process for approval is much quicker because the tests' ability to detect infection needs only to be demonstrated in vitro by the manufacturer. Whether tests developed for diagnostic use may be used to screen blood donors also varies regionally.

However, despite different needs in different regions, there are commonalities. Serologic tests for HBsAg, anti-HCV, anti-HIV, and syphilis are recommended by the WHO.[40] Use of multiplex NAT for HIV, HCV, and HBV is increasingly widespread. Serology testing practices regarding anti-HTLV, antibody to *T. cruzi*, and anti-HBc are variable.

Source plasma

Source plasma (SP) is defined as plasma collected by apheresis and intended for source material for manufacturing use. The products made from SP include intravenous immunoglobulin G (IVIG) and albumin. The manufacturing and purification processes include several steps that inactivate or remove pathogens, often including solvent-detergent (SD) treatment that inactivates lipid-enveloped pathogens. Because of these pathogen reduction processes, testing requirements for source plasma donations differ from those for donors of blood components for transfusion. For example, testing for anti-HBc, anti-HTLV (associated with white cells), and WNV is not required, and NAT testing for HIV, HCV, and HBV may be performed in larger sample pools.

Pathogens that lack a lipid envelope are not susceptible to the SD pathogen reduction treatment commonly used in the manufacturing of plasma derivatives. Incoming plasma intended for manufacturing into plasma derivatives may be tested for some non-enveloped viruses in order to minimize the likelihood that the final product will contain these pathogens. FDA has specifically recommended "in-process testing" to intercept incoming plasma units that contain high titers of parvovirus B19 in order to ensure that the

concentration of this virus in the final manufacturing pool does not exceed 10^4 IU/mL.[41] In-process testing may also be used to intercept units containing hepatitis A, which is also not lipid enveloped. Recently, concern has been raised about the potential contamination of plasma derivatives by hepatitis E, as this virus also lacks a lipid coat and potential transmission by SD plasma has been reported.[42] The need for HEV testing for plasma derivatives is not yet established, as the derivative manufacturing processes may be sufficient to remove or inactivate this virus.

Special considerations

Syphilis

The testing platform methodology and donor reentry guidelines are unique to syphilis.[24] Donor screening tests for syphilis are serologic, and can be broadly categorized as non-treponemal and treponemal assays. Non-treponemal assays are nonspecific tests that detect antibodies reactive against cardiolipin (aka *reagin*), an antibody that is usually found in people recently or currently infected with *Treponema pallidum*, as well as in other biologic conditions such as lupus. The non-treponemal tests include rapid plasma reagin (RPR), the Venereal Disease Research Laboratory (VDRL) test, and the Automated Reagin Test (ART). Because they test for an antibody seen not only in active syphilis but also in many other biologic conditions, they have a high false-positive rate.

More commonly, donor screening is performed using treponemal assays that detect antibody to *T. pallidum*. Treponemal assays include *T. pallidum* particle agglutination, microhemagglutination, and enzyme immunoassays. These assays are more specific for exposure to *T. pallidum*. Because they detect IgG antibody, however, they do not distinguish between current and past infection.

The route for reentry is notably different for syphilis than for the other pathogens mentioned. If the donor tests reactive on a syphilis-screening test, an FDA-cleared treponemal screen different from the test used for initial screening may be used to determine donor eligibility. If the second test is nonreactive, the donor may be immediately reentered. Product disposition varies according to whether the initial reactive donor screen was a non-treponemal test or a treponemal test. If the second test is positive, the donor is deferred indefinitely. The donor may only be reentered 12 months after completion of treatment for syphilis, and must provide written evidence thereof from a physician.

Cytomegalovirus (CMV)

Although varying by geographic and socioeconomic status, in most populations the majority of adults have been infected by CMV. CMV remains in the body after initial infection and has the potential for reactivation. Symptoms of infection in normal immune-competent individuals are mild and self-limited. However, in an immune-compromised individual, CMV infection can have severe manifestations and be fatal. CMV can be transmitted by transfusion of cellular blood components. Therefore, in hospital transfusion settings, immune-compromised patients who have never been exposed to CMV should receive cellular products with a low risk of transmitting CMV virus. There are currently two non-exclusive routes for achieving this status in the United States. The first is serology, and the second is leukoreduction (LR).

In the United States, the testing currently employed for CMV in blood donors is a serology test for IgG and IgM. Because a major proportion of the donor pool would have been exposed to CMV at some point in their lives, most will be positive by this test. Therefore, trying to sustain an inventory with purely CMV-seronegative blood is very difficult, if not practically impossible. However, CMV-seronegative cellular products can be reserved for the most at-risk patients.

An alternative strategy to reduce the likelihood of CMV transmission is LR. After an individual clears a CMV infection, the virus establishes latency in many tissues, including monocytes/macrophages, secretory glands, and kidneys. Reducing the number of potentially CMV-harboring white cells by LR has been shown to reduce the risk of CMV-TTI when compared with non-LR products.[43]

Although both LR and CMV-sero-negative units have been shown to reduce CMV-TTI when compared to sero-positive non-LR units, whether CMV-seronegative products are safer than LR products in regard to CMV-TTI is a topic of great debate. With current LR filters, many studies have found the rate of CMV-TTI to be not significantly different from that of seronegative products.[43–46] One major study[45] showed the rate of CMV-TTI in the LR group was not significantly different, although it was slightly elevated, when compared to that of the seronegative group (2.4% vs. 1.3%). However, this issue is not settled, with many proponents on either side.

West Nile virus

WNV is an RNA virus belonging to the family *Flaviviridae*. Birds are thought to be the primary reservoir, with mosquitos as the vector by which humans acquire the infection. The vast majority (80%) of WNV infections are asymptomatic, with about 20% developing a fever. In a very small number of instances, the infection progresses to a neuroinvasive disease with significant morbidity and mortality.

WNV first appeared in the United States in 1999, and since then has had annually localized epidemics during the summertime. The first WNV-TTI cases were recognized in 2002, which traced the virus to blood donations having viral RNA but not antibodies against it. As a result of these findings, NAT is the only required testing for WNV.

Furthermore, WNV infection is associated with low viral loads, and MP testing has been demonstrated to miss more than 50% of infections.[47–49] In light of these facts, WNV screening by IDT is recommended when WNV is active in the region.[14,49] Consequently, donor centers are required to develop strategies regarding when and how to switch from MP to IDT when WNV activity is high. Determination of WNV activity is accomplished by active communications among regional blood centers whenever one has a positive donor screen for WNV, as well as public health organizations' reports of regional human clinical cases, and avian/animal activity.

Conclusion

Currently, TTI risk reduction from blood and plasma components is achieved primarily through two methods: donor questioning and donor testing. Donor testing broadly falls in two categories: serologic/protein assays and NAT assays, with NAT having shorter window periods. Different countries have slightly varying regulations regarding mandated testing. Furthermore, in certain testing scenarios where a false-positive result is likely the case, there exist well-defined algorithms for donor reentry into the general donor pool. In the Unites States, donor deferral policy and donor reentry are clearly defined.

These testing methods have allowed for great success in reducing TTI. However, a window period nonetheless exists, with its incumbent residual risk. It must be noted that the residual risk associated with window periods only accounts for those pathogens that are known and tested. For those as-yet-unknown and/or untested pathogens, the residual risk is not quantifiable. Therefore, we must remain alert and in contact with public organizations for rapid communication of potentially emerging infectious diseases and strategies for their abatement.

Key references

A full reference list for this chapter is available at: http://www.wiley.com/go/simon/transfusion

1 Carson TH, Ed., *Standards for blood banks and transfusion services*. 29th ed. Bethesda, MD: AABB, 2014.

11 Busch MP, Glynn SA, Stramer SL, *et al*. A new strategy for estimating risks of transfusion-transmitted viral infections based on rates of detection of recently infected donors. *Transfusion* 2005;**45**:254–64.

13 Vermeulen M, Coleman C, Mitchel J, *et al*. Comparison of human immunodeficiency virus assays in window phase and elite controller samples: viral load distribution and implications for transmission risk. *Transfusion* 2013;**53**:2384–98.

29 Kleinman SH, Lelie N, Busch MP. Infectivity of human immunodeficiency virus-1, hepatitis C virus, and hepatitis B virus and risk of transmission by transfusion. *Transfusion* 2009;**49**:2454–89.

CHAPTER 56

Pathogen reduction of blood components and plasma derivatives

Nathan J. Roth

Global Pathogen Safety, CSL Behring, King of Prussia, PA, USA

The pathogen safety of plasma derivative and labile components has been dramatically enhanced over the last 25 years through the implementation of nucleic acid testing (NAT) technologies that effectively screen out units with high virus titers. Additionally, the incorporation of pathogen inactivation (PI) and removal steps into the manufacturing processes of plasma-derived medicinal products has greatly enhanced the safety of the final products against both known and emerging/reemerging viruses. The development of pathogen reduction technologies for labile blood components has proven to be more challenging, but significant advancements have been made over the last decade in the development, commercialization, and routine implementation of pathogen reduction technology (PRT) systems for fresh frozen plasma (FFP) and for platelets. The development of a PRT suitable for whole blood or red cells remains an ongoing challenge.

This chapter discusses the PRTs that are commonly used or under development for the various product classes: (1) labile blood components (whole blood [RBCs], platelets, or FFP); (2) manufactured pooled, solvent–detergent (S/D)-treated plasma; and (3) manufactured plasma-derived medicinal products (PDMPs) such as immunoglobulins, purified clotting factors, and albumin. Each class of product faces unique challenges and incorporates different safety measures in order to prevent transfusion-transmitted infections (TTIs).

PRTs for blood components

Blood component transfusions represent a portal of entry for infectious agents and may contain trace amounts of endogenous bacteria (mostly from the gut or from presymptomatic infections) and/or exogenous bacteria (from the skin). With the volumes generally collected during a donation, trace contaminations are a problem. This is particularly true for platelet products (stored at 22 °C) and in the transfusion of immunocompromised patients. Important interventions to reduce the risk for trace contaminations are careful donor selection, enhanced cleansing of the venipuncture site, use of diversion pouches for the first 15 to 20 mL of a blood collection,[1] and the testing of platelet preparations for the presence of bacteria. Risks for TTIs are escalated by emerging infections combined with increased international air travel.[2] Programs for careful donor selection and extensive laboratory testing pose both organizational and economic challenges in most developing coun-

tries. In addition, the epidemiology of the donor base is less favorable than in most developed countries, the use of whole blood is still dominating, and safe fractionated plasma proteins are mostly unavailable. Therefore, TTIs are a serious problem, causing thousands of infections a year, particularly with hepatitis B virus (HBV), hepatitis C virus (HCV), human immunodeficiency virus (HIV), and malaria. Robust and affordable PRT's for whole blood and blood components would be of great value in these countries. In developed countries, the risk for bacterial and protozoan infections and emerging infectious agents are the main driver for PRTs.

PRTs have been developed and licensed for plasma and platelet components, but the implementation of these systems, although increasing, still remains sporadic and varies widely by country.[3] The development of a suitable PRT for whole blood or RBC components is much more challenging, and although development activities are continuing, to date, no technology is commercially available. The lack of approved PRT systems for whole blood (or for RBCs) may be a significant barrier for the adoption and implementation of PRTs for platelets and plasma.

The goal of PRTs is to provide broad-spectrum inactivation of viral and/or bacterial pathogens that are not routinely tested for by NAT or cultivation methodologies. PI of blood components should inactivate or remove all types of infectious agents, without inducing neo-antigens or reducing the function or lifespan of a blood component. PI should not result in residual toxic substances or involve a risk greater than any TTI associated with the original blood component.[4] Because toxicity may first be revealed after large-scale clinical use, Phase IV postmarketing studies and hemovigilance programs are important.

In general, PRT systems utilize a single type of technology that has a relatively broad-spectrum efficacy against enveloped viruses (including emerging viruses such as West Nile virus [WNV], dengue virus, and chikungunyavirus), vegetative bacteria, and parasites. Arguably, the prophylactic use of these technologies on platelet and plasma components will further improve the safety of the blood supply by preventing window period virus transmission, preventing transfusion transmission of infections during emerging virus outbreaks, and reducing transfusion transmission of cell-associated cytomegalovirus (CMV) and bacterially contaminated components, especially platelets.[5] PRTs that target nucleic acids have the advantage of inactivating residual white blood cells, thereby potentially preventing transfusion-related acute lung injury

Rossi's Principles of Transfusion Medicine, Fifth Edition. Edited by Toby L. Simon, Jeffrey McCullough, Edward L. Snyder, Bjarte G. Solheim, and Ronald G. Strauss.
© 2016 John Wiley & Sons, Ltd. Published 2016 by John Wiley & Sons, Ltd.

(TRALI) and graft-versus-host disease (GVHD). Unlike plasma-derived medicinal products that are produced using manufacturing processes that contain multiple complementary measures with orthogonal modes of action to assure the safety of the final product against cellular pathogens, viruses, and prions (see later in this chapter), PRT systems for labile blood components generally rely on a single type of inactivation technology (which is not universally effective), and therefore each system has inherent limitations that may allow specific pathogens to escape inactivation and removal and transmit disease.[6] Nonetheless, even while recognizing these inherent limitations, PRTs have the potential to significantly reduce the safety gap of untreated components and provide benefit to patients.[7]

PRTs for single-donor plasma and platelets
Methylene blue (MB)-light treatment of FFP

MB, coupled with visible-light treatment, has been used clinically in Europe as a pathogen reduction technology for single-unit FFP for nearly two decades.[8,9] Over 4.4 million units of FFP have been treated and transfused. MB is a positively charged phenothiazine compound with high affinity for negatively charged compounds, such as nucleic acids and lipid bilayers.[10] MB intercalates with nucleic acids or binds to lipids and upon illumination with visible light produces a photodynamic reaction that results in nucleic strand breakage or lipid peroxidation with subsequent modification of surrounding membrane proteins.[11] MB light treatment is broadly effective against enveloped viruses, but inactivation of non-enveloped viruses is virus specific; some non-enveloped viruses (e.g., B19 V) are effectively inactivated, whereas others are nearly completely resistant (e.g., hepatitis A virus [HAV]) (Table 56.1).[8]

Extracellular parasites (*Trypanosoma cruzi*) are susceptible to treatment. MB treatment has no effect upon prions, although leukocyte reduction, if incorporated within the manufacturing process, has been shown have the potential to decrease variant Creutzfeld–Jakob disease (vCJD) infectivity.[12]

MB-treated FFP has not been approved by the US Food and Drug Administration (FDA) for use in the United States, but variations of the technology have been commercially developed for clinical use in Europe by Grifols SA and by Macopharma (Theraflex-MB). Grifols centrally processes MB-treated plasma at an industrial facility near Barcelona, whereas the Theraplex MB-Plasma system is Council of Europe (CE) marked and is intended to be employed at regional blood centers.

MB treatment reduces the potency of some plasma proteins; fibrinogen, factor V, and factor VIII activity are decreased by approximately 10–30%, and the effect on other coagulation factors and inhibitors is smaller.[13,14] No neo-antigenicity after MB treatment has been reported. However, hemovigilance data have raised debate as to whether MB treatment increases, decreases, or has no effect on the rate of adverse events versus quarantined FFP.[15–18] Satisfactory clinical results and efficacy have been reported with MB-treated plasma except for observational studies from Spain that suggest that MB-treated plasma may be less effective in the treatment of thrombotic thrombocytopenic purpura (TTP) than quarantined FFP.[19]

Psoralen-ultraviolet light treatment of FFP and platelets (INTERCEPT System)

Cerus (Concord, CA) has developed a psoralen/ultraviolet-A (UVA)–based PI method (INTERCEPT Plasma or Platelet System)

Table 56.1 Inactivation agents, susceptible pathogens, and modified targets

Inactivation Method	Susceptible Organism	Target/Modification
Methylene blue plus light -Theraflex-MB -Grifols/Biomat MB treated plasma	• Enveloped viruses • Some non-enveloped viruses	Free radical damage of negatively charged nucleic acids and lipid bilayers
S-59 Psoralen plus UVA light -INTERCEPT Plasma -INTERCEPT Platelets	• Enveloped viruses • Intracellular viruses • Some non-enveloped viruses • Vegetative bacteria • Protozoa • Leukocytes	Pyrimidine adducts and cross-links
Riboflavin plus light -MIRASOL Plasma -MIRASOL Platelets -MIRASOL Whole Blood*	• Most enveloped viruses • Intracellular viruses • Some non-enveloped viruses • Vegetative bacteria • Protozoa • Leukocytes	Nucleic acid (guanidine) oxidation
Short UV Light Treatment -THERAFLEX UV-Platelets	• Enveloped viruses • Intracellular viruses • Vegetative bacteria • Leukocytes	Dimerization of nucleic acid pyrimidines
Solvent Detergent + Filtration -VIPS S/D-F Plasma/Cryo	• Enveloped viruses • Intracellular viruses* • Vegetative bacteria* • Protozoa* • Leukocytes*	[4,0]Phospho-lipid bilayer of membranes *Bacteria and cellular debris are removed/reduced by 0.2 u filtration step
S-303 +GSH -INTERCEPT Red Blood Cells (second generation)*	• Enveloped viruses • Intracellular viruses • Some non-enveloped viruses • Vegetative bacteria • Protozoa • Leukocytes	Nucleic acid adducts Some nonspecific modification of membrane/protein nucleophiles

*In preclinical or clinical development.

suitable for the treatment of plasma (recovered or apheresis) and platelets. Because hemoglobin absorbs UVA light, the method is not appropriate for use with red cells. The INTERCEPT treatment system utilizes a synthetic photoreactive psoralen-based derivative (amotosalen, or S59) in conjunction with long-wavelength UV irradiation (UVA). S59 crosses plasma membranes efficiently and intercalates with the RNA and DNA of viruses, bacteria, parasites, and leukocytes. Upon illumination with UVA light, S59 is activated and covalently crosslinks pyrimidine bases, preventing subsequent replication of the nucleic acid. The treatment system is designed to control the concentration of amotosalen and the UV dose to ensure robust PI while minimizing damage to protein and platelet function. After treatment, the residual amotosalen and by-products are removed to below pharmacologically and toxicologically safe levels using an adsorption device integrated as part of the treatment system.[20]

The INTERCEPT system is intended to be implemented under good manufacturing practice (GMP) conditions in blood centers. The systems were granted CE mark for PI of platelets in 2002 and plasma in 2006, and have received regulatory approval for use from a variety of international regulatory bodies, including the PEI (Germany), Swissmedic (Switzerland), and AFSSAPS (France); in 2014, it was approved by the FDA for use in the United States.

The INTERCEPT System is broadly effective against enveloped viruses (including emerging viruses such as chikungunya virus [CHIKV] and dengue virus) and cell-associated viruses (like CMV and HTLV).[20,21] The efficiency with which non-enveloped viruses can be inactivated is variable and virus specific; bluetongue virus and human adenovirus are effectively inactivated, B19 V parvovirus and calicivirus are only moderately inactivated, and HAV and hepatitis E virus (HEV) are resistant.[6,20] The treatment method is also effective against a broad variety of both aerobic and non-aerobic Gram-positive and negative bacteria[22] as well as parasites, including *Plasmodium*, babesia, and *T. cruzi*.[23,24]

The INTERCEPT treatment was proactively employed and may have prevented transfusion transmission of CHKV in the Ile de Reunion epidemic of chikungunya virus (an enveloped virus spread by mosquitoes) in 2006.[25] However, the INTERCEPT treatment system was ineffective in preventing transfusion-associated transmission of HEV (a reemerging non-enveloped virus).[6]

Although INTERCEPT treatment of plasma can moderately affect certain coagulation factors,[26] INTERCEPT-plasma remains clinically efficacious as demonstrated in clinical trials on patients with congenital coagulopathies,[26] those with acquired coagulopathies,[27] and TTP patients requiring therapeutic plasma exchange.[28] An active hemovigilance program of over 7000 transfusions demonstrated high levels of safety and tolerability and a decreased frequency of adverse transfusion reactions compared to untreated plasma.[29]

INTERCEPT treatment of platelets results in some changes in biochemical qualities (e.g., increased P-selectin and CD42b).[30] However, at least 11 clinical trials enrolling more than 1000 patients have been conducted with INTERCEPT platelets that demonstrate efficacy and safety for clinical use.[31–35] In addition, the clinical efficacy has been indirectly confirmed by a retrospective analysis of over 13,000 platelet transfusions from a regional blood center that showed no increased usage of platelet concentrates.[36] No neo-antigenicity, either biochemically or clinically, was observed in clinical trials as a result of INTERCEPT treatment of platelets.

Riboflavin light treatment: Mirasol® PRT System

TerumoBCT (formerly CaridianBCT, Lakewood, CO) has developed the Mirasol Pathogen Reduction Technology (PRT) System for pathogen and leukocyte inactivation in platelet and plasma components. The system utilizes riboflavin (vitamin B$_2$) plus UV light to induce damage to nucleic acids. Riboflavin preferentially associates with nucleic acids and acts as a photosensitizer by mediating an oxygen-independent electron transfer to, primarily, guanine residues upon exposure to light.[37] Damage induced by riboflavin is irreversible because replication and repair processes are impaired due to the guanine base modification.[38] In addition, inactivation can be mediated by direct damage to nucleic acids by UV light or indirectly by damage of membranes, proteins, or nucleic acids by reactive oxygen species created by dissolved oxygen when riboflavin absorbs light.[39]

Riboflavin is a naturally occurring vitamin with a well-known and well-characterized safety profile.[40] Preclinical studies with Mirasol-treated plasma and platelets support a minimal in vitro and in vivo toxicology profile (including chronic administration), and no neo-antigenicity has been reported.[39,41] In vitro studies have shown that Mirasol-treated platelets remain viable and functional throughout storage whether stored in plasma or in platelet additive solutions.[42,43]

The Mirasol PRT System inactivates a wide range of clinically relevant pathogens in both plasma and platelet components. A broad panel of enveloped viruses, including free HIV, intracellular HIV, WNV, and CHIKV, is effectively (4 log$_{10}$), but often not completely, inactivated.[21,40,44] However, certain enveloped viruses such as dengue virus and the model viruses bovine viral diarrhea virus (BVDV) and pseudorabies virus (PRV) appear to be only partially susceptible (~1.5 to 3.5 log$_{10}$ inactivation) to riboflavin–UV treatment and, in side-by-side studies, are inactivated much less efficiently than by INTERCEPT treatment.[21,45] Inactivation of non-enveloped viruses is virus specific; the model parvovirus (PPV) is inactivated effectively, but the relevant human viruses parvovirus B19 V and picornavirus HAV are resistant to treatment (0 to <2 log$_{10}$ inactivation)[40,44] (Table 56.1). Parasites are effectively inactivated by Mirasol treatment.[45–48] A broad range of Gram-positive and Gram-negative bacteria are also susceptible to Mirasol riboflavin treatment.[40,44] In side-by-side laboratory studies conducted using high bacterial spike challenges, Mirasol PRT failed to produce complete inactivation—whereas INTERCEPT treatment inactivated the bacterial challenge to the limit of detection.[49] It can be argued that high bacterial spike challenges may not be as relevant for blood components where bacterial levels are low,[50] but the data suggest a diminished robustness of pathogen inactivation efficacy of Mirasol PRT versus INTERCEPT treatment. Leukocytes are inactivated by the Mirasol PRT system, and therefore, Mirasol treatment should reduce transfusion-associated GVHD and TRALI.[51,52] In Mirasol PRT plasma units, coagulation factor activity is decreased by between ~15% and 35%, whereas coagulation inhibitor functionality is well preserved; a loss in high multimeric vWF has also been observed.[53,54]

The Mirasol PRT system for platelets and plasma received CE mark approval in 2007 and 2008, respectively. The systems are used clinically in various countries in Europe, South America, Africa, and the Middle East.[3] A small, prospective, randomized controlled study of 30 patients who received transfusion of FFP for therapy of congenital or acquired coagulopathies showed that hemostatic effectiveness was retained but larger volumes versus FFP were required.[55] A small randomized controlled clinical trial evaluating the performance and efficacy of platelets treated with the Mirasol PRT (MIRACLE trial) confirmed that there was no increased usage of platelet or red blood cell transfusions in patients receiving Mirasol-treated platelets. In addition, the trial showed that platelet corrected count increments (CCIs) remained stable throughout multiple transfusions of Mirasol-treated platelets.[56]

Theraflex UV light treatment of platelets
Macopharma is developing a UV light PRT system for platelets (the THERAFLEX UV-Platelet system). The system uses low-dose short-wave UV light combined with an efficient agitation system without the need for additional photoreactive compounds.[57,58] UV light is directly absorbed by the nucleic acids of pathogens and leukocytes, resulting in the formation of intra- and inter-pyrimidine dimers that block transcription.

Preclinical studies demonstrate that the Theraflex UV-Platelet system produces a dose-dependent inactivation of bacteria and viruses. Effective inactivation of most enveloped and non-enveloped viruses was achieved at doses of $0.4 \, J/cm^2$. At the proposed treatment dose of 0.2 to $0.3 \, J/cm^2$, small non-enveloped viruses were still effectively inactivated, but larger non-enveloped viruses were inactivated to a lesser degree; HIV was essentially resistant to UV treatment.[59] A broad panel of bacterial species were inactivated by at least 4 logs at the proposed treatment dose of $0.3 \, J/cm^2$; inactivation studies conducted using low-level challenges of bacteria resulted in sterile units followed by treatment and six-day storage.[60] Leukocytes are also inactivated by the treatment procedure.[58]

In vitro studies have shown Theraflex UV-treated platelets show marginal changes in metabolism and activation throughout five-day storage. In an autologous radiolabeled clinical study, recovery and survival were reduced versus untreated platelet concentrates, which is similar to what is observed for other PRT-treated platelets.[61] Additional studies and clinical trials are ongoing.

Red cell pathogen inactivation
To date, no PRT for red cells or whole blood has been licensed for routine use. VI Technologies (VITEX, Watertown, MA) pursued development of INACTINE (e.g., ethylenimine) treated packed RBCs into Phase III clinical trials. Although INACTINE was highly effective at inactivating a broad range of enveloped and non-enveloped viruses, bacteria, protozoa, and leukocytes,[62,63] the Phase III trials were stopped because the treatment caused neo-antigen formation and antibody responses to PEN110-treated red cells.[64]

INTERCEPT Red Blood Cell System
Cerus Corp. (Concord, CA) is developing a second-generation pathogen and leukocyte reduction system for erythrocytes (INTERCEPT for Red Blood Cells) using S303 (an alkylating agent) and glutathione (GSH). S303 is an alkylating agent with three functional components: (1) an acridine anchor that intercalates into nucleic acids, (2) a bis-alkylator group that reacts with nucleophiles, and (3) a small flexible carbon linker that hydrolyzes at neutral pH to yield a nonreactive breakdown product (S300).[65] In the current prototype, after the inactivation step, reagents, and S303 byproducts are removed to toxicologically acceptable levels by centrifugation and removal of the supernatant. S303 readily crosses the membranes of cells and enveloped viruses, allowing it to intercalate with nucleic acids and crosslink them. However, S303 can potentially react nonspecifically with other nucleophiles, including small molecules and proteins. Phase III clinical trials with the first-generation

system were suspended after two patients in a chronic transfusion trial developed antibodies to the acridine moiety of S303 on the RBC surface after exposure to several transfusions.[66–68] The second-generation system has been modified to include GSH to minimize the potential for natural or induced immune responses to S303-treated RBCs.[65] Clinical trials with the second-generation system INTERCEPT RBCs are ongoing.

The second-generation INTERCEPT RBC system is effective at inactivating both enveloped and non-enveloped viruses, although the virus panel studied to date is limited (e.g., B19 V, HAV, and HEV were not included).[69] Inactivation of between 4 and 6 log_{10} of a wide variety of relevant Gram-positive and Gram-negative bacteria was also demonstrated. Residual leukocytes are also inactivated by the INTERCEPT RBC system.[65]

Riboflavin light treatment (Mirasol RBC)
Preliminary studies show promising results with PI of red cells using the Mirasol system adapted for red cells. Pathogen inactivation of viruses and virus susceptibility was similar to that observed for viruses.[70] Pathogen inactivation of bacteria was tested in units spiked with low levels of contamination followed by treatment and storage for seven days. At higher doses, the units tested negative for bacterial outgrowth, but at the proposed dose, some bacterial breakthrough was observed. *In vitro* red cell properties (hemolysis and adenosine diphosphate [ADP] level) were minimally impacted versus untreated controls, and hemolysis remained under 1% over 25 days of storage.[40,70] *In vivo* viability of RBCs from Mirasol-treated whole blood treated at different dose levels was studied in a prospective, single-center, open-label design in normal volunteers,[71] with no serious adverse events reported. Correlative relationships between 24-hour survival/half-life and ADP levels and hemolysis were observed.[72] The data are being used to optimize the Mirasol system for RBCs during further development.

Small-pool S/D treatment and filtration for plasma and cryoprecipitate (VIPS S/D-F)
VIPS SA (Viral Inactivated Plasma Systems, Columbier, Switzerland) has recently developed an S/D-based, easy-to-use system for viral inactivation and sterile filtration of small pools of plasma units (recovered or apheresis) and for small pools of cryoprecipitate. The VIPS Plasma and VIPS Cryo systems are designed for implementation in blood collection establishments. The system is CE marked and is in clinical use in several countries, including Egypt, Thailand, and Indonesia.

The process employs a two-stage viral inactivation step using 1% TnBP and 1% Triton X45. After S/D treatment, the added reagents and lipids are extracted with oil and removed to low levels by passage through an S/D and phthalate adsorption device, followed by passage through a 0.2 sterile filter.[73,74] The methodology has been validated; >90% of plasma coagulation factors, coagulation inhibitors, as well as albumin and immunoglobulin are recovered. S/D treatment (see the "Pooled plasma, S/D treated" subsection) is highly effective at inactivating all extracellular enveloped viruses, but non-enveloped viruses are not inactivated; the process system has been validated to inactivate a wide variety of model and relevant enveloped viruses.[73–76] The sterile filtration step removes bacteria, parasites, leucocytes, cell debris, and plasma microparticles, and it reduces pyrogen.[74] A clinical study using VIPS S/D-F cryoprecipitate FVIII showed a normal pharmacokinetics profile and control of acute and chronic bleeding episodes in hemophilia A patients.[77]

Prion removal

None of the mentioned PRT technologies for blood components eliminate prions. Several companies are developing prion reduction filters for red cell components. A filter employing ligand affinity chromatography has shown significant reduction capacity for exogenously spiked prion spikes,[78] and protection against transmission of vCJD has been verified in ongoing primate transfusion studies.[79]

Pooled plasma, S/D treated

Pooled, S/D-treated plasma (SDPP) is produced in accordance with the EU Pharmacopeia. S/D-treated plasma is prepared using an industrial-scale process in which small manufacturing pools of plasma are created (~60–650 L) by pooling multiple units of recovered or source plasma.[80] Prior to manufacture, the plasma pools are sampled and must test nonreactive for certain virological markers—anti HIV-1 and -2, HBsAg, HCV RNA, HAV RNA, and HEV RNA—by NAT. The plasma pool cannot contain more than 10^4 IU/mL of non-enveloped B19 virus DNA. During the manufacturing process, the plasma pool is incubated in the presence of an S/D mixture (e.g., tributyl phosphate and octoxinol 10 [Triton X-100]) under tightly controlled conditions in order to inactivate enveloped viruses that may be present. The S/D chemicals are subsequently removed to clinically safe levels by either oil or solid phase extraction. The treated product is subsequently sterile filtered into individual doses. The manufacturing process produces standardized biopharmaceutical product with extensive in-process control and without the significant normal variation in plasma protein concentrations observed in single plasma units.

S/D treatment inactivates enveloped viruses by disrupting and destroying the lipid bilayer membranes required for cell adhesion and receptor binding to initiate an infection. Virus validation studies are completed on the S/D manufacturing step to demonstrate that the S/D treatment conditions are robust and effective against a broad variety of enveloped viruses. However, the method does not inactivate non-enveloped viruses and therefore there remains a potential risk for transmission of non-enveloped viruses, especially those that are newly emerging within the population. Therefore, S/D plasma pools (60–650 L) are generally much smaller than those used in the production of fractionated plasma proteins. It is assumed that neutralizing immune antibodies in a plasma pool (i.e., HAV and parvovirus B19) considerably lowers the risk of transmission of non-enveloped viruses already circulating in the population.[81,82] In addition, as an essential regulatory requirement, NAT screening for the non-enveloped viruses HAV, HEV, and parvovirus B19 V assures the safety of S/D-treated plasma. Manufacturers also carefully follow and assess the epidemiology of known and emerging viruses in their donor population.[83]

Prions (transmissible spongiform encephalopathies [TSEs]) are not inactivated by S/D treatment. Octapharma has introduced a prion affinity chromatography step into their S/D manufacturing process without impacting hemostatic quality.[84] The ability of the prion removal step to remove 2.5 to 3 $\log_{10}$ of a surrogate marker of the prion agent has been demonstrated in *in vitro* studies.[85,86]

In Europe, an ABO-independent universal SDPP has been developed by Octapharma by proportionally pooling A, B, and AB plasma. The product (tentatively named Uniplas) is not yet licensed, but has undergone clinical trials in cardiac surgery and liver resection in Europe.[87–89]

Adverse events are less common with SDPP than with ordinary standard plasma components. Particularly important is that there have been no reports of TRALI after transfusion of over five million units of SDPP in Europe.[90,91] Hemovigilance data indicate that febrile, allergic, or anaphylactic reactions are reduced by 70% to 80% with SDPP.[92] These observations are best explained by dilution/neutralization that results from pooling and removal of all cellular components during the S/D treatment process.

Plasma-derived medicinal products

Plasma-derived medicinal products are manufactured from relatively large pools (~2000–4000 L) of plasma. Intermediates from multiple pools of plasma may be combined such that a final container may contain proteins from up to 50,000 individual donations. The pooling of many donations inherently increases the risk that the starting material may be contaminated by an unknown or untested-for virus as compared to individual blood components. However, the pooling process also provides a dilution factor that contributes to safety, and, most importantly, the manufacturing processes of all plasma-derived medicinal products contain steps specifically designed to have a high capacity to inactivate or remove virus. The overall virus safety of plasma-derived medicinal products is achieved by the complementary combination of measures of donor selection, testing of donations and plasma pools, and virus inactivation and removal in the manufacturing process, as demonstrated in virus validation studies. These measures have been highly successful in assuring virus-safe products.

In order to achieve virus-safe plasma-derived products, effective virus reduction steps inherent in the manufacturing process are essential. Usually, a minimum of two distinct effective virus reduction methods are implemented that complement each other in their mode of action. If, for one manufacturing step, a gap is demonstrated in the virus reduction capacity for a range of viruses, a second step covering that gap has to be introduced into the manufacturing process (e.g., dry heat treatment or virus filtration for the reduction of non-enveloped viruses together with S/D treatment for inactivation of enveloped viruses).

Virus inactivation and removal

Following the appearance of HIV transmission by transfusion of blood components and plasma derivatives, a major portion of scientific activity in the plasma industry has been directed at either inactivation (such as pasteurization developed by Norbert Heimburger[93] or S/D treatment developed by Bernard Horowitz[94]) or removal of viruses to ensure product safety. By 1994, the plasma fractionation industry had largely achieved this goal, as indicated by the absence of disease transmission of hepatitis or HIV by any product manufactured by American or European biological producers. After the introduction of second-generation HCV antibody testing, the resulting loss of protection from the antibody in immune globulin products led to transmission of HCV. The introduction of dedicated virus inactivation methods into the manufacturing process of IVIG has prevented such transmission from occurring again.[95]

The success of virus inactivation/removal requires not only validation of the reduction in viral load but also maintenance of the intact therapeutic protein. Techniques such as electrophoresis (especially capillary electrophoresis), size exclusion gel chromatography, isoelectric focusing, or antigen–activity ratio are needed. In addition, nonimmunogenicity must be demonstrated to ensure that neo-antigens have not been introduced.[96,97] Amino acid analysis, cleavage with proteolytic enzymes, circulatory survival in animal models, and measurement of sedimentation and diffusion coefficients, viscosity, circular dichroism, and optical rotary dispersion are used.[98]

The virus validation studies must be performed in dedicated laboratories separate from manufacturing facilities so as not to contaminate the production facility. A process step that removes four logs or more of virus is considered effective when the process step can be reliably performed and is insensitive to modifications within the specifications of the manufacturing process.[99]

Viruses chosen for validation studies should closely resemble the viruses that may potentially be present in contaminated plasma (i.e., transfusion-relevant viruses). To test the ability of the production process to remove viruses in general, they should also represent a wide range of physicochemical properties. For these studies, strains of viruses should be chosen that replicate to high titers in cell culture and can be assayed in an effective, sensitive, and reliable manner in *in vitro* infectivity assays. Routine infectivity assays are currently not available for HBV, HCV, or parvovirus B19. Research infectivity assays for parvovirus B19 have been established in different laboratories,[100,101] and parvovirus neutralization during manufacturing has recently been reported.[102] Consequently, these actual viruses cannot be used for virus validation studies, and, where appropriate, model viruses are used instead.

Virus validation studies should be performed with HIV and HAV as relevant viruses. For those blood-borne viruses that cannot be propagated in cell culture systems, model viruses must be used. Model viruses for HCV include, for example, bovine viral diarrhea virus (a flavivirus) or Sindbis virus (a togavirus). A specific model virus for HBV is not available; therefore, nonspecific model viruses must be used or, potentially, duck HBV but only under situations where a novel inactivation method is employed. A wide range of viruses must be used in virus validation studies. For parvovirus B19, currently only experimental cell culture systems are available; therefore, animal parvoviruses (canine or porcine parvoviruses) are used as model viruses. In case of interaction of human immunoglobulins with viruses used in virus validation studies, the use of model viruses may be essential: HAV can be replaced by porcine or bovine enteroviruses or encephalomyocarditis virus.[99,103]

The virus reduction factor is determined as the difference of the virus load (virus titer × volume) in the spiked starting material and in the final sample. In order to demonstrate a high virus reduction factor, it is often appropriate to detect low virus concentration (i.e., the largest practical sample size should be evaluated for residual virus infectivity). However, the impact of potential cytotoxicity or interference of test matrix (composition of product intermediate) on the accurate determination of a virus titer has to be evaluated and taken into account in the calculation of the virus reduction factor.

In virus validation studies, selected steps (stages) of the manufacturing process are studied to assess and quantitate how effectively they can inactivate or remove a broad-range variety of viruses. These experiments are carried out using a bench-scale version of the commercial manufacturing process with aliquots of starting materials (production intermediate) obtained from the commercial-scale process. The production-scale manufacturing process is closely mimicked in the bench-scale model by tightly controlling key manufacturing parameters (pH, conductivity, flow rates, filter load ratios, etc.). The performance of the bench-scale model is confirmed by comparing key performance characteristics (e.g., filtration time and chromatography profiles) to the full-scale process and by demonstration that the biochemical characteristics (e.g., activity, protein concentration, monomer and aggregate, purity, and

yield) of the resultant output material from the bench-scale model are comparable to those of the production-scale process. The virus validation studies are then performed by deliberately spiking small volumes of high-titer virus into aliquots of product intermediates derived from actual production lots. The virus-spiked product intermediate is then run through the validated bench-scale model of the commercial manufacturing process, and samples are removed for subsequent assay. The amount of virus infectivity removed or inactivated by the manufacturing step is quantified using infectivity assays. The extent of virus removal and inactivation at each individual stage of the production process should be tested at least twice, independently. The results of the virus validation studies (in scaled-down procedures) are predictive for production scale, as the laboratory scale was validated with regard to the comparability of the laboratory scale (model) and full scale (manufacturing), demonstrated in scaled-down validation studies. The demonstration that a step is broadly effective against the wide range of viruses employed in the virus validation studies also provides indirect evidence that the production process can effectively inactivate or remove any novel or emerging virus that could potentially be present.

In addition to providing an accurate reflection of the full-scale manufacturing procedure, scaled-down versions of the production process are also used in so-called robustness studies. These robustness studies evaluate the production parameters that may have an influence on virus inactivation and/or removal. These include parameters such as concentration of protein and other components such as the precipitating agents, temperature, pH, reaction time, amount of stabilizer, temperature for the pasteurization step, and amount of solvent or detergent in S/D treatments. Furthermore, for chromatographic steps, protein concentration, flow rate, washing and elution volume, and resin reuse should be assessed. These robustness studies are performed in the laboratory using parameters in the range of, or even beyond the specifications for, routine production, and assess the impact of these extreme production parameters on the effectiveness of virus reduction steps. The goal of these studies is to demonstrate that the process is robust and effective at removing viruses across the entire potential range of parameters under which the manufacturing process is licensed to be run.

When inactivation processes are validated, the rate of inactivation and the shape of the inactivation curves are assessed. For virus removal, the mass balance of virus infectivity in the starting material versus virus infectivity in the final sample and the final fractions has to be established.

Virus reduction or clearance is achieved during the manufacturing process by removal of viruses. This is accomplished by manufacturing steps designed to purify and concentrate the desired protein, dedicated virus filtration steps, and inactivation of viruses. The inactivation of viruses uses dedicated steps introduced into the manufacturing process.

Virus inactivation

Heat treatment in aqueous solution (pasteurization)

Heating in aqueous solution at 60°C for 10 hours or greater can be a highly effective method for the inactivation of both enveloped and non-enveloped viruses. The effectiveness of inactivation is dependent upon the composition of the solution and the concentration of stabilizers that are used to protect proteins and minimize neo-antigen formation; stabilizers can also protect viruses (especially non-enveloped virus). Stabilizer concentrations are carefully chosen to find conditions that maximize retention of biological activity of the therapeutic molecule while maximizing virus inactivation. All parts of the tank must be heated equally to provide constant temperature in the aqueous solution. The impact of stabilizers and temperature on the virus inactivation capacity for a wide range of viruses must be carefully validated.[104]

The pharmacopoeia method for albumin requires formulation with low concentrations of sodium caprylate alone or with N-acetyl tryptophan as a stabilizer prior to sterile filtration and filling and heat treatment for 60 °C for 10 to 11 hours in the final containers. The safety of the albumin pasteurization method has been demonstrated for decades. An additional contribution to the virus safety of albumin also comes from virus partitioning during ethanol fractionation that contributes to the removal of viruses.[105]

It is possible to pasteurize relatively labile molecules such as factor VIII concentrates in the presence of high concentrations of glycine and sucrose or selected salts. This approach was developed by Heimburger in the late 1970s, resulting in a plasma-derived factor VIII/vWF product with no proven cases of virus transmissions in more than 25 years.

Dry heat

After lyophilization of proteins (in the final container) to remove water, heating at 80 °C for 72 hours or 100 °C for 30 minutes is also an effective virus inactivation step. Higher residual moisture in the lyophilized product can enhance the inactivation of some viruses, but under such conditions protein aggregates increased and the stability of the product was reduced. However, even at residual moisture levels as low as 0.3%, effective inactivation of most viruses can be obtained. In the commercial manufacturing process, the residual moisture is controlled and the process is validated to ensure that each vial remains between predefined limits demonstrated in viral validation studies.[106]

Upper and lower limits of residual moisture should be set based on virus validation studies as well as protein integrity studies and aggregate formation studies. Where such a treatment is applied to the product in its final containers, the variation in residual moisture between vials of product should be within the limits set. Temperature and duration of heating should be monitored throughout the process step.

Vapor heat

Lyophilized (intermediate) products are heated at defined (relatively high) residual moisture (for, e.g., 60 °C for 10 hours followed by 80 °C for 1 hour). Low residual moisture levels of dry heat treatment do not interfere with the success of this method because the product intermediate is further processed to the final product.

S/D treatment

Organic S/D treatment works by disrupting the lipid membrane of enveloped viruses, rendering them unable to bind to and infect cells. This method has been shown to be extremely robust and effective in inactivating a broad range of enveloped viruses, including WNV, HIV, HBV, and HCV.[107] This method does not inactivate non-enveloped viruses. An example of conditions used for virus inactivation is: 0.3% tri(n-butyl) phosphate (TNBP) and 1% ionic detergent (usually either Tween 80 or Triton X-100) at approximately 24 °C for 4 to 6 hours. It is even possible to treat some preparations at 4 °C. Product intermediate has to be filtered to eliminate virus trapped in gross aggregates. Mixing throughout the process is generally used, and homogeneity of distribution of the S/D reagents throughout the S/D treatment process step is assured at the commercial scale through careful validation studies. Every droplet must be treated; solutions are often transferred from one tank to another to ensure that material on the ports, lid, or surfaces of the first tank is subject to the treatment. At the end of the process, the S/D reagents are removed by downstream process steps. In virus validation studies, the key process variables such as the concentration of the S/D compounds, the temperature, and the incubation time as well as the impact of potential lipid content in the product intermediate (because this interferes with the availability of the S/D compounds for virus inactivation) have to be covered.[108]

Octanoic acid (caprylate) treatment

Octanoic acid treatment works by the non-ionic form of octanoic acid disrupting the lipid membrane of enveloped viruses, rendering them unable to bind to and infect cells.[109] Similar to S/D treatment, this method is not effective against non-enveloped viruses. The rapidity and effectiveness of inactivation are dependent upon the amount of free non-ionized octanate present, and therefore octanoic acid concentration, pH, temperature, and protein concentration are all critical variables that need to be controlled during treatment.[110,111]

Low pH

Low pH (approximately 4) has been shown to be an effective method for some immune globulin preparations for the inactivation of enveloped viruses and certain non-enveloped viruses such as human parvovirus B19 V.[113,114] The effectiveness and robustness of a low-pH inactivation treatment are highly dependent upon the exact conditions used (pH, time, temperature, and excipients).

Virus removal by methods for protein purification

Precipitation of proteins can also contribute to the safety of the final product by partitioning away pathogens from the protein of interest. Most often, the precipitate is separated by depth filtration or centrifugation. Because the precipitation conditions are designed to purify or concentrate the protein of interest, these partitioning steps often remove only a small range of different viruses. Careful virus validation studies are required to assess the reliable contribution of such precipitation steps to the overall virus reduction for a final product.

Ethanol, polyethylene glycol (PEG), and caprylate precipitation

At the low temperatures and pH typically used in plasma fractionation processes, the inactivation property of ethanol against enveloped viruses is minimal. However, cold ethanol fractionation of plasma can contribute to virus safety by partitioning viruses away from the therapeutic protein of interest (Figure 56.1).[105] Prior to the incorporation of dedicated virus reduction steps into manufacturing processes, partitioning during fractionation and purification, along with antibody neutralization in plasma pools, was largely responsible for ensuring the safety of immune globulin products. Comparable principles related to ethanol precipitation steps apply to other precipitation principles such as octanoic acid (caprylate) precipitation, PEG precipitation, glycine and NaCl precipitation, or ammonium sulfate precipitation. Although octanoic acid can

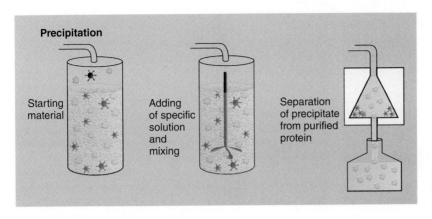

Figure 56.1 A diagram of virus removal by precipitation by ethanol, polyethylene glycol (PEG), caprylate, and so on.

rapidly inactivate enveloped viruses, under some process conditions non-enveloped viruses and certain enveloped viruses can be shown to be precipitated and partitioned (rather than inactivated) by octanoic acid.[114–116] Virus removal by precipitation and depth filtration is virus specific but can contribute significantly to the overall safety of the final product.

Chromatography

Ion exchange, hydrophobic interaction, or affinity chromatography can remove viruses (Figure 56.2).[117,118] When the resin of the chromatography column is reused, efficient sanitization of resins (and column parts) is a necessary step to avoid batch-to-batch contamination.

Virus removal by dedicated manufacturing steps for virus filtration

Virus filtration, also called *nanofiltration* (Figure 56.3), is specifically designed to remove virus. It does so by removing virus based on size while allowing flow-through of the desired protein. Large protein molecules or easily aggregated proteins pose a challenge for this method. Virus filtration using small-pore (~20 nm) or parvovirus-retentive filters is generally a robust and effective means for removing viruses as small as 18–24 nm from process streams, but virus filtration is a complex process. The success depends potentially not only on pore size but also on hydrodynamic forces, adsorption of the virus to the filter surface, and removal of virus aggregated by inclusion in antigen–antibody or lipid complexes.[119] Virus filtration is gentle, but appropriate testing must ensure that shear forces are not damaging the proteins.

Other methods

Besides the established virus reduction factors discussed throughout this section, research into methods such as irradiation, bifunctional hyperoxides, and nucleic acid intercalating substances is ongoing.[120] The suitability of these inactivation methods with respect to modification of proteins has still to be demonstrated. Although UVC irradiation is not used in the manufacturing process of therapeutic proteins (due to the potential for protein modification), utility may be found as a preventative safety step in the treatment of cell culture media entering the production bioreactors for the manufacture of recombinant-derived proteins in mammalian cell lines.[121]

Prions

Prions, the causative agents of human neurodegenerative diseases such as Creutzfeldt–Jakob disease (CJD) and vCJD, cannot be inactivated under conditions used for the manufacture of plasma-derived products without negatively impacting the qualities of the therapeutic protein. However, the manufacturing processes have been shown to contain process steps that have the potential to significantly reduce prion agent infectivity.[122] The prion removal capacity of the manufacturing process can be measured in investigative studies using scale-down models and model infectious agents of TSE using principles consistent with virus validation studies. In such investigative studies, a variety of commonly used manufacturing steps (virus filtration [nanofiltration], octanoic acid and caprylate precipitation, PEG precipitation, and affinity chromatography) were shown to be capable of significantly reducing TSE

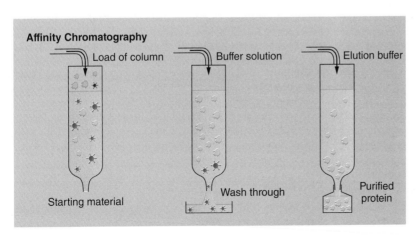

Figure 56.2 A diagram of virus removal by chromatography.

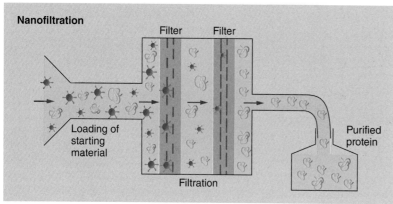

Figure 56.3 A diagram of virus removal by virus filtration nanopore size exclusion.

infectivity. These studies provide reasonable assurance that low levels of TSE infectivity, if present, would be removed by the manufacturing process. There has been one putative report of vCJD (not CJD) transmission of a medium-purity factor VIII concentrate to a hemophiliac patient who did not develop clinical vCJD.[123] The hemophiliac had multiple TSE risk exposures, including exposure to 8Y (BPL) factor VIII concentrate manufactured from UK-sourced plasma, which in at least one lot contained plasma from a preclinical vCJD donor. It should also be noted that the prion removal capacity of the 8Y process was also relatively low versus that of other PDMPs (3.3 log$_{10}$).[124] Importantly, even with heightened surveillance measures in place, there have been no other reports of clinical or nonclinical vCJD (or CJD) transmission by PDMPs manufactured by products that were manufactured from high-TSE-risk UK-sourced plasma.

Manufacturing controls and assessment of final product for virus safety

Each manufacturer must carry out process-specific validation for the licensed manufacturing process used to produce a plasma-derived therapy. The manufacturing process conditions and in-process monitoring for virus inactivation/removal steps must be clearly defined and justified. Segregation of intermediates pre- and postvirus reduction must be assured by the use of closed systems and/or different manufacturing zones with dedicated equipment, air-handling systems, gowning, and restricted personnel movement. Virus reduction is further assured by confirmation of the production records that the conditions validated for the process were rigidly adhered to and that opportunities for cross-contamination and recontamination are prevented.[103]

In general, it is not appropriate to test the final product for viral markers as such tests are not reliable and are difficult to interpret. Testing of final products by NAT is not suitable to demonstrate a safe product due to statistical methods of sampling (Poisson distribution); furthermore, NAT detects genomic sequences and not infectivity of a virus. Virus inactivation techniques such as S/D treatment, octanoic acid treatment, dry heat treatment, and pasteurization disrupt the envelope and/or capsid proteins of the virus but can leave nucleic acid fragments that may be detected by NAT methods but have no bearing on the virus safety of the final product.[103]

An assessment of virus safety in the finished product is a regulatory requirement by some authorities. A probabilistic method is one that has recently been proposed and presented in some detail.[126]

Summary and outlook

The pathogen safety of labile blood components and of manufactured plasma-derived medicinal products has been dramatically enhanced since the 1980s through the implementation of NAT technologies that effectively screen out units with high virus titers. Additionally, the incorporation of multiple orthogonal pathogen inactivation and removal steps into the manufacturing processes of plasma-derived medicinal products has greatly enhanced the safety of the final products against both known and emerging/reemerging viruses. Vigilance, assessment, and verification studies to assess the effectiveness of the virus reduction technologies against emerging pathogens, especially small non-enveloped viruses, is an ongoing responsibility of the manufacturers of plasma-derived therapies. Although the safety of plasma-derived therapies has an excellent history over the last two decades, the development of robust technologies (i.e., 20 nm virus filtration) and the incorporation of these technologies into new and existing manufacturing processes continue.

The development of pathogen reduction technologies for labile blood components has proven to be more challenging, but significant advancements have been made over the last decade in the development, commercialization, and routine implementation of PRT systems for fresh frozen plasma and for platelets. Large-scale studies have proven the clinical effectiveness of some of the PRT system, whereas additional clinical data are needed for others. As these PRT systems gain wider adoption in blood centers, the retrospective evaluations of clinical efficacy based on actual usage will undoubtedly be undertaken. From a pathogen safety perspective, the implementation of PRT technologies to blood components adds an orthogonal layer of safety against many, but not all, potential adventitious pathogens that are not routinely screened for by NAT. Additionally, the inactivation of residual leukocytes by PRTs may have significant clinical and economic advantages. PRT systems designed to be economically feasible and easily implementable in developing countries with more challenging donor epidemiology are being developed and implemented and should have a major impact on patient safety. The development of a PRT suitable for whole blood or red cells remains an ongoing challenge, but promising progress has been made. Broad-scale implementation of PRTs for labile blood components in both developed and developing countries will undoubtedly require positive economic assessments.

Disclaimer

The author works for CSL Behring, a manufacturer of plasma-derived medicinal therapies.

Key references

A full reference list for this chapter is available at: http://www.wiley.com/go/simon/transfusion

4 Epstein JS, Vossal JG. FDA approach to evaluation of pathogen reduction technology. *Transfusion* 2003;**43**:1347–50.

9 Seghatchian J, Struff WG, Reichenberg S. Main properties of the THERAFLEX MB-plasma system for pathogen reduction. *Transfus Med Hemother* 2011;**38**:55–64.

20 Irsch L, Lin L. Pathogen inactivation of platelet and plasma blood components for transfusion using the INTERCEPT blood system™. *Transfus Med Hemother* 2011;**38**:19–31.

36 Cazenave JP, Isola H, Waller C, *et al.* Use of additive solutions and pathogen inactivation treatment of platelet components in a regional blood center: impact on patient outcomes and component utilization during a 3-year period. *Transfusion* 2011;**51**:621–9.

40 Marschner S, Goodrich R. Pathogen reduction technology treatment of platelets, plasma and whole blood using riboflavin and UV light. *Transfus Med Hemother* 2011;**38**:8–18.

56 Cazenave P, Folléa G, Bardiaux F, *et al.* (The Mirasol Clinical Evaluation Study Group). A randomized controlled clinical trial evaluating the performance and safety of platelets treated with Mirasol pathogen reduction technology. *Transfusion* 2010;**50**:2362–75.

57 Seghatchian J, Tolksdorf F. Characteristics of the THERAFLEX UV-platelets pathogen inactivation system—an update. *Transfusion Apheres Sci* 2012;**46**:221–9.

74 El-Ekiaby M, Sayed MA, Caron C, *et al.* Solvent-detergent filtered (S/D-F) fresh frozen plasma and cryoprecipitate minipools prepared in a newly designed integral disposable processing bag system. *Transfus Med* 2010;**20**:48–61.

80 Hellstern P, Solheim BG. The use of solvent/detergent treatment in pathogen reduction of plasma. *Transfus Med Hemother* 2011;**38**:65–70.

95 Tabor E. The epidemiology of virus transmission by plasma derivatives: Clinical studies verifying the lack of transmission of hepatitis B and C viruses and HIV Type 1. *Transfusion* 1999;**39**:1160–8.

CHAPTER 57

Hemolytic transfusion reactions

Robertson D. Davenport[1] & Martin H. Bluth[2]

[1]Department of Pathology, The University of Michigan Medical School, Ann Arbor, MI, USA
[2]Department of Pathology, Wayne State University School of Medicine, Detroit, MI, USA

A hemolytic transfusion reaction (HTR) is the accelerated clearance or lysis of transfused red cells because of immunologic incompatibility. Although they may at times have similar clinical presentations, HTR is distinguished from autoimmune hemolysis or nonimmune causes of shortened survival of transfused red cells. HTR may occur when antigen-positive red cells are transfused to a patient with a preexisting alloantibody, or when a recently transfused patient makes a new alloantibody. The great majority of HTRs are a result of red blood cell (RBC) transfusion. However, HTRs may also result from transfusion of plasma-containing blood components, such as fresh frozen plasma or platelets.

HTRs are classified as acute (AHTR) or delayed (DHTR) reactions, based on whether they occur within 24 hours or after 24 hours of the implicated transfusion. A more important distinction is between intravascular and extravascular hemolytic reactions. Intravascular hemolysis is characterized by hemoglobinemia and hemoglobinuria. In contrast, extravascular hemolysis lacks these dramatic signs, but is characterized by shortened survival of transfused red cells along with the accumulation of hemoglobin breakdown products. Generally, intravascular hemolysis is seen with AHTR, and precipitated by both IgM and IgG antibody isotypes, whereas extravascular hemolysis is usually seen in DHTR, and is principally of the IgG isotype. This distinction is not absolute, however. Occasional acute reactions result in extravascular hemolysis, and some intravascular hemolytic reactions are delayed.

Accelerated clearance of incompatible red cells is an essential feature of HTRs. Transfusion may also stimulate the production of alloantibody without hemolysis. This phenomenon has been termed *delayed serologic transfusion reaction* (DSTR), and it needs to be differentiated from DHTR.[1] DSTR is clinically benign, and is identified during routine type and screen without evidence of hemolysis, but it predisposes to later HTR. Earlier reports of hemolytic reactions have not necessarily differentiated clearly between serologic and true hemolytic reactions.

Incidence

The best estimates of the incidence of HTR are derived from national hemovigilance programs. Older reports have suffered from inconsistency in definition, reliance on passive reporting, use of compatibility testing methods that are less sensitive than current practices, and lack of quality assurance practices. The largest and best established hemovigilance program is the UK Serious Hazards of Transfusion (SHOT). For the reporting year 2013, SHOT reported 17 AHTR out of 2,043,046 RBC units distributed, for a rate of 0.8/100,000 RBC units and 32 DHTR for a rate of 1.6/100,000 RBC units.[2] The Canadian Transfusion Transmitted Injuries Surveillance System (TTISS) for the year 2012 reported 31 AHTR (1.3/100,000 RBC units) and 84 DHTR (3.1/100,000 RBC units).[3] The Irish Blood Transfusion service for the year 2011 reported six AHTR (4.1/100,000 RBC units) and 11 DHTR (7.9/100,000 RBC units).[4] Although there has been expected year-to-year variation in these rates, there have been no substantial differences in the annual occurrence of HTR over the reporting time covered by these hemoviligance programs. These rate estimates are based on the number of units distributed to transfusion services, which are necessarily somewhat greater than the number of units actually transfused, although wastage is low.

The incidence of HTR per transfused patient is harder to estimate. Because most patients receive more than one RBC unit, estimates of the incidence of HTR per transfused patient range from 1:854 to 1:524.[5,6] The population incidence rate of DHTR has been estimated at 1.69 events per 100,000 population per year.[6]

Signs and symptoms

There is a broad range of initial clinical presentations of HTR. The typical progression of intravascular and extravascular hemolysis is shown in Figure 57.1 and Figure 57.2. In all cases, there is an unexpected degree of anemia from the loss of transfused red blood cells. In some cases, particularly with extravascular hemolysis, this is the only clue to HTR. Some reactions, both immediate and delayed, are asymptomatic. In intravascular hemolysis, however, most symptomatic patients experience fever and/or chills. Nausea or vomiting, pain, dyspnea, and hypotension or tachycardia are also common initial symptoms. The reported pain may localize to the infusion site, back, flanks, chest, groin, or head. The cause of pain in HTR is unclear, but is most likely the result of direct stimulation of

Rossi's Principles of Transfusion Medicine, Fifth Edition. Edited by Toby L. Simon, Jeffrey McCullough, Edward L. Snyder, Bjarte G. Solheim, and Ronald G. Strauss.
© 2016 John Wiley & Sons, Ltd. Published 2016 by John Wiley & Sons, Ltd.

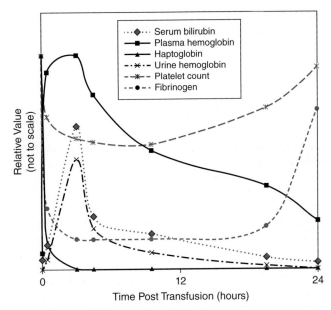

Figure 57.1 Time course of hemolytic and coagulation parameters in intravascular HTR. Source: Duvall *et al.* (1975).[93] Reproduced with permission of Wiley.

nociceptive nerves in perivascular tissue by bradykinin generated from activation of the complement system.[7]

In extravascular hemolysis, fever and/or chills are the most commonly reported initial symptoms. Jaundice also may be an initial sign because elevation of serum bilirubin occurs with both intravascular and extravascular hemolysis. The degree of hyperbilirubinemia depends upon the patient's liver function and rate of red cell destruction. Conjugated and unconjugated bilirubin fractions tend to follow a parallel course, peaking at the same time.[8] Delta bilirubin, a minor albumin-bound fraction, persists past the peak of total bilirubin and is a useful clue to previous hemolysis.

Although HTR typically presents during or shortly after the offending transfusion, the time from transfusion to clinical presentation of DHTR is quite variable. Most delayed reactions present within two weeks after transfusion, but the initial presentation may be up to six weeks later, because of the time required for antibody production.

Complications

Autoantibody is found in about 28% of patients concomitantly with alloantibody, although the reported range is 15% to 53%.[9] Although the half-life of IgG is approximately 3–4 weeks, a positive direct antiglobulin test (DAT) caused by IgG may persist for many months, and there may be evidence of complement deposition on autologous red cells, with a positive DAT caused by C3 persisting for up to 100 days.[10] In most cases, there is no evidence of loss of autologous red cells; however, so-called *bystander hemolysis* can occur. It is not possible to distinguish between autoimmune hemolytic anemia (AIHA) and bystander hemolysis by serologic testing alone.

Patients with sickle cell anemia can present a particular challenge. HTR can precipitate sickle crisis. Factors that contribute to the occurrence of sickle crisis include increased oxygen consumption resulting from fever, the relative loss of circulating hemoglobin A compared to hemoglobin S, and the release of vasoactive mediators causing reduction of local blood flow. HTRs may be particularly severe in patients with sickle cell disease. In such reactions the degree of anemia may actually be greater than before transfusion, probably because of bystander hemolysis of autologous red cells. This phenomenon has been termed the *sickle cell HTR syndrome*.[11] In addition to hemolysis, there is often suppression of erthropoiesis as indicated by a marked drop in the reticulocyte count. Demonstration of an increase in corrected reticulocyte count, increase in the absolute number of hemoglobin-S-containing red cells, or decrease in the ratio of red cell hemoglobin to reticulocyte

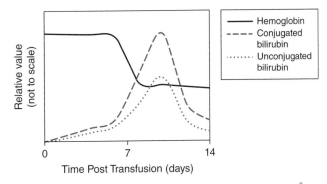

Figure 57.2 Time course of hemolytic parameters in extravascular hemolysis. Source: Cummins *et al.* (1997).[8] Reproduced with permission of Sage.

hemoglobin can indicate the occurrence of hyperhemolysis.[11–13] Pain crisis in a sickle cell patient following transfusion should suggest the occurrence of sickle cell HTR syndrome. Further transfusion in this setting may exacerbate the anemia and even result in fatality. Serologic studies often do not provide an explanation for HTR in these patients, because the causative antibody can be at an undetectable level in the serum during the reaction. In addition, the presence of multiple alloantibodies may make the serologic diagnosis difficult.

Hypotension occurs in some cases of intravascular HTR but is rare in extravascular reactions. Complement activation is likely to be the most important determining factor. The anaphylatoxins C3a, C4a, C5a, and C5a-des-arg are released during immune hemolysis. Additionally, consumption of C1-esterase inhibitor contributes to activation of the kinin pathway, leading to generation of bradykinin.[14] The pro-inflammatory cytokines tumor necrosis factor (TNF) and interleukin-1 (IL1) produced by phagocytes during HTR also may contribute to hypotension and shock.

Impairment of renal function is seen in both intravascular and extravascular HTR, although it is more common in the former. The degree of renal function abnormality varies from an asymptomatic elevation of serum blood urea nitrogen (BUN) and creatinine to complete anuria. Both hypotension and intravascular coagulation contribute to renal impairment. Thrombus formation in renal arterioles caused by disseminated intravascular coagulation (DIC) may cause cortical infarcts. Free hemoglobin contributes to renal injury, causing so-called pigment nephropathy. Experimental evidence indicates that hemoglobin is toxic to renal tubular epithelium cells.[15]

Intravascular hemolysis modulates blood pressure and local blood flow through alterations in the metabolism of the potent physiologic vasodilator nitric oxide (NO). NO can combine with heme and thiol groups of hemoglobin.[16] In oxyhemoglobin, NO causes reduction of ferrous iron (Fe^{2+}) to form ferric methemoglobin [$Hb(Fe^{3+})$]. NO combines with deoxyhemoglobin to form $Hb(Fe^{2+})NO$, but does not cause reduction. Scavenging of NO by free hemoglobin through these pathways results in vasoconstriction and hypertension. NO can also combine with cysteine on the beta-globin chain to form S-nitrosohemoglobin (SNO-Hb). This process is reversible, so SNO-Hb can act as a NO donor with resultant vasodilation. Free hemoglobin reacts with NO much more rapidly than does intraerythrocytic hemoglobin.[17] The effects of intravascular hemolysis may be very similar to the infusion of stroma-free hemoglobin (i.e., hemoglobin-based oxygen carriers [HBOCs]). Indeed, prominent hypertensive effects limited early trials of hemoglobin solutions as a blood substitute.[18]

Disseminated intravascular coagulation occurs in intravascular HTR, but is relatively rare. Rarer still is the occurrence of DIC in extravascular HTR. The production of proinflammatory cytokines is likely to be a major factor in DIC. It can be difficult to distinguish DIC from other causes of coagulopathy, particularly in massive transfusion or liver disease. Uncontrolled bleeding caused by DIC may be the initial manifestation of an acute HTR, particularly in the intraoperative setting. Unfortunately, if HTR is not recognized early in this situation, more incompatible blood may be transfused in an attempt to keep up with blood loss. In one report, nine of 35 patients experiencing HTR while under anesthesia received 4–6 additional units because of excessive bleeding.[19]

Fatality from HTR is rare. For 2013, SHOT reported a mortality rate from HTR of 0.4/1,000,000 components issued.[2] The Canadian TTISS for the period 2006–2012 reported fatal outcome in 8.6% of AHTR and 3.4% of DHTR.[3]

Mortality is dependent on the amount of incompatible red cells transfused. A review of 41 HTRs causing acute renal failure indicated that no deaths occurred among patients receiving less than 500 mL of incompatible blood; there was 25% mortality in the group receiving 500 to 1000 mL and 44% mortality among those receiving greater than 1000 mL of incompatible blood.[19] However, transfusion of even small amounts of incompatible blood is not necessarily safe. At least 12 deaths have been reported to the US Food and Drug Administration (FDA) involving transfusion of less than one unit of blood.[20]

Causes of hemolytic transfusion reactions

Hemolytic transfusion reactions usually result from inadvertent administration of incompatible blood components, or the failure to detect a potential incompatibility. Rarely, incompatible blood components are deliberately transfused before ABO-incompatible marrow infusion or when compatible blood cannot be obtained, with an expectation of possible HTR. Among transfusion-related fatalities from acute hemolysis reported to the FDA during 1976 to 1985, 86% were the result of process errors.[20] Among these errors, 10% occurred in phlebotomy and ordering departments, 33% occurred within the blood bank, and 57% occurred during transfusion administration.

These frequencies are similar to reported transfusion errors in New York State, where 22% occurred in phlebotomy and ordering departments, 32% occurred within the blood bank, and 46% occurred during transfusion administration.[21] More recent figures indicate that non-blood-bank errors account for 56%, blood bank errors account for 29%, and compound errors account for the remaining 15% of transfusion errors.[22] A similar trend in regard to the occurrence of errors was reported by SHOT, which also emphasized that multiple errors are common.[2] In 220 instances in which the wrong blood was transfused, there were three errors in 117 cases, and five errors in nine cases. In part, differences between the FDA and New York figures are accounted for by the inclusion of nonfatal errors in the latter. Serendipitously, a transfusion error may result in administration of compatible blood components, as occurred in a third of the reported New York State events. Although erroneous compatible transfused units do not result in any detrimental clinical sequelae, they are still considered as "never" events and are often required to be reported to governing and/or accrediting bodies.

Misidentification of a pretransfusion sample has been termed "wrong blood in tube" (WBIT). A study covering 62 institutions in 10 countries performed by the Biomedical Excellence for Safer Transfusion Working Party of the International Society for Blood Transfusion has assessed the frequency of WBIT.[23] On the basis of results from over 690,000 samples, it was determined mislabeling occurred in one in every 165 samples. Two countries with national patient identification systems, Sweden and Finland, had miscollection rates too low to quantify. Outside these nations, miscollected samples demonstrating WBIT occurred at a median rate of one in every 1986 samples. The apparent discrepancy between mislabeling and WBIT is because not all mislabeled tubes are miscollected.

The deliberate, physician-guided administration of incompatible blood components may occur in platelet transfusion, urgent transfusion required in patients with multiple alloantibodies or antibodies to high-incidence antigens, or in marrow transplantation.

ABO-incompatible red cells have been successfully administered to patients before major ABO-incompatible marrow transplants in an effort to reduce the titer of isoagglutinins.[24] These patients have predictable, but manageable, reactions. In a retrospective study of 35 patients receiving major ABO-incompatible peripheral blood hematopoietic progenitor cell transplants who were transfused with one ABO-incompatible RBC unit, 23 had no clinical reaction, and four had severe reactions necessitating discontinuation of the transfusion.[25] Some patients who have received incompatible transfusions involving non-ABO antibodies were treated with high-dose intravenous immunoglobulin (IVIG) before transfusion and have not experienced HTR.[26]

High levels of anti-A or anti-B in platelet concentrates, particularly apheresis products, can cause acute hemolysis.[27–30] There is considerable variability in the strength of the implicated antibody, but a high-titer isoagglutinin is usually present in donor plasma when hemolysis occurs. A study of apheresis group O platelets found that 26% had anti-A or anti-A,B titer of 64 or greater, a level that has been associated with HTR.[31] A study of pooled whole-blood-derived platelets found 60% of group O pools had anti-A titer at least 64.[32] Repeated platelet transfusions within a brief period can result in sufficient accumulation of anti-A to cause severe acute hemolysis.[33] However, there is no clear consensus as to what constitutes a critical titer of ABO antibodies. At variance with reports of acute hemolysis, apheresis platelet concentrates are often transfused across ABO groups without adverse consequences. In one study, 16 patients who received both ABO-compatible and -incompatible platelet concentrates were evaluated for evidence of hemolysis.[34] There was no difference between pre-and post-transfusion hemoglobin levels in 24 paired transfusion episodes. Because ABO substance is found on somatic cells in addition to RBC, it is possible that any anti-A or B antibody present in a plasma containing units transfused in to an A or B patient, respectively, may be "diluted out" by binding to antigens present on non-RBC cells thereby avoiding hemolysis.

Diagnosis

Diagnosis of HTR requires clinical suspicion, especially when the transfusion occurred days to weeks previously. The initial laboratory evaluation includes confirmation of the ABO group, a test for free hemoglobin, and a DAT performed on a postreaction blood specimen (Table 57.1). Visual inspection of the postreaction plasma can detect hemoglobin in the range of 20 to 50 mg/dL, equivalent to the lysis of approximately 10 mL of red cells in an adult.[35] It should be remembered that free serum hemoglobin also may be present in nonimmune hemolysis, red cell fragility syndromes, hemoglobinopathies, severe burns, polyagglutination, or infusion of hemoglobin-based oxygen-carrying solutions. A common cause of a false-positive test result for free hemoglobin is drawing a sample through an indwelling catheter using inappropriate technique. Percutaneous intravascular thromboectomy can cause marked hemoglobinemia.[36] A false-negative test result for free hemoglobin may occur if too much time has been allowed to elapse before obtaining the postreaction specimen. A low level of free hemoglobin may be difficult to detect in an icteric specimen.

The DAT may be positive because of the effects of drugs, autoimmune disease, or autoantibodies. If the postreaction DAT is positive, then a test should be performed on a stored prereaction sample. If the prereaction sample is also a positive, then the test is not valid for the purpose of detecting, or excluding, the presence of

Table 57.1 Laboratory investigation of hemolytic transfusion reactions

First-Tier Investigation
- Posttransfusion serum hemoglobin (qualitative)
- Posttransfusion direct antiglobulin test
- Confirmation of posttransfusion ABO-Rh

Second-Tier Investigation
- Repeat pretransfusion ABO-Rh
- Pre- and posttransfusion antibody screen
- Repeat special antigen typing
- Crossmatch with pre- and postreaction specimens

Third-Tier Investigation
- Antibody identification panels on pre- and postreaction samples
- Enhanced antibody screening method: PEG, extended incubation, gel, enzymes
- Red cell eluate on pre- and postreaction samples
- Investigation of transfusion technique and blood storage conditions
- Check of the blood bag, tubing, and segments for hemolysis
- Enhanced crossmatches: PEG, enzymes
- Minor crossmatches of implicated units
- Antibody detection tests on donor units
- Tests for polyagglutination
- Hemoglobin electrophoresis
- Quantitative serum hemoglobin
- Serum bilirubin (conjugated and unconjugated)
- Urine hemoglobin and hemosiderin
- Bacterial culture and Gram stain of blood bags
- Serum BUN and creatinine
- Peripheral blood smear
- Serial hemoglobin, hematocrit and platelet count
- Blood coagulation studies (PT, fibrinogen, FDP)
- DAT on donor units

alloantibody-coated transfused cells and further testing is required. The DAT will be negative if transfused antigen-positive cells have been cleared from circulation. In addition, when small numbers of antibody-coated allogeneic red cells are present, a DAT performed by routine methods may not be sufficiently sensitive. In a study that compared the relative sensitivity of DAT performed with mono-specific IgG antiglobulin technique, flow cytometry, and antibody elution, the DAT could detect 10% antibody-coated cells.[37] Antibody could be detected in the eluate of the samples with as little as 1% antibody-coated red cells present, although in some cases it was not nearly as sensitive. Flow cytometry, however, was consistently the most sensitive method with a detection limit of approximately 1%.[37]

The hemoglobin and antiglobulin tests are useful for screening purposes. However, if either of these is positive, or if there is a strong clinical suspicion, then further testing must be performed. At this point, the implicated blood bags with their attached administration sets should be returned to the blood bank, and all units dispensed to the patient should be returned and quarantined. Units that were transfused within the past 24 hours should also be identified. The ABO grouping and Rh typing of both pre- and postreaction blood specimens should be repeated. Care should be taken to look for mixed-field agglutination. The antibody screen should be repeated on both specimens, and any special antigen typing of donor units should be repeated.

Blood from saved segments or recovered bags and tubing of units transfused within 24 hours should be crossmatched against both the pre- and postreaction specimens. This testing should include a 37 °C reading and an indirect antiglobulin test. If a large number of units have been transfused in the last 24 hours, the blood bank medical director may elect to substitute reconfirmation of ABO grouping of

Table 57.2 Differential Diagnosis of Hemolytic Transfusion Reactions

Alloantibody-induced hemolysis
Delayed serologic transfusion reaction
Autoimmune hemolytic anemia
Cold hemagglutinin disease
Non-immune hemolysis
    Incompatible fluids
    Improper storage
    Malfunctioning blood warmer
    Small needles, high hematocrit
    Improper deglycerolization
    Malfunctioning infusion pumps
    Bacterial contamination
    Mechanical thrombectomy
Hemolytic anemia
    G6PD deficiency
    Congenital spherocytic anemia
Hemoglobinopathies
    Sickle cell disease
    Sickle cell transfusion reaction syndrome
Drug induced hemolysis
Microangiopathic hemolytic anemias
    TTP
    HUS
    HELLP syndrome
Bleeding
Artificial heart valve dysfunction
Paroxysmal nocturnal hemoglobinuria
Polyagglutination
Infections
    Clostridium perfringens
    Malaria
    Babesiosis

donor units. Negative results in these investigations usually rule out HTR, except in unusual circumstances.

Other causes of hemolysis or shortened red cell survival that should be considered in the differential diagnosis of HTR are listed in Table 57.2. Nonimmune hemolysis can have a similar clinical presentation to HTR. Lysis of red cells can be caused by overheating in a blood warmer, or by freezing. Hemolysis can also be caused by inadequate removal of glycerol from frozen red cells or by attempting to force blood through a filter or small-bore needle. The transfusion of outdated blood has been reported to cause hemoglobinuria and transient hemodynamic, pulmonary, and renal changes.[38] Transfusion administered with hypotonic solutions or some drugs may also cause hemolysis.[39] Intravenous dimethylsulfoxide infusion has been reported to mimic HTR.[40] In general, patients tolerate the infusion of hemolyzed blood remarkable well. Often the only sign of an adverse event is hemoglobinuria. However, deaths caused by the transfusion of hemolyzed blood have been reported.[20]

Some hematologic abnormalities, particularly autoimmune hemolytic anemia, can have presentations similar to HTR. Transfusion of blood from donors with glucose-6-phosphate dehydrogenase (G6PD) deficiency can cause hemoglobinemia and hyperbilirubinemia in transfusion recipients.[41] Hemolysis of G6PD deficient donor cells may be particularly marked in the setting of concomitant oxidative medications. However, there is considerable variability in response with some recipients showing no evidence of hemolysis.

Establishing the diagnosis of HTR may be particularly difficult in patients with liver disease, autoimmune hemolytic anemia, sickle cell anemia, or active bleeding. In chronic liver disease there is often

a positive DAT, hyperbilirubinemia, and elevated lactate dehydrogenase (LDH). The clinical and laboratory presentation of AIHA may be identical to HTR. Concern has been raised that transfusion may aggravate hemolysis in AIHA, although one published study has suggested that this is not usually the case even in the face of serologic incompatibility.[42] Characteristically, in both bleeding and AIHA there is proportionate loss of both autologous and transfused red cells. One indication of HTR in these settings is the persistence of transfused red cells that lack the implicated antigen, but the absence of transfused cells bearing the antigen.

Resorption of a hematoma can have manifestations very similar to extravascular HTR. Such patients may have hyperbilirubinemia, elevated LDH, and depressed haptoglobin levels. In addition, the presence in the serum of fibrin degradation products (FDPs) from the hematoma may be confused with DIC. In these patients, as in bleeding patients, persistent circulating antigen-positive red cells and a negative posttransfusion DAT are evidence against the diagnosis of HTR.

The serologic specificity of a red cell antibody is an indication of its clinical significance. However, there is not an absolute correlation between specificity and presence or absence of red cell destruction. The general clinical significance of many red cell antibody specificities is summarized in Table 57.3.

Pathophysiology

The pathophysiologic mechanisms involved in HTR are not well understood. There are essentially three phases: antibody–antigen interaction, phagocytosis and inflammatory cell activation, and

Table 57.3 General clinical significance of red cell antibodies

Blood Group System	*Generally* Clinically Significant* Specificities	*Generally* Clinically Insignificant Specificities
ABO,H	All	-A$_1$ not reactive at 37 °C
Lewis	-Le^a, -Le^a+Le^b	-Le^b
P	-P, -P+P$_1$+Pk (Tj^a)	-P$_1$, -P^k
I/i	-I, -I	-IH, -IA, -IB, -iH, -IP$_1$ not reactive at 37 °C
Rh	All	
Duffy	All	Possibly –Fy6
MNSs	All	-M not reactive at 37 °C
Lutheran	-Lu^b	-Lu^a
Kell	All	
Kidd	All	
Cartwright	-Yt^a, -, -Yt^b	
Diego	-Di^a,- Di^b, -Wr^a	
Colton	-Co^a, -Co3	-Co^b
Dombrock	-Do^a, -Do^b	
Cromer	-Cr^a, -Tc^a	
Augustine	-At^a	
Vel	-Vel	
Lan	-Lan	
Sid		-Sd^a
LW		All
Gerbich		All
Xg		All
Scianna		All
Chido/Rogers		All
Indian	-In^b	-In^a
Cost/York		-Cs^a, -Yk^a, -Yk^b
Knops/McCoy		-Kn^a, -Kn^b
JMH		-JMH
Holly/Gregory		-Gy^a, -Hy
Bg (HLA)		All

* Resulting in hemolytic transfusion reaction or decrease red cell survival.

systemic response. Initially, there is a binding of antibody to red cell antigens, which can result in complement activation. Secondly, immunoglobulin- and complement-coated cells interact with phagocytes, resulting in clearance of red cells and activation of phagocytes. Thirdly, the inflammatory mediators produced in the first two phases act on a variety of cell types, causing a clinical manifestations of HTR.

The course of immune hemolysis is determined by antigen site density, immunoglobulin class of the alloantibody, and activation of complement. ABO antigens are present in high numbers on a red cell surface, approximately 5×10^5 per cell.[35] In contrast, there are 10^3 to 10^4 antigens per cell in the Rh, Kell, Kidd, and Duffy systems. Complement fixation is facilitated by close proximity of antigens that allows bridging of IgG molecules by C1q. However, IgM antibodies can fix complement without a requirement for bridging between molecules. IgM antibodies are common in the ABO system, but relatively unusual as alloantibodies to other antigens. Activation of the classical pathway of complement proceeds from C1q binding through C3 activation. Cleavage of C3 results in C3a liberation into circulation and C3b deposition on the red cell membrane. Activated C3 may then cleave C5 with release of C5a. Assembly of the membrane attack complex then may proceed with resultant intravascular hemolysis. Factor I, also known as C3b inactivator, is the major regulator of C3b activity. Cleavage of membrane-bound C3b by factor I results in the generation of iC3b and release of the small peptide fragment C3c. This terminates the complement cascade because iC3b is enzymatically inactive. iC3b is further degraded into C3dg and C3d by factor I and trypsin-like proteinases.

Erythrophagocytosis results from interaction of immuno-globulin-and/or complement-coated red cells with phagocyte receptors. Cell-bound antibodies promote red cell clearance primarily through interaction of the Fc portion of IgG with specific receptors. Among the IgG receptors, FcγRI principally mediates red cell phagocytosis by monocytes.[43] However, this receptor has a high affinity for monomeric IgG, and is blocked by normal serum concentrations of IgG.[44] FcγRIII appears to be the most important IgG receptor on splenic macrophages in alloimmune and autoimmune red cell clearance, as well as in autoimmune thrombocytopenia.[45–47] Although the IgG is the most common isotype implicated in HTR, other immunoglobulin isotypes (i.e., IgA) have also been reported. The principal complement receptor expressed by macrophages and monocytes, CR3, primarily recognizes iC3b. Receptors for C3a and C5a are present on a wide variety of cells including monocytes, macrophages, neutrophils, platelets, endothelium, and smooth muscle. The physiologic effects of C3a and C5a include oxygen radical production, granule enzyme release, leukotriene production, NO production, and cytokine production. These low-molecular-weight peptides can also produce vasodilation and bronchoconstriction.

Ligation of phagocyte receptors results in cellular activation and production of inflammatory response factors. An experimental model of ABO incompatibility has suggested that monocytes are the leukocyte subpopulation most directly involved in AHTR.[48] Incompatible red cells induce a reduction in CD14 and increase in CD44 expression on monocytes in whole blood. After 24 hours' incubation with incompatible red cells, monocytes showed particularly high levels of CD44. These data demonstrate that monocyte activation is critical in the development of intravascular HTR.

Immune hemolysis stimulates the production of a variety of cytokines that are crucial to the initiation, maintenance, and ultimate resolution of HTR (Table 57.4). ABO incompatibility with

Table 57.4 Cytokines involved in immune hemolysis

Terminology	Biological Activities
Pro-inflammatory cytokines: Interleukin-1 (IL1β) Tumor necrosis factor (TNFα)	Fever Hypotension, shock, death (synergy) Mobilization of leukocytes from bone marrow Activation of T and B cells Induction of cytokines (IL1β, IL6, CXCL8, TNFα, CCL5) Induction of adhesion molecules Induction of procoagulants
Interleukin-6 (IL6)	Fever Acute phase protein response B-cell antibody production T-cell activation
Chemokines: CXLC8	Chemotaxis of neutrophils Chemotaxis of lymphocytes Neutrophil activation Basophil histamine release
CCL5	Chemotaxis of monocytes Induction of respiratory burst Induction of adhesion molecules Induction of IL1β
Anti-inflammatory cytokines: interleukin-1 receptor antagonist (IL1ra, IRAP)	Competitive inhibition of IL1 type I and II receptors

intravascular HTR strongly stimulates production of TNFα and the chemokines CXCL8 (IL8) and CCL2 (MCP-1).[49–52] TNFα is an early response, appearing in plasma within two hours, and has potent proinflammatory effects, including pyrogenic activity, leukocyte activation, stimulation of procoagulant activity, and expression of a large number of gene products related to the inflammatory response. TNFα produced in blood during ABO incompatibility will stimulate endothelial cells to express leukocyte adhesion molecules, chemotactic cytokines, and procoagulant activity.[53] CXCL8 and CCL2 produced in blood during ABO incompatibility appear later than TNFα and reach very high levels. CXCL8 primarily activates neutrophils to undergo the respiratory burst, release granule contents and alter surface adhesion molecules.[54] CCL2 is primarily a chemotactic and activating factor for monocytes.[55]

There is also evidence for the production of cytokines in IgG-mediated extravascular hemolysis.[56–57] There appear to be two categories of cytokine responses in this setting: those produced at high levels (greater than 1 ng/mL by 24 hours), and others produced at lower level (in the range of 100 pg/mL).[56] Low-level cytokine responses include IL1β, IL6, and TNFα. CXCL8 is a high-level response with a time course similar to that of ABO incompatibility. In contrast to the setting of ABO incompatibility, TNFα is produced in a delayed fashion in response to IgG-coated red cells, achieving a level of less than 100 pg/mL. However, cell-associated TNFα can be demonstrated by immunocytochemical staining in monocytes engaged in erythrophagocytosis.

Although the in vitro models employed in these studies are not directly comparable, these findings do suggest a possible reason for the clinical differences between intravascular and extravascular HTRs. In the former case, TNFα is released into systemic circulation where it can have diverse effects on many cell types; in the latter case, TNFα effects may be confined to the site of erythrophagocytosis, primarily the spleen. Both IL1β and IL6 produced by monocytes in response to IgG-coated red cells increase progressively over 24 hours to levels approximating 100 pg/mL. Because IL1β and IL6 are B-cell growth and differentiation factors, the production of these two cytokines promotes the production of red cell allo- and auto-antibodies that are often associated with DHTRs.

IgG-mediated hemolysis also results in the production of the IL1β inhibitor IL1ra.[58] Significant levels of IL1ra appear in a parallel fashion to IL1β. Immunocytochemical staining has demonstrated strong reactivity for IL1ra in monocytes engaged in erythrophagocytosis. Northern blot analysis of mononuclear cell RNA shows that IL1β gene expression precedes that of IL1ra in response to IgG-coated red cells. However, neutralizing antibodies to IL1β do not suppress either IL1ra or IL1β gene expression in this setting. Therefore, it appears that IL1ra production is a primary response to the IgG-coated red cell stimulus, rather than an autocrine phenomenon induced by initial IL1β production. Treatment of mononuclear cells with the steroid dexamethasone inhibits IL1ra production in response to IgG-coated red cells. These data suggest the possibility that the clinical variability of DHTR, and some of the clinical differences from intravascular HTR, may be accounted for, in part, by the relative balance of IL1β and IL1ra production.

Labile blood pressure is a feature of severe HTR, particularly with intravascular hemolysis. Both complement activation products such as C5a and cytokines such as IL1β and TNFα can contribute to hypotension. The common pathway of these mediators is the production of NO by endothelial cells. NO, in turn, causes relaxation of vascular smooth muscle. Hypotension and deposition of thrombi in arterioles, which impair cortical blood flow, are the major factors that contribute to renal failure. In addition, there may be direct effects of inflammatory mediators on the kidneys.

There are several mechanisms by which HTR results in intravascular coagulation. TNFα produced during immune hemolysis can induce tissue factor expression by endothelial cells.[53] Tissue factor is an initiator of the extrinsic pathway that functions as a cofactor for factors VII and VIIa to accelerate the activation of factors IX and X. TNFα and IL1β, acting on endothelial cells, will also decrease the cell surface expression of thrombomodulin. Thrombomodulin is normally present on endothelial cells, and binds thrombin to activate the coagulation inhibitor protein C. Intravascular hemolysis, as in ABO incompatibility, will also induce procoagulant activity in blood leukocytes, largely because of tissue factor expression.[58] This cellular procoagulant is partly inhibited by blocking antibodies to tissue factor and partly dependent of the multifunctional adhesion protein CD11b.

Recently developed transgenic murine transfusion models show promise in further elucidating the mechanisms underlying HTR. Transfusion of human glycophorin A (hGPA)-positive RBC to hGPA negative animals in the presence of IgG or IgM anti-hGPA results in rapid clearance and induces cytokine storm.[59,60] Complement and activating Fc receptors are involved in red cell clearance in this model. Similar clearance of incompatible RBC occurs in a transgenic Fy[b] antigen model.[61] Interestingly, transfusion of transgenic hen egg lysozyme (HEL) positive RBC to passively immunized antigen negative recipients results in disappearance of the HEL antigen from the RBC surface rather the RBC clearance, a phenomenon termed *antigen loss*.[62] This model also showed that alloimmunization to HEL transgenic RBC was increased by viral-like inflammation induced by poly(I:C), but not by bacterial-like inflammation induced by LPS.[63] In a model incorporating HEL-ovalbumin-Duffy antigens, transfusion of 14 days stored RBC enhanced alloimmunization compared to transfusion of freshly collected RBC.[64]

Table 57.5 Therapeutic options in HTR

Therapeutic Intervention	Indication	Typical Dose
Hydration	Prevention of renal impairment Maintain urine output >100 ml/hr	Normal saline and/or 5% dextrose 200 ml/m² /hr
Alkalinization of urine	Prevention of renal impairment Maintain urine pH >7.5	NaH₂CO₃ 40–70 mEq in 1 liter 5% dextrose
Diuresis	Prevention of renal impairment	Mannitol 20% 100 ml/m² * Furosemide 40 to 80 mg
Anticoagulation	Treatment of intravascular coagulation	Heparin 5 to 10 units/kg/hour
Red cell exchange transfusion	Decrease load of incompatible red cells	Exchange of one estimated red cell mass
Plasma or platelet transfusion	Treatment of hemorrhagic complications of DIC	Platelets: 1 unit platelets/10 kg (max. 6 units) or 1 unit Apheresis platelets Plasma: 10 ml/kg fresh frozen plasma
Intravenous Immunoglobulin	Prevention of extravascular hemolysis	400 mg/kg

* Ensure adequate renal function to prevent fluid overload from increased intravascular volume.

Therapy

Patients who have minimal symptoms are best managed by careful observation. However, early vigorous intervention in severe reactions saves lives. Therapeutic options in HTR are summarized in Table 57.5. The severity of HTR is directly related to volume and rate of infusion of incompatible blood. Thus, early recognition, stopping transfusion, and preventing the transfusion of additional incompatible units is the first essential step of treatment. Initial attention must be paid to cardiovascular support. If hypotension is present, fluid resuscitation and pressor support should be considered. Care should be taken to avoid fluid overload, however, especially in patients with impaired cardiac or renal function. Pulmonary artery catheterization is useful in selected patients to guide resuscitation.

Because intravascular hemolysis is an expected consequence of the infusion of ABO-incompatible marrow, some guidance can be obtained from published reports. Isoagglutinin titer clearly influences the clinical response to ABO-incompatible marrow infusion. In general, antibody titers below 64 are associated with mild or no reactions while high titers such as 1024 are associated with significant clinical reactions. The volume of incompatible red cells infused with the marrow also determines the magnitude of the response. One protocol reported to be successful in patients receiving major ABO-incompatible transplants involved preparatory hydration with 5% dextrose in onehalf normal saline with 30 to 40 mEq sodium bicarbonate/L and 15 mEq potassium chloride/L at a rate of 3000 mL/m²/day, and 100 mL/m². Mannitol 20% was given 1 hour before marrow infusion.[65] During marrow infusion, the infusion rate of fluids was increased to 4500 to 6000 mL/m²/day and additional mannitol was given at a rate of 30 mL/m²/hour for the next 12 hours. The rationale for this protocol was to maintain a high rate of urine output and prevent precipitation of hemoglobin in the renal tubules. All these patients had a preinfusion antibody titer no greater than 32. None experienced a clinical reaction to the infusion of approximately 120 to 160 mL of incompatible red cells. Alternatively, red cell depletion of ABO incompatible bone marrow products can prevent AHTR, but with possibly significant loss of hematopoietic progenitor cells and delayed engraftment.[66]

The deliberate transfusion of ABO-incompatible red cells before transplantation has been employed to reduce isoagglutinin titers. In one such protocol, one incompatible RBC unit was given over eight hours on each of two days immediately before transplant.[24] These patients were monitored in an intensive care unit and hydrated with normal saline and 5% dextrose (1:1 ratio) at a rate of 3000 mL/m^2/day. Sodium bicarbonate was administered to maintain the urine pH above 7.0. Of the 12 patients reported in this series, isoagglutinin titers before transfusion ranged from 32 to 1024. One patient developed renal failure requiring hemodialysis for 17 days, but this resolved. In another series of deliberate administration of ABO-incompatible red cells, 35 patients received 50 to 150 mL of incompatible red cells before marrow transplantation.[25] All patients received prednisolone 250 mg, dimethindene 4 mg, and ranitidine 150 mg 30 minutes before the transfusion. No clinical reaction was observed in 23 patients (66%), while severe reactions (chest pain, headache or agues, and/or high changes of heart rate, blood pressure, and/or oxygen saturation) occurred in four patients (11%). The highest pretransfusion titer in this series was 64.

Because the severity and course of HTR are dictated by the load of incompatible red cells in circulation, exchange transfusion with antigen-negative blood may be considered. Although it is not appropriate to expose a patient to added risk of transfusion-related infectious disease if the hemolytic process is well tolerated, with a severe reaction to ABO incompatibility, exchange transfusion might greatly reduce the chance of morbidity or death.

Early treatment of hypotension and DIC are the most important interventions to limit the extent of possible renal impairment. Maintenance of urine output with intravenous fluids and diuretics, such as mannitol or furosemide, early in the course of the reaction has been used successfully. However, if oliguria in the face of normovolemia is present, fluid loading is contraindicated.

The prevention and treatment of DIC are also controversial. Heparin has been advocated by some authors as a treatment for DIC.[67] In addition, heparin may have a direct anticomplement effect, which limits intravascular hemolysis and the sequelae of complement activation.[68] An obvious drawback of heparin therapy, especially in the intraoperative or postoperative patient, is the potential for hemorrhage. Therefore, heparin should be reserved for patients with clear evidence of intravascular coagulation (thrombocytopenia, hypofibrinogenemia, and the presence of FDPs and D-dimers). The use of fresh frozen plasma or platelet concentrates in DIC is also controversial, and transfusion of these components should be limited to those patients with active hemorrhage.

Most extravascular HTRs are not life-threatening and require no acute treatment. However, some patients with extravascular HTR may benefit from intravenous immunoglobulin (IVIG) infusion. A single dose of IVIG, 400 mg/kg infused within 24 hours of transfusion, has been used successfully to prevent transfusion reactions in alloimmunized patients for whom compatible blood was not obtainable.[26,69] Five patients so treated did not experience transfusion reactions and had sustained increases in hematocrit. IVIG, 1 g/kg or 400 mg/kg, has also been used in the treatment of sickle cell HTR syndrome.[70,71]

The selection of blood components for a hemorrhaging patient undergoing HTR is a critical decision. The first consideration is that no patient should be allowed to suffer a fatal hemorrhage while a search for serologically compatible blood is undertaken. Second, red cells lacking known clinically significant antigens to which the patient currently has an antibody should be obtained, if at all possible. For instance, one should not reflexively issue group O-negative red cells to a patient known to have anti-e. When the specificity of the antibody causing the reaction is not known, the results of serologic tests performed up to that point in time must be considered, and clinical judgment exercised. Although the focus of attention in most HTRs is on red cells, care should be taken to avoid transfusion of type-incompatible plasma or platelets that may aggravate hemolysis, especially when ABO incompatibility is a possible cause. Undue haste in both serologic evaluation and decision making must be avoided, because human errors are often committed under pressure.

Future therapies that have not yet been subjected to clinical trials might be directed against inflammatory mediators produced during HTRs. HTRs have a similar clinical presentation to the systemic inflammatory response syndrome (SIRS) (e.g., fever, tachycardia, tachypnea or hypoxemia, and leukocytosis).[72] Cytokine dysregulation is central to the pathophysiology of SIRS, in which elevated levels of TNFα, IL1, and IL6 are associated with mortality.[73,74] These considerations suggest that TNFα or IL1 blockade may be beneficial in the treatment of HTR. Presently, there are three TNFα blocking agents marketed in the United States; etanercept (Enbrel, Amgen), a soluble p75 TNFα receptor fusion protein to the Fc portion of IgG; infliximab (Remicade, Centocor), a chimeric (mouse/human) TNFα antibody; and adalimumab (Humira, Abbott Laboratories), a fully human monoclonal antibody. Anakinra (Kineret, Amgen) is recombinant human IL1ra, which is also approved by the FDA. Unfortunately, clinical trials of these agents in SIRS have been rather disappointing, with most trials not showing improved outcome. Inhibitors of complement show promise in the treatment of HTR. Human recombinant soluble form of complement receptor 1 (sCR1) has been shown to inhibit complement-mediated red cell destruction in vitro and in a mouse model of hemolysis.[75] Since the classical pathway of complement is involved in IgM medicated AHTR, C1 esterase inhibitor (C1-INH) (Berinert, CSL Behring), has potential to prevent intravascular hemolysis.[76] Similarly, eculizumab (Soliris, Alexion Pharmaceuticals), a humanized monoclonal anti-C5, may prevent intravascular hemolysis and C5a production, although not C3b deposition. It should be noted that there are no data at present regarding the safety or effectiveness of drugs that inhibit complement or cytokines in HTR.

Prevention

Much of the activity in blood banks is directed toward the prevention of HTRs. Proper performance of donor unit typing, pretransfusion testing, antibody identification, and crossmatching are critical and are covered in Chapter 16.

Because human errors are the most common cause of severe HTR, administrative systems designed to analyze errors and prevent future recurrence are the most important protective measure. An event-reporting system specifically designed for transfusion services, MERS-TM, has been developed.[77] It allows for the recognition and analysis of errors, determination of patterns of errors, and monitoring for changes in frequency after corrective action is implemented. In one application of MERS-TM, high-severity events with the potential for patient harm were discovered to account for 241 (5%) of the 4670 events over a 47-month period.[78]

Proper identification of the transfusion recipient and pretransfusion blood specimen is the single most important aspect of the prevention of HTR. Every transfusion service must establish and enforce the procedures to be followed in its institution. At a minimum, these procedures should include permanent and unique identification of each patient using a permanent identification method such as a wristband, confirmation of the proper labeling of blood specimens by comparison to the wristband, and confirmation of the patient identification before starting the transfusion. Deviation from institutional policies on patient and specimen identification should be taken very seriously. Use of a special wristband for identification of transfusion recipients may prevent some errors. Such systems generally have a unique identifier on the wristband that is only used by the blood bank. A report of the use of one system over a period of 17 years found that potentially ABO-incompatible transfusions were avoided in five of 411,705 samples typed.[79] A report of the use of another identification system found that of 2198 cases, two potentially ABO-incompatible transfusions were avoided.[80] An alternative system uses bar codes on patient wristbands, blood sample tubes, blood component bags, and nurses' identification badges; and point-of-care reading devices to verify identity.[81] Radiofrequency identification devices also have great promise for reduction error. These tools require investment in information technology, but can be integrated with other systems, such as medication administration, for overall enhancement of patient safety. However, sole reliance on such a device to prevent incorrect administration of blood may undermine other more important steps in proper patient identification.

Confirmation of the recipient's ABO type by point-of-care testing before transfusion is a possible strategy for avoiding AHTR. In principle, seven out of eight ABO-incompatible transfusions could be thus avoided. However, bedside testing is subject to analytic and interpretive errors. At one institution performing bedside ABO confirmation, 13 ABO-incompatible RBC transfusions occurred in eight years.[82] Of these, an error in bedside ABO testing occurred in seven cases. User inexperience is the most important factor in bedside testing errors, although there are device factors as well.[83]

In situations where patient identification error has caused HTR, immediate consideration should be given to the possibility that another patient has been involved in the misidentification and may, too, be at risk of receiving incompatible blood. This is especially likely if there are two patients with similar names or if two samples are received simultaneously from the same patient care location. Identification of such errors can prevent a second hemolytic reaction. Some institutions mandate two separate blood draws for all newly admitted non-O patients at separate time intervals to ascertain and confirm the identity of the patient to mitigate potential hemolytic reactions resulting from incompatible transfusions.

The selection of donor units lacking antigens corresponding to alloantibodies is essential for the prevention of HTR, but whether phenotype matching of donors and recipients is an appropriate strategy for the prevention of alloimmunization and HTR in the nonimmunized patient is controversial. Arguments in favor of this practice have been put forth in the setting of sickle cell disease where, because of ethnic gene pool diversity, there is often a mismatch between the donor and recipient phenotypes. Examination of alloimmunization rates among children in one urban area indicated that children with non-European ethnic origins had a 42.9% incidence of alloimmunization compared to 17.6% in

patients of European ancestry.[84] This was not simply caused by variation in transfusion rates, because the patients of European ethnicity received more transfusions than the others. In another study that compared sickle cell patients to those with other forms of chronic anemia, 30% of the patients with sickle cell anemia were alloimmunized, in contrast to 5% in the group of patients with other forms of anemia.[85] Of the 32 alloimmunized patients with sickle cell anemia, 17 had multiple antibodies and 14 had DHTRs. Although many institutions have not performed phenotype matching for sickle cell patients in the past, it is becoming commonly accepted practice.[86,87]

Phenotype matching may possibly prevent some HTRs in other multitransfused patient populations. In a retrospective study of patients with at lest one red cell antibody who received subsequent transfusions, 21% of 653 patients produced additional antibodies.[88] Patients with hematologic disease or malignancy, warm-reacting autoantibodies, antibodies to high- or low-frequency antigens, and those receiving prophylactic antigen matching were excluded. Of those who formed additional antibodies, 57% did so after one transfusion episode of a median of two RBC units. The authors predicted that matching for Rh, Jk^a, and Fy^a could have prevented the formation of 83% of new antibodies. However, whether prevention of serologic reactions will prevent hemolytic reactions is not clear. In this study, 1% to 10% of potential donors would have been available for 3% of patients and more than 10% of potential donors would have been available for 61% of patients, had phenotype matching been performed. However, the frequency of suitable donors may be different in other locations.

Hemolytic transfusion reactions could be avoided entirely if the responsible antigens on the red cell surface could be removed or camouflaged. Experimental work has suggested that treating red cells with polyethylene glycol (PEG) might be an effective means of camouflaging antigens.[89] PEG modification appears to work by creating a sphere of hydration around the red cell that effectively excludes IgG or IgM from coming into contact with antigenic structures on the membrane surface. PEG-treated red cells have properties of size, shape, intracellular ion content, and oxygen binding that are identical to untreated red cells. However, PEG-treated red cells have a low shear viscosity compared to normal red cells. This also may be advantageous in sickle cell disease in which increased blood viscosity within capillaries can result in occlusive crises.

The effectiveness of PEG modification is dependent on the molecular weight and branching characteristics of PEG molecules and the chemistry of covalent attachment.[90] Use of a dichlorotriazine derivative of 5-kD PEG results in complete inhibition of direct agglutination by anti-D. However, such cells are still agglutinated by anti-D in the indirect antiglobulin test. A and B epitopes are partially, but not completely, masked. In contrast, red cells coated with branched chain 10-kD PEG after treatment with succinimidylpropionate-modified 20-kD PEG are not agglutinated by anti-A, anti-B, and anti-D. Treatment of red cells with maleimidophenyl-PEG 5 kD and 20 kD can inhibit agglutination by Rh and ABO antibodies.[91] However, the approach may be limited by the occurrence of anti-PEG in many individuals.[92]

Group A and group B red cells can be converted to group O cells by enzymatic cleavage of terminal determinant saccharides with α-N-acetylgalactosaminidase or α-D-galactosidase.[93–95] The use of such technology for large-scale conversion of red cells raises the possibility that acute HTRs from ABO incompatibility may be completely avoidable in the future. However, there are issues with regard to completeness of antigen removal and the possibility of exposure of neoantigens by enzymatic treatment. Treatment of red cells with α-N-acetylgalactosaminidase results in rapid loss of A epitopes binding *Dolichos biflorus* lectin.[93] Inhibition of complement-mediated hemolysis is somewhat slower. However, the epitopes of A antigen that react with human source anti-A are relatively resistant to enzymatic degradation. Additionally, there are differences in the enzymatic sensitivity of A epitopes on the red cell membrane. Glycosphingolipids with short oligosaccharide chains display the greatest resistance to enzymatic treatment.

Work on enzyme-converted group O (ECO) red cells from group B red cells has advanced to the stage of the clinical trials.[96,97] An initial trial of a two-unit transfusion of ECO RBCs to group O subjects demonstrated good 24-hour posttransfusion survival (95%), with a half-life of 29.5 days.[96] There was no clinical or laboratory evidence of hemolysis. A subsequent study with larger volume transfusions had similar results. Subjects who received a second transfusion did not show evidence of alloimmunization or increase in anti-B titer.[97] In another study, occasional serologic incompatibility with enzyme-converted red cells was seen, as well as transient positive DAT and increases in anti-B titer after transfusion. However, no adverse effects of whole unit transfusion were seen, and normal posttransfusion red cell survival was demonstrated in the face of incompatibility.[98] A screening technique has recently been used to discover several novel exoglycosidases with high specific activity for the removal of A and B determinants at neutral pH.[99] Complete conversion of whole RBC units from group A and group B to group O, as indicated by no reactivity with licensed typing reagents, was achieved with low enzyme concentrations. Clinical trials are ongoing to assess the safety and efficacy of this promising product.

Summary

Although the prevention of HTRs continues to be a major focus in transfusion medicine, advances in serology and transfusion service practices have significantly reduced their incidence. Simultaneously, advances in the understanding of the pathophysiology of HTRs have given us insights to help guide the management of patients undergoing reactions. It is conceivable that technological advances in red cell modification and oxygen-carrying solutions will significantly change red cell transfusion practice in the future and virtually eliminate the occurrence of HTR. Until such time, however, HTRs will remain a major adverse consequence of blood transfusion.

Disclaimer

The authors have disclosed no conflicts of interest.

Key References

2 Bolton-Maggs PHB (Ed.), Poles D, Watt A, Thomas D on behalf of the Serious Hazards of Transfusion (SHOT) Steering Group. The 2013 Annual SHOT Report (2014). http://www.shotuk.org/wp-content/uploads/74280-SHOT-2014-Annual-Report-V12-WEB.pdf

11 Petz LD, Calhoun L, Shulman IA, *et al*. The sickle cell hemolytic transfusion reaction syndrome. *Transfusion* 1997;**37**:382–92.

23 Dzik W, Murphy M, Andreu G, *et al*. An international study of the performance of sample collection from patients. *Vox Sang* 2003;**85**:40–7.

26 Kohan AI, Niborski RC, Rey JA, *et al*. High-dose intravenous immunoglobulin in non-ABO transfusion incompatibility. *Vox Sang* 1994;**67**:195–8.

56 Davenport RD, Burdick M, Moore SA, Kunkel SL. Cytokine production in IgG mediated red cell incompatibility. *Transfusion* 1993;**33**:19–24.

77 Callum J, Kaplan H, Merkley L, *et al*. Reporting of near-miss events for transfusion medicine: Improving transfusion safety. *Transfusion* 2001;**41**:1204–11.

88 Schonewille H, van de Watering L, Brand A. Additional red blood cell alloantibodies after blood transfusions in a nonhematologic alloimmunized patient cohort: Is it time to take precautionary measures? *Transfusion* 2006;**46**:630–5.

CHAPTER 58

Febrile, allergic, and nonimmune transfusion reactions

Emmanuel A. Fadeyi & Gregory J. Pomper

Department of Pathology, Wake Forest University School of Medicine, Winston-Salem, NC, USA

This chapter reviews a variety of acute, nonhemolytic, and non-infectious transfusion reactions, the most common of which are febrile, nonhemolytic transfusion reactions (FNHTRs) and allergic reactions. Other acute, nonhemolytic reactions are reported less frequently and include transfusion-related acute lung injury (TRALI) and anaphylactic or anaphylactoid reactions. Additional acute adverse effects can occur in massive transfusion because of the large volume of blood components transfused over a short period. The complications of massive transfusion include dilutional coagulopathy, hypothermia, citrate toxicity, and electrolyte disturbances, among others. Some patients cannot tolerate the acute increase in intravascular blood volume caused by transfusion and experience the complications of transfusion-associated circulatory overload (TACO). Acute reactions can be caused by the toxicity of chemicals that leach into blood components from blood storage containers or filters or by chemicals added to improve storage conditions, such as dimethyl sulfoxide (DMSO). Other reactions are caused by endogenous mediators generated in the blood during filtration, processing, or storage, such as bradykinin-mediated hypotensive reactions. It is important that these complications of transfusion be recognized by patient care teams and blood bank personnel, and that appropriate treatments and preventive measures be instituted for patient safety and well-being.

Febrile nonhemolytic transfusion reactions

Description

An FNHTR is commonly defined as an increase in body temperature of 1 °C or more that occurs during or within several hours of transfusion and is unrelated to hemolysis, sepsis, or other known causes of fever. The use of a 1 °C increase in body temperature as a threshold for defining an FNHTR avoids undue concern over small fluctuations in body temperature unrelated to transfusion that do not justify discontinuation of transfusion and follow-up investigation. Many FNHTRs begin with the patient feeling uneasy and experiencing chills. In mild reactions, the signs and symptoms do not progress. Chills with or without an increase in body temperature can be classified as an FNHTR if other possible causes of chills are unlikely and the time course of the reaction correlates with the transfusion. In the most severe reactions, patients may experience rigors (severe shaking chills) or a fever elevation of 2 °C or more over baseline. Although signs and symptoms usually are

limited to chills and fever, some patients may also rarely experience more severe symptoms such as headache, nausea, and/or vomiting.

The fever of FNHTR usually persists no more than 8 to 12 hours after the start of transfusion. If fever persists 18 to 24 hours or longer, it is unlikely to be transfusion related. Generally, FNHTRs are self-limited and have no sequelae. However, elderly patients, patients with compromised cardiovascular status, or critically ill patients are at risk of cardiorespiratory complications associated with FNHTR. Because fever increases oxygen demand and consumption an estimated 13% for every 1 °C over 37 °C and shivering increases oxygen demand approximately 300%, FNHTRs can aggravate preexisting cardiac, pulmonary, and cerebrovascular insufficiency. Therefore, prompt recognition and antipyretic management of FNHTRs can be very beneficial.

An FNHTR almost always is associated with transfusion of cellular blood components, such as red cells, platelets, and granulocyte preparations and less commonly with noncellular components, such as plasma and cryoprecipitate. The incidence of FNHTR varies widely and median rates have been reported as higher for platelets (4.6%) than for red cells (0.33%).[1]

The reaction risk of blood components, however, varies according to numerous factors, such as method of preparation of the blood component (e.g., leukocyte reduction, storage time, medications, patient and donor characteristics, monitoring practices, and many others). These factors vary among different geographic regions and medical centers. In addition, rates based on reactions reported to blood banks are lower than those based on systematic surveillance of responses to all transfusions. A recent study demonstrated that the rate of reported FNHTR were low for prestorage-leukocyte reduced pooled platelets compared to poststorage-leukocyte reduced pooled platelets.[2]

Longer platelet storage times are also associated with higher rates of FNHTR.[3-5] Reactions also are more frequent among certain recipients, such as multitransfused patients or multiparous women who have developed leukocyte or platelet alloantibodies.

Etiology

An FNHTR appears to be part of the systemic inflammatory response syndrome (SIRS) provoked in transfusion recipients by the immune challenge of transfusing foreign cells or infusing soluble inflammatory mediators present in stored blood components. The term *systemic inflammatory response syndrome* was coined to describe the constellation of observed body responses to various

Rossi's Principles of Transfusion Medicine, Fifth Edition. Edited by Toby L. Simon, Jeffrey McCullough, Edward L. Snyder, Bjarte G. Solheim, and Ronald G. Strauss.

insults, such as infection, trauma, burns, and ischemia. It is defined as the presence of two or more of the following: body temperature more than 38 °C or less than 36 °C; heart rate more than 90 beats/minute; tachypnea (respiratory rate >20 breaths/minute or $PaCO_2$ less than 32 mm Hg); and white cell count more than 12,000/μL or less than 4×10^9/L, or more than 10% immature neutrophils (band forms). Although a mild FNHTR may not completely fulfill these criteria, FNHTR is nevertheless an inflammatory response.

Exogenous pyrogens such as lipopolysaccharide (LPS) and pyrogenic cytokines initiate a series of responses leading to hyperthermia. These responses include rapid muscle contractions that cause shivering, rigors, and an increase in heat generation. Heat conservation is achieved through cutaneous vasoconstriction, which also contributes to the sensation of a chill. Perceived chills lead to behavioral changes that can further increase body temperature. For example, the patient may cover up, and the result is inhibition of heat dissipation.

An FNHTR appears to have two possible underlying causes: (1) the more "classical" pathway of infused antigens, such as leukocytes, that stimulate the in vivo generation of cytokines in the recipient; and (2) the infusion of pyrogenic cytokines or other inflammatory response mediators (e.g., activated complement proteins, LPS, or neutrophil-priming lipids) that accumulate in the plasma portion of cellular blood components during storage.[5–6] A third cause of fever, infusion of blood components contaminated with bacteria or bacterial products, will produce a febrile response, but it is not usually categorized as an FNHTR but rather as a bacterial septic reaction, if recognized. The common pathway by which these different stimuli induce posttransfusion fever has been attributed to an increase in circulating pyrogenic cytokines in the recipient, such as interleukin-1β (IL1β), IL6, and tumor necrosis factor α (TNFα). Pyrogenic cytokines induce fever by mediating upregulation of the thermostatic set point for body temperature in the thermoregulatory center of the hypothalamus. This mechanism is supported by the association of febrile reactions with a specific cytokine polymorphism *IL1RN*2.2* genotype.[7] Severe nonhemolytic transfusion reaction have also being linked to inflammatory cytokines and chemokines generated by mononuclear cells in donor blood by HLA Class II antibody containing plasma unit.[8] Recently, research has led investigators to a more complex model of fever generation, building on a model where cytokines principally induce fever to one where central nervous system stimulation by prostaglandin E2 (PGE2) is pivotal. Alternative hypotheses have resulted from the finding that a febrile response to LPS occurs even with blockade of either IL1 or TNFα and that the presence of circulating cytokines lags behind the development of fever.[9] Research has found that LPS-induced C5a production via complement activation results in rapid peripheral PGE2 production.[10] In addition, LPS binds to toll-like receptor 4 and induces cytokine production, leading to a two-phase rapid and delayed febrile response. Hyperthermic stimuli compete with hypothermic stimuli to achieve a central thermal balance point that may elevate or decrease based upon physiologic stimuli.[11] Central to the febrile response is the presence of EP3 prostaglandin receptors that bind PGE2 in the hypothalamus (Figure 58.1).[12] These newer models of the fever response provide possible explanations for why FNHTRs continue to occur despite prestorage leukocyte reduction that minimizes cytokine accumulation in storage. Clinical evidence supports the hypothesis that febrile reactions can be caused by noncytokine hyperthermic stimuli present in cellular transfusion products.[13] More research is needed for the development of more targeted

antipyretic medications that may eventually lead to the extinction of FNHTRs.

Alloimmunization to leukocytes or platelets

Transfusion recipients at greatest risk of an FNHTR are those with leukocyte or platelet antibodies who receive transfusions with blood components containing large numbers of passenger leukocytes or platelets.[14–15] Less frequently, donor antibodies to leukocytes, present in the plasma portion of blood components, are associated with FNHTRs. The implicated antibodies most often have HLA specificity, although they also may be platelet- or granulocyte-specific. A minimum of approximately 1×10^7 leukocytes per unit of red blood cells (RBCs) appears necessary to cause an FNHTR, although this number varies among individuals.[16–17] The role of donor leukocytes in FNHTR is supported by the finding that decreasing the leukocyte content of blood components below this threshold reduces the incidence of FNHTRs.

A variety of mechanisms are possible by which antibody–leukocyte or antibody–platelet interactions cause fever. For example, donor monocytes may be activated and secrete pyrogenic cytokines when recipient antibodies bind to them. An alternative explanation is that immune complex formation between recipient antibodies and donor leukocytes or platelets leads to generation of activated complement components such as C5a, which stimulate the production of PGE2.

Storage-generated cytokines

Antibodies to leukocytes or platelets do not appear to account for all FNHTRs, particularly those caused by platelet transfusions. For example, some patients with no history of transfusion or pregnancy experience an FNHTR to their first transfusion of platelets.[18] It is unlikely that these reactions are mediated by recipient leukocyte or platelet antibodies because these recipients have no previous exposure to foreign cells. In addition, the rate of FNHTRs to platelet transfusion increases with increasing blood bank storage time of the transfused platelet concentrate.[3–5] This indicates that time-dependent change occurs in the platelet concentrate during storage that has a role in stimulating an FNHTR in some patients. Furthermore, febrile reactions still occur with the use of prestorage leukocyte reduction. In some cases, this is the result of inappropriate filter use or filter failure. However, this observation also supports the possibility that a substance or substances in the plasma portion of blood components not removed by filtration may be responsible for mediating at least some FNHTRs. The discovery that pro-inflammatory cytokines accumulate in the plasma portion of platelet concentrates may account for many of these findings.

A variety of leukocyte-derived, pro-inflammatory cytokines, including IL1β, IL6, IL8, tumor necrosis factor-α (TNFα), macrophage inflammatory protein-1α (MIP1α), and growth-related oncogene-α (GROα), are generated and accumulate in the plasma portion of platelet concentrates during storage.[19–21] Extracellular levels of these cytokines generally increase with increasing component storage time and are roughly proportional to the passenger leukocyte content of the blood component bag. Prestorage or early-storage leukocyte reduction (within one to two days of collection) prevents or greatly reduces generation of these cytokines. Because they have pyrogenic activity, many of these cytokines (if present in high enough concentration) can induce febrile responses in transfusion recipients. Elevated levels of IL1β, IL6, and TNFα in the plasma portion of platelet concentrates correlate positively with the occurrence of an FNHTR. Some studies have shown that IL6 levels

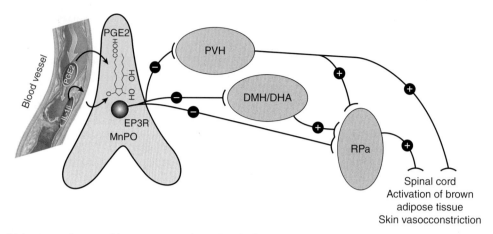

Figure 58.1 A model for neuronal action of the EP3 receptors (EP3Rs) in the fever response after systemic immune challenge. In response to lipopolysaccharides or cytokines, prostaglandin E2 (PGE2) is generated by macrophages of the liver and lung and endothelial cells lining venules in the brain. PGE2 is transported or diffuses across the blood–brain barrier and acts on EP3Rs in the median preoptic area (MnPO). These are hypothesized to be GABAergic neurons that inhibit thermogenic systems in the hypothalamic paraventricular nucleus (PVH), the dorsomedial nucleus/dorsal area (DMH/DHA), and the raphe pallidus nucleus in the medulla (RPa). These thermogenic nuclei activate sympathetic preganglionic neurons in the spinal cord, resulting in cutaneous vasoconstriction and activation of brown adipose tissue that ultimately raise body temperature. Source: Lazarus et al. (2007).[12] Reproduced with permission of Nature Publishing.

in the plasma portion of platelet concentrates correlate best with the occurrence of FNHTR. In one study, chills, fever, or both occurred more frequently after infusion of the plasma portion of the platelet concentrates than after infusion of the cellular portion containing platelets and leukocytes.[19] The plasma portions that caused an FNHTR contained higher levels of IL1β and IL6 than did those that did not cause chills or fever. These data support the role of the plasma portion of platelet concentrates as a source of inflammatory mediators and as a possible stimulus of FNHTR in some transfusion recipients. Although levels of a variety of pro-inflammatory cytokines in the plasma portion of platelet concentrates correlate with the occurrence of FNHTRs, it is unknown which, if any, of these actually mediate FNHTRs.

Platelet-derived cytokines, such as CD40L (CD154), CCL5 (RANTES), transforming growth factor β1 (TGF-β1), CXCL4 (platelet factor 4; PF4), CXCL8 (IL8), and MIP1α are present in the plasma portion of platelet concentrates and apheresis platelets. All platelet-derived cytokines accumulate during platelet storage and CD40L has been associated with clinical FNHTRs.[22] These cytokines are not known to be directly pyrogenic, but they stimulate the synthesis of pro-inflammatory mediator, IL1β, IL6, IL8, and TNFα. Because RANTES can activate basophils and mast cells and stimulate histamine release, it may play a role in mediating some allergic reactions (see the "Allergic Reactions" section).[23]

Some pro-inflammatory cytokines, such as IL1β and IL8, have been detected in the supernatant portion of stored RBCs, although at much lower levels than in platelet concentrates.[24] Because the cold storage temperature of RBC units, 1–6 °C, has an inhibitory effect on cellular metabolism, the capacity of passenger leukocytes in RBC units to synthesize and secrete cytokines is less than those in platelet concentrates. As a result, the levels of cytokines in RBC units appear to be too low to mediate significant physiologic reactions.

The stimulus for cytokine generation during storage of blood components remains unknown. Measurements of cytokine messenger RNA levels and total cytokine levels (intracellular plus extracellular) in platelet concentrates indicate that accumulation of leukocyte-derived cytokines is caused in part by new synthesis

and secretion. The stimulus for synthesis and secretion of leukocyte-derived cytokines may be, for example, contact activation of monocytes after these cells interact with the plastic of the storage containers or tubing.[25] Other possibilities include the direct stimulatory effects of C5a on PGE2 or the stimulatory effects of activated complement components on monocytes or other leukocytes in the blood component bag. The presence of platelet derived cytokines (e.g., CD40L, RANTES, and TGF-β1) in the plasma portion of platelet concentrates likely results from their release from preexisting stores, because the biosynthetic activity of platelets is limited.

Bacterial contamination of blood components

An FNHTR may result from infusion of a blood component contaminated with bacteria or bacterial products such as LPS. Unless a Gram's stain and bacterial cultures are performed, mild septic transfusion reactions characterized by only fever and chills are likely to be classified clinically as FNHTR.[26–27]

Transfusion reactions caused by contaminating bacteria, whether mild or severe, are manifestations of the SIRS, described earlier. Pro-inflammatory cytokines (such as IL1β, IL6, IL8, and TNFα) are implicated in the pathogenesis of SIRS associated with sepsis.[28] If bacterial contamination of blood components has occurred, the greatest source of cytokines is likely the transfusion recipient's cells stimulated by the infused bacteria or bacterial products. However, cytokine production by leukocytes in the component bag during storage stimulated by bacteria or bacterial products also may contribute to the reaction.

Diagnosis

As a routine part of the transfusion procedure, the vital signs of transfusion recipients (pulse, temperature, and respiratory rate and oxygen percent saturation) should be measured immediately before transfusion and at intervals during and soon after transfusion. The patient should be watched closely, particularly in the first 30–60 minutes of transfusion, for the onset of chills, shivering, or rigors, which often precede a fever.

A transfusion reaction is a possibility if chills, fever (1 °C or more over pretransfusion temperature), or both develop any time during transfusion or up to several hours after the transfusion has ended. A febrile response to transfusion, however, is not specific for an FNHTR. For example, a fever may be the early manifestation of a more serious acute hemolytic, septic, or TRALI transfusion reaction. When a patient has a febrile reaction to transfusion, an evaluation to rule out hemolysis and possibly bacterial contamination should be undertaken promptly. Nursing staff should stop the transfusion immediately and notify the physician caring for the patient. They should verify that the identity of the transfusion recipient, based on the patient's identification bracelet and verbal confirmation with the recipient, if possible, matches that of the intended recipient, as indicated on the blood component tag. All containers and transfusion sets should be sent to the laboratory along with a posttransfusion blood specimen and a report that summarizes the clinical reaction. The clinical team should also have verbal communication with the blood bank staff to ensure that the postreaction blood specimen, component bag, and infusion set are received by the blood bank as soon as possible.

Investigation of a febrile reaction in the blood bank generally begins with a recheck of the records for clerical errors. The posttransfusion serum/plasma must be visually evaluated for hemolysis and should be compared with the pretransfusion specimen. A direct antiglobulin test must be performed on the posttransfusion blood specimen and ideally on a pretransfusion specimen for comparison. The ABO grouping of the patient sample and the donor unit should be repeated. When suggested by the preliminary serologic results, the crossmatch may be repeated for RBC transfusions to confirm patient–donor compatibility. The results of these tests confirm or exclude a hemolytic transfusion reaction as the basis for the fever. When a septic reaction is highly suspected, for example if the patient arrives with a high fever (2 °C or more) or accompanying hypotension, the bag contents should be examined by means of a Gram's stain and culture for bacterial contamination. Blood cultures also should be obtained from the transfusion recipient's posttransfusion blood specimen to correlate bacteremia with the same organism that may be detected in the blood component bag. Most blood banks do not test for HLA-specific, platelet-specific, or granulocyte-specific antibodies in the recipient's serum as possible causes of an FNHTR. Identification of these antibodies and pyrogenic cytokines is reserved for specialized laboratories and does not play a role in the immediate evaluation of most reactions.

The patient is examined by the primary team and the blood bank physician to determine whether associated symptoms or circumstances can explain the fever, such as drug reactions, sepsis, or other inflammatory conditions unrelated to transfusion. The time course of the development and resolution of fever should be examined in relation to the transfusion. In cases in which the transfusion recipient has a fever at the start of transfusion or is experiencing intermittent spiking fevers, a posttransfusion increase in body temperature can be difficult to interpret. In such cases *possible FNHTR* may be the most definitive diagnosis that can be made. An FNHTR is a diagnosis of exclusion, arrived at by means of eliminating the possibility of immune hemolysis, bacterial contamination of the blood component, TRALI, or other causes of fever unrelated to transfusion.

Treatment

The transfusion should be stopped immediately. The intravenous line should be kept open with normal saline solution to provide ready access for the possible infusion of crystalloid and intravenous medication in case the fever is a sign of a more serious hemolytic or

septic reaction. Most patients, however, should be reassured that febrile transfusion reactions usually are harmless and that the fever typically responds to antipyretic therapy. The antipyretic agent of choice is acetaminophen (adults, 325 to 650 mg orally; children, 10 to 15 mg/kg orally or rectally). Aspirin and nonsteroidal antiinflammatory drugs are contraindicated in the treatment of many transfusion recipients, such as those receiving platelets. Unless the patient has signs of an allergic reaction, such as urticaria, erythema, or pruritus, antihistamines are not indicated in the management of FNHTR. However, it is not unusual for physicians to prescribe both an antipyretic and an antihistamine in combination for mild reactions.

Patients occasionally develop rigors (severe shaking chills) after a transfusion and meperidine had been a mainstay therapy for many years. Because shivering can increase oxygen demand significantly, it is important to control the shaking chills, particularly for patients with cardiac or respiratory insufficiency. When administered to adults at doses of 25 to 50 mg intravenously, meperidine remains a very effective treatment for rigors. Meperidine is effective in rapidly arresting rigors through mechanisms not clearly understood. Unfortunately, meperidine has fallen out of favor with some hospitals because of unacceptable central nervous system toxicities and other downsides. Use of meperidine is generally contraindicated in the care of patients with renal failure because of accumulation of the proconvulsant metabolite normeperidine. Use of meperidine also is contraindicated in the care of patients who have taken monoamine oxidase inhibitors within the previous 14 days because of the risk of serotonin syndrome (excess serotonin activity). Toxicities secondary to metabolite accumulation, short half-life, and higher equianalgesic dose compared to morphine has decreased interest but was used in 36% of cases.[29] On the basis of anecdotal evidence, morphine may be slightly less efficacious for the treatment of rigors, but its safety profile is more acceptable when given as a onetime dose of 2 to 4 mg intravenously.

After symptoms of an acute febrile reaction have been treated and the patient has been stabilized, any unused portion of the blood component should be returned to the blood bank and not transfused, even if blood bank testing rapidly rules out hemolysis. A new device that has been FDA approved for the detection of bacteria in both whole blood–derived platelets and apheresis PLT products is the Pan Genera Detection (PGD) test, which can detect 10^3 to 10^5 colony-forming units per ml and may be more sensitive than the Gram stain.[30] The use of Gram's stain helps detect heavily contaminated units (with detection limits not less than 10^6 organisms per mL), and lower levels of contamination may be missed. If the febrile reaction is caused by bacterial contamination of the component bag, restarting transfusion of the same component can cause a severe and even fatal septic transfusion reaction as more bacteria or bacterial products are infused. For this reason, a new blood component unit should be used if transfusion is still needed after the patient's condition has been stabilized. Hemolysis of either donor or recipient red cells usually is not significant because of the small amount of red cells and plasma in platelet preparations. The transfusion should generally not be restarted for at least 30 minutes as a precaution to allow other possible signs or symptoms of a serious reaction to develop. High transfusion-related fevers, such as a 2 °C increment or more, are more likely to be associated with septic reactions and should preclude restarting the transfusion. However, lesser fevers do not rule out bacterial contamination of the blood component. If the transfusion is restarted, the patient should be made as comfortable as possible with appropriate antipyretic therapy, as described earlier. The transfusion should proceed slowly and the patient observed closely for further signs of a reaction or further temperature elevation throughout the transfusion, which should be stopped if symptoms recur. Restarting transfusion of a blood component that has caused an FNHTR should not be routine.

Prevention
Premedication
Premedication with acetaminophen but not diphenhydramine should be considered for patients with a history of FNHTR. Patients who have no history of FNHTR do not need premedication. Despite a number of studies showing no benefit to premedication in preventing transfusion reactions, the practice remains common in many institutions.[31] A prospective, randomized, double-blind controlled trial of acetaminophen and diphenhydramine pretransfusion medication versus placebo showed that pretransfusion medication may decrease the risk of FNHTR to leukoreduced blood products.[32] Premedication with the glucocorticoid hydrocortisone sodium succinate (adults, 100 mg intravenously) may be useful in the care of reaction prone patients when an antipyretic agent alone is ineffective. Glucocorticoids have anti-inflammatory effects that may help prevent or reduce the severity of FNHTRs. For example, they inhibit the enzyme phospholipase A_2, thereby blocking production of arachidonic acid and its metabolites such as PGE2, a key mediator of fever. Glucocorticoids also inhibit synthesis of pyrogenic cytokines, such as IL1 and IL6. A variety of glucocorticoids other than hydrocortisone are available. However, hydrocortisone has the advantage of being a short-acting glucocorticoid (biologic half-life, 8 to 12 hours), and it induces a shorter period of immunosuppression than do many other glucocorticoid preparations. Because glucocorticoids generally act through changes in gene expression, hydrocortisone should be administered at least 4 to 6 hours before transfusion so that its anti-inflammatory action has time to take effect.

Rate of infusion
Slowing the speed of infusion of a blood component can possibly prevent or decrease the severity of FNHTR. The rate of increase in body temperature in FNHTR caused by leukocyte alloimmunization appears to be directly related to the rate of infusion of leukocytes in the blood components.[17] A slower rate of infusion is of theoretic advantage in decreasing the severity of reactions caused by bacterial contamination or storage-generated cytokines. Slower infusion avoids a sudden bolus of bacterial toxins or cytokines that may provoke an immediate and possibly massive inflammatory response.

Leukocyte reduction
The prophylactic transfusion of leukocyte-reduced components in the treatment of patients receiving repeated transfusions is effective in avoiding alloimmunization to leukocytes, which is one of the major causes of FNHTR. Leukocyte-reduced blood components ideally should be transfused to such patients beginning with the first transfusion. Leukocyte reduction is effective in the care of patients already alloimmunized to leukocytes, because FNHTRs in these patients are directly related to the number and rate of infusion of passenger leukocytes. The threshold number of white cells associated with the development of an FNHTR generally ranges from 0.25×10^9 to 2.5×10^9.[17] The removal of approximately 90% of leukocytes (10^{10}), which usually leaves less than 5×10^8 white cells

per RBC unit, is sufficient to prevent most FNHTRs.[16,33] For that reason, leukocyte reduction for the purpose of preventing FNHTRs often is defined as decreasing the passenger leukocytes to less than 5×10^6 per transfusion. Leukocyte reduction of blood components can be performed either at the time of component preparation (prestorage leukocyte reduction) or immediately before transfusion (poststorage leukocyte reduction). Poststorage leukocyte reduction by means of filtration can be performed in the blood bank before distribution of the component for transfusion or during administration of blood components. The latter often is called *bedside leukocyte reduction*.

Leukocyte-reduced RBC units have in the past been prepared by various poststorage techniques, including simple centrifugation with buffy coat removal, saline washing, and deglycerolization of frozen RBCs.[34–35] Saline-washed and frozen deglycerolized RBCs are rendered leukocyte reduced because approximately 1 to 2 $\log_{10}$ leukocytes are removed by repeated centrifugation and washing steps on automated cell washers. Filtration of RBCs units through microaggregate filters designed to remove microaggregate debris more than 40 microns in diameter after an extra centrifugation step or after centrifugation and cooling (spin, cool, filter) also has been shown to reduce leukocytes in RBC units sufficiently to reduce the incidence of FNHTRs.[36–39]

High-efficiency leukocyte reduction filters for red cells and platelets have been developed that are capable of removing both microaggregate debris and nonaggregated leukocytes.[40] These leukocyte reduction filters can remove 3 or more log (99.9% or more) leukocytes, thereby decreasing the leukocyte content to approximately 1×10^6/unit or less. Despite their efficacy in leukocyte reduction, the use of bedside leukocyte reduction filters has had variable and sometimes disappointing results in reducing the incidence of FNHTRs to platelet concentrates.[41] This may be the result of causes of FNHTR other than leukocyte antibodies in the transfusion recipient. For example, storage-generated, extracellular cytokines in the component bag that either are not removed or are inadequately removed by means of poststorage filtration are now believed to mediate some reactions. As a result, the practice of prestorage leukocyte reduction is increasingly replacing poststorage leukocyte reduction. Prestorage leukocyte reduction not only removes leukocytes but also removes leukocytes before they have a chance to release cytokines that can accumulate extracellularly in blood component bags during storage. Prestorage leukocyte reduction has also yielded conflicting results on the efficacy of leukocyte reduction to mitigate FNHTRs.[42]

Prestorage leukocyte reduction of platelet concentrates or RBC units is achieved by use of blood component containers with in-line leukocyte reduction filters in a closed system between the primary collection bag and satellite containers. Prestorage leukocyte-reduced platelets also can be prepared with some automated apheresis instruments equipped with centrifugation chambers designed to minimize leukocyte collection (so-called *process leukocyte reduction*). Because some data indicate that only approximately 15% of patients who experience an FNHTR will have a similar reaction to the next transfusion, some blood banks provide a leukocyte-reduced component (either prestorage or bedside leukocyte reduced) only when a patient has had two or more documented febrile reactions.[43] This practice is cost-effective but has the disadvantage of subjecting some patients to two uncomfortable reactions before a preventive measure is taken. Prestorage leukocyte reduction by means of filtration is a more efficient and cost-effective way to eliminate extracellular leukocyte-derived cytokines while reducing passenger leukocytes. Moreover, in evaluations of plasma removal from platelet concentrates to reduce the risk of FNHTR, this technique still is associated with FNHTR in a relatively large percentage of recipients. Neither leukocyte reduction nor poststorage plasma removal has been effective in eliminating all FNHTRs to platelet transfusions.

Allergic reactions

Description

An allergic reaction can be classified as an immediate hypersensitivity response consisting of transient localized or generalized urticaria, erythema, and pruritus. More serious allergic reactions can be complicated by hypotension and angioedema of the face and larynx. Allergic reactions can be categorized as those that have only cutaneous manifestations and usually are mild, resolving soon after administration of antihistamines. If other organ systems—cardiovascular, respiratory, or gastrointestinal—are involved beyond mild hypotension, particularly if the reaction is serious enough to necessitate treatment beyond antihistamines, the reaction would be considered *anaphylactic* or *anaphylactoid* (see the "Anaphylactic and Anaphylactoid Reactions" section). Allergic and anaphylactic reactions, however, are part of a continuum. Allergic reactions occur during or soon after transfusion of plasma-containing blood components. Atopic individuals—those with other known allergies—appear at greater risk of allergic reactions. A large retrospective review of reported transfusion reactions noted that 17% of all reactions in a nine-year period were allergic and 1% of reactions were very severe.[44] Other papers report allergic reaction rates of approximately 0.19% for red cells and 0.53% for platelet transfusions.[42,45]

Etiology

Allergic reactions are mediated by recipient immunoglobulin E (IgE) or non-IgE antibodies to proteins or other allergenic soluble substances in the donor plasma. The result of the hypersensitivity reaction is secretion of histamine from mast cells and basophils, which mediates cutaneous reactions by increasing vascular permeability.

Although the source of histamine in allergic reactions is believed in many cases to be the transfusion recipient's mast cells and basophils, it has been hypothesized that histamine generated by leukocytes in stored cellular blood components may play a role. Several studies have shown that histamine accumulates in the plasma portion of platelet concentrates and RBC units with increasing storage time. However, histamine is not synthesized during storage but rather it leaks into the extracelluar plasma or may be due to calcium ions (Ca^2+) influx-inducing activity toward mast cell in patients prior to transfusion.[46–48] These data are consistent with the observation that allergic transfusion reactions also are more common with increasing storage time of blood components.[49] Several of the chemokines that accumulate in the plasma portion of platelet concentrates during blood bank storage, such as IL8, RANTES, and MIP1α, can recruit and activate basophils and stimulate histamine release. Therefore, it is theoretically possible that the infusion of storage generated donor cytokines during transfusion may contribute to the onset of allergic reactions among transfusion recipients. Consistent with this hypothesis, the biologic activity of RANTES is present at higher levels in apheresis platelets that cause allergic reactions.[48] In a recent study that measures the concentration of allergic agonists such as C5a, brain-derived neurotrophic factor (BDNF), and CCL5 (RANTES) in apheresis platelets showed that high levels of these agonists were associated with allergic transfusion reactions.[49] Therefore levels of acute inflammatory mediators and growth or chemotactic factors of basophils and mast cells do not appear to be associated with allergic transfusions reactions according to the study. However, the study only evaluated 20 platelet transfusions with associated allergic transfusion reactions.[49]

Allergic (and anaphylactic) reactions have been reported after infusion of antibodies in donor plasma, such as penicillin antibody infused into recipients receiving penicillin or related antibiotics, and after infusion of drugs in donor plasma, such as penicillin infused into recipients already sensitized to penicillin.

Diagnosis

Urticaria is readily diagnosed clinically by the presence of the cutaneous wheal-and-flare reaction. Because allergic symptoms usually are mild and are not characteristic of hemolytic transfusion reactions, serologic blood bank investigations to rule out hemolysis usually are unrevealing. Isolated, mild urticarial reactions not accompanied by other signs and symptoms necessitate minimal diagnostic evaluation. If the reaction is severe, has atypical manifestations, or is accompanied by fever (uncharacteristic of allergic reactions), a more elaborate laboratory evaluation to rule out a hemolytic or septic transfusion reaction is indicated. In the diagnosis of an allergic reaction as transfusion related, it is important to rule out, if possible, urticarial drug reactions that may be circumstantially attributed to transfusions. Careful attention to the timing of onset of urticaria relative to the transfusion may help avoid this confusion. Administration of medications should generally be discouraged in the peritransfusion period to avoid such confusion.

Even mild allergic reactions should be reported to the blood bank. Monitoring allergic reactions and correlating reactions with any newly implemented changes in blood component collection, processing, storage, or filtration are important in detecting new and unexpected causes of reactions. In the care of patients with repeated allergic reactions, notification of the blood bank allows the blood bank medical director to consult on measures to manage or prevent such reactions in the future.

Treatment

The patient can be treated with a first-generation, H_1-blocking antihistamine (adults, 25 to 50 mg diphenhydramine intravenously or orally). If the sedating side effects of first-generation antihistamines must be avoided, newer, less sedating antihistamines are available for oral administration (adults, cetirizine 10 mg orally, loratadine 10 mg orally, or fexofenadine 60 mg orally); however, parenteral antihistamines are preferred in the management of acute reactions because of their more rapid bioavailability. An H_2 blocker, such as cimetidine (adults, 300 mg intravenously) or ranitidine (adults, 50 mg intravenously), may be added to the H_1 blocker to speed resolution of the reaction. Combining H_1 and H_2 antagonists has given better results in treating patients with allergic reactions in nontransfusion settings than has use of an H_1 antagonist alone.[51–52] For reactions characterized by only localized urticaria, such as a few hives, the transfusion can be temporarily discontinued while an antihistamine is administered. The transfusion can be resumed in approximately 30 minutes if the urticaria has cleared and if no further symptoms occur. For patients with generalized urticaria or a more serious allergic reaction accompanied by facial or laryngeal edema or hypotension, the transfusion should be discontinued and the infusion set with any untransfused blood returned to the blood bank. If laryngeal edema causes breathing difficulties or if hypotension is severe, epinephrine (adult dose, 0.2 to 0.5 mL of 1:1000 solution [0.2 to 0.5 mg] subcutaneously) can be administered.

Prevention

Transfusion recipients often are given routine premedication with an antihistamine such as diphenhydramine in an effort to prevent or reduce the severity of allergic transfusion reactions, even when they have had no previous reactions. The value of this approach is uncertain, because few patients have allergic reactions. At least two randomized double-blind placebo-controlled studies of premedication using diphenhydramine and acetaminophen have failed to show a benefit of premedication to reduce reactions.[53–54] When premedication is restricted to patients who have had two or more previous allergic reactions, overall reaction rates do not increase. Accordingly, premedication with an antihistamine should probably be reserved for recipients who have had a previous allergic reaction. For patients with repeated reactions not eliminated by premedication with an H$_1$ blocker alone, a combination of H$_1$ and H$_2$ blockers has been shown more effective.[51–52]

Should premedication not prevent repeated allergic transfusion reactions, another option is to reduce the plasma content of transfused blood components. This can be achieved in RBC and platelet preparations with automated saline "washing."[55–56] However, washing or plasma removal steps generally should be reserved for patients with two or more serious allergic reactions (e.g., those that include angioedema or hypotension) that are not prevented with premedication with both H$_1$ and H$_2$ blockers, because cell washing is time-consuming and can delay transfusion. Patients with two or more severe allergic reactions can undergo testing for IgA deficiency to rule out a relative deficiency of IgA, because this has been reported to cause both a severe allergic and anaphylactic reactions.[57]

Anaphylactic and anaphylactoid reactions

Description

Anaphylactic reactions are serious and potentially life-threatening immediate hypersensitivity reactions to allergens in the plasma of transfused blood components.[58] These reactions can have a rapid onset beginning as early as seconds to minutes after the start of the transfusion, and can occur with small transfused volumes. Anaphylactic reactions are differentiated from other allergic (urticarial) transfusion reactions by their systemic nature and severity. These reactions generally affect multiple organ systems, as evidenced by cutaneous, respiratory, cardiovascular, and gastrointestinal effects. The symptom complex often includes the rapid onset of laryngeal edema and bronchospasm with stridor, wheezing, coughing, and respiratory distress. Other symptoms include generalized urticaria, erythema, tachycardia, hypotension, nausea, vomiting, diarrhea, and cramping abdominal or pelvic pain. Severe reactions can proceed rapidly to shock, syncope, respiratory failure, and death. Fatal anaphylactic reactions are less common than are fatal hemolytic or septic reactions.

Etiology

Anaphylactic reactions occur when an allergen present in plasma is transfused to a patient who through previous sensitization has an IgE directed against that allergen.[59] Immunoglobulin E is bound by

means of Fc receptors to mast cells and basophils. The binding of allergen to cell-bound IgE results in cross-linking of IgE and Fc receptors. This cross-linking activates the mast cells and basophils to secrete preformed mediators, such as histamine, as well as newly synthesized mediators, such as leukotrienes, prostaglandins, cytokines, and platelet-activating factor (PAF) (Figure 58.2).[60] PAF induces downstream production of nitric oxide (NO) through inducible and possibly constitutively expressed NO synthase.[61] As a potent vasodilator, NO is believed to be the principal compound causing hypotensive and cardiovascular collapse during anaphylaxis, although the exact mechanism remains under debate.

Anaphylactoid reactions are acute hypersensitivity reactions that are clinically identical to anaphylaxis but are not mediated by IgE antibodies or IgE involvement cannot be established. For example, immune complexes involving antibodies other than IgE may result in complement fixation and generation of the anaphylatoxins C3a, C4a, and C5a, which activate basophils and mast cells. Some cytokines secreted by monocytes as part of the inflammatory

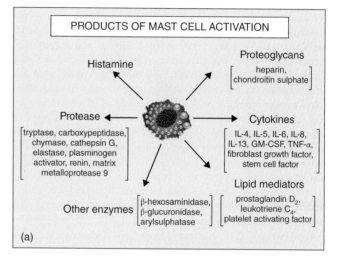

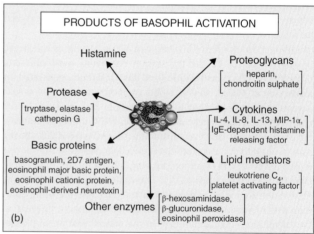

Figure 58.2 (A) Mast cell with its activation products. (B) Basophil with its activation products. Note that currently only two products of mast cell activation (histamine and total tryptase) and one product of basophil activation (histamine) can be measured in clinical laboratories as markers of acute anaphylaxis events. Used with permission from Simons et al. (2007).[60] IL, interleukin; GM-CSF, granulocyte macrophage colony-stimulating factor; TNFα, tumor necrosis factor alpha; MIP, macrophage inflammatory protein.

cascade initiated by non-IgE immune complex formation also can directly activate basophils and mast cells and initiate anaphylactoid reactions. Moreover, IgG4 subclass antibodies can bind to Fc receptors of mast cells and basophils and, in a manner analogous to that of IgE, mediate cellular activation and degranulation after binding of allergen. The term *anaphylactoid* is sometimes used to describe mild or clinically atypical anaphylactic reactions. However, *anaphylactoid* is better used to differentiate the mechanism of the reaction, not its clinical severity or presentation.

The best documented anaphylactoid reactions have resulted from the transfusion of donor plasma containing IgA to IgA deficient recipients who have produced a class-specific IgG anti-IgA antibody that reacts with all IgA subclasses. Less commonly, patients with normal total IgA levels have a subclass-specific IgA deficiency and may make an anti-IgA of restricted specificity. Although IgA deficiency is relatively common (approximately one case among 700 persons), anaphylactoid reactions occur only among some IgA-deficient transfusion recipients, because not all make anti-IgA. Anaphylactic or anaphylactoid reactions have been documented among patients with deficiencies of other plasma proteins, such as complement, von Willebrand factor, and haptoglobin.[62–63] In an analogous manner, these patients produce an antibody to the missing factor that reacts with transfused, plasma-containing blood components. Angiotensin-converting enzyme (ACE) inhibitors are drugs commonly prescribed to treat hypertension. Patients taken ACE inhibitors have been reported to have anaphylactoid reactions during online extracorporeal apheresis such as plasma exchange.[64] In most anaphylactic or anaphylactoid reactions, however, the allergen is never identified, nor is evidence obtained to differentiate anaphylactic from anaphylactoid mechanisms.

Diagnosis

Anaphylactic and anaphylactoid reactions are diagnosed from clinical signs and symptoms.[65] The cutaneous signs and symptoms and the often rapid onset of the reaction help differentiate anaphylactic reactions from acute hemolytic and septic transfusion reactions. Serum β-tryptase levels may be measured to confirm an anaphylactic reaction, because it is a marker for mast cell degranulation. However, no laboratory measurement is available in time to meaningfully affect recognition and management of an anaphylactic reaction.

Recipient IgA levels should be measured in a pretransfusion blood specimen to determine if the recipient is IgA deficient. Although the results of tests for IgA deficiency do not affect diagnosis or management of the reaction at hand, it is important for avoiding future reactions.[58] Testing should be performed on a specimen drawn before transfusion, because IgA deficiency can be masked by any IgA provided by the transfusion. Recipient anti-IgA also can be measured, especially for rare cases in which the anti-IgA is subtype-specific and total IgA levels are within the reference range. Although IgA is the most commonly known allergen in anaphylactoid reactions, in most anaphylactic and anaphylactoid reactions, the offending allergen is not IgA and is never identified.

Treatment

Anaphylactic and anaphylactoid reactions are managed identically.[65] Severe reactions are true medical emergencies and should be managed by experienced critical care staff, if possible. The patient should be placed in an intensive care unit as soon as it is practical without jeopardizing emergency care. Once anaphylaxis is evident clinically, 1:1000 epinephrine solution (1 mg/mL) should be administered subcutaneously in a dose of 0.2 to 0.5 mL for adults (0.01 mL/kg of body weight for children). The dose may be repeated every 15 to 30 minutes as needed. Intravenous crystalloid or colloid solution should be administered as needed to support the patient's blood pressure. For example, 500 mL to 1 L of normal saline solution can be administered in the first 15 to 30 minutes. Further infusion should be titrated to blood pressure. If the systolic blood pressure is less than 60 mm Hg, intravenous epinephrine in a dose of 1 to 5 mL of a 1:10,000 solution (0.1 mg/mL) for adults and 0.1 mL/kg for children, is administered over 2 to 5 minutes by means of intravenous push. An epinephrine drip (1 to 4 µg/minute) may be started, and administration of other pressors, such as dopamine, can be considered. Blood pressure, pulse, and urine output should be monitored. It may be necessary to monitor the effectiveness of fluid replacement and pressor infusion through measurement of central venous pressure.

Respiratory distress is managed with supplemental oxygen. The patient's upper airway may have to be secured with endotracheal intubation if obstruction from laryngeal edema is imminent. Stridor is a sign of laryngeal edema. Endotracheal intubation and mechanical assistance with ventilation are indicated if the $PaCO_2$ increases to more than 65 mm Hg. When intubation is difficult or impossible because of laryngeal obstruction, cricothyrotomy or tracheostomy is an option. Wheezing caused by obstruction of small bronchi and bronchioles by increased mucus production and smooth muscle contraction can be managed with nebulized albuterol or metaproterenol and intravenous aminophylline.

Urticaria, angioedema, or gastrointestinal distress is managed with an antihistamine (adults, 50 mg diphenhydramine intravenously; children, 1 to 2 mg/kg intravenously). H_2-blocking antihistamines may be added as an adjunct to H_1 blockers. Glucocorticoids, such as hydrocortisone, 200 mg given intravenously every six hours, are also administered because they reduce late-phase inflammatory responses. Glucocorticoids, however, are not expected to be of benefit in the initial management of anaphylaxis because of their delayed onset of action.

Prevention

Patients with IgA deficiency who have already had an anaphylactic reaction or who are known to have anti-IgA should receive transfusion of RBC and platelet preparations that have been saline-washed with an automated cell washer.[54,57] If plasma transfusion is necessary, only IgA-deficient donors should be used. Patients who have anaphylactic reactions to any other known plasma allergen also should be treated with transfusion of saline-washed RBCs or platelet preparations. Because anaphylactic reactions can be induced by very small amounts of allergen, washing must be extensive. Washing and saline replacement by means of automated cell washers have been shown generally successful in removing IgA sufficiently to prevent recurrences of anaphylactoid reactions.

If a patient has had one anaphylactic reaction of unknown causation, the next transfusion need not necessarily be performed with washed RBCs or platelets, because the reaction might have been donor specific. The next transfusion may be administered slowly with vigilance after premedication with both H_1 and H_2 blockers and a glucocorticoid. The patient care team should be prepared to respond to an anaphylactic reaction. The patient ideally should be in a critical care unit with monitoring at the time of transfusion and with a critical care physician and nurses in attendance. Some blood banks with the capability of automated cell washing, nevertheless, may choose to provide saline-washed

RBCs and platelet concentrates for future transfusions after a single anaphylactic reaction as a precautionary measure, particularly if the patient is not expected to receive many more transfusions.

Complications of massive and rapid transfusion

Massive transfusion is defined as the replacement of one blood volume within a 24-hour period. For practical purposes for adults of average size, this is roughly equivalent to 10 units of RBCs with any accompanying crystalloid, colloid, platelet, or plasma infusions. An infusion of greater than four units of RBCs in an hour and ongoing use anticipated could also be regarded as a massive transfusion. The possible complications include citrate toxicity, electrolyte imbalance (hyperkalemia from transfusion of older RBCs, hypocalcemia from citrate toxicity), circulatory overload, and hypothermia. Recipients of massive transfusions are at increased risk of hemolytic transfusion reactions (including ABO incompatibility), FNHTR, and allergic reactions because of the number of units they receive. Reactions can be more severe with massive transfusion because rapid infusion means the implicated unit often has been completely administered before the onset of symptoms. The large number of units transfused in a short time complicates the investigation of transfusion reactions, because each transfused component must be investigated.

The lethal triad of severe trauma consists of hypothermia, acidosis, and coagulopathy. "Damage control" resuscitation methods have been developed to directly address the coagulopathy of trauma. The coagulopathy of trauma develops because of severe injury and is already present when a patient presents for emergency medical care. Trauma coagulopathy is not caused by the resuscitation efforts of emergency medical interventions as traditionally understood.[66] Recent advances in trauma research have shown that early application of damage control resuscitation can greatly improve survival through an application of a 1:1 plasma–red cell ratio from patient presentation.[67] In well-coordinated trauma centers, massive transfusion protocols now provide six units of plasma, six units of RBCs, six whole blood–derived platelet concentrates (or one apheresis platelet) or four units of plasma, four units of RBCs, and one unit of apheresis platelets. Aggressive damage control transfusion has been associated with a number of risks including hyperkalemia. Despite these risks, retrospective studies have shown that the application of early, aggressive transfusion support improves overall survival in this severely injured population that would otherwise have very poor prognosis.

Rapid transfusion can also occur during therapeutic apheresis and red cell exchange apheresis (erythrocytapheresis). During apheresis procedures, as many as 10–20 units of fresh frozen plasma or 4–8 units of RBCs can be transfused over 1.5–2 hours. Although any acute transfusion reaction can occur during apheresis-associated transfusion, citrate toxicity in particular is a common but usually mild complication.

Citrate toxicity

Rapid blood transfusion can cause a transient decrease in the level of ionized calcium because of the calcium-chelating properties of the citrate anticoagulant in stored blood components.[68] The clinical presentation of citrate-induced symptoms is also termed *citrate toxicity*. Citrate toxicity can occur whenever large volumes of plasma that contain citrate are transfused, such as during massive transfusion, plasma exchange, or other apheresis procedures.[69–71]

Citrate infusion can induce hypocalcemia, hypomagnesemia, and other electrolyte imbalances, and these imbalances are associated with clinical symptoms. Apheresis procedures can produce a unique clinical paradox of urinary calcium excretion in the setting of hypocalcemia.[70,72] Hypocalcemia is a recognized complication of liver transplantation, in which large amounts of plasma are transfused. However, the precise mechanism of hypocalcemia is not well understood and may not be caused entirely by citrated plasma.[73,74]

Citrate ordinarily is rapidly metabolized to bicarbonate in mitochondria-rich tissue, such as liver, skeletal muscle, and kidney.[68] In the routine transfusion of blood components, patients with normal liver function usually tolerate the citrate infusion without significant complications. However, patients with liver or renal failure or parathyroid dysfunction are at greater risk of citrate toxicity when they receive rapid transfusions of plasma or plasma-containing blood components. Citrate anticoagulates blood by binding divalent cations such as calcium, thus hypocalcemia is a primary symptom. Other divalent cations such as magnesium and zinc can also be bound by citrate, but the contribution of hypomagnesemia to clinical symptoms is less pronounced.[75] During apheresis, citrate is administered as acid–citrate–dextrose formula A (ACD-A) in constant proportion to the whole blood flow rate. Healthy plateletpheresis donors receive relatively large doses of citrate, and many experience mild symptoms of the citrate effect, but the symptoms usually do not progress because of the short duration of the procedure. Donors of peripheral blood stem cells (PBSCs), however, receive smaller doses of citrate per unit of time but usually experience more severe citrate toxicity because of the longer duration of the procedure. Paresthesia caused by transient hypocalcemia is common in apheresis. It typically occurs after the initial infusion of the priming solution (if citrate is used) or later as apheresis progresses. Apheresis practitioners should be aware that peripheral paresthesia caused by hypocalcemia can be masked in patients with a preexisting neuropathy as a result of chemotherapy (vincristine) or as part of a neurologic condition.

Citrate toxicity is recognized clinically because of the signs and symptoms of hypocalcemia. It can be confirmed by measuring the plasma-ionized calcium level in the patient. Symptoms of hypocalcemia include peripheral and perioral paresthesia (Chvostek and Trousseau signs can occasionally be elucidated), muscle spasm, cramping, nausea, vomiting, cardiac arrhythmia, bradycardia, hypotension, and, if severe, tetany. An electrocardiogram (ECG) can show prolongation of the QT interval with hypocalcemia, but the relation is not linear with the ionized calcium level, and ECG findings are an unreliable guide to calcium therapy.

Mild citrate toxicity during transfusion or apheresis is managed or prevented in part by means of slowing the rate of transfusion or reinfusion. When slowing the infusion rate is impossible or ineffective and the patient has signs and symptoms of hypocalcemia, calcium supplementation is indicated. The best guide to determining a need for calcium supplementation is measurement of the patient's ionized calcium levels, if results can be obtained rapidly. Calcium replacement during apheresis should generally be given when a patient has symptoms, when the patient's clinical condition may exacerbate citrate effects, or when prolonged large-volume leukapheresis is expected to cause citrate toxicity. Infusion of calcium itself, however, is associated with development of ventricular arrhythmia and even cardiac arrest. Therefore, intravenous calcium replacement for the management or prophylaxis of apheresis-induced citrate toxicity should be administered only by experienced apheresis staff. Under no circumstances should calcium be added directly to a unit of blood, because it causes clots to form in the bag.

Citrate toxicity during apheresis is related to the citrate concentration of the reinfused blood or colloid solution, the infusion rate, the blood volume of the patient, and the total time over which the citrate is infused.[76] It is difficult to establish a definitive safe rate of citrate infusion because of the large number of variables involved. However, citrate dosages of up to 1 mg/kg/minute given during plateletpheresis usually are well tolerated. A safe rate of calcium replacement for controlling citrate toxicity during PBSC apheresis is 0.5 to 0.6 mg of calcium ion for every 1.0 mL of infused ACD-A.[77,78] These dosages have been successful for prophylaxis against citrate toxicity during large-volume leukapheresis. To avoid excessive volume during PBSC apheresis, administration of a concentrated calcium solution (calcium chloride or calcium gluconate) is appropriate. Care must be taken to coordinate the calcium infusion with whole blood flow during the apheresis procedure to avoid the potential for catheter thrombosis. Calcium administration should be halted soon after interruptions in whole blood flow.

Electrolyte disorders

Because of inhibition of sodium–potassium–adenosine triphosphatase in red cell membranes by the cold storage temperature of RBC units, extracellular potassium accumulates with increasing blood bank storage times. Extracellular potassium increases at the rate of approximately 1 mEq/day during the first three weeks of RBC storage in citrate–phosphate–dextrose–adenine-1 (CPDA-1).[79] Potassium levels in additive solution-1 (Adsol) units are markedly higher on Day 7 of storage (17 mmol/L) than on Day 0 (1.6 mmol/L). The increase is even greater by Day 42 (46 mmol/L).[80] Total extracellular volume in additive solution is less than half of that in CPDA-1 blood; this must be taken into account when the amount of transfused extracellular potassium is considered.

Hyperkalemia resulting from massive transfusion of older RBC units with an elevated amount of extracellular potassium can cause significant cardiac complications and possibly death in some patients.[81] Acidosis can contribute to hyperkalemia, and severely injured patients presenting with a potassium level greater than 4 mmol/L are at increased risk. Other patients at risk of hyperkalemic complications are neonates and those with renal failure. The diagnosis of hyperkalemia is made by means of measurement of potassium in the serum and observation of ECG changes, which include peaked T waves, prolongation of the PR interval, and ventricular arrhythmia.[82] In neonatal transfusions, hyperkalemia can be avoided by use of fresh RBC units (less than seven days old) or older units that have been saline-washed to remove the extracellular fraction containing the potassium.[83,84] However, transfusion of older RBC units does not place neonates at risk of hyperkalemia if small-volume transfusions (10 to 15 mL/kg) are given slowly.[85]

Hypokalemia can also develop during massive transfusion or large-volume apheresis.[70,86]

As the anticoagulant citrate in blood components is metabolized to bicarbonate, the blood can become alkalotic, producing hypokalemia. The degree of hypokalemia may be sufficient to necessitate infusion of potassium if symptoms develop. However, the use of newer RBC additive solutions such as Adsol has helped to decrease the effect of hypokalemia. RBC units are plasma-reduced before the addition of additive solution, which itself contains no additional citrate. Therefore, most of the citrated plasma is removed from additive solution RBC units during production. Animal studies have shown fewer physiologic aberrations during massive transfusion

with Adsol RBCs than with CPDA-1 units.[87] The complications of hypokalemia, therefore, are more likely when large numbers of units of plasma rather than RBC units are transfused. Posttransfusion hypokalemia can also be due to potassium uptake by transfused old RBCs.

Hypothermia

Hypothermia, defined as a core body temperature of less than 35 °C, may be caused by rapid infusion of large quantities of cold (1 °C to 10 °C) blood or RBC units. Hypothermia during massive transfusion has been shown to induce cardiac arrhythmia and arrest.[88] Hypothermia is a known independent risk factor for early coagulopathy, multiple organ failure (MOF) development, and mortality.[89] Even smaller quantities of cold blood can be cardiotoxic if transfused into central venous lines, because the newly infused cold blood can reach the heart before sufficient warming has occurred. Data published in the early 1960s showed that massive transfusion at a rate of approximately one unit every 5–10 minutes was sufficient to lower the temperature of an esophageal probe behind the right atrium to nearly 30 °C.[88] The resulting decrease in sinoatrial node temperature was associated with the development of ventricular fibrillation.

For most routine transfusions given at a standard rate of administration, blood does not have to be warmed.[90] The patient may experience minor chills, but this is easily remedied by warming the patient, as with extra blankets. Transfusion of cold RBC units through central venous lines, however, should be avoided. Indications for warming blood include rapid transfusion, which are generally considered to be more than 50 mL/kg/hour for an adult and more than 15 mL/kg per hour for a child, and exchange transfusion for infants. Because blood warming during certain massive transfusions sometimes delays infusion and impedes resuscitation, it is not always practical. Warming blood for transfusion in the treatment of patients with cold agglutinin disease has a theoretic basis but is debatable because supportive outcome data are lacking.

If blood has to be warmed, an approved warming device should be used and the temperature must be kept below a point where hemolysis occurs.[90] Care must be taken when warming up blood because warming to a temperature above 42 C may cause hemolysis.[91] Infusion of thermally injured cells can induce disseminated intravascular coagulation and shock. Heating blood with a device other than an approved blood warming device, such as a commercial microwave oven, is unacceptable. Blood that has been warmed but not used should not be reissued for another patient because of the increased risk of bacterial proliferation at warmer temperatures.

The maximum flow rate that can be achieved with commercially available blood warmers is 850 mL/minute; however, most can provide a rate of only 150 mL/minute. Most recent research has focused on comparisons between commercial warming devices and the comparison studies usually evaluate warming capability in the rapid transfusion setting.[92] Most of the available federally approved blood warming devices safely warm blood and other intravenous fluids across a range of flow rates. However, although little recent data exist correlating the clinical benefits of warming blood, many emergency centers and trauma services use such devices routinely without incident.

An alternative to using mechanical blood warmers that circumvents such flow limitations is rapid admixture with warm or hot saline solution immediately before transfusion.[90,93] This technique immediately warms a unit of RBCs, yet does not cause significant hemolysis. However, it necessitates that warmed saline solution be available at all times in trauma care and requires attention to technique to avoid the direct infusion of hot saline solution into the patient.

Reactions attributed to microaggregate debris

Microaggregate debris ranges in diameter from 20 to 120 microns and consists of nonviable platelets, white cells, and strands of fibrin that form in blood during storage.[94,95] Because of their size, microaggregates are not removed from transfused blood with the standard 170- to 260-micron screen filters. A variety of adverse events have been attributed to the presence of microaggregate debris after large-volume and massive transfusion.

Studies in the 1960s showed that patients undergoing open heart surgery with cardiopulmonary bypass experienced postperfusion syndrome during the postoperative period. This symptom complex consisted of cerebral and renal dysfunction attributed in part to occlusion of end-organ capillaries with microaggregate debris. Cotton wool (Swank) microaggregate blood filters capable of retaining particles or debris with a size of 40 microns or more appeared to eliminate many of these reactions. During the Vietnam War, some soldiers who underwent massive transfusion experienced respiratory distress syndrome (shock lung). At autopsy, the cause was presumed to be the material found in soldiers' lungs that was positive on a periodic acid–Schiff (PAS) test. Because microaggregate debris stains PAS-positive, this was taken at the time as evidence of the pathologic nature of microaggregate debris.

During the 1970s and 1980s, studies were undertaken to determine whether removal of microaggregate debris from blood was clinically significant.[94] Several studies showed that microaggregate filtration of up to 6 units of blood during either hip or cardiac surgery provided no benefit. Collins et al.[96] concluded that the underlying clinical condition rather than the infusion of the microaggregate debris in blood led to the development of the respiratory distress syndrome reported earlier among patients undergoing massive transfusions. Microaggregate blood filters today are used mostly in conjunction with cardiopulmonary bypass pumps and reinfusion of shed autologous blood collected during or after surgery. With the widespread adoption of leukocyte reduction filtration, routine leukocyte-reduced red cell transfusions are no longer complicated by microaggregate debris because these filters can remove not only leukocytes, but also the larger microaggregate particles. Current studies are investigating the utility of washing stored blood to remove microaggregate debris that accumulates during storage.[97]

Circulatory overload

Hypervolemia, termed TACO, is a possible consequence of transfusion in the care of patients with cardiac insufficiency, renal impairment, or already expanded blood volumes, such as patients with chronic anemia. Moreover, patients with restricted blood volumes (e.g., infants and small children) are at risk of TACO if transfused blood is not reduced to an amount proportional to body mass and intravascular blood volume. The reported incidence of TACO varies widely depending on the method of data collection used. The risk of TACO increases with rapid infusion. The 2011 US Food and Drug Administration report on transfusion-related mortality indicated that TACO was the second most commonly reported cause of death next to TRALI, accounting for an average of 15% of reported deaths between 2007 and 2011.[98]

Circulatory overload increases central venous pressure, causes congestion of the pulmonary vasculature, and decreases lung compliance, manifesting as dyspnea, tachycardia, acute hypertension, and in the extreme, pulmonary edema and left- or right-sided heart failure. Other signs and symptoms of circulatory overload include tachypnea, dry cough, chest or throat tightness, jugular venous distention, and pulmonary rales. Laboratory measurements of circulatory overload include PaO_2, atrial natriuretic peptide and B-type natriuretic peptide (BNP).[99,100] B-type natriuretic peptide (BNP), and N-terminal pro-BNP (NT-pro-BNP) are cardiac neurohormones specifically secreted from the ventricles in response to volume expansion and pressure overload.[101] BNP has a reported 81% sensitivity for detecting circulatory overload in the appropriate clinical setting. However, BNP and NT-pro-BNP testing did not reliably distinguish TACO from TRALI and possible TRALI in a cohort of transfused critically ill patients.[102] Diagnosing TACO can be difficult and confounded by other concomitant pathology. There is no accepted clinical definition of TACO and the symptoms of TACO can overlap significantly with other transfusion reactions such as TRALI (Table 58.1).[103,104] Some rapid methods of differentiating the overlapping symptoms include blood pressure, response to diuretic therapy, white cell count, and heart auscultation for an S3 (third heart sound).

If symptoms of overload appear, the transfusion should be stopped, and intravascular volume reduction through diuresis should be instituted as needed (e.g., administration of 40 mg furosemide intravenously). The patient should be placed in an upright (reverse Trendelenburg) position, if possible, with supplemental oxygen as necessary.

Rapid transfusion of any blood component into a patient who is not actively hemorrhaging produces no benefit and can cause harm.

Table 58.1 Features in TRALI and TACO

Feature	TRALI	TACO
Body temperature	Fever can be present	Unchanged
Blood pressure	Hypotension	Hypertension
Respiratory symptoms	Acute dyspnea	Acute dyspnea
Neck veins	Unchanged	Can be distended
Auscultation	Rales	Rales, S3 may be present
Chest radiograph	Diffuse, bilateral infiltrates	Diffuse, bilateral infiltrates
Ejection fraction	Normal, decreased	Decreased
PA occlusion pressure	18 mmHg or less	Greater than 18 mmHg
Pulmonary edema fluid	Exudate	Transudate
Fluid balance	Positive, even, negative	Positive
Response to diuretic	Minimal	Significant
White count	Transient leukopenia	Unchanged
BNP	<200 pg/mL	>1200 pg/mL
Leukocyte antibodies	Donor leukocyte antibodies present, crossmatch incompatibility between donor and recipient	Donor leukocyte antibodies may or may not be present, positive results can suggest TRALI even with true TACO cases

The typical patterns that would be expected for cases of transfusion-related acute lung injury (TRALI) or transfusion-associated circulatory overload (TACO) are represented. A given case of TRALI or TACO may lack some of the typical features. Also, a case of TRALI may have some features suggesting TACO or vice versa, and TRALI and TACO can be present together. The best strategy is to develop a full clinical profile of the case using the feature list above, and determine which diagnosis is most supported. BNP, brain natriuretic peptide; PA, pulmonary artery.

As a general guide, infusion should be at a rate not to exceed 2 to 4 mL/kg/hour, and the rate should be lower (~1 mL/kg/hour) for patients at high risk of circulatory overload.[105] In neonates, a slower blood infusion rate increases the hematocrit and decreases cardiac demand without affecting pulmonary artery pressure. More rapid infusion rates are associated with decreased lung compliance and increased pulmonary airflow resistance.[106,107]

For patients with volume overload caused by medical reasons existing before transfusion, furosemide can be given prophylactically, and transfusion should proceed slowly. The rate of transfusion can be even further slowed, if necessary, by dividing a unit of RBCs or another component into smaller aliquots and transfusing a portion at a time over as much as four hours, the maximum allowable time a blood component should be kept outside blood-bank-monitored storage. For RBCs and thawed plasma, the unused portion can be stored in the blood bank at 1 °C to 6 °C for up to 24 hours while the initial aliquot is administered. Platelet aliquots can be sampled from a single apheresis platelet unit, and with this practice, donor exposures can be minimized. It is important that transfusion of all or part of a blood component be completed within four hours and that any unused portion be stored under regulated blood bank conditions because of concerns about increased risk of bacterial contamination during improper storage. RBC units, apheresis platelets, and whole blood–derived platelet pools can be further concentrated by means of centrifugation and plasma removal, if other measures to prevent volume overload are inadequate.

Toxic reactions resulting from blood manufacture or processing

Hypotensive reactions

Hypotension may accompany various transfusion reactions including hemolytic and allergic reactions, septicemia, and TRALI, but isolated hypotension as a primary manifestation has not been considered a unique type of transfusion reaction. In the past several years, there have been several reports of transfusion reactions characterized primarily by hypotension, and it now appears that such reactions do require a separate category of transfusion reactions.[108] Hypotension has been reported among patients receiving bedside, leukocyte-reduced platelets who are also medicated with ACE inhibitors.[109] These reactions appear to be caused by generation of bradykinin in transfused blood just as it is being passed through negatively charged leukocyte reduction filters. The mechanism is believed to involve the formation of activated factor XIIa when factor XII, a contact factor, is exposed to the negatively charged filter surface. The filter surface can mimic exposed, negatively charged subendothelium, which is the natural activating stimulus for the contact factors of the intrinsic coagulation pathway after blood vessel damage in vivo. Factor XIIa converts prekallikrein to kallikrein, which cleaves high-molecular-weight kininogen to form bradykinin. The biologic activity of the infused bradykinin is prolonged in transfusion recipients who are also receiving ACE inhibitors (e.g., captopril and enalapril), which inhibit kininase II, the enzyme that breaks down bradykinin. The combination of bradykinin generation just as the blood is being infused with inhibition of the transfusion recipient's ability to break down bradykinin produces prolonged bradykinin activity conducive to hypotensive reactions.

These reactions are less likely with use of prestorage leukocyte-reduced blood components, because the bradykinin is broken down rapidly in the component bag during storage before transfusion. Although hypotensive reactions have been reported more frequently with negatively charged bedside leukocyte reduction filters, they also have been rarely reported with positively charged filters. This can be explained in part by the possibility that patients taking ACE inhibitors may be more prone to hypotensive reactions in general because of their relative inability to rapidly break down bradykinin generated in vivo by any allergic mechanism. Hypotensive reactions to bedside leukocyte reduction among patients taking ACE inhibitors can be prevented by use of prestorage leukocyte-reduced blood components or by means of temporary discontinuation of ACE inhibitor treatment.

Apheresis procedures are also associated with hypotensive reactions and the literature has described hypotensive reactions in both adult and pediatric apheresis patients.[110,111] Apheresis may contribute to hypotensive reactions through several mechanisms including the potentiation of bradykinin-mediated effects by albumin and secondary to hypocalcemia.[111,112] Data suggest that calcium infusions can mitigate some atypical apheresis reactions, while withholding ACE inhibitor medications 24 to 48 hours before apheresis may also contribute to lessening reactions.

Ocular reaction to leukocyte-reduced blood components: red eye syndrome

Some patients receiving transfusions of RBCs prestorage leukocyte reduced with a specific filtration system (LeukoNet Prestorage Leukocyte Reduction Filtration System, HemaSure, Marlborough, MA) sustained bilateral conjunctival erythema (red eye syndrome).[113] The conjunctival erythema occurred within 24 hours of transfusion. Resolution occurred spontaneously within 2 to 21 days with a median duration of five days. The implicated prestorage leukocyte reduction system has been discontinued, and red eye syndrome has not been reported with other leukocyte reduction filters.[114] The red eye symptoms are hypothesized to be an allergic or toxic reaction to cellulose acetate derivatives that leached from the filter membrane.

Plasticizer toxicity

Plasticizers are chemicals used to make rigid polyvinyl chloride plastics more malleable. The traditional plasticizer for blood storage bags is di(2-ethylhexyl)phthalate (DEHP), which leaches over time from the plastic into the blood and blood components with increasing exposure. The DEHP metabolite, mono(2-ethylhexyl)phthalate (MEHP), also accumulates during storage.[115] Infusion of blood that contains DEHP results in deposition of DEHP in various tissues; the greatest accumulation is in body fat. Results of some studies with animals have suggested that DEHP is toxic and may even be carcinogenic in large quantities.[116] Other studies with animals have shown that MEHP is associated with formation of peroxisomes, indicating tissue alteration and toxicity. Although there have been no reports of transfusion-related plasticizer toxicity among humans, results of some in vitro experiments suggest that high concentrations of MEHP have a negative inotropic effect and can cause irregular contractions in isolated human myocardial cells. Some clinical data have described the production of antiplasticizer IgE in transfusion recipients and the incorporation of plasticizer into red cells during storage.[117] Despite the possible adverse effects of DEHP plasticizers, other data indicate that these substances stabilize red cell membranes and improve the morphologic features of platelets during storage.[118,119] No good evidence exists, however, of actual improvement in posttransfusion outcomes as the result of these effects.

Formulations for plastic blood bags are being developed with plasticizers other than DEHP that have a decreased capacity to leach into plasma. For example, one polyvinyl chloride–based material is made with plasticizer butyryl tri-n-hexyl citrate (BTHC). Although BTHC also leaches into blood components, it does so at a significantly slower rate than does DEHP. It also provides an antihemolytic effect similar to that of DEHP.[120] Studies have shown this citrate-based plasticizer is suitable for storage of both RBCs and platelets.[121]

Dimethyl sulfoxide toxicity during infusion of cryopreserved progenitor cells

DMSO is a versatile solvent that has been used as the principal cryopreservative for mononuclear cells since the 1950s. It is widely used as a cryopreservative for marrow and PBSCs used in human hematopoietic progenitor cell transplantation. Despite this, DMSO is not approved by the FDA as a pharmacologic agent for intravenous administration, and guidelines for intravenous administration are obscure. Toxicologic studies, however, have established the general safety of intravenous DMSO infusion.[122,123] The metabolism of DMSO yields a characteristic harmless odor, described as a malodorous garlic or sulfur-like smell. Because of the exceptional solvent properties of the compound, DMSO is distributed throughout all tissues after administration. The two metabolites of DMSO are dimethyl sulfdioxide and dimethyl sulfide (DMS). Dimethyl sulfdioxide is an odorless compound excreted by the kidney, and DMS is excreted through the lungs and through other tissues and contributes to the characteristic odor.

The clinical toxicity of DMSO in marrow transplantation has been studied. Anaphylactoid symptoms attributable to the release of histamine and other mediators are common. Other toxic clinical signs and symptoms include hemolysis with hemoglobinuria, hyperosmolality, increased serum transaminase values, nausea, vomiting, abdominal cramping, fever, chills, tachypnea, cough, diarrhea, flushing, and headache.[124,125] Patients who have been conditioned with chemotherapy or who have smaller body mass (<70 kg), seem more likely to experience nausea and vomiting after infusion of DMSO-preserved cells. Cardiovascular toxicities include decreased heart rate and bradycardia, occasionally increased heart rate and tachycardia, ectopic heartbeat, heart block, hypotension, hypertension, and other lesser blood pressure changes.[124,126] Some studies, however, raise the question whether there is any significant cardiovascular toxicity of DMSO.[127] It is possible that some adverse effects attributed to DMSO may be caused by the cellular infusion itself.

The mechanism of the clinical toxicities associated with DMSO infusion has not been well established. Histamine receptor binding of DMSO, histamine release, direct vagal tonic effects, cold thermal vagal responses, and renal failure secondary to hemolysis explain many of the symptoms observed during cryopreserved cellular infusion.[124,128] Increases in thrombin-antithrombin complex, β-thromboglobulin, platelet factor 4, and von Willebrand factor caused by DMSO have been described.

Several measures can be taken to prevent or reduce DMSO toxicity. Antihistamine prophylaxis is recommended routinely before any administration of DMSO. Intravenous DMSO should be given as a 10% to 40% solution to avoid local irritation. The recommended maximum daily dose of DMSO is 1 g/kg/day. Slowing an infusion containing DMSO or increasing the time between infusions of multiple aliquots greatly diminishes DMSO-related toxicity, which appears to be a dose-dependent but short-lived response. However, because DMSO is toxic to thawed mononuclear cells, hematopoietic progenitor cells can tolerate exposure to 10% DMSO for only as long as 1 hour.[129] This limits how much the infusion rate can be slowed. Antiemetics and sedatives can help to ameliorate symptoms, and cellular products can be carefully washed before infusion to remove DMSO and other substances.

Reactions in special transfusion settings

Granulocyte transfusion reactions

Granulocyte transfusions remain in use as a treatment option for neutropenic patients because of improved granulocyte collection yields after donor treatment with steroids and granulocyte colony-stimulating factor (G-CSF). Febrile nonhemolytic transfusion reactions after granulocyte transfusion are common. Severe reactions can be accompanied by pulmonary complications (e.g., TRALI, dyspnea, pulmonary infiltrates, and hypoxia), hypotension, and even cardiovascular collapse.[130] In a recent study of dexamethasone- and G-CSF-stimulated granulocyte transfusions, 37% of patients (7% of transfusions) experienced chills, 32% of patients (7% of transfusions) experienced a fever, and 11% of patients (2% of transfusions) experienced hives or itching during a course of therapy.[131] Oxygen desaturation of greater than 3% occurred in 7% of transfusions, and severe desaturation of greater than 6% occurred in three of 11 patients experiencing oxygen desaturation. In addition, granulocyte transfusions carry further risk of leukocyte alloimmunization and cytomegalovirus infection.[132]

Concurrent administration of amphotericin B and granulocytes has been linked to severe pulmonary reactions, although the association has not been confirmed and remains in doubt. In a study that examines one hundred and ninety-five series of granulocyte transfusions in 144 patients demonstrated no severe pulmonary toxicity from concomitant administration of granulocytes and amphotericin B.[133] Dyspnea as a side effect of granulocyte transfusion was equally common among patients receiving amphotericin B and those in a matched control group not receiving amphotericin B. It is safe to administer granulocyte transfusion and amphotericin B simultaneously without pulmonary toxicity.

Nevertheless, it is prudent to separate amphotericin B administration and granulocyte therapy by at least 6 hours to avoid confusion about the cause of a severe reaction, which can occur with either of these reaction-prone treatments. Because of the relatively high rate and severity of febrile, pulmonary, and allergic reactions, it is prudent to give premedication with acetaminophen and diphenhydramine to recipients of granulocyte transfusions. Hydrocortisone may be added as premedication in the treatment of patients with severe reactions who otherwise cannot tolerate granulocyte transfusion, although the immunosuppressive effects of this agent are unwelcome among patients who need granulocyte transfusions to fight serious and life-threatening infections. Granulocyte concentrates should be transfused slowly.

Autologous transfusion reactions

A variety of reactions to autologous blood occur despite the complete compatibility. In a study involving 596 hospitals, the rate of reported FNHTRs to autologous blood was 0.12% and the rate of allergic reactions was 0.01% per transfused unit.[134] Such rates are approximately fivefold to 10-fold lower than those reported for allogeneic units. The cause of autologous transfusion reactions has not been clearly established. Mechanisms in many

Table 58.2 Transfusion Reaction Summary

Type	Cause	Signs and Symptoms	Treatment	Prevention
Febrile, nonhemolytic frequency of FNHTRs before leukocyte-reduction 0.33–0.37% in (red cells), 0.45 to 2.18% in (platelets) after leukocyte reduction 0.15–0.19% (red cells), 0.11 to 0.15% (platelets)	Recipient antibodies against leukocytes or platelets antigens in donor blood components; cytokines in plasma or supernatant portion of stored components; undetected bacteria contamination of blood component	Chills, fever (>1 °C increase in body temperature); rigors in severe reactions	Stop transfusion, notify physician and blood bank, maintain IV line, monitor vital signs; physician may order acetaminophen	Premedicate with acetaminophen (or glucocorticoid for refractory cases); give leukocyte-reduced RBCs
Allergic overall frequency of 0.11%	Allergen is a soluble substance in donor plasma	Localized or generalized urticaria, erythema and pruritus; if severe, may have laryngeal or facial angioedema, and hypotension	Hold transfusion, notify physician, monitor vital signs; physician may order antihistamines or restart of transfusion if mild urticaria clears and no other symptoms in 30 minutes	Premedicate with H$_1$ blocking antihistamine; add H$_2$ blocker or glucocorticoid for refractory cases; consider washed RBCs and platelets for repeated or severe reactions
Anaphylactic or anaphylactoid	Recipient antibodies to a soluble substance in donor plasma; infusion of plasma with IgA into IgA-deficient recipient with IgG anti-IgA antibodies	Urticaria, flushing, angioedema, stridor, wheezing, tachycardia, hypotension, shock, abdominal pain, diarrhea, pelvic pain	Stop transfusion; maintain IV line; notify physician and blood bank, monitor vital signs; physician may order antihistamines, epinephrine, oxygen, IV crystalloid, or glucocorticoids	Premedicate with antihistamines and glucocorticoid; transfuse washed RBCs and platelets for recurrent reactions; use IgA deficient donors or washed RBCs and platelets for sensitized patients with IgA deficiency
Transfusion-associated circulatory overload (TACO)	Blood volume too large or infusion too fast for compromised cardiovascular system	Dyspnea, orthopnea, systolic hypertension, headache, peripheral edema, coughing, cyanosis	Slow or stop transfusion; keep IV line open; notify physician; monitor vital signs and input and output; physician may order diuretics and oxygen	Transfuse slowly; use split units; consider premedication with diuretics; carefully monitor aged, debilitated, cardiac or pediatric patients
Hypothermia	Core body temperature <35 °C caused by rapid infusion of cold blood products, such as RBCs, FFP, cryoprecipitate	Decreased body temperature, chills, cardiac arrhythmia (ventricular fibrillation)	Slow or stop transfusion; use an approved blood warmer, blankets, and other patient warming techniques (warm lavages, lamps)	Transfuse slowly, use an approved blood warmer
Citrate toxicity	Excessive infusion of citrate during apheresis procedure or massive or rapid transfusion; patients with liver failure are at increased risk	Perioral or peripheral paresthesia, tingling, buzzing, teeth chattering, bed or chair moving, cramps, nausea, vomiting, arrhythmia, bradycardia, hypotension, prolongation of QT interval, tetany	Slow or stop transfusion; slow or stop apheresis procedure; give IV calcium chloride or gluconate (for PBSC apheresis: 0.5 mg Ca^2+/1.0 mL ACD-A), or check ionized Ca^2+ and dose per results; monitor relief of symptoms; consider hypomagnesemia	More likely in pediatric and lightweight patients (<70 kg) and patients with liver dysfunction, renal failure, or less skeletal muscle; observe patients closely for any symptoms, give IV calcium (for PBSC apheresis: 0.5 mg Ca^2+/1.0 mL ACD-A).
Electrolyte disorder	Hyperkalemia: transfusion of older blood components or massive transfusion of RBCs	Hyperkalemia: cardiac arrhythmia, ECG changes—peaked T waves, prolongation of PR interval (if severe, flat or lost P wave), widened QRS, ventricular arrhythmia	Hyperkalemia: give calcium to protect against cardiac effect, alkalinize blood, D50 plus insulin, sodium polystrene sulfonate; dialysis	Hyperkalemia: give fresh products (<7 days old), or washed products
	Hypokalemia: massive or rapid transfusion of citrate and metabolic alkalosis	Hypokalemia: cardiac arrhythmia, ECG changes—ST depression, U waves	Hypokalemia: give potassium	Hypokalemia: give Adsol-preserved RBCs (not Nutricel).
Hypotensive	Bradykinin generation with use of negatively charged bedside leukocyte reduction filters in patients taking angiotensin-converting enzyme (ACE) inhibitors; apheresis procedures using albumin, especially in patient's taking ACE inhibitors; see also citrate toxicity	Hypotension; sometimes also flushing, respiratory distress, nausea, abdominal pain, and loss of consciousness	Stop transfusion, notify physician and blood bank; support blood pressure.	Avoid use of bedside leukocyte reduction filters in patients taking ACE inhibitors; use prestorage leukocyte-reduced components or discontinue ACE inhibitor before transfusion or apheresis procedure; if during apheresis, correct electrolyte disorder such as hypocalcemia
DMSO toxicity	Cryopreservative for bone marrow, PBSCs, Cord blood, donor lymphocyte infusions, or any frozen cellular component; toxicity with DMSO >1.0 g/kg/day	Flushing, nausea, vomiting, abdominal cramping, throat tightness and cough, hypotension, hypertension, arrhythmia, fever, chills, headache, hemoglobinuria, hyperosmolality, increased liver enzymes	Antihistamines; antiemetics; slow or stop the infusion; supportive care; wait between infusions for symptoms to clear	Antihistamines; washed or plasma or volume depleted cellular infusions; antiemetics

IV, intravenous; RBCs, red blood cells; FFP, fresh frozen plasma; PBSC, peripheral blood stem cell; ACD-A, acid–citrate–dextrose–adenine; D50, dextrose 50% in water; ECG, electrocardiogram; DMSO, dimethyl sulfoxide.

Table 58.3 Overlapping Signs and Symptoms of Transfusion Reactions

Sign or Symptom	Possible Reaction	Most Likely > Less Likely Blood Component*
Fever, chills, rigors	Febrile nonhemolytic	Platelets (especially septic)
	Septic Acute hemolytic TRALI	>RBCs > plasma
Urticaria, pruritus	Allergic	Plasma > platelets > RBCs
	Anaphylactic	
Dyspnea	TACO TRALI Anaphylactic	Any
Hypotension	Septic Hypotensive Acute hemolytic Anaphylactic	Platelets > plasma > RBCs

* Granulocytes would very likely cause febrile reactions and dyspnea. However, granulocytes are not listed in the table because they are infrequently transfused compared to other blood components.
RBCs, red blood cells; TRALI, transfusion-related acute lung injury; TACO, transfusion-associated circulatory overload.

cases presumably are the same as for allogeneic transfusions. For example, autologous units can be contaminated with bacteria as can allogeneic units, and contamination leads to febrile reactions or septic complications.[135] Because autologous donors are patients, not healthy volunteers, they may have various medical problems that put them at increased risk of bacteremia.

Accumulation of inflammatory mediators in blood component bags during storage, released from passenger leukocytes or platelets, may result in the infusion of pyrogenic substances. Autologous leukocytes, rather than allogeneic leukocytes, can also generate endogenous pyrogens. Allergic reactions may be provoked by histamine generation during storage of blood components or by chemicals leached from blood storage containers or filters. Moreover, autologous transfusions may contribute to volume overload and hypervolemic reactions through mechanisms identical to allogeneic transfusions.

Summary

A variety of acute, nonhemolytic, and noninfectious reactions are reported after transfusion (Table 58.2). Many of these reactions have an immune basis and represent inflammatory or allergic responses to infused cells (e.g., many FNHTRs) or plasma (e.g., some FNHTRs, allergic, and anaphylactic reactions). Although urgent transfusion can be lifesaving, it is important to recognize that a large volume of blood components given too quickly can itself have adverse chemical or physical effects, such as hypothermia, hyperkalemia, hypokalemia, hypocalcemia, and circulatory overload. Some reactions also are caused by unintended consequences of blood storage conditions or processing, such as generation of

bradykinin by the contact of blood with some filter surfaces, leaching of toxic chemicals from filters or containers, and use of the chemical DMSO during hematopoietic progenitor cell preservation. It is important that these reactions and toxicities be recognized rapidly by the patient care team and blood bank personnel so that appropriate treatment and preventive measures can be instituted quickly. Care providers who administer transfusions must recognize that some symptoms of transfusion reactions, such as fever, are nonspecific and may be early manifestations of potentially life-threatening reactions, such as hemolysis or sepsis (Table 58.3). For that reason, the guiding rule regarding most transfusion reactions is to err on the side of conservatism and stop the transfusion immediately. Transfusion of a blood component that causes a reaction before complete infusion should not be restarted, with the possible exception of mild urticarial reactions. Several strategies are available to prevent repeated reactions among patients who are reaction-prone. These include leukocyte reduction for the prevention of FNHTR, cell washing for the prevention of allergic and anaphylactic reactions and possibly some FNHTRs, and various premedication regimens.

Disclaimer

The authors have disclosed no conflicts of interest.

Key References

A full reference list for this chapter is available at: http://www.wiley.com/go/simon/transfusion

2 Wang, RR, Triulzi DJ, Qu L, et al. Effects of prestorage vs poststorage leukoreduction on the rate of febrile nonhemolytic transfusion reactions to platelets. *Am J Clin Pathol* 2012; **138** (2): 255–9.

7 Addas-Carvalho, M, Salles TS, Saad ST. The association of cytokine gene polymorphisms with febrile non-hemolytic transfusion reaction in multitransfused patients. *Transfus Med* 2006; **16** (3): 184–91.

33 Bordin JO, Heddle NM, Blajchman MA. Biologic effects of leukocytes present in transfused cellular blood products. *Blood* 1994; **84**: 1703–21.

42 King KE, Shirey RS, Thoman SK, et al. Universal leukoreduction decreases the incidence of febrile nonhemolytic transfusion reactions to RBCs. *Transfusion* 2004; **44**: 25–9.

49 Savage, WJ, Savage JH, Tobian AA, et al. Allergic agonists in apheresis platelet products are associated with allergic transfusion reactions. *Transfusion* 2012; **52** (3): 575–81.

54 Wang SE, Lara PN Jr., Lee-Ow A, et al. Acetaminophen and diphenhydramine as premedication for platelet transfusions: A prospective randomized double-blind placebo-controlled trial. *Am J Hematol* 2002; **70**: 191–4.

57 Anani, W, Triulzi D, Yazer MH, et al. Relative IgA-deficient recipients have an increased risk of severe allergic transfusion reactions. *Vox Sang* 2014; **107** (4): 389–92.

98 US Food and Drug Administration Fatalities reported to FDA following blood collection and transfusion. 2012. http://www.fda.gov/BiologicsBloodVaccines/SafetyAvailability/ReportaProblem/TransfusionDonationFatalities/ucm302847.htm

99 Fiebig EW, Wu AH, Krombach J, et al. Transfusion-related acute lung injury and transfusion-associated circulatory overload: mutually exclusive or coexisting entities? *Transfusion* 2007; **47**: 171–2.

CHAPTER 59

Transfusion-related lung injury

Ulrich J. Sachs[1] & Jonathan P. Wallis[2]

[1]The Platelet and Granulocyte Laboratory, Institute for Clinical Immunology and Transfusion Medicine, Justus Liebig University, Giessen, Germany
[2]Department of Haematology, Freeman Hospital, Newcastle upon Tyne, UK

Respiratory compromise related to transfusion may be divided broadly into cardiogenic and noncardiogenic. Acute noncardiogenic pulmonary edema occurring immediately after transfusion of donor plasma known to contain leukoagglutinins was first clearly described by Brittingham in 1957.[1] Scattered case reports of *allergic pulmonary edema* or *anaphylactic pulmonary edema* followed. In 1985, Popovsky and Moore[2] published the first prospective study of this complication that they termed *transfusion-related acute lung injury* (TRALI). They reported a much higher incidence of the complication than had previously been considered likely, and following their report, increasing numbers of individual cases and small case series were published. With the development of hemovigilance schemes in the late 1990s, it became apparent that TRALI was not only an important cause of transfusion-related morbidity but also, with the reduction in infective complications of transfusion, a leading cause of transfusion-related mortality. In the first decade of this century, a better understanding of the pathophysiology led to successful preventative strategies. The increased understanding and interest in TRALI led also, via active hemovigilance schemes, to improved recognition of cardiogenic dyspnea due to volume overload, now generally termed *transfusion-associated circulatory overload* (TACO).

TRALI: clinical features

Clinical reports of TRALI describe a sudden deterioration in lung function closely related to blood transfusion. The changes occur rapidly and generally begin within two hours and nearly always within six hours of the subsequently implicated transfusion. A small number of reports suggest that the onset may rarely be delayed until 12 hours or more after transfusion.[3] The conscious patient describes a tightness in the chest, feels short of breath, develops a dry cough, and may also experience nausea, dizziness, and rigors. On examination, the patient is hypoxic, is often hypotensive, and has tachypnea and tachycardia. Widespread crepitations are heard on auscultation of the chest. Rigors and fever are commonly reported but are not always present, and fever may develop only some hours after the transfusion.

On intubation, or on suction of the already ventilated patient, a typical finding is of a copious frothy tracheal exudate, much like lightly whipped egg white. The nature and quantity of this exudate are often remarked on by attending anesthetists, and it may be considered one of the hallmarks of severe TRALI. Arterial blood gasses show hypoxia and hypercapnia that are often severe. Chest X-rays show nodular shadowing typically in the "bat's wing" pattern of acute respiratory distress syndrome (ARDS) (Figure 59.1). Physiologic measurements such as pulmonary artery wedge pressure or esophageal Doppler study of the left atrium show systemic hypovolemia that may be marked. Further diagnostic tests of value are described in this chapter.

These cases represent the severe end of the spectrum of the disorder. Most early published reports describe severe cases such as these, but with more knowledge of the condition many milder cases are being recognized. Milder cases are proportionately less dramatic.

Recovery of respiratory function starts as early as six hours after the onset in milder cases, but in some cases deterioration may continue until 24 hours or beyond.

Some authors have reported a slightly different clinical picture in which the chief signs are rigors and fever with transient respiratory dysfunction, hypertension rather than hypotension, and occurrence usually within 30 minutes of transfusion. Pulmonary edema is not always demonstrated radiologically, and recovery is within 1 or 2 hours. These reactions have typically been associated with cellular blood components. It has been suggested that these cases may represent a different and non-antibody-related etiology (discussed further in this chapter) from the "classical" severe cases.[4] However, a similar spectrum of mild to moderate reactions of this nature has also been documented with transfusion of plasma containing antibody to a neutrophil antigen, anti-HNA-2.[5]

Acute lung injury with noncardiogenic pulmonary edema is common among critically ill patients and is generally considered to have a multifactorial pathogenesis. Many sick patients receive transfusion, especially after multiple trauma. There is evidence that TRALI is a significant contributor to acute lung injury (ALI) and that plasma-rich components from female donors are particularly implicated. The relationship between ALI and TRALI is further discussed in this section.

Pathophysiology

It is now understood that many cases of TRALI, including the most severe cases, are due to an antibody–antigen interaction between donor and donation. Other mechanisms have been postulated and may be contributory to antibody-related cases or to other causes of

Rossi's Principles of Transfusion Medicine, Fifth Edition. Edited by Toby L. Simon, Jeffrey McCullough, Edward L. Snyder, Bjarte G. Solheim, and Ronald G. Strauss.
© 2016 John Wiley & Sons, Ltd. Published 2016 by John Wiley & Sons, Ltd.

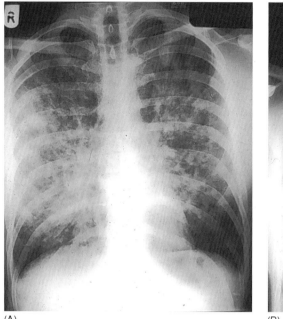
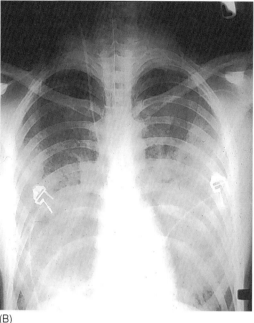

(A)   (B)

Figure 59.1 Chest X-rays from a 33-year-old man with severe TRALI, taken 2 hours (A) and 24 hours (B) after onset of symptoms, following transfusion of FFP containing HLA class II antibodies. Note the "bat's wing" pattern of edema with sparing of the lung bases, the air bronchograms clearly visible on the first radiograph, and the more confluent airspace shadowing but still with basal sparing in the second X-ray.

lung damage. It has been suggested, and is a helpful distinction, that TRALI should be clearly divided into antibody-related and non-antibody-related lung damage.

Acute lung injury

ALI is the result of a capillary endothelial leak that allows fluid to pass from the pulmonary vessels, initially into the interstitial space and subsequently into the alveolar space. Because this edema is distinct from hydrostatic edema caused by cardiac failure or volume overload, it is sometimes known as *nonhydrostatic edema*. Numerous stimuli have been suggested to contribute to the likelihood of developing nonhydrostatic pulmonary edema, including sepsis, trauma, aspiration of gastric contents, disseminated intravascular coagulation, and high tidal volume ventilation. In some cases of TRALI, the transfusion appears to be the only probable cause of the lung injury, whereas in other cases it may be only one of several possible factors present. Histopathology, clinical findings, and experimental work have helped elucidate the nature of the stimulus from the transfused blood and the mechanism of the lung damage.

Histopathology

Histopathologic findings from fatal TRALI cases are consistent with those for early ARDS, showing interstitial and intra-alveolar edema[2,3,6–10] and extravasation of neutrophils into the interstitial and air spaces (Figure 59.2).[3,6,7,10] Hyaline membranes and destruction of the pulmonary architecture have been reported.[6,7] A consistent finding in TRALI is the presence of increased numbers of neutrophils within the pulmonary capillary vasculature and small pulmonary vessels.[9,10] On electron microscopic pictures, neutrophils were degranulated and focally in direct contact with denuded stretches of the capillary wall. A positive correlation has been reported between capillary leukostasis and desquamated epithelial cells, and between the degree of capillary leukostasis and the amount of proteinaceous fluid within the alveolar air spaces.[10]

From these observations, it appears that the neutrophil is central to the occurrence of lung damage. After sequestration in the early stages of TRALI, neutrophils and endothelial cells of the pulmonary microvasculature establish close contact. Activation of the neutrophils leads to endothelial damage and capillary leakage. The transit of proteinaceous fluid from the vessels into the air spaces results in acute pulmonary edema. In the later stage, especially of severe

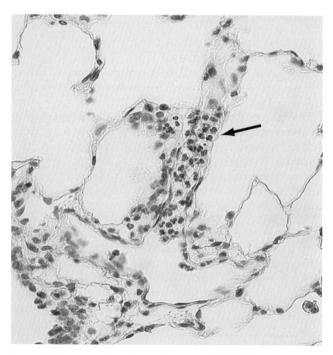

Figure 59.2 Sections of lung from a fatal case of TRALI. Note the presence of granulocytes in the capillaries (arrow indicates neutrophils).

TRALI, neutrophils extravasate from the capillary into the alveoli and induce further pulmonary injury.

Evidence for an antibody-related etiology

The relationship between TRALI and leukocyte antibodies in donor plasma was first noted by Brittingham, who reported that leukoagglutinins present in the plasma of a multitransfused patient induced an acute pulmonary reaction when transfused to a volunteer.[1] Severe pulmonary edema was similarly induced in a healthy volunteer who received an experimental gamma globulin concentrate, deliberately prepared from plasma that contained leukocyte- and, in particular, monocyte-reactive antibodies.[11] It is likely that this preparation contained high levels of HLA class II antibodies. In addition to these cases of TRALI resulting from experimental transfusion of plasma containing leukocyte antibodies, there are numerous case reports of TRALI in which a transfused unit has been found to contain antibodies reactive with recipient leukocytes. In two large series of TRALI, where pulmonary infiltrates were apparent in chest X-rays, leukocyte antibodies in the donor of a transfused blood component were detected in 61% to 89% of cases.[2,12]

Animal models have provided confirmation of this antibody-mediated mechanism of TRALI. Severe vascular leakage was reproduced in isolated rabbit lungs by application of HNA-3a antibodies in an ex vivo rabbit lung model.[13] From this experiment, it was concluded that leukoagglutinating antibodies and concomitant complement activation are capable of causing TRALI. Other animal experiments have confirmed that antibodies are capable of causing TRALI but suggest that complement is not a prerequisite for TRALI induced by antibodies to CD177 (HNA-2), because the induction of TRALI was found to be dependent on the density of the cognate antigen and occurred in a complement-free environment.[14] Alternative mechanisms leading to TRALI have been proposed and are discussed in this chapter, but the available evidence demonstrates that donor leukocyte antibodies reacting with recipient antigens are the predominant mechanism. Large clinical studies were able to corroborate these experimental findings, as were hemovigilance data obtained in countries in which plasma from female donors (or female donors with a history of pregnancy) was no longer used for clinical transfusion.[15–19]

Specificities of antibodies identified as causing TRALI

Antibodies to HLA class I and II antigens and to neutrophil antigens have all been clearly implicated as causing TRALI. Evidence from hemovigilance schemes and laboratories specializing in TRALI investigation has shown that the majority of cases (75–90%) are associated with HLA antibodies, and that with improved detection techniques about 50% of these are directed against HLA class II antigens.[20] Antibodies to neutrophil antigens are found in about 10–25% of cases. Interestingly, in three large clinical studies that investigated donor-related risk factors for TRALI patients, HLA class I antibodies were not identified as risk factors.[15–17] In contrast, two of the three studies calculated an odds ratio of 3.08–3.2 for HLA class II positive units and of 1.71–4.85 for units from donors who produced a positive test with granulocytes in the laboratory.[15,17]

Mechanisms of lung damage in TRALI
Priming and activation of neutrophils

The dogma that TRALI is mediated by activated neutrophils has lost some of its cogency during recent years, mainly because TRALI could still be precipitated in animals depleted of neutrophils.[21–23] It appears reasonable to consider neutrophils as major, but not sole, mediators in a process that also includes monocytes and the endothelium. Neutrophils activated by injurious agents will respond by the de novo synthesis of a range of highly toxic reactive oxygen species (ROS) and the release of preformed granular enzymes, proteins, and neutrophil extracellular traps (NETs).[24,25] Neutrophils may be activated directly by one sufficiently strong stimulus, but the process often requires two or more stimuli. The first or "priming" stimulus will potentiate the response to a second or "activating" stimulus. A large percentage of patients who develop TRALI are sick, and there is in vivo evidence that surgical procedures and active infections induce neutrophil priming.[26–28] In response to priming agents, neutrophils undergo polarization, a process that leads to "stiffening" of the cell.[29] This "stiffening" augments mechanical retention of neutrophils within the pulmonary capillary bed and prolongs their passage through the lungs (discussed further in this chapter).[30] Prolonged, close contact between neutrophils and the endothelium provides a micro-environment in which transmembrane receptors and released mediators of each cell type can interact closely. Sequestered neutrophils, having been primed in the circulation, and endothelial cells can be activated by exogenous stimuli present in the blood bag. These transfused stimuli include antibodies, cytokines, and bioactive lipids (also discussed further here).

Antibodies to neutrophil antigens involved in TRALI cases are able to prime and activate neutrophils in some cases without additional stimuli,[14,31–33] explaining why even completely healthy individuals can develop TRALI if the antibody stimulus is sufficient.[11]

Aspects of neutrophil passage through the pulmonary microvasculature

The alveolar capillary bed is a complex interconnecting network of short capillary segments. The path of a neutrophil from arteriole to venule crosses up to eight or more alveolar walls and encounters more than 50 capillary segments. Approximately half of these pulmonary capillaries are narrower than the diameter of a spherically shaped neutrophil (Figure 59.3). This forces neutrophils to slow and to deform before passing through the narrow capillary segment. The transit time of neutrophils through the pulmonary microvasculature is mainly affected by their deformation time, and slow transit accounts for significant accumulation of neutrophils in the lungs.[34] The pulmonary circulation normally contains about 30%, the "marginated pool," of the total blood neutrophil pool. The stimulus-induced decrease in deformability appears to be more important than selectin-mediated rolling, a key mechanism of neutrophil adhesion within other capillary beds, but changes in surface receptors in primed neutrophils will also lead to molecular adhesion to endothelial cells.[34–36] Under physiologic conditions, primed and locally trapped neutrophils migrate from the capillaries into the alveoli as part of a local inflammatory reaction. In TRALI, the primed and trapped neutrophil encounters a further activation signal in the form of transfused antibody or other transfusion stimulus, activates its microbicidal arsenal, and induces endothelial damage.

Activation of pulmonary endothelial cells

TRALI can also be triggered by activated pulmonary endothelium. In addition to constitutively expressed surface receptors, activated endothelial cells upregulate surface membrane receptors that

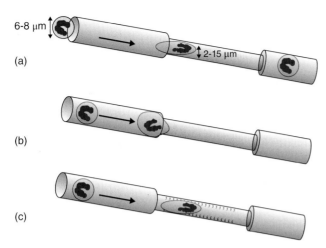

Figure 59.3 The neutrophil's passage through the pulmonary microvasculature. Approximately 50% of all pulmonary capillaries surrounding the alveoli have a smaller diameter than the spheric neutrophil. (A) In order to pass through the capillary, neutrophils are forced to pause, deform, and assume a "sausage shape" that allows transit of the capillary. (B) Neutrophil priming is associated with a decrease of deformability (called *stiffening*), which results in local trapping of the cell and a prolonged overall transit time. (C) Activation of the endothelial cells of the capillaries results in the upregulation of surface ligands, which also results in local trapping of the cell and a prolonged overall transit time.

facilitate neutrophil adhesion and priming. Primary activation of endothelial cells has been suggested as the mechanism responsible for TRALI induction after infusion of bioactive lipids.[37,38] More recently, antibodies recognizing proteins present on the endothelial surface (i.e., HNA-3a) were shown to directly interfere with endothelial function,[22] indicating that barrier breakdown leading to lung edema does not necessarily involve the activation of neutrophils. These experimental data are in line with a clinical observation in which a HLA-B44-negative patient transfused with blood containing anti-HLA-B44 antibodies developed a "half-sided" TRALI in his recently transplanted, HLA-B44-positive lung only.[39] These antibodies must have either reacted with transplant endothelium or, possibly, donor-type (alveolar) macrophages.

Activation of monocytes

The question of whether white blood cells other than neutrophils might contribute to TRALI was raised when investigators tried to unravel the mechanism behind HLA class II–induced TRALI. In contrast to HNA and HLA class I, HLA class II antigens are usually not present on neutrophils (or endothelial cells), but are present on monocytes. Kopko *et al.* suggested a monocyte-dependent mechanism, where HLA class II antibodies bind to monocytes, induce the release of neutrophil-activating mediators, and finally induce neutrophil activation and TRALI.[40] Using human plasma with anti-HLA-DR7 and -DR52 specificity and human neutrophils and monocytes in an ex vivo rat lung model, Sachs *et al.* showed that HLA class II antibodies can induce TRALI via such a multistep pathway, including the initial activation of monocytes and the release of interleukin-8 (IL8).[41] Subsequently, experiments in mice delineated that monocytes may also be involved in HLA class I–mediated TRALI, because depletion of these cells suppressed HLA class I antibody–mediated TRALI, as did the blockage of MIP2 receptors, the murine analog of IL8.[21,23]

Platelets and TRALI

The extent to which platelets participate in TRALI is still unresolved. Both blockage of platelet function by aspirin and immune-mediated platelet depletion were recorded to suppress TRALI in a murine model,[42,43] but other experiments using different methods of platelet depletion have failed to confirm this,[21] indicating that the process of elimination itself rather than the absence of platelets could mediate protection. There are also conflicting data on the involvement of platelets in neutrophil extracellular trap formation.[24,25] Whether platelets are present in alveolar capillary wall lesions (e.g., as neutrophil–platelet aggregates) is also unresolved.[21,44]

Neutrophil, monocyte, and endothelial cell interplay

The interplay between neutrophils, monocytes, endothelial cells, and, possibly, platelets—regardless of whether it has primarily been started by neutrophil, monocyte, or endothelial cell activation—contributes largely to lung damage. Neutrophils respond to monocyte- and/or endothelial cell–derived mediators by activating and expressing integrins and by releasing pro-inflammatory mediators and granule contents. Released mediators activate endothelial cells, which, in turn, mobilize selectins, upregulate adhesion proteins, and produce inflammatory mediators; thereby, they enhance neutrophil and platelet adhesion and neutrophil, platelet, and monocyte activation. It is within this interplay that the lung barrier breaks down and allows transit of proteinaceous fluid and, later, of neutrophils into the alveolar space. At least in the experimental setting, other blood cells seem to act as attenuators in this complex process.[45,46]

Mechanisms of lung injury by different mediators in transfused blood components

The exact pathway leading to lung damage associated with transfusion depends on the nature of the antibody or other stimulus and the interplay between it and the cellular components.

Antibodies to human neutrophil antigens

Serologic workup of TRALI patients identified antibodies to human neutrophil antigens in a number of cases.[47–49] In hemovigilance schemes, they were detected in approximately 10% of cases before preventive measures were installed. As discussed above, the ability of these antibodies to induce TRALI has been shown in ex vivo models of lung injury.[13,14] HNA antibodies, particularly those of HNA-2 and HNA-4a specificity, are capable of directly activating neutrophils, which appears to be the mechanism by which they induce TRALI (Figure 59.4A).[14,31,50] Of note, antibodies against HNA-3a can interact directly with endothelial cells, because their cognate antigen CTL-2 is expressed not only on neutrophils but also on endothelial cells of the lungs.[22] Binding of anti-HNA-3a to endothelial cells leads to the production of ROS within the endothelium, as a consequence of which endothelial cells loosen their contacts and allow fluid to shift to the alveolar spaces (Figure 59.4E). It is suggested that this direct mechanism of TRALI induction accounts for the high rate of fatal cases of TRALI associated with HNA-3a antibodies.[51] The activation of endothelial cells by direct binding of HNA-3a antibodies leads also to cellular activation and neutrophil recruitment, indicated by the fact that these antibodies can induce (milder) TRALI in a murine model in the absence of neutrophils, but induce more severe TRALI when neutrophils are present,[22] corroborating the idea that once the process is started, multiple players become involved.

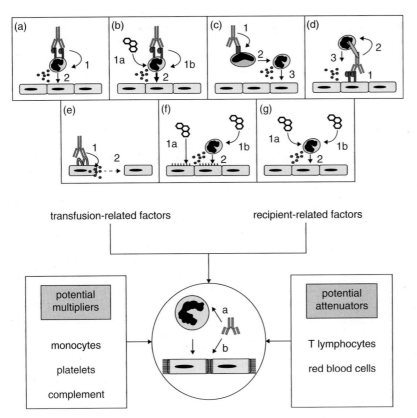

Figure 59.4 Proposed mechanisms of TRALI. The activation of neutrophils and the subsequent release of toxic agents that harm the endothelium, predominantly ROS, are key mechanisms in TRALI. Epidemiological, clinical, and experimental data show that most TRALI reactions are induced by antibodies present in a transfused blood component. These antibodies may recognize epitopes on the surface of (A, B) the neutrophil, (C) the monocytes, or (D, E) endothelial cells. Binding of HNA or HLA class I antibodies to neutrophils causes direct activation of the cell. (C) Binding of antibodies, especially of HLA class II antibodies, to monocytes has been proposed to induce the release of mediators that activate the neutrophil. (D) Experimental data demonstrate that neutrophils may also be activated indirectly when HLA class I antibodies are bound to the endothelium of the lung, where they can recruit neutrophils via their Fc receptors binding to the Fc parts of these antibodies. (E) Further evidence indicates also direct endothelial effects of antibodies, such as Anti-HNA-3a. (F, G) Biologically active substances other than antibodies (e.g., bioactive lipids and CD40L derived from cellular blood components) are thought to cause some cases of TRALI. These substances are usually too weak to activate neutrophils directly, but may induce TRALI in concert with other factors that activate endothelial cells or neutrophils. See text for details.

Antibodies to HLA class I antigens

HLA class I antibodies are frequent in the donor population, and the presence of such antibodies in transfused plasma can be anticipated to be a common cause of TRALI. The cognate antigens are expressed on all cell types that are discussed to play a role in TRALI. It is well documented that HLA class I antibodies can directly bind to neutrophils and prime oxidases in both humans and rats.[52,53] In line with this, there are numerous anecdotal reports of TRALI associated with HLA class I antibodies, especially of anti-HLA-A2 specificity, which is directed against a frequent HLA antigen. However, HLA class I antibodies were not associated with increased risk of TRALI in several observational studies.[15–17]

Most TRALI experiments in animals were performed with anti-MHC (major histocompatibility complex) class I antibodies. Of note, only one out of several tested monoclonal MHC class I antibodies induces TRALI in mice when infused (anti-H2K[d], clone 34.1.2s), and results obtained with these experiments, albeit highly informative, should be interpreted carefully, especially when it comes to their impact on transfusion medicine. An elegant study performed in mice by Looney and coworkers[42] presented in vivo data on the mechanism of endothelial cell–dependent TRALI (Figure 59.4D). Transfusion of an MHC class I monoclonal antibody to mice expressing the cognate antigen induced TRALI and acute peripheral blood neutropenia. Mice lacking neutrophils and mice lacking the Fcγ-receptor were resistant to MHC class I antibody–induced TRALI. Transfer of wild-type neutrophils into FcRγ[−/−] mice restored TRALI following antibody infusion. This model is consistent with binding of the antibody directly to endothelial cells, in the first vascular bed encountered after injection, and recruitment of neutrophils through binding of the immunoglobulin Fc portion to the neutrophil Fcγ receptor. The protection observed in FcRγ[−/−] mice argues against direct

neutrophil activation by the antibody. The idea of Fc-receptor-dependent trapping has been challenged by numerous findings from other investigators, all performed with the same monoclonal antibody as inducer of TRALI. A major aspect is that depletion of monocytes abrogates TRALI in this model,[21,23] indicating that monocyte activation needs to be considered as a crucial step in anti-MHC class I–induced murine TRALI.

As outlined above, direct neutrophil binding of HLA class I antibodies was demonstrated for humans and rats,[52,53] and evidence that HLA class I antibodies can also cause TRALI by direct binding to neutrophil antigens comes from case reports of "inverse TRALI." In one well-documented case, infusion of human granulocytes caused severe lung injury in a patient who had class I antibodies.[54] The antibodies cannot have reacted with the native endothelial cells but did react in vivo with the donor granulocytes, in keeping with a mechanism of TRALI by direct activation of neutrophils (Figure 59.4A and 59.4B). In summary, different experimental findings reported for HLA class I antibodies make it very likely that numerous activation steps must generally come together before the reaction commences in a patient. This may involve antibody binding to neutrophils, endothelial cells, and monocytes. The fact that human antibodies—in contrast to the monoclonals used in animal studies—are polyclonal and differ in their binding characteristics and avidity may explain the lack of a clear association of HLA class I antibodies and TRALI in studies of donor risk factors.

Antibodies to HLA class II antigens

In contrast to HNA and HLA class I, HLA class II antigens are usually not present on neutrophils (or endothelial cells), but on monocytes. Neutrophils and endothelial cells may express HLA class II upon stimulation, but HLA class II antigen expression was not found on vascular endothelium of pulmonary capillaries or intravascular neutrophils in a patient who experienced fatal TRALI caused by an HLA class II antibody.[55] Although a direct mechanism between HLA class II antibodies and the other two cell types cannot formally be excluded, monocytes appear currently as major target cells for these type of antibodies (Figure 59.4C).[40,41,56] It is unlikely that transfused antibodies have direct access to the alveolar space through an intact endothelium in sufficient concentration to induce release of cytokines and subsequent activation of neutrophils and/or endothelial cells, but where there is already some damage to the pulmonary endothelium, such a reaction may exacerbate ALI.

It remains possible that detection of antibodies to HNA and HLA could be surrogates for antibodies to as-yet-unknown antigens on other cell types (e.g., on monocytes). Alloantibodies to these or other cells might explain some apparently antibody-negative cases.

Inverse TRALI: transfusion of neutrophils

In most cases of TRALI, antibodies or neutrophil-priming agents present in the blood component are causative for the pulmonary reaction. However, TRALI, as described above, has also been reported in alloimmunized patients receiving blood components that contain neutrophils. Viable neutrophils may still be present in other blood components, and Popovsky and Moore estimated that 6% of observed TRALI cases were caused by antibodies present in the recipient.[2] As universal leukocyte reduction has been introduced in many countries, inverse TRALI caused by leukocytes in platelet concentrates (PCs) and red blood cells (RBCs) must nowadays be considered as a rare constellation; it will remain of particular relevance to patients receiving granulocyte transfusions.[54,57]

Non-antibody mediators of TRALI

Bioactive lipids

Blood components may accumulate intermediate metabolic products, such as bioactive lipids, during storage. These substances are breakdown products of membrane lipids, including lyso-phosphatidylcholines (lysoPCs), which can prime respiratory burst reactions of the neutrophil. Because these neutrophil-priming agents do not develop in stored acellular plasma, their generation is dependent on the presence of blood cells. RBCs are known to alter significantly during their shelf life (see also Chapter 9), and this blood component is a candidate mediator of antibody-negative TRALI. Indeed, administration of supernatant from stored (but not from fresh) human RBCs caused TRALI in an ex vivo and later also in an in vivo animal model of TRALI (Figure 59.4F and 59.4G).[37,52] However, in a syngeneic rat model of RBC transfusions by Vlaar et al., these findings could not be reproduced: RBCs were prepared from donor rats and transfused after storage. When rats were pretreated with LPS, there was no difference in the histopathology score or cytokine levels after the transfusion of fresh (day 0) and old (day 14) rat RBCs. When red cells and supernatant were transfused separately, the supernatant induced lung inflammation but no lung edema, and lysoPCs were not involved in the inflammatory reaction.[58]

Biologically active breakdown products were also investigated in the setting of platelet transfusions. In a cross-species study, supernatant of aged human platelets, but not of fresh platelets, caused ALI in an ex vivo rat lung model.[38] In a syngeneic rat model, whole aged rat platelet suspensions, but not fresh ones, led to neutrophil adherence and some edema in lung. However, when LPS was used to mimic patient-related risk factors, stored platelets no longer induced TRALI despite an increased lysoPC content.[59]

In summary, there is currently no clear evidence on whether lysoPCs (or other bioactive lipids[60]) are involved in TRALI or not. It should be noted that cumulative data from three large clinical trials are not supportive for a role of RBC storage time and/or lysoPC content as relevant risk factors for TRALI.[15–17]

CD40 ligand (CD40L)

CD40L is another neutrophil-priming breakdown product. It is a platelet-derived pro-inflammatory mediator found in cell-associated and soluble (sCD40L) forms. It may be found in PCs and accumulates during storage.[61] sCD40L binds to CD40, which is present on the surface of monocytes, macrophages, and neutrophils.[62] This CD40L–CD40 interaction induces neutrophil priming, which was suspected to be associated with TRALI after platelet transfusions because its concentration in transfused PCs that were involved in TRALI cases was found to be significantly higher than in control units. In vitro, human microvascular endothelial cells preincubated with LPS experienced severe damage when sCD40L-primed neutrophils were added, whereas unprimed neutrophils did not induce such damage.[62] In a rather complicated murine experiment, others have questioned the role of CD40L in TRALI.[63] In line with these animal experiments and in contrast to other case reports, patients with TRALI after cardiac surgery did not differ in their sCD40L levels from controls.[64] In summary, the contribution of CD40L to TRALI is still incompletely defined.

Immunoglobulins

Normal IgG has been postulated to activate neutrophils in a patient with osteopetrosis being treated with gamma interferon and granulocyte and monocyte colony-stimulating factor.[65] The patient had very low levels of endogenous IgG1 and IgG2 and developed severe lung injury shortly after transfusion of platelets from an untransfused male donor. No leukocyte antibodies could be found in either donor or recipient. It is suggested that transfused IgG binding to the neutrophils, which were already primed by interferon and stimulating factor, was sufficient to cause neutrophil activation and lung injury. This case may be considered a good example of "multiple-hit" TRALI.

Reports of lung injury following intravenous IgG infusion are rare and seem to be associated with high doses or concentrates prepared intentionally with a high level of leukocyte antibodies.[11,66] It is possible that antibodies are both diluted and neutralized during the preparation of the pooled product, as suggested for pooled viricidally treated plasma.[67,68]

Multiple-hit/threshold theory of TRALI causation

Where the stimulus to endothelial and neutrophil activation is sufficient, lung damage can occur in an otherwise healthy individual with no other likely cause of lung injury. Evidence for this comes from reports of TRALI in transfused volunteers as described here and also from reports where plasma has been used for clinical reasons in otherwise healthy individuals. These cases are a minority, and most patients receiving transfusion and especially transfusion of plasma have significant comorbidities, some or many of which may also result in priming or activation of neutrophils or damage to pulmonary endothelial cells. It has been suggested that TRALI will be more common in such patients. Early reports noted that most patients with TRALI had recently undergone surgery and suggested that this in itself was a sufficient second stimulus in many cases. Some experimental evidence for the "two-hit" or "multiple-hit" theory has been provided by studies on bioactive lipids described

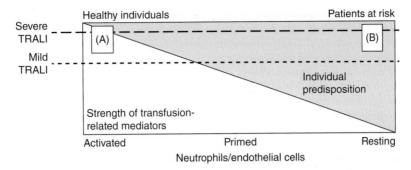

Figure 59.5 The Bux–Sachs TRALI threshold model. The TRALI threshold model proposes that a certain threshold must be overcome to commence a TRALI reaction. The threshold of mild TRALI, in which oxygen supply is sufficient, is lower than that of severe TRALI, in which patients require mechanical ventilation (horizontal lines). In order to overcome this threshold, numerous factors must act in concert. These factors can be summarized as strength of exogenous transfusion-related mediators (light box) and individual predisposition of the patient (gray box). The individual predisposition covers both constitutive (genetic) factors and dynamic or acute influences (i.e., acute infection or trauma). A strong exogenous transfusion-related mediator, such as a strong activatory neutrophil-specific antibody, will precipitate a TRALI reaction even if the influence of the individual predisposition is low (example A, in an otherwise healthy recipient). In contrast (example B, an individual "at risk," e.g., a septic patient with an activated pulmonary endothelium), a relatively mild exogenous transfusion-related mediator with low neutrophil-priming activity will be sufficient to overcome the threshold. Source: Bux and Sachs (2007).[69] Reproduced with permission of Wiley.

here.[37] The multiple-hit theory has been further developed by Bux and Sachs,[69] who suggest that neutrophil and endothelial cells are central to the pathogenesis of TRALI and that activation of these cells requires sufficient stimuli from one or more sources to reach a certain threshold, at which point full activation and lung damage will ensue (Figure 59.5). Depending on the magnitude of the neutrophil or endothelial cell response, the lung damage can be mild or severe with corresponding clinical effects.

Transfusion-associated circulatory overload

TACO has become increasingly recognized through hemovigilance schemes. In contrast to TRALI, the essential pathogenesis is of increased pulmonary capillary pressure leading to hydrostatic pulmonary edema. Patients particularly at risk are the small and elderly, those with preexisting cardiac disease, and those with relative fluid overload such as some patients with dialysis-dependent renal failure. Obstetric cases are also reported and may be related in part to the raised circulating volume during pregnancy and the cardiac effects seen in preeclampsia. Transfusion of any fluid, crystalloid, or colloid can lead to cardiac overload. Where

blood transfusion is involved, all components have been implicated, and unlike TRALI there is no overrepresentation of high-volume plasma component transfusion. There is no clear evidence that red cells themselves are implicated by pathophysiological mechanisms other than intravascular volume. It remains possible that stored red cells with relatively poor oxygen delivery characteristics may contribute to cardiac ischemia and thus cardiogenic edema, but there is no clear evidence in favor of this hypothesis.

TACO: definition

The hemovigilance working party of the International Society of Blood Transfusion revised their definition of TACO in 2014 to better capture the range of cases whereby there is volume overload usually with radiographic pulmonary edema resulting from transfusion of blood components (Table 59.1).[70]

TACO: epidemiology

Heart failure and pulmonary edema brought on or worsened by transfusion have been recognized for many years. Patients with severe anemia due to vitamin B_{12} deficiency were particularly

Table 59.1 International Society of Blood Transfusion definition of TACO (2014)[70]

Cases of TACO are characterized by acute or worsening respiratory distress within 6 hours of transfusion (some cases may occur up to 12 hours), with the following features:

Primary Features
- Evidence of acute or worsening pulmonary edema with bilateral infiltrates
- An enlarged cardiac silhouette on chest imaging

Enlarged heart contour should always be present if looked for.
- Evidence of fluid overload

Evidence of fluid overload could be: a positive fluid balance; a response to diuretic therapy combined with clinical improvement.

Features to Support Diagnosis Are
- Elevated BNP or NT-pro BNP to more than 1.5 times pretransfusion value (if available)
- Increase in mean arterial pressure or increased pulmonary wedge pressure; typically the mean arterial pressure is raised, often with widened pulse pressure; however, hypotension may occur (in cases of acute cardiac collapse).

Confirmed cases (definite imputability) should show at least two primary features or one in combination with two supportive features. Cases with only one primary feature (e.g., without chest imaging) may be reported as possible or probable TACO depending on supporting features.

In ICU, patients who may be receiving positive pressure ventilation with varying degrees of PEEP (positive end expiratory pressure) pulmonary edema may be difficult to diagnose at higher levels of PEEP or indeed become apparent if PEEP is reduced or removed.

Source: International Society of Blood Transfusion (2015).[70] Reproduced with permission of ISBT.

known to be susceptible to sudden cardiac decompensation after transfusion. The rising incidence of cardiac overload due to transfusion was first highlighted by hemovigilance data from Quebec in 2010.[71] Subsequently, with increased recognition and reporting, it has emerged as a major cause of transfusion-related morbidity and mortality in many countries, including Ireland and the United Kingdom. Reports from the UK hemovigilance system (SHOT UK) show an increase in reports from three in 2007 to 96 in 2013, the latter being an incidence of the order of one in 10,000 blood components transfused.[18] In Ireland, over 10 years the reported rate was seen to increase from one in 42,000 to one in 6268 units of red cells transfused.[72] Prospective surveys suggest a higher rate still, perhaps as much as 1%.[73,74] The incidence per unit is higher after red cell transfusion than with plasma or platelets alone, although this may be due to the patient's underlying illness and indication for transfusion rather than a specific effect of component type. Morbidity and mortality may be difficult to ascribe only to blood transfusion in a vulnerable patient who may also receive other fluids, but there is no doubt that transfusion appears to be a key factor in many cases. The majority of patients developing TACO are elderly with a history of cardiac disease, respiratory disease, renal failure, or a combination of these conditions. A small number have no known cardiorespiratory comorbidities. Patients are typically elderly with known cardiac failure, but younger previously fit patients may also be affected.[72] Others have identified

an unexpectedly high incidence in obstetric patients, perhaps related to the expanded blood volume seen in pregnancy.[18] Cases have also been reported in children.

TACO: diagnosis

Diagnosis is by identification of hydrostatic pulmonary edema as in Figure 59.6 and accompanying text on the differential diagnosis of TRALI/ALI and TACO/cardiac failure. Hypertension is characteristic of TACO, whereas hypotension is characteristic of TRALI. It is not impossible for a patient to have both volume overload due to incautious fluid management and a capillary leak whether due to TRALI or to ALI from other causes.

TACO: treatment

Treatment is that of cardiac failure or volume overload, putting the patient in an upright position, and giving oxygen and diuretics, fluid restriction, and even phlebotomy. Continuous positive airway pressure or even mechanical ventilation may be necessary, and in patients with marked renal failure dialysis with removal of fluid may be used.

TACO: prevention

Avoidance of unnecessary transfusion is the best preventive measure for TACO. Although the risks of transfusion are well known in anemia due to vitamin B_{12} deficiency, a more common cause of

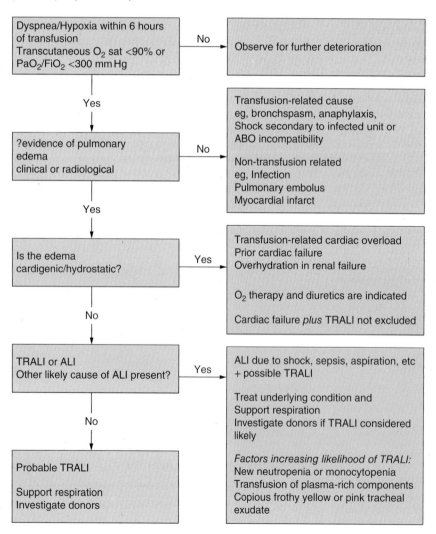

Figure 59.6 Flow chart for diagnosis of TRALI.

anemia is iron deficiency. TACO has been reported following transfusion of such patients. Transfusion is rarely necessary in the absence of active bleeding and should be avoided in patients with easily correctable chronic anemia. Pretransfusion assessment for risk factors for TACO such as low body weight and the comorbidities mentioned, especially fluid overload and poorly controlled heart failure, may allow a careful transfusion protocol with diuretic cover and close observation. In "at-risk" patients, top-up transfusions should be restricted to no more than one unit of red cells at a time, or in small patients of no more than 4 mls/kg body weight of plasma reduced or optimal additive red cells, in order to achieve a rise in hemoglobin of 1 g/dL. There is no prospective or retrospective evidence for or against the use of fresher red cells in this circumstance.

Hypertension, tachypnea, tachycardia, and reduced oxygen saturation are all signs of cardiac overload. Early recognition may allow reduction in transfusion rate, discontinuation of transfusion, or use of oxygen and diuretics to halt or reverse the developing volume overload.

Transfusion-associated dyspnea (TAD)

TAD is defined by increased breathlessness not meeting the criteria for TRALI or TACO or an allergic reaction and occurring within 24 hours of transfusion. Respiratory distress should be the most prominent clinical feature and should not be explained by the patient's underlying condition or any other known cause. It is important to record and classify such reactions, but given the uncertainty as to whether there is a specific pathophysiology, their clinical usefulness in managing transfusion is uncertain.

ALI and transfusion in critically ill patients

Clinical evidence for the theory that "multiple hits" may result in TRALI has been provided by studies involving critically ill patients who are known to be susceptible to ALI. Numerous retrospective studies have suggested a relationship between the amount of blood transfused and morbidity and mortality. All these studies are beset by the difficulty in allowing for the confounding factor of how much blood the patient required also being a marker for the severity of the illness. The Transfusion Requirements in Critical Care (TRICC) trial of transfusion triggers was both prospective and randomized, and it found a significantly higher incidence of pulmonary edema and a higher incidence of ALI in patients receiving more transfusion where the standard component was relatively plasma rich.[75] Gajic et al.[76] studied the clinical associations with ALI developing in patients during mechanical ventilation that was required for management of critical illness. They found a strong association with transfusion of plasma, but not with red cell transfusion, the age of transfused red cells, the leukocyte content of transfused red cells, or platelet transfusion. Further studies identified transfusion of female plasma as being particularly associated with development of ALI in keeping with an antibody type of mechanism.[77] A prospective study in intensive care patients comparing male donor and parous female plasma found similar results.[78] The incidence of ALI associated with transfusion in these studies was of the order of 1 in 50 to 200 units of female plasma transfused, a far higher incidence than the reported incidence of TRALI in other circumstances. These findings are in keeping with the Bux–Sachs threshold model of TRALI in which highly susceptible patients subject to multiple toxic insults to neutrophils and endothelial cells develop lung damage after a relatively mild additional stimulus from transfusion.

Diagnosis and differential diagnosis

Respiratory dysfunction

The development of new respiratory dysfunction caused by pulmonary edema in association with recent transfusion should be considered as evidence of possible TRALI. Significant respiratory dysfunction consistent with ALI can be defined as a decrease in transcutaneous oxygen saturation to less than 90% or an arterial pO_2 of less than 60 mm Hg while breathing room air, or a PaO_2–FiO_2 ratio of less than 300 mm Hg.

Pulmonary edema can be demonstrated by clinical examination and chest X-ray. Alternative causes of sudden respiratory dysfunction, without edema, include transfusion-related problems such as allergic reactions with bronchospasm, shock associated with a bacterially infected unit or with ABO incompatibility, and causes unrelated to the transfusion such as cardiac arrythmias, infection, and pulmonary embolus (Figure 59.6).

Distinguishing between hydrostatic and nonhydrostatic pulmonary edema

Once pulmonary edema is demonstrated, it is necessary to determine whether it is cardiogenic (hydrostatic) or caused by increased capillary permeability as in TRALI and other forms of ALI (nonhydrostatic). Cardiogenic pulmonary edema may be caused by TACO or by factors unrelated to transfusion, such as simple overhydration, especially in renal failure.

Radiology

Radiographic appearances of edema from increased pulmonary capillary permeability are often characteristic with patchy or nodular shadowing; they are mainly peripheral but spare both the apices and the costophrenic angles, and have the appearance of air bronchograms. This pattern is sometimes likened to a bat's wing. In contrast, cardiogenic edema typically shows upper lobe venous distension and edema in the perihilar and basal areas. Edema in overhydration or renal failure is typically perihilar, and shows no air bronchograms. In severe TRALI or in later stages, the radiologic appearances may progress to a complete white-out of the lung fields.

Physiologic measurements

Physiologic measurements are aimed primarily at assessing the cardiac status. Measurement of the left atrial pressure or volume may be by pulmonary artery wedge pressure through a Swan–Ganz catheter, via esophageal Doppler ultrasound, or by transthoracic echocardiography. High left atrial filling pressure or volume suggests cardiogenic pulmonary edema or fluid overload. Normal or low pressure or volume is in keeping with noncardiogenic pulmonary edema. Low levels indicate hypovolemia, a common finding in TRALI. Electrocardiography may also be helpful in detecting cardiac strain patterns or evidence of infarction.

Prior or new cardiac failure does not exclude the possibility of TRALI, because both may be present in the same patient. However, cardiac failure does indicate that the use of diuretics, which are otherwise contraindicated in TRALI, may be beneficial.

Laboratory tests

A serum level of B-type natriuretic peptide (BNP) of <250 pg/mL is consistent with ALI rather than cardiac failure, whereas a level of >250 pg/mL or a twofold increase from a previous level is consistent with cardiac failure.[74] A low level is not completely specific for ALI nor very sensitive, as many patients with ALI also have cardiac dysfunction. A high level may also be seen in renal failure.

A protein concentration in the pulmonary edema of greater than 70% of the serum protein is strong evidence in favor of a capillary-to-alveolar leak as seen in ALI from any cause.

Implicating transfusion as a cause of nonhydrostatic edema

Consensus definition of TRALI

A consensus definition of TRALI was agreed upon in 2004.[79] A clinical diagnosis of TRALI is considered where a new episode of ALI has occurred within six hours of a blood component or derivative transfusion. Where no other cause of ALI is found, the diagnosis of TRALI is considered probable whatever further tests show. Where another possible cause of ALI is present, the diagnosis of TRALI can only be considered possible (Table 59.2). These criteria are useful but do not include laboratory tests. Many cases of TRALI will be in patients with competing etiologies for ALI. Further recipient and donor investigation can help determine, often in retrospect, the probability that the lung injury was wholly or partly due to transfusion.

Laboratory tests

Changes in circulating leukocytes

Leukopenia, in particular neutropenia and monocytopenia occurring within the first hour after the transfusion and possibly present before the development of clinical lung injury, is supportive of transfusion as opposed to other causes of ALI. The neutropenia is often followed by neutrophilia 5–6 hours later.[1,80] Monocytopenia is common, may be absolute, and may be more persistent than the neutropenia.[80,81] Neither change is completely specific or sensitive. The degree of neutropenia is likely to be greater with neutrophil-specific antibodies such as anti-HNA-2, and with neutrophil-agglutinating antibodies such as anti-HNA-3a and anti-HLA-A2, whereas monocytopenia alone is most likely to be seen with HLA class II antibodies.[81] Neutropenia is seen without evidence of lung damage with some neutrophil-specific antibodies.[5,82]

Table 59.2 2004 Consensus conference definition of TRALI

I. TRALI criteria
A. ALI
  1. Acute onset
  2. Hypoxemia
    a. Research setting:
      i. PaO$_2$/FiO$_2$ ≤300, or
      ii. SpO$_2$ <90% on room air
    b. Nonresearch setting:
      i. PaO$_2$/FiO$_2$ ≤300, or
      ii. SpO$_2$ <90% on room air, or
      iii. other clinical evidence of hypoxemia
  3. Bilateral infiltrates on frontal chest radiograph
  4. No evidence of left atrial hypertension (i.e., circulatory overload)
B. No preexisting ALI before transfusion
C. During or within 6 hours of transfusion
D. No temporal relationship to an alternative risk factor for ALI
II. Possible TRALI
A. ALI
B. No preexisting ALI before transfusion
C. During or within 6 hours of transfusion
D. A clear temporal relationship to an alternative risk factor for ALI

Source: Kleinman et al. (2004).[79] Reproduced with permission of Wiley.

Donor tests

To implicate a particular donation as a cause of antibody-related TRALI requires leukocyte typing of the recipient and antibody testing of the donors (discussed in this chapter). Samples for neutrophil and HLA typing should be taken early from the patient in case death ensues. The finding of a donor–recipient antibody–antigen match is of value in donor management and will make the diagnosis of TRALI more likely than a negative investigation, especially where only a small number of units have been transfused. Such matches also occur in patients without TRALI, and are of increasing statistical likelihood where a large number of units have been transfused. A positive match does not prove that TRALI has occurred.

Management and outcome

Management of the patient

The mainstay of treatment is respiratory support, either with oxygen alone or with oxygen and continuous positive airway pressure by mask or mechanical ventilation. In severe cases with systemic hypovolemia, there must be adequate fluid replacement in addition to positive pressure ventilation. This will often require central venous pressure or left atrial volume monitoring. Additional strategies such as high-frequency ventilation and prone ventilation can be of value. Diuretics are contraindicated, because they have been clearly reported to worsen the hypovolemia and hypotension in several cases.[83] Only where there is concomitant fluid overload from cardiac failure or other causes are diuretics indicated. The use of corticosteroids after the insult is of uncertain value. When the diagnosis is made within six hours and the lung damage is severe, use of high-dose steroids might in theory limit further damage by inhibition of neutrophil activation. Prednisolone, methylprednisolone, and dexamethasone have all been used, but there is no useful clinical evidence regarding efficacy. When the diagnosis is made later, they are unlikely to be of value. In intractable cases for which maximal ventilation is insufficient, extracorporeal membrane oxygenation has been used to support the patient until recovery.[84] The use of plasmapheresis with the intent of removing the causative antibody has been reported.[11] Further transfusions should be given if clinically indicated, but plasma-rich products from female donors should be avoided.

Clinical course and outcome

Most patients begin to improve by 24 hours after the initial injury. Milder cases improve as early as six hours. Chest X-rays usually show clearance of edema by 48–96 hours. Nearly all patients who recover do so without any long-term lung damage. Other organ damage such as acute renal failure is seen in more severe cases, although it is not clear whether this is all due to hyopoxia and hypovolemia or whether there is damage to capillary beds in organs other than the lungs.[80] Mortality in different published series varies between 5% and 30%. This depends in part on how cases are ascertained. Where patients receiving transfusion were assessed prospectively for the complication, the incidence was higher, presumably because of recognition of milder cases, but the mortality was low (6%). Where reports depend on a physician recognizing and reporting the condition, the incidence is lower but mortality higher. As an example, the hemovigilance scheme in the United Kingdom reported seven deaths out of 28 possible, probable, or likely cases reported in 2002, a mortality of 25%.[85] Mortality is more likely in patients receiving larger volumes of single-donor plasma (including fresh frozen plasma [FFP]) rather than RBCs and more likely in patients with more comorbidities.

TRALI in neonates and children

TRALI has been reported in children with the same features as noted in adults, including leukopenia, nonhydrostatic pulmonary edema, and hypovolemia. Some of the published reports ascribed death of the child partly or wholly due to the transfusion reaction.[65,86,87] Age range of cases is from 0 months to 16 years, but only a few neonatal cases have been reported,[57,88] and no neonatal cases have been reported to the UK hemovigilance scheme over 10 years. Use of blood components is more common in neonates than older children, and neonates also receive larger volumes of single-donor plasma relative to their weight. It is possible that neonates are in some way less susceptible to TRALI.

Directed donations and TRALI

A particular feature of pediatric TRALI is its occurrence after the use of directed donations from the mother. This practice has been documented to cause TRALI and can be expected to be high risk by virtue of the high probability of the mother having leukocyte antibodies that will match her child's antigen specificity.[89] By the same rationale, directed donations from a wife to a husband, or of a leukocyte-containing component from a child to a mother or a husband to a wife, will be particularly likely to cause TRALI.

Donor investigation

Strategies of donor investigation vary among blood centers. The dual aim of investigation is to help establish the diagnosis and to allow appropriate management of implicated donors. A typical scheme adapted from Su and Kamel[90] is shown in Figure 59.7. Investigation of donors is undertaken only when a diagnosis of TRALI is considered probable or possible. Donations transfused within the six hours before the development of lung injury are considered to be under suspicion. Where the number of possibly implicated donors is small (four or fewer), all donors should be investigated. Where the number of possibly implicated donors is greater, the high-risk donors with a history of pregnancy or transfusion are initially investigated. If a donor or donors are found

with an antibody that matches a cognate antigen, investigations of the lower risk donors are not undertaken. If no donor is implicated in the initial investigation, further lower risk donors can be tested in those cases that are considered to be probable TRALI. A further selection policy is to initially investigate only those donors of plasma-rich components. Investigations are undertaken at a qualified laboratory with adequate sensitivity for HLA class I and II antibodies, and HNA antibodies. Recipient HLA and HNA typing may be performed prospectively or only when a donor antibody is found. Tests for recipient antibodies may be undertaken when the lung injury followed transfusion of granulocyte concentrate, or following non-leukocyte-reduced component transfusion in which no donor–recipient antibody–antigen match can be identified. When a non-antibody mechanism is suspected, or if an antibody-related etiology has been largely excluded, tests on the residual donation for abnormal lipids or other bioactive substances may be carried out at a research or reference center.

Management of implicated donors

Management of implicated donors varies among countries and centers. It is possible to permanently defer all donors who are implicated in a case of TRALI by virtue of having leukocyte antibodies of any specificity. This would undoubtedly exclude many donors unnecessarily, and the logical extension of such a policy is that all donors with leukocyte antibodies should be deferred whether or not they have been possibly implicated in a case of TRALI. Alternatively, only those donors with antibody matching a recipient antigen are excluded from future donation. This policy assumes that some feature of the antibody in that donor makes them more likely to have caused TRALI in the index case, and thus to cause TRALI with further donations. Finally, it is possible to defer donors who are either possibly or definitely implicated only from donation of plasma-rich components. In addition, some centers automatically defer permanently any donor found to have anti-HNA-3a because of the high frequency of the antigen in the recipient pool (95%) and the common association with severe TRALI. As more countries restrict the manufacture of plasma-rich components to male or nulliparous untransfused female donors, the policy of donor management will become less contentious.

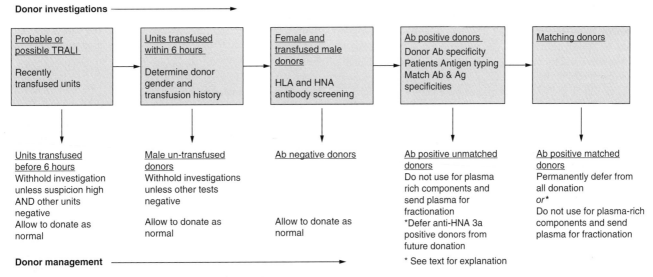

Donor investigations ⟶

| Probable or possible TRALI

Recently transfused units | Units transfused within 6 hours

Determine donor gender and transfusion history | Female and transfused male donors

HLA and HNA antibody screening | Ab positive donors
Donor Ab specificity
Patients Antigen typing
Match Ab & Ag specificities | Matching donors |

Units transfused before 6 hours
Withhold investigation unless suspicion high AND other units negative
Allow to donate as normal

Male un-transfused donors
Withhold investigations unless other tests negative

Allow to donate as normal

Ab negative donors

Allow to donate as normal

Ab positive unmatched donors
Do not use for plasma rich components and send plasma for fractionation
*Defer anti-HNA 3a positive donors from future donation

Ab positive matched donors
Permanently defer from all donation
or
Do not use for plasma-rich components and send plasma for fractionation

* See text for explanation

Donor management ⟶

Figure 59.7 Flow chart for investigation and management of donors.

Incidence and epidemiology

Variables affecting the incidence of TRALI

The frequency of reported TRALI depends upon variables affecting the donors, the recipients, and the physicians. Antibody-associated TRALI, which is the common and severe form, is nearly always associated with blood donations from female donors with a history of pregnancy and is both more common and more severe with transfusion of plasma-rich products, such as FFP or apheresis platelets. HLA antibodies have been found in approximately 15% of all female donors but are more common in those who have had more pregnancies and more recent pregnancies,[91,92] and they are even more common with more sensitive tests.[93] Human neutrophil antibodies are less common. Therefore, incidence of TRALI will depend in part on the donors used by the local blood center. Policies to reduce the number of components containing antibodies are discussed further in this chapter.

Lookback studies for regular donors of blood whose antibody-containing plasma has been implicated in a case of TRALI show that many cases of TRALI are either overlooked or unreported. In addition, infusion of an antibody to a recipient with a matching antigen does not necessarily result in TRALI.[94,95] Both inherited and acquired recipient variables and details of the transfusion will affect the likelihood of developing clinically apparent TRALI. Inherited variables have not been defined but will almost certainly include polymorphisms in the immune response pathways. The presence of high levels of soluble HLA antigens in the recipient's plasma may be protective.[96] Acquired recipient variables include the presence of other lung insults and other forms of comorbidity, as discussed. Transfusion variables include the titer and specificity of antibody, the volume of plasma infused, and the speed of infusion. Plasma-reduced RBCs transfused over 90 minutes rarely cause TRALI, whereas FFP given over 15 minutes—a more than 50-fold higher rate of plasma transfusion—is not uncommonly implicated.

Finally, the likelihood of diagnosing and reporting TRALI depends heavily on the physician's knowledge of the condition.

Reported frequency of TRALI

One single-hospital prospective study estimated frequency for all blood components transfused without any donor selection as 1 in 5000 units.[2] A retrospective single-hospital study estimated the incidence as 1 in 7900 units of FFP only.[80] Hemovigilance data from voluntary reports in the United Kingdom found a reported incidence of approximately 1 in 30,000 units of FFP transfused.[85] Retrospective studies of ALI/TRALI in critically ill patients and a single prospective trial of TRALI after FFP infusion found that as many as 1 in 50 to 200 units of plasma from parous female donors could cause some respiratory dysfunction when compared to plasma from male donors.[74,78]

It is not possible to give a single figure for incidence, but the chance of female donor plasma containing an antibody matching a recipient antigen is greater than 1 in 50. Severe and clinically distinct TRALI probably occurs about 1 in 2500 to 4000 units of female donor plasma transfused. ALI in which transfusion is a contributory factor in a critically ill patient may be much more common.

Prevention

The majority of severe TRALI cases have an antibody-related etiology. Therefore, prevention is largely aimed at reducing the likelihood of transfusion of the causative antibodies. There are several strategies to be considered.

Avoidance of unnecessary transfusion of plasma

This includes unjustified transfusion of plasma components such as FFP and unnecessary transfusion of plasma associated with RBCs. Use of FFP varies considerably among countries, and it has been demonstrated that use to correct minor coagulopathies is both ineffective and unnecessary.[97,98] Avoidance of unnecessary transfusion of FFP will reduce the potential for transfusion of units containing antibody. RBCs in additive solution containing less than 20 mL residual plasma are uncommon causes of TRALI, and in those recorded cases there have usually been multiple antibodies in the donor plasma matching cognate antigens in the recipient. Whole blood donations, particularly from high-risk donors (parous female or previously transfused donors), can be processed into RBCs in additive solution with minimal remaining plasma. Similarly, use of platelet additive solutions will reduce the volume of plasma with platelets.

High-risk donor exclusion

The most straightforward form of this policy is to exclude donations from all female donors from production of plasma-rich components. Some individual blood centers have followed such policies locally for some years.[99] The effectiveness of this intervention was demonstrated in the United Kingdom, where such a policy was instituted nationally in 2003. An active hemovigilance scheme clearly showed a 66% decrease both in the incidence of probable TRALI and in associated deaths over the next three years (Figure 59.8).[100] Further developments of this policy include excluding only females with a history of pregnancy and excluding any donor with a history of transfusion or organ grafting. Evidence of the efficacy of excluding female donor plasma comes from many countries, including those of North America and the Netherlands, Germany, and Australia.

Antibody testing

By testing donors for HLA and HNA antibodies, it is possible to exclude all donors with detectable antibodies, or those with antibodies of certain specificities or titer, either from all blood donation or just from donation of apheresis plasma-rich components. This strategy is attractive in that unnecessary exclusion of valuable donors is avoided but it also depends on the sensitivity and specificity of the antibody tests. It has been used with apparent success in some centers.[101]

Use of pooled plasma

Pooled solvent/detergent-treated plasma does not appear to cause TRALI. It is hypothesized that this is because of dilution of antibodies, neutralization of HLA antibodies by soluble HLA antigens in the plasma of other donors, and subsequent removal of the immune complexes in the processing.[67,68] Extensive use of solvent/detergent-treated plasma in Europe has not been associated with TRALI.[102,103]

Nonantibody TRALI and inverse TRALI

Leukocyte reduction reduces the production of cellular activation or breakdown products that have been implicated in TRALI. It also will prevent the rare but distinct cases of inverse TRALI related to bystander granulocyte transfusion.

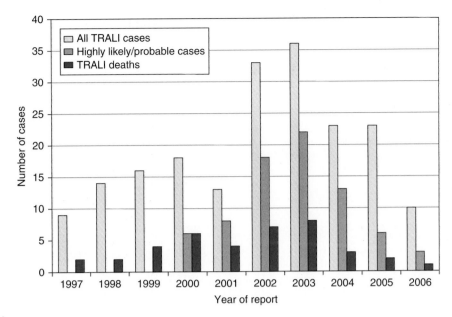

Figure 59.8 Cases of TRALI reported to the UK hemovigilance scheme from 1996 to 2006. After 1998, all cases were considered by an expert panel and classified as highly likely, probable, possible, or unlikely. From 1996 to 2003, case ascertainment rose steadily with increasing knowledge of the condition among physicians. From October 2003, a policy to procure FFP from male donors only was introduced. Following the change, there was a decrease in reports, and a marked decline in highly likely or probable TRALI and in deaths from TRALI (note that cases were recorded by the year that the report was made, and that many cases documented for 2004 occurred in 2003). Source: Data from Dr. C Chapman on behalf of SHOT UK (http://www.shotuk.org). Reproduced with permission.

Conclusion

It has taken over 50 years for the full extent of TRALI to be appreciated. It is now recognized as one of the major but preventable adverse outcomes of transfusion. Preventive strategies through female donor exclusion have proved highly effective. Concerns about loss of donor plasma for transfusion have not proved a major problem partly because more rational and evidence-based use of plasma is reducing demand. TACO typically occurs in patients with cardiac failure, expanded blood volume due to pregnancy, renal failure, or other causes. With the reduction in TRALI-related deaths and introduction of hemovigilance schemes, it has emerged as an important cause of transfusion-related morbidity and mortality.

Disclaimer

The authors have disclosed no conflicts of interest.

Key references

A full reference list for this chapter is available at: http://www.wiley.com/go/simon/transfusion

13 Seeger W, Schneider U, Kreusler B, *et al.* Reproduction of transfusion-related acute lung injury in an ex vivo lung model. *Blood* 1990;**76**:1438–44.

15 Gajic O, Rana R, Winters JL, *et al.* Transfusion-related acute lung injury in the critically ill: prospective nested case-control study. *Am J Respir Crit Care Med* 2007;**176**:886–91.

22 Bayat B, Tjahjono Y, Sydykov A, *et al.* Anti-human neutrophil antigen-3a induced transfusion-related acute lung injury in mice by direct disturbance of lung endothelial cells. *Arterioscler Thromb Vasc Biol* 2013;**33**:2538–48.

37 Silliman CC, Voelkel NF, Allard JD, *et al.* Plasma and lipids from stored packed red blood cells cause acute lung injury in an animal model. *J Clin Invest* 1998;**101**:1458–67.

41 Sachs UJ, Wasel W, Bayat B, *et al.* Mechanism of transfusion-related acute lung injury induced by HLA class II antibodies. *Blood* 2011;**117**:669–77.

43 Looney MR, Nguyen XJ, Hu Y, *et al.* Platelet depletion and aspirin treatment protect mice in a two-event model of transfusion-related acute lung injury. *J Clin Invest* 2009;**119**:3450–61.

72 Piccin A, Cronin M, Brady R, *et al.* Transfusion-associated circulatory overload in Ireland: a review of cases reported to the National Haemovigilance Office 2000 to 2010. *Transfusion* 2015 Jun;**55** (6):1223–30.

CHAPTER 60

Transfusion-associated graft-versus-host disease

Eric A. Gehrie,[1] Edward L. Snyder,[1] & Alex B. Ryder[2]

[1]Department of Laboratory Medicine, Yale School of Medicine, Yale University; and Blood Bank, Yale-New Haven Hospital, New Haven, CT, USA
[2]Department of Pediatrics and Department of Pathology, University of Tennessee Health Science Center, La Bonheur Children's Hospital, TN, USA

Transfusion-associated graft-versus-host disease (TA-GVHD) is a rare but almost uniformly lethal complication of blood transfusion. Although the graft-versus-host disease (GVHD) that occurs after allogeneic bone marrow transplantation and TA-GVHD share some clinical similarities, GVHD after bone marrow transplant is not uncommon and often responds positively to immunosuppression.[1] The much rarer TA-GVHD, however, in contradistinction to bone marrow GVHD, is associated with destruction of the recipient's bone marrow, does not respond to immunosuppressive therapy,[1] and is generally fatal.[2] Because there are no effective treatments for TA-GVHD, management of this complication focuses almost entirely on prevention by irradiation of cellular blood components (whole blood, red blood cells [RBCs], granulocytes, and platelets) that are intended for susceptible recipients. Over the past 10–15 years, the use of irradiation in high-risk situations has reduced the incidence of TA-GVHD in the Western world and Japan to almost undetectable levels. In this chapter, we review the pathophysiology and incidence of TA-GVHD, characteristics of blood transfusion recipients that make them susceptible to the development of TA-GVHD, and strategies to prevent, diagnose, and treat TA-GVHD.

Pathophysiology of TA-GVHD

The development of TA-GVHD requires infusion of viable allogeneic donor ("nonself") lymphocytes, which subsequently engraft, proliferate, and attack recipient ("self") tissues. Unlike GVHD, in which the transplanted donor hematopoietic cells in the engrafted marrow are the cells that mediate the attack on host (recipient) tissues, TA-GVHD results in destruction of both the host tissues and host bone marrow by donor T lymphocytes that engraft in the recipient following transfusion. It is the host bone marrow aplasia that occurs only in TA-GVHD that drives its lethality.

The biologic basis for the differentiation of "self" and "nonself" is based on immune recognition of specific cell surface proteins, most importantly human leukocyte antigens (HLA), which are expressed on the surface of both immune and non-immune cell types. In most situations, transfused donor lymphocytes are identified by the host immune system due to their expression of "non-self" HLA proteins. The recognition of "non-self" HLA proteins by the host immune system usually leads to attack and death of donor lymphocytes contained in the transfused unit of blood or platelets. However, in rare situations, transfused donor lymphocytes are not recognized as "non-self" by the recipient immune system. If the transfused donor lymphocytes are sufficiently viable to engraft and proliferate within the recipient, TA-GVHD can result.

Partially because TA-GVHD is exceptionally rare, the precise circumstances needed to induce TA-GVHD are not known. Transfusion-associated microchimerism (TA-MC) is a condition that occurs after transfusion of cellular blood components, in which a small number of donor allogeneic lymphocytes proliferate within a host and remain detectable for years. TA-MC is associated with perhaps 10% of patients transfused after sustaining traumatic injury, but is not known to have any clinical sequelae.[3] Distinguishing the factors that influence why T-lymphocyte engraftment sometimes results in severe disease (TA-GVHD), and sometimes results in no disease manifestations (TA-MC), is the subject of ongoing investigation.

In many cases, the presence of severe acquired or congenital immune deficiency in the transfusion recipient serves as a prerequisite to the development of TA-GVHD. TA-GVHD, however, has also been reported to occur in the absence of a recognized immune deficiency, particularly in situations where the blood donor is homozygous for HLA antigens for which the recipient is heterozygous.[2] In this scenario, all HLA antigens expressed by the donor are also expressed by the host, but the host expresses HLA antigens that are not expressed by the donor. This can result in *unidirectional tolerance*, where donor lymphocytes are spared from attack by the host immune system, whereas host tissues are left vulnerable to attack by donor lymphocytes and their progeny (Figure 60.1).

Incidence of TA-GVHD

At present, TA-GHVD is an extremely rare phenomenon. In the United Kingdom, more than 40 million cellular blood components have been transfused since 1999 (Table 60.1). During that interval, there has been only one case of reported TA-GVHD. Similar data compiled by the US Food and Drug Administration (FDA) identified only three cases of fatal TA-GVHD in the United States from 2005 to 2013, during which time almost 150 million cellular blood components were transfused (Table 60.2). In both the United Kingdom and the United States, widespread use of blood component irradiation in at-risk populations has contributed to the low incidence of TA-GVHD.

In Japan, there is substantially less HLA diversity than in the United States or the United Kingdom. In addition, Japan has a high rate of directed-donor blood collections where relatives donate

---

Rossi's Principles of Transfusion Medicine, Fifth Edition. Edited by Toby L. Simon, Jeffrey McCullough, Edward L. Snyder, Bjarte G. Solheim, and Ronald G. Strauss.
© 2016 John Wiley & Sons, Ltd. Published 2016 by John Wiley & Sons, Ltd.

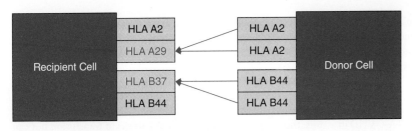

HLA A2

HLA A29

Recipient Cell

HLA B37

HLA B44

HLA A2

HLA A2

Donor Cell

HLA B44

HLA B44

← Immune Attack on Recipient Cell Mediated by Detection by Donor Cell of "non-self" HLA type

Figure 60.1 Unidirectional tolerance occurs when donor lymphocytes mediate an attack on host tissues while simultaneously being viewed as "self" by the host immune system. In this example, recipient cells expressing HLA A29 and HLA B37 antigens are attacked by donor lymphocytes that do not express these antigens; however, donor-derived HLA A2 and HLA B44 expressing cells are not targeted by the recipient immune system because these antigens are also expressed by recipient cells. Scenario depicted similar to a case report by Benson et al.[49]

Table 60.1 UK reports of cellular blood component infusions and TA-GVHD to the serious hazards of transfusion hemovigilance network, 1996–2013

Year	Number of RBCs Transfused (UK)	Number of Platelets Transfused (UK)	Reports of TA-GVHD (UK)	Reference
2013	2,043,046	312,140	0	[34]
2012	2,146,783	311,737	1 (Fatal)	[14]
2011	2,162,137	301,628	0	[35]
2010	2,180,781	246,962	0	[36]
2009	2,209,153	266,312	0	[37]
2008	2,174,256	258,419	0	[38]
2007	2,235,638	255,474	0	[39]
2006	2,316,152	259,654	0	[40]
2005	2,428,934	258,528	0	[41]
2004	2,607,410	264,539	0	[42]
2003	2,678,098	251,741	0	[43]
2001–2002	2,679,925	251,451	0	[44]
2000–2001	2,706,307	250,259	1 (Fatal)	[21]
1999–2000*	2,737,572	249,622	0	[45]
1998–1999	2,386,475	259,025	4 (All fatal)	[20]
1997–1998	2,750,000	330,000	4 (All fatal)	[19]
1996–1997	2,430,000	252,000	4 (All fatal)	[18]
Total	40,872,667	4,579,491	14	

*Universal leukodepletion introduced in 1999.

blood for other family members.[4,5] As a result, Japan has historically had a higher rate of TA-GVHD, and a large proportion of TA-GVHD case reports are published by Japanese authors.[4,5] Indeed, in Japan prior to the routine irradiation of blood components, TA-GVHD had a calculated expected incidence of 1 in 874 transfusions when donor and recipient were unrelated, and 1 in 102

Table 60.2 Reports of TA-GVHD to US FDA compared to annual estimates of transfusion of cellular blood components, 2005–2013

Year	Number of RBCs Transfused (US)	Number of Platelets Transfused (US)	Number of Reports of Fatal TA-GVHD to FDA	Reference
2013	NR	NR	0[16]	[16]
2012	NR	NR	0[16]	[16]
2011	13,785,000	2,169,000*	1[16]	[16, 46]
2010	NR	NR	1[16]	[16]
2009	NR	NR	0[16]	[16]
2008	15,014,000	2,021,000*	0[17]	[17, 47]
2007	NR	NR	0[17]	[17]
2006	14,650,000	1,731,000*	0[17]	[17, 48]
2005	NR	NR	1[17]	[17]
Total	130,347,000 (est)	17,763,000 (est)	3	

*Apheresis equivalent units.
NR, Not reported; est, estimate.

when donor and recipient were a mother–child pair.[4] Routine irradiation of cellular blood components was introduced in Japan in 1998, and there have been no published reports of TA-GVHD in Japan between 1999 and 2013.[2] Similar scenarios are found in other countries where there is substantially less HLA diversity among the donor–recipient population.

Clinical scenarios associated with TA-GVHD

Patients without recognized immunodeficiency syndromes

Prior to the widespread irradiation of cellular blood components in Japan, the rate of TA-GVHD in Japan was higher than in Western Europe or the United States. The Japanese medical literature describes numerous cases of TA-GVHD in patients without a recognized immunodeficiency.[6] Uchida et al. reported that, among 66 confirmed cases of TA-GVHD in Japan from 1992 to 1999, 65 of the patients were not considered by the study authors to be immunosuppressed.[2] The majority of these patients received transfusions either during the treatment of solid tumors or for surgical or traumatic bleeding episodes.[2] Similarly, Juji et al. reported 96 cases of TA-GVHD among immunocompetent Japanese undergoing cardiac surgery between 1981 and 1986.[7]

There are several factors that appear to play a role in the pathogenesis of TA-GVHD among patients without recognized immunodeficiency syndromes. One contributing factor is likely the relative HLA homogeneity in Japan, where many of the cases were reported. A study of 655 Japanese found the frequency of the most common HLA haplotype to be 7.5%, and the second most common HLA haplotype had a frequency of 5%. In contrast, the same study found the frequency of the most frequent HLA haplotype among US Caucasians to be only 4%, and the most common HLA haplotype among Italians was identified in only 2.2% of the population.[4] It is likely that the lack of HLA diversity among the Japanese population resulted in unidirectional tolerance more frequently in Japan than in other parts of the world, helping to explain the historically high levels of TA-GVHD in Japan prior to widespread irradiation of cellular blood components. However, the calculated incidence of TA-GVHD based on HLA similarity is much lower than the actual incidence of TA-GVHD,[1,8] indicating that a lack of HLA diversity is likely only one of many factors that influence the pathogenesis of TA-GVHD.

Another factor that may contribute to TA-GVHD in some patients is trauma or major surgery, particularly cardiac surgery.[9] Although the mechanism of immune suppression, if any, contributing to TA-GVHD in these patient populations is not known, it has been reported that hospitalized patients, compared to healthy volunteers, are less likely to generate antibodies after exposure to allogeneic, minor blood group antigens via transfusion.[10] Consequently, it is possible that although hospitalization and surgery help to prevent alloimmunization, they simultaneously increase the risk of developing TA-GVHD. This hypothesis may also help explain the reported relatively high (10%) incidence of TA-MC seen after transfusion following a traumatic injury.[3]

Besides cardiac surgery and HLA similarity between donor and recipient, other factors that have been associated with TA-GVHD in immunocompetent individuals have also been described, including transfusion of recently collected (<72 hours old) blood,[6] use of blood collected from first- or second-degree relatives,[6] and use of nonirradiated cellular blood products.[11] These factors likely enhance the probability of developing TA-GVHD by either enhancing the viability or dose of transfused lymphocytes (e.g., using fresh or non-leukoreduced or non-irradiated blood components) or increasing the likelihood of HLA similarity between donor and recipient (e.g., using blood from close family relations). A murine model of TA-GVHD has been described.[1]

TA-GVHD in immunosuppressed patients

Although cases of TA-GVHD are reported among patients without recognized immunodeficiency, many more reported cases involve patients who are profoundly immunosuppressed.[8] Among immunosuppressed patients, those considered at highest risk for the development of TA-GVHD include patients with severe T-cell immunodeficiency syndromes (e.g., severe combined immunodeficiency or DiGeorge syndrome), patients undergoing allogeneic or autologous bone marrow transplant, patients diagnosed with Hodgkin's lymphoma or aplastic anemia on immunosuppressive therapy, neonates, a fetus receiving intrauterine transfusions, and patients being treated with purine analogs (fludarabine, cladribine, or deoxycoformicin) or alemtuzumab (anti-CD52).[8,12,13] Although rare cases of TA-GVHD have been reported in patients after organ transplantation, undergoing treatment for solid tumors, or with either non-Hodgkin's lymphoma or acute leukemia (without stem cell transplantation), the risk is generally considered to be lower compared to the first groups listed above.[12,13] No cases of TA-GVHD attributed only to immunodeficiency caused by HIV/AIDS (in the absence of other conditions listed above) have been reported in the medical literature to date.[12,13] National guidelines from the United Kingdom and Australia address the importance of ensuring that all cellular blood products used in high-risk settings are appropriately irradiated.[12,13]

In a recent case report in 2011 in the United Kingdom, two intrauterine transfusions were administered to a fetus (hemoglobin 4.4 g/dL) at 21 weeks gestation who was anemic due to a maternal parvovirus infection. The transfusions were performed using a total of 33 mL of non-leukoreduced, nonirradiated blood that had been collected from the mother.[14,15] Although cellular blood components (including whole blood) intended for intrauterine transfusions are generally leukoreduced and irradiated in the United Kingdom, these product modifications were not made in this case due to the emergent need for the transfusions. At 32 weeks gestation, the fetus was delivered hydropic and pancytopenic. Two months after birth, a bone marrow biopsy revealed an aplastic marrow, and maternal engraftment was detected by chimerism studies. HLA typing performed on the mother found her to be HLA homozygous and showed unidirectional tolerance for her child. The neonate was diagnosed with TA-GVHD and died despite attempted allogeneic stem cell transplantation using stem cells collected from the mother.

Diagnosis of TA-GVHD

The most common signs and symptoms of TA-GVHD are fever, erythema, pancytopenia, bone marrow aplasia, diarrhea, and hepatitis; these generally occur within 1–2 weeks of transfusion but can be seen up to 30 days after transfusion.[2,5] The case fatality rate for TA-GVHD approaches 100%.[2,14,16–21] The diagnosis of TA-GVHD requires a high degree of clinical suspicion, particularly given the relatively long latency period between transfusion and the development of symptoms (up to 30 days). In addition, if patients are critically ill at the time of their transfusion, it may be difficult to differentiate the clinical signs of TA-GVHD from their underlying illness. For these reasons, TA-GVHD may be underdiagnosed.[22] Nonetheless, a diagnosis of TA-GVHD should be considered in any patient with fever, erythema, neutropenia, diarrhea, and hepatitis within 30 days of a transfusion with nonirradiated cellular blood products (whole blood, RBCs, granulocytes, or platelets). It is notable that reports of TA-GVHD have never been attributed to transfusions with plasma, cryoprecipitate, factor concentrates, albumin, intravenous immunoglobulin, or previously frozen, deglycerolized RBCs. This is presumably due to the absence of sufficient viable donor lymphocytes in these products.[12]

If TA-GVHD is suspected clinically, donor lymphocytes can be differentiated from host lymphocytes by measuring differences in restriction fragment length polymorphisms or numbers of short tandem repeats between the donor and the host. These tests can be performed using molecular assays that are routinely utilized to detect donor–recipient chimerism in patients who have undergone allogeneic stem cell transplantation.[22] One strategy is to biopsy both affected and unaffected patient tissues and to compare the results to samples obtained from the blood donor (if available).[12] In older reports, detection of the Y chromosome was used to diagnose TA-GVHD resulting from a blood transfusion from a male donor to a female recipient.[23] Today, this approach is considered to be relatively insensitive in most circumstances, and would be of no use in cases of TA-GVHD suspected in male recipients, in patients who have undergone a sex-mismatched stem cell transplant, or in cases involving transfusion of a blood component collected from a female donor.

Prevention of TA-GVHD

Although the introduction of universal leukoreduction is associated temporally with a reduction in the reported incidence of TA-GVHD, cases of TA-GVHD have been reported in patients receiving leukoreduced (but nonirradiated) cellular blood transfusions.[24] In addition, the minimum dose of lymphocytes required to cause TA-GVHD in humans is not precisely known, and it may be influenced by factors that are not likely to be fully known prior to transfusion. These factors include the degree of HLA match between donor and recipient, the viability of the remaining transfused lymphocytes, and the degree of immunosuppression of the recipient. Consequently, leukoreduction alone is not considered to be sufficient prophylaxis against TA-GVHD; irradiation of cellular blood components is the only widely recognized method to prevent TA-GVHD in all cellular blood components.[12]

In the United States, in order to render lymphocytes contained in RBCs, platelets, granulocytes, or whole blood incapable of engraftment, it is an AABB Standard that for blood component irradiation, 25 Gy must be directed at the center of the blood component being irradiated, with a minimum of 15 Gy at any part of the bag.[25] Of note, standards in the United Kingdom require a minimum dose of 25 Gy, with no more than 50 Gy delivered to any portion of the bag.[12] Special, radiation-sensitive labels are used to verify and permanently document that a blood product was irradiated. The expiration date of irradiated RBCs is shortened to 28 days from the date of irradiation, or the product's original expiration, whichever comes first.[25] In contrast, platelet component expiration is not affected by irradiation. Blood products that are inadvertently irradiated more than once, or at a dose not in accordance with standards, usually need to be discarded, unless the medical director of the facility determines otherwise.

It must be noted that bone marrow, peripheral blood stem cells, or donor lymphocytes infused as part of a hematopoietic stem cell transplant program must *never* be irradiated.

Most blood banks or blood centers use ^{137}Cs, ^{60}Co, or X-rays as a source of ionizing radiation to provide the required dose of radiation.[26] In order to remove sources of ionizing radiation from hospital blood banks or blood centers that could be used for domestic terrorism, the US government is reviewing the possibility of eliminating irradiators that use ^{137}Cs or ^{60}Co and replacing them with X-ray-based irradiators.

In the future, γ irradiation may be one of several acceptable ways to prevent TA-GVHD. Pathogen inactivation systems using amotosalen[27,28] or riboflavin[29,30] and ultraviolet (UV) light have shown promise in inactivating lymphocytes and potentially preventing TA-GVHD. At present, however, pathogen inactivation systems are not available for use with RBCs, whole blood, or granulocytes and are not widely used in the United States for prevention of TA-GVHD in platelets. This is an area that may rapidly change in the future, given recent (2014) regulatory action in the United States licensing amotosalen/UV-A light systems for pathogen reduction of fresh frozen plasma (FFP) and platelets. Special tags that are sensitive to UV light can be used to label usints of plasma or platelets that have been pathogen inactivated using amotosalen and UV light.

Due to the rarity of cases of TA-GVHD, and the limited availability of irradiation in hospitals in some rural areas of the United States, there is not universal consensus on the specific medical conditions that require the use of irradiated cellular blood products. Some of the most common indications for irradiation are summarized in Table 60.3. In some areas of the world where cellular blood product irradiation is not universal, patients with TA-GVHD risk factors are occasionally transfused with non-irradiated blood.[31] Fortunately, the incidence of TA-GVHD is still very low among patients with risk factors who should have received irradiated blood. For example, in the United Kingdom between 2006 and 2010, there were 389 instances where patients inadvertently received nonirradiated cellular blood components (when irradiation was indicated). This cohort included 178 patients undergoing purine analog therapy, 68 patients with lymphoma (including Hodgkin's lymphoma), and 44 patients undergoing stem cell transplant. None of these patients developed TA-GVHD as a consequence of their transfusion, although the reason for this lack of negative outcomes is unclear. Possible explanations include lack of HLA similarity between donors and recipients, or decreased lymphocyte viability due to the storage time of the blood component before transfusion. Regardless, if a patient at risk for TA-GVHD is transfused with a nonirradiated cellular blood component, they should be monitored for signs of TA-GVHD for 30 days.

Table 60.3 Stratification of risk for development of TA-GVHD based on medical condition, component infused, and medication exposures

Highest Risk Association	Lower-Risk Association	No Known Risk
Medical Conditions -Stem cell transplant -Aplastic anemia -Neonatal status -Intrauterine status -Hodgkin's lymphoma -Severe cellular immunodeficiency syndromes	**Medical Conditions** -Acute leukemia -Solid organ transplantation -Solid tumors -Non-Hodgkin's lymphoma -T cell malignancies -Patients undergoing trauma resuscitations or cardiac surgery	**Medical Conditions** -HIV/AIDS -Congenital humoral immunodeficiencies
Blood Components -Nonirradiated whole blood -Nonirradiated RBCs -Nonirradiated platelets -Nonirradiated granulocytes -Nonirradiated cellular components used for intrauterine transfusions -Nonirradiated "fresh" (<72 hours from collection) cellular blood components -Nonirradiated cellular components collected from first- or second- degree relatives, or in transfusion within population with limited HLA diversity (e.g., Japan)		**Blood Components** -Plasma -Clotting factor concentrates -Cryoprecipitate -Albumin -Intravenous immunoglobulin -Irradiated whole blood -Irradiated RBCs -Previously frozen, deglycerolized RBCs -Irradiated platelets -Irradiated granulocytes -Freeze-dried plasma
Medications -Purine analogs (e.g., fludarabine, cladribine, and deoxycoformicin) -Purine antagonists (e.g., clofarabine) -Alemtuzumab (anti-CD52)	**Medications** Other cytotoxic or immunomodulatory agents (e.g., ATG or rituximab)	**Medications** Noncytotoxic, nonimmunomodulatory agents (e.g., antibiotics)

Treatment of TA-GVHD

There are only rare reports of patients surviving TA-GVHD. In one case, recovery was attributed to treatment with OKT3 and cyclosporin A.[32] Another case of atypical TA-GVHD resolved spontaneously, although the patient had a maculopapular rash, which is not classic for TA-GVHD.[33] However, overall, one of the distinguishing characteristics of TA-GVHD, compared to post–bone marrow transplant GVHD, is that TA-GVHD does not usually respond to immunosuppressive therapy.[1] Unfortunately, treatment is supportive and the case fatality rate approaches 100%.

Conclusion

TA-GVHD is a rare but almost uniformly fatal consequence of transfusion with cellular blood components. Although the incidence of TA-GVHD in the United States, the United Kingdom, and Japan has become very low in the past 10–15 years, there are still sporadic case reports. Therefore, vigilance—in terms of both avoidance of unnecessary transfusions and irradiation of blood components given to high-risk patients who are susceptible to TA-GVHD—must continually be borne in mind.

Key references

A full reference list for this chapter is available at: http://www.wiley.com/go/simon/transfusion

2 Uchida S, Tadokoro K, Takahashi M, Yahagi H, Satake M, Juji T. Analysis of 66 patients definitive with transfusion-associated graft-versus-host disease and the effect of universal irradiation of blood. *Transfus Med* 2013 Dec;**23**(6):416–22.

4 Ohto H, Yasuda H, Noguchi M, Abe R. Risk of transfusion-associated graft-versus-host disease as a result of directed donations from relatives. *Transfusion* 1992 Sep;**32**(7):691–3.

12 Treleaven J, Gennery A, Marsh J, *et al.* Guidelines on the use of irradiated blood components prepared by the British Committee for Standards in Haematology blood transfusion task force. *Br J Haematol* 2010 Jan;**152**(1):35–51.

13 Australian and New Zealand Society of Blood Transfusion (ANZSBT). *Guidelines for prevention of transfusion-associated graft-versus-host disease (TA-GVHD).* Sydney, Australia: ANZSBT, 2011.

14 Bolton-Maggs PHB (Ed.), Watt A, Thomas D, Cohen H; Serious Hazards of Transfusion (SHOT) Steering Group. *The 2012 annual SHOT report.* Manchester, UK: SHOT, 2013.

CHAPTER 61

Transfusional iron overload

Sujit Sheth

Department of Pediatrics, Weill Cornell Medical College, New York, NY, USA

Introduction

Tissue iron overload inevitably results in patients who receive regular red blood cell (RBC) transfusions for congenital or acquired anemias. Iron is initially sequestered in normal storage sites, namely the liver and monocyte–macrophage (reticuloendothelial) system, but as these tissues become increasingly saturated, iron begins to deposit in other organs such as the endocrine glands and the heart. The body lacks an effective means of eliminating this excess iron, and without therapy, cirrhosis, heart disease, diabetes, and other disorders develop; death is usually the result of cardiac failure. Transfusional iron overload, with its resulting morbidity and mortality, is an important health issue in patients of all ages. Children with thalassemia major (TM), or other inherited disorders such as Diamond–Blackfan anemia (DBA), congenital dyserythropoietic anemia (CDA), and congenital aplastic anemia, are dependent on regular red cell transfusions to maintain their well-being. Children with sickle cell disease (SCD) who are found to be at increased risk of stroke based on transcranial Doppler (TCD) evaluation, or who have developed silent infarcts in the brain, may be placed on a regular transfusion program to reduce the risk of progressive neurologic disease.[1,2] Adults with severe aplastic anemia (SAA) or myelodysplasia syndrome (MDS) may also become dependent on regular red cell transfusions. In addition, with chemotherapeutic regimens becoming more intense and myelosuppressive, patients undergoing treatment for various forms of cancer, particularly leukemias and lymphomas, may also receive a large number of red cell transfusions. Transfusions around stem cell transplantation may lead to iron overload when the indication is nonhematologic, or worsen premorbid transfusional hemochromatosis. With advances in the medical management of many of the conditions enumerated above, including improved chelation regimens, patients also have a better survival probability, thus increasing the number of individuals in whom transfusional iron overload requires close medical attention. Most long-term experience in the management of transfusional iron overload comes from studies in patients with TM. We now understand that the pathophysiology of iron loading is different based on the underlying condition, and consequently the management must be adapted to minimize complications of iron toxicity. Recently, there has been much debate on the relevance of transfusional iron overload in MDSs without consensus on who requires treatment or on the benefits of such therapy.[3] There are no uniform guidelines for assessment and management, and individual tailoring of therapy is recommended.

Pathophysiology

Iron is an essential nutrient required by every cell. It is present in the human body in hemoglobin, myoglobin, and several mitochondrial respiratory enzymes. It serves as a carrier for oxygen and electrons and acts as a catalyst for a variety of oxygenation reactions. It is able to perform these functions in part because of its ability to reversibly and readily cycle between its ferrous and ferric forms. This very property also makes it potentially toxic, capable of producing free radicals, which can cause cellular damage (Figure 61.1).

The normal body iron concentration is approximately 40–50 mg Fe/kg body weight ($\sim$4–5 g in total); women have lower amounts, and men somewhat higher.[4] Three-quarters of this iron, about 30 mg Fe/kg, is contained in the circulating red cell compartment as hemoglobin, and approximately 5–6 mg Fe/kg is present in functional form in a variety of heme compounds (myoglobin and cytochromes) and iron-dependent enzymes. The remainder (5 mg Fe/kg in women and 10–12 mg Fe/kg in men) is held in reserve in the two primary storage forms, ferritin and hemosiderin, in the liver, bone marrow, spleen, and muscle, readily available when required for erythropoiesis. Normally, iron balance is maintained by controlling iron absorption: Iron stores and iron absorption are reciprocally related so that as stores increase, absorption declines, and these processes are closely managed by the iron regulatory "hormone" hepcidin,[5] which plays a critical role in iron metabolism. It regulates the absorption of iron from the gastrointestinal tract through its effect on levels of ferroportin, the protein responsible for transporting iron out of the enterocyte. Red cells are normally broken down by cells of the monocyte–macrophage system, and the iron contained in hemoglobin is usually returned via transferrin to the erythroid precursors in the bone marrow, for recycling into new red cells. Hepcidin controls the release of iron from macrophages, an effect also mediated by ferroportin. In the normal host, when the body has adequate or increased amounts of iron, hepcidin is upregulated, iron absorption from the intestine is inhibited, and iron is sequestered in its storage sites, the macrophages and hepatocytes. The body lacks any effective mechanism for the excretion of excess iron. Iron exchange is limited so that the adult male absorbs and loses only about 0.01 mg Fe/kg/day.

Rossi's Principles of Transfusion Medicine, Fifth Edition. Edited by Toby L. Simon, Jeffrey McCullough, Edward L. Snyder, Bjarte G. Solheim, and Ronald G. Strauss.

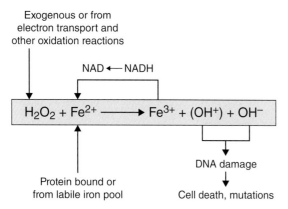

Figure 61.1 Iron-induced oxidative tissue damage caused by free radicals generated through the Fenton reaction.[92] These reactive oxygen species (ROS) affect all tissues, but the heart and endocrine organs may be particularly susceptible.

Iron overload may result from repeated blood transfusion, excessive iron absorption from the gastrointestinal tract, or a combination of these processes.[4] In patients with severe congenital anemias, such as the thalassemias, DBA, or CDA, death from severe anemia in infancy is averted by a regular transfusion program that, if adequate, allows for normal growth and development during the first decade of life. Individuals with MDS or SAA usually begin transfusions later in life. As in normal individual, macrophages process senescent red cells (transfused in these patients) and extract iron from heme. With no effective means for the excretion of this iron, there is gradual tissue accumulation of this iron, which eventually exceeds the body's capacity for safe storage. As the amount of iron increases, there is virtually no change in the amount that is contained within the functional or transport (transferrin-bound) pools, and almost all of the excess iron is stored. Initially, the iron is sequestered in the cells of the monocyte–macrophage system, but with continued accumulation, iron spills over and is deposited in other tissues, usually the liver (hepatocytes), heart, pancreas, and other endocrine organs. Transfusion-dependent individuals may be broadly categorized as those having ineffective erythropoiesis, such as individuals with thalassemia, some MDS, or some forms of sideroblastic anemia; those with effective erythropoiesis, such as individuals with sickle cell anemia or hereditary spherocytosis; and those with decreased or absent erythropoiesis, such as patients with other myelodysplastic syndromes, SAA, or DBA. The "effectiveness" of erythropoiesis, with the ability to incorporate iron into hemoglobin in mature red bleed cells, is a critical determinant of the pathophysiology of iron loading in transfusion-dependent patients. Once transfused red cells are phagocytosed by macrophages, hepcidin levels determine the fate of iron released from heme. If hepcidin levels are high, more iron remains sequestered in these storage cells, and less is released for potential deposit in other tissues. Iron stored in the hepatocyte is similarly retained. In contrast, if hepcidin levels are low, more iron is released from these cells and may be available for deposition in other parenchymal tissues. Thus, hepcidin helps determine the partition and internal redistribution of the excess iron between the monocyte–macrophage and parenchymal sites,[5] another crucial factor in tissue toxicity.

Ineffective erythropoiesis and, to a lesser degree, anemia result in a downregulation of hepcidin expression and result in enhanced absorption of iron from the intestine.[6] Patients with TM or thalassemia intermedia (TI), paradoxically, have relatively low levels of hepcidin even in the presence of iron overload, as a result of their marked ineffective erythropoiesis. In patients with SCD, who have intact erythropoiesis, hepcidin expression varies inversely with erythropoietic drive,[7] with untransfused patients excreting less hepcidin in the urine. Similarly, patients with DBA or SAA, who have almost no erythropoiesis, likely have appropriately elevated hepcidin levels when iron loading occurs. Thus, patients with TM or TI not only have higher iron burdens because of increased intestinal absorption, but also have a greater risk of parenchymal tissue deposition than the latter groups. In fact, patients with TI who have received very few or no red cell transfusions may have profound iron overload as a result of marked hepcidin inhibition[8] as a result of their ineffective erythropoiesis. In patients with TM or TI, regular transfusion suppresses ineffective erythropoiesis to some extent, and hepcidin levels may rise somewhat, but they remain inappropriately low in relation to the higher body iron burden, resulting in iron loading through gastrointestinal absorption. A newly described hormone, erythroferrone (ERFE), has been shown in mice to suppress hepcidin expression.[9] When erythropoiesis is active, even if ineffective, maturing erythroid precursors may produce ERFE, which could suppress hepcidin leading to iron mobilization from stores and deposition in tissues. In thalassemic mice, another growth differentiation factor (GDF15) has been identified, which is secreted during erythroblast maturation and suppresses hepcidin production.[10] Its role in human disease is not completely clear. Therefore, variability in the hepcidin response to the underlying erythropoietic status produce differences in the partition and distribution of the excess iron, even when the volume of red cells transfused is similar. This likely explains the variability of iron deposition in different transfusion dependent conditions.

Although hepcidin levels are critical in modifying the pathophysiology of iron loading in transfusion-dependent patients, several other variables are important in determining the morbidity related to the increased body iron burden. These include (1) the age at which transfusion therapy began, (2) the duration of transfusion therapy, and (3) the initiation and maintenance of effective chelation. Additional modifying factors include other genetic determinants, alcohol use, coexisting viral hepatitis, and other drugs and medications that the patient may be taking. The complex interplay between the underlying disorder and these factors in each individual plays a key role in the pathophysiology of iron toxicity.

Even though the body has the ability to safely store increased amounts of iron, deposition in nonstorage tissues eventually occurs as the body iron burden rises. Without treatment, patients with thalassemia, who begin transfusions in infancy, develop growth retardation, diabetes, and other endocrine disturbances in the first decade of life, and death owing to iron loading of the myocardium occurs during the second decade. Patients with SCD, who receive regular transfusions to prevent the occurrence of strokes, may begin these transfusions later in childhood, and may already achieve normal growth and sexual maturation before the threshold for tissue damage is reached. A comparative study of regularly transfused patients with TM and SCD with similar transfusional iron burdens showed that the latter group had fewer cardiac and endocrine complications.[11,12] The SCD group began regular transfusions at a later age, and had been transfused for approximately half as long as the thalassemia patients, possibly contributing to the observed differences in clinical manifestations. It has been reported that patients with DBA who begin transfusions in early infancy may have higher cardiac iron burdens and may be at higher risk for cardiac mortality.[13] Patients with MDS who begin transfusions in adulthood may not have any endocrine abnormalities, although the iron may contribute to some extent to the diabetes or sexual dysfunction that these older individuals may have. These observations emphasize the relevance of the age at which transfusions are begun, particularly with regard to growth, development, and sexual maturation. As the duration of transfusion increases, severe iron loading may occur in all transfusion-dependent patients who are not effectively chelated, and diabetes and cardiac disease may develop, the latter remaining the major cause for morbidity in all of these patients.

In recent years, there has been much interest and some controversy surrounding iron overload in patients with MDS, specifically the role in pathophysiology and the need for treatment. The major cause of siderosis in these individuals is mostly red cell transfusions, but ineffective erythropoiesis may play some role. Iron deposition in the different organs is not as consistent as it may be in TM, and the role of iron in organ dysfunction is also not clear. Excess iron has been demonstrated in the liver after just 20 units of packed RBCs, and in the heart after 75 units.[14] Iron has been demonstrated in the pituitary and pancreas of these individuals as well,[15] and although hepcidin levels are variable, they are usually lower in low-risk MDS patients.[16] However, removal of iron may improve trilineage erythropoiesis and reduce transfusion requirements,[17,18] with postulated mechanisms including reduction in oxidative stress, increase in erythropoietin, and inhibition of nuclear factor κB (NF-kB).[19]

Iron overload has also been described in the setting of stem cell transplantation, with several studies showing that the incidence of iron overload in these patients is generally high,[20] with higher burdens conferring a poorer prognosis on patients with MDS or acute myeloid leukemia undergoing transplantation,[21] possibly related in part to an increased risk of invasive fungal infections.[22] More prospective studies related to iron in this setting are underway.

As the body accumulates iron from transfused red cells, chelation therapy is usually begun to prevent deposition and damage to parenchymal tissues. Just as the rate of uptake of iron by these tissues is influenced by transfusion parameters and hepcidin levels, the variability of the chelation regimen also plays an important role. The timing of initiation, choice of chelator and dosing, and compliance with the regimen are some of these variables. When transfusion and chelation are occurring simultaneously, there is likely a complex and dynamic balance between transfusional iron loading and chelator-induced iron purging.[23] Different organs may take up iron at different rates and likely have different thresholds for when tissue damage occurs. It has been demonstrated that in transfused and chelated patients with thalassemia and SCD, the relationship the liver iron concentration and myocardial iron levels is nonlinear and variable.[24]

In summary, the pathophysiology of iron metabolism in the condition underlying the transfusion-dependent anemia, as well as the factors directly related to the initiation, intensity, duration and effectiveness of both the transfusion regimen and the chelation regimen, contribute to the pathology of transfusional iron overload.

Storage iron is present in the body predominantly in two high-molecular-weight forms, ferritin and hemosiderin. Both forms are stained on pathological specimens by Prussian blue, via the Pearl's reaction. Hemosiderin is insoluble and is deposited in aggregates of varying sizes, whereas ferritin is soluble and more homogeneously distributed within cells. Under physiologic conditions, iron is distributed approximately equally between these storage forms, but as the body's iron load increases, the proportion stored as hemosiderin increases dramatically. A small amount of iron is present in a low-molecular-weight intracellular pool, likely the most toxic form of iron, because of its propensity for producing free radicals, which cause oxidative damage. It is likely that the ferritin fraction is in closer equilibrium with the low-molecular-weight iron pool.[25] As the magnitude of iron excess grows, some stored iron may be mobilized into the circulation from macrophages or hepatocytes. As transferrin is increasingly saturated, some plasma non-transferrin-bound iron (NTBI) may appear. This iron may be more easily taken up by parenchymal tissues that do not normally store iron, leading to toxicity. Thus, it is critical to ensure that effective chelation therapy is ongoing to bind this iron and prevent its entry into cells, thereby avoiding organ damage.

Histopathological examination of the liver in mild transfusional iron overload reveals predominant Kuppfer cell iron deposition, with preserved hepatocyte architecture and no fibrosis. As iron loading continues, the hepatocytes also demonstrate increased iron uptake, and there is some disruption of the architecture and some scarring and fibrosis. Until this point, these changes are reversible with appropriate chelation. With massive overload, there is bridging fibrosis and progression to cirrhosis, which may or may not be reversible.[26] Myocardial iron distribution is heterogeneous, with more in the left heart than the right, the ventricles than the atria, and the epicardium than the endocardium.[27] It has been suggested, based on studies in the iron-loaded gerbil model, that iron in myocardial fibers may cause impaired repolarization of the myocytes,[28] which interferes with generation and orderly propagation of the electrical impulse and may lead to a variety of arrhythmias. With progressive loading, fibers may not contract normally, and a restrictive cardiomyopathy with impaired filling and diastolic dysfunction may result, eventually leading to congestive heart failure. Heart failure is reversible in part, and with improved chelation, cardiac function may be recovered substantially.[29,30] Therefore, long-term monitoring of transfused and chelated patients should include serial measurement of myocardial iron deposition as well as the liver iron concentration.

Transfusional iron burden

The total amount of iron that enters the body via red cell transfusion may be estimated. As the magnitude of the iron burden is critical in the development of complications, it is of great importance to maintain accurate records, in each patient, of the amount of red cells transfused. The total amount of transfused red cells is calculated as the total amount of blood in milliliters multiplied by the hematocrit of each unit (as a percentage) divided by 100. Each milliliter of red cells contains 1.08 mg of iron, and the total amount of iron introduced (K_{in}) is calculated as

$$K_{in} = (\text{total amount of red cells transfused, in mL}) \times 1.08.$$

Alternatively, if the exact volume is not available, the iron burden may be estimated from the number of units transfused. Each unit of transfused red cells contains 200–250 mg of iron. Using one of these methods, the total iron burden may be calculated. Transfusion-dependent patients usually require 200–300 ml/kg/yr of blood, an amount equivalent to 0.25–0.40 mg Fe/kg/day.

With no physiologic means of excreting this excess iron, and the inapplicability of phlebotomy in patients who are regularly transfused, these individuals must receive iron chelation therapy in order to facilitate excretion. A minimum chelator-induced excretion of

0.25–0.40 mg Fe/kg/day would maintain iron balance in such individuals. Higher levels of excretion would be necessary to produce a negative iron balance.

Iron balance may be monitored during chelation therapy to assess the efficacy of such treatment. The total body iron (Us) at any point in time t may be extrapolated from the liver iron concentration (in mg Fe/g dry weight) using the formula published by Angelucci et al.:[31]

$$Us(t) = 10.6 \times \text{liver iron concentration} \times (\text{body weight in kg})$$

For patients who are being chelated as well, there is an ongoing change in the body iron balance as the iron entering the body through transfused red cells is removed by the chelator. In these situations, it is important to monitor the total body iron excretion between measurements of liver iron concentration. This may be calculated based on the amount of red cells transfused (Kin = iron introduced in mg) and on the changes in total body iron between measurements of liver iron concentrations at baseline ($t0$) and a later time (t), expressed as milligrams of iron excreted per day.[32]

$$\text{Total body iron excretion} = (Kin + [Us(t0) - Us(t)])/(t - t0)$$

Clinical features

Although iron deposition in tissues begins soon after the initiation of regular transfusions, signs and symptoms of iron toxicity usually occur after a few years of iron loading, when the usual storage sites for iron have been almost saturated, and there is deposition in other tissues that do not normally store iron. Organs suffer damage, often irreversible, resulting in significant morbidity and sometimes an early death, commonly as a result of cardiac failure.[33,34] A cross-sectional study of patients with thalassemia born after 1970 in Italy found that 7% had heart failure, 6% diabetes, 11% hypothyroidism, and 55% hypogonadism.[35] A third of these patients had died, the cause of death in 68% being heart failure. Such data are not available for other transfusion-dependent conditions or MDS.

Liver disease of transfusional iron overload may be manifested as hepatomegaly; abnormalities in function; fibrosis, which may lead to scarring, bridging fibrosis and micronodular regeneration, and cirrhosis; and hepatocellular carcinoma.[36,37] Patients may be asymptomatic, or have mild to moderate icterus with progression, symptoms, and signs of cirrhosis and hepatic failure.

Heart failure remains the leading cause of mortality in transfusional iron overload. Unfortunately, symptoms do not appear until the myocardium has large amounts of deposited iron, and routine testing by conventional echocardiography and Holter monitoring early in the course almost always yields normal results. With progressive deposition, patients manifest symptoms. Early signs may include a variety of arrhythmias, including supraventricular or ventricular tachycardias, premature of extra systoles, heart block, and atrial fibrillation. Contractile dysfunction affects diastole early,[38] likely the reason that conventional echocardiography, which assesses mainly systolic function, indicates "normal" function. The onset of cardiac failure is late, and often sudden, and it is an ominous sign. Both complications are often refractory to treatment. Therefore, prevention of myocardial iron loading should be one of the main thrusts of therapy.

In patients who begin receiving transfusions in early childhood, the developing endocrine organs are particularly susceptible to iron deposition if effective chelation is not initiated at the appropriate time. The anterior pituitary is most often involved, resulting in slow growth, delayed sexual maturation, and often infertility, the latter being the result of direct iron deposition in the gonads as well. Supplemental growth hormone or sex hormone therapy is often required to treat these complications. The pancreatic islet cells are also susceptible to the toxic effects of iron. Impaired insulin secretion and abnormal glucose tolerance usually precede the development of insulin-dependent (type 1) diabetes and may occur in highly loaded individuals at any age.[39,40] Older males may experience dysfunction in sexual performance, and females may develop secondary amenorrhea related to gonadal iron deposition and disturbances in sex hormone secretion. Thyroid dysfunction, although uncommon, may also manifest at any age.[36]

Other manifestations include arthropathy and skin pigmentation, which are directly related to iron deposition in these tissues. Patients with marked hemosiderosis appear bronzed initially, and with progression may appear darker, or grayish. Complicating the manifestations of iron toxicity are the clinical signs and symptoms of chelator side effects, which are described further in this chapter.

Measurement of iron burden

The goal of therapy for individuals with transfusional iron overload is to maintain iron balance at low levels of tissue iron, thereby preventing the development of overload and complications. When there is little or no ineffective erythropoiesis, simply keeping track of the volume of packed red cells transfused would provide a measure of the body iron burden in transfused patients who are not being chelated. Different tissues load iron at different rates, and the balance between loading via transfusion and removal by chelation is also a determinant in the differential deposition of iron. Thus, monitoring iron deposition in any one organ is not representative of the others. The ideal means of monitoring iron overload would be to periodically assess tissue iron levels in each of the different organs affected using a technique that is safe, accurate, noninvasive, and valid over a wide range of concentrations. Magnetic resonance (MR)-based methods meet almost all of these criteria, and have become accepted as the standard for these tissue iron measurements, although access to centers offering them is still limited.

The reference method for assessing the liver iron concentration (LIC) (normal <1.6 mg/g dry weight) has been the quantitative chemical estimation of nonheme iron in liver tissue obtained by biopsy. To obtain accurate results by this method, several requirements must be met: The patient should not have cirrhosis or focal lesions, the biopsy must weigh at least 1 mg dry weight (dw) (or 4 mg wet weight), and it should be processed using strictly iron-free methods. Serial biopsies would ideally allow monitoring of not only the rate of iron loading and the efficacy of chelation therapy in the liver, but also detection of the development of, and rate of progression of, fibrosis or scarring. Because liver biopsy is an invasive procedure with considerable risks, biopsy is only recommended now for the monitoring of progression of fibrosis or hepatitis.

Instead, magnetic resonance imaging (MRI) techniques have been developed to noninvasively measure the liver iron concentration. Hemosiderin and ferritin iron affect the relaxation of hydrogen atoms present in the nuclei of tissue water molecules. Initial limitations in the technology have been overcome, and more sensitive instruments capable of measuring more rapid signal decay (very short relaxation times) are now used to quantify hepatic and cardiac iron concentration. Two widely used MRI techniques are (1) a gradient echo T2-based sequence, which measures the signal intensity ratio of liver to skeletal muscle;[41] and (2) a stimulated spin-echo R2-based sequence scan (www.resonancehealth.com/

rh_ferriscan; Ferriscan).[42] Correlation between these magnetic measurements and tissue iron content as assessed by biopsy has improved over time, and this method now provides a safe, accurate, and noninvasive means of assessing LIC.[41–43] The relationship between estimates of liver iron concentration by MR methods and the serum ferritin has been variable.

The liver iron concentration (LIC) has been used as an indicator of the body's total iron burden. In patients with TM, who had been cured by stem cell transplantation, phlebotomy was used as a means of removing excess iron that had accumulated from years of red cell transfusions. A serial decline in the liver iron concentration correlated well ($R = 0.98$; $P < 0.001$) with the amount of iron removed by phlebotomy, supporting the idea that the liver iron concentration is a reflection of the total body iron load.[25] It has also been demonstrated that whereas patients with thalassemia who had liver iron concentrations of 6–13 mg Fe/g dw had an almost twofold risk of progression of fibrosis, in those with liver iron concentrations of 13–41 mg Fe/g dw, the hazard rate was almost 9.[44] Furthermore, coexisting infection with the hepatitis C virus (HCV) independently increased the risk for progression of fibrosis threefold. These observations confirmed the results of previous studies that had reported that LIC >7 mg Fe/g dw is associated with an increased risk of hepatic fibrosis, diabetes, and other complications of iron overload. Based on these data, it has been suggested that maintaining LIC in the "ideal range" of 3–7 mg Fe/g dw in regularly transfused and chelated patients should minimize iron deposition in non-storage parenchymal sites and prevent significant toxicity.[45] In addition, individuals who are heterozygous for hereditary hemochromatosis may be asymptomatic with LIC in that range. However, more recently it has been suggested that maintaining LIC closer to the upper limit of normal is more ideal in TM patients, but there are only limited data to support this.[46] Because correlation between hepatic and cardiac iron concentrations is not satisfactory,[24] independent assessment of myocardial iron should be performed.

Although the liver iron concentration can be measured directly by biopsy or noninvasive means, direct quantification of myocardial iron is not feasible. A surrogate for cardiac iron burden, myocardial T2* (decay of transverse magnetization as a result of spin–spin relaxation and magnetic field inhomogeneity) [normal>230 milliseconds], also measured by MRI, has been shown to correlate with function[47–50] and is currently used in several centers. Iron concentrations in the myocardium are much lower than those in the liver, and the iron is distributed heterogeneously in different areas of the heart. A multi-echo spin-echo T2* technique is the most widely used method of assessing myocardial iron. All individuals with clinical cardiac disease had T2* measures of <20 msec, and all subjects with T2* values above 20 msec had normal cardiac function.[47] An algorithm has been developed to assess risk for iron-induced cardiac disease, and abnormalities in both contractile and electrical function, based on T2* values.[50]

More recently, methods for assessing iron deposition in other tissues such as the pancreas and anterior pituitary have been described with some correlation with endocrine function in these two organs.[51,52] However, these techniques are not universally available, and current ideal monitoring includes periodic assessment of hepatic and myocardial iron deposition only. Such serial measurements would be an accurate and reliable means of monitoring the progression of iron loading and the efficacy of chelation therapy.

Magnetic biosusceptometry has been validated to be a safe, accurate, and noninvasive method of quantitatively measuring the liver iron concentration over a wide range of body iron burdens. The principle is that storage iron (both hemosiderin and ferritin) is paramagnetic: That is, when a steady magnetic field is applied, these molecules will induce a field change that is proportional to the number of iron atoms present. An extremely sensitive sensor, or SQUID (superconducting quantum interference device), measures this response. A strong linear correlation ($R = 0.99$) between liver iron concentration determined by biopsy, and by SQUID susceptometry, has validated this technique,[53] but use of this method has been limited because of the complexity and high cost of building, installing, and maintaining the instrument. Currently, only four centers around the world are using this technique. Other limitations include use in individuals who are obese, are very small, or have metal implants or devices that may not be removed prior to the study. In addition, susceptometric methods cannot be used to quantify iron in other organs that may be loaded with iron, such as the heart, pancreas, and other endocrine organs. A new high-transition temperature device, cooled using liquid nitrogen and with better resolution of the signal from surrounding tissues, is under development.[54]

Traditionally, the serum ferritin level has been used as an indirect estimate of the body iron burden. Although several studies have shown a significant correlation between the serum ferritin level and the liver iron concentration estimated by biopsy in patients with thalassemia,[55,56] the coefficient of correlation in most studies was poor, with marked scatter around the correlation line. A recent study in patients with SCD also showed poor correlation between serum ferritin levels and the liver iron concentration measured in biopsy tissue in patients with SCD.[57] There are several reasons for this variability in the serum ferritin level, which do not necessarily reflect a change in the body iron burden. Ferritin is well-known to be an acute phase reactant, and serum levels may be increased by infection, inflammation, hepatic dysfunction, tissue injury, or hemolysis, and decreased when there is chronic hypoxia or a deficiency of ascorbic acid. Thus, it is at best an indirect marker of iron overload; and, although it is practical and easy to measure, it is not reliable as an indicator of the total body iron burden or as a parameter for the monitoring of chelator efficacy, and does not in any way inform of the differential iron loading that may exist between the liver and the heart.

Without the wide availability of noninvasive measures of hepatic and cardiac iron, there is still reliance on the serum ferritin level as a means of monitoring the iron burden and the efficacy of chelation. However, it may actually be misleading in individual patients, remaining stable in the face of rising body iron burden and ongoing deposition in the heart and endocrine organs. Similarly, measurements of serum iron, transferrin or transferrin saturation, and urinary iron excretion do not provide a reliable indication of the level of body iron stores. Plasma non-transferrin-bound iron (NTBI) has been suggested to be a marker of the "toxic iron pool," but its measurement is very complex and is currently still used largely for research purposes only.[58,59] These limitations in serum measurements of iron-related moieties underscore the need for assessment of iron in specific tissues.

As discussed in this chapter, there is variability in iron deposition between the heart and the liver, as a result of the changing balance between transfusional iron loading and chelation.[23,24] Thus, optimal monitoring of iron burden should include assessment of both the hepatic iron concentration by biopsy, magnetic resonance, or susceptometry as well as myocardial iron using the surrogate T2* estimate. These noninvasive monitoring methods are not yet widely available, but special effort should be devoted to securing such testing for patients in order to chelate them effectively and prevent the development of complications.

Management

The primary goal of chelation therapy is to prevent tissue deposition of excess iron, thereby preventing organ damage and resulting morbidity and mortality. Maintaining safe levels of tissue iron requires achieving a balance between the amount of iron entering the body and that being removed by chelation. Unlike in patients with hereditary hemochromatosis, phlebotomy to remove excess iron is not an option for those with transfusion dependence, although it may become an option after the patient has successfully undergone stem cell transplantation, or once therapy has been completed in case of patients treated with intensive chemotherapy regimens. If transfusion therapy is ongoing, iron-overloaded patients must be treated with a chelating agent capable of sequestering iron and permitting its excretion from the body. As discussed previously, a minimum chelator-induced excretion of 0.25–0.40 mg Fe/kg/day is necessary to maintain iron balance in regularly transfused individuals. In less regularly transfused individuals, such as those on intensive chemotherapy regimens or those with thalassemia intermedia or sickle cell syndromes, a lower daily iron excretion rate may be tolerated. Monitoring the rate of iron loading by keeping a record of units transfused, as well as periodic assessments of tissue iron levels, is extremely helpful in tailoring chelation therapy. The ideal chelator should form a high-affinity 1:1 uncharged complex with iron; be able to chelate intracellular iron; be orally effective, with a long half-life, high chelator efficiency, and low toxicity profile; and be effective in removing iron from, and preventing deposition in, all organs that may be affected by long-term usage. Such a chelator is not yet available. Chelators in current use are described in brief in the "Chelation Therapy" section; more detailed reviews of chelation are available elsewhere.[60]

Chelation therapy
Chelating agents

Three iron chelators are in clinical use currently. One of these, deferoxamine, has been the mainstay for approximately four decades; and the other two, deferiprone and deferasirox, have been approved for clinical use in the past 10 years. Table 61.1 shows a comparative evaluation of these agents.

Deferoxamine B mesylate (DFO, Desferal®)

Deferoxamine B mesylate (DFO, Desferal; Figure 61.2), a naturally occurring trihydroxamic acid produced by *Streptomyces pilosus*, was first introduced almost 40 years ago and has been found to be a generally safe and effective means of managing iron overload, ameliorating or preventing iron-induced organ damage, and reducing morbidity and mortality. In fact, patients with TM who were effectively chelated survived significantly longer than those whose chelation was ineffective.[61] Deferoxamine is a hexadentate chelator that forms a charged 1:1 complex with iron that does not readily enter or leave cells and is excreted almost equally by the liver in bile and by the kidneys. Unfortunately, deferoxamine is not absorbed intact when taken orally and has a very short half-life (approximately 15 minutes); it must be administered by subcutaneous infusion using a portable syringe pump over 8–12 hours daily for maximal chelation efficiency.[62] It has been shown that levels of NTBI (the form of iron that more easily enters parenchymal cells) rise in the plasma within 16 hours of the end of the infusion,[62] and maintaining chelator levels in the body is critical to prevent toxic effects of this iron. Patients who receive the drug in this manner often have pain, swelling, and redness at the site of infusion, and may develop injection abscesses. Rare toxicities occur when deferoxamine is present in excess of chelatable iron, including effects on hearing (usually high-frequency hearing loss) and vision (leading to blindness in severe instances).[62,63] For all of these reasons, compliance with this regimen is not very good, and morbidity from organ deposition and dysfunction is often the result. The dosage range for deferoxamine is between 30 and 50 mg/kg administered over 8–12 hours by subcutaneous infusion 5–7 times a week.[63] In severely loaded individuals, such as those with iron-induced cardiac disease,[29] it may be administered by continuous intravenous infusion, although dosing above 50 mg/kg/day does not increase iron excretion further[62] and may result in toxicity. Although cardiac function may improve relatively quickly (2–3 months), such continuous therapy may have to be continued for many months or even years before there is a substantial decline in the liver iron concentration or improvement in the myocardial T2*.[30] A recent review by the Cochrane Collaboration concluded that deferoxamine is still the recommended first-line agent for chelation in patients with thalassemia.[64]

Deferiprone (1,2-dimethyl-3-hydroxypyridin-4-one, DFP, L1)

Deferiprone (Figure 61.2) is a bidentate chelator that forms an uncharged 3:1 complex with iron, enabling it to easily cross

Table 61.1 Chelators in current clinical use

	Desferrioxamine	Deferasirox	Deferiprone
Structure, iron binding (chelator:iron)	Hexadentate, (1:1)	Tridentate, (2:1)	Bidentate, (3:1)
Half-life	20–30 min	10–16 hours	1.5–2.5 hours
Route of administration, frequency	Parenteral IV or SQ, usually SQ over 8–12 hours, 5–7 nights per week	Oral, once daily	Oral, in 3 divided doses
Iron excretion	Urinary and fecal	Mostly fecal	Mostly urinary
Dose range	30–60 mg/kg	10–40 mg/kg	75–100 mg/kg
Usual chelation application	First or second choice as single agent, or in combination	Usual first choice now, and in combination	Usually second choice, and in combination
Reported efficacy	Efficient hepatic and cardiac iron removal	More efficient clearance of hepatic iron, also effective in cardiac iron removal	More efficient in removing cardiac iron, less so for hepatic iron clearance
Adverse events	Local and allergic reactions, optic neuritis, sensorineural hearing loss	Gastrointestinal upset, rash, hepatic and renal toxicity, proteinuria	Neutropenia/agranulocytosis, gastrointestinal upset, arthralgia/arthropathy, hepatotoxicity
Dose adjustment required if	Impaired renal function	Hepatic or renal toxicity	Hepatotoxicity or neutropenia

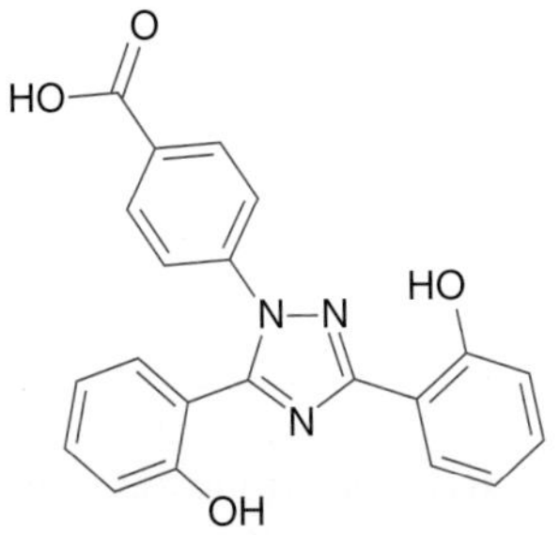

Figure 61.2 Chemical structure of the different chelator molecules.

Deferasirox (Exjade®)
Tridentate (2:1); low MW

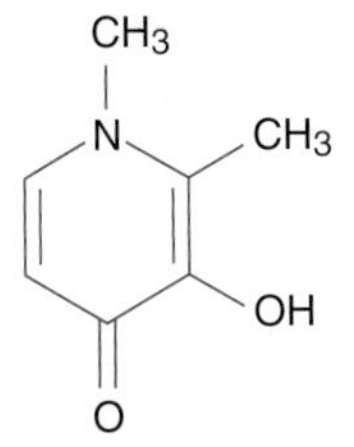

Deferiprone (Ferriprox®, Kelfer®)
Bidentate (3:1); low MW

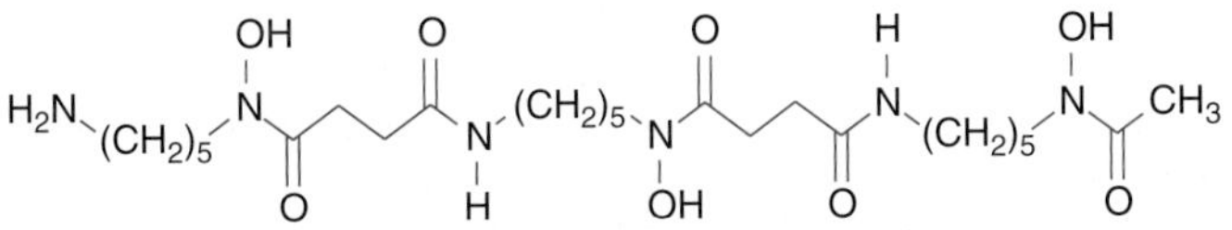

Deferoxamine (Desferal®)
Hexadentate (1:1); high MW

membranes and remove toxic iron from cells. It is effective orally, but has a short half-life (<2 hours) and must be taken 3–4 times a day. Most of the chelated iron is excreted in the urine. It is less effective than deferoxamine in reducing the liver iron concentration, but it has been suggested to have greater effectiveness in removing myocardial iron.[65] A retrospective study comparing TM patients who had been treated with deferiprone long term showed that there were significantly fewer cardiac events as compared with patients who had been treated with deferoxamine alone.[34] Serious idiosyncratic complications have been reported with its use, including neutropenia (up to 5%) and agranulocytosis (up to 0.5%), the development of an erosive arthropathy (from 5 to >20%), and the development of a neurologic syndrome of cerebellar and psychomotor retardation.[66] In spite of adherence to the suggested weekly monitoring of blood counts, one death from agranulocytosis has been reported.[67] Although a Canadian study described progression of hepatic fibrosis in several patients who were on this drug long term,[68] a subsequent study did not confirm this finding.[69] Deferiprone is prescribed at 75–100 mg/kg/day divided into three doses, with careful monitoring of blood counts every week. The ability of this drug to move across the cell membrane led to the idea of using it in combination with deferoxamine, with deferiprone acting as a siphon to bind iron and transport it extracellularly. Although one study showed that patients treated with combination deferoxamine and deferiprone showed significantly greater improvements in T2* than those on deferoxamine alone,[70] the significance of this finding is limited by the small number of subjects and the short duration of evaluation. Although approved for use as an iron chelator, a recent independent review by the Cochrane Collaboration[71] concluded that deferiprone is a second-line agent for iron chelation in thalassemia.

Deferasirox (ICL 670Q, Exjade®, DFX)
Deferasirox (Figure 61.2) is a tridentate N-substituted bis-hydroxyphenyltriazole chelator that forms a 2:1 complex with iron that is primarily excreted in bile. With a plasma half-life of 12–16 hours, once-daily administration means the drug is present in the circulation throughout the day, enabling constant effective scavenging of iron. At the suggested starting dose of 20 mg/kg, most patients are not able to achieve negative iron balance, although this dose appears adequate to maintain iron balance in well-chelated individuals.[72] At higher doses, it is able to cause negative iron balance (reduction in liver iron concentration) but may result in a higher incidence of hepatic and/or renal toxicity. Other side effects include gastrointestinal upset, rash, and, rarely, neutropenia.[72] Patients who are on this agent should have careful monitoring of hepatic and renal function, and appropriate dose adjustments should be made. Studies have shown that deferasirox is able to consistently remove myocardial iron as well as deferoxamine, and higher doses of 30–40 mg/kg/day may be an effective way of reducing the cardiac iron burden and improving function.[73] Because it is the most conveniently administered iron chelator, with once-daily dosing, it has become the first choice of many hematologists for initiating chelation. However, a recent Cochrane Collaboration review[74] concluded that there was not enough evidence to support this in thalassemia, and stated, "If a strong preference for deferasirox is expressed, it could be offered as first-line option to individual patients after a detailed discussion of the potential benefits and risks." Deferasirox has been used with good efficacy in patients with SCD,[75] but there are as yet no long-term studies of this agent in patients with MDS and transfusional iron overload.

Newer agents in the desferrithiocin family[76,77] have shown promise in the animal model. These are tridentate chelators that initially showed significant nephrotoxicity in the rodent and primate models, but, with structural modifications, these have not been an issue. Phase I/II human trials have been initiated, with little human data available to date.

Initiation of chelation
Without data to support a lower range, the optimal range recommended for maintaining the liver iron concentration is 3–7 mg Fe/g dw,[78] as discussed previously. When this range is reached after regular transfusion, chelation therapy should be initiated. There are no immediate clinically apparent consequences of not instituting chelation when the patient reaches this range, or even higher levels of iron overload, because such complications usually result at higher

levels and after more prolonged loading. The goal of therapy is to prevent these complications, and chelation should be instituted well before they occur. Based on calculations in the "Transfusional Iron Burden" section, the range for initiation of chelation is usually reached after approximately 15 transfusions (or a total of ~180 ml/kg of packed RBCs). If records of transfused volumes are not available, the liver iron concentration, as measured by biopsy or noninvasive methods such as MRI or SQUID, should be used in making the decision. Usually in children in whom iron is required for growth, aggressive chelation could potentially reduce the amount of available iron, and a conservative liver iron concentration of 4–5 mg/g dw is usually used as the threshold for initiating chelation (Table 61.2). In the past, a serum ferritin level of 1000 ng/ml was used as the threshold for initiation of chelation, and some models have been proposed more recently[79] to suggest that 800 ng/ml should be the threshold in non-transfusion-dependent thalassemia patients. However, the correlation between the liver iron concentration and serum ferritin was not strong. An MRI assessment of LIC is strongly recommended if possible so as to provide a baseline to which subsequent measures could be compared to evaluate efficacy of the chelation regimen. Cardiac and endocrine organ iron deposition occurs late, and initial measurements are not indicated. Although an oral chelating agent would be much preferred by patients compared to a parenterally administered one, as discussed previously, there is still not enough experience or data with regard to the long-term use of deferasirox or deferiprone as a first-line agent, and these agents are only recommended if deferoxamine is contraindicated. However, given the complexity of parenteral administration of deferoxamine and the ease of administration and proven efficacy of deferasirox, an increasing number of hematologists are initiating chelation with the latter. Deferiprone remains the choice for patients who have tried one of the others and have had to discontinue because of toxicity.

There is much controversy as to when patients with MDS should begin chelation, or if they even need chelation.[3,80,81] Several centers have reported their experience,[82–84] but good data to inform the development of a guideline are lacking. Some studies are underway to gather such information, and there are likely to be some clearer directions in the future. With preexisting bone marrow disease, deferoxamine or deferasirox may be the safer options, but some centers have used deferiprone[85] with success.

Compliance

Compliance with chelation therapy is the primary determinant of morbidity and survival in such patients, and the responsibility of the medical team caring for such patients in reinforcing this cannot be emphasized enough. If compliance with chelation is poor, iron loading exceeds removal and iron accumulates first in the liver and then in the other parenchymal tissues, including the heart. A meta-analysis of 18 studies of patients with thalassemia confirmed that noncompliance results in significant cardiac and endocrine morbidity, and increased risk of death from heart disease.[86] When transfusion and chelation are begun in early childhood, it is usually the responsibility of the parent to ensure that the chelation regimen is followed. In adolescence and young adulthood, when this responsibility shifts to the patient, various distractions and life-changing events may result in poor compliance. Often, a lack of physical symptoms in spite of significant iron overload lulls such individuals into a false sense of wellness and invulnerability. This is a particularly critical time for all caregivers to monitor these patients very carefully. Similarly, older individuals who have begun regular transfusion later in life may feel that it is unnecessary to chelate because the onset of symptoms may be several years later. Education and constant reinforcement are necessary to ensure compliance and reduce morbidity and mortality. Providing patients with accurate estimates of their tissue iron levels may be a powerful motivator, especially when achievable targets for LIC and cardiac T2* are set.

Patients on chelation should be vigilant for symptoms and signs of infection, particularly if they have undergone splenectomy. Because almost all microorganisms require iron to thrive, mobilization of iron sequestered in stores could allow such microbes to run rampant. Therefore, chelation should be temporarily suspended if there is any suspicion of a bacterial or fungal illness, until this is appropriately managed.

Table 61.2 Guidelines for chelation therapy

	Current Guidelines For Chelation
Initiation of Chelation	
When to begin	LIC 3–7 mg Fe/g dry weight, or
	Total transfusion volume ~180 mL/kg packed red cells, or ~15 transfusions
Choice of chelator	Deferoxamine (Desferal®) 35–40 mg/kg by subcutaneous infusion over 8–12 hours 5–7 times/week
	Deferasirox (Exjade®) 20–30 mg/kg/day on empty stomach, daily
Intensification (in conjunction with expert consultation and advice)	
Indication	1. LIC >15 mg Fe/g dry weight, with T2* >20 msec, no clinical cardiac disease
	2. LIC 3–15 mg Fe/g dry weight, with T2* 10–20 msec, no clinical cardiac disease
	3. LIC >15 mg Fe/g dry weight, with T2* 10–20 msec
	4. LIC 3–15 mg Fe/g dry weight, with T2* <10 msec
Regimen	Deferoxamine 50 mg/kg/day
	For 1 and 2: by subcutaneous infusion over 8–12 hours daily
	For 3 and 4: by continuous infusion via central venous catheter
	Deferasirox
	For 1 and 2: 30–40 mg/kg/day
	For 3 and 4: 40 mg/kg/day
	Combination therapy (see table 3)
	Multiple combinations are in use. Usually deferasirox or deferiprone added to a lower dose/less frequent base deferoxamine regimen

LIC, Liver iron concentration.

Table 61.3 Combination chelation therapy

Combination	Deferasirox (DFX) and add desferrioxamine (DFO)	Desferrioxamine (DFO) and add deferiprone (DFP) OR deferiprone and add desferrioxamine	Deferasirox (DFX) and add deferiprone (DFP)
Documented efficacy	Improvement in both LIC and cardiac T2*	Improvement in cardiac T2*, cardiac function (LVEF), and decrease in LIC	Unknown
Synergy	Unknown	Yes	Unknown
Indication	Rising LIC despite DFX at max dose, or DFX dose limited by toxicity	Worsening cardiac T2* despite DFO/DFP at max dose, or to reduce DFO infusions per week	POSSIBLY for worsening cardiac T2* despite DFX at max dose, or DFX dose limited by toxicity
Regimens described	DFX 20–30 mg/kg with DFO 30–40 mg/kg, simultaneously or sequentially	DFO 30–40 mg/kg with DFP 75–100 mg/kg, in a variety of combinations	DFX 20–40 mg/kg with DFP 75–100 mg/kg, concomitantly or alternating

Intensification of chelation

Noncompliance resulting in a positive iron balance and a rise in the liver iron concentration, or shortening of the T2*, would necessitate changes in the chelation regimen to prevent progression of organ damage. The compliance record should be closely examined, and consultation with an expert in the management of iron overload should be obtained, before intensification of chelation is undertaken. Dosage of deferoxamine may be increased to a maximum of 50 mg/kg/day, beyond which there seems to be no additional increment in urinary iron excretion.[62] Higher doses have also been associated with the development of a pulmonary syndrome.[87] Increasing the frequency of subcutaneous administration to seven days per week is a more effective strategy (Table 61.2). For patients with symptomatic heart disease, continuous intravenous chelation with deferoxamine at 50 mg/kg/day has been shown to be effective in reversing heart failure, improving cardiac function, and reducing the liver iron concentration more effectively[18] (Table 61.2). Generally, an indwelling catheter is required, because deferoxamine may cause sclerosis of peripheral veins. Close monitoring for toxicity and efficacy is necessary. Because noncompliance is the primary cause of severe loading, this regimen may not be acceptable to the patient. Studies using 40 mg/kg of deferasirox have shown some efficacy. Various combinations of chelators have been used with reported efficacy in the thalassemias,[29,49,70,88,89] but there are little data in other conditions. However, these reports have not consistently shown efficacy or benefit of a single combination. Some

recommendations are made in Tables 61.2 and 61.3. Longer prospective studies with larger numbers of patients are required before a specific combination therapy can be recommended. Intravenous deferoxamine as described above should be considered the base of the regimen for any patient with a severe iron burden, corresponding to a liver iron concentration above 15 mg Fe/g dw even in the absence of clinical cardiac deposition, and for those with myocardial T2* values below 10 ms.

Monitoring while on chelation

Once chelation is begun, regular non-invasive assessment of iron deposition in the heart (MRI T2*) and liver (MRI R2 or SQUID) every 12–18 months is recommended (Table 61.4) to ensure the efficacy of chelation and give warning of rising levels, which may be associated with significant iron toxicity. When chelation is being initiated, an MR-determined LIC is helpful to establish a baseline, which would help evaluate the success of ongoing chelation. A cardiac T2* is usually not necessary for a few years after chelation has been initiated if compliance is good and the LIC remains in the desired range. If, however, the LIC rises due to ineffective chelation and intensification of the regimen is being considered, a cardiac T2* should be obtained. Given the discordance between LIC and cardiac iron loading while on transfusion and chelation,[24] cardiac T2* should be obtained regularly for monitoring. As previously discussed, higher LIC values predispose to progression of fibrosis,[44] and keeping the LIC in the ideal range of 3–7 mg Fe/g dw is important to prevent this from occurring. A liver

Table 61.4 Recommended comprehensive evaluation of regularly transfused and chelated individuals

System	Test	Frequency
Monitoring of iron load	LIC by biopsy, MRI or SQUID	Every 12–18 months. More frequently if high iron burden and on intensive chelation
	Cardiac T2*	
Cardiovascular	MRI for assessment of function (echocardiograhy with tissue Doppler if MRI not possible)	Annually
	Holter monitoring	Annually
Hepatobiliary	Bilirubin levels and AST/ALT monitoring	Every transfusion visit if on deferasirox or if active HBV or HCV infection. Less frequent if on deferoxamine.
	HBV, HCV serology	Annually
Hematologic	CBC with differential	Weekly if on deferiprone
Renal	BUN and serum creatinine	Every transfusion visit if on deferoxamine or deferasirox
Endocrine	Thyroid and parathyroid function	Annually
	Bone Density	Annually
	Glucose tolerance	Annually
	hGH, testicular and ovarian function	Based on age and clinical indications
Other	HIV serology	Annually
	Vision and hearing	Annually if on deferoxamine
	Pulmonary function	Every 2 years

LIC, Liver iron concentration; SQUID, magnetic susceptometry.

biopsy may be indicated if there is coexisting hepatitis, or liver dysfunction suggestive of fibrosis or progression to cirrhosis. Adjustments in the chelation regimen should preferably be based on changes in the LIC or the cardiac T2*. More frequent measurements may be indicated after such changes have been made to ensure optimal efficacy of the regimen.

In addition to monitoring iron burden and adherence to chelation therapy, organ function must also be monitored for the development of abnormalities related to the transfusion and chelation regimen (Table 61.4). The ideal method for assessing cardiac function is magnetic resonance assessment of chamber dimensions, ventricular filling, and ejection fractions. This would provide indicators of systolic as well as diastolic function. Conventional echocardiography does not provide adequate assessment of diastolic function, and it is suboptimal because cardiac dysfunction in iron-induced cardiac disease is mainly diastolic and systolic function is preserved until late in the course of the iron-induced restrictive cardiomyopathy. Normal results often lead to a false sense of well-being and noncompliance with chelation. Serial measurements may provide useful information on trends and may signal the need for closer evaluation by MRI.[90] Despite preserved global function, tissue Doppler echocardiography–detected regional wall motion abnormalities may represent an early sign of cardiac disease.[91] These special echocardiographic techniques may be of limited use, but annual magnetic resonance–based cardiac function assessment, performed at the same time as T2* measurement, is the ideal method of monitoring. Holter monitoring for development of arrhythmias is also recommended annually. Regular assessment of hepatic and renal function should also be part of comprehensive care. In addition to screening for transfusion-associated viral infections, frequent assessment is also indicated to monitor for chelator toxicity. Comprehensive annual endocrine evaluations, including thyroid and parathyroid function, bone density assessment, glucose tolerance, and gonadal function testing, are recommended, especially for growing children and adolescents. Vision and hearing should be evaluated annually in patients on deferoxamine. Testing of pulmonary function is also recommended, although not as frequently. Monitoring for chelator toxicity should also be followed, as shown in Table 61.4.

Summary

Iron overload is a significant cause of transfusion-related morbidity and mortality. With improved survival of patients with inherited or childhood transfusion-dependent anemias, older individuals with marrow failure, and cancer patients who have undergone intensive chemotherapeutic treatments or stem cell transplantation, the prevalence of this entity is likely to continue to grow. There is evidence to suggest that reduction of iron burden in individuals with MDS and patients undergoing stem cell transplantation may be beneficial and result in better outcomes. More research is underway in those fields. Newer technologies are now available for the noninvasive assessment of the body iron burden, making it easier to quantify the amount of excess storage iron in different tissues and to monitor the efficacy of chelation regimens. New oral drugs have made it easier for patients to be compliant with the chelation therapy that must be instituted in order to prevent tissue iron deposition and ameliorate the toxicity that would result from such deposition. As more information becomes available on the long-term use of deferasirox and deferiprone, combination therapy with deferoxamine may change the way chelation is prescribed. Research continues on the development of newer oral chelators. These developments hold promise for a new era of effective diagnosis, monitoring, and treatment of transfusional iron overload.

Key references

A full reference list for this chapter is available at: http://www.wiley.com/go/simon/transfusion

3 Temraz S, Santini V, Musallam K, et al. Iron overload and chelation therapy in myelodysplastic syndromes. *Crit Rev Oncol Hematol* 2014 Jul;**91**(1):64–73.

4 Brittenham GM. Disorders of iron homeostasis: iron deficiency and overload. In: Hoffman R, Benz EJ Jr, Silberstein LE, et al., Eds. *Hematology: basic principles and practice.* 6th ed. Philadelphia: Elsevier Saunders; 2012: chap. 34.

5 Ganz T. Systemic iron homeostasis. *Physiol Rev* 2013 Oct;**93**(4):1721–41.

20 Majhail NS, Lazarus HM, Burns LJ. Iron overload in hematopoietic cell transplantation. *Bone Marrow Transpl* 2008;**41**(12):997–1003.

29 Porter JB, Wood J, Olivieri N, et al. Treatment of heart failure in adults with thalassemia major: response in patients randomised to deferoxamine with or without deferiprone. *J Cardiovasc Magn Reson* 2013;**15**:38.

35 Borgna-Pignatti C, Cappellini MD, De Stephano P, et al. Survival and complications in thalassemia. *Ann NY Acad Sci.* 2005;**1054**:40–7.

38 Wood JC, Enriquez C, Ghugre N, et al. Physiology and pathophysiology of iron cardiomyopathy in thalassemia. *Ann NY Acad Sci* 2005;**1054**:386–95.

43 Wood JC, Enriquez C, Ghugre N, et al. MRI R2 and R2* mapping accurately estimates hepatic iron concentration in transfusion-dependent thalassemia and sickle cell disease patients. *Blood* 2005;**106**(4):1460–5.

49 Carpenter JP, He T, Kirk P, et al. On T2* magnetic resonance and cardiac iron. *Circulation* 2011;**123**(14):1519–28.

78 Brittenham GM. Iron-chelating therapy for transfusional iron overload. *N Engl J Med* 2011;**364**:146–56.

CHAPTER 62

Immunomodulatory and pro-inflammatory effects of allogeneic blood transfusion

Eleftherios C. Vamvakas,[1] José O. Bordin,[2] & Morris A. Blajchman[3]

[1]Department of Pathology, Cedars-Sinai Medical Center, Los Angeles, CA, USA
[2]Department of Hematology and Transfusion Medicine, Universidade Federal de São Paulo, São Paulo, Brazil
[3]Departments of Pathology and Medicine, McMaster University, Hamilton, ON, Canada

Introduction

The question we confront is whether observations of immunologic consequences of allogeneic blood transfusion (ABT) represent only laboratory curiosities or clinically relevant alterations in the recipient's immune function—the so-called immunomodulatory effect of ABT.[1] The constellation of all such ABT-associated laboratory and clinical findings is known as *transfusion-related immunomodulation* (TRIM). Initially, the term TRIM encompassed effects attributable to ABT by means of immunologic mechanisms only; however, more recently, the term has been used more broadly to encompass additional effects that could be related to ABT by means of both immunomodulatory and pro-inflammatory rather than only immunomodulatory mechanisms.[2]

ABT may either cause alloimmunization or induce tolerance. ABT introduces a multitude of foreign antigens into the recipient, including human leukocyte antigen cell surface receptor (HLA-DR) antigens found on the donor's dendritic antigen-presenting cells (APCs). The presence or absence of autologous HLA-DR antigens on the donor's white blood cells (WBCs) plays a decisive role in whether alloimmunization or immune suppression will ensue following ABT.[3] Transfusions sharing at least one HLA-DR antigen with the recipient will induce tolerance, whereas fully HLA-DR-mismatched transfusions lead to alloimmunization.[4] In addition to the degree of HLA-DR compatibility between donor and recipient, the immunogenicity of cellular or soluble HLA antigens found in transfused blood components depends on the viability of the donor dendritic APCs and the presence of the required co-stimulatory signals for the presentation of the donor antigens to the recipient's T cells. Nonviable APCs and/or absence of the requisite co-stimulatory signals result in T-cell unresponsiveness.[5–7] Thus, when a multitude of antigens is introduced into the host by ABT, the host response to some of these antigens is often decreased, and immune tolerance (or TRIM) ensues.[8] Several immune-function alterations have been documented in association with ABT (Table 62.1).[9,10]

All these ABT-related laboratory immune alterations could potentially be associated with clinical effects. Evidence from a variety of sources indicates that ABT enhances the survival of renal allografts.[11] In addition, other possible effects are increase of the recurrence rate of resected malignancies and the incidence of postoperative bacterial infections, reduction of the recurrence rate of Crohn's disease[12] and the risk of fetal loss in women with recurrent spontaneous abortions (RSAs), activation of infections with cytomegalovirus (CMV) or human immunodeficiency virus (HIV), and increased short-term (up to 3 months post transfusion) mortality from all causes.[13,14]

Different biologic mechanisms may be involved in each of these purported clinical manifestations of TRIM, and the clinical evidence supporting each of the aforementioned hypotheses must be examined on its own merits.[13,15] The specific constituent(s) of allogeneic blood that mediate(s) the TRIM effect(s) also remain(s) unknown, and published literature has suggested that TRIM effects may be mediated by one or more of the following: (1) soluble HLA class I peptides that circulate in allogeneic plasma; (2) soluble biologic response modifiers released in a time-dependent manner from WBC granules or membranes into the supernatant fluid of red-blood cell (RBC) or platelet concentrates during storage; and/or (3) allogeneic mononuclear cells (Figure 62.1).[15]

Beneficial clinical TRIM effects

Enhanced survival of renal allografts

The only clearly established TRIM effect is beneficial: the enhanced survival of renal allografts in patients who have received pretransplant ABT.[11,17] In both observational studies and randomized controlled trials (RCTs), patients transfused with allogeneic blood have been shown to have a significantly better renal-allograft survival than untransfused patients, regardless of the number of HLA-A, HLA-B, and HLA-DR locus mismatches between recipient and donor.[11,18] This is true also when there is a common HLA haplotype, or shared HLA-B and HLA-DR antigens between donor and recipient.[19] The TRIM effect has further been reported to be associated with allografts between HLA-identical siblings.[20]

The ABT-related enhancement of renal-allograft survival has been confirmed by animal data and clinical experience worldwide.[18] In the past, it was a standard policy in many renal-transplant units to deliberately expose patients on transplant waiting lists to one or more allogeneic RBC transfusions. Subsequently, the beneficial effect of pretransplant ABT was thought to be less important with the advent of cyclosporine and other potent

Table 62.1 Documented immune function alterations in association with ABT

- Decreased T-helper (CD4) cell count
- Decreased helper/suppressor (CD4/CD8) T-lymphocyte ratio
- Decreased lymphocyte response to mitogens
- Reduction in delayed type hypersensitivity
- Decreased natural-killer (NK) cell function
- B-cell activation
- T-cell activation
- Hypergammaglobulinemia
- Decreased cytokine (IL2, interferon-γ) production
- Suppression of lymphocyte blastogenesis
- Decreased monocyte and macrophage phagocytic function
- Increased production of anti-idiotypic antibodies

immunosuppressive drugs, and, as a consequence, many centers discontinued its use.

However, a multicenter observational study, reporting on 58,036 renal allografts from cadaveric donors after the advent of cyclosporine, indicated that patients who had received ABT were still more likely to have a successful renal allograft than those who had not.[21] This study reported that the one-year renal-allograft survival of patients receiving pretransplant ABT was 3–5% better than that of those who did not receive ABT. Similar results were also reported for patients who received renal allografts from living-related donors.[22] The beneficial effect of pretransplant ABT in the outcome of cadaveric renal allografts was confirmed by a RCT conducted at 14 transplant centers.[23] Patients were randomly assigned to receive either three pretransplant, *non-WBC-reduced* RBC transfusions or no ABT. The renal-allograft survival was significantly higher in the 205 transfused patients than in the 218 untransfused subjects (90%

vs. 82% at 1 year, $p = 0.02$; 79% vs. 70% at 5 years, $p = 0.025$). The beneficial effect of ABT was found to be independent of age, gender, underlying disease, prophylaxis with lymphocyte antibodies, or the presence of preformed lymphocytotoxins.[23]

There have been two more RCTs[24,25] that compared types of pretransplant ABTs given to prolong graft survival. Both studies were small, enrolling 52 and 144 patients, respectively. The first RCT[24] compared non-WBC-reduced and WBC-reduced RBCs and found no difference in graft survival. However, the WBC-reduced RBCs administered in this 1985 RCT did not meet the current European WBC reduction standard ($<10^6$ WBCs/unit), and all transfused RBC components may have been equally effective in mediating the ABT effect. The other RCT[25] compared recipients of one HLA-DR-mismatched ABT, one HLA-DR-matched ABT, and no ABT. There was no difference in graft survival at one year or five years. The risk of acute rejection in patients who had received an HLA-DR-shared ABT was lower than that observed in the other two groups (19% vs. 33%), but this difference did not attain statistical significance in this small RCT. The three available RCTs[23–25] have employed different study designs and have addressed different clinical questions, so that the integration of their results in a meta-analysis is not possible owing to the clinical heterogeneity of the studies.

In observational studies, recipients of non-WBC-reduced whole blood or RBCs have had better one-year cadaveric-allograft survival than patients given WBC-reduced blood components such as frozen-thawed-deglycerolized RBCs. Such data indicate that allogeneic WBCs are involved in eliciting this beneficial TRIM effect.[26] However, the mechanism(s) involved in the ABT-related enhancement of renal allograft survival remain(s) to be elucidated. An experimental-animal model has suggested that the beneficial effect of donor-specific ABT might be related to the type of transplanted organ. Whereas ABT appears to lead to permanent acceptance of all

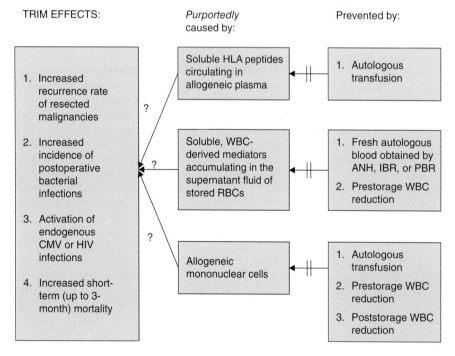

Figure 62.1 TRIM effects, postulated mediators of TRIM, and preventive strategies that could be effective if the TRIM effects were mediated by each corresponding mediator. The purported deleterious TRIM effects are mediated by an unknown constituent(s) of allogeneic blood that may (or may not) include one (or more) of the mediators shown in the figure. Stored autologous blood, obtained by preoperative autologous blood donation (PABD), is replete with WBC-derived soluble mediators because both autologous and allogeneic WBCs deteriorate equally during storage, releasing such mediators. Fresh autologous blood, transfused within hours of collection and processing, is free of WBC-derived soluble mediators and can be procured by acute normovolemic hemodilution (ANH), intraoperative blood recovery (IBR), or postoperative blood recovery (PBR). WBC-reduction filters do not retain WBC-derived soluble mediators, accounting for the difference between prestorage and poststorage WBC reduction in abrogating the TRIM effects mediated by such mediators. Source: Vamvakas (2006).[16] Reproduced with permission of American Society for Clinical Pathology.

renal allografts, this benefit was not observed with pancreas, skin, or heart allografts.[27] ABT administered during the actual operation for renal transplantation has not been shown to affect subsequent allograft survival.[17] In observational studies, patients who receive more than 10 RBCs have a better one-year allograft survival than patients who receive only one or two RBC units. However, patients who receive more than 10 RBCs appear to have a poorer overall allograft survival than those who receive fewer than 10 RBC units.[28]

Such data suggest that multitransfused patients often develop cytotoxic antibodies and are thus at greater risk for earlier and more severe allograft-rejection episodes.[22] Along these lines, Solheim[29] has discerned another potential benefit from pretransplant ABTs, which is especially relevant in settings where there is a shortage of organs for transplantation. When several prospective recipients on a renal-transplant list produce crossmatch-negative results with an available organ, pretransplant ABTs could help identify high-responder patients (i.e., patients most likely to form cytotoxic antibodies in response to pretransplant ABTs, and also most likely to reject a transplanted kidney because of formation of cytotoxic antibodies after a negative crossmatch). Transplant surgeons could thus channel the scarce organ away from such patients, and give it to a patient in whom it is most likely to survive.[29]

A recent Agency for Healthcare Research and Quality (AHRQ) review of all available clinical evidence[30] suggested that pretransplant ABT has a neutral to beneficial effect on graft rejection, graft survival, and patient survival compared with no ABT. However, such benefits were reported mostly in studies conducted before the introduction of modern immunosuppressive drugs and solid-phase technology to detect formation of cytotoxic antibodies. In addition, the strength of the evidence was low.

Three other recent reviews of the clinical literature concluded that pretransplant ABTs place patients at increased risk of forming cytotoxic antibodies, and that the ensuing HLA alloimmunization reduces renal allograft survival and increases wait time for transplantation.[31–33] By searching the MEDLINE, Embase, and Cochrane Library datasets for English-language publications between January 1984 and March 2011, the latest analysis[33] captured 180 studies and data from publicly available registries. The authors noted that implementation of universal WBC reduction had not decreased HLA alloimmunization in patients receiving renal allografts to any significant extent.[34] Although a recent study again reported a beneficial effect of pretransplant ABT with current immunosuppression protocols such as cyclosporine,[35] most current evidence appears to indicate that improvements in graft survival comparable to those previously ascribed to the beneficial "ABT effect" are now attainable without pretransplant ABTs. For this reason, the graft outcome risk–benefit ratio has now become too high to justify consideration of pretransplant ABTs when these can be avoided.[31–33]

In summary, the beneficial ABT effect in renal transplantation is established, and it used to be clinically relevant before the advent of cyclosporine and similar immunosuppression regimens. Before 1984, the demonstration of this beneficial ABT effect had led to the consideration of pretransplant ABT(s) as a strategy to improve renal allograft survival in transplant recipients. However, with the rapid improvement in peri-transplant immunosuppression therapy, the additional effect of ABT became marginal. For this reason, the relevance of such pretransplant ABT protocols in clinical practice diminished because of the improvements in HLA technology and the remarkable advances in targeted and safe immunosuppression. Alloimmunization to HLA antigens can occur despite the use of WBC-reduced blood components. Therefore, in the modern era, the use of pretransplant ABTs should be avoided whenever possible. When ABT is necessary in patients awaiting renal transplantation, WBC-reduced blood components must be given to reduce the risks of HLA alloimmunization and CMV transmission.

Reduced risk of RSAs

Transfusion of allogeneic WBCs has been proposed as a form of immunotherapy for the prevention of RSAs.[36,37] In this setting, the fetus represents a semi-allogeneic graft to its mother, and maintenance of a pregnancy depends on immunologic equilibrium between the implanted fetus and the maternal immune response to the fetus. When the genetic parents share HLA antigens, this balance may be altered and maternal blocking antibodies may not be formed, predisposing the pregnant woman to RSAs. Different transfusion protocols of allogeneic WBCs have been used at various centers to reduce the risk of RSAs, employing WBCs obtained from either sexual partners or third-party donors. Such WBCs have been administered intravenously, intracutaneously, or as an intradermal injection of mononuclear cells obtained by gradient separation. WBC-containing blood products have included pooled buffy coats, single-donor buffy coats, or RBC suspensions containing WBCs.

The American Society for Reproductive Immunology (ASRI) conducted a worldwide collaborative individual-patient-data (IPD) meta-analysis to examine the efficacy of immunotherapy with allogeneic WBCs in patients with a history of RSAs[38] and concluded that such treatment was effective. The effect was small, with only 8–10% of affected women benefiting from the treatment. In contrast to the ASRI data, a recent multicenter RCT[39] that enrolled 183 women with a history of three or more spontaneous abortions reported a nonsignificant decrease in live-birth rate in patients randomly assigned to immunotherapy as compared with controls (36% vs. 48%). However, the size of this RCT was likely inadequate to establish a clinically relevant treatment effect. Thus, the efficacy of transfusions of allogeneic WBCs for the treatment of patients with RSAs remains to be established.

Reduced risk of recurrence of Crohn's disease

Several observational studies have examined whether postoperative recurrence in patients with Crohn's disease (which is immune-mediated) can be reduced by the perioperative administration of ABT. Pooled data from the available studies suggest that the recurrence rate in transfused and untransfused patients is similar: 37.5% versus 40.5%.[12,40–43] However, such integration of the reported data may be inappropriate, because the available studies are observational and medically heterogeneous (i.e., using different follow-up periods and surgical interventions). Nonetheless, an IPD meta-analysis of 622 patients with Crohn's disease found no effect of perioperative ABT on subsequent need for surgical intervention, independent of age, gender, disease location, or extent of the resection.[44] Because many factors affect the risk of recurrence in patients with Crohn's disease, a large RCT is needed to clarify the role of ABT, if any, in modulating Crohn's disease activity in patients with this disorder.

Deleterious clinical TRIM effects

Increased recurrence of resected malignancies

If ABT has a beneficial effect in renal transplantation, where immunosuppression is beneficial because it may prevent allograft rejection, ABT could also have deleterious effects in situations where impairment of the recipient's immune function can be detrimental. In 1981, eight years after the first report of the beneficial effect of pretransplant ABT on renal allograft survival,[11] Gantt[45] voiced his concern that perioperative ABT for curative resection of a malignancy might provoke recurrence of cancer. Thus, if the host's immune response to a tumor contributes to controlling the tumor's growth, the impairment of the host's immunity, due to ABT, would impair this defense mechanism and facilitate tumor growth.

More than 100 observational studies of ABT and cancer recurrence have been reported,[46] and their *unadjusted* results (i.e., their findings before adjustment for the effects of confounding factors) were subjected to five meta-analyses.[46–50] When the available results were integrated for seven cancer sites, there was agreement between the five overviews on the magnitude and statistical significance of the risk of cancer recurrence, death due to cancer recurrence, or overall mortality in transfused compared with untransfused patients. A statistically significant adverse clinical outcome was found among transfused (compared with untransfused) patients for all cancer sites evaluated except for cervix.[46] Brand and Houbiers[46] and Vamvakas[48] ascribed this summary TRIM effect (detected across the unadjusted analyses of the observational studies) to the effects of confounding factors, whereas recent meta-analysts[49,50] portrayed the summary TRIM effect as a real deleterious effect of ABT.

Not finding an adverse effect of ABT when the unadjusted results of the observational studies of cervical cancer are integrated is puzzling.[46] Virus-associated cancers (e.g., cervical cancer) are considered immunogenic, and, should ABT exercise a TRIM effect, the TRIM effect should be apparent specifically in cervical cancer (as opposed to cancers from other investigated sites). By the time of the meta-analysis of Brand and Houbiers,[46] the association between ABT and cervical cancer recurrence had been investigated in six observational studies that had included more than 1000 women. Although the low overall recurrence rate in the six studies precluded a definitive conclusion, no adverse ABT effect was detected across the six studies.[46] These results were possibly due to the fact that, in the development of cervical intraepithelial neoplasia, the expression of HLA class I molecules on malignant cells is specifically down-regulated. Human papillomavirus–specific cytotoxic cells (whose function might potentially be suppressed by ABT) may thus not be effective against cervical cancer cells because of this reduction in class I HLA molecule expression.[46]

Observational studies reporting a significant ABT effect on cancer recurrence continue to be reported,[51] including current reports of a dose-dependent ABT effect mediated by *WBC-reduced* RBCs.[52] The demonstration of a dose-dependent ABT effect in patients receiving WBC-reduced RBCs versus no ABT in the current era[52] parallels the demonstration of a dose-dependent ABT effect in patients receiving non-WBC-reduced RBCs versus no ABT in the numerous (now historical) observational analyses of the 1980s and 1990s.[46–50] Although they do not rule out the existence of an adverse TRIM effect, the current observations[52] link the dose-dependent ABT effect to illness severity necessitating ABT, rather than to a TRIM effect promoting cancer recurrence and mediated by allogeneic WBCs. Similarly, the ABT effect attributed to non-WBC-reduced RBCs in the numerous (now historical) observational analyses of the 1980s and 1990s[46–50] was not confirmed by the available RCTs of perioperative ABT and cancer recurrence, which are discussed in the "TRIM Effects Mediated by Allogeneic Mononuclear Cells" section.

Increased risk of postoperative bacterial infection

Approximately 40 observational studies,[53–58] which had compared the risk of postoperative bacterial infection between transfused and untransfused patients undergoing gastrointestinal surgery, orthopedic operations, cardiac surgery, or various other surgical procedures, seemed to indicate that patients receiving perioperative ABT (compared with those not receiving ABT) had a higher risk of developing postoperative bacterial infection.[53] The studies also indicated that patients receiving transfusion generally differed from those not receiving transfusion in several prognostic factors that predisposed to adverse clinical outcomes.[54] Based on these two sets of observations, some authors concluded that ABT has a direct deleterious effect on the recipient, causing an increased risk of postoperative bacterial infection.[53] Other investigators concluded that clinical need for ABT can be a surrogate marker for a variety of adverse prognostic factors and that the other variables that generated the need for ABT in the published studies also determined the subsequent clinical outcome.[54]

Currently, the controversy over TRIM is focused on differing interpretations[55–58] of the findings of the available RCTs of perioperative ABT and postoperative infection. Hitherto, there have been 22 RCTs[59–80] that compared the risk of postoperative infection and/or mortality between patients randomly assigned to receive non-WBC-reduced allogeneic versus autologous or WBC-reduced allogeneic RBCs. Three of these RCTs[60–62,81] also compared the risk of cancer recurrence between the two randomization arms. Nineteen RCTs were conducted in the perioperative setting; three enrolled HIV-seropositive patients,[72] all hospitalized patients,[75] or trauma patients.[80]

Based on an integration of the results of all nine RCTs published or reported through 2002[59,62,64,68–70,73,76–77] and comparing the risk of postoperative infection between patients randomly assigned to receive non-WBC-reduced versus WBC-reduced ABT in the event that they needed perioperative transfusion, two meta-analyses[55,66] concluded that non-WBC-reduced ABT is associated with postoperative infection. In contrast, a third meta-analysis[57] that integrated the findings of all 12 RCTs published or reported through 2005[59,62,64,68–70,73,76–80] found no association between non-WBC-reduced ABT and postoperative infection. Similarly, no association between ABT and postoperative infection was detected when the findings of RCTs[60,61,65,66,74] comparing recipients of allogeneic and autologous RBCs were integrated.[82]

Two principal reasons for the disagreements between the three meta-analyses[55–57] are (1) the inclusion in the analysis of all 12 RCTs available today versus the nine initially published RCTs; and (2) the integration (or not) of the results of all 12 (or nine) RCTs despite extreme medical heterogeneity. Medical heterogeneity included such factors as the RBC product transfused to the non-WBC-reduced arm (i.e., non-buffy-coat-reduced versus buffy-coat-reduced allogeneic RBCs or whole blood), the RBC product transfused to the WBC-reduced arm (i.e., WBC-reduced RBCs or whole blood filtered before or after storage), the transfusion dose, the surgical setting (gastrointestinal, cardiac, or other), the types of postoperative infections evaluated, the criteria for diagnosing postoperative infection, and the frequency of postoperative infection recorded in each study.[58]

One would expect (1) more of a TRIM effect in association with the transfusion of non-buffy-coat-reduced (compared with buffy-coat-reduced) allogeneic RBCs, because the buffy-coat-reduced RBCs used in Europe contain only about one-third of the donor

WBCs found in the non-buffy-coat-reduced RBCs used in North America; (2) a greater reduction of a TRIM effect(s) attributable to the transfusion of prestorage- (compared with poststorage-) filtered, WBC-reduced allogeneic RBCs, because of the removal of WBC-derived soluble mediators through prestorage (but not poststorage) filtration (Figure 62.1); and (3) more of a TRIM effect in cardiac (compared with other) surgical settings, because in cardiac surgery allogeneic mononuclear cells and/or WBC-derived soluble mediators might serve as a second inflammatory insult that compounds the diffuse inflammatory response to the extracorporeal circuit.[83]

Therefore, one would not expect all 12 RCTs available today (or all nine initially published RCTs) to have targeted the same TRIM effect. In contrast, depending on their design, these 12 (or 9) RCTs probably targeted TRIM effects that varied in magnitude and/or nature, making the integration of all 12 (or all 9) RCTs by a meta-analysis inappropriate. For example, RCTs administering RBCs filtered before storage to the WBC-reduced arm[62,68,70,73,76–80] investigated TRIM effects mediated by both WBC-derived soluble mediators and allogeneic mononuclear cells (Figure 62.1), whereas RCTs transfusing RBCs filtered after storage to the WBC-reduced arm[59,64,68,69] investigated only TRIM effects mediated by allogeneic mononuclear cells. Meta-analyses should integrate only results from subsets of RCTs that are medically sufficiently homogeneous to justify the assumption that all combined studies have targeted a TRIM effect that is *biologically* similar.[58] Results from meta-analyses of such homogeneous subsets of RCTs are presented in the "TRIM Effects Mediated by Allogeneic Mononuclear Cells" section.

Blumberg *et al.*[56] had earlier attributed the disagreements between the three meta-analyses[55–57] to the reliance on the intention-to-treat principle in the meta-analysis that did not detect an adverse TRIM effect of ABT[57] versus the use of results from "as-treated" analyses in the two meta-analyses that reported a deleterious TRIM effect.[55,56] Intention-to-treat analyses often have reduced statistical power to detect a treatment effect compared with "as-treated" analyses.[56] However, both intention-to-treat and "as-treated" analyses demonstrated a deleterious TRIM effect when the analysis integrated the findings of *all* nine initially published RCTs; whereas neither the intention-to-treat nor the "as-treated" analysis showed an association between non-WBC-reduced ABT and postoperative infection when the analysis integrated the results of *all* 12 RCTs available today (Table 62.2).[58]

Increased risk of short-term (up to 3 months posttransfusion) mortality

An association between non-WBC-reduced ABT and short-term (up to 3 months posttransfusion) mortality from all causes was described in the RCT of van de Watering *et al.*[68] This RCT had been designed to investigate an association between non-WBC-reduced ABT and postoperative infection but instead observed an association between non-WBC-reduced ABT and mortality. The association between ABT and mortality was reported as a data-derived hypothesis,[68] and the authors postulated that non-WBC-reduced ABT may predispose to multiple-organ failure (MOF), which might predispose to mortality. These investigators undertook another RCT that confirmed the association between ABT and mortality but did not find an association between non-WBC-reduced ABT and increased MOF.[73]

Several preclinical[84–88] and clinical[83,89–102] observations have supported the hypothesis that ABT in general, and non-WBC-reduced ABT in particular, may be associated with MOF. The mechanisms underlying the development of MOF are unclear, but most evidence suggests that tissue injury is mediated by reactive oxygen species and proteolytic enzymes released from activated neutrophils.[100–102] Silliman *et al.*[84] proposed that ABT may exercise a neutrophil-priming effect mediated by bioactive lipids that accumulate during storage. They postulated that rapidly deteriorating WBCs in stored RBCs release cytotoxic enzymes that may act on fragmented RBC membranes to produce mediators that are responsible for neutrophil priming and endothelial-cell activation (Figure 62.2).

These investigators[84–86] demonstrated that plasma obtained from stored RBCs primes neutrophils for superoxide production and enhanced cytotoxicity, and also activates pulmonary endothelial cells in a dose- and age-dependent fashion. The length of RBC storage was important in these studies, because no evidence of neutrophil priming was obtained when plasma stored for short periods was used. Silliman *et al.*[87] also showed that lipids from the plasma supernatant of RBCs stored for 42 days cause acute lung injury in isolated pulmonary models. Similarly, Chin-Yee *et al.* reported that plasma supernatant from stored RBCs activates neutrophils.[88] In that study, WBC reduction of the RBC units abrogated the effect.[88]

Based on this observation that ascribes a neutrophil-priming effect to ABT (Figure 62.2), it is possible that the reported[68,73]

Table 62.2 Meta-analyses of RCTs of non-WBC-reduced ABT and postoperative infection: impact of the method of analysis and the number of RCTs included in the analysis

| | Method of Analysis | | | | | |
| | Intention-to-Treat[+] | | | "As-Treated"[+] | | |
Number of RCTs Included in the Analysis[†]	Number of Patients Analyzed	Summary OR	95% CI	Number of Patients Analyzed[‡]	Summary OR	95% CI
9 RCTs[59,62,64,68–70,73,76–77] published or reported through 2002[55,56]	5017	1.38	1.03–1.85[*]	3265 (65.1%)	1.56	1.06–2.31[*]
12 RCTs[59,62,64,68–70,73,76–80] published or reported through 2005[57]	6290	1.24	0.98–1.56	4460 (70.1%)	1.31	0.98–1.75

[+] The intention-to-treat analyses included all patients randomly assigned preoperatively to receive non-WBC-reduced or WBC-reduced ABT in the event that they needed perioperative transfusion. The "as-treated" analyses retained only those patients from each randomization arm who ended up receiving transfusion during or after surgery.

[†] Integration of all nine (or all 12) RCTs, as shown in this table, is inappropriate because of the extreme medical heterogeneity of the studies (see text). Therefore, readers should resist the temptation to assign a medical or biological meaning to the figures presented in the table. Instead, readers are referred to Figures 62.4 and 62.5, which depict the results obtained when medically homogeneous subsets of these RCTs[59,62,64,68–70,73,76–80] were integrated.

[‡] The percentage of all randomized patients that was included in the "as-treated" analyses is given within parentheses.

[*] Statistically significant adverse TRIM effect (p < 0.05).

Source: Vamvakas (2007).[58] Reproduced with permission of Wiley.

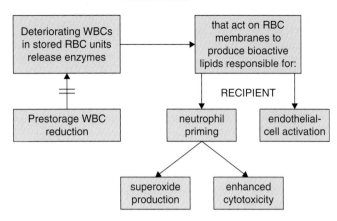

DONOR UNIT

Figure 62.2 Proposed mechanism leading from the accumulation of bioactive lipids in the supernatant fluid of stored non-WBC-reduced RBCs to the development of multiple-organ failure (MOF) in the recipient.[84–88]

association between ABT and short-term mortality could in fact reflect a "pro-inflammatory" rather than an "immunomodulatory" effect of ABT covered under the general concept of adverse TRIM effects,[2] which may include effects attributable to ABT by either immunomodulatory or pro-inflammatory mechanisms, or by a combination of these mechanisms.

In the study of Johnston et al.,[90] patients receiving allogeneic RBCs had a significantly higher risk of MOF than recipients of polymerized hemoglobin. Neutrophils obtained from recipients of RBCs demonstrated priming, as evidenced by increased beta-2 integrin expression, superoxide production, and elastase release. Neutrophils obtained from recipients of polymerized hemoglobin showed no evidence of priming. Studies investigating the benefits obtained from placing a WBC reduction filter in the arterial line of the cardiopulmonary bypass circuit[91–93] suggested that non-WBC-reduced ABT may provoke cardiac and/or pulmonary failure. Furthermore, associations between ABT and prolonged mechanical ventilation[94,95] or MOF[89,96–99] were reported by some, but not all,[103,104] observational studies.

Eleven RCTs, comparing recipients of non-WBC-reduced versus WBC-reduced allogeneic RBCs, and reporting on cancer recurrence, postoperative infection, or mortality as the primary outcome, have presented information on short-term (up to three months posttransfusion) mortality from all causes.[64,67,68,70,73,75–80] Because WBC reduction filters do not retain soluble mediators, if ABT exercised the described WBC-dependent neutrophil-priming effect that is mediated by bioactive lipids that accumulate during storage (Figure 62.2), allogeneic RBCs that are WBC-reduced before storage should abrogate this effect; but allogeneic RBCs that are WBC-reduced after storage should confer no benefit. Despite this theoretical prediction, no increase in mortality in association with non-WBC-reduced ABT was detected either across the subset of RCTs transfusing RBCs filtered before storage to the WBC-reduced arm, or across the subset of RCTs transfusing RBCs filtered after storage to the WBC-reduced arm.[57]

However, across five RCTs conducted in cardiac surgery[68,73,76,78,79] that had transfused RBCs filtered before storage to the non-WBC-reduced arm, non-WBC-reduced ABT was associated with a 72% increase in postoperative mortality (summary odds ratio [OR], 1.72; 95% confidence interval [CI], 1.05–2.81; $p < 0.05$; see Figure 62.3). The TRIM effect in these studies could be associated with factors prevalent in the setting of patients undergoing cardiac surgery. For example, bioactive lipids that accumulate during the storage of non-WBC-reduced RBCs and/or allogeneic

mononuclear cells may represent a second inflammatory insult that may compound the diffuse inflammatory response associated with the cardiopulmonary bypass circuit, which may predispose recipients to MOF and mortality.[83]

Insights into the mechanism(s) of the TRIM effect(s) in cardiac surgery and trauma

During cardiac surgery, exposure to the extracorporeal bypass circuit, hypothermia, and reperfusion injury can generate a systemic inflammatory response syndrome (SIRS) that is counteracted by a compensatory anti-inflammatory response syndrome (CARS).[105] Any intervention by biologic response modifiers (e.g., soluble mediators) contained in stored non-WBC-reduced RBCs (e.g., as described under the "Mediators Originating in WBC Granules" section) during an already-existing inflammatory cascade could thus produce an imbalance in the SIRS–CARS equilibrium toward SIRS. An overwhelming SIRS causes a dormant state of cell metabolism referred to as *multiple-organ dysfunction syndrome* (MODS), which can ultimately lead to MOF and death.[105] However, an association between non-WBC-reduced ABT and MOF has not been reported by any RCT, and the mechanism by which non-WBC-reduced ABT (but not WBC-reduced ABT) is associated with increased mortality in cardiac surgery remains unknown.[2] In the completed cardiac-surgery RCTs (Figure 62.3), non-WBC-reduced ABT was not associated with any particular cause of death, yet the aggregate mortality was higher in the non-WBC-reduced arm than in the WBC-reduced arm.[2]

Bilgin et al.[106] investigated the pro- and anti-inflammatory cytokine profiles in patients participating in their cardiac-surgery RCT that compared recipients of buffy-coat-reduced versus WBC-reduced allogeneic RBCs.[73] Patients who developed postoperative infection had higher interleukin-6 (IL6) concentrations, and patients who developed MODS had higher IL12 concentrations, in the subgroup of subjects who received more than three non-WBC-reduced RBC units. These findings supported the authors' thesis that non-WBC-reduced ABT amplifies an inflammatory response that is a "second hit" superimposed upon the ongoing SIRS induced by cardiac surgery. Such a "second-hit" inflammatory response may subsequently lead to a more profound CARS, which amounts to transfusion-induced immunosuppression predisposing to enhanced susceptibility to postoperative infection.

Bilgin et al.[107] also presented a combined observational analysis of the data from the two Dutch RCTs[68,73] conducted in cardiac surgery. After adjusting for confounding factors in the combined data set, it was the *plasma* (rather than the RBC) transfusions that were associated with higher mortality in patients undergoing open-heart surgery. Non-WBC-reduced RBC transfusion was also significantly associated with postoperative infection.[107] The authors concluded that, although it is difficult to separate the effects of the concomitantly administered allogeneic blood components (non-WBC-reduced or WBC-reduced RBCs, platelets, and plasma), future ABT studies in cardiac surgery should consider the possible adverse effects of all these various transfused blood components.[107]

All platelets transfused in the two Dutch RCTs[68,73] in cardiac surgery had been WBC-reduced. Bilgin et al.[107] underscored the independent effect of WBC-reduced platelet transfusions on mortality observed in their observational combined analysis. Platelets expressing CD4L upon activation (in the extracorporeal circuit as well as during storage of the platelet components) are presumed to represent a vital link between coagulation and inflammation. As such, they may enhance microthrombi and venous thrombo-embolism, in particular under changing rheological conditions such as those that occur in cardiac surgery. Both thrombi and infection play a pivotal role in the development of MODS and mortality.

The link between plasma and platelet transfusion and mortality found in the latest cardiac-surgery analysis of Bilgin et al.[107] is an observational finding that needs to be examined in future studies. Although this finding[107] is indicative of a TRIM effect in cardiac surgery independent of allogeneic WBCs and not abrogated by WBC reduction, it should be borne in mind that an observational analysis cannot establish an effect of platelet and/or plasma transfusion that is independently associated with postoperative complications; instead, any demonstrated effect of platelet and/or plasma transfusion may be simply a marker of the effect of the concomitantly administered non-WBC-reduced RBC transfusions. The established finding from cardiac-surgery RCTs (Figure 62.3) thus remains that non-WBC-reduced (compared with WBC-reduced) RBC transfusion increases short-term postoperative mortality. Therefore, cardiac surgery is an established indication for WBC reduction.

More recently, there have been challenges[108,109] to the two-hit SIRS–CARS model postulated by Bilgin et al.[105] to account for the mechanism of the TRIM effect(s) in cardiac surgery. Jackman et al.[109] studied immunomodulation in transfused trauma patients and delineated distinct roles of trauma and ABT in inducing immune modulation post injury. They demonstrated broad shifts in the expression of soluble immune mediators following traumatic injury and ABT, including *early* anti-inflammatory responses in contrast with the *later* anti-inflammatory (hence, immunomodulatory) responses envisioned by the SIRS–CARS model.

Xiao et al.[110] found that, of the 20,720 genes investigated, expression of 16,820 (>80%) was significantly altered in blood WBCs after blunt trauma, appropriately naming this response a "genomic storm." Early responses involved an increase in the expression of genes regulating innate immunity, microbial recognition, and inflammation, but also in anti-inflammatory mediators such as those involved with the IL10 signaling pathway. Jackman et al.[109] found a similar scope of responses at the protein level, with the levels of 31 out of the 41 measured serum proteins significantly altered following trauma. Taken together, these studies[109,110] demonstrate that the immune response to traumatic injury is incredibly broad, with significant changes observed in a majority of the genes and proteins assessed. Moreover, in contrast with the SIRS–CARS model of inflammation after trauma, these

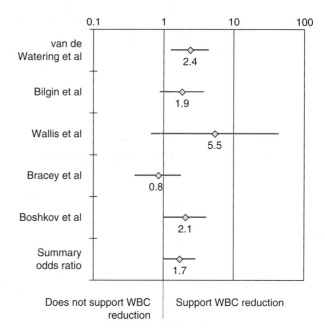

Figure 62.3 Postoperative mortality in cardiac-surgery patients. Randomized controlled trials (RCTs) investigating the association of non-WBC-reduced allogeneic blood transfusion (ABT) with short-term (up to three months posttransfusion) mortality from all causes and conducted in the setting of cardiac surgery.[68,73,76,78,79] For each RCT, the figure shows the odds ratio (OR) of short-term mortality in recipients of non-WBC-reduced versus WBC-reduced allogeneic RBCs, as calculated from an intention-to-treat analysis; and the summary OR across the depicted RCTs, as calculated from a meta-analysis.[57] A deleterious ABT effect (and thus a benefit from WBC reduction) is demonstrated by an OR >1, provided that the effect is statistically significant (p < 0.05; i.e., provided that the associated 95% CI does not include the null value of 1).

findings[109,110] indicate that immunosuppression occurs *immediately* after injury, coincident with some proinflammatory elements. In fact, most of the largest anti-inflammatory responses, at both the RNA and protein levels, were seen at the earliest time points examined. Such an early response was mirrored in the mouse model of Jackman et al.,[109] with similar cytokine profiles seen at four hours after traumatic blood loss.

Although the major immunological event for transfused trauma patients appears to be the injury, ABT does influence this response.[109,110] Xiao et al.[110] found approximately 400 genes whose expression was dependent on the volume of blood transfused, most of which were downregulated in response to ABT. Jackman et al.[109] found that, following adjustment for other clinical variables such as injury type and severity, seven of 41 proteins measured were significantly different between patients receiving modest ABT versus no ABT. An additional three proteins measured were significantly higher among those receiving ≥5 RBCs compared with the modest ABT group.[109]

Studies "before-and-after" WBC reduction

In the late 1990s, Canada and many western European countries implemented universal WBC reduction of cellular blood components by means of prestorage filtration. It became possible to compare the risk of infection or mortality in recipients of non-WBC-reduced RBCs before implementation of WBC reduction with the risk of infection or mortality in recipients of WBC-reduced

RBCs after implementation of WBC reduction. Such observational studies cannot establish causal relationships. Five studies have reported data on the risk of infection and/or short-term mortality.[111]

A large Canadian study included 9525 patients undergoing cardiac surgery, 1731 patients undergoing orthopedic surgery, and 3530 patients admitted to the intensive care unit (ICU). A statistically significant ($p = 0.04$) decrease in short-term mortality (from 7.0% to 6.2%) after WBC reduction was found but without a concomitant reduction in the risk of postoperative infection. The data-derived hypothesis offered was that the observed decrease in the number of deaths was not mediated through suppression of the recipient's immune function, but through a pro-inflammatory microvascular effect of transfused WBCs that affects several organ systems. This hypothesis was buttressed by the findings of a companion before-and-after study in premature infants.[113] In that setting, the implementation of universal WBC reduction coincided with a reduction in several secondary morbidity outcomes from several organ systems (i.e., bronchopulmonary dysplasia, retinopathy of prematurity, and necrotizing enterocolitis)—an observation consistent with a diffuse pro-inflammatory microvascular effect of allogeneic WBCs.

However, when all before-and-after studies were considered together in a meta-analysis,[111] and the findings of the unadjusted analyses from five studies were integrated, there was an unadjusted association of WBC reduction with a decreased risk of postoperative infection. This association did not persist when findings from the multivariate analyses of the three observational studies that had adjusted for the effects of confounding factors were integrated. There was neither an unadjusted nor an adjusted association of WBC reduction with decreased short-term mortality.[111]

Effect of the length of RBC storage

If bioactive lipids or other soluble mediators accumulating in a time-dependent manner during storage were associated with adverse outcomes, an association between prolonged storage of transfused non-WBC-reduced allogeneic RBCs and increased risk of occurrence of these adverse outcomes should be seen (because the longer the non-WBC-reduced allogeneic RBCs are stored, the higher the level of such soluble mediators that they will contain). Also, the RBC storage lesion (Chapter 9) occurs in both the non-WBC-reduced and the WBC-reduced units, generating considerable numbers of nonfunctioning RBCs removed from the recipient's circulation within 24 hours of the transfusion. This places a considerable burden on the reticuloendothelial system of a multitransfused recipient that could interfere with the host's response to bacteria and other challenges. After RCTs from 1993 to 2004 of non-WBC-reduced versus WBC-reduced ABT reported no adverse TRIM effect(s) vis-à-vis cancer recurrence and postoperative infection (with the exception of cardiac surgery), investigation focused on the possible deleterious effects of the transfusion of "old" (versus "fresh") RBCs.

The Age of Blood Evaluation (ABLE) RCT[114] enrolled approximately 2500 intensive-care unit (ICU) patients in Canada to detect a 5% absolute risk reduction (from 25% to 20%) in the mortality of ICU patients associated with transfusion of fresh (versus old) RBCs. Patients were randomly assigned to receive RBCs stored for ≤7 days versus RBCs issued per standard blood-bank policy (which issues for transfusion the longest-stored compatible RBC unit available in the inventory). The Red Cell Duration Study (RECESS)[115] intended to compare 1434 US cardiac-surgery patients randomly assigned to receive RBCs stored for ≤10 versus ≥21 days. The study evaluated change in the multiple-organ dysfunction score (MODS; from preoperative to highest composite MODS, adjusted for baseline MODS). The Age of Red Blood Cell in Premature Infants (ARIPI) RCT[116] recruited 450 premature neonates in Canada and allocated them to receive RBCs stored for <7 days versus RBCs issued per standard blood-bank policy. ICU patients, cardiac-surgery patients, and premature neonates were considered to be most vulnerable to any deleterious effect. These three RCT failed to show a difference between the study cohorts who received fresh versus old RBC transfusions. However, also in Canada, Heddle et al.[117] are simultaneously conducting a "pragmatic" RCT that admits all hospitalized transfused patients to detect an adverse effect of old RBCs in an unselected population not restricted to ICU patients, cardiac-surgery patients, or neonates. This last RCT[117] is intended to enroll 25,000 patients to detect a 15% reduction in mortality in association with transfusion of fresh (compared with old) RBCs.

In 1999, Vamvakas and Carven[118] reported specifically on the TRIM effect of RBC storage. In an observational study of patients undergoing cardiac surgery, 54 of 416 (13.0%) patients developed postoperative pneumonia. Among 269 patients given RBCs, the risk of pneumonia increased by 1% per day in the mean storage time of the transfused RBCs ($p < 0.005$). In an analysis of all patients, the risk of pneumonia increased by 5% per unit of non-WBC-reduced allogeneic RBCs and/or platelets received, although this difference did not attain significance ($p = 0.06$).[118] No association of the length of RBC storage was detected with such surrogate and nonspecific indicators of postoperative morbidity as the postoperative length of hospitalization, the postoperative length of stay in the ICU, and the length of endotracheal intubation after the day of operation.[119]

Numerous observational studies were published subsequently and have been critically reviewed.[120–123] These observational studies attributed to the transfusion of old (rather than fresh) RBCs such common (and nonspecific) adverse outcomes as a greater risk of mortality and organ failure (often analyzed by means of such surrogate variables as length of hospitalization and length of stay in the ICU) in addition to in-hospital infection. Furthermore, various other mechanisms were proposed to account for the postulated deleterious effect(s) ascribed to old RBCs. These include procoagulant[124] and/or immune[125] effects of old (versus fresh) RBCs secondary to the development of microparticles in old blood, increased iron load from hemolyzed stored RBCs,[126] and/or depletion of nitric oxide[127] or S-nitrosylated hemoglobin[128] in stored RBCs causing reduced ability of the transfused RBCs to induce vasodilation (thereby resulting in inadequate blood flow and impaired oxygen delivery).[129]

Further mechanisms were proposed by Cata et al.[130] These authors attributed the TRIM effect(s) primarily to the effect(s) of RBC storage, proposed mechanisms to account for a continuing deleterious effect of stored RBCs after the implementation of WBC reduction, and focused especially on the tumor-promoting effect(s) of stored RBCs (whether WBC-reduced or not).[130] They proposed that transfusion of allogeneic blood components (RBCs, but also platelets and fresh frozen plasma) is associated with a pro-inflammatory burden of bioactive substances in the recipient. The extent of this pro-inflammatory load in the recipient seems to be proportional to the length of storage of the transfused RBCs. Many of these bioactive substances have the potential to directly and indirectly affect the innate immune function (natural-killer [NK] cell activity) in the recipient—a key protective mechanism for local tumor control and also directed against metastatic spread in the surgical patient. The question therefore is whether the acute inflammatory burden produced by the perioperative ABT in the immuno-suppressive environment of anesthesia and surgical trauma creates a pro-tumor environment for the establishment of distant metastases.[130]

Cytokine concentrations are significant in stored WBC-reduced RBC units.[131] Exposure of WBC-reduced stored RBC supernatant to whole blood triggers release of IL6, IL10, and tumor necrosis factor-α (TNFα),[132] reduces lipopolysaccharide-induced release of TNFα,[133] and induces regulatory T-cell (Treg) activation.[134] Treg cells (comprising some 1–2% of circulating CD4-positive T-helper cells that coexpress a very high density of the IL2 receptor-α [CD25[hi]]) inhibit IL2 production and suppress the functions of T-helper type 1 (Th1) responses by CD4 and CD8 T cells.[135–137] The activation of Treg cells is antigen nonspecific, because they can be activated by lipopolysaccharide and can become immuno-suppressive through the Toll-like receptor-4 pathway.[138]

Furthermore, a recent animal study[139] found that RBCs (rather than WBCs) are implicated in the cancer-promoting effects of both autologous and allogeneic blood transfusions, with prolonged storage of the transfused RBCs enhancing tumor progression. However, clinical studies have hitherto suggested that neither prolonged RBC storage[140–142] nor administration of non-WBC-reduced (versus WBC-reduced) RBCs[143,144] is associated with any increased risk of cancer recurrence.

All this evidence[131–139] suggests that administration of stored blood components may be more deleterious than the administration of fresh blood components from a proinflammatory/immu-nomodulatory perspective and that universal WBC reduction may not abrogate the proinflammatory/immunomodulatory effects of ABT.[130] If the association of old (versus fresh) RBCs with the *common* adverse outcomes investigated in the recently com-pleted[114–116] or still ongoing[117] RCTs of the effect of the length of RBC storage were shown to be causal, the allowed storage period of RBCs would have to be promptly reduced, and increased reliance would have to be made on patient blood management (PBM) approaches because the patient's own freshly shed blood is the freshest blood possible.[145] Prompt policy intervention would be required because the effect of old (versus fresh) RBCs on *common* adverse outcomes reported from some observational studies[146–150] *far* exceeds the risks from the reduction in inventory and the need to recruit additional first-time donors, as well as the cost of producing more RBC units to make up for the expected increase in outdated units after the allowed RBC storage period is reduced. Thus, the question of whether old blood is less safe than fresh blood was appropriately the most critical issue facing transfusion medicine in 2011.[151] However, the results of three of the four RCTs undertaken in the United States or Canada have been consistently negative.

The negative findings of the RCTs of RBC storage[114–116] had been correctly predicted by all four critical reviews of the available observational clinical studies.[120–123] These reviews questioned the soundness of the clinical evidence adduced to justify the under-taking of RCTs. More specifically, in observational studies, any effect of RBC storage appeared to be a surrogate factor for the number of RBC units transfused, which in turn was a surrogate factor for illness severity predisposing to a need for transfu-sion.[122,152–154] Thus, in the ABLE RCT,[114] 37.0% of patients receiv-ing fresh RBCs had died at 90 days, as compared with 35.3% of patients receiving old RBCs. The hazard ratio for death in recipients

of fresh (compared with old) RBCs was 1.1 (p = 0.38). There were no significant differences between the randomization arms in any of the secondary outcomes. In the RECESS,[115] the main change in MODS was an increase of 8.5 and 8.7 points, respectively, in recipients of fresh versus old RBCs (p = 0.44). Seven-day mortality was 2.8% versus 2.0%, respectively (p = 0.43); 28-day mortality was 4.4% versus 5.3% (p = 0.57). Adverse outcomes did not differ significantly between the randomization arms. In the ARIPI RCT,[116] the relative risk of the primary outcome (a composite of major neonatal morbidities) was exactly 1.00. Thus, a slight, non-significant trend favored old RBCs as the better component to transfuse in the ABLE RCT,[114] and fresh RBCs in the RECESS,[115] with no difference whatsoever observed in the ARIPI RCT[116]: exactly what is expected when no clinical difference exists between old and fresh RBCs.

TRIM effects mediated by soluble molecules circulating in allogeneic plasma

Soluble HLA molecules

Soluble HLA proteins and immunoreactive HLA peptides are possible mediators of the TRIM effect(s). Nonpolymorphic peptides derived from HLA class I molecules might induce antigen-non-specific immunosuppression, whereas polymorphic HLA class I peptides have antigen-specific immunomodulatory effects.[155] It also seems possible that allogeneic plasma containing soluble HLA antigens may enter the recipient's thymic circulation, producing clonal deletion of the recipient's T cells that are directed against the allogeneic donor antigens.[156]

Factor VIII concentrates

In vitro studies have indicated that low-molecular-weight compo-nents found in factor VIII concentrates may inhibit the proliferative responses of peripheral blood mononuclear cells to phyto-hemagglutinin.[157] In these studies, high-purity factor VIII concen-trates reduced the induction of T-cell-activation molecules such as the IL2 receptor (CD25), the transferrin receptor (CD71), CD38, the CD11a–CD18 ratio, and HLA-DR antigen expression.[157] This inhibitory action of factor VIII concentrates was at least partly due to their contamination by transforming growth factor (TGF)-β.[158]

Autoantibodies

Some people spontaneously produce large amounts of neutralizing autoantibodies to a number of growth factors (e.g., granulocyte-macrophage colony-stimulating factor) or cytokines (e.g., IL1, IL6, and interferon-α).[159] The autoantibodies in question are detectable in immunoglobulin preparations and in plasma for transfusion. Therefore, if such donors donate blood, large amounts of neutral-izing autoantibodies to growth factors or cytokines may be trans-ferred to recipients by transfusion. In the plasma of transfusion recipients who had received plasma from donors with high titers of high-affinity neutralizing autoantibodies to IL6 (0.1% of normal donors), Hansen *et al.*[159] demonstrated a 500-fold or greater increase in the concentration of complexed IL6/autoantibody to IL6, as compared with free IL6 detectable in the patients' plasma prior to the transfusion.

When these autoantibodies reach a certain level, they may render a donor (or the recipient of plasma from such a donor) cytokine-deficient, but overt clinical sequelae of such cytokine deficiency have not been reported. Hansen et al.[159] christened this phenomenon *transfusion-related inhibition of cytokines* (TRICK). Depending on the cytokine or growth factor involved, TRICK could conceivably increase the transfusion recipient's susceptibility to infection or delay hematopoietic recovery after stem cell transplantation.

Evidence from RCTs

One RCT[76] design permitted examination of the hypothesis that soluble plasma molecules circulating in allogeneic plasma may mediate TRIM effects. Wallis et al.[76] randomized 597 patients undergoing cardiac surgery to receive plasma-reduced, buffy-coat-reduced, or WBC-reduced allogeneic RBCs. Plasma-reduced RBCs are equivalent in WBC content to the buffy-coat-rich RBCs used in North America. The highest risk of postoperative infection was observed in the plasma-reduced arm, in which the incidence of postoperative infection was 17.1%, as compared with 10.8% in the buffy-coat-reduced arm and 11.3% in the WBC-reduced arm ($p = 0.20$). Although the difference between the three arms was not significant, plasma removal did not appear to confer a benefit with regard to the prevention of TRIM (i.e., allogeneic plasma did not mediate TRIM).

TRIM effects mediated by WBC-derived soluble mediators

Mediators originating in WBC granules

Biologic response modifiers accumulating in blood components during storage have been implicated in the pathogenesis of TRIM.[160] These mediators are contained in intracellular WBC granules, and are released in a time-dependent manner as the WBCs deteriorate.[161] Nielsen et al.[161] reported that the concentration of histamine, eosinophil cationic protein, eosinophil protein X, myeloperoxidase, and plasminogen activator inhibitor-1 increase 3- to 25-fold in the supernatant fluid of RBC components between days 0 and 35 of storage. Histamine, eosinophil cationic protein, and eosinophil protein X have been shown to inhibit neutrophil function, thereby contributing to the development of immunosuppression and tissue damage.[162,163]

Soluble HLA molecules and Fas ligand

Soluble HLA molecules are present in the serum or plasma of healthy individuals. The liver is the main source of soluble HLA molecules found in the circulation. High levels of these molecules have been found in the serum or plasma of transplanted patients and patients with a variety of conditions, including inflammatory, autoimmune, and infectious diseases. Soluble HLA molecules are also found in the supernatant fluid of stored RBCs and platelets, in direct proportion to the length of storage and the number of cells present. The biological significance of these molecules has not been fully established, although it has been reported that they may be involved in the downregulation of the immune response and/or induction of tolerance.

Ghio et al.[164] and Puppo et al.[165] found soluble Fas-ligand (sFasL) and soluble HLA class I molecules in the supernatant plasma of RBC and random-donor platelet units. The sFasL content of either 30-day stored RBCs or 5-day stored platelets was approximately 20 ng/ml. The infusion of sFasL in transfused blood components may bind the Fas molecule expressed on the NK and cytotoxic T-cells of the recipient, thus preventing the binding of the Fas

molecule on these immune cells to the Fas-ligand on virus-infected cells. Therefore, the infusion of sFasL in transfused blood components may impair the function of NK and cytotoxic T-cells in the recipient, thus preventing apoptosis of virus-infected cells.[166,167] Ghio et al.[164] and Puppo et al.[165] demonstrated the functional capacity of sFasL molecules in stored blood components by culturing Jurkat cells in the presence of plasma supernatant from stored RBCs. Jurkat cells express Fas, and are thus susceptible to the effects of sFasL present in transfused blood components. In this in vitro experiment, sFasL from the plasma supernatant of stored RBCs triggered apoptosis of the Jurkat cells, which was measured by flow cytometry.

These authors[164,165] also documented the accumulation of soluble HLA class I molecules in stored RBCs and platelets, although the concentrations achieved were only 4 ng/ml in 30-day stored RBCs and five-day stored platelets. Furthermore, stored supernatant plasma was shown to exercise an immunosuppressive effect in functional experiments, inhibiting the cytotoxic activity of lymphocytes known to be cytotoxic for cells infected with Epstein–Barr virus (EBV). This was not a nonspecific effect, as the cytotoxic activity of lymphocytes was restored after the stored supernatant plasma was depleted of soluble HLA class I molecules. However, only supernatant plasma from stored non-WBC-reduced (as opposed to WBC-reduced) cellular blood components inhibited the cytotoxic activity of lymphocytes directed against EBV-infected cells. Similarly, prestorage WBC reduction prevented the accumulation of sFasL in stored RBCs.

Apoptotic WBCs

Innerhofer et al.[168,169] reported that impaired proliferative T-cell responses, decreased CD3+ counts, and a state of inappropriate immune activation, along with a diminished cytolytic response, occur even after transfusion of WBC-reduced RBCs containing a median residual WBC count of 0.03×10^6 WBCs/unit (i.e., a count far below the qualifying 5×10^6 limit). This suggests that not only transfused, intact, immunologically competent WBCs but also transfused, apoptotic, or necrotic WBCs could be important in provoking TRIM responses. Finally, activation of complement components[170] and formation of anaphylatoxins[171] have also been reported during storage, but their significance in the context of TRIM is uncertain.

Evidence from animal models

If soluble biologic response modifiers and remnants of apoptotic or necrotic WBCs accumulating in blood components during storage were shown to be responsible for some of the adverse TRIM effects of ABT, WBC reduction procedures intended to prevent such TRIM effects should be performed before storage, prior to WBC deterioration and prior to the release from WBC membranes or granules of soluble biologic response modifiers (Figure 62.1). The available WBC reduction filters do not retain soluble biologic response modifiers and are also ineffective in removing WBC fragments. Therefore, both biologic response modifiers and the remnants of apoptotic or necrotic WBCs can be expected to persist in a blood component filtered after storage, and the importance of the timing of WBC reduction as regards the TRIM effects has been demonstrated in experimental animals.[172]

Bordin et al.[172] showed that ABT promotes tumor growth of established animal tumors and that the tumor-growth-promoting effect of ABT can be ameliorated by prestorage (but not by poststorage) WBC reduction. These authors[172] used outbred

New Zealand White (NZW) rabbits with established tumors as blood recipients, and outbred California Black rabbits as allogeneic blood donors. "Syngeneic" donor blood was collected from NZW rabbits who were littermates, or siblings, of the transfusion recipients. Non-WBC-reduced allogeneic, poststorage WBC-reduced allogeneic, prestorage WBC-reduced allogeneic, or syngeneic RBCs were transfused on days +4 and +9 after the infusion of syngeneic epithelial tumor cells. All rabbits were killed 28 days after the infusion of the tumor cells, and the number of pulmonary tumor nodules was counted. Rabbits that received non-WBC-reduced allogeneic, poststorage WBC-reduced allogeneic, prestorage WBC-reduced allogeneic, or syngeneic RBCs had a median of 50.0, 39.0, 20.0, and 17.5 pulmonary nodules, respectively. The difference between non-WBC-reduced allogeneic and prestorage WBC-reduced allogeneic or syngeneic transfusion was highly significant ($p < 0.0001$), but the difference between non-WBC-reduced allogeneic and poststorage WBC-reduced allogeneic transfusion was only marginally significant ($p = 0.06$).

Evidence from RCTs

With respect to infection, a recent theory[173,174] attributes the purported susceptibility of transfused patients to infection to a sustained inhibition of neutrophil chemotaxis caused by TGFβ. TGFβ renders neutrophils insensitive to chemotactic stimulation. Inhibition of chemotaxis is caused by both exogenous TGFβ, contained in the supernatant of transfused blood components,[173] and endogenous TGFβ produced by the recipient's neutrophils in response to sFasL and soluble HLA molecules found in the transfused supernatant.[174]

However, the results of meta-analyses of medically homogeneous subsets of RCTs that reported on postoperative infection contradicted the theory that attributes the TRIM effect to WBC-derived soluble mediators that accumulate during storage.[57,58] Among nine RCTs transfusing RBCs WBC-reduced before storage to the WBC-reduced arm,[62,68,70,73,76–80] no TRIM effect was detected (summary OR, 1.06; 95% CI, 0.91–1.24; $p > 0.05$).[57] If the TRIM effect were mediated by WBC-derived soluble mediators, prestorage filtration should have abrogated an increased infection risk associated with non-WBC-reduced ABT, because it would have removed the allogeneic WBCs from the components given to the WBC-reduced arm of the studies before WBCs could release mediators into the supernatant fluid. Accordingly, a deleterious TRIM effect associated with non-WBC-reduced ABT would have been expected in this analysis, but the meta-analysis detected no such effect (Figure 62.4).

In contrast, among four RCTs[59,64,68,69] that transfused RBCs filtered after storage to the WBC-reduced arm, there was a more than twofold increase in the risk of infection in association with non-WBC-reduced ABT (summary OR, 2.25; 95% CI, 1.12–4.25; $p < 0.05$; Figure 62.5). If the TRIM effect were mediated by WBC-derived soluble mediators, poststorage filtration should not have abrogated an increased infection risk associated with non-WBC-reduced ABT, because it would not have removed such mediators from the supernatant fluid of the stored RBCs given to the WBC-reduced arm of the studies. Thus, the large TRIM effect detected in this analysis (Figure 62.5) may be due to the inclusion of three early RCTs[59,64,69] that had reported an unusually large TRIM effect.[58] These RCTs administered blood components that are no longer used in Western Europe or North America (allogeneic whole blood,[59] poststorage-filtered allogeneic whole blood,[59] or poststorage-filtered allogeneic RBCs[64,69]).

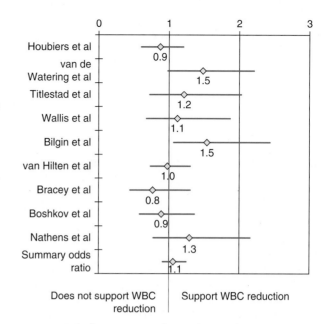

Figure 62.4 Risk of postoperative infection after transfusion of prestorage-filtered WBC-reduced RBCs. Randomized controlled trials (RCTs) of ABT and postoperative infection administering prestorage-filtered allogeneic RBCs to the WBC-reduced arm.[62,68,70,73,76–80] The figure shows the odds ratio (OR) of postoperative infection in recipients of non-WBC-reduced versus WBC-reduced allogeneic RBCs, as calculated from an intention-to-treat analysis of each study; and the summary OR across the depicted RCTs, as calculated from a meta-analysis.[57] A deleterious ABT effect (and thus a benefit from WBC reduction) is demonstrated by an OR >1, provided that the effect is statistically significant ($p < 0.05$; i.e., provided that the associated 95% CI does not include the null value of 1).

TRIM effects mediated by allogeneic mononuclear cells

The only established TRIM effect (i.e., the beneficial effect of pretransplant ABT on renal allograft survival) appears to require viable WBCs. Patients awaiting renal transplantation derived less immunologic benefit from pretransplant RBC transfusions that are WBC-reduced, washed, or frozen-thawed. Mincheff et al.[175] implicated the dendritic APCs of the allogeneic donor in the induction of a state of anergy in the recipient, proposing that during refrigeration APCs lose their ability to deliver co-stimulation. These investigators hypothesized that, following ABT, the recipient's T cells are stimulated by allogeneic donor APCs in the absence of co-stimulation, and this interaction induces a state of anergy in the recipient's T cells.

Evidence from animal models

Animal data suggest that the TRIM effects are most likely mediated by transfused allogeneic mononuclear cells.[176] Kao[177] induced immune suppression in mice receiving donor WBCs free of plasma and platelets. A recent theory[178] proposes that donor dendritic cells expressing both alloantigen and the OX-2 (CD200) co-stimulatory molecule are required for the production of the TRIM effect.

CD200 is a transmembrane protein of the immunoglobulin superfamily that is expressed on various cell types, including a subpopulation of dendritic cells and some T and B cells.[179] Its receptor (CD200R or OX-2R) appears only on myeloid dendritic cells and some T cells. The interaction between CD200 and its receptor provokes a tolerance signal that leads to suppression of classical T-cell-mediated responses and the generation of

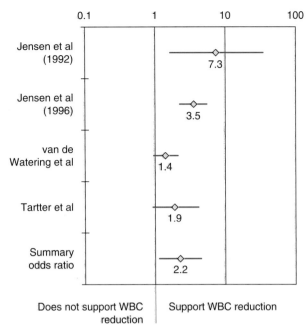

Figure 62.5 Risk of postoperative infection after transfusion of poststorage-filtered WBC-reduced RBCs or whole blood. Randomized controlled trials (RCTs) of ABT and postoperative infection administering poststorage-filtered allogeneic RBCs or whole blood to the WBC-reduced arm.[59,64,68,69] The figure shows the odds ratio (OR) of postoperative infection in recipients of non-WBC-reduced versus WBC-reduced allogeneic RBCs or whole blood, as calculated from an intention-to-treat analysis of each study; and the summary OR across the depicted RCTs, as calculated from a meta-analysis.[57] A deleterious ABT effect (and thus a benefit from WBC reduction) is demonstrated by an OR >1, provided that the effect is statistically significant ($p < 0.05$; i.e., provided that the associated 95% CI does not include the null value of 1).

γδ-suppressor T cells. Thus, CD200-deficient mice have reduced ability to downregulate activation of APCs. The absence of down-regulatory signals in such mice results in exaggerated inflammatory responses and increased susceptibility to autoimmune encephalitis and collagen-induced arthritis. The interaction between CD200 and its receptor suppresses macrophage function, prolongs allograft survival, and prevents allogeneic fetal loss in a mouse model of cytokine-triggered abortions.[180]

Clark *et al.*[178] demonstrated ABT-induced tumor growth in a murine model that employed BALB/c mice as allogeneic donors and C57Bl/6 mice as blood recipients. The recipient mice received a tail vein injection of syngeneic FSL10 fibrosarcoma cells, followed by transfusion of 50–200 μL of allogeneic blood. Pulmonary tumor nodules were counted three weeks after the FSL10 cell infusion. There was a dose–response relationship between the volume of transfused allogeneic blood and the number of pulmonary tumor nodules, along with proliferation of TGFβ-positive suppressor T cells in the spleen.

The tumor-growth-promoting effect of ABT was mediated by donor myeloid dendritic cells that expressed both CD11c and CD200 on their surface, because it could be blocked by monoclonal antibodies to either CD11c or CD200. (The effect could not be blocked by antibodies to CD200R, or by antibodies to other molecules participating in these interactions, an observation that implicated the subset of donor myeloid dendritic cells expressing both CD11c and CD200 in the pathogenesis of TRIM.) The

interaction between the donor CD200 and its receptor on the recipient's T cells induced proliferation of γδ-suppressor T cells that released cytokines, especially TGFβ. Physiological concentrations of TGFβ stimulated proliferation of FSL10 fibrosarcoma cells in vitro. As TGFβ can also suppress host defenses against infectious agents,[181] it could be the basis of the TRIM effect with regard to both postoperative infections and tumor growth, at least as regards sarcomas.

Bordin and Blajchman[182] reviewed the findings of animal models of ABT and cancer recurrence and reported that 17 published models had found stimulation of tumor growth by ABT, as compared with three models that had reported inhibition of tumor growth and four models that had found no effect. Data from both inbred and outbred animal models have indicated that ABT accelerates tumor growth and enhances formation of metastatic nodules.[172,183–186] Allogeneically transfused mice inoculated intramuscularly with either syngeneic malignant melanoma (B16) or mastocytoma (P815) cells developed larger tumors than did syngeneically transfused mice.[183] Similar results were obtained when syngeneic B16 tumor cells were infused intravenously and the numbers of pulmonary nodules enumerated.[183,184] Experiments performed to investigate the effect of the tumor–cell dose showed that the ABT effect was only evident when small numbers (1.25–2.5×10^5) of tumor cells were inoculated into the host animal. The effect was not evident when large numbers of tumor cells were inoculated, suggesting that the tumor burden had a strong bearing on whether the ABT effect became manifest.

Studies in both inbred (mice) and outbred (rabbits) animals have shown that ABT has a tumor-growth-promoting effect when administered prior to the infusion of syngeneic tumor cells.[172,185] In the murine model, male C57Bl/6J mice (MHC type H-2b) were blood recipients, Balb/c mice (MHC type H-2d) were allogeneic donors, and the tumor cells were syngeneic (H-2b) methyl-cholanthrene-induced fibrosarcoma cells.[185] To better replicate the situation seen clinically, the enhancement of tumor growth by ABT has been investigated in animals (mice and rabbits) that received such syngeneic and allogeneic transfusions subsequent to the inoculation of the tumor cells, and the data indicated that ABT enhanced tumor growth also in animals with established tumors.[172] Using inbred animals (mice) only, another series of investigations provided similar evidence indicating that ABT given after tumor-cell engraftment enhanced tumor growth.[186] Is was also shown that animals with either non-established or established tumors receiving non-WBC-reduced ABT developed significantly larger numbers of pulmonary nodules than did animals given WBC-reduced ABT.[172,185]

Finally, the tumor-growth-promoting effect of ABT can be adoptively transferred to naive animals by spleen cells harvested from allogeneically transfused animals.[185] In these experiments, the number of pulmonary nodules observed in animals that had received spleen cells from allogeneically transfused animals was significantly higher than that observed in animals that had received spleen cells from animals transfused with syngeneic blood. Importantly, the ABT effect could not be adoptively transferred to naive animals that received spleen cells derived from animals transfused with prestorage-WBC-reduced allogeneic blood.

The *clonal deletion* seen in recipients of ABT refers to the removal of lymphocytes that promote the clearance of transfused alloantigens. Interactions between Fas and FasL are involved in the clonal deletion of T cells and the downregulation of cytotoxic T-cell activity. In a murine model, Hashimoto *et al.*[187] investigated the possibility of splenic-lymphocyte deletion secondary to ABT-related augmentation of apoptosis. These investigators demonstrated that non-WBC-reduced ABT upregulated the expression of Fas and FasL on CD4+ as well as CD8+ splenic T cells and could thereby promote their apoptosis. The ABT-related immune alterations could be partially prevented by WBC reduction of the transfused blood, as CD8+ splenic cells from mice receiving non-WBC-reduced ABT showed higher expression of Fas and FasL than cells from mice receiving WBC-reduced ABT.

The data regarding the TRIM effect in animal models of infection are contradictory. Moreover, a variety of experimental conditions such as the anesthesia, presence of shock or trauma, type of surgery, blood volume, as well as timing and transfusion frequency have all been reported to have an impact on the results.[188–192] In a series of studies in experimental animals, Waymack *et al.* have demonstrated that allogeneically transfused animals had immune impairment and a poorer response to a septic challenge than did syngeneically transfused animals.[188–191] In a burn model, these investigators observed that rats given ABT had higher mortality than did rats given syngeneic blood or saline.[192] In a rat bacterial-peritonitis model, a significant adverse effect on survival was associated with ABT.[189] In another study, ABT was associated with marked immune impairment to a bacterial challenge immediately after the transfusion.[193]

Moreover, ABT and, in particular, transfused allogeneic WBCs adversely affected host resistance to a gut-derived infection with *Escherichia coli* in a murine model.[194] In addition, in a cecal ligation and puncture murine model, ABT greatly increased susceptibility to infection. These studies also indicated that spleen cells of allogeneically transfused mice produced increased quantities of the Th2 cytokines (IL4, IL10, and lesser amounts of IL2), probably leading to increased antibody production and a decreased cell-mediated response.[195] In contrast, in murine experiments using a bacterial-peritonitis model that compared syngeneic with ABT, the latter was shown not to influence overall survival of animals challenged with *E. coli*.[196] Although a clear negative effect of shock was detected, no adverse effect of transfusions, either syngeneic or allogeneic, was observed in a rat model.[197]

Microchimerism

HLA compatibility between donor and recipient may result in the persistence of allogeneic donor WBCs, including dendritic APCs, in the recipient. Such long-term engraftment and survival of small numbers of donor cells (microchimerism) have been proposed as a possible mechanism of TRIM.[198] Microchimerism could cause the downregulation of the recipient's immune response, resulting in tolerance to donor alloantigens and allograft survival. Microchimerism results in the release of IL4, IL10, and TGFβ from Th2 lymphocytes.[199] These cytokines have been shown to inhibit the production of Th1 cells and to deactivate cytotoxic T cells, thereby suppressing allograft rejection. Along similar lines, ABT was shown to cause a shift in peripheral T-cell cytokine secretion toward that of the Th2 phenotype, and to downregulate Th1 cytokine secretion. Impairment of Th-1 cytokine secretion results in impairment of various functions of cellular immunity (including antigen processing, macrophage activation, the T-cell cytotoxic function, and the neutrophil and monocyte cytocidal activity) that are supported by Th1 cytokines, such as IL2, IL12, and interferon-γ.[200]

In 1995, Lee *et al.*[201] employed quantitative allele-specific polymerase chain reaction methods to demonstrate a 1000-fold

expansion of allogeneic donor WBCs in the recipient's circulation 3–5 days following transfusion in otherwise healthy adults undergoing elective orthopedic surgery. The allogeneic WBCs were cleared from the circulation within two weeks. The finding was verified in a canine transfusion model, and—as expected—irradiation of blood products abrogated the allogeneic donor WBC expansion phase. However, in 1999, the same group documented high-level and long-lasting WBC microchimerism among selected victims of traumatic injury who had received a large number of very fresh units of blood during resuscitation.[202] In some of these trauma patients, up to 3–4% of circulating WBCs were of donor origin as long as two years following transfusion. Analysis of lymphocyte subsets using immunomagnetic bead enrichment showed that both lymphoid and myeloid lineages were represented.

Long-term transfusion-associated microchimerism appears to be a common, albeit only recently recognized, complication of ABT[203] that has hitherto been demonstrated only in trauma patients.[202] Injury produces an immunosuppressive and inflammatory milieu in which very fresh blood components, containing WBCs capable of replication, are often transfused in large quantities. Transfusion-associated microchimerism is present in approximately half of transfused, severely injured patients at hospital discharge.[203] In approximately 10% of the patients, the chimerism associated with a single blood donor may increase in magnitude over months to years, representing up to 2–5% of circulating WBCs.[202,203] Nonetheless, in other patient populations, such as those infected with HIV, ABT-induced microchimerism is transient.[204]

Microchimerism is detected also following administration of WBC-reduced allogeneic RBCs.[205] Utter *et al.*[206] examined a subgroup of the trauma patients enrolled in the RCT of Nathens *et al.*[80] that had randomized patients to receive non-WBC-reduced or WBC-reduced allogeneic RBCs filtered before storage. Nine of 32 (28%) patients in the non-WBC-reduced group developed microchimerism, as compared with 13 of 35 (37%) patients in the WBC-reduced group ($p = 0.43$).[206] Several months after the transfusion, subjects with transfusion-associated microchimerism were no more likely than subjects without transfusion-associated microchimerism to have at least one symptom suggestive of chronic graft-versus-host disease (64% versus 76%, respectively), indicating that transfusion-associated microchimerism is prevalent in this patient population but unlikely to be associated with symptoms.[206] Fresland *et al.*[207] also reported that microchimerism after ABT could be induced by transfusion of RBCs WBC-reduced by prestorage filtration.

The only significant predictor of transfusion-associated microchimerism to date is the length of storage of transfused RBCs, with "fresh" (compared with "old") RBCs associated with a higher risk of microchimerism.[208] Reed *et al.* reported a significantly ($p < 0.05$) different RBC storage time between non-transfusion-associated microchimerism recipients (21 ± 8.3 days) versus transfusion-associated microchimerism recipients (16.1 ± 6.2 days).[203] Similarly, the minimal length of RBC storage was a median of 13 days in non-transfusion-associated microchimerism recipients compared to a median of five days in transfusion-associated microchimerism recipients ($p < 0.005$).[203] Nonetheless, transfusion-associated microchimerism has also been observed with older RBCs (stored for 22 days).[207] If transfusion-associated microchimerism were related to TRIM effects in trauma, and were also associated with transfusion of "fresher" RBCs, it is important to appreciate that it would be the transfusion of fresh (as opposed to old) RBCs that would be logically associated with adverse TRIM effects in trauma. Nonetheless, no adverse clinical effects have hitherto been observed in the small number of completed studies of transfusion-associated microchimerism,[208] indicating any TRIM effects in trauma are not related to transfusion-associated microchimerism.

Evidence from RCTs

One RCT[72] was specifically designed to test a possible TRIM effect of allogeneic mononuclear cells. The Viral Activation Transfusion Study (VATS)[72] transfused unmodified allogeneic RBCs stored of <2 weeks (and thus containing relatively undamaged allogeneic mononuclear cells) to the non-WBC-reduced arm. The two study arms were controlled for comparable duration of storage of the transfused RBCs. There was no difference between the study arms in the HIV or CMV viral load or the length of survival. Median survival was 13.0 months in recipients of prestorage-filtered allogeneic RBCs, as compared with 20.5 months in recipients of non-buffy-coat-reduced allogeneic RBCs ($p = 0.12$). Thus, the VATS results have impugned the theory attributing the TRIM effect to allogeneic mononuclear cells. No other RCT transfusing fresh components to the non-WBC-reduced arm has been reported, and the effect of fresh components has not been studied in the context of more "traditional" TRIM effects (i.e., cancer recurrence or postoperative infection).

Despite the convincing evidence provided by animal models for a relationship between transfusion of allogeneic mononuclear cells and tumor recurrence, no RCT of ABT and cancer recurrence has transfused fresh non-WBC-reduced RBCs to the non-WBC-reduced arm to test for the effect of immunologically competent allogeneic mononuclear cells seen in animal models. Moreover, no RCT of ABT and cancer recurrence has enrolled patients with sarcomas—tumors whose growth is stimulated by TGFβ[178]—or patients with tumors for which the immune response plays a major role. (These include skin tumors, such as melanomas, keratoacanthomas, and squamous and basal-cell carcinomas; and certain virus-induced tumors, notably Kaposi's sarcoma and certain lymphomas.[209])

Instead, the three available RCTs[60,62,81] of ABT and cancer recurrence enrolled patients with colorectal cancer—a tumor that is not sufficiently antigenic to render an impairment of the host's immunity capable of facilitating tumor growth, and whose cells have not been shown to be stimulated by TGFβ. The existence of a specific immune response to colorectal cancer cells has not been established. Although it is possible to generate cytotoxic T cells in vitro that recognize antigens expressed by colorectal cancer cells,[210,211] the relevance of these cytotoxic cells in tumor growth may be limited because of a loss of the expression of HLA molecules and adhesion molecules on the colorectal cancer cells.[212,213] Furthermore, if the ABT cancer-promoting effect were mediated by allogeneic WBCs, the dose of ABT used in each of the three available RCTs[60,62,81] could have been insufficient for causing the adverse effects because all three RCTs had administered buffy-coat-reduced RBCs to their non-WBC-reduced arm.

Thus, these 3 RCTs[60,62,81] permit very limited inference with regard to the biologic significance of the TRIM mediators discussed in this chapter. No adverse TRIM effect of ABT on cancer recurrence is detected across the three studies (Figure 62.6). The summary OR of cancer recurrence in recipients of non-WBC-reduced allogeneic compared with the autologous or WBC-reduced allogeneic RBCs is 1.04 (95% confidence interval [CI], 0.81–1.35; $p \gg 0.05$).[214] A fourth RCT[144] was recently reported in gastrointestinal cancer.

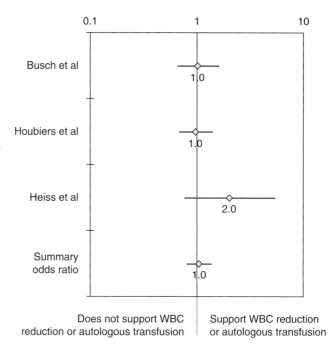

Figure 62.6 Cancer recurrence after transfusion. Randomized controlled trials (RCTs) investigating the association of non-WBC-reduced allogeneic blood transfusion (ABT) with cancer recurrence in colorectal cancer.[60,62,81] For each RCT, the figure shows the odds ratio (OR) of cancer recurrence in recipients of non-WBC-reduced versus WBC-reduced allogeneic or autologous RBCs or whole blood, as calculated from an intention-to-treat analysis; and the summary OR across the depicted RCTs, as calculated from a meta-analysis.[214] Each OR is surrounded by its 95% confidence interval (CI). A deleterious effect of ABT (and thus a benefit from autologous transfusion or WBC reduction) is demonstrated by an OR >1, provided that the effect is statistically significant ($p < 0.05$; i.e., provided that the associated 95% CI does not include the null value of 1).

Between patients randomly assigned to receive non-WBC-reduced versus WBC-reduced ABT, there was no difference in survival or cancer recurrence.[144]

Summary and conclusions

TRIM encompasses the laboratory immune aberrations that occur after ABT (Table 62.1) and their established or purported clinical effects. TRIM is a real biologic phenomenon resulting in at least one established beneficial clinical effect in humans (the enhanced survival of renal allografts), but deleterious clinical TRIM effects have not yet been confirmed. Initially, TRIM encompassed effects attributable to ABT by immunomodulatory mechanisms (e.g., cancer recurrence, postoperative infection, or virus activation); more recently, TRIM has also included effects attributable to ABT by pro-inflammatory mechanisms (e.g., multiple-organ failure or mortality).

The mechanism(s) of the TRIM effect(s) remain(s) elusive, and it is possible that a large number of biologic mechanisms underlie these effect(s). The infusion of foreign antigen in either soluble or cell-associated form has been shown to induce immune suppression, anergy, as well as clonal deletion in studies in experimental animals. However, most studies evaluating proposed mechanisms have been done in rodents, and their findings may not be applicable to the human immune system.[215] Support for the theory that TRIM is due to the allogeneic WBCs has come mainly from data from animal models. These have shown that animals receiving allogeneic buffy-coat leukocytes develop significantly more pulmonary tumor nodules than do animals given either plasma or prestorage-WBC-reduced whole blood.[172] It is possible that prestorage WBC reduction may prevent the accumulation of soluble mediators that are actively synthesized and released by WBCs during RBC storage, and that such WBC-derived soluble mediators are involved in the immunomodulation observed following ABT. However, storage lesions of RBCs and platelets occur even when the units have been WBC-reduced prior to storage (WBC removal only slightly improves these storage lesions—see Chapters 9 and 24).

The totality of the evidence from RCTs does not demonstrate the kind of deleterious TRIM effect that would justify universal WBC reduction specifically for prevention of this effect (i.e., a TRIM effect manifest across all clinical settings and transfused RBC products), although universal WBC reduction may be justified on the basis of other WBC-related adverse effects.[176] Non-WBC-reduced ABT is associated with an increased risk of short-term (up to three months post transfusion) mortality from all causes specifically in cardiac surgery. Even in this setting, the reasons for the excess deaths attributed to non-WBC-reduced ABT remain elusive. The initial hypothesis suggested that non-WBC-reduced ABT may predispose to MOF, which, in turn, may predispose to mortality.[68] However, hitherto, no cardiac-surgery RCT has demonstrated an association between non-WBC-reduced ABT and MOF.

The TRIM effect seen in cardiac surgery deserves further study to pinpoint the cause(s) of the excess deaths, but RCTs comparing recipients of non-WBC-reduced versus WBC-reduced RBCs in cardiac surgery are not likely to be performed. We believe that WBC reduction of all cellular blood components transfused in cardiac surgery is appropriate based on the accumulated evidence on the adverse TRIM effect(s) in this specific clinical setting. Where selective WBC reduction is practiced, WBC reduction of all cellular components transfused in cardiac surgery should be added to the other established indications for selective WBC reduction.

The evidence for the existence of some TRIM effects may not be available because the requisite studies have not been conducted. An effect of the transfusion of allogeneic mononuclear cells would be expected to increase tumor recurrence, based on the convincing findings from experimental animals. However, no available RCT has transfused fresh non-WBC-reduced RBCs to the non-WBC-reduced arm to specifically study the effect of allogeneic mononuclear cells. Moreover, no available RCT has enrolled patients with a tumor whose growth would be expected to be stimulated by ABT. A possible adverse TRIM effect of allogeneic mononuclear cells has similarly not been adequately investigated in the areas of post-operative infection and mortality.

Indeed, in many cases, the preclinical studies were conducted and the hypotheses about mechanisms formulated after clinical studies (including RCTs) had already presented data-derived hypotheses to account for unexpected ABT effects. Because it has not been possible to conduct further RCTs after the hypotheses about TRIM mediators (Figure 62.1) were crystallized, we may never know whether some adverse TRIM effects exist (or not) in humans, because we have been unable to test for them in RCTs. Moreover, it is possible that the available RCTs have targeted outcomes that did not capture the true nature of the ABT effect. If this effect were "pro-inflammatory" rather than "immunomodulatory," it would have been expected to result not in clinical impairment of the recipient's

immunity, but in multiple-organ dysfunction. MOF and related outcomes were not studied in most completed RCTs.

Following a great interest in TRIM in the 1990s and the early years of the twenty-first century (when the adverse TRIM effects were debated as the primary reason for implementing *universal* [as opposed to selective] WBC reduction in North America—if not in both North America and Western Europe), remarkably few clinical studies on the adverse TRIM effects (and even the mechanisms of these effects) appeared in the last seven years. This is partly due to the fact that each country's policy decisions vis-à-vis implementing universal WBC reduction had already been made in the early years of the 21st century;[216,217] it is also partly due to the funding of research into the deleterious effects of stored RBCs in lieu of research into the *bona fide* TRIM effects.

It remains unclear whether deleterious clinical TRIM effects of ABT truly exist, and—in the event that they do—whether they are mediated, directly or indirectly, by allogeneic WBCs. The question of whether universal WBC reduction should be discontinued and selective WBC reduction reintroduced was posed after no new research was reported to justify the policy decisions made in favor of WBC reduction in the early years of the twenty-first century (when there was an implicit expectation that adverse TRIM effects would later be established[111]). Some US transfusion medicine experts have argued against such a change in clinical practice on the grounds that patients and clinicians would not agree with the change.[218] Whereas ardent believers in TRIM have continued to argue in favor of universal WBC reduction,[219] Bilgin, van de Watering, and Brand[220] presented a concise and sobering review of the evidence from RCTs that separated experimental evidence from speculation, conviction, faith, and belief.

Based on the stark absence of any adverse ABT effect in RCTs outside the setting of cardiac surgery, these authors concluded that reversal to the use of buffy-coat-reduced RBCs (with restriction of WBC reduction to its established selective indications) is a "safe option."[220] The data presented in this chapter support the scientific merits of this position,[220] which is further supported by the latest results from the three-year follow-up[221] of 2016 patients randomized to receive "liberal" versus "restrictive" ABT in the RCT of Functional Outcomes in Cardiovascular Patients Undergoing Surgical Hip Fracture Repair (FOCUS) trial.[222] Over three years of follow-up, 841 (42%) patients died. Long-term mortality did not differ between the "liberal" and "restrictive" ABT arms of the RCT (hazard ratio, 1.09; 95% CI, 0.95–1.25), and causes of death did not differ either, providing no support for the hypothesis that a liberal transfusion strategy (and thus ABT) has an adverse effect on long-term mortality or affects the causes of death.[221]

Key references

A full reference list for this chapter is available at: http://www.wiley.com/go/simon/transfusion

2   Vamvakas EC, Blajchman MA. Transfusion-related immunomodulation (TRIM): an update. *Blood Rev* 2007;**21**:327–48.

11   Opelz G, Sengar DP, Mickey MR, *et al*. Effect of blood transfusions on subsequent kidney transplants. *Transplant Proc* 1973;**5**:253–9.

13   Vamvakas EC, Blajchman MA, eds. *Immunomodulatory Effects of Blood Transfusion*. Bethesda, MD: AABB Press, 1999.

68   van de Watering LMG, Hermans J, Houbiers JGA, *et al*. Beneficial effect of leukocyte depletion of transfused blood on post-operative complications in patients undergoing cardiac surgery: A randomized clinical trial. *Circulation* 1998;**97**:562–8.

73 Bilgin YM, van de Watering LMG, Eijsman L, *et al.* Double-blind, randomized controlled trial on the effect of leukocyte-depleted erythrocyte transfusions in cardiac valve surgery. *Circulation* 2004;**109**:2755–60.

112 Hébert PC, Fergusson D, Blajchman MA, *et al.* Clinical outcomes following institution of the Canadian universal leukoreduction program for red blood cell transfusions. *JAMA* 2003;**289**:1941–9.

114 Lacroix J, Hebert PC, Fergusson DA, *et al.* Age of transfused blood in critically-ill adults. *N Engl J Med* 2015;**372**:1410–18.

115 Steiner ME, Ness PM, Assman DJ, *et al.* Effects of red-cell storage duration on patients undergoing cardiac surgery. *N Engl J Med* 2015;**372**:1419–29.

122 Vamvakas EC. Meta-analysis of clinical studies of the purported deleterious effects of "old" (versus "fresh") red blood cells: Are we at equipoise? *Transfusion* 2010;**50**:600–10.

172 Bordin JO, Bardossy L, Blajchman MA. Growth enhancement of established tumors by allogeneic blood transfusion in experimental animals and its amelioration by leukodepletion: the importance of timing of the leukodepletion. *Blood* 1994;**84**:344–8.

185 Blajchman MA, Bardossy I, Carmen R, Sastry A, Singal DP. Allogeneic blood transfusion-induced enhancement of tumor growth: two animal models showing amelioration by leukodepletion and passive transfer using spleen cells. *Blood* 1993;**81**:1880–82.

Index

This index uses letter-by-letter alphabetization, ignoring spaces and hyphens. Page numbers in **bold** indicate tables; page numbers in *italics* indicate figures.

Rossi's Principles of Transfusion Medicine, Fifth Edition. Edited by Toby L. Simon, Jeffrey McCullough, Edward L. Snyder, Bjarte G. Solheim, and Ronald G. Strauss.
© 2016 John Wiley & Sons, Ltd. Published 2016 by John Wiley & Sons, Ltd.

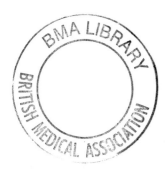